Volume 3

Pediatric

Orthopedics

SECOND EDITION

MIHRAN O. TACHDJIAN, M.S., M.D.

Professor of Orthopedic Surgery,
Northwestern University Medical School
Attending Orthopedic Surgeon and Former Head
Division of Orthopedics
Children's Memorial Hospital
Chicago, Illinois

1990
W.B. SAUNDERS COMPANY
Harcourt Brace Jovanovich, Inc.
Philadelphia ■ London ■ Toronto ■ Montreal ■ Sydney ■ Tokyo

W. B. SAUNDERS COMPANY
Harcourt Brace Jovanovich, Inc.

Independence Square West
Philadelphia, PA 19106

Library of Congress Cataloging-in-Publication Data

Tachdjian, Mihran O.

Pediatric orthopedics.

Includes bibliographies and index.

1. Pediatric orthopedia.   I. Title. [DNLM: 1. Orthopedics—in
infancy & childhood. WS 270 T117p]

RD732.3.C48T33 1990   617'.3   87–13006

ISBN 0–7216–8726–1 (set)

Listed here is the latest translated edition of this book together with the language of the translation and the publisher.

Spanish (*1st Edition*)–Nueva Editorial Interamericana S.A. de C.V., Mexico 4 D.F., Mexico

Editor: Edward H. Wickland, Jr.
Developmental Editor: Kathleen McCullough
Designer: Bill Donnelly
Production Manager: Bill Preston
Manuscript Editors: Ruth Barker, Constance Burton, Tina Rebane
Mechanical Artist: Karen Giacomucci
Illustration Coordinator: Peg Shaw
Indexer: Julie Schwager

Volume 1 ISBN   0–7216–8722–9
Volume 2 ISBN   0–7216–8723–7
Volume 3 ISBN   0–7216–8724–5
Volume 4 ISBN   0–7216–8727–X
Pediatric Orthopedics   Complete Set ISBN   0–7216–8726–1

Last digit is the print number: 9   8   7   6   5   4   3   2

Dedicated With Love to
My Wife
Vivian B. Tachdjian

Preface

During the past 18 years, great strides have been made in pediatric orthopedics. A new edition of this book is long overdue. The gestation period of such an *Arbeit* has been prolonged because of the tremendous amount of labor involved in writing a single-author book. The objectives and format of the textbook have not changed from the first edition. I have attempted to present a thorough and comprehensive treatise on the affections of the neuromusculoskeletal system in children.

I have expressed my preferred methods of treatment and surgical procedure based upon my personal experience and the privilege of association with the leaders in pediatric orthopedics throughout the world who have participated in the faculty of the Pediatric Orthopedic International Seminars, which I have directed annually since 1972. The names of the faculty appear in the acknowledgments in the following pages.

The illustrations and operative plates are all original; the majority represent the superb artistry of Mr. Ernest Beck, to whom I am greatly indebted. I also wish to acknowledge Miss Patricia Piescinski for her beautiful drawings.

I wish to thank the entire staff of the W.B. Saunders Company, particularly Miss Ruth Barker, Mr. Albert Meier, Mrs. Kathleen McCullough, and Mr. Edward H. Wickland, Jr.

I would also like to express my gratitude to Mrs. Mikie Boroughf, who assisted in the preparation of this book.

A question frequently posed to me over the years has been, "How do you write such an extensive book?" Every word has been handwritten in my illegible handwriting, readable only by Mrs. Lynn Ridings, without whose assistance and editorial support this work would not have been possible.

MIHRAN O. TACHDJIAN, M.D.

Acknowledgments

I would like to give special thanks to the following people for their help in writing certain sections of this book: Ellen Chadwick, M.D., and Stanford Shulman, M.D.—infectious diseases; Ramiro Hernandez, M.D.—CT scan of the hip; James Donaldson, M.D.—ultrasonography in congenital dislocation of the hip; Andrew Poznanski, M.D.—assistance in imaging findings in various skeletal disorders, especially bone dysplasias; Steven Hall, M.D.—orthopedic aspects of pediatric anesthesia; David McLone, M.D., and Thomas Naidich, M.D.—neurosurgical aspects of myelomeningocele and spinal dysraphism; Dror Paley, M.D.—Ilizarov limb lengthening; George Simons, M.D.—complications of talipes equinovarus; David H. Sutherland, M.D.—gait; and Mary Weck, R.P.T.—physical therapy for cerebral palsy.

I also wish to express my gratitude to the members of the faculty of the Pediatric Orthopedic International Seminars over the past 18 years.

Robert Abrams, M.D.
James Aronson, M.D.
Marc Asher, M.D.
R. Kirklin Ashley, M.D.
Henry H. Banks, M.D.
Riad Barmada, M.D.
Melvin H. Becker, M.D.
Henri Bensahel, M.D.
Anthony Bianco, M.D.
Eugene E. Bleck, M.D.
Prof. Alexander Bliskunov
Walter P. Blount, M.D.
J. Richard Bowen, M.D.
David W. Boyer, M.D.
Robert Bright, M.D.
Prof. Dieter Buck-Gramcko
Wilton H. Bunch, M.D.
Aloysio Campos da Paz, Jr., M.D.
S. Terry Canale, M.D.
Henri Carlioz, M.D.
Nils Carstam, M.D.
Prof. Robert Cattaneo

Mr. Anthony Catterall, F.R.C.S.
Prof. Paul L. Chigot
Eldon G. Chuinard, M.D.
Robert G. Chuinard, M.D.
Stanley M.K. Chung, M.D.
Sherman S. Coleman, M.D.
Mr. Christopher L. Colton, F.R.C.S.
Clinton L. Compere, M.D.
James J. Conway, M.D.
Henry R. Cowell, M.D.
Alvin H. Crawford, M.D.
Burr H. Curtis, M.D.
Prof. George Dall, F.R.C.S.
Prof. G. DeBastiani
Prof. Julio dePablos
Luciano Dias, M.D.
Harold M. Dick, M.D.
Alain Dimeglio, M.D.
James Donaldson, M.D.
John Dorst, M.D.
James Drennan, M.D.
Denis S. Drummond, M.D.

Prof. Jean Dubousset
Mr. Denis M. Dunn, F.R.C.S.
Peter M. Dunn, M.D.
Robert E. Eilert, M.D.
Richard E. Eppright, M.D.
John J. Fahey, M.D.
Albert B. Ferguson, Jr., M.D.
J. William Fielding, M.D.
Mr. John Fixsen, F.R.C.S.
Victor Frankel, M.D.
Nicholas Giannestras, M.D.
Prof. Alain Gilbert
J. Leonard Goldner, M.D.
Neil E. Green, M.D.
William T. Green, M.D.
Paul P. Griffin, M.D.
Donald Gunn, M.D.
John E. Hall, M.D.
Judith G. Hall, M.D.
John E. Handelsman, M.D.
Robert Hensinger, M.D.
Ramiro Hernandez, M.D.
Charles Herndon, M.D.
John A. Herring, M.D.
M. Mark Hoffer, M.D.
Walter A. Hoyt, Jr., M.D.
Mr. J. Rowland Hughes, F.R.C.S.
Prof. Sean P. F. Hughes
Prof. Gabriel Abramovich Ilizarov
Roshen Irani, M.D.
Francois Iselin, M.D.
Preston James, M.D.
Prof. Lutz F.H. Jani
Ali Kalamchi, M.D.
William J. Kane, M.D.
Buni'chiro Kawamura, M.D.
Theodore E. Keats, M.D.
Armen S. Kelikian, M.D.
Hampar Kelikian, M.D.
Mr. J.A. Kenwright, F.R.C.S.
Ara Y. Ketenjian, M.D.
Eugene Kilgore, M.D.
Richard E. King, M.D.
Prof. Predrag Klisiç
Steven Kopits, M.D.
Warren G. Kramer, M.D.
Mr. Douglas Lamb, F.R.C.S.
Prof. Anders F. Langenskiöld
Loren Larsen, M.D.
Franco Lavini, M.D.
Richard E. Lindseth, M.D.
Mr. George Lloyd-Roberts, F.R.C.S.
John E. Lonstein, M.D.
Wood Lovell, M.D.
G. Dean MacEwen, M.D.
John B. McGinty, M.D.
Douglas W. McKay, M.D.
Mr. Brian McKibbin, F.R.C.S.
David McLone, M.D.
John E. Madewell, M.D.
Roger A. Mann, M.D.
Prof. P.G. Marchetti
Prof. S. Matsuno

Peter L. Meehan, M.D.
Malcolm B. Menelaus, M.D.
Michael Michelson, M.D.
Lee W. Milford, M.D.
Edward A. Millar, M.D.
Mr. George P. Mitchell, F.R.C.S.
Prof. Giorgio Monticelli
Raymond T. Morrissy, M.D.
Colin F. Moseley, M.D.
Alf S. Nachemson, M.D.
Ann Nachemson, M.D.
John J. Niebauer, M.D.
John A. Ogden, M.D.
Michael B. Ozonoff, M.D.
Lauren M. Pachman, M.D.
Dror Paley, M.D.
Arsen Pankovich, M.D.
Arthur M. Pappas, M.D.
Klausdieter Parsch, M.D.
Sir Dennis Paterson
Hamlet A. Peterson, M.D.
Guillermo de Velasco Polo, M.D.
Ignacio V. Ponseti, M.D.
Melvin Post, M.D.
Jean-Gabriel Pous, M.D.
Andrew K. Poznanski, M.D.
Charles T. Price, M.D.
Mercer Rang, M.D.
Mr. A.H.C. Ratliff, F.R.C.S.
Inge Reimann, M.D.
L. Renzi-Brivio, M.D.
B. Lawrence Riggs, M.D.
Veijo A. Ritsila, M.D.
John M. Roberts, M.D.
Charles Rockwood, M.D.
Robert B. Salter, M.D.
Robert L. Samilson, M.D.
Shahan K. Sarrafian, M.D.
Michael F. Schafer, M.D.
William L. Schey, M.D.
Keith Schroeder, M.D.
Mr. W.J.W. Sharrard, F.R.C.S.
Stanford T. Shulman, M.D.
Robert S. Siffert, M.D.
Michael A. Simon, M.D.
George W. Simons, M.D.
Clement B. Sledge, M.D.
Wayne O. Southwick, M.D.
Donald P. Speer, M.D.
Prof. Renato Spinelli
Jurgen Spranger, M.D.
Lynn T. Staheli, M.D.
Stanko Stanisavljevic, M.D.
Herbert H. Stark, M.D.
Howard Steel, M.D.
David H. Stulberg, M.D.
Y. Sugioka, M.D.
David H. Sutherland, M.D.
Alfred B. Swanson, M.D.
Prof. W. Taillard
David J. Thompson, M.D.
Georges R. Thuilleux, M.D.
Dietrich Tonnis, M.D.

Levon K. Topouzian, M.D.
Miguel Ferrer Torrelles, M.D.
Prof. Naoichi Tsuyama
Prof. Raoul Tubiana
Vincent J. Turco, M.D.
Prof. M.V. Volkov
Prof. Heinz Wagner
Prof. Isidor Wasserstein
R.S. Watanabe, M.D
Hugh G. Watts, M.D.
Prof. B.G. Weber
Stuart L. Weinstein, M.D

Prof. S. L. Weissman
Dennis R. Wenger, M.D.
G. Wilbur Westin, M.D.
Harvey White, M.D.
Mr. Peter Williams, F.R.C.S.
John C. Wilson, M.D.
Robert Winter, M.D.
Miss Ruth Wynne-Davies, F.R.C.S.
Yasuo Yamauchi, M.D.
Prof. Eduardo Zancolli
Seymour Zimbler, M.D.

Preface to the First Edition

This work was undertaken upon the invitation of its publisher and begun with interest and great personal involvement that have never faltered. Now that its manuscript is complete, I must seize the occasion of this prefatory statement to answer the reader's natural question: Why was it done?

I began with the perhaps-simplistic idea of providing a detailed technical presentation of surgical treatment of disorders of the neuromuscular and skeletal systems in children. I intended to write primarily for the orthopedic surgeon but I hoped also to interest physicians and surgeons of other specialties involved in the care of children.

I had no sooner set out on what proved a long and tortuous path than I began to appreciate that one cannot describe the techniques of surgery without considering also the biological principles of surgery, the dynamics of trauma, and the rationale for surgical intervention. That rationale is itself dependent upon knowledge of neuromuscular physiology and of the biomechanics of motion. One cannot speak of the management of disorder or of the amelioration of congenital defect without understanding disease process and the genesis of musculoskeletal anomaly. The surgeon who operates well performs not only with skill but also with reason; and that reason rests upon a diagnostic acumen fortified by physical examination, pathology, radiology and accurate classification. Similarly, the evaluation of surgery cannot be set out without attention to its possible complications and its aftercare.

On reflection, I realize the project I have undertaken is more ambitious than I had originally envisioned. And so I have written a long and complex book. Its very length and complexity must mean occasional omission and even error. I have tried to guard against them by citing for each important statement significant findings from the vast literature of pediatric orthopedics; but the opinions I have expressed concerning preferred methods of treatment and surgical procedure arise from personal experience and from the privilege of having learned and worked at fine teaching centers.

In another and perhaps more important way I have departed from original intent. I decided to omit chapters on the hand and on orthotics and prosthetics in the conviction that these highly individual subjects should be treated intensively and thoroughly in separate monographs.

I wish to express gratitude to John Dusseau, Editor of the W. B. Saunders Company, for the confidence he invested in me. Without his support, advice, and encouragement, this work would have been impossible.

I wish to express thanks also to the Trust Under Will of Helen Fay Hunter–Crippled Children's Fund, and to Mr. Carl A. Pfau and the Harris Trust and Savings Bank Trustees for their generous support.

The kind indulgence of the Board of Directors of Children's Memorial Hospital in allowing me the necessary time to complete this work is greatly appreciated. I also wish to thank certain of my professional colleagues and members of the orthopedic staff for their sincere cooperation during preparation of this manuscript.

With the exception of a few that have been reproduced from other works, the illustrations and operative plates are all original. The majority represent the superb artistry of Mr. Ernest Beck, to whom I am greatly indebted. I also wish to thank medical artists Wesley Bloom, Jean McConnell, Diane Nelson, and Laurel Schaubert. The diligent work of Miss Helen Silver and Mr. John Kelley of the Photography Department, Children's Memorial Hospital, must be particularly acknowledged.

The entire staff of W. B. Saunders Company, particularly Miss Ruth Barker and Mr. Raymond Kersey, are to be commended for their meticulous work during the preparation and production of the printed book.

Finally, I wish to thank Miss Eleanor Lynn Schreiner, who, in her role as my personal editor, has prepared and finalized the entire manuscript as it has been written during the past four years. Without her assistance and meticulous attention to clarity, this task would have been difficult, if not impossible, to achieve. For her unselfish dedication I shall always be grateful.

I shall conclude in the hope that if the reader learns as much from reading as the writer has from writing this monograph, its attendant trouble and trial will have been amply repaid in the better care of children.

MIHRAN O. TACHDJIAN

Contents

VOLUME 1

1

2

Congenital Deformities 104

V O L U M E   2

3

4

VOLUME 3

5

6

VOLUME 4

7

8

Volume 3

5. The Neuromuscular System

GENERAL CONSIDERATIONS

Levels of Affection

The neuromuscular system may be affected at various levels, each of which is characterized by changes in motor function peculiar to the site and extent of involvement.

At the *spinomuscular level*, motor activity is simple; the impulses arising in the anterior horn cells of the spinal cord are transmitted through the peripheral nerves to the myoneural junctions and then to the individual muscles. In disorders at the spinomuscular level, the loss of motor power is focal and segmental, with complete paralysis of the muscles or muscle groups that are supplied by a peripheral nerve or by the anterior horn cells in the spinal cord. Muscular paralysis is flaccid or hypotonic, with reaction of degeneration, atrophy, fibrillations, and fasciculations. The deep tendon and superficial reflexes are diminished or absent. Pyramidal tract signs, abnormal involuntary movements, and ataxia are absent. There may be trophic changes in the skin, nails, and bone.

Pathologic processes at the spinomuscular level may be further classified into various sublevels. When the disease originates in the anterior horn cells, as in poliomyelitis, the *spinal level* of the motor system is affected. Other examples of diseases at the spinal level are progressive spinal muscular atrophy of

Werdnig-Hoffmann type, progressive bulbar palsy, syringomyelia, and intramedullary neoplasm. The loss of function of the anterior horn cells and the motor nuclei of the brain stem results in clinical findings of flaccid paralysis, atrophy, areflexia, reaction of degeneration, and fasciculations.

At the *neural level* of the motor system, the peripheral nerves and nerve roots are affected, common examples of which are obstetrical brachial plexus palsy and progressive neural muscular atrophy (Charcot-Marie-Tooth disease). In affections of nerves, sensory fibers are usually involved, with resultant sensory changes such as anesthesia or hyperesthesia. Otherwise, the clinical findings are similar to those of spinal level affections; i.e., there is flaccid paralysis, atrophy, reaction of degeneration, and areflexia as a result of loss of conduction of motor impulses. In the absence of sensory changes it is difficult to distinguish between diseases of the peripheral nerves, anterior roots, and anterior horn cells.

When the pathologic process arises at the myoneural junction, as in myasthenia gravis and familial periodic paralysis, then it is a disease at the *myoneural level*. In diseases of primarily muscular origin, the motor system is involved at the *muscular level*. The muscular dystrophies are familiar examples of disturbance of the muscular level in diseases at the spinomuscular

Table 5–1. Differentiation of Motor Disorders at Various Levels of Neuromuscular Function*

	Spinomuscular			Extrapyramidal	Pyramidal	Cerebellar	Psychomotor
	Muscular	Neural	Spinal				
Loss of motor power	Focal-segmental Usually proximal and axial muscle groups Complete	Focal-segmental Usually distal limb musculature Complete	Focal-segmental Usually distal limb musculature Complete	Generalized Entire limb and movements Incomplete	Generalized Entire limb and movements Incomplete	None Ataxia may simulate loss of power	No true loss Bizarre, may simulate any type
Tone	Flaccid	Flaccid	Flaccid	Rigid	Spastic	Hypotonic (ataxia)	Normal or variable, may be increased
Atrophy	Present	Present	Present	Absent	Minimal (due to disuse and chronic paresis)	Absent	Absent
Fasciculations	May be present	Absent	May be present	Absent	Absent	Absent	Absent
Reaction of degeneration	Present	Present	Present	Absent	Absent	Absent	Absent
EMG							
Interference pattern	Normal until late in disease	Reduced	Reduced				
Fibrillation potential	Not usually present	Present	Usually present				
Action potential	Short duration	Prolonged with normal or polyphasic potentials	Prolonged with occasional giant potentials				
Evoked sensory and mixed nerve potentials	Normal	Absent, diminished amplitude, or prolonged conduction time	Normal				

Reflexes							
Deep	Diminished and preserved until late	Absent early	Absent early	Normal or variable	Hyperactive	Diminished or pendular	Normal or increased range
Superficial	Diminished	Absent	Absent	Normal or increased	Diminished or absent	Normal	Normal or increased
Pyramidal tract response	No	No	No	No	Yes	No	No
Sensory deficit	Absent	Usually present	Absent	Absent	May be present (stereognosis or other cortical)	Absent	Absent
Trophic disturbance	Present	Present	Present	Absent	Usually absent	Absent	Absent
Ataxia	Absent	Absent	Absent	Absent	Absent	Present	Absent (may simulate ataxia)
Abnormal movements	Absent	Absent	Absent	Present	None	May be present (intention tremor and ataxia)	May be present
Associated movements	Normal	Normal	Normal	Absence of normal associated movements	Presence of pathologic associated movements	Normal	Normal

*Adapted from DeJong, R. N.: The Neurological Examination. 3rd edition. New York, Hoeber Medical Division, Harper & Row, 1967, p. 382; and Farmer, T. W.: Pediatric Neurology. New York, Hoeber Medical Division, Harper & Row, 1964, p. 612.

level. Paralysis is flaccid, but reflexes persist until the late stages, when marked atrophy has occurred. There is loss of contractibility without loss of excitability; i.e., the muscle fibers have degenerated and have been replaced by fibroadipose tissue, but the peripheral nerves and anterior horn cells are normal.

In disorders of the motor system at the *extrapyramidal level*, there is generalized involvement of the muscles of the limbs and trunk. The muscle tone is hypertonic. Atrophy, fasciculations, and reaction of degeneration are absent. Motion of the limbs is hyperkinetic, with loss of associated or automatic movements. The deep tendon and superficial reflexes are normal. There are no pyramidal tract responses and no sensory deficit. Athetoid cerebral palsy is a common example of a disease at the extrapyramidal level.

At the *pyramidal* or *corticospinal level* of involvement, motor deficit arises from affection of motor nuclei of the cerebral cortex. Paresis is usually generalized and associated with hypertonicity or spasticity of muscles. Pyramidal tract signs and pathologic reflexes are usually present. There is usually some atrophy that is not focal; it is caused by chronic paralysis and disuse. Fasciculations, trophic disturbances, reaction of degeneration, and abnormal movements are absent. The deep tendon reflexes are hyperactive and the superficial reflexes are diminished or absent. Spastic cerebral palsy illustrates the pyramidal level of motor involvement.

Cerebellar level lesions are characterized by loss of coordination and control, or ataxia. There is no real loss of motor power. Fasciculations, reaction of degeneration, atrophy, and trophic disturbances are absent. The deep tendon reflexes may be diminished or pendular, but the superficial reflexes are normal. Pyramidal tract responses cannot be elicited.

The *psychomotor level* of motor performance is the highest level of neuromuscular activity, at which volitional movements are initiated and affected by integration, memory, and symbolization. Paralysis caused by hysteria is an example of psychomotor disturbance. Loss of motor power is bizarre, with no actual paralysis. There is no real neurologic deficit. There are no fasciculations, no atrophy, and no true ataxia.

Differential features of various levels of motor function are illustrated in Table 5–1.

Neuromuscular System as a Functional Unit

Muscles are the expressive unit of the neuromuscular system and the moving force of the body. Muscles whose contraction directly produces a specific action are classified as *agonists* or *primary movers* (protagonists). An example is the biceps brachii in flexion of the elbow. Those muscles that oppose the agonists must be relaxed for contraction of the agonists (these are called *antagonists* or *moderators*), as, for example, the triceps brachii is in flexion of the elbow.

A motor action, even in an apparently simple motion, is quite complex. It involves the *muscles of fixation*, which stabilize the adjacent joints and afford a firm base for muscle action. The action of *synergists* is to assist the agonists and to reduce to a minimum all unnecessary motions. The execution of a motor movement requires the coordinated action of all four physiologic muscle groups—the contraction of the agonists and the relaxation of the antagonists as well as the associated function of the synergists and the muscles of fixation. Loss of function of any of these muscle groups will result in disturbance of motor performance.

Responses of Muscles

The responses of muscles to injury and disease are predictable. Muscles that are not used atrophy. The rapidity of development of such disuse atrophy is well illustrated by the atrophy of the quadriceps femoris that follows a painful lesion of the knee or immobilization of the knee in an above-knee cast. With progressive resistive exercises, muscles hypertrophy. Painful stimuli will cause protective spasm of a muscle, which, when maintained in its shortened position for a period of time, will tend to develop myostatic contracture. The antagonist muscles to those in spasm are weakened by being maintained in their longer, stretched position and by inhibition of their function and recovery.

Muscular action affects bone growth. In the growing skeleton, muscle imbalance will cause deformity in the direction of action of the stronger muscle. Muscles are very sensitive to ischemia, as illustrated by Volkmann's ischemic contracture. Chronic systemic disease causes generalized muscle weakness and increased fatigability.

Affections of the Brain and Spinal Cord

CEREBRAL PALSY

Definition

Cerebral palsy is difficult to define, as it is not a single disease entity but, rather, a convenient category denoting a wide spectrum of conditions having certain common characteristics. The generally accepted criteria of the symptom complex of cerebral palsy are as follows:

1. It must be due to a fixed, nonprogressive brain lesion or lesions. No active disease should exist at the time of diagnosis. Thus, transient disorders or those that are the result of a progressive disease of the brain or spinal cord are excluded.

2. The original lesion must occur prenatally, at birth, or early in the postnatal period. The exact limits of this early period are not agreed upon, and it is best to avoid arbitrary age limits. The interference with the developing central nervous system by the early fixed lesion is the significant pathologic feature.

3. In certain children, the primary disorder involves the musculoskeletal system and lack of motor control is the greater handicap, whereas in others, mental retardation, convulsions, sensory disturbance, speech impediments, or defects of hearing, language, or eyesight may be the more important difficulty. The concern of the orthopedic surgeon is the disorder of movement and posture and the deformation of the musculoskeletal system.

The term *cerebral palsy* has certain administrative usefulness. The foregoing criteria of this category of disease should, however, be carefully examined, as conditions such as Friedreich's ataxia, progressive hereditary paraplegia, or amaurotic familial idiocy should not be included under the heading of "cerebral palsy." There are numerous syndromes and nonfixed brain lesions that manifest themselves in hypertonia or hypotonia with or without spasticity, athetosis, and rigidity or ataxia.

The orthopedic surgeon should obtain an appropriate neurologic consultation prior to treating musculoskeletal deformities of the cerebral palsy patient. This author has encountered a number of children with brain tumors, spinal cord tumors, and other treatable progressive lesions of the central nervous system that have been misdiagnosed as cerebral palsy.

Classification

The differing approaches of clinicians and therapists concerned with the diagnosis and treatment of cerebral palsy are reflected in the various classifications they have used.[3, 213, 248]

During the past 25 years, the ones most commonly employed are essentially modifications of Phelps's description of the clinical manifestations of cerebral palsy, which consists primarily of helpful suggestions to therapists and others concerned with the practical management of these patients.[408, 410, 413] Phelps based his classification primarily on the state of muscle tone, the presence or absence of involuntary movement, and the topographical distribution of motor deficits, taking into account etiologic factors, the presumed site of neuropathologic changes, and associated sensory defects (Table 5–2).

The defect of a classification that defines categories primarily in terms of changes in muscle tone is that the muscle tone of individual

Table 5–2. American Classification of Cases of Cerebral Palsy*

Spastic	
Aspastic	
Spastic	
Monoplegia	
Hemiplegia	
Paraplegia	
Triplegia	
Quadriplegia	
Basilar	
Athetosis	
Tension	Rotatory
Nontension	Emotional release
Dystonic	Tremor
Flail	Unclassified
Arm, neck	Paraplegia
Deaf	Quadriplegia
Shudder	Monoplegia
Hemiathetoid	Recovered
Cerebellar release	
Rigidity	
Intermittent	
Continuous	
Miscellaneous	
Hemiplegia	
Paraplegia	
Triplegia	
Quadriplegia	
Tremor	
Intention	
Constant	
Ataxia	
Cerebellar	
Eighth nerve	

*Based on that of Phelps by Hellebrandt, F. A.: Trends in the management of cerebral palsy. Lectures in Medical College of Virginia (unpublished manuscript). 1950–1951.

patients varies greatly with maturation and may alter considerably from day to day—and even from hour to hour—according to position, posture, state of alertness or fatigue, environmental temperature, and emotional state.

Perlstein and Minear have attempted to produce more comprehensive descriptive classifications by considering the site of pathologic change, clinical manifestations, topographical description, severity of motor involvement, muscle tone, and etiology (Tables 5–3 and 5–4).[352, 394, 395]

Crothers and Paine, stressing that the characteristic signs in cerebral palsy manifest themselves only gradually, have offered a more explicit neurologic classification (Table 5–5).[122]

Ingram and Balf have suggested a classification by neurologic syndromes based on that of Freud, with modifications made necessary by advances in knowledge since his time (Table 5–6).[15, 256]

Classification of cerebral palsy is difficult but very important. There is no general agreement. In the care of the child with cerebral palsy, the orthopedist is part of a multidisciplinary team. The neurologist or pediatrician may be using any one of the foregoing classifications, and the orthopedic surgeon should be familiar with their vocabulary.

The distribution of paralysis is described according to the number of limbs involved. If a patient has one limb involved, the condition is termed *monoplegia*; if two limbs on the same side are affected, *hemiplegia*; if two lower limbs, *paraplegia*; if three limbs, *triplegia*; or if four limbs, *quadriplegia* or *tetraplegia*. There is little agreement about the use of the terms *diplegia* and *double hemiplegia*. The term "cerebral diplegia" or "diplegia" is employed by some authors to describe the condition of patients with more or less symmetrical paralysis, dating from birth or shortly afterward, which is more severe in the lower than in the upper limbs.[117, 172, 255] *Double* or *bilateral hemiplegia* is used when there is asymmetry of involvement between the two sides.

Pure paraplegia, i.e., involvement of the lower limbs with absolutely no affection of the upper limbs, is rare. Often these patients have moderate spasticity of the lower limbs and minimal involvement of the upper limbs with dysfunction of fine motor movements. The term "spastic diplegia" is more accurate for this type of cerebral palsy. Most of these children are

Table 5–3. *Classification of Cerebral Palsy by Perlstein, 1952**

By Clinical Symptoms	Topographical Involvement of Extremities	By Muscle Tone	Severity	Etiology
Spastic conditions	Paraplegia	Isotonic	Mild	Prenatal
				Hereditary
Dyskinesias	Diplegia	Hypertonic	Moderate	Static
Choreas	Quadriplegia or tetraplegia	Hypotonic	Severe	Progressive
		—	—	Acquired in utero
Athetoids	Hemiplegia	—	—	Infection
Dystonia	Triplegia	—	—	Anoxia
Tremors	Monoplegia	—	—	Cerebral hemorrhage
Rigidity	Double hemiplegia	—	—	Rh factor
Ataxia	Limited to both upper extremities	—	—	Metabolic disturbance
				Gonadal irradiation
				Natal factors
				Anoxia
				Cerebral hemorrhage
				Trauma
				Pressure change, etc.
				Postnatal factors
				Trauma
				Infections
				Toxic causes
				Vascular accident
				Anoxia
				Neoplasms and developmental defects

*From Perlstein, M. A., and Barnett, H. E.: Nature and recognition of cerebral palsy in infancy. J.A.M.A., *148*:1389, 1952.

Table 5–4. *Classification of Cerebral Palsy (Minear, 1956)**

Physiologic (motor)		Physical status	
Spastic		Physical growth evaluation (Wetzel Grid or other)	
Athetotic		Developmental level (Gesell)	
Tension	Ataxic	Bone age	
Nontension	Tremor	Contracture	
Dystonic	Atonic (rare)	Convulsive seizures	
Tremor	Mixed	Posture and locomotive behavior patterns	
Rigidity	Unclassified	Eye-hand behavior patterns	
		Visual status	
Topographical		Sensory	
Monoplegia	Quadriplegia	Amblyopia	
Paraplegia	Diplegia	Field defects	
Hemiplegia	Double hemiplegia	Motor	
Triplegia		Auditory status	
		Pitch range loss	
		Decibel loss	
Etiologic		Speech disturbances	
Prenatal			
Hereditary		Functional capacity (degree of severity)	
Acquired in utero		Class I.	Patients with cerebral palsy with no practical limitation of activity
Natal			
Anoxia		Class II.	Patients with cerebral palsy with slight to moderate limitation of activity
Postnatal			
Trauma (subdural hematoma, skull fractures, wounds, contusions of the brain)		Class III.	Patients with cerebral palsy with moderate to great limitation of activity
Infections (meningitis, encephalitis, brain abscess)		Class IV.	Patients with cerebral palsy unable to carry on any useful physical activity
Toxic causes (lead, arsenic, coal tar derivatives, streptomycin, etc.)			
Vascular accidents		Therapeutic	
Anoxia (carbon monoxide poisoning, strangulation, high altitudes, deep pressure anoxia, hypoglycemia)		Class A.	Patients with cerebral palsy not requiring treatment
Neoplastic or late development defects (brain tumors, hydrocephalus, brain cysts, internal hydrocephalus)		Class B.	Patients with cerebral palsy who need minimal bracing and minimal therapy
		Class C.	Patients with cerebral palsy who need bracing and apparatus, and the services of a cerebral palsy treatment team
Supplemental		Class D.	Patients with cerebral palsy limited to such a degree that they require long-term institutionalization and treatment
Psychological evaluation			
Degree of mental deficiency, if any			

*Adapted from Minear, W. L.: A classification of cerebral palsy. Pediatrics, *18*:841, 1956.

Table 5–5. *Classification of Cerebral Palsy Patients by Types (Crothers and Paine, 1959)**

Spastic monoplegia		
Spastic hemiplegia		
Prenatal or natal	right	left
Postnatal	right	left
Spastic tetraplegia		
Symmetrical		
Asymmetrical		
Spastic triplegia		
Spastic paraplegia		
Extrapyramidal cerebral palsies, not mixed		
Kernicterus		
Mixed types		
Cerebral palsy plus cord injury		

*Adapted from Crothers, B., and Paine, R. S.: The Natural History of Cerebral Palsy. Cambridge, Mass., Harvard University Press, 1959.

the product of premature birth. When a patient has only paraplegia, spinal cord pathology should be ruled out.

Almost all the cerebral palsy patients with quadriplegia have involvement of their trunk, head, and neck, with abnormal posturing and disorders of movement. Currently, the term "total body involved" is used to classify this type of cerebral palsy.[59]

Etiology and Pathology

The nonprogressive brain lesion in cerebral palsy may be due to birth injury, developmental malformations, or damage acquired postnatally. Etiologic diagnosis is circumstantial in the majority of patients. Pathologic findings are available in only a few patients, and even then, one has difficulty in determining the primary underlying cause. Ingram and Crothers and Paine have given a critical etiologic analysis of their own cases as well as a comprehensive review of the literature.[122, 256]

BIRTH INJURY

Little first described three types of paralysis that could occur as a result of abnormal birth, denoting them as "hemiplegic rigidity," "paraplegia," and "generalized rigidity," as well as a condition characterized by "disordered movement."[319–321] These would now be considered forms of cerebral palsy.

Birth injury is direct or indirect damage incurred during pregnancy or during labor and the process of delivery. It must be differentiated from abnormalities of the brain that are due to genetically determined developmental malformations dating from early pregnancy, and others caused by a variety of teratogenic insults. Cerebral palsy due to birth injury should also be distinguished from postnatal or acquired cerebral palsy, the consequence of insults sustained by the infant following birth.

Abnormalities of pregnancy, labor, and delivery may cause "hypoxic," "traumatic," or "toxic" damage to the brain.

Table 5–6. *Classification of Cerebral Palsy in Childhood (Ingram, 1955; Balf and Ingram, 1956)**

Neurologic Diagnosis	Extent	Severity
Hemiplegia	Right Left	Mild Moderately severe Severe
Bilateral hemiplegia		Mild Moderately severe Severe

Diplegia
  Hypotonic
  Dystonic
  Rigid or spastic
	Paraplegic
	Triplegic
	Tetraplegic
		Mild
		Moderately severe
		Severe

Ataxia	Unilateral Bilateral	Mild Moderately severe Severe

Dyskinesia
  Dystonic
  Choreoid
  Athetoid
  Tension
  Tremor
	Monoplegic
	Hemiplegic
	Triplegic
	Tetraplegic
		Mild
		Moderately severe
		Severe

Other		

*Adapted from Ingram, T. T. S.: A study of cerebral palsy in the childhood population of Edinburgh. Arch. Dis. Child., 30:87, 1955, and Balf, C. L., and Ingram, T. T. S.: Problems in the classification of cerebral palsy in childhood. Brit. Med. J., 2:163, 1955.

Hypoxia. In the last trimester of pregnancy, probable causes of fetal hypoxia are (1) antepartum hemorrhage due to placenta previa or other causes, with the attendant disturbance in placental nutrition; (2) pre-eclamptic toxemia (infarction of placentae of toxemic mothers tends to be more extensive than in mothers without toxemia, and there is greater decline of the oxygen saturation of the umbilical vein in pregnancy complicated by pre-eclampsia, as compared with normal pregnancies);[579] (3) postmaturity; and (4) maternal causes of anoxemia such as cardiopulmonary disease.

Hypoxic damage to the fetus during labor and delivery may be caused by umbilical cord prolapse or torsion, or both, resulting in obstruction of circulation to the cord.

Neonatal apnea is not only the end result of many different forms of fetal injury but is also a cause of further hypoxic damage in the newborn infant. The common causes of a failure to breathe after birth are prematurity and hypoxia during pregnancy or delivery. There may be poisoning or structural damage to the respiratory center, or the air passages may be obstructed as a result of the infant's premature efforts to breathe before delivery. Other neonatal complications that may cause hypoxia in the period immediately following birth include the following: persistent atelectasis due to immaturity, bronchial obstruction, or the baby's failure to expand the lungs; or hindrance of pulmonary respiratory exchange by hyaline membrane formation, pulmonary edema, intrauterine pneumonia, or aspiration of gastrointestinal contents.

Traumatic Birth. In recent years, the tendency has been to attribute less importance to trauma as an etiologic factor in birth injury and to emphasize the dangers of hypoxia. However, there is quite adequate evidence to suggest that subdural hemorrhage is predominantly the result of birth trauma. The forms of abnormal labor and delivery that are especially prone to cause subdural hemorrhage are prolonged labor because of disproportion or malpresentation, precipitate delivery, forceps delivery, breech extraction, and version and extraction. Subdural hemorrhage most often results from tears of the dural ligaments that involve either the tributaries of the sagittal sinus or the great cerebral vein itself. Tears are especially liable to occur when undue or oblique stresses are placed on the tentorium cerebelli or the falx.[252]

Toxic Injury. Fetal damage may be caused by toxic agents that operate during late pregnancy, labor, and delivery. These include (1) conditions that act by causing toxic accumulations of naturally occurring substances (e.g., rhesus incompatibility, producing an excess of bilirubin and ammonia in the fetus; maternal uremia, causing an excess of nitrogenous waste products to accumulate; or diabetes, in which an excess of a variety of hormonal substances that are damaging to the fetus are produced); and (2) the presence of abnormal tissues that cause injury to the developing brain, such as in syphilis, rubella, cytomegalovirus, and toxoplasmosis; in these maternal infections, secondary infection of the fetus is quite common. Cocaine, heroin, and marijuana can cross the placental barrier and cause damage to the central nervous system of the fetus. Alcohol adversely affects the development of the fetal cerebrum. Smoking during pregnancy causes fetal growth retardation.

DEVELOPMENTAL MALFORMATIONS

Findings that suggest developmental malformations as a possible cause of cerebral palsy are (1) known family history of cerebral palsy, congenital malformations, or neurologic disease (excluding mental retardation) in siblings, parents, uncles, aunts, or cousins; (2) births of patients after apparently uncomplicated pregnancy, labor, and delivery that were not thought to have been likely to cause gross hypoxia or trauma; (2) associated congenital malformations of patients, excluding those possibly secondary to cerebral palsy; (4) patients' having extremely small heads with an occipitofrontal circumference of less than one percentile for age.

The problem of etiologic diagnosis of developmental malformations as a cause of cerebral palsy is complex, and positive diagnostic criteria are difficult to establish. Clinically, developmental malformations might be responsible for a significant proportion of patients with bilateral hemiplegia and ataxic diplegia.

Experimental work and clinical observations have shown that a number of agents are likely to provoke developmental abnormalities in the unborn child, usually in the first three months of pregnancy. The connection between roentgen irradiation and congenital fetal defects is well established.[365, 597] The most frequent neurologic manifestations are diplegia and ataxia, often complicated by epilepsy. Rubella in the early months of pregnancy tends to produce offspring with congenital cataracts and abnormalities of other systems, with the brain being affected in a significantly high proportion of

Table 5–7. *Neurologic Sequelae of Various Causes of Cerebral Palsy*

Etiologic Factors	Neurologic Sequelae
Prematurity	Spastic paraplegia
Breech delivery	Athetoid or spastic paraplegia
Toxemia of pregnancy	Spastic hemiplegia or quadriplegia
Birth trauma	Spastic hemiplegia or quadriplegia
Anoxia	Athetosis
Rh factor and kernicterus	Athetosis with deafness and paralysis of supravergence
Maternal rubella	Spasticity, with deafness or auditory aphasia, cataract, and congenital heart disease
Precipitate or cesarean delivery	Spastic quadriplegia, ataxia, or rigidity
Placenta previa and abruptio	Athetosis

cases; spastic paraplegia and athetosis may be the presenting clinical picture.

CAUSES OF ACQUIRED CEREBRAL PALSY

Well-recognized causes occurring in postnatal life include intracranial trauma, cerebral embolism, arterial thrombosis, intracranial abscess, venous thrombosis of the lateral sinus, meningitis, and viral encephalitides.

Perlstein and Barnett state that there is a statistically significant correlation between certain etiologic factors and specific clinical syndromes. In general, brain damage caused by anoxia is usually followed by extrapyramidal syndromes, whereas that caused by primary trauma and hemorrhage results in pyramidal affections. A list of some of the more common neurologic sequelae of various etiologic factors is given in Table 5–7.[395]

Blumel, Eggers, and Evans, in a study of 100 cerebral palsy patients, reported the chief causes to be trauma at birth (13 per cent), anoxia (24 per cent), prematurity (32 per cent), congenital defects (11 per cent), and postnatal causes (7 per cent).[61] More than one agent may be operative in producing cerebral palsy, and for the most part, the possible causes cannot be definitely identified.

In the past, the teaching has been dogmatic, it being said that spasticity is the result of damage to the motor cortex or pyramidal tracts, that athetosis is caused by lesions of the basal ganglia, that ataxia is due to damage or disease of the cerebellum or its connections, and that tremor and rigidity are the sequelae of more widespread lesions of the central nervous system. The gradual accumulation of more reliable and accurate information has failed to show a definite correlation between the pathologic findings and clinical features.[117] Generally, destructive, infectious, or vascular lesions will produce unilateral or asymmetrical paralysis, whereas developmental malformations will result in symmetrical involvement, although two or more destructive injuries could produce symmetrical paralysis.

Neurophysiologic Considerations

For a basic understanding of the musculoskeletal manifestations of brain damage in children, it is imperative to have a clear knowledge of the following fundamentals of the pathophysiology of the central nervous system.

SPASTICITY

Spasticity may be defined as a state of increase in tension of a muscle when it is passively lengthened, which is caused by an exaggeration of the muscle stretch reflex. It occurs in association with lesions of the cerebrum and descending pathways of the so-called pyramidal level of function. In the past, spasticity has been ascribed to the loss of, or release from the normal inhibiting action of, the pyramidal cortex on the anterior horn cells. Recent work indicates that spasticity results from an imbalance of the inhibitory and fasciculatory centers in the midbrain and brain stem reticular formations, with consequent alteration of the alpha and gamma motor neuron balance.

Increased tension of a spastic muscle may be demonstrated on rapid passive movement of a part of a limb; initially there is a free interval, but increasing resistance is met with "blocking" and limitation of further movements. On moving the part of the limb to its original posture, there is absence of resistance. If passive movement of the limb is performed slowly, it is comparatively free. If the part is moved abruptly or suddenly, this "blocking" may be felt from the beginning of the passive movement, following which the muscle resists to a certain point and then relaxes. This "clasp knife" type of waxing and waning resistance of spasticity is distinguished from rigidity; in rigidity, resistance to passive movement is not intermittent, remaining constant throughout the movement. Rigidity is not velocity sensitive.

Objective means for accurate measurement of the degree of spasticity are not available. Thus far, clinical evaluation remains the most reliable method. The degree of hypertonicity and the range of motion of spastic limbs may vary between examinations and among different examiners. On palpation a spastic muscle may be hard, or it may be soft and flabby, depending not so much on the actual amount of spasticity as on the degree of contraction or relaxation at the time of palpation. The degree of electrical neuromuscular activity of a spastic muscle depends on whether the muscle is relaxed or stimulated.

In spasticity, the deep tendon reflexes are exaggerated and pathologic reflexes such as the Babinski and Hoffmann signs are present. On sudden dorsiflexion of the ankle or rapid distal movement of the patella, one may elicit *clonus*—alternate spasm and relaxation of the agonist and antagonist muscles.

Testing of motor power is difficult in spasticity, but it is important and an attempt should be made. In general, there is associated motor weakness of the antagonist muscle groups. For example, when triceps surae muscle is spastic, there will be motor weakness of the antagonist anterior tibial muscle. The patient may have partial or no voluntary cerebral control over the anterior tibial muscle. A spastic muscle may have varying degrees of motor weakness. In muscle examination, both the motor power and the physiologic status should be assessed. Motor power is graded by the standard that was accepted by the National Foundation for Infantile Paralysis, and the same abbreviations are used: zero, *0*; trace, *T*; poor, *P*; fair, *F*; good, *G*; and normal, *N*. For physiologic status, the author uses the following notations and abbreviations: S for spastic (stretch reflex); H for hypotonic; C0 for cerebral zero (i.e., the patient has no voluntary control over the muscle); and *IN* for innervation normal. Cerebral zero muscles may be stimulated to function by patterning; for example, a C0 anterior tibial may be stimulated to dorsiflex the ankle by flexion of the hip-knee against resistance. Table 5–8 shows motor strength combinations of muscles in cerebral palsy patients.[547]

Table 5–8. *Physiologic Status Variations in Motor Strength of Muscles in Cerebral Palsy*

Physiologic Status	Motor Strength
Innervation normal *(IN)*	P to N
Spastic *(S)*	P to N
Hypotonic *(H)*	0 to G
Cerebral zero *(0C)*	0 to G

In the motor evaluation of a child with spasticity, the following pitfalls should be borne in mind. Tension athetosis should be distinguished from spasticity. Tension athetosis is produced by the intentional effort of the athetoid patient to prevent any undesired motion of the athetoid limb. By shaking the limb, this voluntary tension can be released. The spastic limb cannot be shaken loose because the exaggerated stretch reflex of a spastic muscle is involuntary and will occur whenever it is stretched by sudden passive elongation. It is also essential to differentiate between voluntary resistance of a normal muscle and exaggerated stretch reflex of a spastic muscle.

Spastic paralysis has a certain predilection for specific groups of muscles, with any variations depending upon the disease syndrome. In perinatal spastic paralysis, for example, the spasticity is more marked in the flexor muscles of the upper limb. The shoulder is adducted, flexed, and medially rotated; the elbow is flexed; the wrist and fingers are flexed; and the thumb is adducted in the palm. In the lower limb in spastic paraplegia, the hip is adducted, flexed, and medially rotated; the knee is flexed; and the ankle is held in plantar flexion. In acquired spastic cerebral palsy, the deltoid muscle may be spastic and hold the shoulder in abduction; and in the foot and ankle, the anterior tibial muscle may be spastic, posturing the foot in inversion.

ABNORMAL MOVEMENTS OR HYPERKINESIA

These may be defined as involuntary contractions of the voluntary muscle caused by lesions in various parts of the motor system—the motor cortex and its descending pathways, the basal ganglia, the midbrain and brain stem centers, the cerebellum and its connections, the spinal cord, the peripheral nerves, or the muscles themselves. Hyperkinesia is frequently present in the extrapyramidal type of cerebral palsy and must be regarded as a sign of disease and not as a disease entity. The character of the disordered movement depends both on the site of the lesion and on the type of pathologic change.

In the clinical study of hyperkinesia, one should observe the part and extent of the body involved, analyze the pattern and rhythmicity of the movement, and describe its various components.

Gait analysis, electromyography, and video records are of great value in recording hyperkinesias and evaluating effects of various modalities of treatment.

The more common forms of hyperkinesia seen in cerebral palsy are described next.

ATHETOSIS

Athetosis may be defined as a fluctuation of posture superimposed upon a persistent attitude; there are "swings" of movement from one posture to another, such as from hyperextension of the fingers and wrist and pronation of the forearm to full flexion of the fingers and wrist and supination of the forearm, caused by release of two opposing actions.[133]

Clinically, athetosis is characterized by involuntary writhing or squirming movements that are irregular, coarse, relatively continuous, and somewhat rhythmic. They are intensified by voluntary motion or tension and disappear during sleep. Coordination is very poor. There is marked impairment of voluntary movements. In the limbs, the distal portions (i.e., the hands, fingers, and toes) are more markedly affected. The face, neck, and trunk may be involved. Facial grimacing is slower and more sustained than in chorea. There may be associated hypertonicity of the musculature or some muscle weakness.

Tension may develop to control involuntary motions. The state of tension is not constant and can be released by repeated rapid passive flexion and extension of the joints of the involved limb. As was emphasized earlier, tension in athetosis must be distinguished from spasticity, in which the exaggerated stretch reflex is constantly present, and also from rigidity, in which a lead pipe–like resistance of the muscle is found. In athetosis, the deep tendon reflexes are usually normal and the plantar response is flexor.

Undulating and writhing movements of the limbs may also be present when there is loss of position sense in conditions such as peripheral nerve disease or posterolateral sclerosis. These become more marked when the eyes are closed. Muscle tone is usually not increased. This is called pseudoathetosis and is not a true hyperkinesia.

In athetosis, the predominant pathologic changes are in the basal ganglia, especially the caudate nucleus and putamen, although there may also be cortical involvement. It may be associated with status marmoratus or with brain changes resulting from erythroblastosis fetalis, kernicterus, or infantile encephalitis. Acquired athetosis may occur later in life as a result of disease or trauma.

Various clinical types of athetosis have been described by Phelps, such as rotatory, shudder, flair, tension, nontension, hemiathetosis, neck and arm, deaf athetosis, balance release, and emotional release.[413]

In dystonic movements usually seen in dystonia musculorum deformans, there is excessive muscular tone in certain muscle groups. It involves larger portions of the body, producing distorted postures of the limbs and trunk. There may be dysarthria, facial grimacing, and torticollis.

Tremor may be defined as a series of involuntary, rhythmic, purposeless, oscillatory movements that result from alternate contraction of agonist and antagonist groups of muscles that have reciprocal innervation. Muscles of fixation and synergists also play a part in the movement of tremor. One may distinguish tremors according to their rate, amplitude, rhythmicity, relationship to rest and movement, etiology, and underlying pathologic change.

Tremors may be elicited by asking the patient to hold his fingers extended and separated with his arms outstretched, to draw circles, or to perform slow movements. Tremors should be observed at rest and on activity.

The type of tremor seen frequently with lesions of the basal ganglia and extrapyramidal structures is *resting, static,* or *nonintention tremor,* which is slow, coarse, and compound in type. It is present with inactivity when the limb is in an attitude of repose or static posture and becomes less marked with activity. It is independent of voluntary movement and may disappear temporarily while the part is engaged in some voluntary effort. The tremor may involve the hands, feet, lips, mandible, or head.

If there is involvement of the cerebellar efferent pathways and their connections with the thalamus, the tremor encountered may be of the *intention, motor,* or *kinetic* type. It is absent while the patient is resting but reappears with activity.

Toxic tremors such as those seen in hyperthyroidism are fine and are usually rapid. *Psychogenic tremors* are of medium amplitude and rate. There is also a *physiologic normal tremor,* which may be brought out by placing the limb in a position of tension or by performing voluntary movements at the slowest possible rate.

ATAXIA

Lesions of the cerebellum produce loss of coordination and control, or ataxia, in which kinesthetic sense is destroyed. The various disturbances of equilibrium, muscle function, and movement seen in cerebellar disease are as follows:

1. There is *loss of posture and balance* both with the eyes open and with the eyes closed. With midline lesions, there is a wide-based, staggering, and unsteady gait that resembles that seen in alcoholic intoxication. The patient is unable to walk tandem or to follow a straight line on the floor. He may sway backward, forward, or to either side. In unilateral cerebellar disease, there is persistent swaying or deviation toward the affected side. In standing, the patient tends to fall toward the side of the lesion. On attempting to walk a straight line, he turns toward the involved side.

The cerebellar ataxic gait should be distinguished from the gait of sensory ataxia. The latter is also referred to as the gait of spinal ataxia, as it results most frequently from interruption of the proprioceptive pathways in the spinal cord. It is seen in conditions such as peripheral neuritis, brain stem lesions, tabes dorsalis, and posterolateral and multiple sclerosis. There is loss of position sense. The patient does not appreciate motion of the parts of the body, particularly of the joints and muscles of the lower limbs. Spatial orientation is disturbed, with loss of awareness of position of his feet and legs in space. If the patient walks with his eyes open, keeps his eyes on the floor watching his feet, and thus correlates visual impulses with proprioceptive ones, the gait may not be too abnormal. When the eyes are closed, the patient staggers and is unsteady, his feet seem to shoot out, and he may be unable to walk. With severe involvement, the patient walks with a broad base and the gait is irregular and jerky, even when his eyes are open. He stamps his feet in two phases, first on the heel and then on the toes, with a slapping sound or "double tap." An experienced clinician may diagnose the condition by hearing the patient walk.

2. *Asynergy and dyssynergy*—in which there is loss or disturbance of coordinated action between various groups of muscles or several movements that normally act synchronously—are present. There may be decomposition of movement.

3. There is *dysdiadochokinesia or adiadochokinesia*—in which alternate movements, such as successive pronation and supination of the forearms or opening and closing of the hands, are carried out slowly, irregularly, and clumsily. The patient is unable to terminate one movement and follow it immediately by its diagrammatic opposite because of a disturbance of reciprocal innervation of agonists and antagonists.

4. There is *dysmetria*—loss of ability to gauge the distance, speed, or power of movement. The patient may overshoot the desired point or stop before it is reached.

5. The muscles are *hypotonic* and tire easily.

6. *Intention type tremor* is commonly seen.

7. The *muscles of phonation are synergic*, with the result that speech is slurred, jerky, or explosive in type.

8. *Nystagmus* is usually present.

9. *Hyporeflexia* is common, probably caused by hypotonicity of the flexor and extensor muscles and loss of the restraining effect that they normally exert upon each other.

RIGIDITY

Rigidity is caused by diffuse damage to the brain. It is a state of fairly steady increased muscular tension equal in degree in agonist-antagonist groups such as flexor and extensor muscles in a limb, with resistance to passive movement in all directions and present throughout the entire range of motion. Resistance to passive motion is present on either slow or rapid movement of the limb. The muscles are firm, prominent, and tense. If the resistance to passive movement is continuous, it is referred to as waxy resistance, lead-pipe resistance, or flexibilitas cerea; if the resistance to passive motion is discontinuous, interrupted at regular intervals in a jerky fashion, the muscles giving way in a series of steps as if the manipulator were moving a limb attached to a heavy cogwheel or pulling it over a ratchet, the rigidity is referred to as *cogwheel rigidity*.

Prevalence

The reported prevalence of cerebral palsy varies in different countries between 0.6 and 5.9 per 1000 births. In Western countries, the birth prevalence rate is about 2.0 per 1000. With improved obstetrical care and increasing cases of prophylactic cesarean section, and exchange transfusion for Rh incompatibility, the prevalence of cerebral palsy is declining in the United States. In Britain, Ingram reports 2.5 per 1000.[255] Stanley reported the incidence of cerebral palsy in Western Australia to be 1.6 per 1000 live births.[520]

Hagberg et al. studied the epidemiologic trends and the changing panorama of cerebral palsy in Sweden. They studied 773 patients born with cerebral palsy between 1959 and 1978. This 20-year span was divided into five four-year periods. In the first three periods (1959 to 1970), the incidence of cerebral palsy decreased from 1.9 to 1.4 per 1000, but in the last period (1975 to 1978) the incidence of cerebral palsy increased to 2.0 per 1000. The decreasing and increasing trends were in spastic and ataxic diplegia—the premature type of cerebral palsy. Perinatal risk factors were responsible for the changing pattern, especially in the low birth weight surviving babies.[205]

Clinical Features

There are certain differences in the clinical findings between perinatal and acquired cerebral palsy, but they are not so important that they should be considered separately. The common types of cerebral palsy are here described briefly to facilitate understanding of the total problem involved in the management of the child with cerebral palsy. The reader is referred to the works of Crothers and Paine, Ingram, Illingworth, Denhoff and Robinault, and Woods for a more detailed description.[122, 132, 248, 256, 590]

SPASTIC HEMIPLEGIA

Certain authors distinguish between "hemiplegia" and "hemiparesis" on the basis that hemiplegia is more severe than hemiparesis and is of sudden onset, whereas others use the two terms interchangeably, as the late pictures of the two conditions are quite similar.

Side of Involvement. Hemiplegia is slightly more frequent on the right side (56 per cent, Hood and Perlstein, 1956; 59 per cent, Ingram, 1964).[238, 256] The majority of people have a natural right-handed preference; thus right hemiplegia constitutes a great disadvantage. Clinically, when the dominant side is affected, reading and writing difficulties, aphasia, and behavioral disturbances occur more frequently.

Musculoskeletal Manifestations. The evolution of physical findings in hemiplegia has been examined experimentally in monkeys by studying the reorganization of motor functions in a cerebral cortex deprived of motor and premotor areas in infancy.[290, 291, 567] The sequence of events is as follows: The initial acute findings are flaccid paralysis and absence of movement of the affected side. Soon, within hours or days, automatic movements recover if they ever appear. Spasticity will take weeks or even months to develop.

Byers and Tizard observed a similar sequence of clinical findings in human infants with hemiplegia.[87, 565] Initially, the affected limb is relatively flaccid, motionless, and hyporeflexic (often a diagnosis of a lesion of the brachial plexus is made). Soon it passes through a period

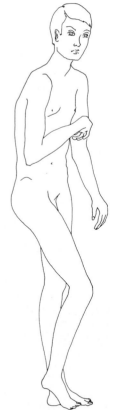

FIGURE 5–1. Posture of the upper limb in spastic cerebral palsy.

of reflex activity, but this stage is seldom observed clinically. Then it progresses to the period of hypertonus and hyperreflexia with the typical spastic hemiplegia posture and the tendency to contractural deformities in that position.

In congenital hemiplegia, the arm is adducted and medially rotated at the shoulder; the elbow is flexed, the forearm pronated, the wrist and fingers flexed, and the thumb adducted in the palm (Fig. 5–1). In some hemiplegics the upper limb is minimally involved; in these cases, spasticity may be difficult to detect until the child is asked to slap the hand of the examiner and incoordination is displayed; or when he runs and the upper limb assumes the posture of elbow flexion, forearm pronation, and wrist-finger flexion. The spasticity increases under stress. In the lower limb the hip is adducted, slightly flexed, and medially rotated. The knee is flexed because of spasticity of the hamstrings. The spastic child tends to stand on his toes (Fig. 5–2). When he touches the heel on the floor, the heel is usually everted and the knee may be hyperextended because of the spasticity

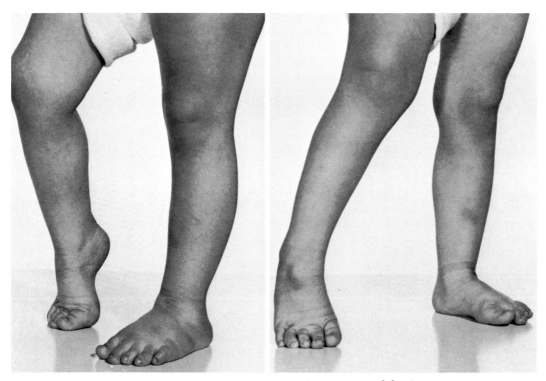

FIGURE 5–2. Right spastic hemiplegia showing equinus deformity.

of the gastrocnemius soleus muscle. The gait may be toe-toe, toe-heel, or plantigrade on the affected side, depending on the severity of involvement. On weight-bearing on the hemiplegic leg, there is an abductor lurch with a contralateral drop of the pelvis; the Trendelenburg test may be positive.

Spastic hemiplegia is seldom diagnosed at birth. The usual history obtained is that the mother observed the baby to be dominantly right- or left-handed. In fact, a strong hand dominance under 12 months of age should make one very suspicious of contralateral hemiplegia or some other abnormality. In other patients, the clenched fist or lack of use of the hemiplegic upper limb, or the equinus posture of the foot and ankle, may be the first abnormal finding noted by the parents. Occasionally, these abnormalities may escape attention, and hemiplegia is diagnosed when the child begins to walk and is seen to have a toe-toe or toe-heel gait on the affected side.

Motor development, in general, is slightly delayed. About one third of hemiplegics are walking by 18 months of age, two thirds by two years, and 90 per cent by three years.

All children with spastic hemiplegia show a varying degree of underdevelopment and atrophy of the involved upper and lower limbs. The severely involved and functionally poor limbs have the greatest amount of shortening and atrophy.

Reflex Examination. In congenital hemiplegic children, the asymmetrical tonic neck reflex, the grasp reflex, and the sucking reflex tend to persist on the affected side after they have already disappeared on the contralateral normal side. The plantar response tends to remain extensor in the hemiplegic foot as it becomes flexor in the opposite normal foot.

Sensory Disturbances. Sensory defects are quite common in cerebral palsy. Tizard, Paine, and Crothers, in a detailed study of the sensory function of 106 cerebral palsied children with congenital or postnatally acquired hemiplegia, found 57 patients (53.8 per cent) with sensory disorders.[566] Tachdjian and Minear reported an incidence of 41.7 per cent in 96 children with different types of cerebral palsy.[548] The most common sensory defects are astereognosis, impaired two-point discrimination, and impaired position sense. These are perceptual functions that are affected by lesions of the somatosensory cortices. Hemianopsia, usually homonymous on the hemiplegic side, is present in about 25 per cent of the cases.

A *modality* is a distinct subjective response to stimulation. *Perception* is an elaboration of sensation involving the synthesis of information of several modalities or a temporal pattern of single modality. Stereognosis, for example, is a perception based mainly upon the fusion of the modalities of touch and proprioception. The parietal lobes are the primary somatosensory cortices, with the thalamus being their sensory gateway. The postcentral gyrus area is primarily a sensory center, whereas the precentral gyrus is primarily motor. Both are closely united by connecting neurons to form a *sensorimotor functional unit*. Stimulation of the postcentral gyrus produces most sensory responses, but stimulation of the precentral gyrus will also produce some sensory responses. The reverse is true for motor responses.

Permanent sensory defects produced by cortical lesions are only discriminative and have a strong spatial element—for example, defects in stereognosis, two-point discrimination, topognosis, and identification of numbers traced lightly on the skin. Perceptions of temporal pattern (vibratory sensibility) are affected less frequently by cortical lesions unless they extend into the white matter. Any permanent damage of crude or simple sensations such as touch, pain, and temperature implies subcortical damage.

In the pathogenesis of sensory defects in the hands of children with cerebral palsy, there are two factors to consider: (1) organic brain lesions in the parietal cortices, the thalamus, or both; and (2) inexperience in using the hand. It is hard to determine which of these two plays the greater role in a specific case.

Epilepsy. Seizures are frequent in spastic hemiplegia (Perlstein and Hood, 43 per cent; Illingworth, 35 per cent).[248, 396] The seizures may be of late onset.[267] They are more frequent in children with acquired hemiplegia than in those with congenital hemiplegia. In the series of Crothers and Paine, 29 per cent of the patients with congenital hemiplegia and 55 per cent of those with postnatally acquired hemiplegia were epileptic at the time of examination.[122] The types of seizure seen are the generalized grand mal, the focal or jacksonian, and less commonly, myoclonic jerks and petit mal. The presence of seizures seems to correlate unfavorably with the intellectual development and general prognosis.

Intelligence and Speech Development. The degree of intellectual impairment varies greatly in spastic hemiplegia from the apparently normal to the grossly subnormal and untestable. In general, the greater the severity of hemiplegia, the greater is the degree of mental impairment, but this is by no means constant. Ingram reported that 41 per cent (28 of the 68 tested patients) had I.Q.'s below 70, and only 23 (33 per cent) were above 85.[256] Specific impairments found in hemiplegic patients are the inability to deal with written symbols, difficulty of organization and retention of memory, and perceptual problems, such as the failure to correctly visualize masses in space and to delineate horizontal and vertical directions and the third dimension.

Severe dysarthria is rare in spastic hemiplegia, but minor articulatory abnormalities are common. Hood and Perlstein found the mean age of verbalizing single words to be 22.4 months in patients with hemiplegia on the right side as compared with 20.5 in those with hemiplegia on the left, and the mean age of saying sentences to be 32.8 and 28.8 months, respectively.[238]

Prognosis. All hemiplegics are able to walk independently in time and to perform activities of daily living. They attend regular school and participate in peer group activities. All of them have one normal hand, and they are able to participate in some type of occupation, although they cannot perform work requiring skilled use of both upper limbs. Abnormalities of behavior, mental retardation, and epilepsy are the principal obstacles to competitive performance in adult life.

SPASTIC DIPLEGIA

Spastic diplegia is the most common type of cerebral palsy in North America. In about two thirds of the cases the cause is prematurity; other etiologic factors are hypoxia, rubella, encephalitis, head trauma, and cerebral embolism. The condition is characterized by moderate to marked spasticity of the lower limbs, with minimal involvement of the upper limbs. The hips show adduction-flexion–medial rotation spasticity and contracture; the ankles, equinus deformity; the feet, valgus deformity with oblique or vertical tali; and the knees, varying degree of flexion or extension spasticity and contracture. The upper limbs have minimal spasticity, as shown by pronator teres spasticity, mild spasticity of the elbow flexors, and incoordination of fine motor activities of the fingers and thumb. In general, motor function of the hands and upper limbs is adequate. The trunk is grossly normal with deficiency of anterior and/or posterior equilibrium reactions. Perceptual and visual-motor deficits with esotropia are usually present. On neurologic examination the deep tendon reflexes in the lower limbs are exaggerated—the Babinski sign is positive. Infantile automatism is absent.

Prognosis for independent walking is good for children with spastic diplegia; they usually walk by four years of age. About 80 per cent of the spastic diplegic children are community walkers; about 18 per cent require external support for ambulation (crutches or walker); only 2 per cent of these children are nonwalkers.

Intellect and speech are usually normal or slightly impaired. Ordinarily, children with spastic diplegia attend regular school, and as adults, they live independently—with appropriate education and vocational guidance they are gainfully employed. It is vital for these patients to adjust to life within the parameters of their intellectual and physical capabilities. Preventive psychologic counseling is indicated for some patients. Anxiety neurosis can be a problem in adolescence and adult life when these individuals are pushed to achieve tasks that they are incapable of performing. An overzealous physical therapy program in order to walk "normally" can be deleterious. The family and society should provide positive support to these patients.

SPASTIC QUADRIPLEGIA WITH TOTAL BODY INVOLVEMENT

In almost all the patients, spastic quadriplegia originates prenatally or at the time of birth, but there is usually a delay of several weeks or months before the classic picture is apparent. Ingram has proposed three stages in the evolution and gradual development of the final picture—the hypotonic stage, the dystonic stage, and a third stage in which rigidity and spasticity are present together in varying degrees in different patients.[255, 256]

The Hypotonic Stage. Paucity of movement is the striking clinical feature. Unless seizures or other marked neurologic findings are present, these children are thought to be normal and the condition is rarely diagnosed. The duration of the hypotonic stage usually varies between six weeks and six months, although it may be much longer. In general, the longer its duration, the greater the severity of involvement.

The Dystonic Stage. On examination, there is constant muscular rigidity that is more severe in the lower limbs. Sudden extension of the neck and head will produce a typical dystonic posture: The shoulders are adducted and medially rotated, the elbows extended, the forearms pronated, the wrists and fingers flexed,

and the thumbs adducted in the palm. In the lower limbs, the hips are extended, adducted, and medially rotated; the legs scissored; the knees extended; the ankles in equinus position; and the toes flexed. When the child is held in vertical position, rigidity is markedly increased in the limbs. The generalized dystonic attacks are present between 2 and 12 months.

The Rigid-Spastic Stage. The phase of predominant rigidity evolves gradually from the stage of dystonia.

Within a period of several weeks or months the spastic state insidiously appears. The posture and physical findings are similar to those in hemiplegia except that they are bilateral and usually the legs are more severely affected than the arms. The face is expressionless. There is a tendency to drool, and defects in speech are common. Visual disturbances and strabismus are present in some patients. Seizures are a frequent manifestation. Disturbance of hand sensation, so common in spastic hemiplegia, is relatively less so in spastic quadriplegia. Mental impairment is great in these children. It is rare that they have nearly normal intelligence.

About one third of patients with spastic quadriplegia fail to achieve standing balance for independent walking. Contractural deformities of the lower limbs provide a poor base for the development of balance (Fig. 5–3). For the sake of convenience and brevity, the musculoskeletal abnormalities are discussed later under *Treatment*.

Pure spastic *paraplegia* without involvement of the upper extremities is rare. One should be cautious in entertaining such a diagnosis in young children, for the majority of these patients have arm involvement at a later age.

Triplegia is almost always a variant of asymmetrical quadriplegia.

EXTRAPYRAMIDAL CEREBRAL PALSY

In the past this disorder constituted the second largest classification of cerebral palsy; at present its prevalence is decreased with improved obstetrical care and prevention of blood incompatibility. The presenting clinical picture is one of marked retardation of motor development. Most of the children are seen between 6 and 12 months of age because of a delay in achieving head and neck control or sitting balance.

At this stage of the disease, the infant will be found to be hypotonic, with an expressionless facies and an open, drooling mouth. The deep tendon reflexes are normal, but immature re-

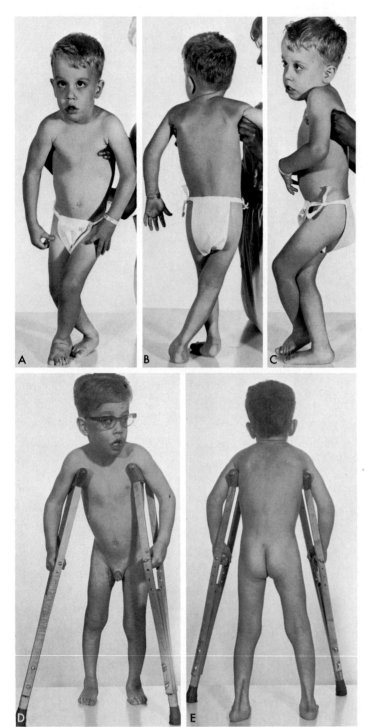

FIGURE 5–3. *Spastic quadriplegia with total body involvement.*

A to **C.** At four years of age. The marked scissoring of the hips and equinus deformity of the ankles provide a poor base upon which balance can develop. Note the pes valgus.

D and **E.** Following correction of contractural deformities by adductor myotomy and heel cord lengthening the patient is able to stand and walk with the assistance of crutches.

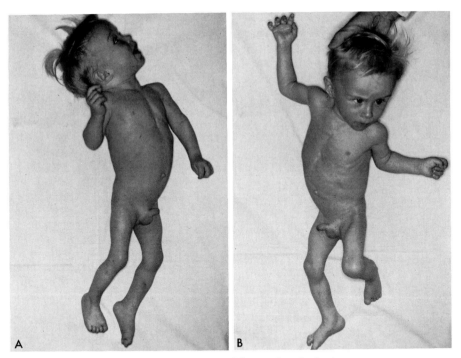

FIGURE 5–4. Extrapyramidal type of cerebral palsy.

A two-year-old infant with tension athetosis. Note the persistence of asymmetrical tonic neck reflex in **A**.

flexes such as the asymmetrical tonic neck reflex persist. Between 12 and 18 months of age, the hypotonia in the limbs is gradually replaced with varying degrees of tension. Soon involuntary movements develop. When the infant is placed prone in the mother's lap, an emotionally and posturally secure position, the tension and involuntary motions decrease or disappear, but when placed supine on the examination table, an insecure posture, tension athetosis, becomes marked (Fig. 5–4). The reciprocal action of the agonist and antagonist muscles is lost in the slow, purposeless, involuntary movements, interfering with functional activities. In pure extrapyramidal cerebral palsy, there is no evidence of spasticity and contractural deformities do not usually develop.

The rate of development of balance and postural reflexes is very variable. Uncontrolled involuntary movements may hinder function in these children to the extent that sitting, walking, or effective use of the hands may be impossible during their entire life. As handwriting is impossible, these patients are taught to use an electric typewriter. Substitution for hand function by the mouth may enable the child to perform such activities as turning the pages of a book or holding a pencil steady.

Often these children ambulate by creeping, or pivoting on the abdomen or buttocks.

Patients with extrapyramidal involvement are the most intelligent group of those with cerebral palsy. Hearing loss is common in these children, although other sensory defects, such as astereognosis, are quite rare.

Kernicterus as a cause of extrapyramidal cerebral palsy is becoming less and less frequent because of effective prophylaxis. In the Crothers and Paines series, it constituted 4.3 per cent of all cases of cerebral palsy and 19 per cent of those of the extrapyramidal type.[122]

In the differential diagnosis one should consider Werdnig-Hoffmann disease, amyotonia congenita, and birth injury to the spinal cord. In the neonate, the generalized flabbiness of the muscles, the labored abdominal respirations with intercostal retraction, and the absence of deep tendon reflexes may suggest amyotonia congenita. In neonatal spinal cord injury, there is a level of anesthesia distal to a certain segment, crossed extension reflex, and a respiratory pattern similar to that in amyotonia congenita.

Mixed cerebral palsy with involvement of both extrapyramidal and pyramidal systems is not uncommon. In some of these children, a diagnosis of spastic quadriplegia will be made in the first year of life, and then, later on, signs of extrapyramidal tract involvement will develop. Others will begin as pure athetoids and will develop spasticity later.

Management

GENERAL PRINCIPLES

Generalizations concerning treatment of cerebral palsy that are applicable to all affected children cannot be made. Many disciplines are involved, including pediatrics, neurology, orthopedic surgery, physical therapy, occupational therapy, psychology, speech therapy, audiology, sociology, and vocational counseling.

The care of children with cerebral palsy extends over a period of many years. In the course of this multidisciplinary treatment, the patient must be evaluated as an individual, as a member of the family, and as a future member of the community. The child with cerebral palsy will mature to become an adult with cerebral palsy. The problems and physical handicaps persist for the life span of the patient.

The problem is a dynamic one, changing with the growth, development, and maturation of the central nervous system. As the child grows, he acquires higher levels of performance and greater skills; however, with skeletal growth and muscle imbalance, various deformities may develop.

As was stated before, a great variety of conditions are included under the term "cerebral palsy." Each child should be carefully and thoroughly assessed to determine his individual difficulties. Vagaries must be avoided. An attempt should be made to find out why a child cannot do a certain task and what the implications of this failure are for his present disability and future performance. It is important to think in terms of doing something *for* the patient and not *to* the patient.

The objectives of management of cerebral palsy, in order of priority, are as follows: first, *communication*—speech and language; second, *use of upper limbs*—i.e., activities of daily living such as feeding, toilet needs, dressing, household maintenance, and writing; and third, *ambulation-walking*.

The orthopedic surgeon's primary concern is the care of the musculoskeletal system, helping to achieve the maximum potential of locomotion as well as functional use of the upper limbs, with the ultimate aim of normalizing performance of daily activities to the greatest possible degree. Frequently, because he sees the patient more often than do the other specialists, the orthopedic surgeon may be undertaking most of the patient's care. It is important that he be aware of his limitations and seek the help of other disciplines, as other problems involving speech, sight, hearing, and mentality, most certainly affect orthopedic management. This concept of *total care* must constantly be borne in mind.

SURGICAL MANAGEMENT

Surgery has a definite role in the management of cerebral palsy. It can prevent and correct deformity and improve function. In the past, conservative management of cerebral palsy has been overemphasized, and the role and value of operative treatment overlooked. In 1942, Green and McDermott evaluated their experience with surgical treatment of cerebral palsy and pointed out the principles to be followed.[196] The importance of the role of surgery has also been delineated by Baker, Banks and Green, Bost, Chandler, Eggers, Keats, McCarroll, Phelps, Silver, Samilson, Bleck, and others.*

The following factors determine the result of surgery and should be carefully assessed preoperatively:

TYPE OF CEREBRAL PALSY

It is in the spastic type of cerebral palsy that operative measures are most useful. In the other forms of cerebral palsy, such as athetoid, rigid, ataxic, or tremor, soft-tissue operations on the limbs are seldom indicated.

The active movements of athetoid children are distorted because of a lack of voluntary control of the involved muscle or muscle groups. If a deforming athetoid muscle is transferred or lengthened, the athetosis may shift to other muscles of similar function, resulting in the same deformity. For example, when in a patient with flexion athetosis of the wrist flexors (but not of the finger flexors), the flexor carpi ulnaris muscle is transferred to the dorsum of the wrist, persistent flexion athetosis of the finger flexors may then develop owing to shifting of the athetosis to the flexor digitorum profundus and sublimis muscles. Less frequently, the athetosis may be transferred to the wrist flexors, and severe extension deformity of the wrist may develop. Neurectomy and tendon lengthening or transfer operations are likely to be followed by a recurrence of the original

---

*See References 9–14, 59, 102, 103, 149–152, 277–288, 329, 414, 416, 417, 468, 505, 508.

deformity or, at times, the development of an opposite deformity. In pure athetosis there is no constant spasm of the muscles, and myostatic contractures do not usually develop.

In the cerebral palsied child with extrapyramidal involvement, surgery is indicated mainly in certain fixed deformities, and the operation should be primarily limited to bony procedures such as arthrodesis of the wrist. Surgery, however, should be performed only after carefully assessing its anticipated results by using plaster or plastic splints or orthoses over a period of time. Because plaster of Paris cast fixation is usually not tolerated by athetoid patients, it is wise to test preoperatively to determine whether such a problem exists and whether it can be overcome by using tranquilizing relaxant drugs such as diazepam (Valium) or chlordiazepoxide (Librium).

REFLEX MATURATION AND MOTOR LEVEL DEVELOPMENT

There is a great variation in severity, extent of involvement, and prognosis in cerebral palsy. The asymmetrical tonic neck reflex and the Moro and grasp reflexes normally disappear between four and six months of age. One should note whether they are still present at the age of two years. Does the child have good sitting and standing balance? Does he crawl? Is there reciprocal motion between his upper and lower limbs? What degree of control and function does he have in his upper limbs?

In the retarded child, one should note the rate of maturation of his neurophysiologic and motor systems. What is his potential for further improvement with growth and development? Are his deformities interfering with his already precarious balance and hindering his stance and locomotion? It must be remembered that the nursing and perineal care of a retarded child may be greatly simplified by a simple lengthening or myotomy of the hip adductors. Surgical procedures are also performed prior to attainment of the desired level of motor and neurophysiologic maturation to prevent deformities, primarily hip dislocation. Prevention of hip dislocation is, in fact, the principal indication for surgery before evidence of sitting balance has developed. Even though these children will never be able to walk, they will be much more comfortable when seated with support and have much less difficulty with nursing care than if their hips were dislocated.

Prognosis for Walking. Bleck studied the locomotor prognosis in cerebral palsy by performing the following seven tests and assigning one point if the automatism was present or the normal postural reflex was absent: (1) asymmetrical tonic neck reflex—one point; (2) neck righting reflex—one point; (3) Moro reflex—one point; (4) symmetrical tonic neck reflex—one point; (5) extensor thrust—one point; (6) parachute reaction (should be present)—one point if absent; (7) foot placement reaction (should be present)—one point if absent. The prognosis for walking was poor when the score was two points or more; it was guarded ("might walk") when the score was one point; and it was good when the score was zero. The accuracy of prediction of motor prognosis was 94.5 per cent. Crutch walkers were considered as functional walkers in this study.[55] According to Bleck, walking ability reaches a plateau by the age of seven years.[55] Previously, Beals had found that motor performance in children with spastic diplegia reaches a plateau at seven years of age.[34] Sutherland et al. demonstrated that major determinants of gait, linear measurements, and gait electromyelograms are of the adult type at the age of seven years.[538]

Inability to sit alone after the age of four years is a poor prognostic sign—the probability is great that the child will be a nonwalker. Mental retardation is not a factor in the ability to walk.[356a] Intelligence, however, has a definite effect on upper limb functions. In general, when a cerebral palsy child cannot reach for an object and bring it to his mouth or is unable to cross the hand over the midline of the trunk, prognosis for upper limb function is poor. Also, astereognosis is a poor prognostic sign.

ADEQUACY OF POSTOPERATIVE CARE

The feasibility of *adequate* and *meticulous postoperative care* should be determined. Several factors influence this, namely:

Age of Patient. He should be old enough to cooperate in the postoperative period to obtain the maximum benefit from the surgery. Usually this age range is from four to six years.

Level of Intelligence. In order to be able to cooperate with his physical therapist during the postoperative training period, the child should possess a reasonable mentality. Will he be trainable after his operation? What is his span of attention? Is he able to communicate? Mental retardation is not a contraindication to surgery, but in sophisticated procedures, such as tendon transfers, postoperative cooperation is crucial. The motivational factor often determines the difference between success and failure.

Associated Defects. When planning surgical procedures consider the presence of associated defects, such as vision problems, deafness, sensory disorders, and seizures. Control of seizures by phenytoin (Dilantin) can cause osteopenia and increased susceptibility to fractures.

Home and Family Situation. Is it adequate and conducive to good follow-up care? Are the parents sufficiently intelligent? How interested are they in the child? How faithfully have they kept their appointments? What has been their past performance with conservative management? In the preoperative period it is imperative to indoctrinate the patient and his family concerning exercises and night support. They should be well prepared for an aggressive postoperative training program.

TYPE AND TIMING OF SURGICAL PROCEDURES

In the past, it has been emphasized that soft-tissue procedures should not be performed during the growth period because the deformities will recur. The results of Green and Banks[19, 20, 195] have shown, however, that if the patients receive adequate postoperative care with a well-supervised program of exercises and night supports, the recurrence of deformities can be prevented. Unless a surgeon is willing to supervise minute details of postoperative care, he should never operate on these children.

Bone operations, such as triple arthrodesis, should be delayed until age ten years, in order to avoid interference with skeletal growth.

Surgical procedures and physical therapy should be planned so that they interfere minimally with the patient's education. It is best, whenever possible, to perform operations during vacation periods. Physical therapy programs should be realistic and goal oriented. The parents and child should be informed in order to prevent unrealistic expectations.

The parents should realize that the motor handicap of cerebral palsied children can be substantially improved by surgery, but that, unless the child's involvement is minimal, he will never be completely normal. The objective of surgery is to improve function. A patient who has no potential for walking or standing and transfer should not have surgical procedures performed on the feet.

INTERDEPENDENCE OF THE FOOT, ANKLE, KNEE, HIP, AND TRUNK

In the treatment of deformities of the foot and ankle in neuromuscular diseases it is imperative to determine the posture and balance of the trunk.[9] The foot, ankle, knee, hip, and trunk are interdependent.

The prerequisites for a stable upright posture in stance are plantigrade feet and ankles; extended knees and hips; and trunk, head, and neck balanced and centered on the supporting base (Fig. 5–5).

The spine-pelvis-hip should be considered as a unit. Pelvic obliquity may be caused by a scoliotic curve, or the pelvic obliquity may cause the scoliosis. The hip on the high side of the pelvis is unstable, and it may progressively dislocate. The contralateral hip should be assessed for abduction contracture. Any muscle that crosses, inserts, or originates on the pelvis may cause rotation or altered inclination. In cerebral palsy, translatory rotation of the lower limbs is deranged or lost.

The hip and knee mark the two ends of one bone—the femur; the knee and ankle are connected by the tibia and fibula (Fig. 5–6). The ankle, knee, and hip should be treated as one functional unit. The posture of each depends upon that of the others; they reflect and affect each other. Deformity and muscle weakness at

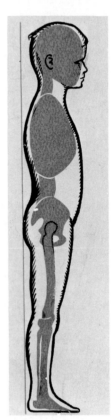

FIGURE 5–5. *Requisites for stable upright posture in stance.*

Requirements are (1) plantigrade feet and ankles, (2) slightly hyperextended knees, (3) extended hips, and (4) trunk-head-neck balanced and centered on the supporting base.

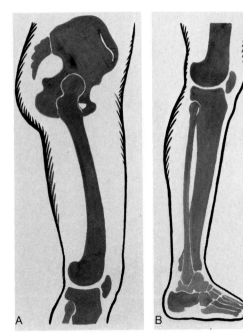

FIGURE 5–6. *Interdependence of the hip, knee, and ankle.*

A. The hip and knee mark the two ends of one bone—the femur. The hip, femur, and knee should be treated as a functional unit. **B.** The knee and ankle are connected by the tibia and fibula. The knee, tibia, and ankle should be treated as one functional unit.

one level influence stability at the adjacent levels, requiring compensatory adaptations to achieve independent stance and gait. Each level should be assessed both individually and in relation to adjacent levels.

Hip flexion deformity will affect the posture of the trunk, knees, and ankles. First, to achieve balance, lordosis of the lumbar spine is increased excessively (Fig. 5–7A). If the hip flexion deformity exceeds the degree that can be accommodated by lumbar lordosis, the trunk leans forward; this posture, with the knees in extension, requires support by crutches or walker to achieve balance (Fig. 5–7B). The knees flex to restore balance, and their flexed posture exerts more than normal strain on the antigravity muscles, demanding strong action on the part of the gluteus maximus, triceps surae, and quadriceps femoris (Fig. 5–7C).

When the ankles are fixed in equinus position and there are no compensatory accommodations at the hip and knee, the center of gravity of the trunk is posterior to the base of support (Fig. 5–8A). It is brought over the feet by flexion of the hips (Fig. 5–8B). Therefore, one method of compensating for fixed equinus deformity is by

hip flexion. Another is by hyperextension of the knees (Fig. 5–9). In calcaneus deformity of the feet (e.g., due to overlengthening of the triceps surae), the center of body weight falls posterior to the ankle axis. This is compensated for by bringing the body weight forward by excessive knee flexion and reducing body height; the tibia tilts forward because control by the triceps surae is lacking, and as a result the posture in both stance and gait is unstable (Fig. 5–10).

KINETIC ELECTROMYOGRAPHY AND GAIT ANALYSIS

The usefulness of kinetic electromyography and gait analysis in preoperative and postoperative assessment of the upper and lower limbs is well shown by Perry, Hoffer, Simon, Sutherland, and others.[227, 405, 510, 534] It is beyond the scope of this textbook to discuss gait analysis—the reader is referred to the excellent textbook of Sutherland and cited literature.[92, 105, 403–405, 534, 537]

NONOPERATIVE METHODS OF MANAGEMENT

Physical Therapy*

In combination with orthopedics, physical therapy can be very beneficial to the individual with cerebral palsy in improving motor function and achieving maximum motor potential. Many "methods" or "systems" of physical therapy are described in the literature, such as the Phelps, Kabat and Knott, Fay, Doman and Delacato, Bobath neurodevelopmental, Rood, Ayres sensory integration, and Vojta methods.[7a, 7b, 62—88, 138, 162, 163, 271a, 271b, 449]

For a critical assessment of these various "systems of therapy" the reader is referred to Bleck.[59] These systems of therapy are "philosophies" of management that the physical and occupational therapist applies to his or her methods of treatment.

The goals of physical therapy are the following: *first*, to enable the cerebral palsied child *to stand*. Even in the severe total body involved child, standing is important, as it will facilitate care of the child in dressing and transferring to the bathroom, chair, or bed. This makes a definite difference as the child gets older and heavier and the parents begin to age; it may prevent institutionalization of the adolescent. Almost all patients with cerebral palsy with appropriate support and physical therapy can be taught to stand. The *second goal is mobility*

---

*Written with Mary Weck, P. T., Senior Physical Therapist and Former Head of Physical Therapy Department, Children's Memorial Hospital, Chicago, Illinois.

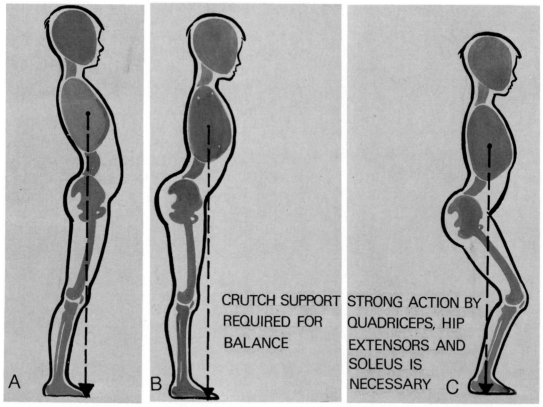

CRUTCH SUPPORT REQUIRED FOR BALANCE

STRONG ACTION BY QUADRICEPS, HIP EXTENSORS AND SOLEUS IS NECESSARY

A   B   C

FIGURE 5–7. Hip flexion deformity; its effect on posture of the trunk, knee, and ankle.

A. Excessive lumbar lordosis develops to achieve balance. **B.** If hip flexion deformity exceeds the amount accommodated by lumbar lordosis, the trunk leans forward; with knees in extension, crutch support is required for stability of balance. **C.** With knees flexed and trunk tilted backward, balance is regained. This exerts excessive strain on the antigravity muscles—gluteus maximus, triceps surae, and quadriceps.

and ambulation. Walking can be subclassified into various grades: (1) *community walker;* (2) *household walker*—the individual can get about the house with or without external support but requires a wheelchair outside the house; (3) *physiologic walker*—The individual can walk with the assistance of a physical therapist or parents for short periods; otherwise a wheelchair is required for mobility; (4) *nonwalker*—the patient is wheelchair dependent for all activities. Nonwalkers can be subclassified as (a) *independent transfer*—assistance is not necessary to get in and out of wheelchair; (b) *transfer with assistance;* and (c) *totally dependent*—those who must be lifted in and out of the chair.

It is vital that a physical therapy program be goal oriented and realistic. For example, all hemiplegic and most spastic diplegic children with cerebral palsy will be able to walk with appropriate orthopedic measures and physical therapy; whereas walking by children with total body involvement is almost impossible or non-

functional. In the quadriplegic child, therapeutic efforts should be directed toward mobility in the wheelchair. Sitting can be classified as follows: (a) by *ability*—propped, hand dependent or hand free; (b) by *pattern of deformity*—windswept hips and pelvis or asymmetrical slouch; and (c) by *severity of deformity*—beyond surgery, amenable to surgery, or no surgery.[431] Seating is assessed in special seating clinics.[176]

The hemiplegic or spastic diplegic child is instructed to stand with his center of gravity located over his base of support and to take normal reciprocal steps in walking; these children should be discouraged from using a walker or crutches and dragging themselves around from one place to another, leaning forward and displacing their center of gravity anteriorly.

When the center of gravity of a normal individual with an intact central nervous system is displaced anteriorly, he assumes an equinus posture with his feet-ankles; when his center of gravity is displaced posteriorly, his feet will assume a plantigrade position. It is important

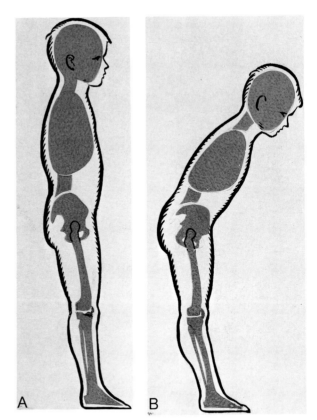

FIGURE 5–8. Compensation for fixed equinus deformity of the ankle by hip flexion.

A. When there are no compensatory accommodations at the hip and knee, the center of gravity of the body is posterior to the feet. **B.** The hips flex to bring the body to a position overlying the feet.

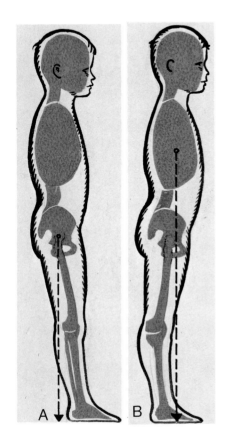

FIGURE 5–9. Hyperextension of the knees to compensate for fixed equinus deformity of the ankle.

A. When the equinus deformity of the ankle is fixed and there is no compensatory accommodation at the hip and knee, the center of gravity is posterior to the base of support. **B.** One method of aligning the trunk and bringing the center of gravity over the feet is by knee hyperextension. Note that the hips are in neutral position or slightly hyperextended.

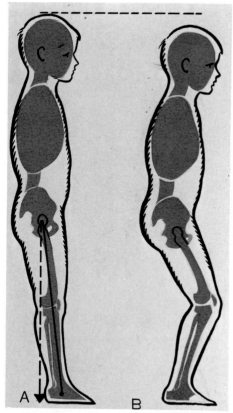

FIGURE 5–10. *The effect of calcaneus deformity of the ankle on posture of the hip and knee.*

A. In pes calcaneus (due, for example, to overlengthening of the triceps surae) the center of body weight falls behind the ankle axis. **B.** To compensate, body weight is brought anterior to the ankle axis by greater knee flexion, height is diminished, and the tibia falls forward because of lack of control by the weak triceps surae. The posture in both stance and gait is unstable.

for the child with cerebral palsy that physical therapeutic efforts be directed to maintain his center of gravity normally aligned over his base of support and to develop motor strength of his trunk extensors, gluteus maximus, quadriceps femoris, and abdominal muscles. The child is instructed to achieve postural control and develop appropriate movement patterns. The trunk is aligned over his pelvis and his pelvis posteriorly over his feet. He is instructed to do a lateral shift, which will free a foot for a smooth step.

Mobility without ambulation is achieved by the use of wheelchairs that are lightweight and either motorized or manually operated. The use of a wheelchair allows the cerebral palsied child to go out and keep up with other children in the neighborhood and partake in play activities.

Psychologically this is very important; it motivates the child to get out of the wheelchair and walk short distances.

The *third* goal of physical therapy is to *prevent contractural deformity of joints and bony deformities*. This is achieved by performing range of joint motion exercises, elongating shortened muscles several times daily. It is vital that range of motion exercises be *gentle*, prolonged, and maintained. The joints are kept out of deformity by appropriate splinting at night. Muscle strengthening exercises are performed, providing resistance by gravity and body weight. The child is positioned appropriately, such as prone at night, to keep the parts out of deformity.

Physical therapy plays an important role in postoperative habilitation and training programs. Recurrence of original deformity is prevented by strengthening the elongated muscle and developing cerebral control and motor strength of its antagonist muscle; for example, following heel cord lengthening, active exercises are performed to strengthen triceps surae as well as anterior tibial muscle. Range of motion exercises are performed to maintain full range of ankle motion.

Plaster of Paris Cast Immobilization and Inhibitory Splinting. The concept of "inhibitive casts" was introduced by Yates and Mott in 1977.[593] It was based on the theory that immobilization in cast reduces muscle hypertonicity. According to Duncan, early balance of the infant is enhanced by inborn supportive reflexes, righting reaction, and four superficial foot reflexes. There are four specific areas on the plantar aspect of the foot that respond to skin stimulation: (1) head of the first metatarsal, (2) head of the second metatarsal, (3) ball of the foot, and (4) sole of the heel. Pressure on the ball of the foot by displacing the center of gravity anteriorly will stimulate the toe grasp reflex with contraction of the toe flexors followed by muscle contraction of triceps surae, hamstrings, glutei, and trunk extensors; these muscle actions will checkrein progressive forward displacement of the center of gravity.[144a] It was proposed by Duncan and Mott that "inhibitive casts" control reflex-induced foot deformity by decreasing hypertonicity of cocontracting muscles.[144b] Mott and Yates reported the results in 111 children—68 per cent were predicted to be nonwalkers; following 3 to 12 months of treatment with "inhibitory casts" 14 per cent were walking independently, 20 per cent were cruising or walking with aids, and 14.4 per cent were walkers. The mean follow-up was eight years. Surgery or orthosis was required in 23 per cent. These results were not duplicated by other authors. In a prospective study of 34 children reported by Watt and associates, range of ankle dorsiflexion improved immediately and five weeks after cast application, but at six months post casting, it deteriorated to the precast range. They found no improvement in the neurodevelopmental milestones and no changes in the ankle clonus Babinski response or quadriceps reflex.[584a] In the experience of Sussman, the so-called inhibitive casts were not inhibitive; they served more as rigid ankle-foot orthoses.[533b] They cause muscle atrophy.[585a] The triceps surae muscle and its antagonist muscle (anterior tibial) atrophy; after immobilization is discontinued, both agonist and antagonist muscle groups regenerate and regain motor strength—recovery of triceps surae is greater than that of anterior tibial. Unless appropriate splinting is applied and a physical therapy program instituted, the equinus deformity will recur.

"Inhibitory casts" or splints should not be employed where there is fixed contracture of triceps surae because they will cause rocker-bottom deformity of the foot with vertical plantar flexed talus and dorsolateral displacement of the talocalcaneonavicular joint. This author recommends lengthening of the triceps surae.

When there is fixed equinus deformity of the ankle and heel cord lengthening is contraindicated because of the young age of the patient or weak triceps surae motor strength and risk of developing calcaneus deformity, a stretching dorsiflexion cast can be applied for one or two weeks to elongate the triceps surae. Prior to cast application the parents should be aware of the great possibility of pressure sores and blisters while the cast is on. Following removal of the cast, a rigid ankle-foot orthosis is used part of the day, and a knee-ankle-foot orthosis at night, to maintain the correction and prevent recurrence of the deformity.

When the equinus is dynamic, i.e., when there is no fixed contracture of triceps surae, a rigid ankle-foot orthosis is utilized part time in conjunction with an intensive physical therapy program. However, it is crucial that standing lateral radiograms of the foot-ankle be made with the orthosis on to ensure that the talus is not vertical and that a rocker-bottom deformity is not caused by the orthosis. Prolonged and continuous wear of the ankle-foot orthosis is not recommended, as it will cause marked muscle atrophy.

Orthosis. In the past, "bracing" of children with cerebral palsy was very popular and widely employed. Orthosis did not enhance walking and development of normal posture; also, it did not prevent development of structural deformity of bones and joints (such as hip dislocation).[209a, 498b]

This author recommends the use of orthotics in selected cases: UCBL (University of California Biomechanics Laboratory) foot orthoses to control oblique or vertical plantar flexed talus; supramalleolar orthosis (SMO) for mild dynamic equinus; and ankle-foot orthosis (AFO) for moderate dynamic equinus (often an ankle joint is provided, limiting plantar flexion but allowing dorsiflexion). Knee-ankle-foot and hip-knee-ankle-foot orthoses are used only as night splints to maintain joints in neutral position. Cable-twisters are not effective in correcting medial rotation gait.

In the upper limb, opponens splints are used to keep the thumb out of adduction-flexion in the palm; elbow-wrist-hand orthoses are used at night to maintain the forearm in supination and the elbow in slight flexion.

Biofeedback devices have been tried as therapeutic modalities. In the experience of this author they are not effective in preventing or correcting deformities of the musculoskeletal system. They do no harm.[59]

Drug Therapy for Muscle Relaxation. Many drugs have been tried in the past; however, in time they were found to be ineffective. At present, diazepam (Valium) is the most commonly used medication as a muscle relaxant in spastic cerebral palsy; it acts on the cerebral cortex and appears to diminish startle response and anxiety. This author recommends its use in the postoperative period in the total body involved cerebral palsy patient with severe spasticity. It provides relief of painful muscle spasms, making the patient more comfortable. Its routine use in the nonsurgical patient is not recommended.

When diazepam is ineffective in providing relief from painful muscle spasm, dantroline sodium (Dantrium) may be given orally; however, it is hepatotoxic, and liver function should be monitored by determination of SGOT blood levels.

The Hip

The common deformities of the hip in cerebral palsy are adduction, flexion, and medial rotation; occasionally the hips are in extension, abduction, and lateral rotation. With growth the biologically plastic skeleton of the child will respond to the forces of muscle imbalance with consequent development of coxa valga, increased anteversion of the femoral neck, acetabular dysplasia, subluxation, and eventual dislocation of the hip.

The type of deformity depends upon the degree and distribution of involvement and the type of cerebral palsy. Spasticity is the major deforming force; therefore, the hip deformities are common in spastic cerebral palsy. The greater the severity of involvement, the greater the hip deformity. In general, the child with spastic hemiplegia has minimal or no hip problems, whereas the diplegic cerebral palsy child with predominant involvement of the lower limbs and minimal involvement of the upper limbs has moderate hip deformities, which often interfere with efficacy of gait. The quadriplegic child with severe spasticity of all four limbs, who is unable to ambulate and has total body involvement, has disabling deformities of both hips, often with subluxation or dislocation that interferes with his sitting balance.

In pure athetosis, hip deformities are rare; in mixed cerebral palsy (spastic and athetoid), hip deformities do develop and pose difficult problems in management.

ADDUCTION-FLEXION DEFORMITY

Adduction deformity of the hip is caused by spasticity and contracture of the hip adductors (adductor longus, adductor brevis, adductor magnus, and pectineus), the gracilis, and the medial hamstrings (semitendinosus and semimembranosus muscles).

Gait analysis of cerebral palsy patients with adducted hips has shown overactivity of the hip adductors and the gracilis or medial hamstrings, or both.

Electromyographic examination shows continuous activity of the hip adductor muscles during both stance and swing phases of gait. It is important to distinguish between limitation of hip abduction caused by overaction and pull of the hip adductors and that caused by the gracilis and medial hamstrings. The two deforming components are differentiated by performing passive hip abduction with the hips in extension, first with the knees in extension and then with the knees in 90 degrees of flexion; the latter (flexed posture of the knees) relaxes the gracilis and medial hamstring muscles (Fig. 5–11). Any asymmetry of involvement between the right and left sides should be carefully noted at this time.

To determine further the degree of contrac-ture of the gracilis muscle (one of the major forces in the production of hip adduction deformity), Phelps has suggested the following maneuver: The patient is placed in prone position with the hips in maximum abduction and the knees in 90 degrees of flexion; if the gracilis muscle is shortened upon passive full extension of the knee, the hip will automatically adduct. The degree of hip adduction is noted.[414] Electromyographic studies have shown, however, that the Phelps gracilis test can be positive for either the gracilis or the medial hamstrings.[219]

In gait, hip adductor spasticity causes close approximation of the knees and thighs and a short stride length. *Scissoring* is a term used to describe the severe adduction posture of the hips when the patient is upright; when walking, one limb crosses over the other. True scissoring must be distinguished from approximation of the knees for stability and balance.

Flexion deformity of the hip is primarily caused by spasticity and contracture of the iliopsoas and secondarily by the rectus femoris muscles. The overactivity of these muscle groups in gait in cerebral palsy patients with flexed hip posture has been demonstrated by gait analysis. To distinguish between the two forces, the *Thomas test* is performed with the knee in extension and then in flexion (Figs. 5–12 and 5–13). When the rectus femoris is the cause, hip flexion deformity is increased with the knee in flexion and decreased with the knee in extension; when it is due to the iliopsoas muscle, however, the position of the knee has no effect on the degree of hip flexion contracture. Palpation for tautness of the muscle fibers of the iliopsoas and pelvic origin of the rectus femoris muscles is also of some assistance. In the *Ely test* or *prone rectus test* the child is placed prone with the hip and knee in extension. On passive flexion of the knee, if the test is positive, the pelvis will elevate from the table. The degree of knee flexion when the pelvis begins to rise and the maximum elevation of the pelvis are recorded. It has been shown by electromyographic studies that the prone rectus test can be positive for any of the hip flexors. In the two-joint muscle, the tests are not positive for any one muscle (Fig. 5–13). Often it is the iliopsoas muscle that is the principal deforming force in the causation of hip flexion deformity.

Other spastic muscles that may contribute to flexion deformity of the hip, particularly in stance, include the following: (1) tensor fasciae latae, (2) sartorius (flexing the hip to 90 degrees of flexion), (3) pectineus, (4) adductors longus

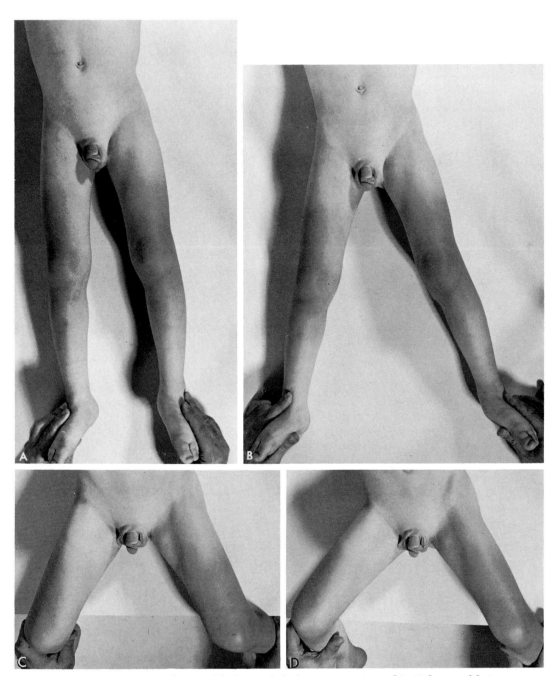

FIGURE 5–11. Passive abduction of the hips with the knees in extension and in 90 degrees of flexion.

Flexion of the knee will relax the gracilis and medial hamstring muscles, enabling differentiation between limitation of hip abduction caused by spasticity and contracture of the hip adductors and that due to the gracilis and medial hamstrings. **A** and **C** show the range of motion when the spastic muscles grab; **B** and **D** demonstrate the maximum range of passive hip abduction.

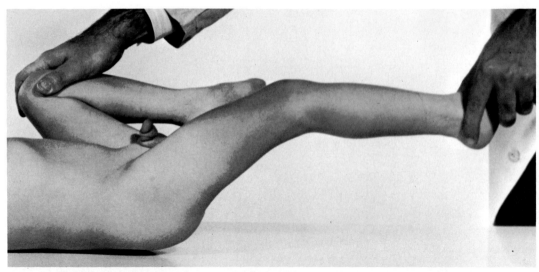

FIGURE 5–12. Thomas test demonstrating flexion deformity of the hip in spastic cerebral palsy.

Deformity is primarily caused by spasticity and contracture of the iliopsoas and rectus femoris muscles. To distinguish between the two components, the Thomas test is performed with the knee in extension and then in flexion. If flexion contracture of the hip is due to spasticity of the iliopsoas muscle, the degree of hip flexion deformity is not altered by a change in position of the knee.

and brevis (flexing the hip from hyperextension to 20 degrees of flexion), and (6) gracilis (flexing to 30 degrees of flexion).

In stance and gait a flexed attitude of the hip may be secondary to flexion deformity of the knee or equinus deformity of the ankle; also, when balance is poor, the spastic child will flex his knees and hips to lower his center of gravity. "Jump position" is a term referring to the posture of a spastic child who stands with his knees and hips flexed and the ankles in equinus position (Fig. 5–14).

One of two radiographic methods may be used for accurate determination of the degree of hip flexion deformity in stance; with the patient standing as erect as possible, a true lateral of the lumbar spine, pelvis, and proximal femur is made. In the *Milch method*, a line is drawn from the ischial tuberosity to the anterior superior iliac spine and a second line is drawn parallel along the axis of the femoral shaft. The angle formed by the intersection of these two lines is the *pelvic-femoral angle*, which normally measures 55 degrees. In the *Fick method* the sacrofemoral angle is the angle formed between the lines drawn across the superior surface of the first sacral vertebra and the axis of the femoral shaft. In the normal child and adolescent the sacrofemoral angle measures 50 to 65 degrees. In flexion deformity of the hip the longitudinal axis of the femoral shaft moves proximally toward the horizontal line drawn on top of the first sacral vertebra; therefore, the

sacrofemoral angle diminishes to less than 50 degrees.[53] These radiographic methods of mensuration of hip flexion deformity are ordinarily impractical for routine use, as the spastic child has poor balance and often requires the support of walkers or parallel bars for standing and walking. Inspection of the standing posture of the patient and the Thomas test are of more clinical value.

The *stretch reflex of rectus femoris* is elicited as follows: With the patient in prone position, the patient's buttocks are sharply slapped—this evokes hip flexion by contraction of rectus femoris causing the pelvis to rise off the table (Fig. 5–15).[522] This test should be performed with a certain degree of trepidation. The test may be objectionable to the parents and patient. Contracture and degree of spasticity of the rectus femoris are best tested by the Ely test (see Fig. 5–13A and B).

MEDIAL ROTATION DEFORMITY OF THE HIPS

Several factors should be considered in the pathogenesis of this condition. It is principally caused by spasticity and myostatic contracture of the muscles that medially rotate the hip; these are the gluteus minimus and anterior portion of gluteus medius, tensor fasciae femoris, medial hamstrings, and anterior portion of the hip adductors. Gait analysis can be of help in defining the pathogenically active muscle.[105, 405, 537, 576]

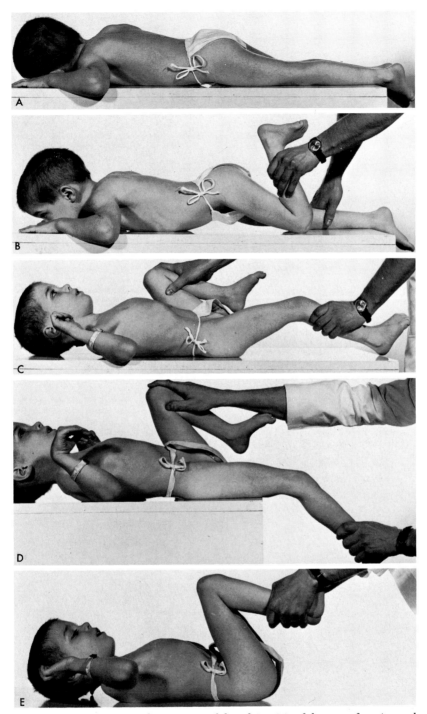

FIGURE 5–13. Spasticity and contracture of the pelvic origin of the rectus femoris muscle.

A and **B.** Positive Ely test. The child is placed in prone position with the hip and knee in extension. On passive flexion of the knee the pelvis will elevate from the table. **C.** On the Thomas test 35 degrees of flexion of the hip is demonstrated. To distinguish between the iliopsoas and rectus femoris as causes of flexion contracture of the hip, the Thomas test is performed with the knee in extension and then in flexion. If flexion contracture of the hip is due to spasticity of the iliopsoas muscle, the degree of hip flexion deformity is not altered by a change in position of the knee. **D.** Spasticity and contracture of the rectus femoris is demonstrated by sudden passive flexion of the knee with the hip in extension. Note the lumbar lordosis to compensate for fixed flexion contracture of the hip. **E.** The degree of passive knee flexion is near normal when the hip is flexed, relaxing the pelvic origin of the rectus femoris muscle.

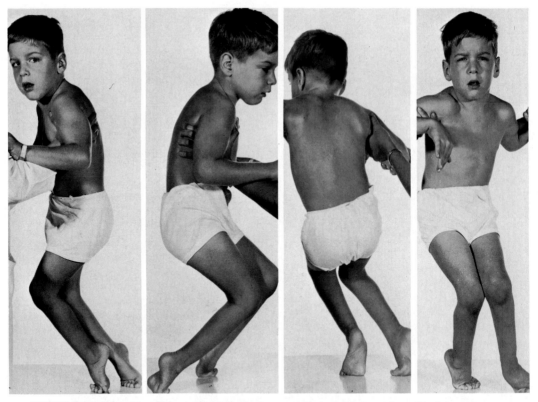

FIGURE 5–14. A five-year-old boy with cerebral palsy—spastic quadriplegia with total body involvement.

Note the severe flexion, medial rotation, and adduction contracture of the hips, flexion deformity of the knees, and equinus deformity of the ankles and feet. It is obvious that the severity of the deformities prevents the child from walking and interferes with his already precarious balance. He was treated by bilateral adductor myotomy, obturator neurectomy (anterior branch), and heel cord lengthening; this was followed six months later by fractional lengthening of the hamstrings. The patient is able to ambulate now with minimal support of crutches.

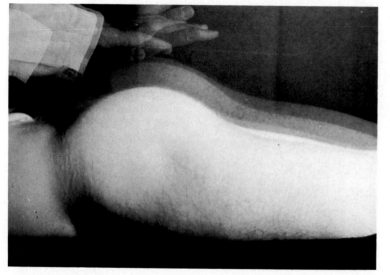

FIGURE 5–15. Steel's technique for testing stretch reflex of rectus femoris.

The response is elicited by sharply striking the buttocks of the patient, who is in prone posture with the hips and knees in extension. The resulting stretch and contraction of the spastic rectus femoris will suddenly elevate the pelvis from the table. (From Steel, H. H.: Gluteus medius insertion advancement for correction of internal rotation gait in spastic cerebral palsy. J. Bone Joint Surg., 62-A:919, 1980. Reprinted by permission.)

Excessive femoral antetorsion is another pathogenic factor in medial rotation deformity of the hip. When walking on level ground, from the onset of swing phase until midstance, the pelvis, femur, and tibia rotate medially. At midstance, they suddenly rotate laterally and continue to do so until toe-off as swing phase begins. The gluteus medius contracts at the onset of stance until midstance. Medial rotation of the entire limb takes place in the early stance phase activity of gluteus medius.

During clinical examination, the various pathogenic factors are assessed. The patient walks with medially rotated lower limbs with the patellae facing medially. The stride angle, i.e., the angle of the foot from the line of progression, is negative. The patient toes-in and may trip and fall down. Often, medial rotation deformity of the hip is associated with hip abductor muscle weakness, and the patient walks with gluteus medius limp and Trendelenburg lurch. Next, passive lateral rotation of the hip is performed with the patient in prone position with the hip in extension and the knee in 90 degrees of flexion. It is best to test range of motion of one hip at a time. Passive lateral rotation of the hip is performed suddenly to determine the degree of lateral rotation at which the spastic muscles grab, and then gradually and steadily to note the absence or presence of fixed deformity. Steel elicits the stretch reflex of gluteus medius–minimus as follows: The patient is placed in prone position with the hip in extension and neutral position as to abduction-adduction and rotation, and the knee is flexed 90 degrees. With one hand the examiner stretches the upper thigh-hip and with the other hand pushes the leg sharply toward the opposite limb into lateral rotation. In the presence of stretch reflex of gluteus medius–minimus the leg will bounce back into medial rotation; in the normal subject the leg will come to rest where it was lying (Fig. 5–16).[522]

Bony deformities of the hip are usually acquired. Coxa valga and increased anteversion of the femoral neck develop first, followed by dysplasia of the acetabulum and gradual progressive levering of the femoral head out of the acetabular socket. The dynamic imbalance between the spastic hip adductors and weakened hip abductors combined with spastic hip flexors is the prime deforming force in the causation of coxa valga. With loss of hip abductor power, growth from the greater trochanteric apophysis is not normally stimulated, and valgus deformity of the femoral neck results from disparity of relative growth between the capital femoral epiphysis and the greater trochanteric apoph-

ysis. Absence of normal weight-bearing forces is another factor in the pathogenesis of coxa valga.

Brooks and Wardle studied the effect of muscle action on the shape of the femur by performing experiments on ten decalcified femora. The effect of iliopsoas action alone on femoral shape was that of valgus deformity, a posterior deflection of the neck, an untwisting of the upper diaphysis, and an increased anterior curvature of the shaft. The tendency to femoral deformity produced by an iliopsoas force was abolished by a gluteal force acting at the greater trochanter when these forces are in the ratio of 5:3, respectively.[78]

HIP SUBLUXATION AND DISLOCATION

The *prevalence* of hip subluxation or dislocation in cerebral palsy varies, from 2.6 to 28 per cent depending upon the age of examination, severity of involvement, type of cerebral palsy, and method of management of the child (Table 5–9). In the experience of this author, in an unselected group of cerebral palsy patients, the prevalence was 4.2 per cent; this probably represents an average representative figure.[548]

Dislocation of the hip occurs more frequently in the nonambulatory patient with the spastic type of cerebral palsy. It is more common in the quadriplegic and diplegic patients, being rare in the hemiplegic.

Howard et al. studied the natural history of spontaneous dislocation of the hip in 102 patients with cerebral palsy. The incidence of hip dislocation was 59 per cent in patients with bilateral hemiplegia and severe involvement of the upper limbs, whereas in those with diplegia and minimal involvement of the upper limbs only 6.5 per cent were affected. These investigators substantiated the strong correlation between stability of the hip and the patient's ability to walk. In the pure athetoid child dislocation of the hip is uncommon, but in the mixed cerebral palsy patient (spastic and athetoid) it does occur relatively more frequently.[243]

Table 5–9. *Prevalence of Hip Subluxation and Dislocation in Cerebral Palsy*

Author	Year	Percentage
Gherlinzoni and Pais[181]	1950	4.6
Mathews, Jones, and Sperling[346]	1953	2.6
Tachdjian and Minear[548]	1956	4.2
Pollock and Sharrard[425]	1958	23
Phelps[416]	1959	17
Samilson et al.[479]	1972	28

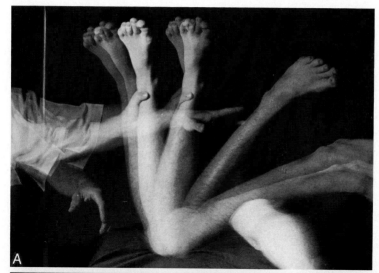

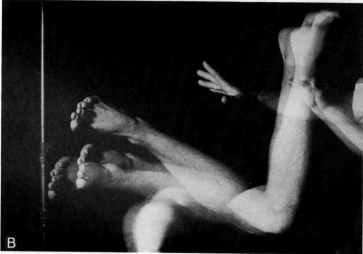

FIGURE 5–16. The gluteus medius and minimus stretch reflex.

Place the patient supine with the hip extended to neutral and the knee flexed at right angles; next, suddenly push the leg toward the opposite limb into lateral rotation. **A.** If the gluteus medius and minimus muscles are spastic, the leg will bounce back rapidly into medial rotation. **B.** Normal gluteus medius and minimus muscles. Note the leg rests where it was pushed. (From Steel, H. H.: Gluteus medius insertion advancement for correction of internal rotation gait in spastic cerebral palsy. J. Bone Joint Surg., 62-A:919, 1980. Reprinted by permission.)

Pathogenesis. Dislocation of the hip in cerebral palsy is paralytic, but congenital dislocation does occur. Paralytic dislocation of the hip is a gradual process, usually developing late in childhood, at around five to seven years of age. Congenital hip dysplasia does occur in cerebral palsied children; its prevalence is similar to that in the general population. The congenital nature of hip instability is suggested if the subluxation or dislocation develops during the first two years of life, and when there is dysplasia of the acetabulum (Fig. 5–17). Paralytic dislocation of the hip is characterized by relative ease of reduction and absence of acetabular dysplasia in its early stages.

The following factors lead to dislocation of the hip in cerebral palsy: (1) *muscle imbalance* between strong and contracted hip adductors versus weak hip abductors, and strong hip flexors versus weak hip extensors. Muscle imbalance between hip flexors and extensors and flexion deformity alone do not dislocate the hip; the combination of strong hip adductors and flexors is the potent pathogenic factor in hip instability.

(2) *Excessive femoral antetorsion with coxa valga* develops early in spastic cerebral palsy; however, the femoral neck–shaft angle is normal in most spastic children in the early stages of hip instability. The valgus appearance is apparent, owing to the increased femoral antetorsion; on making an anteroposterior radiogram of the hip in full medial rotation, the actual coxa valga is minimal.[35] The abnormal configuration and development of the upper femur is primarily due to muscle imbalance—the abnormal pull of the iliopsoas causes excessive antetorsion. Another factor to consider is the lack

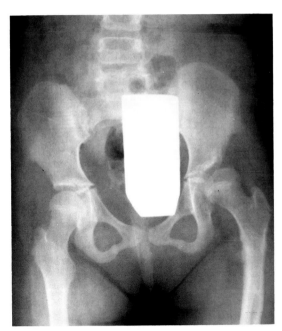

FIGURE 5–17. Congenital dysplasia of the left hip in a child with cerebral palsy.

Note the marked dysplasia of the acetabulum.

of weight-bearing and diminished or absent muscle forces of the glutei on the greater trochanteric apophysis.[317, 416, 479]

(3) *Acetabular insufficiency* is not a problem in the early stages of subluxation; however, if dislocation persists for several years, acetabular insufficiency will gradually develop.

(4) *Retention of neonatal reflexes* may be a significant factor. Asymmetrical trunk incurvation (or Galant's reflex) will cause a long thoracolumbar C curve of the spine and will force the hips into "windblown" position; the hip on the high side of the pelvis is in an unstable position with functional coxa valga, especially if there is associated muscle contracture of the iliopsoas. Persistent strong crossed extension reflex will force the neonatal and infant hip into continued extended posture, which may dislocate the hip. The pathogenetic factor of forced hip extension in hip stability is well shown in congenital hip dislocation—the same mechanism acts in the cerebral palsied child. Positive supporting reaction and abnormal persistence of asymmetrical tonic reflex are other neonatal reflexes that may force the hip into unstable extended position.

The center of the movement of the hip moves distally toward the lesser trochanter when there is a dynamic imbalance between the strong hip flexors-adductors versus weak hip extensors and abductors (Fig. 5–18). Adduction-flexion posture of the hip exerts an anterolateral force on the hip capsule, which stretches; abnormal forces gradually dislocate the hip posteriorly. Initially the hip is subluxated with the femoral head riding laterally and superiorly; then it is dislocatable on adduction of the hip and reducible on adduction-abduction of the hip. Eventually the hip is dislocated and irreducible.

Anterior dislocation occurs very occasionally. Often it is iatrogenic, the result of overzealous surgical release of the hip flexors and adductors. A latent undetected extensor thrust may be a factor. The hip abductors and extensors become overactive, and fixed abduction lateral rotation contracture of the hips will dislocate the femoral heads anteriorly. This makes sitting difficult, and the hips gradually become painful. In mixed cerebral palsy, unilateral or bilateral extension lateral rotation contracture of the hip may be present on rare occasion, and the hips may dislocate anteriorly without previous surgical intervention.

Clinical Features. Dislocation of the hip in cerebral palsy should be suspected when there is marked limitation of hip abduction, a positive Galeazzi sign, prominence of the greater trochanter, and asymmetry of the skin folds of the thigh. Radiograms of the hips should be made to confirm the diagnosis. Widening of the medial joint space is the earliest sign of lateral displacement of the femoral head; soon Shenton's line is broken, indicating superior subluxation. Eventually, if the displacement goes untreated, the femoral head will be totally dislocated out of the acetabulum. With persistence of dislocation, posterior and superior insufficiency of the acetabulum will develop.

The hip may be painful during the process of progressive displacement out of the acetabulum, i.e., during the stages of subluxation and when dislocatable. The parents will note that the child is uncomfortable when the hip is moved passively. Once the hip is totally dislocated and spontaneously irreducible, pain is not a symptom until later on, when degenerative arthritis develops.

In the ambulatory patient, walking may be impaired. Sitting balance may be a problem. Pelvic obliquity develops, particularly in unilateral dislocations or when involvement is asymmetrical. Scoliosis develops in the majority of patients. In the etiology of scoliosis, in addition to dislocation of the hip, pelvic obliquity, and loss of sitting balance, neurologic impairment is an important factor. Because of associated extreme adduction contracture of the hips, perineal care is difficult or may be impossible; this

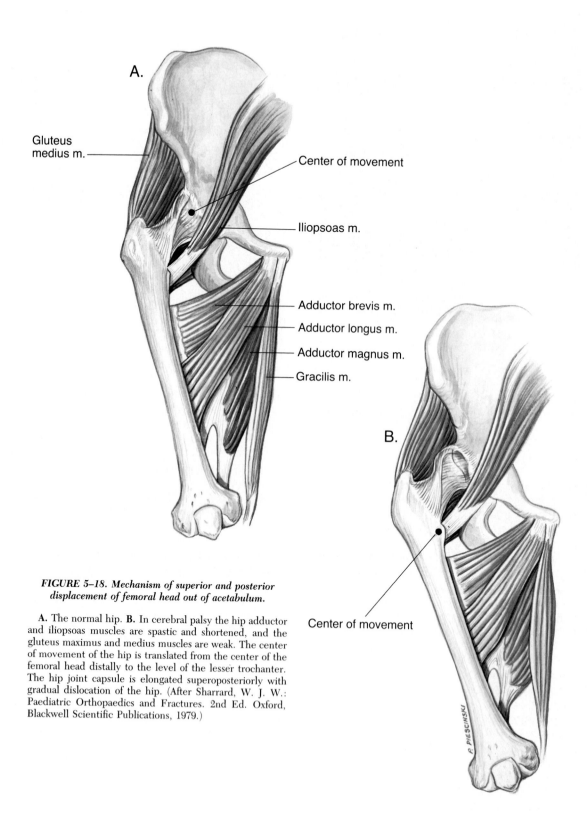

FIGURE 5–18. *Mechanism of superior and posterior displacement of femoral head out of acetabulum.*

A. The normal hip. **B.** In cerebral palsy the hip adductor and iliopsoas muscles are spastic and shortened, and the gluteus maximus and medius muscles are weak. The center of movement of the hip is translated from the center of the femoral head distally to the level of the lesser trochanter. The hip joint capsule is elongated superoposteriorly with gradual dislocation of the hip. (After Sharrard, W. J. W.: Paediatric Orthopaedics and Fractures. 2nd Ed. Oxford, Blackwell Scientific Publications, 1979.)

often is the major complaint of the parents. Excessive pressure on the ischium leads to decubitus ulcers. Stress fractures of the femur are common; when the hip is dislocated, the long lever arm with a relatively fixed fulcrum causes spiral fracture of the femoral shaft or supracondylar fracture of the femur when a bedridden osteoporotic cerebral palsied child is turned over.

TREATMENT

Conservative measures consist of *gentle* passive stretching and range-of-motion exercises to prevent the development of contractural deformity. The hip adductors, flexors, and medial rotators are elongated by gentle manipulation several times a day. Splints or bivalved hip spica casts that hold the hips in abduction, lateral rotation, and extension are used at night. Prone posturing is important. The same splint may be used during the day for standing for short periods. In the preoperative period, routine use of the bivalved night cast is not recommended, as it is usually not well tolerated by the severely spastic child. As a rule, hip abduction orthoses are not effective in preventing hip subluxation or adduction contracture. The primary indication for these hip-positioning devices (bivalved abduction plaster casts or polypropylene splints) is to maintain range of motion obtained by soft-tissue release and to prevent the patient from assuming flexed and asymmetrical posture at night. They should extend distally to include the foot and leg and not terminate above-knee, as the supracondylar area of the femur is a common site of fracture in the osteoporotic nonambulatory patient.

Orthoses (total control) to support the hips and lower limbs for standing and ambulation were used extensively in the past. These devices are not satisfactory substitutes for good balance; they interfere with development of gait, cause disuse atrophy of muscles, and may be a factor in early development of scoliosis. Their use has been gradually discarded. When the child has good sitting balance, reciprocal motion between the upper and lower limbs, and adequate upper limb function, the deformities of the lower limbs are assessed to determine whether surgical intervention is indicated. Often the scissor-like deformity and the equinus position of the feet prevent the child from walking. Prerequisites for surgical intervention of the lower limbs are weight-bearing and demonstration of potential for locomotion. The exception to this rule occurs when the hips begin to develop subluxation; in such an instance,

surgical intervention is indicated, even prior to the development of sitting balance. It is paramount to prevent dislocation of the hip, as these patients will have much less difficulty with hygienic care, will have a wider and more secure base for assisted sitting, and will be much more comfortable than if their hips were dislocated.

Hip Flexion-Adduction Deformity. Adductor myotomy is often performed in combination with fractional lengthening of the iliopsoas tendon when there is flexion contracture of the hip. The operative technique and postoperative care for adductor myotomy and fractional lengthening of the iliopsoas tendon are described and illustrated in Plate 58. In the past this author used to perform neurectomy of the anterior branch of the obturator nerve. Neurectomy causes fibrosis of the innervated muscle; postoperatively there is increased risk of permanent contracture of the fibrosed muscle. For the past ten years this author has discontinued neurectomy of obturator nerves. It is still used by other surgeons; therefore, it is illustrated for the sake of completeness.

If the pelvic origin of the rectus femoris is very spastic, it may be a factor in the causation of hip flexion deformity. In such an instance, hip flexion contracture will be increased when the knee is flexed during performance of a Thomas test. The pelvic origin of rectus femoris is sectioned in a separate longitudinal incision (Fig. 5–19).

Transfer of the Origin of the Adductor Longus and Gracilis Posteriorly to the Ischium with Release of the Adductor Brevis. The objective of this procedure is to correct adduction, flexion, and medial rotation deformity of the hip. Initially the procedure was developed in 1955 by Garrett for paralytic dislocation of the hip, particularly in myelomeningocele; later both Garrett and Perry recommended the procedure for cerebral palsy patients. Stephenson and Donovan had the first published reports on adductor transfer in cerebral palsy.[525] The indications for the operative procedure are essentially the same as for adductor myotomy. The operative technique of posterior transfer of hip adductors is as follows (Fig. 5–20):

The patient is placed in supine position with a sandbag under the buttocks, and both lower limbs, perineum, pelvis, and lower abdomen are thoroughly prepped and draped. Both hips are placed in 90 degrees of flexion and maximal abduction and lateral rotation. A horizontal skin incision is made beginning 2 cm. superior to the adductor longus and extending 1 cm. pos-

Text continued on page 1644

Adductor Myotomy of Hip and Neurectomy of Anterior Branch of Obturator Nerve (Banks and Green)

OPERATIVE TECHNIQUE

A. With the patient in supine position, both lower limbs and hips are prepared and carefully draped to allow full manipulation of the hips. Meticulous attention should be paid to avoiding contamination from the perineal area. In the groin, the prepared area should be proximal enough to include the origin of the adductor longus muscle. With both hips in flexion, abduction, and lateral rotation, a longitudinal incision is made over the posterior border of the adductor longus, beginning about ½ inch below the pubis and extending distally for about 3 inches.

B. The subcutaneous tissue and deep fascia are incised in line with the skin incision. Any bleeding vessels are clamped and coagulated.

C. With a blunt instrument or finger, the interval between the adductor longus (anteriorly) and the adductor brevis (posteriorly) is developed.

D. Next, the adductor longus is retracted forward and the anterior branch of the obturator nerve is identified. The motor branches to the adductor longus, adductor brevis, and gracilis muscles are isolated. It is best to identify these nerves positively by gently pinching with a smooth forceps or by using a nerve stimulator and observing the contraction of the corresponding muscles.

E. These motor branches are individually clamped distally with hemostats and dissected proximally to their origin, where they are sectioned, an approximately 2 cm. segment of the nerve being excised. The posterior branch of the obturator nerve should not be damaged.

F. The adductor longus is then sectioned transversely in its tendinous portion over a blunt instrument close to its origin from the pubis. The adductor brevis is divided obliquely at a lower level to minimize the extent of dead space (the author uses a coagulation knife, sectioning the muscle over a nonconductive object such as plastic tubing). Next, the gracilis muscle is isolated in the posteromedial portion of the wound. With the knees in extension, it is sectioned obliquely in an opposite direction to that of the adductor brevis and at a lower level.

Plate 58. Adductor Myotomy of Hip and Neurectomy of Anterior Branch of Obturator Nerve (Banks and Green)

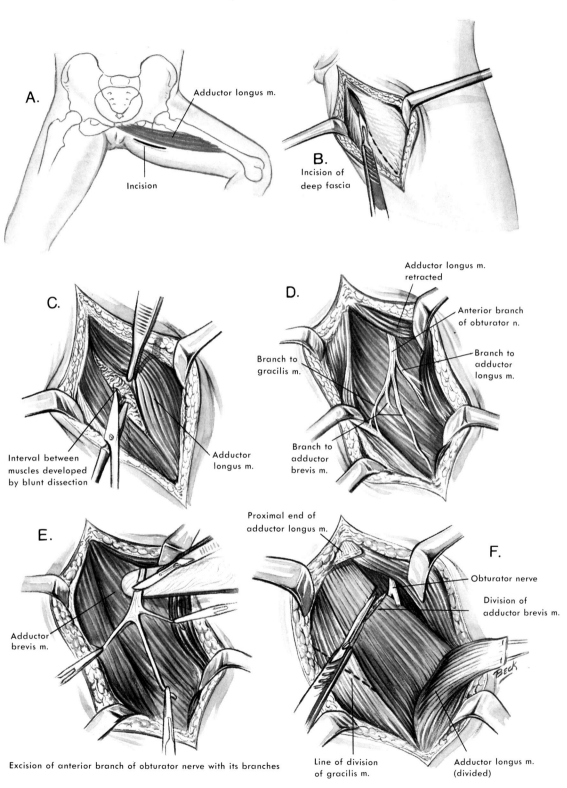

A.

Adductor longus m.

Incision

B.

Incision of deep fascia

C.

Interval between muscles developed by blunt dissection

Adductor longus m.

D.

Adductor longus m. retracted

Anterior branch of obturator n.

Branch to gracilis m.

Branch to adductor longus m.

Branch to adductor brevis m.

E.

Adductor brevis m.

Excision of anterior branch of obturator nerve with its branches

F.

Proximal end of adductor longus m.

Obturator nerve

Division of adductor brevis m.

Line of division of gracilis m.

Adductor longus m. (divided)

1639

Adductor Myotomy of Hip and Neurectomy of Anterior Branch of Obturator Nerve (Banks and Green) (Continued)

G. At this time, the degree of correction obtained is checked by abducting both hips in extension. If there is still some limitation to complete hip abduction, the most anterior fibers of the adductor magnus may be divided.

H. If iliopsoas lengthening is indicated, the hips are again flexed, laterally rotated, and abducted. This position of the hip rotates the proximal femur, bringing the lesser trochanter anteriorly and making it more accessible. The interval between the pectineus and adductor brevis is developed and widened by blunt dissection to expose the lesser trochanter and the iliopsoas tendon. If the pectineus muscle is hypertrophic and covers the iliopsoas tendon, it may be released or retracted medially with the adductor brevis.

I. A small periosteal or staphylorrhaphy elevator is inserted deep to the iliopsoas tendon, bringing it into view. With a curved hemostat the iliopsoas tendon is dissected free of its adjacent tissues. Care should be taken not to injure the sciatic nerve. Next, with the elevator under the iliopsoas tendon, two transverse incisions are made 1.5 to 2 cm. apart, dividing only its tendinous fibers, not its muscle fibers. The hip is hyperextended and the tendon is lengthened 2 to 4 cm.

An alternative method of lengthening the iliopsoas (not illustrated) is at the pelvic brim. Its advantages are that the resultant weakening of the motor power of the hip flexors is less than that of lengthening the iliopsoas at its insertion. Also, it obviates the risk of injury to the medial circumflex femoral vessels. Its disadvantages are that it requires a separate iliac incision and there is risk of injury to the femoral nerve. This author has extensive experience with fractional lengthening of the iliopsoas near its insertion; loss of power of the hip flexors and inadvertent injury to the circumflex vessels has not been a problem.

J. All bleeding vessels should be clamped and coagulated, establishing complete hemostasis. The author routinely uses suction tubes, which are connected to a Hemovac. The deep fascia is not sutured. Only subcutaneous tissue and skin are closed.

K. A plaster of Paris hip spica cast is applied with the hips in full abduction and extension and in 10 to 15 degrees of lateral rotation. If there is flexion contracture of the knees, the patellae should be well padded. Toe-to-groin casts joined by an abduction bar should not be used, as pelvic obliquity may result.

POSTOPERATIVE CARE

One or two days after operation, the suction catheters are removed. The period of immobilization in solid casts varies. Ordinarily in three to four weeks, the solid casts are removed and bilateral long leg bivalved hip spica casts are made, in which the hips are kept in the desired amount of abduction, extension, and lateral rotation. In the presence of subluxation or dislocation of the hip, immobilization in a solid cast is continued for two to three months. When the patient is cooperative and has a good motor picture, the casts may be bivalved and exercises instituted as early as the fifth to seventh postoperative day.

Active hip abduction, adduction, and extension exercises are performed, first in the supine position. The range of motion of joints is maintained by gentle passive stretching exercises. As muscle strength increases, exercises are performed, first against gravity and then against resistance. As soon as functional range of motion in the weight-bearing joints is developed, standing and walking are allowed under supervision, and appropriate external support; reverse walkers may be used. Forward flexion of the trunk should be avoided. Gait training is continued until as normal a gait pattern as is possible is obtained. External support is discontinued when good balance is present. Some patients, especially severe quadriplegics, have to use reverse walkers for support indefinitely.

The length of time that bivalved casts should be worn at night is variable. As a rule, they are used for at least six months to a year. They are not discontinued until the patient has effective full active abduction of the hips against gravity. If there is any tendency to recurrence of contracture, bivalved night casts are reapplied.

Plate 58. Adductor Myotomy of Hip and Neurectomy of Anterior Branch of Obturator Nerve (Banks and Green)

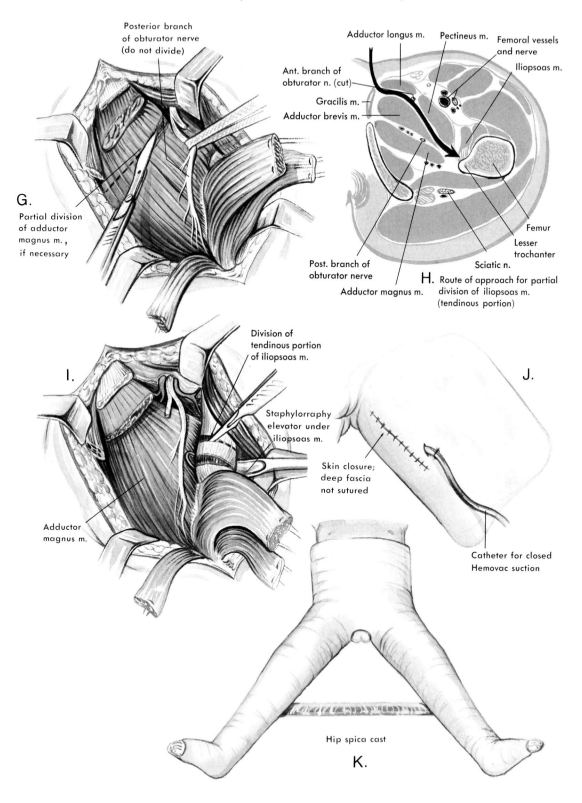

G. Partial division of adductor magnus m., if necessary

Posterior branch of obturator nerve (do not divide)

Adductor longus m.

Pectineus m.

Femoral vessels and nerve

Iliopsoas m.

Ant. branch of obturator n. (cut)

Gracilis m.

Adductor brevis m.

Post. branch of obturator nerve

Adductor magnus m.

Femur

Lesser trochanter

Sciatic n.

H. Route of approach for partial division of iliopsoas m. (tendinous portion)

I.

Division of tendinous portion of iliopsoas m.

Staphylorraphy elevator under iliopsoas m.

Skin closure; deep fascia not sutured

Adductor magnus m.

J.

Catheter for closed Hemovac suction

Hip spica cast

K.

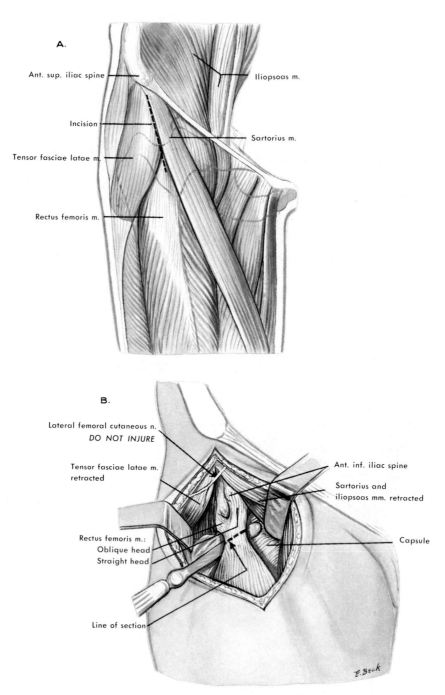

FIGURE 5–19. *Rectus femoris release at its origin.*

A. Longitudinal incision between sartorius and tensor fasciae latae. **B.** Section of the oblique and straight heads near their origin. It is important not to injure the lateral femoral cutaneous nerve. The capsule of the hip joint should not be divided.

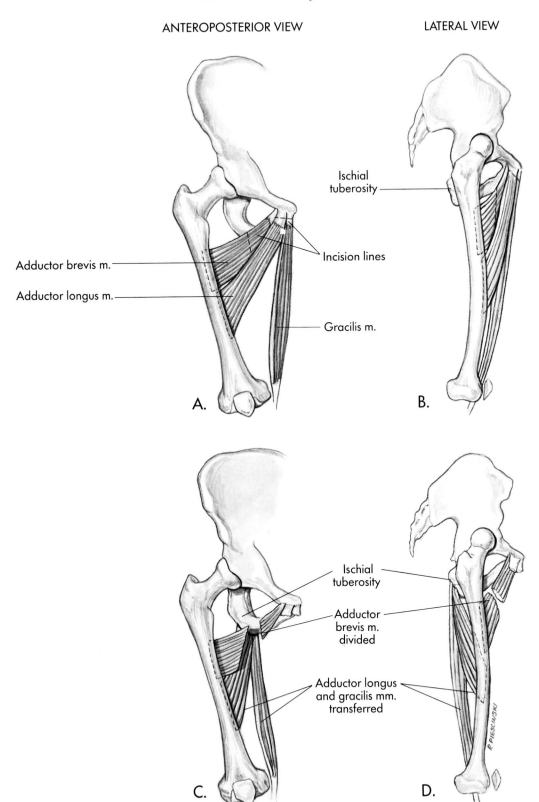

ANTEROPOSTERIOR VIEW   LATERAL VIEW

Ischial tuberosity

Adductor brevis m.

Adductor longus m.

Incision lines

Gracilis m.

A.

B.

Ischial tuberosity

Adductor brevis m. divided

Adductor longus and gracilis mm. transferred

C.

D.

FIGURE 5–20. *Posterior transfer of hip adductors to ischium.*

    A and **B.** Anteroposterior and lateral views showing the line of division of the gracilis and adductor longus muscles at their origin and the line of myotomy of the adductor brevis. **C** and **D.** The adductor longus and gracilis muscles transferred to the ischium, and the adductor brevis divided.

terior to the ischial tuberosity, parallel to the inguinal crease. Subcutaneous tissue is divided in line with the skin incision. The surgeon must pay attention to the veins; they are clamped and coagulated as necessary. Meticulous hemostasis is crucial during the entire procedure. The fascial dissections are longitudinal in plane. The tendinous attachment of the adductor longus is identified, and the interval between the pectineus and iliopsoas is carefully developed by blunt dissection. The anterior branches of the obturator nerve are identified, and the nerve supply to the adductor longus and gracilis is left intact; motor function of the transferred muscles should be preserved. A heavy nonabsorbable suture is placed in the tendinous portion of the adductor longus; then, using sharp scalpel and electrocautery, the adductor longus tendon is detached subperiosteally from its origin on the pubic ramus. The adductor brevis is sectioned obliquely using cutting current electrocautery. Then the gracilis muscle is detached subperiosteally from its origin on the pubic ramus. It is vital to maintain the thick, fibrous periosteal attachment of the origin of the adductor longus and gracilis tendons. By blunt dissection the adductor longus and gracilis muscles are mobilized distally, preserving their neurovascular supply. Then by blunt dissection the anteroinferior aspect of the ischial apophysis is exposed. The adductor magnus is left intact. By means of a clamp the adductor longus and gracilis tendons are held against the anteroinferior aspect of the ischial tuberosity and sutured firmly to the apophysis of the ischium with nonabsorbable sutures. If necessary, the transferred tendons may be anchored with a few sutures to the tendons of adductor magnus to relieve tension on bone. The wound is thoroughly irrigated with automatic pulsating irrigation. Suction catheters are placed, and the wound is closed in the usual fashion. A bilateral hip spica cast is applied with each hip in 25 to 35 degrees of hip abduction, neutral extension, and slight lateral rotation. Four weeks postoperatively the cast is removed, and active exercises are begun. The patient is allowed to ambulate six weeks postoperatively.

There is controversy in the literature as to whether the complex surgical procedure of posterior transfer of the hip adductor achieves a better functional result than the relatively simple hip adductor myotomy. Stephenson and Donovan, in a follow-up study of 87 patients, reported 48 per cent good and 35 per cent fair results (i.e., 83 per cent had improvement in their gait or walked for the first time following the procedure); the results were poor in 17 per cent. None of the patients, however, was worsened by the procedure, and in no case did an abduction contracture develop.[526] Couch et al. reported the results in 28 patients—excellent in 16 and good in 11, with one failure.[118] They stressed that the procedure should be carried out only in ambulatory or near-ambulatory patients. In the nonambulatory patient they recommended simple adductor myotomy, obturator neurectomy, and iliopsoas lengthening for prevention of a "hip at risk" for subluxation. With the hip in flexion the hip adductors are strong medial rotators of the hip; by attaching the transferred tendons of the adductor longus and gracilis to the ischium, their function as medial rotators of the hip is negated. Suturing of the tendons to the posterior part of the tendon of the adductor magnus will not relieve the medial rotation gait pattern.[115]

Griffin et al. performed a thorough study of the results of posterior transfer of hip adductors in six patients by pre- and postoperative clinical assessment, videotape recordings of gait, and electromyographic gait analysis. Gait improved and endurance increased in all six patients; postoperatively all six were community ambulators. The average increase in the degree of hip abduction was 35 degrees. Hip flexion contracture was less, but increase in hip extension strength was not observed. The transferred adductors were active through at least two thirds of stance and rarely caused activity before the onset of double support. Unanticipated changes in activity in muscles not operated upon were found; this was also noted in earlier reports by Perry et al.[202, 405] It was the opinion of Griffin et al. that in comparing the adductor transfer group with the adductor myotomy–obturator neurectomy group, the adductor transfer patient walks with a less broad-based gait and has more security, less trunk shift, a longer single support phase in stance, and more endurance than a patient who has undergone other procedures. Postoperative management is less demanding because there is less need for prolonged use of abduction splints at night to prevent contractures—the muscle fibrosis that follows denervation does not occur in adductor transfer patients.[202]

Root and Spero compared the results of 98 adductor transfers in 50 patients with 102 adductor myotomies with or without obturator neurectomy in 52 patients. The groups were similar with regard to severity of their disease, age, and associated concomitant surgery. Functional change, change in passive motion of the hip, and change in stability of the hip were determined in assessing results. In their experience, although the adductor transfer operation takes longer and is associated with a higher incidence of postoperative drainage, the overall improvement in these patients is greater and is maintained better than that after adductor myotomy with or without neurectomy. The transferred muscle provides greater pelvic stability, decreases hip flexion contractures, and reduces instability of the hip. In reviewing these data, it is difficult to determine whether the better function following the transfers is due solely to the transfers or also to associated procedures performed simultaneously or later (e.g., pelvic and femoral osteotomy in 29 patients and hamstring release in 22 patients).[456]

Reimers and Poulsen compared the before-and-after results of two groups of patients—36 adductor transfers and 29 adductor myotomies. There was no significant difference in the results of the two series; they found no proven advantage of the adductor transfer over adductor myotomy. Because adductor transfer is a more complex operation and fraught with greater postoperative complications (particularly wound infection) they favored adductor myotomy over adductor transfer.[440]

This author does not recommend posterior transfer of the hip adductors because the procedure is more difficult and takes longer to perform; often the transferred tendons detach postoperatively with hip abduction; the probability of postoperative wound infection and drainage is definitely greater; an abnormal hollow in the upper medial thigh created by the procedure is cosmetically objectionable, and the postoperative results of adductor transfer over simple adductor myotomy are not better. In some patients with adductor transfer, exaggerated lumbar lordosis is a definite problem.

Intrapelvic obturator neurectomy in spastic cerebral palsy was advocated by Chandler because, after neurectomy of the obturator nerve, some adductor power remains, as the pectineus is innervated by the femoral nerve and the ischial origin of the adductor magnus by the sciatic nerve.[103] The operative technique is as follows:

A transverse incision is made in the abdomen just above the symphysis pubis, parallel with one of the distal transverse skin creases. The subcutaneous tissue and fascia are divided in line with the skin incision. The wound flaps are retracted proximally and distally, exposing the two rectus abdominis muscles. The sheath of one of the rectus muscles is split longitudinally in its lateral third and reflected, and the margin of the muscle is identified. The rectus abdominis muscle is retracted medially and, with the operator's index finger used as a blunt dissector, the peritoneum and bladder are pushed posteriorly and held so with a retractor. Again, with the index finger, the obturator nerve is palpated and its course identified within the pelvic wall as it enters the neural foramen of the obturator fascia. The obturator nerve is dissected free of its accompanying vessels with a nerve hook and is delivered out into the wound. One should be cautious not to tear accompanying vessels. The nerve is stimulated for positive identification. Nonabsorbable sutures are placed around the nerve, 1 cm. apart, and the nerve in between is excised. The deep retractors are removed, allowing the bladder and peritoneum to fall into place. The rectus sheath is closed. The opposite obturator nerve is resected following the same technique, and the wound is closed in the usual manner. A bilateral long leg hip spica cast is applied, immobilizing the lower limbs with the hips in 110 to 120 degrees of combined abduction, neutral extension, and 10 to 15 degrees of lateral rotation.

In three to four weeks, the hip spica cast is removed and active and passive exercises are begun. The same general principles of care are followed as outlined for adductor myotomy of the hips.

This author does not recommend intrapelvic obturator neurectomy because abduction deformity of the hip with loss of active hip adduction, which is a very disabling complication, may occur. In such an instance, Pollock recommends transfer of the origin of the hamstrings to the inferior ramus of the pubis and their insertion to the medial femoral condyle to "make" it a hip adductor.[421] In some cases, fibrosis of hip adductors may develop and cause recurrent fixed adduction contracture.

Paralytic Dislocation of the Hip. In cerebral palsy (with the exception of congenital hip dislocation) this is an acquired deformity, and it can almost always be prevented. In infancy, appropriate physical therapy is in order. The hip adductor and flexors are gently passively elongated without eliciting stretch reflex. Prone posturing at night in bivalved cast or splint with the hip in abduction is vital. In some cases, standing with the hips in abduction and medial rotation for 30 to 60 minutes several times a day is appropriate. The objective is to prevent development of flexor-adductor contracture of the hips. Traction and passive stretching exercises are not tolerated by cerebral palsy patients—they elicit the stretch reflex.

Increasing adduction-flexion contractures of the hip (especially if in the radiogram there is a break in Shenton's line and widening of the medial joint space indicating beginning subluxation of the hip) require adductor myotomy and iliopsoas lengthening to prevent progressive subluxation and eventual dislocation of the hip.[547]

In the *subluxated hip*, adductor myotomy and iliopsoas lengthening are performed to correct muscle imbalance as an etiologic factor of subluxation. Excessive femoral antetorsion is almost always present in these hips; however, one should refrain from derotation osteotomy of the femur. Simple soft-tissue release is often adequate to control the subluxation. If there is associated acetabular dysplasia, the age of the patient is a factor in modality of treatment. In the child under four years of age, simple soft-tissue release should always be performed first with appropriate splinting at night; with weight-bearing with or without orthosis during the day and an adequate physical therapy regimen, the acetabulum will develop and the hip will stabilize. Significant acetabular dysplasia in the young child indicates congenital hip subluxation. In the child four years of age and older, presenting hip dysplasia may require a bony procedure for stabilization; often derotation osteotomy of the proximal femur and occasionally derotation-varization are required. Innominate osteotomy is rarely necessary. CAT scan studies should be performed preoperatively to determine the exact degree of femoral torsion and acetabular torsion. In the cerebral palsied child, acetabular antetorsion is usually normal; therefore, Salter's derotation innominate osteotomy of the acetabulum is not indicated. The problem is often superior and posterior deficiency of the acetabulum, and the procedure of choice is either Chiari's medial displacement osteotomy of the innominate bone, with or without shelf, or Staheli's acetabular augmentation. In the older patient, this author favors Chiari's osteotomy (with combined shelf if necessary) to correct acetabular dysplasia and provide stability to the hip. In his experience, the results with the Chiari procedure have been excellent.

Acetabular augmentation is favored by other authors. Zuckerman et al. reported the results of 20 acetabular augmentations performed in 17 cerebral palsied patients with progressive instability. The average follow-up was 41.5 months, with a range of 24 to 147 months. The results were rated good in 18 hips, fair in one, and poor in one. In 19 patients, the hip became stable. The CE angle increased from a preoperative mean of minus 17 degrees to a follow-up mean of 50 degrees. The range of motion of the hips was not altered significantly postoperatively. The only complication was a supracondylar fracture of the femur that was incurred after cast removal. In the one poor result, in which the hip was not stabilized (it redislocated posteriorly), the patient had mixed cerebral palsy (spastic-athetoid) and retroversion of the proximal femur because of a previous overzealous derotation osteotomy, and the acetabular augmentation shelf did not extend far enough posteriorly.[600]

In the severely subluxated hip with marked dysplasia of the acetabulum it is important to correct both sides, i.e., by derotation osteotomy of the femur (with femoral shortening if indicated) and innominate osteotomy with Chiari's or acetabular augmentation.

The Dislocated Hip. The problems of the completely displaced high-riding femoral head are complex. Each patient should be individually assessed. Among the factors to consider are (1) the status of the articular cartilage of the hip joint. Have degenerative changes in the femoral head developed? (2) Is there significant pain? (3) The degree of shallowness and inadequacy of the acetabulum; (4) the presence or absence of fixed pelvic obliquity; (5) the presence or absence of scoliosis. Is there fixed spine deformity combined with pelvic obliquity? (6) The ambulatory status of the patient. Is there interference with locomotion owing to progressive dislocation of the hip? (7) What is the sitting posture? Is the unilateral dislocated hip interfering with the sitting ability of the patient? (8) Are there problems with perineal care and personal hygiene owing to severe adduction flexion contracture of the hips?

Some surgeons recommend withholding surgery until there is significant pain, limited sitting ability, or problems with perineal hygiene; when this stage is reached, resection of the femoral head-neck is performed. This author disagrees with this view and recommends early aggressive surgical management. Open reduction should be performed with subtrochanteric femoral shortening and soft-tissue release of hip adductors, often combined with Chiari's medial displacement innominate osteotomy with or without acetabular augmentation shelf. Traction should not be employed because it is ineffective in reducing such hips and is not tolerated by the cerebral palsied child.

Fixed pelvic obliquity should be corrected

first; unless this is performed and a level pelvis provided, the hip on the high side of the pelvis will be unstable and will redislocate. The pelvic obliquity may be suprapelvic, infrapelvic, or both. Suprapelvic fixed pelvic obliquity due to scoliosis is corrected first by spine fusion to the pelvis. Infrapelvic obliquity due to abduction contracture of the contralateral hip should be corrected by soft-tissue release.

First, myotomy of the adductor longus and brevis and gracilis is carried out through a medial approach; it is best not to release the iliopsoas at this time through the medial approach because of the hazard of inadvertent division of medial circumflex vessels. Next, the hip joint is exposed through an anterolateral surgical approach, and a subtrochanteric femoral shortening is performed through a separate lateral incision. The amount of femoral shortening is equal to the degree of superior displacement of the femoral head—femoral shortening should be adequate. If in doubt, one should excise a larger segment. Excessive femoral antetorsion is corrected by laterally rotating the distal femoral segment. Internal fixation is achieved by a six-hole "AO" or "DSP" plate. Do not cause femoral retrotorsion! The iliopsoas tendon is lengthened after femoral shortening—it is preferable to perform it at the level of anterior iliac spines instead of at its insertion.

Often there is superior and posterior deficiency of the acetabulum in long-standing dislocation of the hip. Stability to the hip is provided by Chiari's medial displacement innominate osteotomy; this may be combined with an acetabular augmentation shelf procedure, particularly in its posterior aspect. For details of the operative technique the reader is referred to Chapter 2 in the section on congenital dislocation of the hip. Illustrative cases are shown in Figures 5–21 and 5–22. Some surgeons may prefer to correct dysplasia of the acetabulum by double innominate osteotomy or simple shelf acetabular augmentation.

This combined procedure, i.e., adductor release, open reduction, femoral shortening, and innominate osteotomy, is extensive. The patient should be in good medical condition. The operation should be performed by an experienced, capable pediatric hip surgeon, in a children's hospital with excellent anesthesia and intensive care departments that specializes in the care of such patients. If the hip is subluxated or dislocated and painful, if the acetabulum is shallow, and if the patient has no potential for ambulation, a Schanz abduction osteotomy is performed. This will relieve the pain, abduct the lower limb, provide good sitting support, and facilitate perineal care (Fig. 5–23).

Resection of the Head-Neck Femur. One may

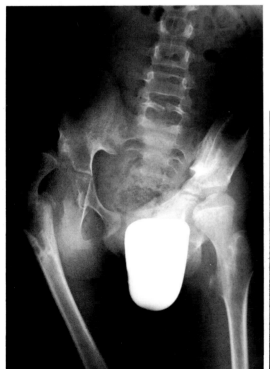

A

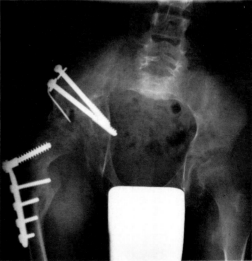

B

FIGURE 5–21. *Paralytic dislocation of the left hip in severe spastic cerebral palsy.*

A. Preoperative radiogram. **B.** Postoperative radiogram following open reduction with femoral shortening, capsular plication, and Chiari's pelvic osteotomy and shelf acetabuloplasty.

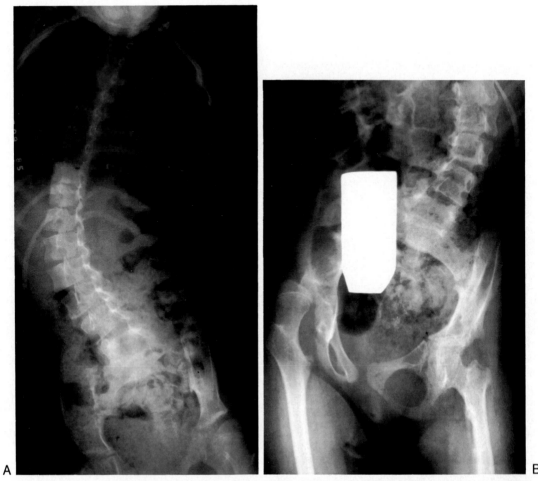

A   B

FIGURE 5–22. *Paralytic dislocation of the left hip with severe scoliosis.*

A. Anteroposterior view of the spine showing right dorsolumbar scoliosis (long C-curve). Note the left hip subluxation.
B. Anteroposterior view of the left hip—note the progressive subluxation.

consider the Girdlestone procedure in a patient who is confined to wheelchair or bed with severe pain due to marked degenerative changes.[182] The experience of this author with the Girdlestone procedure and Castle's muscle interposition arthroplasty modification has been disappointing. The greater trochanter migrates cephalad; relief of pain is temporary; soon the hip becomes painful. It is best to consider hip arthrodesis or total hip arthroplasty.

Root et al. presented the results of eight hip fusions in cerebral palsy patients with painful subluxated or dislocated hips with marked degenerative changes; six had successful arthrodesis with relief of pain and return to preoperative functional level of performance. Pseudarthrosis developed in two hips that were managed by surgical revision, one by a second arthrodesis and the other by total hip replace-

ment. Root and colleagues recommended hip fusion in unilateral hip disease in patients who are unable to ambulate and in young active ambulatory patients. They also presented the results of 15 cases of total hip arthroplasty in cerebral palsied patients with a painful dislocated hip. In 13 of the 15 patients the pain was relieved and function restored to the preoperative level of performance commensurate with their neuromuscular disability. In the remaining two, the results were failure, requiring reoperation.[455]

Anterior Dislocation. This rare, often iatrogenic problem is treated by soft-tissue release of glutei and hamstrings (proximally) to correct the abduction-extension contracture of the hips. If these releases fail to provide stable reduction of the hips, a subtrochanteric femoral shortening is performed with derotation to correct

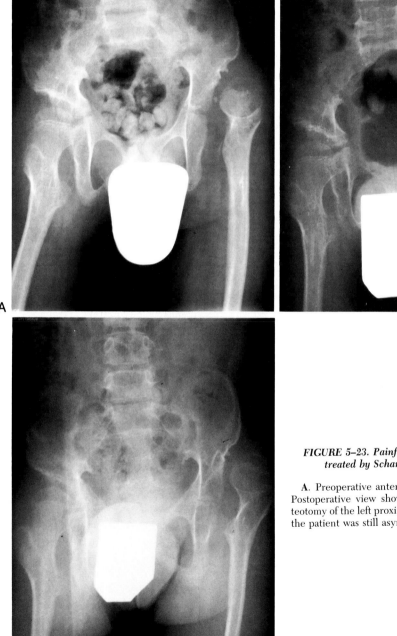

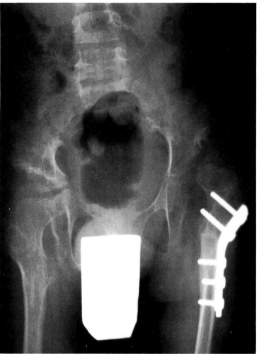

FIGURE 5–23. Painful subluxation of the left hip treated by Schanz abduction osteotomy.

A. Preoperative anteroposterior view of the hips. **B**. Postoperative view showing the Schanz abduction osteotomy of the left proximal femur. **C**. Two years later—the patient was still asymptomatic.

excessive femoral antetorsion. Do not create retrotorsion! If the problem is associated with anterior deficiency of the acetabulum, innominate osteotomy with acetabular augmentation shelf is performed to provide anterior coverage of the femoral head. If all these measures fail, as a last resort, one may have to resect the femoral head-neck through an anterior approach. The objective is to allow functional range of hip flexion for sitting and to relieve pain (if present).

Medial Rotation Deformity of the Hip. This is often associated with adduction-flexion deformity of the hip; following adductor myotomy and musculotendinous lengthening of the iliopsoas, the hip spica cast should hold the hips in extension and 15 to 20 degrees of lateral rotation. During postoperative physical therapy and gait training, efforts are directed toward passive and active exercises to promote lateral rotation of the hip—often release of hip adduction-flexion contracture will correct medial rotation deformity of the hip.

When limitation of lateral rotation of the hip with medial foot progression angle is present in the absence of hip flexion-adduction deformity, the following operative procedures are available to correct the deformity: (1) Steel's anterior advancement of the tendinous insertion of the gluteus medius–minimus from the greater trochanter to the anterior aspect of the upper femoral shaft; (2) posterior transfer of the tensor fasciae latae and sartorius muscles; (3) posterolateral transfer of the semitendinosus tendon to the anterior aspect of the lateral femoral condyle; (4) medial transfer of the rectus femoris; and (5) lateral rotation osteotomy of the femur. In the literature, Durham described division of the gluteus minimus and anterior fibers of the gluteus medius muscle fibers.[145] The Durham procedure should not be performed, as it will further weaken the abductor power and lateral stability of the hip joint.

In the preoperative assessment one should determine the muscle or muscles responsible for medial rotation deformity of the hips: Is it hyperactivity of the gluteus medius–minimus, medial hamstrings, or anterior hip adductors? When the hip is in adduction and flexion, the iliopsoas may aggravate medial rotation; however, ordinarily it is not a primary deforming force. Electromyography studies and gait analysis will delineate abnormal activity of the deforming muscles and assist in decision making.[522, 537]

Is there associated hip abductor muscle weakness and Trendelenburg lurch? Often, medial rotation gait is associated with gluteus medius limp. In such cases, muscle tendon transfers are sometimes performed to correct hip medial rotation and increase motor strength of hip abductor muscles.

What is the position of the knee in gait? When medial rotation gait is combined with knee flexion in walking, hyperactivity of the medial hamstrings may be the causative factor, and one should consider semitendinosus transfer or lengthening of the medial hamstrings. This author does not recommend semitendinous transfer because simple lengthening is effective and is a simpler procedure. Or, is the knee in extension with spasticity of the rectus femoris and marked limitation of knee flexion? In such a case, medial transfer of the rectus femoris may be indicated.

Is there excessive femoral antetorsion? Clinically this is tested by determining range of lateral rotation of the hip with the hip in extension and the patient prone or supine. When there is excessive femoral antetorsion, lateral rotation of the hip will be limited and there will be excessive medial rotation of the hip in extension. With the patellae facing straight forward and the hip extended, the lateral surface of the greater trochanter will be situated more posteriorly than normal. One may approximately determine the degree of femoral antetorsion by drawing an imaginary line between the prominent lateral surface of the greater trochanter and the center of the hip joint.[317]

Before surgery it is best to determine the exact degree of femoral antetorsion by CAT scan studies. When the degree of femoral antetorsion is greater than 45 degrees, consideration should be given to derotation osteotomy of the femur. The femoral neck–shaft angle is determined. In severe coxa valga, varization osteotomy is indicated.

Posterior Transfer of Tensor Fasciae Latae and Sartorius Muscles. In 1923, Legg transferred the origin of the tensor fasciae latae from the anterior portion of the ilium to the posterior third to improve the power of hip abduction in patients with anterior poliomyelitis.[310] Barr, in 1943, advocated the Legg procedure for treatment of flexion medial rotation deformity of the hip in spastic paralysis.[26] Green added the sartorius muscle to the tensor fasciae latae to increase the motor strength of the abductors and lateral rotators.[20, 196] This author added proximal advancement of the gluteus medius–minimus muscles to restore normal physiologic length of the elongated hip abductor muscles. Indications are medial rotation gait with gluteus medius lurch in an ambulatory spastic cerebral palsy patient who is ten years of age or older. It is vital to have a motivated patient who is cooperative with the postoperative exercise program. The hip should be concentrically reduced and stable; the degree of femoral antetorsion should be less than 40 degrees; and there should be no flexion and adduction contracture of the hip. The operative technique is described in Plate 59. In his experience, the author has found posterior transfer of tensor fasciae latae and sartorius muscles and proximal advancement of gluteus medius–minimus muscles to be very effective in correction of medial rotation gait and gluteus medius lurch in spastic cerebral palsy.

Steel's Anterior Advancement of the Tendinous Insertion of Gluteus Medius–Minimus from the Greater Trochanter to the Anterior Aspect of the Upper Femoral Shaft.[522] The objective of this operative procedure is to correct medial rotation gait in spastic cerebral palsy when it is caused by a hyperactive gluteus medius–minimus complex with a positive stretch reflex. By advancing the insertion of gluteus medius–minimus anteriorly the function of these muscles is changed from that of medial rotators of the hip to that of lateral rotators. By also distally advancing these muscles, their resting length is not altered and their function as hip abductors is not compromised. The operative technique is described and illustrated in Plate 60.

Electromyography studies of normal subjects by Steel demonstrated that gluteus medius–minimus acted as medial rotators of the hip in the first 25 per cent of the stance phase (from 0 to 15 per cent of the gait cycle) and then as hip abductors until nearly the end of the stance phase. In the last 25 per cent of the swing phase, gluteus medius–minimus acted as medial rotators of the hip. Steel also noted during the very beginning of the stance phase, when medius-minimus are functioning as medial rotators, their fibers are lengthening; this lengthening-contraction phenomenon in spastic cerebral palsy was shown by EMG to elicit a stretch reflex.

Requisites for Steel's gluteus medius–minimus advancement operation are (1) passive range of hip abduction and lateral rotation of at least 30 degrees, and (2) absence of stretch reflex or contracture of the rectus femoris muscle. Steel stresses the importance of releasing both heads of the rectus femoris if a rectus stretch reflex or contracture is present because this will cause flexed posture of the hips in gait and impair the success of gluteal advancement.

Rectus femoris and hip adduction contracture release can be performed simultaneously with Steel's advancement procedure.

Posterolateral Transfer of Semitendinosus Tendon to the Anterolateral Aspect of the Femur. This procedure was described by Baker as the "barber pole" or stripe transfer.[14] The semitendinosus tendon is routed through a subcutaneous tunnel, converting its action from a medial rotator to a lateral rotator of the hip.

In the electromyographic and gait analysis studies of Sutherland et al., it was shown that medial rotation of the hip occurred just prior to heel strike and continued through the greater portion of the stance phase. The medial hamstring contracted in definite synchrony with the medial rotation motion of the hip. The results of seven medial hamstring transfers were graded as good or excellent in five, fair in one, and poor in one.[537]

In the experience of this author the results of medial hamstring transfer have not been satisfactory. It is imperative to select the patients carefully and to perform the procedure after EMG gait analysis.

Derotation Osteotomy of the Femur. When medial rotation deformity of the hip is fixed because of structural bony deformity and marked antetorsion of the proximal femur in the patient over ten years of age, lateral rotation osteotomy of the femur may be indicated. Simple derotation osteotomy is transverse and is preferably performed at the subtrochanteric level. Internal fixation is best achieved with large DSP plates and with seven or eight screws. Secure fixation is crucial. Hip spica cast immobilization provides additional support.

Coxa valga may be associated with increased antetorsion. In such an instance, derotation osteotomy is performed at the intertrochanteric level and combined with varization. The method of internal fixation used is a matter of individual preference.

Following varization osteotomy, the already weakened hip abductors can be further relaxed. In such an instance, the gluteus medius and minimus muscles are tightened by transplanting their insertion on the greater trochanter down the femoral shaft.

In lateral rotation of the distal fragment of the hip in patients over 15 years of age with severe fixed flexion–internal rotation deformity, the hip should be tilted into extension to correct the fixed flexion deformity.

Occasionally, genu recurvatum is the accompanying deformity, and it is indicated to carry out the rotational osteotomy at the supracondylar level so that the distal femoral segment

Text continued on page 1660

Posterolateral Transfer of Tensor Fasciae Latae and Sartorius and Proximal Advancement of Gluteus Medius and Minimus

OPERATIVE TECHNIQUE

The patient is placed supine with a small sandbag under the buttocks of the operated hip tilting him 20 degrees toward the opposite hip. The lower abdomen, the pelvis, and the entire lower limb are prepared and draped to allow free motion of the hip.

The range of abduction of the hip is tested. A vital requisite for the posterolateral transfer of the tensor fasciae latae and sartorius is full range of hip abduction; if it is limited by spastic contracted hip adductors, an adductor myotomy is performed first.

A and **B.** The incision begins at the junction of the posterior and middle thirds of the iliac crest and extends forward to the anterior superior iliac spine, and then is carried distally into the thigh for about 7 to 10 cm. in the groove between the tensor fasciae latae and the sartorius muscle. The subcutaneous tissue and superficial and deep fasciae are incised over the iliac crest, and the fascia lata is divided in line with the skin incision. The lateral femoral cutaneous nerve is identified, mobilized by sharp dissection, and protected by retracting with a vascular tape.

C. The groove between the tensor fasciae latae laterally and sartorius and rectus femoris medially is opened by blunt dissection and the deep fascia is divided. The ascending branches of the lateral femoral circumflex vessels cross the midpoint of the intermuscular groove; they are identified, isolated, and protected from inadvertent injury.

Plate 59. Posterolateral Transfer of Tensor Fasciae Latae and Sartorius and Proximal Advancement of Gluteus Medius and Minimus

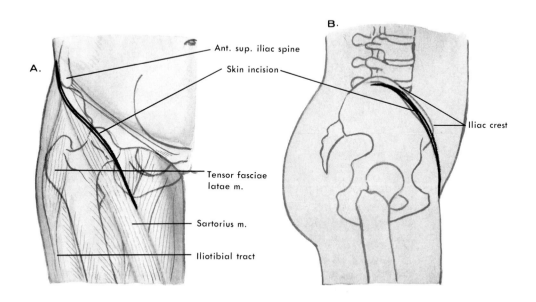

A.

Ant. sup. iliac spine

Skin incision

Tensor fasciae latae m.

Sartorius m.

Iliotibial tract

B.

Iliac crest

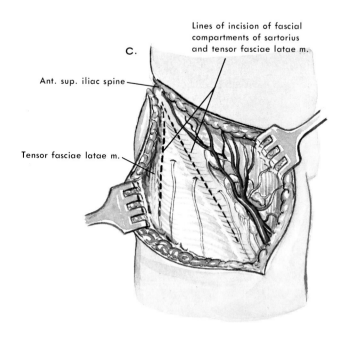

Lines of incision of fascial compartments of sartorius and tensor fasciae latae m.

C.

Ant. sup. iliac spine

Tensor fasciae latae m.

Posterolateral Transfer of Tensor Fasciae Latae and Sartorius and Proximal Advancement of Gluteus Medius and Minimus (Continued)

D and **E.** The origin of the sartorius is detached from the anterior superior iliac spine, and its free end is marked with 0 Tycron suture. The sartorius is reflected distally and medially by blunt dissection; the muscle is freed and mobilized distally as far as possible without disturbing its nerve supply from the femoral nerve. **F.** Next, with a scalpel the cartilaginous iliac apophysis is sharply divided into lateral one third and medial two thirds down to bone from the junction of its posterior and middle thirds to the anterior superior iliac spine. With a broad periosteal elevator, the lateral part of the iliac apophysis and the tensor fasciae latae and the gluteus medius and minimus are subperiosteally stripped and reflected as a continuous sheet to the superior rim of the acetabulum. It is not necessary to extend the dissection posteriorly to the greater sciatic notch. With a periosteal elevator, the medial half of the cartilaginous iliac apophysis with the periosteum on the inner wall of the ilium is stripped in a continuous sheet for a distance of 3 cm.

Then the intermuscular interval between tensor fasciae latae anteriorly and gluteus minimus posteriorly is identified and gently developed. The boundary between the two muscles is not definite; a Bovie electrocautery knife is used to separate the two muscles. The nerve and blood supply by the superior gluteal nerve and vessels should not be disturbed.

Plate 59. Posterolateral Transfer of Tensor Fasciae Latae and Sartorius and Proximal Advancement of Gluteus Medius and Minimus

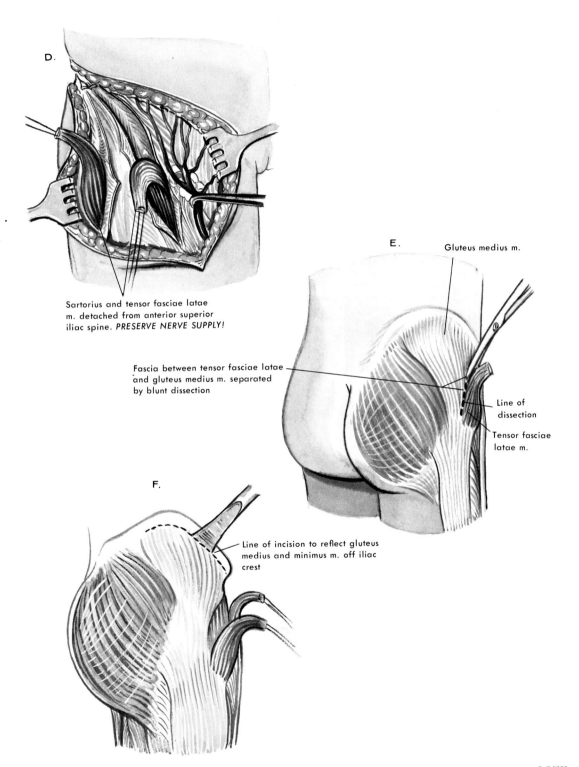

D.

Sartorius and tensor fasciae latae
m. detached from anterior superior
iliac spine. *PRESERVE NERVE SUPPLY!*

Fascia between tensor fasciae latae
and gluteus medius m. separated
by blunt dissection

E.

Gluteus medius m.

Line of
dissection

Tensor fasciae
latae m.

F.

Line of incision to reflect gluteus
medius and minimus m. off iliac
crest

Posterolateral Transfer of Tensor Fasciae Latae and Sartorius and Proximal Advancement of Gluteus Medius and Minimus (Continued)

G. Then with a power drill, four holes are made in the middle third of the iliac crest, two for the reattachment of sartorius and tensor fasciae latae, and two for the proximal advancement of gluteus medius and minimus.

H. The hip is fully abducted. The tensor fasciae latae is firmly reattached to the iliac crest as far posteriorly as possible in the posterior part of the middle third of the iliac crest, and the sartorius is reattached to the anterior part of the middle third of the iliac crest.

I. With the hip in full abduction the gluteus medius and minimus are reattached to the inner aspect of the iliac crest. The medial two thirds of the iliac apophysis is resutured to the gluteal fasciae and muscles over the iliac crest.

The procedure is usually performed bilaterally in the cerebral palsied child with spastic diplegia.

J. The wound is closed in the usual fashion. A bilateral long-leg hip spica cast is applied with the hips in 40 degrees of abduction, neutral extension, and 15 degrees of lateral rotation.

POSTOPERATIVE CARE

The cast is bivalved four to six weeks after surgery (the length of time depending upon the age and size of the patient and security of fixation of the muscle tendon transfers), and a physical therapy program is begun. Active assisted exercises are performed to develop hip abduction, lateral rotation, and flexion. It is important for these patients to sleep prone in a bivalved hip spica cast or splint. Standing with assistance is allowed when the transferred tensor fasciae latae and sartorius are fair in motor strength. Walking is begun gradually. Meticulous postoperative care is crucial for success.

Plate 59. Posterolateral Transfer of Tensor Fasciae Latae and Sartorius and Proximal Advancement of Gluteus Medius and Minimus

G.

Four 3/16″ drill holes below sectioned cartilaginous apophysis of ilium. Holes emerge on inner wall of ilium

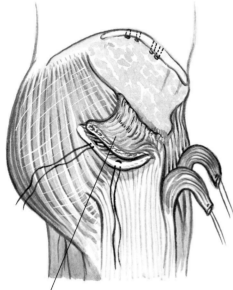

Gluteus medius and minimus m. reflected distally to level of hip capsule

H.

Sartorius and tensor fasciae latae m. attached to whip sutures through drill holes to middle third of iliac crest

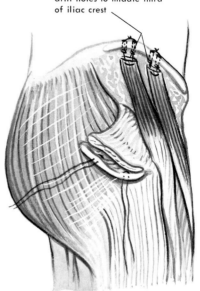

I.

Gluteal mm. advanced proximally and attached by whip sutures through drill holes to inner wall of iliac crest—overlapping tensor fasciae latae and sartorius m.

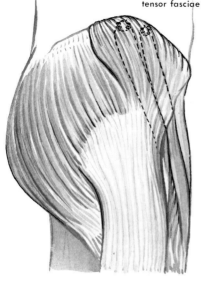

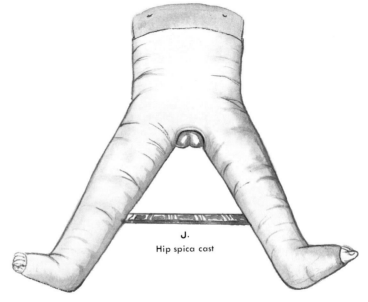

J.

Hip spica cast

Steel's Anterior Advancement of the Gluteus Medius and Minimus Insertion for Correction of Medial Rotation Gait

OPERATIVE TECHNIQUE

The operation is performed with the patient in supine posture. The pelvis and both lower limbs are prepared and draped. One should be able to manipulate the lower limbs freely during surgery without contamination of the wound. There should be complete surgical access to the hip adductor region superomedially, to the iliac crest, and to 5 cm. posterior to the greater trochanter.

A. A curvilinear incision (slightly convex anteriorly) is centered over the lateral aspect of the greater trochanter. It begins at the anterior border of gluteus maximus far enough superiorly to expose the muscle bellies of the gluteus medius and minimus; it is extended distally curving anteriorly toward the greater trochanter, and posteriorly toward the linea aspera of the femur for a distance of about 5 cm. By palpation, identify the fascia overlying the gluteus medius-minimus muscle bellies. The deep fascia lying between the gluteus maximus posteriorly and tensor fasciae latae anteriorly is divided. Next, carefully develop the plane between the gluteus minimus and hip joint capsule. Both gluteus medius and minimus should be transposed as one functional unit, taking great care to preserve their nerve and blood supply. Do not confuse the plane between the gluteus medius and minimus with the interval between minimus and hip joint capsule.

B. The conjoined tendons of gluteus medius and minimus are detached from their insertion to the tip of the greater trochanter with a piece of the trochanteric apophysis and bone; one may use a sharp osteotome or an electric saw. The apophyseal growth plate of the greater trochanter should not be disturbed.

C. Next identify the intertrochanteric and subtrochanteric surfaces of the femur anteriorly and elevate the origin of vastus intermedius and reflect distally. Exposure should be adequate to accommodate the detached greater trochanteric wafer. The femoral cortex is roughened with a gouge.

D. At this point the hip is abducted and laterally rotated to within 10 degrees of maximum. (If the hip adductors are taut, they are released by myotomy at this time.) Next, the tendons of gluteus medius-minimus are anchored with a wafer of trochanteric bone to the anterior surface of the roughened femur by use of a cancellous screw, a staple or staples, or crisscross threaded Steinmann pins. The vastus intermedius is resutured over the new insertion of gluteus medius-minimus to bone. The fasciae latae and the wound are closed in layers. A double hip spica cast is applied, including the foot and leg.

POSTOPERATIVE CARE

The hip spica cast is removed in six weeks, and the hip is mobilized and ambulation commenced. The internal fixation device is removed two to three months postoperatively.

Plate 60. *Steel's Anterior Advancement of the Gluteus Medius and Minimus Insertion for Correction of Medial Rotation Gait*

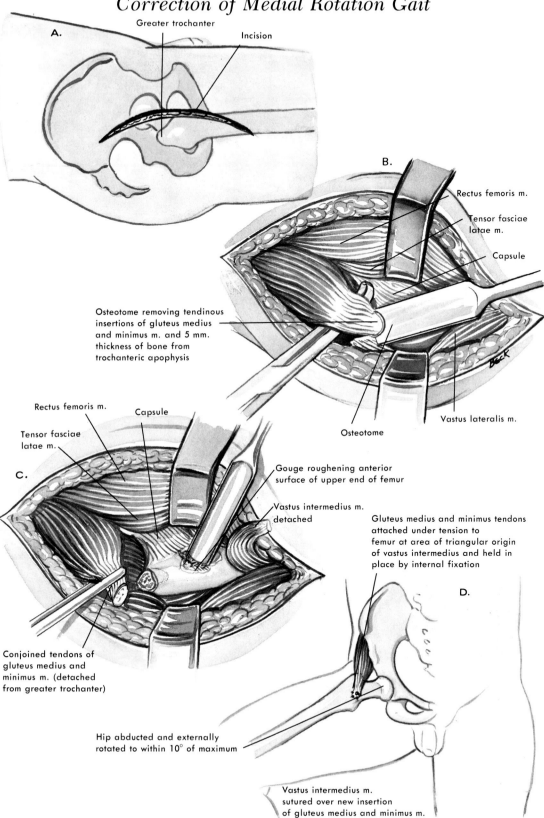

A.

Greater trochanter

Incision

B.

Rectus femoris m.

Tensor fasciae latae m.

Capsule

Osteotome removing tendinous insertions of gluteus medius and minimus m. and 5 mm. thickness of bone from trochanteric apophysis

Osteotome

Vastus lateralis m.

Rectus femoris m.

Capsule

Tensor fasciae latae m.

C.

Gouge roughening anterior surface of upper end of femur

Vastus intermedius m. detached

Gluteus medius and minimus tendons attached under tension to femur at area of triangular origin of vastus intermedius and held in place by internal fixation

D.

Conjoined tendons of gluteus medius and minimus m. (detached from greater trochanter)

Hip abducted and externally rotated to within 10° of maximum

Vastus intermedius m. sutured over new insertion of gluteus medius and minimus m.

1659

can be tilted posteriorly. Overcorrection should be avoided.

In general, femoral osteotomy in an ambulatory cerebral palsy patient should be approached with caution. These patients will develop marked disuse muscle atrophy and regress in their motor level of function. It may take up to one year for an adolescent cerebral palsy patient to regain his preoperative level of motor performance. This should be made very clear to the family and patient before surgery. At present this author favors mid-diaphyseal simple transverse derotation osteotomy and internal fixation with an intramedullary interlocking rod with screws proximally and distally to control rotation. The limbs are not immobilized in cast. The patient is allowed to ambulate with assistance a few days postoperatively. Rehabilitation is much faster with this method.

PROBLEMS AND COMPLICATIONS

Pelvic obliquity following adductor myotomy of the hips is a frequent problem: It may cause lumbar scoliosis and subluxation of the adducted hip on the high side. One should take the following measures to avert this complication. Bilateral long leg casts should not be used following adductor myotomy, as they permit the pelvis to tilt. It is important to immobilize the hips in a bilateral long leg hip spica cast. Failure to recognize asymmetry of involvement is another cause; on the less affected side, adductor myotomy should be performed to a lesser extent. Even if the preceding precautions are taken, pelvic obliquity may still result because of differences in recovery of hip abductor power following adductor myotomy. In the postoperative muscle re-education period this can usually be detected. Pelvic obliquity is managed by splinting of the hips in appropriate position, with the abducted hip in relative adduction and the adducted hip in abduction. Exercises are performed to elongate the shortened hip abductors, and active exercises are carried out to increase motor strength of the antagonist muscles.

Abduction–lateral rotation and extension contracture of the hips is often caused by overzealous myotomy of the hip adductors and flexors. The result is inability to sit; in the severe case the hips may subluxate anteriorly. In the preoperative assessment these patients often display a strong startle reflex, with the upper limbs assuming an abducted laterally rotated posture. In such cases, caution should be exercised in the extent of hip adductor myotomy. If the hips are not subluxating, an adductor myotomy should not be performed; if the hips are unstable, only the adductor longus and gracilis muscles should be divided. Neurectomy of the anterior branch of the obturator nerve should not be performed.

Loss of ability to flex the hip may occur if the iliopsoas muscle is completely detached. It is important to fractionally lengthen the iliopsoas at its musculotendinosus junction and not completely section the muscle.

Hematoma or wound infection may occur because of the proximity of the incision to the perineum. Strict adherence to sterile technique and use of routine closed Hemovac suction is crucial to prevent this complication.

Disuse bone atrophy and stress fracture are common sequelae of hip spica immobilization. It is crucial that these children be upright and weight-bearing, with the hip spica cast on, to prevent osteoporosis. Prolonged immobilization should be avoided as much as possible. Active isometric exercises are performed while the patient is in cast. When removing the hip spica cast, one should be very gentle, especially at the knee, as the fractures often occur in the supracondylar region of the femur.

The Foot and Ankle

The triceps surae muscle comprises the gastrocnemius, a three-joint muscle (knee, ankle, and subtalar); and the soleus, a two-joint muscle (ankle and subtalar). The coordinated, harmonious action of the triceps surae with its principal antagonist, the anterior tibial, is necessary to have a normal heel-toe gait with adequate push-off. In the majority of children with spastic cerebral palsy, this normal gait pattern is lost because of equinus deformity of the ankle and foot, which may be *functional*—a result of spasticity and exaggerated stretch reflex of the triceps surae without myostatic shortening—or it may be *fixed*—because of permanent shortening of the triceps surae muscle.

Equinus deformity may be caused by contractural involvement of both the soleus and the gastrocnemius muscles, or it may be due to contracture of the gastrocnemius alone. These two types of involvement can be differentiated by passive dorsiflexion of the ankle joint, first with the knee flexed and then with it extended. The gastrocnemius portion of the triceps surae originates from the femoral condyles and is, therefore, relaxed when the knee is passively flexed. If the equinus deformity is chiefly due to contracture of the gastrocnemius, it disappears. With the knee extended, the part played by the gastrocnemius is tested (Fig. 5–24). Care should be taken to apply the dorsiflexion force to the hindfoot and not to the forefoot, as the latter brings the peroneal, tibialis posterior, and toe flexor muscles into play (Fig. 5–25). Contracture of the gastrocnemius is the primary cause of equinus deformity in spastic cerebral palsy.

The gait pattern may be toe-toe if the body weight of the child is unable to overcome the exaggerated stretch reflex of the calf muscles (Fig. 5–26); or, depending upon the degree of involvement, the gait may be toe-heel or plantigrade (planting the foot as a unit). A taut triceps surae muscle may prevent dorsiflexion of the ankle, and the tibia, acting as a lever, thrusts the knee into recurvatum when the heel

touches the floor. More frequently, however, the knee is held in flexion by the spastic hamstrings and a stretched-out, poorly functioning quadriceps muscle. The spastic gastrocnemius muscle plays a lesser role in producing flexion deformity of the knee. On plantar flexion of the foot, the gastrocnemius is relaxed, any persistence of knee flexion deformity most probably being caused by the hamstrings.

In equinus deformity, the hindfoot is often forced into valgus position when the heel touches the floor, resulting from the bowstring effect of the triceps surae on the ankle and subtalar joints. With rigid resistance to dorsiflexion of the foot, the calcaneus rotates underneath the talus and is displaced posterolaterally (Fig. 5–27). With loss of support of the susten-

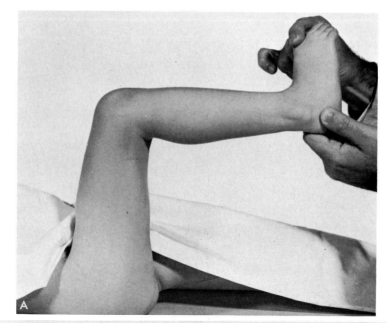

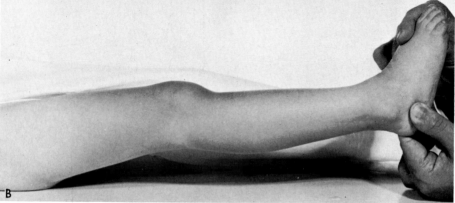

FIGURE 5–24. *Testing spasticity and contracture of triceps surae muscle by passive dorsiflexion of the ankle.*

A. With the knee in flexion, the gastrocnemius muscle is relaxed and equinus deformity is caused by contracture of the soleus muscle. **B.** With the knee in extension the parts played by both the gastrocnemius and soleus are tested.

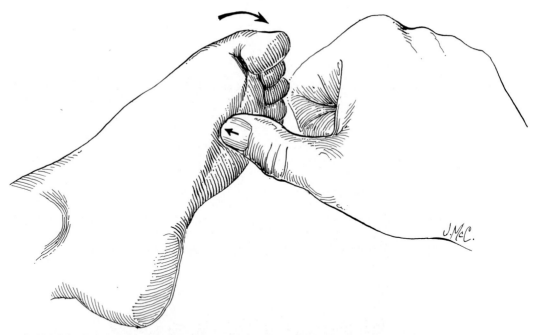

FIGURE 5–25. Spasticity of toe flexors shown by dorsiflexion of the foot by pressure over the metatarsal head.

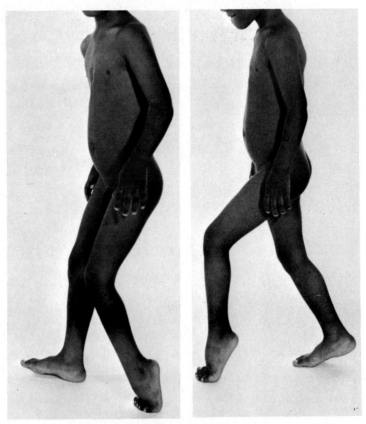

FIGURE 5–26. Toe-toe gait in spastic hemiplegia.

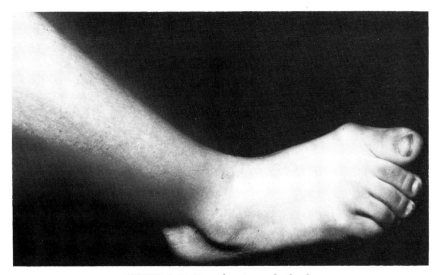

FIGURE 5–27. Pes valgus in cerebral palsy.

Spasticity of peroneal muscles increases the deformity.

taculum tali beneath the head of the talus, the talus drops into a vertical position. Dorsiflexion occurs in the midfoot, and a rocker-bottom deformity results; the calcaneus is still in equinovalgus position. The stress of weight-bearing is on the head of the talus (the midfoot) and not on the heel. This valgus deformity is increased when the peroneal muscles are spastic.

Less often, the foot position is equinovarus, owing to spastic posterior tibial and toe flexor muscles (Fig. 5–28). On weight-bearing or passive dorsiflexion of the ankle, the posterior tibial stands out as a taut band in its groove behind the medial malleolus; the toes may be curled. In stance, the varus deformity is usually more marked in the forefoot, and on walking, these children toe in. Functional or fixed medial rotation deformity of the hip or tibia vara, or both, will aggravate the toeing-in.

In acquired cerebral palsy, the anterior tibial muscle may be spastic; these children usually have varying degrees of varus deformity of both the hindfoot and the forefoot, and a plantigrade gait.

It is essential to perform a muscle test prior to determining the type and extent of surgery; determine the motor strength of the overactive muscle and its antagonist. Often, voluntary active contraction of the anterior tibial muscle cannot be elicited with the knee in extension (Fig. 5–29). The child is asked to dorsiflex the ankle with the knee in extension and flexion. The gastrocnemius portion of the triceps surae is relaxed when the knee is flexed. If the

anterior tibial does not contract with the knee flexed, the child is asked to flex the hip and knee against resistance. This maneuver (called synkinesia, "confusion" or automatic reflex, or Strümpell test) will cause the anterior tibial muscle to contract, bringing the ankle and foot into dorsiflexion. In order to prevent recurrence of equinus deformity, it is essential to develop active voluntary function of the anterior tibial in gait in the postoperative period.

The effect of hip and knee flexion contracture on equinus deformity of the foot should be assessed, for if it is not corrected, the equinus deformity is likely to recur (Fig. 5–30).

CONSERVATIVE MANAGEMENT

Initially, all children should have a trial period of nonoperative treatment. The surgeon should condition the patient and his family for future care and indoctrinate them concerning exercises and night support.

Conservative measures consist of passive manual elongation of the gastrocnemius-soleus muscles with the knee in extension, active exercises to develop function of the anterior tibial muscle, wearing of a bivalved cast or plastic splint at night to hold the foot and ankle in dorsiflexed neutral position, the part-time use of inhibitory cast or orthoses during the day, and gait training.

A bivalved removable above-knee cast or plastic splint is an effective means of night support that prevents the foot from resting in equinus and maintains it in neutral position. A

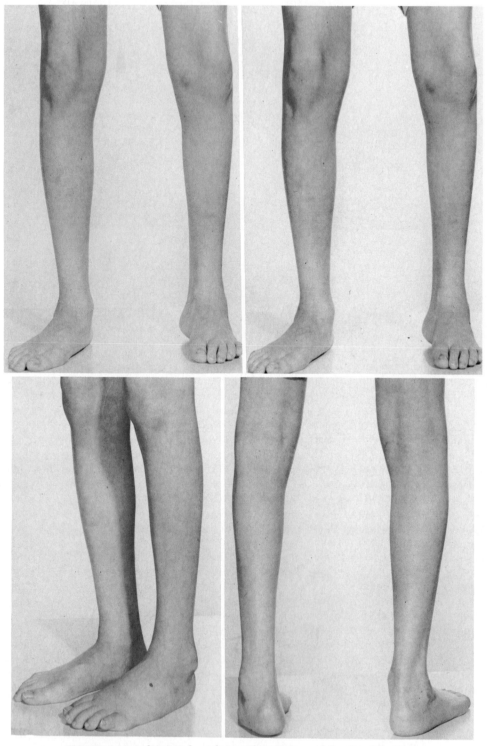

FIGURE 5–28. *Left spastic hemiplegia with equinovarus deformity of the foot.*

Note the taut posterior tibial tendon behind the medial malleolus.

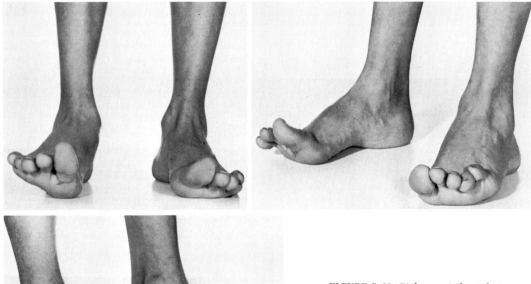

FIGURE 5–29. Right spastic hemiplegia.

Cerebral zero anterior tibial muscle is demonstrated. Note on active voluntary dorsiflexion of the ankle the anterior tibial muscle does not contract on the right side.

bivalved cast is more comfortable than a night brace and should fit the limb snugly. Its purpose is support, not correction. A common pitfall is to make the cast in maximal dorsiflexion at the ankle; this will not be tolerated and will cause a pressure sore on the heel. Initially, it is advisable to place the knee in 5 to 15 degrees of flexion, the ankle being in neutral or 5 to 10 degrees of plantar flexion. As equinus deformity lessens, each subsequent bivalved cast is made with the ankle in more dorsiflexion, as tolerated.

To control the contracture of the gastrocnemius muscle, the night orthosis should be above-knee, holding the knee in extension. A below-knee orthosis does not control the gastrocnemius and the commonly associated contracture of the hamstring muscles.

In order to ensure effective use of day orthoses, the shoe should be high-topped and should fit snugly. Often in hemiplegia, because of the smaller size of the foot, it may be necessary to obtain mismated shoes. To secure the forefoot in the shoe, an extra strap may be used over the dorsum of the foot, or one may have to lace the shoes in the reverse direction with the bow at the base of the tongue.

Stretching or wedging plaster casts to correct fixed equinus deformity are not tolerated well by cerebral palsied children; they should be used only in selected cases, if at all.

SURGICAL TREATMENT

Equinus Deformity. Operative correction of equinus deformity is indicated if a toe-toe or toe-heel gait persists following an adequate period of conservative management. In stance, if the heel goes into marked valgus position and the talus into plantar flexion because of shortening of the spastic gastrocnemius muscle, heel cord lengthening should be considered to prevent development of fixed valgus and rocker-bottom deformity of the foot. Correction of functional equinus deformity may also be indicated. If overactivity and exaggerated stretch reflex of the gastrocnemius and soleus cause equinus deformity of the foot when walking, heel cord lengthening is indicated, despite the fact that the foot can be passively dorsiflexed to neutral position.

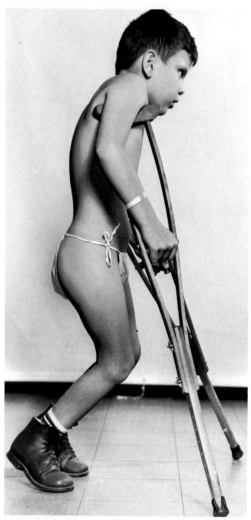

FIGURE 5–30. *Equinus posture of the ankles and feet secondary to flexion contracture of the knee and hip.*

flexors inhibit the action of the gluteus maximus, which is the most important antigravity muscle. The triceps surae muscle can be hyperactive to compensate for hip extensor muscle weakness. Often, equinus deformity is lessened following hip flexor release and acquisition of control over the gluteus maximus.

The purpose of Achilles tendon lengthening is to correct fixed myostatic contracture of the triceps surae, alter the point at which stretch reflex of the triceps surae is elicited, develop voluntary control over and motor strength in the cerebral zero anterior tibial muscle, and establish dynamic muscle balance between dorsiflexors and plantar flexors of the ankle. The key to success is the adequacy of postoperative care. It is imperative that the parents realize that surgery is only the initial stage of treatment. The child should be at least three years old; tendo Achillis lengthening should not be performed in a child under two years of age.

During the past 150 years, various techniques for elongating the triceps surae muscle have been described in the literature. The type of procedure employed is not so important; the result obtained is related to the selection of patient and the adequacy of postoperative care. The author prefers sliding lengthening of the heel cord, the White procedure, as advocated by Banks and Green.[19, 586] Because anatomic continuity of the heel cord is not disturbed, one can control the amount of lengthening, allowing relatively early mobilization. The operative procedure of sliding heel cord lengthening is described and illustrated in Plate 61, and the postoperative care is shown in Figures 5–31 through 5–34.

Subcutaneous tenotomy of the tendo Achillis was performed by Delpech in 1816 and popularized by Stromeyer (Fig. 5–35).[130, 531] The initial results in cerebral palsy were excellent; however, because of poor postoperative care the long-term results were discouraging. This author does not recommend subcutaneous lengthening of the heel cord because it is difficult to control the degree of lengthening. The same is true for Z-lengthening; it should not be performed to correct equinus deformity in spastic cerebral palsy (Fig. 5–36).

Vulpius and Stoffel, in 1913, described an operation to correct spastic equinus deformity. In their procedure the aponeurotic tendon of the gastrocnemius and soleus was divided transversely just below the middle of the leg, leaving the underlying muscle fibers intact. By forceful dorsiflexion of the ankle, the segments of the aponeurotic tendon were separated, but conti-

Before surgery the child must have good sitting and potential for standing balance and should be able to walk, at least with the assistance of appliances. The potential for independent or assisted gait is an absolute preoperative requisite. Second, the triceps surae is lengthened only when its motor strength is fair plus or better. Heel cord lengthening should not be performed if the triceps surae motor strength is only fair or less because the result will be a calcaneus deformity, which is more disabling than equinus deformity. Third, hip flexion deformity should be corrected prior to correction of equinus deformity. The author recommends caution and restraint in simultaneous multilevel surgery; i.e., do not lengthen the heel cord and hip flexors (iliopsoas and rectus femoris) at the same time. Spasticity and contracture of the hip

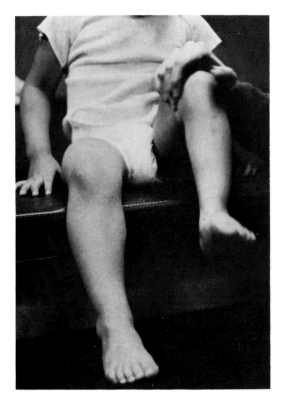

FIGURE 5–31. Active exercises to stimulate reflex function of cerebral zero anterior tibial muscle.

Ankle dorsiflexion is performed with the knee and hip in flexion and manual resistance against the thigh.

nuity of the soleus muscle fibers was not disturbed.[578] Later, one or two V-shaped incisions were made instead of transverse incisions (Fig. 5–37). Compere and Schnute popularized the Vulpius procedure in the United States, and Baker further modified it, using a tongue-in-groove lengthening (Fig. 5–38).[9] In both the Vulpius and the Baker operations, aponeurotic lengthening of the soleus is often also performed.

When equinus deformity is primarily caused by contracture of the gastrocnemius muscle, Silfverskiöld recommends lowering or recession of the gastrocnemius muscle heads below the level of the knee joint and partial neurectomy of the tibial motor nerves to the gastrocnemius muscle to further decrease its motor power (Fig. 5–39). This procedure does not disturb the soleus muscle, which retains its function for effective push-off in gait.[504]

In 1950, Strayer described recession of the gastrocnemius muscle in its distal portion. The gastrocnemius tendon is divided transversely at its junction with the conjoined gastrocnemius-soleus tendon. The foot is dorsiflexed to neutral position, and the retracted proximal part of the

gastrocnemius tendon is resutured to the underlying soleus (Fig. 5–40).[529] In 1958, Strayer reported on distal gastrocnemius recession in 23 patients, in 16 of whom the results were good or excellent.[530]

Silver and Simon, in 1959, reported their experience with the proximal gastrocnemius recession of Silfverskiold in 66 children, on whom 110 operations were done. In addition, they performed neurectomy of one head of the gastrocnemius. The equinus deformity recurred in five cases; on their evaluation, the failures were attributed to muscle imbalance and weakness of the dorsiflexor muscles of the foot.[505]

The advantage of the Strayer and Silfverskiöld procedures is that they preserve soleus function for push-off in gait; there are, however, definite disadvantages to each. The Silfverskiöld operation removes the posterior dynamic support to the knee provided by the gastrocnemius, with the result that genu recurvatum is a potential complication. This procedure should not be

Text continued on page 1674

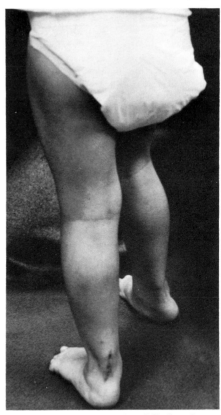

FIGURE 5–32. Following tendo Achillis lengthening the patient is raised to upright posture when the gastrocnemius-soleus muscles are fair in motor strength.

It is important to maintain the hips in extension, contracting the gluteus maximus muscle, and to prevent the knees from going into flexion. Flexion of the knee will overstretch the triceps surae muscle.

Sliding Lengthening of the Heel Cord

A. With the patient preferably in prone position, a posteromedial incision about 7.5 cm. long is made just medial to the tendo Achillis. The subcutaneous tissue and tendon sheath are divided in one plane so that the latter remains attached to subcutaneous tissue and can be reconstructed effectively later on. It is not necessary to disturb the deep surface of the tendon or to dissect around the sheath.

B. The rotation of fibers of the tendo Achillis is studied next, as it varies greatly. The tendon usually rotates about 90 degrees on its longitudinal axis between its origin and insertion, so that the fibers that occupy a medial position proximally twist laterally as they approach their insertion on the calcaneus and are posterior to those fibers that proximally occupied a lateral position. Straight Keith needles may be used to mark rotation of fibers.

The Achilles tendon is then transversely sectioned at two levels. The site of division must be chosen according to the degree of rotation of fibers. Usually the anteromedial half to two thirds of the tendon is divided distally near its insertion and then the posteromedial half of its fibers is divided in the proximal end of the wound.

C. The foot is then passively dorsiflexed with the knee in extension. The medial portion of the tendon will slide on the lateral portion, lengthening the tendon in continuity. (A third incision, midway between the others, is indicated at times if stretching does not occur easily; its site can be readily determined by palpation.) There is no fraying of the tendon as in the Z-plasty type of tendon lengthening. The actual amount of lengthening depends upon the degree of equinus deformity. At the end of the procedure the foot should rest comfortably in neutral position or 5 degrees of dorsiflexion. Correction beyond this point should be avoided, as it may cause calcaneus deformity. The pneumatic tourniquet is released and all bleeding vessels are clamped and coagulated.

D. The sheath, including a small portion of the subcutaneous tissues, is meticulously closed over the lengthened Achilles tendon.

E. The lower limb is immobilized in a well-padded above-knee cast with the knee in full extension or 5 degrees' flexion (but no hyperextension) and the foot-ankle in neutral position or 5 to 10 degrees of dorsiflexion. It is essential to mold the plaster cast well, particularly at the ankle, heel and the knee.

POSTOPERATIVE CARE

The cast is removed three to four weeks following surgery, and a bivalved cast or splint is manufactured for night use. The foot should be in neutral position and the knee in five degrees of flexion. If there is any asymmetry or involvement of the trunk, it is best to manufacture a hip spica cast with the hips in 20 to 25 degrees of abduction and 5 degrees of lateral rotation and the knee-ankle-foot as above. Active and gentle passive exercises are performed to increase range of motion of the ankles, feet, and knees to develop motor strength of agonist and antagonist muscles, particularly the anterior tibial and triceps surae. When the joints have functional range of motion and the motor strength of the muscles is at least poor plus or, preferably, fair, the patient is allowed to ambulate, initially with support and then independently. It is vital that the knees not assume a flexion posture and that the hips be in extension and the trunk not carried forward. Calcaneus posture of the feet and ankles and crouch posture at the knees and hips should be avoided.

Plate 61. Sliding Lengthening of the Heel Cord

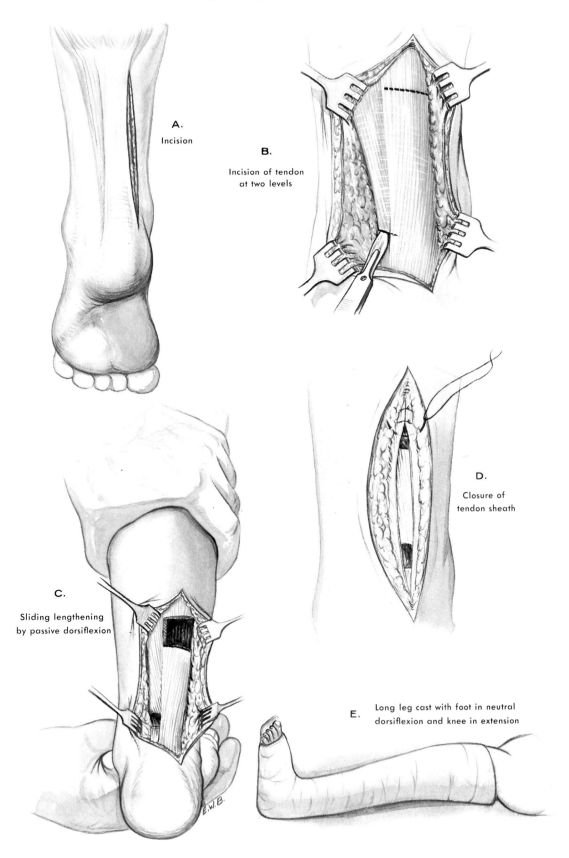

A.
Incision

B.
Incision of tendon
at two levels

C.
Sliding lengthening
by passive dorsiflexion

D.
Closure of
tendon sheath

E. Long leg cast with foot in neutral
dorsiflexion and knee in extension

E.W.B.

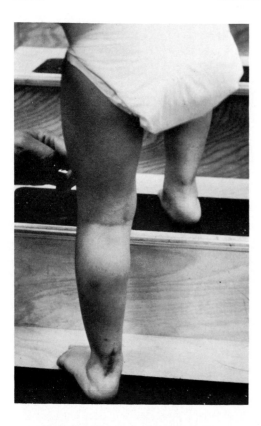

FIGURE 5–33. *In the postoperative period following tendo Achillis lengthening, the triceps surae muscle should be protected from overstretching.*

When the child is taught to climb up and down steps, the knees should be supported to ensure that they do not flex.

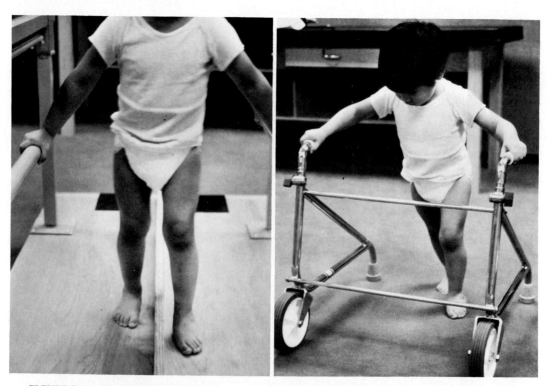

FIGURE 5–34. *During gait training the triceps surae is protected by having the child hold onto parallel bars.*

At home, the older child may use a walker for support. The hips should be in extension, as shown in this patient. In order to prevent hip flexion contracture, this author recommends a reverse walker.

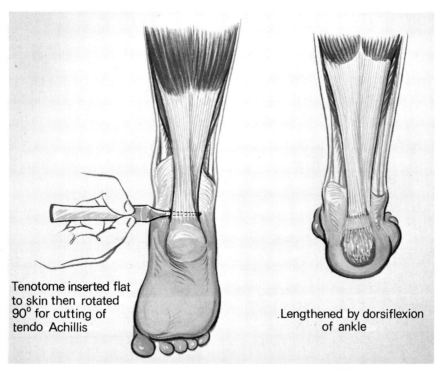

Tenotome inserted flat
to skin then rotated
90° for cutting of
tendo Achillis

Lengthened by dorsiflexion
of ankle

FIGURE 5–35. Subcutaneous lengthening of tendo Achillis.

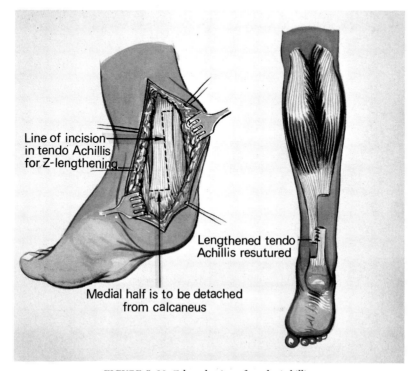

Line of incision
in tendo Achillis
for Z-lengthening

Lengthened tendo
Achillis resutured

Medial half is to be detached
from calcaneus

FIGURE 5–36. Z-lengthening of tendo Achillis.

This procedure should not be performed to correct equinus deformity in spastic cerebral palsy.

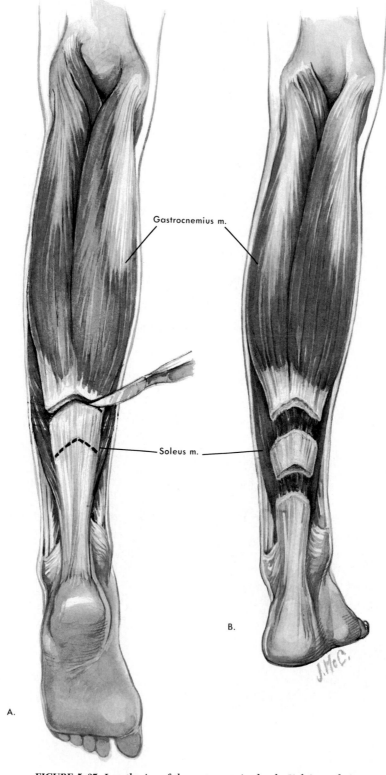

Gastrocnemius m.

Soleus m.

A.

B.

J.McC.

FIGURE 5–37. Lengthening of the gastrocnemius by the Vulpius technique.

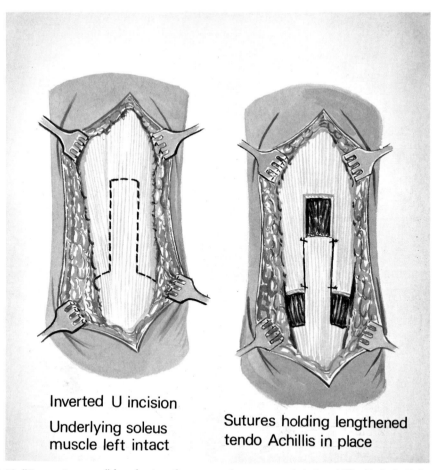

Inverted U incision

Underlying soleus
muscle left intact

Sutures holding lengthened
tendo Achillis in place

FIGURE 5–38. "Tongue-in-groove" lengthening of gastrocnemius aponeurosis in its middle third, the Baker technique.

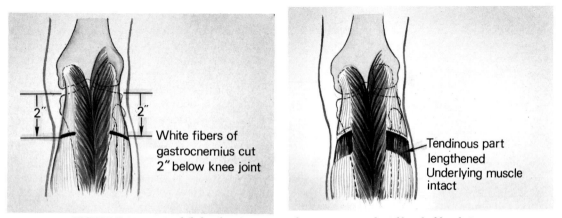

White fibers of
gastrocnemius cut
2" below knee joint

Tendinous part
lengthened
Underlying muscle
intact

FIGURE 5–39. Proximal (below-knee) recession of gastrocnemius, the Silfverskiöld technique.

Silfverskiöld combined this procedure with neurectomy of the motor branch of the tibial nerve to the gastrocnemius.

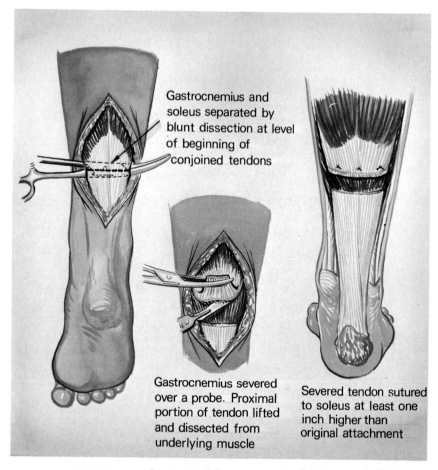

Gastrocnemius and soleus separated by blunt dissection at level of beginning of conjoined tendons

Gastrocnemius severed over a probe. Proximal portion of tendon lifted and dissected from underlying muscle

Severed tendon sutured to soleus at least one inch higher than original attachment

FIGURE 5–40. Distal recession of the gastrocnemius, the Strayer technique.

performed when the hamstrings need to be lengthened at a later date or when, in gait, the knee goes into hyperextension when the heel touches the floor. Following the Strayer procedure, in which it is completely freed from the soleus, the gastrocnemius muscle may retract proximally as a small functionless knot in the upper calf. For these reasons, the Strayer procedure is not advocated.

Fractional lengthening of the gastrocnemius above the knee was described by Green and McDermott in 1942, and later by Baker in 1954 and 1956 (Fig. 5–41).[9, 11, 196] Its only indication is for a mild equinus deformity with fixed flexion contracture of the knee when the hamstrings are being lengthened.[196] It should not be employed as a primary procedure.

In 1913, Stoffel described neurectomy of the motor branches of peripheral nerves for the correction of spastic contractures.[528] Since then, division of motor nerves to one or both heads of the gastrocnemius to correct equinus defor-

mity has been advocated by numerous surgeons. This author does not recommend neurectomy of motor branches of the tibial nerve because it produces fibrosis of the triceps surae muscle with consequent myostatic contracture and recurrence of fixed equinus deformity. Tibial neurectomy should be performed only when there is severe ankle clonus on weight-bearing that hinders walking. It is imperative that one distinguish the clonus caused by the gastrocnemius from that caused by the soleus. When it diminishes or disappears on flexion of the knee, the clonus is caused primarily by the gastrocnemius; when the clonus is unaltered by changes in the position of the knee, the soleus is its chief cause. Motor branches of the tibial nerve to the spastic muscle causing the clonus are the ones to be resected. This author recommends that after the motor nerve is sectioned, it be reimplanted in the muscle to prevent fibrosis. The tendo Achillis is usually not lengthened at the same time, although, on occasion, it may

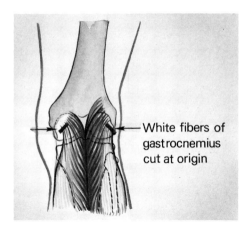

White fibers of
gastrocnemius
cut at origin

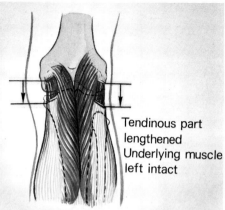

Tendinous part
lengthened
Underlying muscle
left intact

FIGURE 5–41. *Proximal (above-knee) recession of gastrocnemius, technique of Green (1942) and Baker (1954).*

ment of the heel cord from point C (the posterior tuberosity of the calcaneus) to point D (the upper surface of the calcaneus immediately behind the subtalar joint) the power of the triceps surae is diminished by 48 per cent according to the calculations of Pierrot and Murphy.[418] On push-off the fulcrum in the foot moves distally to the first metatarsal head (point A), weakening the push-off power by the ratio of

$$\frac{C + D}{AC} = 0.15 \pm 0.02$$

Text continued on page 1680

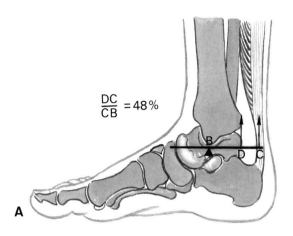

$$\frac{DC}{CB} = 48\%$$

A

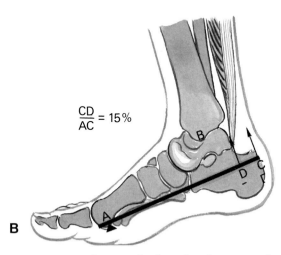

$$\frac{CD}{AC} = 15\%$$

B

FIGURE 5–42. **The principle of anterior advancement of the heel cord for correction of pes equinus due to spastic cerebral palsy.**

A. The power of the triceps surae is reduced to 48 per cent when the Achilles tendon is transferred from C to D. **B.** The power of push-off of the triceps surae is reduced to only 15 per cent with transfer of the heel cord from C to D. (Redrawn from Pierrot, A. H., and Murphy, O. B.: Heel cord advancement—a new approach to the spastic equinus deformity. Orthop. Clin. North Am., 5:118, 1974.)

have to be done later. The operative technique of neurectomy of motor branches of the tibial nerve is described and illustrated in Plate 62.

Anterior advancement of the heel cord was originally described by Estève of Paris in 1936.[155] Murphy of Lexington, Kentucky, independently introduced the procedure in the United States in 1959.[418] The principle of anterior advancement of the tendo Achillis from the posterior tuberosity to the dorsum of the calcaneus immediately posterior to the subtalar joint is to shorten the lever arm and weaken the triceps surae without changing the resting length of the muscle. Murphy proposed that skeletal growth would not affect the end result and that permanent correction could be achieved without the use of splints and orthotic devices. The principle of the operation is illustrated in Figure 5–42. The axis of ankle motion is the midportion of the body of the talus. The triceps surae muscle acts on the ankle joint and foot through a lever system, the fulcrum of which is located at point B in the midportion of the body of the talus. On anterior advance-

Neurectomy of Motor Branches of Tibial Nerve to Gastrocnemius

A. The patient is placed in prone position with a pneumatic tourniquet on the proximal thigh. A transverse incision 5 to 7 cm. long is made immediately proximal to the popliteal crease in line with the flexion creases of the skin.

B. The deep fascia is divided and the tibial nerve, lying superficial to the vessels, is exposed. The first branch is cutaneous; it is not disturbed. The next two branches are the motor nerves to the gastrocnemius. One branch emerges from the medial side and enters the medial head close to its origin; just prior to disappearing into the muscle, it divides into three branches. The other branch emerges from the lateral side and similarly enters the lateral head close to its origin, but it divides into only two branches. The motor branch to the soleus muscle emerges distal to that of the gastrocnemius. It is best to stimulate each branch to determine which is the principal cause of clonus.

C. The appropriate motor branches are resected by dividing them proximally at their origin and distally at their entrance into the muscle. The wound is closed in layers in the usual manner. The limb is immobilized in a long leg cast with the foot at 5 to 10 degrees of dorsiflexion at the ankle and with the knee in full extension. The cast is removed in three weeks; the postoperative care is similar to that after heel cord lengthening. (Some surgeons apply only a pressure dressing and allow the patient to walk when he is comfortable and when the wound is healed.)

Plate 62. Neurectomy of Motor Branches of Tibial Nerve to Gastrocnemius

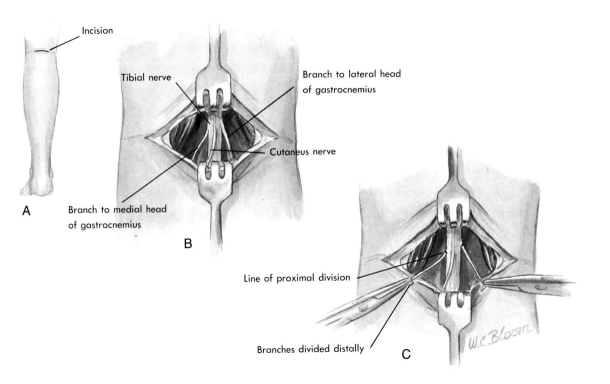

Incision

Tibial nerve

Branch to lateral head of gastrocnemius

Cutaneus nerve

Branch to medial head of gastrocnemius

A

B

Line of proximal division

Branches divided distally

C

W.C.Bloom

Anterior Advancement of Tendo Achillis for Correction of Spastic Equinus Deformity (Murphy Technique)

OPERATIVE TECHNIQUE

A. With the patient in prone position, a posteromedial incision is made about 1 cm. medial to the tendo Achillis; it begins at the os calcis and extends proximally for a length of 7.5 to 10 cm. The subcutaneous tissue and tendon sheath are divided in one plane in line with the skin incision.

B. The Achilles tendon is identified and isolated by sharp and blunt dissection to its insertion. It is detached from the calcaneal tuberosity as far distally as possible to preserve length. Caution is exercised to avoid injury to the calcaneal apophysis.

C. Next, a Bunnell pull-out wire suture is placed on the distal end of the tendo Achillis. The flexor hallucis longus tendon is identified, mobilized, and retracted medially. The upper surface of the calcaneus is exposed. A 0.6-cm. drill hole is made from the superior part of the calcaneus immediately posterior to the subtalar joint to exit on the plantar aspect of the non-weight-bearing area of the calcaneus. With a curet the drill hole is enlarged, if necessary.

D. The pull-out wire and Achilles tendon are passed through the drill hole and are tied over a sterile, thick felt pad and a button on the plantar aspect of the foot with the ankle in 15 degrees of plantar flexion. It is vital that the heel cord be routed anterior to the flexor hallucis longus. If attention is not paid to this important detail the Achilles tendon will reattach itself to its original insertion. The tourniquet is released, and after complete hemostasis the wound is closed. An above-knee cast is applied with the ankle joint in 15 degrees of plantar flexion and the knee in 10 degrees of flexion.

POSTOPERATIVE CARE

The cast and pull-out wire are removed in four to six weeks. Physical therapy is begun to restore ankle motion and develop strength of the anterior tibial and triceps surae muscles. Other details of postoperative care follow the same principles outlined for tendo Achillis lengthening.

Plate 63. Anterior Advancement of Tendo Achillis for Correction of Spastic Equinus Deformity (Murphy Technique)

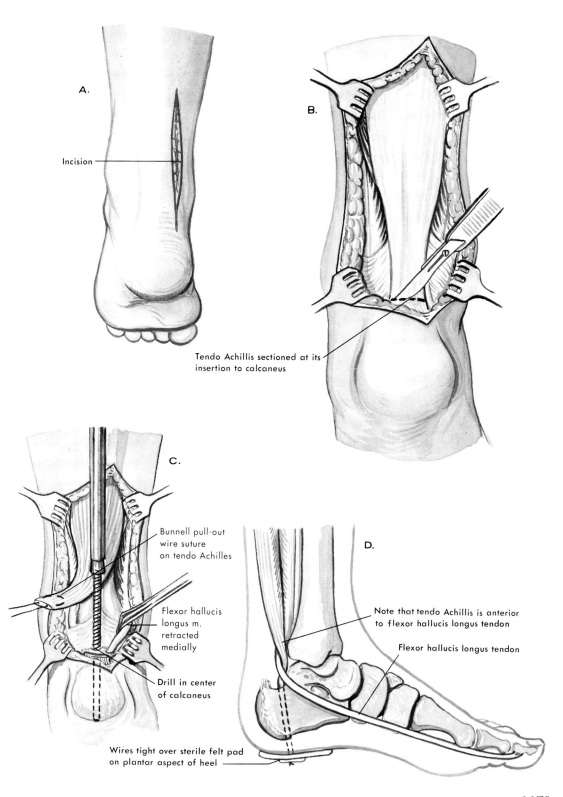

A.

Incision

B.

Tendo Achillis sectioned at its insertion to calcaneus

C.

Bunnell pull-out wire suture on tendo Achilles

Flexor hallucis longus m. retracted medially

Drill in center of calcaneus

Wires tight over sterile felt pad on plantar aspect of heel

D.

Note that tendo Achillis is anterior to flexor hallucis longus tendon

Flexor hallucis longus tendon

Therefore, the advantage of anterior advancement of the heel cord is that it decreases resistance to ankle dorsiflexion by 48 per cent. This author considers anterior advancement of the tendo Achillis to correct equinus deformity in spastic paralysis when the triceps surae muscle is of fair motor strength. The operative technique is described in Plate 63.

Throop and associates reported the results of 79 anterior advancements of the tendocalcaneus; in 17.7 per cent they were excellent (heel-toe gait, good push-off, no hyperextension of the knee); in 72.2 per cent, good (flat foot-strike with or without push-off, no hyperextension of the knee); and in 10.1 per cent, poor (toe-heel gait, recurrence of equinus deformity, calcaneus gait). Totaled, the percentages of excellent and good results show that the operation was satisfactory in 89.9 per cent. The indication for the Murphy procedure was given as the presence of dynamic equinus angulation with no more than 15 per cent of fixed equinus deformity.[563]

If by 6 to 12 months following heel cord lengthening the patient is unable to develop voluntary control over a cerebral zero anterior tibial muscle, this author recommends shortening the stretched-out and elongated muscle by plication or excision of a segment at its distal attachment and transferring a neurophysiologically normal and strong extensor hallucis longus to the base of the first metatarsal, rerouting it through the anterior tibial muscle to promote reflex stimulation of and voluntary control over it. This procedure is a modification of that of Alfonso Tohen.[567] If any equinus deformity is present, it should be corrected by a stretching below-knee walking cast. It should be possible to passively dorsiflex the ankle joint to at least 20 degrees beyond neutral prior to surgery. The details of operative technique are illustrated in Plate 64.

Valgus or varus deformity associated with the equinus foot is usually caused by an imbalance of the muscles of inversion and eversion—the tibialis posterior and the peroneal muscles. Treatment of these deforming spastic muscles may be carried out at the same time as correction of equinus deformity; however, one must be cautious not to overcorrect and cause a reverse deformity.

Pes Varus. When the spastic posterior tibial muscle is causing pes varus, it may be lengthened at the same time as the heel cord. This is particularly indicated when there is continuous activity of the posterior tibial muscle as shown by dynamic electromyography during gait analysis (see below). It is not necessary to make a separate incision. Through the posteromedial incision for heel cord lengthening, the posterior tibial muscle and tendon can be exposed above the medial malleolus in the distal third of the leg immediately posterior to the tibia. At two levels, 5 cm. apart and well above the site where muscle fibers terminate on the tendon, two incisions are made over the tendinous portion of the posterior tibial muscle but not into the muscle fibers themselves. The proximal incision is transverse, and the distal one oblique. The sliding lengthening of the tendon is obtained by forcing the foot into valgus position and by gentle stretching between two moist sponges (Fig. 5–43).

Total section with release of the posterior tibial tendon should be avoided, as it will cause marked valgus deformity in the growing foot. One should remember the adage—in spastic cerebral palsy under every varus foot there is potential for valgus deformity. Baker recommends freeing the sheath of the posterior tibial tendon behind the medial malleolus and allowing it to be displaced anterior to the malleolus.[11] The author does not advise this procedure because, in its new transposed position, the posterior tibial muscle still acts as an invertor of the foot, causing calcaneovarus deformity.

Anterior transfer of the posterior tibial tendon through the interosseous route for the correction of nonstructural varus deformity of the hindfoot in spastic paralysis has been described by several authors. Williams reported the results in 53 feet in 42 patients as follows: (1) Of 28 patients who had required below-knee orthoses, 23 were able to discard them postoperatively; (2) 38 patients had improved gait with plantigrade position of the foot and decrease in toeing-in; (3) 24 feet showed improved shoe wear; (4) 27 feet demonstrated voluntary control over the transferred tibialis posterior; and (5) 23 feet had active contraction of the transfer in gait. (6) In seven feet all the muscles of the lower leg were in spasm, including the transferred tibialis posterior; in these patients the feet were frozen at right angles to the leg, but function was remarkably good. (7) Of the 53 feet, 5 needed further surgical procedures to obtain an acceptable result—these consisted of triple arthrodesis in three, lengthening of the transfer to correct spastic calcaneus deformity in one, and shortening of the transfer to overcome a drop foot in one. The overall rating of the transfers in the 42 patients was good in 22, fair in 14, and poor in 6. Williams regarded

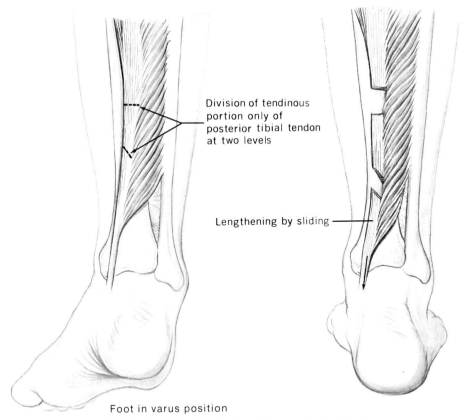

Division of tendinous
portion only of
posterior tibial tendon
at two levels

Lengthening by sliding

Foot in varus position

FIGURE 5–43. Sliding lengthening of the posterior tibial tendon.

anterior transfer of the tibialis posterior as "one of the most reliable and successful operations in cerebral palsy."[589]

This author does not share Williams's enthusiasm. It is very difficult to train an out-of-phase transfer in a child with brain damage. The results are unpredictable, and not infrequently, a reverse deformity may develop. When the procedure is combined with heel cord lengthening, calcaneovalgus or calcaneus deformity is a common complication.

More definitive preoperative assessment by kinetic electromyography synchronized with three-plane motion pictures in gait and with force plate measurements is available in special centers. Perry and Hoffer have utilized preoperative and postoperative dynamic electromyography as an aid in planning tendon transfers in children with cerebral palsy.[403]

In the gait of a normal person, there is habitual phasic activity of groups of muscles working automatically during portions of the stance and swing phases. In cerebral palsy this selective and habitual phasic muscle control is disturbed because primitive modes of muscle action persist in the form of patterns of activity

that respond to posturing of the trunk and limbs, to different rates of stretch, and to residual perinatal reflexes. Muscle grading in cerebral palsy is difficult because of the "patterning" or stretch activation of the muscles, but electromyography will show their activity during different phases of gait. By applying this information in addition to the basic principles of tendon transfer learned in poliomyelitis—a muscle of normal or good motor strength, ample tendon excursion, a direct line of pull, normal range of joint motion, and meticulous postoperative training—one can achieve the desired function in cerebral palsy.

Perry and associates recommend anterior transfer of the posterior tibial tendon for pes varus when the muscle is active only in the swing phase preoperatively; it is a prerequisite that there be full range of passive motion of the ankle and hind part of the foot. (When there is equinus deformity, anterior transfer of the posterior tibial tendon should be preceded by heel cord lengthening.) On the other hand, if the tibialis posterior is active continuously in both swing and stance phases of gait, they recommend lengthening and not transfer because the

Text continued on page 1686

Extensor Hallucis Longus Rerouting Through Anterior Tibial Tendon and Shortening of Anterior Tibial Muscle

OPERATIVE TECHNIQUE

A. A Longitudinal incision about 7 cm. long is made over the dorsum of the foot. It starts at the base of the proximal phalanx of the big toe and extends proximally to the first cuneiform bone. Subcutaneous tissue is divided in line with the skin incision; wound margins are undermined and gently retracted. Injury to the superficial vessels and sensory nerves is avoided.

B. The extensor hallucis longus tendon is identified and detached from its insertion as far distally as possible. The stump is sutured to the tendon of the extensor hallucis brevis with the big toe held in marked dorsiflexion to prevent plantar drop of the hallux postoperatively. (It is described in Plate 106). The tendon of the extensor hallucis longus is dissected free of its sheath as high as possible. Then a second incision is made over the course of the anterior tibial tendon in the distal third of the leg. The tendons of the extensor hallucis longus and the anterior tibial are identified. The extensor hallucis longus is pulled into the proximal wound by gentle traction.

C. With a scalpel, three slits of appropriate size are made in the anterior tibial tendon. The extensor hallucis longus tendon is rewound by passing through these slits and then delivered into the distal wound with an Ober tendon passer.

Plate 64. Extensor Hallucis Longus Rerouting Through Anterior Tibial Tendon and Shortening of Anterior Tibial Muscle

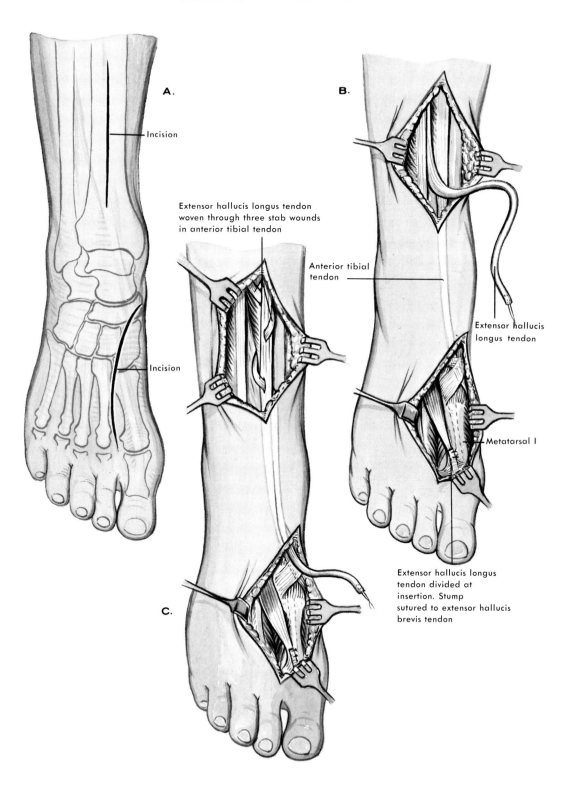

A.

Incision

Incision

B.

Extensor hallucis longus tendon woven through three stab wounds in anterior tibial tendon

Anterior tibial tendon

Extensor hallucis longus tendon

Metatarsal I

Extensor hallucis longus tendon divided at insertion. Stump sutured to extensor hallucis brevis tendon

C.

Extensor Hallucis Longus Rerouting Through Anterior Tibial Tendon and Shortening of Anterior Tibial Muscle (Continued)

D. The extensor hallucis longus tendon is sutured to the insertion of the anterior tibial muscle with the ankle in neutral position or 10 degrees of dorsiflexion. Any excess of the extensor hallucis longus tendon is either excised (as illustrated) or, if it is long enough, reattached to its insertion. Next, the lax anterior tibial tendon is shortened by plication and suturing to the capsule of the first metatarsal-cuneiform joint.

E. Another way of shortening the anterior tibial tendon is by excising an appropriate segment distally and suturing the cut ends together. The tourniquet is released, and after complete hemostasis the wound is closed in layers in the usual fashion. The foot and ankle are immobilized in a below-knee walking cast.

POSTOPERATIVE CARE

Three weeks after surgery the cast is removed and an above-knee splint is made that maintains the ankle at 5 to 10 degrees of dorsiflexion and the knee in neutral extension; the splint is worn at night. During the day a dorsiflexion-assist below-knee orthosis is used. Active assisted exercises are performed to develop function in and cerebral control over the cerebral zero anterior tibial muscle. Gentle passive exercises are carried out to maintain range of ankle motion. During the day periods of gait training without orthosis are carried out to activate the anterior tibial muscle function. The dorsiflexion-assist orthosis is gradually discontinued over a period of three to six months. Persistent and meticulous physical therapy and night splinting are vital.

Plate 64. Extensor Hallucis Longus Rerouting Through Anterior Tibial Tendon and Shortening of Anterior Tibial Muscle

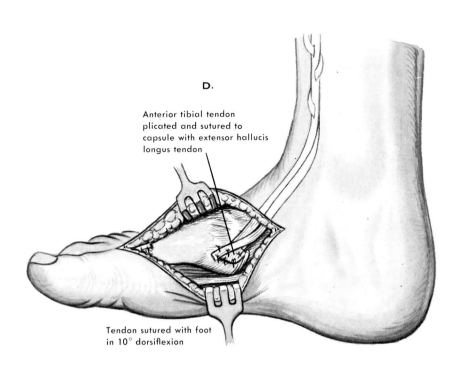

D.

Anterior tibial tendon plicated and sutured to capsule with extensor hallucis longus tendon

Tendon sutured with foot in 10° dorsiflexion

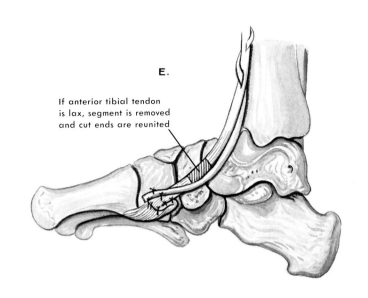

E.

If anterior tibial tendon is lax, segment is removed and cut ends are reunited

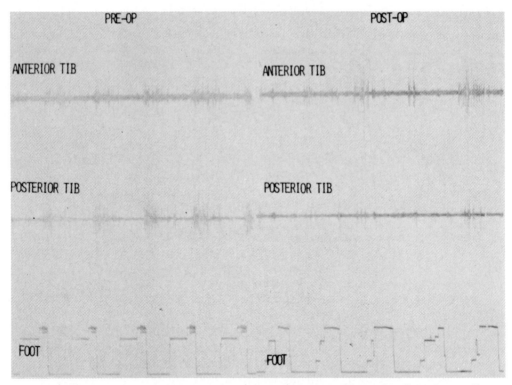

FIGURE 5–44. Preoperative and postoperative dynamic electromyographic studies of anterior transfer of posterior tibial tendon in spastic cerebral palsy.

Note that the muscle is active during the swing phase of gait both before and after anterior transfer. (From Perry, J., and Hoffer, M. M.: Preoperative and postoperative dynamic electromyography as an aid in planning tendon transfers in children with cerebral palsy. J. Bone Joint Surg., 59-A:532, 1978. Reprinted by permission.)

transfer frequently becomes a tenodesis. In three children the phase action of the posterior tibial muscle was reversed (i.e., it was active during the swing phase); the tendon was transferred anteriorly, and all three transfers functioned automatically (Fig. 5–44). Two children had continuous activity of the posterior tibial muscle, which was lengthened at its musculotendinous junction (Fig. 5–45).[404]

As a general rule this author does *not rec-ommend* anterior transfer of the posterior tibial tendon in spastic paralysis unless the facilities of a gait analysis laboratory are available and dynamic electromyography demonstrates that the muscle is active only during the swing phase of gait. He employs it then only if the ankle and hind part of the foot have full passive range of motion, i.e., the varus posture of the foot is not fixed. The child should be intelligent and of an age to be motivated to cooperate during the postoperative training period. The indication for transfer is drop foot due to ankle dorsiflexor insufficiency, provided that the aforementioned requisites are met. Otherwise, it is safer and much simpler to lengthen the

tibialis posterior when there is continuous activity in both swing and stance phase of gait or to perform split posterolateral transfer of the posterior tibial muscle.

Split posterior tibial tendon transfer is recommended by Green and Griffin when the posterior tibial muscle is diphasic, the anterior tibial muscle weak, and the peroneals weak or absent. Through a posteromedial incision, the posterior tibial tendon is split longitudinally into halves, leaving the anteromedial half attached to the navicular. The posterolateral half is passed laterally, anterior to the neurovascular bundle and the long flexors, into the sheath of the peroneus brevis tendon, and sutured as far distally as possible into the peroneus brevis near its insertion (Fig. 5–46).[193] In the experience of Green et al., the results were excellent in all 16 patients.[193] Kling et al. assessed the results of 37 split posterior tibial tendon transfers in cerebral palsy patients with equinovarus. The follow-up was a mean of eight years with a range of 4 to 14 years. The results were excellent in 30, good in 4 and poor in 3. None of the patients developed a calcaneal or calcaneo-

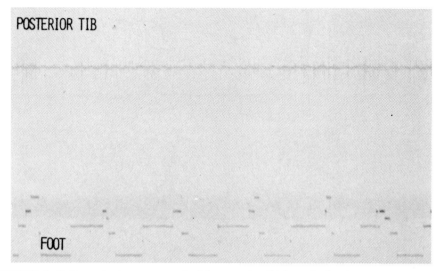

FIGURE 5–45. *Dynamic electromyograph of the posterior tibial muscle showing continuous activity in both phases of gait.*

A preoperative study. This muscle is lengthened at its musculotendinous junction; it should not be transferred anteriorly. (From Perry, J., and Hoffer, M. M.: Preoperative and postoperative dynamic electromyography as an aid in planning tendon transfers in children with cerebral palsy. J. Bone Joint Surg., 59-A:532, 1978. Reprinted by permission.)

valgus deformity. The poor results were seen in those with recurrent deformity.[295]

In the experience of this author, the subtalar joint mobility is decreased or lost following split posterior tibial tendon transfer. This may be a disadvantage in some patients, whereas in others, the provision of subtalar joint stability may be desirable.

In the adolescent patient the hindfoot varus deformity may be severe and fixed; in such cases, soft-tissue procedures will not correct it, and a bony procedure is required. The author recommends a Dwyer lateral calcaneal close-up wedge osteotomy (see Plate 109 in Chapter 7) or, preferably, lateral displacement osteotomy of the calcaneus. It is wise to precede or combine it with soft-tissue release, such as lengthening of the posterior tibial tendon, in order to prevent recurrence of deformity. Fixed hindfoot and midfoot varus in the skeletally mature patient is treated by triple arthrodesis.[257]

Transfer of Tibialis Anterior. In acquired spastic paralysis the anterior tibial muscle may be hyperactive, pulling the foot into varus posture. The anterior tibial tendon may be transferred laterally to the base of the second or third metatarsal—never more laterally—to change the action of the muscle from varus dorsiflexion to pure dorsiflexion. In perinatal spastic cerebral palsy, calcaneovarus deformity of the foot may develop as a complication of overlengthening of the tendo Achillis, with con-

sequent poor function of the triceps surae and overactivity of the tibialis anterior; these cases present another indication for lateral transfer of the tibialis anterior. In mixed (spastic-athetoid) cerebral palsy, the anterior tibial muscle may be hyperactive; in such cases it is best to refrain from transferring the anterior tibial muscle, as a reverse deformity may develop.

Split anterior tibial tendon transfer has been performed extensively at Rancho Los Amigos Hospital, Downey, California, on adults with cerebrovascular accidents and also on spastic children. Hoffer and associates presented the results of 21 split anterior tibial tendon transfers in 16 children. Gait improved in all patients; all 16 had required braces before surgery, and only 7 required them postoperatively. The fixed deformities were released in 15 feet (12 patients). Twenty of the 21 transfers functioned with force equal to that noted in their spastic patterns preoperatively. Deformities recurred in two feet.[228]

Perry and Hoffer later reported the results of four split anterior tibial tendon transfers for treatment of varus posture of the foot. All four patients required braces preoperatively, and after surgery they all became brace-free and had balanced foot posture. Preoperative dynamic electromyography had shown continuous activity of the anterior tibial during gait, and the postoperative electromyograms did not show any change. The feet improved because

Text continued on page 1692

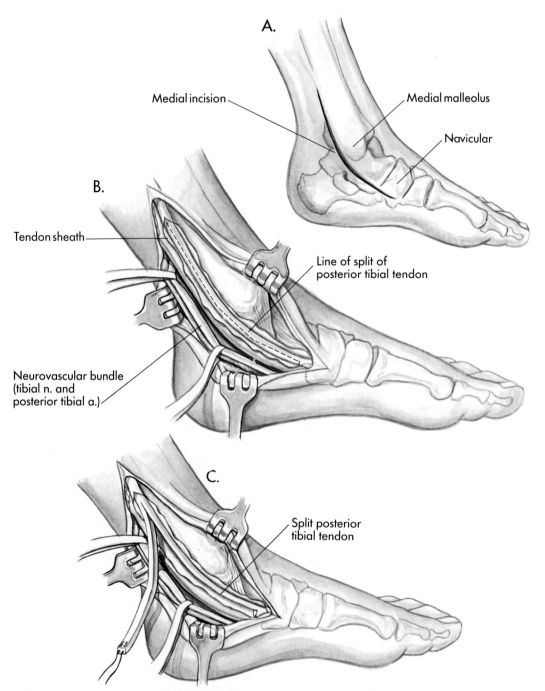

FIGURE 5–46. Surgical technique of the split posterior tibial tendon transfer.

A. Line of medial incision. **B.** Medial view of the foot and ankle. The sheath of the posterior tibial tendon is incised, and the plantar half of the tendon is divided and dissected free from its insertion into the navicular. It is vital to obtain as much length as possible. **C.** The posterior tibial tendon is split longitudinally and proximally to its musculotendinous junction; the dorsal portion of the tendon is left intact attached to the navicular. Do not divide the retinaculum of the ankle. Note that the neurovascular bundle and long toe flexors are gently retracted posteriorly.

Illustration continued on opposite page

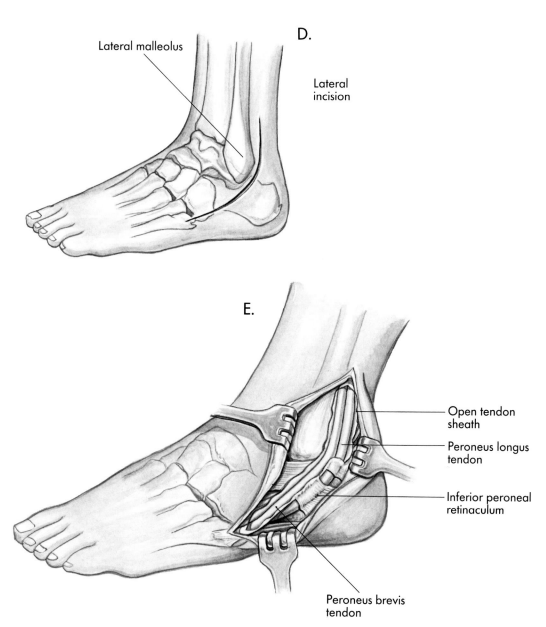

FIGURE 5–46 Continued. Surgical technique of the split posterior tibial tendon transfer.

D. Lateral view of the foot and ankle showing the line of the skin incision. **E.** The peroneus brevis and longus tendons are identified, and the tendon sheath is opened, exposing the peroneal tendons.

Ilustration continued on following page

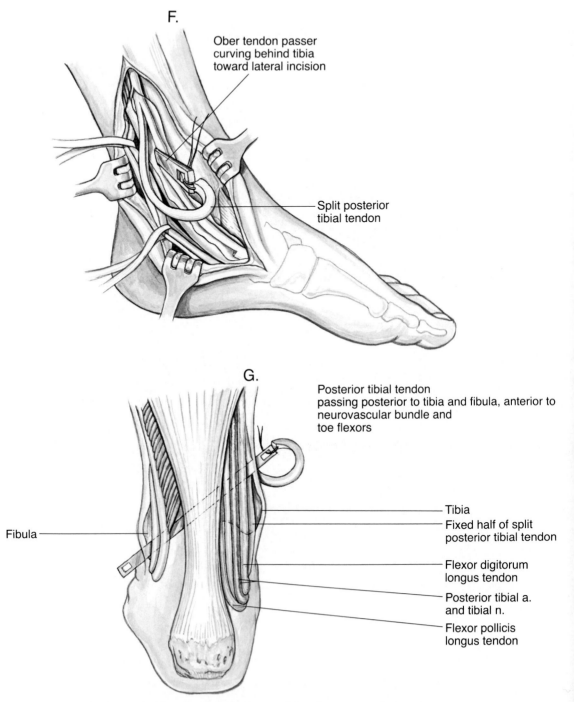

F.

Ober tendon passer
curving behind tibia
toward lateral incision

Split posterior
tibial tendon

G.

Posterior tibial tendon
passing posterior to tibia and fibula, anterior to
neurovascular bundle and
toe flexors

Fibula

Tibia

Fixed half of split
posterior tibial tendon

Flexor digitorum
longus tendon

Posterior tibial a.
and tibial n.

Flexor pollicis
longus tendon

FIGURE 5–46 Continued. Surgical technique of the split posterior tibial tendon transfer.

F and G. The split half of the posterior tibial tendon is transferred to the lateral side of the foot, passing anterior to the neurovascular bundle, long toe flexor tendons, and flexor digitorum longus. It is inferior to the lateral malleolus and deep to the peroneus brevis tendon.

Illustration continued on opposite page

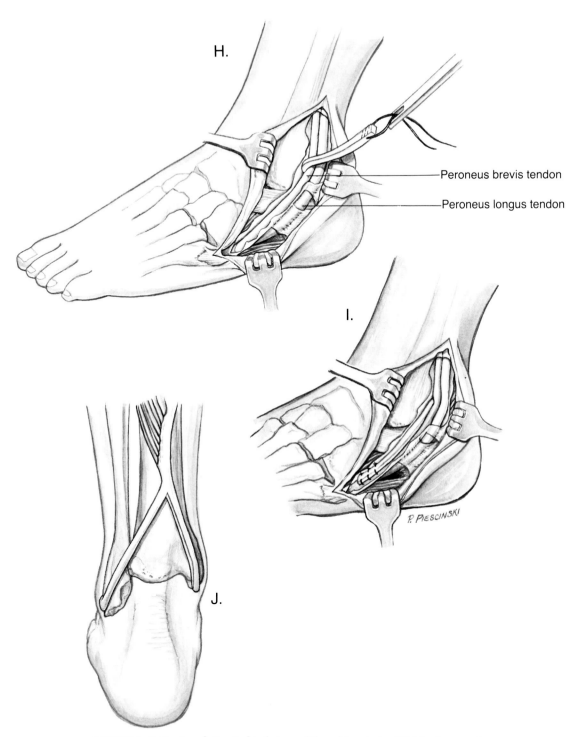

H.

Peroneus brevis tendon

Peroneus longus tendon

I.

P. PIESCINSKI

J.

FIGURE 5–46 Continued. *Surgical technique of the split posterior tibial tendon transfer.*

H and **I.** The split posterior tibial tendon is brought out into the peroneus brevis tendon sheath, the tension on it is adjusted, and it is sutured to the tendon as far distally as possible. It is best to weave it through the peroneus brevis tendon.

J. Posterior view of the ankle and hindfoot, showing the direction of the tendon transfer. It is oblique from its musculotendinous junction above toward the tip of the lateral malleolus distally and laterally. The continuous contraction of the spastic posterior tibial tendon provides mechanical stability and control of the hindfoot in neutral position or five degrees of valgus inclination.

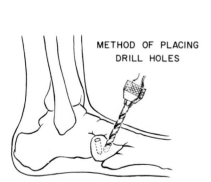

METHOD OF PLACING
DRILL HOLES

CUBOID

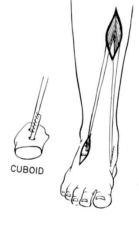

**FIGURE 5–47. Split anterior tibial tendon
transfer in the treatment of spastic
varus hindfoot.**

(From Hoffer, M. M., Reiswig, J. A.,
Garrett, M. M., and Perry, J.: The split
anterior tibial tendon transfer in the treatment of spastic varus hindfoot in childhood.
Orthop. Clin. North Am., 5:32, 1974. Reprinted by permission.)

the force of the anterior tibial tendon was balanced.[403] In a further ten-year follow-up report of 27 feet by Hoffer et al., the results were satisfactory, with one recurrent mild dynamic varus and two recurrent equinus deformities. These investigators recommended split anterior tibial tendon transfer to be combined with heel cord lengthening to correct equinus and posterior tibial lengthening when associated with hindfoot varus and posterior tibial muscle showed continuous activity on dynamic gait electromyography.[221]

The technique of split anterior tibial tendon transfer is relatively simple (Fig. 5–47; also see Plate 98, Chapter 7). An incision 5 to 7 cm. long is made over the dorsomedial aspect of the foot, centered over the medial cuneiform. The anterior tibial tendon is identified and split into halves; the medial half is left anchored to the base of the first metatarsal. The lateral half of the tendon is sectioned, dissected free, and tagged with a whip suture. A second longitudinal incision, 7 cm. long, is made over the anterior aspect of the distal third of the leg, lateral to the crest of the tibia. With an Ober tendon passer the lateral half of the tendon is delivered to the proximal wound. A third longitudinal incision is made on the dorsolateral aspect of the foot, 5 cm. long and centered over the cuboid. The lateral half of the anterior tibial tendon is delivered into the third wound deep to the extensor retinaculum with an Ober tendon passer. With a 7/64-inch drill, two holes are made in the cuboid at converging angles. The holes are joined at their depth with a small curet. The dorsal roof of the cuboid should be preserved. The lateral half of the split anterior tibial tendon is passed through the hole and sutured to itself with the ankle in 5 to 10 degrees of dorsiflexion. The wounds are closed

in the usual fashion, and a below-knee cast is applied. Weight-bearing with the cast is permitted within a few days; the cast is removed at four weeks. The patient is immediately fitted with an ankle foot orthosis, with the ankle joint at 5 degrees of dorsiflexion. Plastic splints are worn at night to hold the ankle in slight dorsiflexion. Active and passive exercises are performed to develop anterior tibial muscle function and to maintain range of ankle motion. Use of the ankle-foot orthosis during the daytime is gradually discontinued at six months.[228]

The split anterior tibial tendon transfer acts as a balanced yoke, and leaving its medial half attached to the base of the first metatarsal preserves its action as dorsiflexor of the first metatarsal. This author recommends split anterior tibial tendon transfer when the peroneus longus is functioning, as the action of the medial half of the anterior tibial tendon will counterbalance the plantar flexing action of the peroneus and prevent the development of forefoot equinus (anterior cavus) deformity. The posterior tibial muscle, if contracted, can be fractionally lengthened at the same time. The procedure should not, however, be combined with simultaneous heel cord lengthening. It is best to stage the two operations to ensure success of the outcome.

Pes Valgus. It is more common in spastic diplegia than in spastic hemiplegia; in the latter, pes varus is the more common foot deformity.[40]

Etiology. Valgus deformity of the foot is commonly associated with contracture of the triceps surae because the height of the foot is reduced when the hindfoot is everted, and the tendo Achillis is relatively lengthened. The valgus deformity is severe when there is a dynamic muscle imbalance between the evertors and invertors of the foot, i.e., the peroneal muscles are spastic and strong, and the anterior and posterior tibial muscles are cerebral zero or weak. Spasticity and contracture of the long toe extensor muscle will aggravate the valgus deformity of the mid- and forefoot.

Dynamic electromyographic studies will disclose various patterns of muscle activity. (1) The peroneal muscles may be hyperactive in both swing and stance phases with hypoactive or electrically silent posterior tibial muscle; (2) there may be hyperactive peroneal muscles with normal activity or hyperactivity of posterior tibial muscle; (3) extensor digitorum longus may be of normal activity or hyperactive; occasionally the long toe extensors may be hyperactive. It is advisable to perform gait analysis with dynamic electromyography prior to tendon transfers to correct valgus deformity of the foot.[40b, 511a]

Ligamentous hyperlaxity (due to defective cross-linking of collagen) is another cause of pes valgus.[40b]

In pes valgus the calcaneus and talus are plantar flexed and the talonavicular and calcaneocuboid joints are subluxated laterally to a varying degree; the head of the talus is prominent on the medial-plantar aspect of the foot. In childhood, valgus deformity of the foot is flexible, i.e., normal articular relationship of the talocalcaneonavicular and calcaneocuboid joints can be restored by passive plantar flexion and inversion of the foot. In the adolescent and skeletally mature foot, the valgus deformity may be fixed. With weight bearing on the medial aspect of the midfoot, secondary hallux valgus with painful callosity over the first metatarsal head may develop.

In early childhood, management of valgus foot is approached conservatively. Supportive shoes with a Thomas heel, a 1/8- to 3/16-inch medial heel wedge, an extended medial heel counter, and a 3/8-inch longitudinal arch support may be fitted. It should be explained to the parents, that such "orthopedic" shoes simply support the foot—they do not correct the deformity. Gentle passive exercises to elongate the contracted triceps surae and peroneal muscles are performed several times a day. The hypotonic posterior tibial and anterior tibial muscles are strengthened by active exercise. Splints are worn at night to hold the ankle and foot in neutral position. In severe pes valgus, UCBL (University of California Biomechanics Laboratory) foot orthoses are prescribed. Supramalleolar orthosis is indicated when equinus and valgus deformities are marked and the talus is plantar flexed into vertical position. It is important to make anteroposterior and lateral standing radiograms of the foot with the orthotics on to determine whether plantar flexion of the talus and sagging of the talonavicular cuneiform joints are corrected by the orthosis.

Surgical correction of equinus deformity, however, should not be long delayed, as fixed pes valgus may develop that may require extensive bony procedures for correction. Conversely, premature surgery should not be performed. A sliding heel cord lengthening is performed at the appropriate time. The distal portion of the tendo Achillis is sectioned in its lateral half to decrease the eversion pull of the triceps surae. This is combined with fractional lengthening of the peroneal muscles at their musculotendinous junction through a separate incision over the middle third of the fibula when the peroneals are spastic and a deforming force. In the postoperative period, a UCBL shoe insert is used to support the foot. Passive and active exercises are performed as already described.

The results of peroneus brevis fractional lengthening (intramuscular tenotomy) were reported in 30 cases of spastic pes valgus by Nather et al; the hindfoot valgus decreased in 14, was unchanged in 12, and increased in 4; the greater improvement was noted in the mild cases.[369] Peroneus brevis musculotendinous lengthening is recommended by this author when valgus deformity of the foot is mild or moderate; in severe cases it is not adequate to correct the valgus deformity. It is carried out in combination with other surgical procedures, such as heel cord lengthening, medial displacement osteotomy of the calcaneus, and extra-articular subtalar Grice arthrodesis.

Perry and Hoffer recommend lengthening of the peroneus longus or brevis when the muscles are active continuously throughout both the stance and the swing phases of the gait cycle. On the other hand, if the peroneus brevis or longus is active only during the stance phase, they transfer the tendon of the hyperactive muscle posteromedially through the sheath of the tibialis posterior to the navicular. In two such transfers the muscle activity of the transferred peroneus brevis remained unchanged postoperatively. In the personal experience of this author, the results of posteromedial transfer of the peroneals have not been satisfactory.

By the time the child is eight to ten years of age, if the pes valgus persists and its severity is of such a degree that it interferes with shoe wear, balance, and locomotion, a subtalar extra-articular arthrodesis is performed (Fig. 5–48).

Text continued on page 1698

Extra-Articular Arthrodesis of the Subtalar Joint (Grice Procedure)

OPERATIVE TECHNIQUE

A. A 2½-inch long and slightly curved incision is made over the subtalar joint, centering over the sinus tarsi.

B. The incision is carried down to the sinus tarsi. The capsules of the posterior and anterior subtalar articulations are identified and left intact. The operation is extra-articular. If the capsule is opened inadvertently, it should be closed by interrupted sutures.

The periosteum on the talus corresponding to the lateral margin of the roof of the sinus tarsi is divided and reflected proximally. The fibrofatty tissue in the sinus tarsi with the periosteum of the calcaneus corresponding to the floor of the sinus tarsi and the tendinous origin of the short toe extensors from the calcaneus is elevated and reflected distally in one mass.

C. The remaining fatty and ligamentous tissue from the sinus tarsi is thoroughly removed with a sharp scalpel and curet.

Plate 65. *Extra-Articular Arthrodesis of the Subtalar Joint (Grice Procedure)*

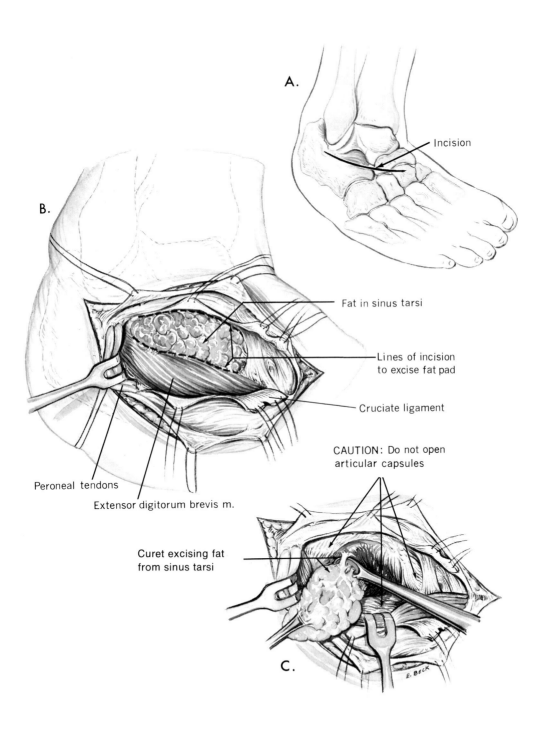

A.

Incision

B.

Fat in sinus tarsi

Lines of incision to excise fat pad

Cruciate ligament

CAUTION: Do not open articular capsules

Peroneal tendons

Extensor digitorum brevis m.

Curet excising fat from sinus tarsi

C.

E. BECK

Extra-Articular Arthrodesis of the Subtalar Joint (Grice Procedure) (Continued)

D. Next the foot is manipulated into equinus position and inversion, rotating the calcaneus into its normal position beneath the talus and correcting the valgus deformity. Broad straight osteotomes of various sizes (¾ to 1¼ inches or more) are inserted into the sinus tarsi, blocking the subtalar joint and determining the length and optimum position of the bone graft and the stability that it will provide. The long axis of the graft should be parallel with that of the leg when the ankle is dorsiflexed into neutral position, and the hindfoot should be 5 degrees valgus or neutral, but never varus. Even a slight degree of varus deformity of the heel seems to increase with growth.

E. The optimum site of the bone graft bed is marked with the broad osteotome. A thin layer of cortical bone (⅛ to 3⁄16 inch) is removed with a dental osteotome from the inferior surface of the talus (the roof of the sinus tarsi) and the superior surface of the calcaneus (the floor of the sinus tarsi) at the marked site for the bone graft. It is best to preserve the most lateral cortical margin of the graft bed to support the bone block and to prevent it from sinking into soft cancellous bone.

F. A bone graft of appropriate size can be taken from the anteromedial surface of the proximal tibial metaphysis as a single cortical graft, which is then cut into two trapezoidal bone grafts with their cancellous surfaces facing each other. Lately the author prefers to use fibular bone grafts with the cortices intact. The corners of the base of the graft are removed with a rongeur so that it is trapezoidal in shape and can be countersunk into cancellous bone, preventing lateral displacement after operation.

The bone graft is placed in the prepared graft bed in the sinus tarsi by holding the foot in varus position. An impacter may be used to fix the cortices of the graft in place. The longitudinal axis of the graft should be parallel with the shaft of the tibia with the ankle in neutral position.

With the foot held in the desired position, the distal soft-tissue pedicle of fibrofatty tissue of the sinus tarsi, the calcaneal periosteum, and the tendinous origin of the short toe extensors are sutured to the reflected periosteum from the talus. The subcutaneous tissue and skin are closed with interrupted sutures, and an above-knee cast is applied.

POSTOPERATIVE CARE

The cast is removed eight to ten weeks after operation. Radiograms are taken; if there is solid healing of the graft, gradual weight-bearing is allowed with the protection of crutches. Active and passive exercises are performed to strengthen the muscles and to increase the range of motion of the ankle and of the knee.

Plate 65. Extra-Articular Arthrodesis of the Subtalar Joint (Grice Procedure)

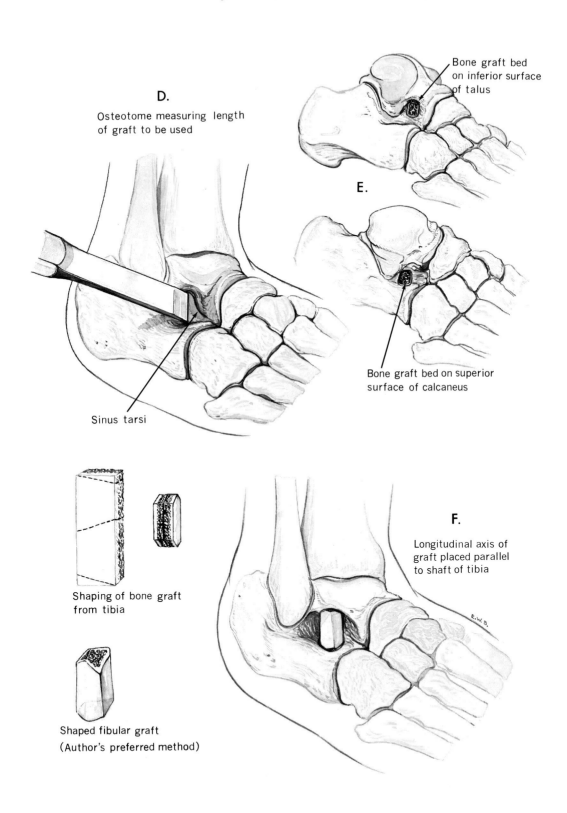

D.

Osteotome measuring length of graft to be used

Bone graft bed on inferior surface of talus

E.

Sinus tarsi

Bone graft bed on superior surface of calcaneus

Shaping of bone graft from tibia

Shaped fibular graft (Author's preferred method)

F.

Longitudinal axis of graft placed parallel to shaft of tibia

E.W.B.

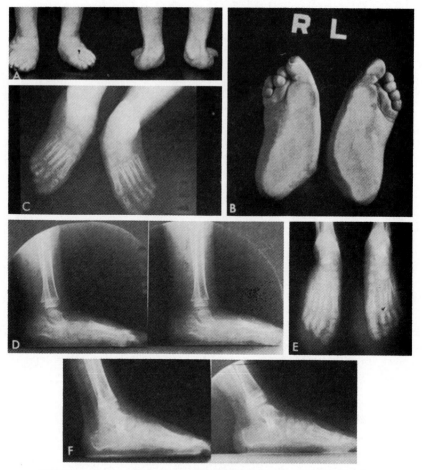

FIGURE 5–48. Equinovalgus deformity of the feet in spastic cerebral palsy.

A. Severe valgus foot deformities at age three years and three months. **B.** Plantar view of feet. **C** and **D.** Weight-bearing radiograms of feet preoperatively. **E** and **F.** Weight-bearing radiograms of feet eight months after bilateral heel cord lengthening and subtalar bone block arthrodesis. Note incorporation of talocalcaneal bone graft.

Illustration continued on opposite page

This will control the alignment of the foot and will help to avoid a triple arthrodesis later when growth is complete. The operative technique of extra-articular subtalar arthrodesis (Grice procedure) is described in Plate 65.

In the experience of this author, with early, preventive soft-tissue surgery, the alignment of the foot can be controlled in most cases, obviating the need for a Grice procedure.

Several end-result studies of the Grice extra-articular arthrodesis in cerebral palsy have appeared in the literature.* Banks and his colleagues reported long-term results of Grice subtalar arthrodesis in 72 valgus feet in 44 patients with cerebral palsy; the results were

excellent in 43 feet (as shown in Figure 5–48), good in 15, fair in 8, and poor in 6. Overcorrection and hindfoot varus deviation was the most significant complication; the heel varus deformity was minor in five feet and marked in three feet.[18a] It is vital to determine the degree of correction by intraoperative radiograms before closure of the wound. Threaded Steinmann pins or cancellous bone screws should be used for internal fixation; they give the graft greater stability and allow immobilization of the limb with the foot in neutral position and the knee in extension to prevent hamstring contracture postoperatively. Results of Grice subtalar arthrodesis have been reported in the literature by the other authors; they have not been as successful as Banks. It is well documented that the Grice procedure corrects valgus deformity of the hindfoot and restores the height of the

*See References 12, 77, 79, 104, 134, 193, 200, 201, 281, 287, 331, 347, 358a, b, 386, 387, 423, 426, 448, 462a, 490, 518.

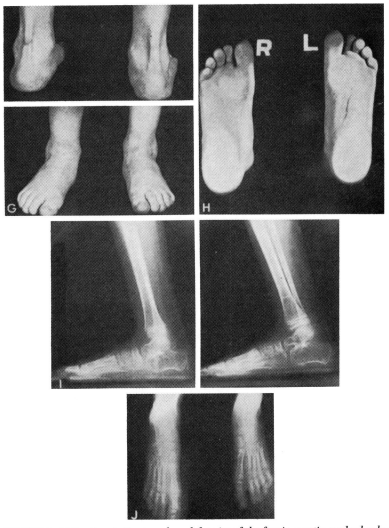

FIGURE 5-48 Continued. Equinovalgus deformity of the feet in spastic cerebral palsy.

G. Weight-bearing photographs of feet three years and six months postoperatively. H. Plantar weight-bearing views of feet three years and six months postoperatively. I and J. Weight-bearing radiograms three years and six months postoperatively. (From Banks, H., and Panagakos, P.: The role of the orthopedic surgeon in cerebral palsy. Pediatr. Clin. North Am., *14*:495, 1967. Reprinted by permission.)

longitudinal arch. When the graft is extra-artic-ular, it will interfere minimally with the growth of the foot. On the other hand, the Grice procedure does not correct fixed valgus or varus deformity of the mid- or forepart of the foot; it does not improve pes planus due to ligamentous relaxation and sagging of the talonavicular or naviculocuneiform joint. There are also draw-backs of which one should beware: The Grice arthrodesis does cause loss of lateral mobility of the hindfoot and may cause difficulty in walking on rough terrain; it also exerts excessive liga-mentous strain on the ankle joint.

When performing a Grice extra-articular sub-talar arthrodesis one should follow certain basic dicta rigidly:

1. Equinus deformity should be corrected first; failure to do this will result in fusion of the calcaneus to the talus with the heel in fixed equinus position and the foot in abduction and eversion. Upon weight-bearing the talus will tilt into valgus position in the ankle mortise. It is imperative that one determine preoperatively whether the calcaneus can be restored to its normal position beneath the talus; this is done by making lateral radiograms of the foot after it

has been passively manipulated into an equinus position and inversion. When there is contracture of the triceps surae muscle, it is essential to make a lateral radiogram of the foot and ankle with the foot in inversion and the ankle in maximal forced dorsiflexion. Equinus deformity is corrected by heel cord lengthening, but the procedure should *not be combined* with the Grice procedure. Prolonged immobilization in a cast will cause marked atrophy of the triceps surae and result in calcaneus deformity. Stage the two operations. If it is impossible to place the calcaneus in a normal position beneath the talus, the Grice procedure should not be performed.

2. Always determine the stability of the body of the talus in the ankle mortise preoperatively by making weight-bearing stress radiograms of the ankle. Determine the level of the lateral malleolus. Is there valgus deviation of the ankle? The distal fibular growth plate should be level with the ankle joint. In paralyzed limbs the fibula is frequently underdeveloped, the distal fibular physis being at the same level or a more proximal level than that of the tibia.[337] Removal of a bone graft from the ipsilateral tibia will definitely accelerate growth of that bone and further increase the disparity in length between the fibula and tibia.[244, 386] It is better to use an iliac bone graft if there is already a valgus deformity of the ankle.[104] If fibular bone graft is used, it should, however, be taken at the junction of the proximal and middle thirds of the shaft. The excised segment of the fibula should not be too long, and the periosteum should be meticulously closed to ensure union. When bilateral extra-articular subtalar arthrodesis is performed, an autogenous fibular bone graft should be taken from each leg. A common tendency is to take a long segment of the fibula from one leg to use for both feet; this, however, will result in nonunion of the fibula, a high-riding lateral malleolus, and valgus deformity of the ankle. This author strongly recommends the use of iliac bone for grafts. When there is marked valgus deformity of the ankle, it is corrected by supramalleolar osteotomy of the tibia in the skeletally mature patient, as described in the section on myelomeningocele. In the younger adolescent, medial epiphyseodesis of the distal tibia is performed at the appropriate skeletal age to correct ankle valgus.

3. Avoid overcorrection and varus deformity by taking intraoperative radiograms. After the graft is placed in the sinus tarsi, the position of the heel is carefully inspected clinically and on radiographic views. The hindfoot should never be fused in varus position.

4. Malposition or shifting of the bone graft in the sinus tarsi should be recognized and corrected in the operating room.

5. Internally fix the subtalar joint by a single cancellous screw.

6. The dynamic balance of muscles that act on the foot should be restored, and contractural deformities should be corrected by appropriate musculotendinous lengthenings. Invertor-evertor muscle imbalance may cause recurrence of deformity in the growing foot. Overzealous correction should, however, be avoided.

7. Detect pseudarthrosis early. The bone graft may fail to unite to the talus or calcaneus, or pseudarthrosis may occur in the middle, or the entire bone graft may be resorbed. The incidence of pseudarthrosis has been greatly reduced by the use of autogenous fibular or iliac bone graft, rather than homologous "bone bank" bone; it will still develop in a certain percentage of cases, however, and it is important that it be detected and revised or corrected—by insertion of another graft, if necessary. Otherwise, the correction will be lost and the os calcis will be united to the talus with the foot in fixed planovalgus position.

Modifications of Grice Extra-articular Arthrodesis. Batchelor performed subtalar arthrodesis by inserting an autogenous fibular graft from the neck of the talus across the sinus tarsi into the calcaneus with the hind part of the foot held in neutral position. The subtalar joint is not exposed.[30, 490]

The technique of the operation is as follows: Under tourniquet hemostasis a 4-cm.-long longitudinal incision is made over the dorsomedial aspect of the foot in line with and centered over the neck of the talus. (The tendency is to place the incision too far anterior.) The neck of the talus is exposed after it has been identified under image intensification. The calcaneus is inverted into neutral position or 5 degrees of valgus, but not varus, deviation. A smooth Steinmann pin is drilled through the body of the talus into the calcaneus, transfixing the subtalar joint. The pin also serves as a guide for the drill. Under image intensification control, a 9-mm. drill is driven through the neck of the talus plantarward, posteriorly, and slightly laterally. As the electric drill passes through the inferior cortex of the talus one can feel the ease with which it traverses the sinus tarsi until it meets the resistance of the cortex of the superior surface of the calcaneus. Its position is checked under an image intensifier and, if it is correct, the drill is advanced for an additional 2 or 3 cm. and then is withdrawn. Larger burrs are used, if necessary, until the

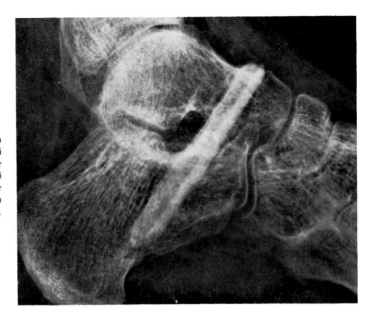

FIGURE 5–49. Batchelor subtalar extra-articular arthrodesis.

Note a fibular bone graft is inserted from the neck of the talus across the sinus tarsi into the calcaneus with the hindpart of the foot held in neutral position. The sinus tarsi is not opened. (From Brown, A.: A simple method of fusion of the subtalar joint in children. J. Bone Joint Surg., *50-B*:370, 1968. Reprinted by permission.)

hole is large enough for the fibular graft. The fibular bone graft of desired length is taken from the junction of the proximal and middle thirds of the fibula. One end of the graft is trimmed to a point and is gently tapped through the hole made in the talus and calcaneus. The position of the graft is double-checked with anteroposterior and lateral radiograms of the foot. Inferiorly, it should be well down into the calcaneus. Its superior surface should be flush with the superior surface of the neck of the talus; any excess bone is resected from the graft (Fig. 5–49). The Steinmann pin is removed, and the tourniquet is released. After complete

hemostasis the wound is closed. An above-knee cast is applied; it is exchanged for a walking cast in two weeks. The total period of cast immobilization is eight weeks. Brown reported the results of the Batchelor extra-articular subtalar arthrodesis in 23 feet in 20 patients (9 of whom had cerebral palsy). Stability with survival of the graft was maintained in 17 patients for at least four years. Fracture of the graft occurred in two patients, both heavy boys 15 years old or over (Fig. 5–50). Brown does not advocate the procedure for patients over the age of 11 or 12 years.[79]

Seymour and Evans presented the results in

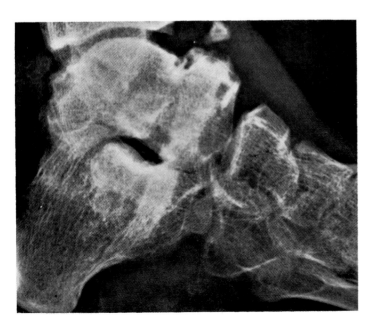

FIGURE 5–50. Fracture of the fibular bone graft in Batchelor extra-articular subtalar arthrodesis.

(From Brown, A.: A simple method of fusion of the subtalar joint in children. J. Bone Joint Surg., *50-B*:370, 1968. Reprinted by permission.)

27 feet in 16 patients (5 had cerebral palsy and 10 had myelomeningocele). Follow-up periods ranged from 9 to 20 months. Avascular necrosis of the talus did not develop in any case. In two of the five cerebral palsy patients the pes valgus persisted. In the myelomeningocele group there were three failures. In one patient, both grafts broke down. Seymour and Evans accord the Batchelor procedure two advantages over the Grice operation. First is the simplicity of insertion and retention of the graft with the Batchelor technique. In the Grice procedure, insertion and retention of the graft in the sinus tarsi may be difficult, necessitating its placement under some compression, which may lead to overcorrection. Second, the fixation of the foot after insertion of the graft is stable and firm, permitting tendon transfers without fear of loss of alignment of the subtalar joint.[490]

Hsu, Yau, O'Brien, and Hodgson studied valgus deformity of the ankle resulting from fibular resection for a graft in Batchelor type subtalar fusion in children, of whom 30 had poliomyelitis and 2 had cerebral palsy. They divided the patients into two groups: Group A, whose grafts were taken from the lower third of the fibula (28 legs in 25 patients), and Group B, whose grafts were taken from the middle third of the fibula (9 legs in 7 patients). In Group A, 20 of the 28 fibulae failed to regenerate fully, and fibular pseudarthrosis resulted; in 16 of these patients there was definite upward migration of the distal epiphysis of the fibula in relation to the tibia. In Group B, eight of the nine legs showed regeneration of the fibula, and seven of these had no valgus inclination of the ankle mortise. When a segment of the fibula is resected from its lower third, the main blood supply of the periosteum is disrupted; hence the bone fails to regenerate to fill the defect. On the other hand, the middle third of the fibula is surrounded by muscle origins and is richly endowed with muscular and periosteal vascular anastomoses, making its regeneration more likely after removal of the fibular segment and interruption of the nutrient arterial blood supply.[244]

Dennyson and Fulford modified the Batchelor operation by using a metal screw instead of a bone peg for internal fixation of the subtalar joint and a cancellous graft instead of cortical bone to obtain osseous union.[134] The experience of this author with the Batchelor technique of subtalar fusion is limited. Problems with fractures of the graft with its potential for causing upward migration of the distal fibular epiphysis and development of a valgus ankle outweigh the "simplicity" of the operation. The Grice operation is, therefore, recommended over the Batchelor technique for extra-articular arthrodesis of the subtalar joints in children. However, the subtalar joint should be fixed internally with a cancellous screw or threaded Steinmann pins.

Calcaneal Osteotomy to Correct Hindfoot Valgus Deformity. Dwyer's open-up lateral wedge osteotomy of the calcaneus with insertion of a tibial bone graft has been used by Silver and Simon for correction of hindfoot valgus deviation. They reported the results in 73 feet in 42 patients (bilateral deformities in 31 and unilateral deformity in 11). In 61 operations, homogenous autoclaved tibial bone was used for the graft; the homogenous bone appeared to be as satisfactory as autogenous bone. The results in 56 feet were good (neutral position of hindfoot); in 7, fair (mild residual valgus deformity); and in 6, poor. In the poor category, there were four feet in which overcorrection produced varus deformity requiring subsequent calcaneal wedge osteotomies; in two feet there was recurrence of marked valgus deformity requiring repeat calcaneal osteotomy with homogenous bone grafts and Achilles tendon lengthening. "In retrospect the Achilles tendon lengthenings should have been done during the first operation." According to Silver, Simon, and Lichtman, the advantage of calcaneal osteotomy is that it improves the weight-bearing alignment of the foot and retains approximately 50 per cent of subtalar motion. The flexibility imparted by the subtalar motion decreases the stress on the midtarsal joints and the foot, making possible better locomotion on uneven terrain.[506]

Dwyer's calcaneal osteotomy creates a compensatory deformity in the calcaneus to mask the primary site of the deformity above, i.e., at the talocalcaneonavicular joint. This author strongly recommends that soft-tissue procedures (tendo Achillis and peroneal lengthening) be performed first, that postoperatively the feet be supported by UCBL foot orthoses, and that a meticulous physical therapy program be carried out to restore function and dynamic balance of muscles controlling the foot and ankle. Then weight-bearing radiograms of the feet are carefully studied; if the anteroposterior talocalcaneal angle is markedly divergent (i.e., greater than 25 degrees) and the *talus is plantar-flexed*, Dwyer's calcaneal osteotomy should not be performed. The site of deformity is the subtalar joint, and it should be stabilized by Grice subtalar extra-articular arthrodesis.

Horizontal osteotomy through the base of the posterior articular process of the calcaneus with lateral wedge grafts was used by Baker to correct hindfoot valgus deviation (Fig. 5–51). It provides normal contact between the talar and calcaneal articular surfaces, restores normal talocalcaneal alignment, and places the sustentaculum tali under the talus to provide support for the talus. The hindfoot pronation is corrected without interfering with subtalar motion. It does not create a bone block. The results in 31 feet treated by this osteotomy with an average follow-up observation of two years were as follows: In 21 feet the alignment was satisfactory, in 8 feet there was persistent mild valgus deformity, and in 2 feet there was moderate varus deformity.[14]

The operation is performed through a 5- to 7-cm. longitudinal incision over the sinus tarsi. The subcutaneous tissues are divided in line with the skin incision. The contents of the sinus tarsi are not cleaned out. The peroneal tendons and fibular collateral ligaments are identified and retracted posteriorly with a blunt dissector, thereby providing adequate exposure. The calcaneus is stabilized by firmly holding it during the osteotomy. The line and depth of osteotomy is determined by lateral radiograms of the foot with two Kirschner wires inserted parallel to the posterior talocalcaneal joint. With a sharp, thin osteotome or oscillating saw, an osteotomy through the base of the posterior articular process of the calcaneus is performed through the *horizontal plane*. Do not enter the subtalar joint! The osteotomy extends to, but not through, the medial cortex, which should be preserved as a hinge. Next, osteotomes of different widths (1 to 2 cm.) are inserted into the osteotomy site to determine the width of the bone graft. Anteroposterior radiograms of the foot are made with the osteotome in place to check the restoration of normal alignment between the talus and calcaneus. The anteroposterior talocalcaneal angle should be 15 degrees. Autogenous bone wedges of correct width are then taken from the ilium and inserted into the osteotomy site. The wedges are based laterally. The osteotomized segments are fixed internally with a threaded Steinmann pin. Overcorrection should be avoided. The dorsoplantar radiogram of the foot is repeated, and the anteroposterior talocalcaneal angle is measured; it should be 15 degrees. The wounds are closed, and an above-knee cast is applied. The Steinmann pin is removed at six weeks, and the total period of immobilization is two months. This author recommends medial displacement osteotomy of the

os calcis instead of Baker's horizontal osteotomy; it is as effective and is simpler, and bone grafting is not required.

Triple arthrodesis is indicated to relieve symptoms and to correct the deformity of severe valgus deviation in the skeletally mature foot that is painful, fixed by osseous deformation, and causing serious problems in shoe wear and fitting.

Pes Calcaneus. Overlengthening of the tendo Achillis will result in calcaneus deformity of the foot and ankle (Fig. 5–52). Another cause is lengthening of a triceps surae muscle whose motor strength is fair or less. When the hips and knees have significant flexion deformity, the feet are forced into dorsiflexion, and calcaneus deformity will develop. With weakness of the triceps surae the fibula will fail to develop and will be short in relation to the tibia; the lateral malleolus will be elevated, and the ankle mortise will assume a valgus tilt. Functionally, calcaneus deformity of the ankle is more disabling than equinus deformity.

Pes calcaneus can be prevented if certain basic dicta are followed: (1) Correct hip flexion deformity first, and then at a later stage lengthen the Achilles tendon; (2) lengthen the triceps surae *only* when its motor strength is normal or good; (3) do not overlengthen the tendo Achillis; and (4) provide meticulous postoperative care as outlined in the section on Achilles tendon lengthening.

Initially, treatment of calcaneus deformity is conservative: splinting at night with the ankles in plantar flexion, passive and active exercises to elongate shortened weak plantar flexors, and protection of the ankles with orthoses that prevent dorsiflexion beyond neutral position. The knees should be supported so that they do not flex in stance and gait. The hip flexors should be elongated by passive exercises. The gluteus maximus should be strengthened by active exercises and pelvic tilt. Sleeping prone is of great help.

Surgical correction is indicated in the severe, persistent case. The author recommends splitting the tendo Achillis and suturing the lateral half or two thirds of it to the distal fibular metaphysis. Additional Mersilene strips are used to reinforce the tenodesis. Fixed bony deformity is corrected by posterosuperior displacement osteotomy of the os calcis.

Deformities of the Forefoot and Toes. Metatarsus varus may be congenital, postural, or spastic in type. The congenital type is treated by manipulation and cast, whereas the postural type will correct itself spontaneously or respond

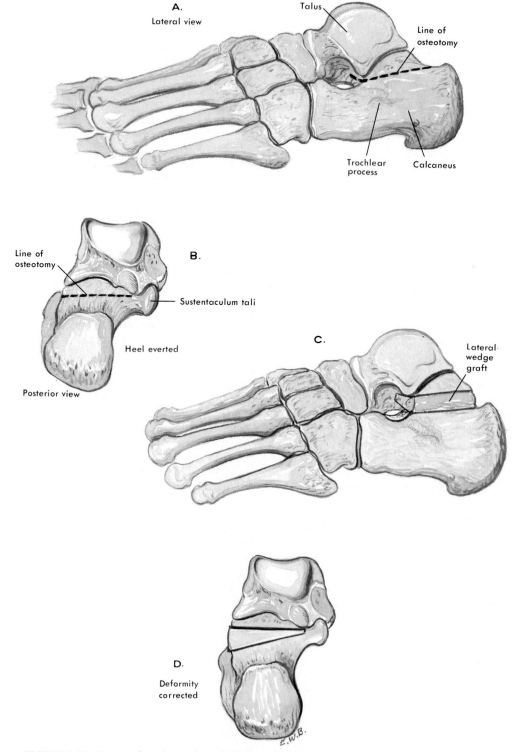

FIGURE 5–51. *Horizontal osteotomy through the base of the posterior articular process of the calcaneus with lateral wedge graft (Baker procedure).*

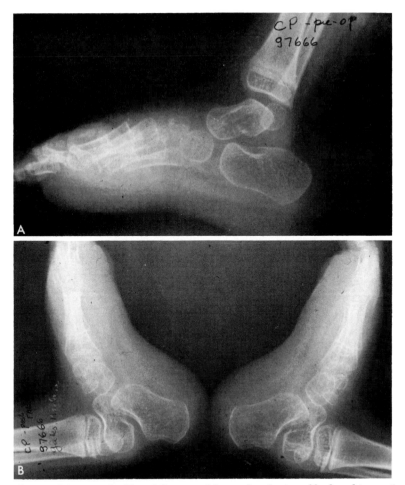

FIGURE 5–52. *Calcaneus deformity of ankle and foot caused by overlengthening of heel cord in spastic cerebral palsy.*

A. Preoperative lateral radiogram. **B.** Lateral radiogram of the ankles and feet two years after excessive heel cord lengthening.

to passive manipulation alone. The spastic metatarsus varus is usually associated with hallux varus and is caused by hyperactivity of the abductor hallucis. It is treated conservatively by manipulation and splinting; if conservative measures fail, the abductor hallucis is lengthened fractionally at its musculotendinous junction. When the hallux is in normal position or slightly valgus, it is best to release the abductor hallucis muscle at its origin.

Hallux valgus is caused by spasticity and contracture of the adductor hallucis. This is treated by sectioning of the adductor hallucis tendon near its insertion on the lateral side of the base of the proximal phalanx of the great toe. If it is associated with significant metatarsus primus varus, osteotomy of the base of the first metatarsal may be indicated.

Hammer or mallet toe in spastic cerebral palsy is usually caused by hyperactivity of the

long or short toe flexors, or both. If it does not respond to passive elongation exercises, proper shoes, and metatarsal support, it is treated by fractional lengthening of the long toe flexors in the distal part of the leg or sectioning of the short toe flexors. Severe fixed hammer toes require transfer of the long toe extensors to the metatarsal necks and fusion of the proximal interphalangeal joints. Neurectomy of the motor branches of the plantar nerves to intrinsic muscles of the foot is not recommended.

The Knee

The knee joint should not be regarded as an isolated problem in cerebral palsy, since it is affected by deformities of the hip or ankle. The mechanism of the knee joint is complex because of the pressure of "two-joint" muscles, i.e., the hamstrings, which extend the hip and flex the knee; the gastrocnemius, which plantar flexes the ankle and flexes the knee; and the quadriceps (direct head of rectus femoris), which extends the knee and flexes the hip.

Disabilities of the knee encountered in spastic paralysis are (1) flexion deformity, which may be fixed or functional; (2) extensor contracture due to spasticity of the quadriceps; (3) genu recurvatum; and (4) loss of complete active extension of the knee due to elongation of the patellar tendon.

FLEXION DEFORMITY

Flexion deformity is frequently present. It is imperative that one determine whether flexion deformity of the knee is *primary*, caused by spasticity and contracture of the hamstrings; *secondary*, to compensate for equinus deformity of the ankle and flexion deformity of the hip; or *functional*, to lower the center of gravity to achieve balance such as seen in triceps surae motor weakness following excessive heel cord lengthening.

Assessment. One should carefully study the active and passive range of motion of the hip, knee, ankle, and foot, determining at which point the spastic muscles grab. The conventional method of testing spasticity and contracture of the hamstrings is by straight-leg raising: The patient's leg with the knee in *complete extension* is passively raised from the examining table with one hand, while the examiner's other hand steadies the pelvis and keeps it flat on the table. When the pelvis begins to tilt, the angle between the lower limbs and examination table is measured and recorded (Fig. 5–53). This method of testing hamstring tautness is accurate if the knee can be fully extended. In the pres-

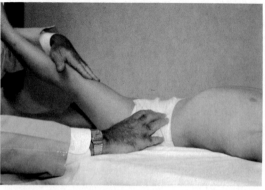

FIGURE 5–53. Method of determining hamstring tautness by straight leg raising.

The knee should be in complete extension and the pelvis should be stabilized. The angle between the lower limb and the examination table is measured.

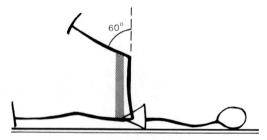

FIGURE 5–54. Holt's method of determining hamstring contracture.

The contralateral hip is in extension, the tested limb is flexed to 90 degrees at the hip, and the knee is extended passively. The angle between the anterior aspect of the leg and thigh determines the degree of hamstring contracture. Bleck measures the angle on the popliteal surface between the leg and thigh.

ence of knee flexion contracture, this author recommends the method described by Holt; the hip of the tested lower limb is flexed 90 degrees, and then the knee is extended passively.[236] The degree of loss of complete knee extension is noted. In the Holt method the angular deficit between the anterior aspects of the leg and thigh is measured (Fig. 5–54).

An alternative way is to measure the popliteal angle between the posterior aspects of the leg and thigh.[56] The degree of fixed flexion deformity of the knee is determined by passive extension of the knee with the hip *in extension* (not flexion).

The location of the patella should be determined: Is it riding high owing to elongation of the patellar tendon? Are the patellar retinacula contracted? Is there quadriceps lag? What is the degree of fixed flexion deformity of the knee? One should perform a complete muscle test in order to assess any imbalance between flexors and extensors of the knee. Stance and gait must be analyzed.

The ability of the patient to extend the knee fully in stance is noted. Does the knee assume increasing flexion attitude during walking? In the swing phase of gait the distance between the origin of the hamstrings from the ischial tuberosity and their insertion into the tibia becomes greater; as a result, when the lower limb is swung foward, the pelvis rotates simultaneously. The stride is short (Fig. 5–55).

The sitting posture is compromised in hamstring tautness; because the hamstrings are hip extensors, they restrict the degree of hip flexion. The patient will have difficulty sitting on the floor with the knees in extension; he has to flex his knees to diminish the pull of the hamstrings on the ischium and pelvis. In moderate hamstring contracture, when the patient sits, his lumbar spine assumes a kyphotic posture.

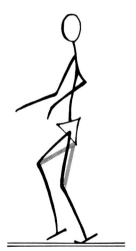

FIGURE 5–55. *Pathologic gait as a result of hamstring contracture.*

The knee is in flexion, the foot is in equinus posture, and the length of the stride is short. (Redrawn after Reimers, J.: Contracture of the hamstrings in spastic cerebral palsy. J. Bone Joint Surg., 56B:102, 1974.)

In severe hamstring contracture the patient tends to slide down the chair and has to be strapped down with the knees in flexion (Fig. 5–56).

Dynamic electromyography of the hamstring muscles in gait will disclose prolonged and out-of-phase contractions throughout most of the stance phase. The abnormal hamstring activity is often associated with prolonged and out-of-phase action potentials of the quadriceps femoris muscle. Energy requirements of gait are increased with flexion deformity of the knee.

Radiograms of the knee are taken to detect the presence of any structural bony changes in the proximal end of the tibia and the distal end

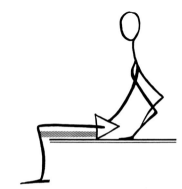

FIGURE 5–56. *Effect of hamstring contracture on sitting posture.*

Note the resultant lumbar kyphosis. (Redrawn after Reimers, J.: Contracture of the hamstrings in spastic cerebral palsy. J. Bone Joint Surg., 56B:102, 1974.)

of the femur, and the position of the patella. In moderate or severe flexion deformity of the knee the patella will be riding high.

Treatment. Conservative measures in the treatment of flexion contracture of the knee consist of prone posturing with the hips and knees in extension, gentle passive manual elongation of the hamstrings to prevent permanent shortening, active exercises to increase the motor strength of the quadriceps, and the use of a bivalved night cast or plastic orthosis that holds the knee in extension and the ankle at neutral position. Crawling should not be allowed, and other modalities of locomotion should be available, such as motorized wheelchairs. These nonoperative measures can often prevent the development of fixed flexion deformity of the knee. They should always be carried out prior to surgical intervention.

Surgical procedures about the knee should be performed with great caution. Hamstring lengthening is *contraindicated* in the presence of *hip flexion* and *equinus deformity*. One third of the hip extensor torque is provided by the hamstrings.[581] *Hip flexion deformity* due to spasticity and contracture of the iliopsoas inhibits function of the gluteus maximus. Length ening of hamstrings, particularly proximally, further weakens hip extensor strength. Consequently, hip flexion deformity develops, which progressively increases by the unbalanced action of the spastic, taut iliopsoas. The hamstrings provide posterior stability to the pelvis. Weakening of this posterior pelvic support by proximal hamstring release will tilt the pelvis forward and result in excessive low lumbar lordosis and dorsolumbar kyphosis. The lordosis is aggravated by the hip flexion deformity. The functional disability may be quite marked, with loss of ability of the patient to walk without crutches. *Genu recurvatum* is a disturbing deformity that may follow hamstring lengthening. This is often caused by *equinus deformity* due to a taut soleus muscle; the gait is toe-heel, and at heel strike the proximal end of the tibia is pulled posteriorly by the shortened soleus. Another cause of genu recurvatum is the weakening of the motor strength of the lengthened hamstrings. The motor strength of the hamstrings may be adequate for knee flexion during the swing-through phase of gait but not strong enough to maintain muscle balance during stance and to prevent genu recurvatum.[142] The combination of excessive lumbar lordosis and genu recurvatum is very disabling functionally. Therefore, it is evident that hamstrings should not be lengthened in the presence of equinus

Text continued on page 1712

Fractional Lengthening of Hamstrings

OPERATIVE TECHNIQUE

A. The patient is placed in prone position with a pneumatic tourniquet high on the proximal thigh. A 3 to 4 inch-long midline incision is made, starting just proximal to the popliteal crease. The subcutaneous tissue is divided and the incision carried to the deep fascia. The posterior femoral cutaneous nerve will be in the proximal aspect of the wound and should not be damaged.

B. The deep fascia is incised and the hamstring tendons are identified by blunt dissection. It is imperative to divide the tendon sheath of each hamstring tendon separately and mark it with 000 silk sutures for meticulous closure later.

C. In the lateral compartment of the wound, the biceps femoris tendon is exposed. It should be gently dissected away from the common peroneal nerve, which lies on its posteromedial surface. A blunt instrument, such as a staphylorrhaphy probe or a joker, is passed deep to the biceps tendon.

D. With a sharp knife, the tendinous portion of the biceps femoris is incised transversely at two levels, 3 cm. apart, leaving the muscle fibers intact. The tendon is lengthened in continuity by straight leg raising with the knee in extension.

Plate 66. Fractional Lengthening of Hamstrings

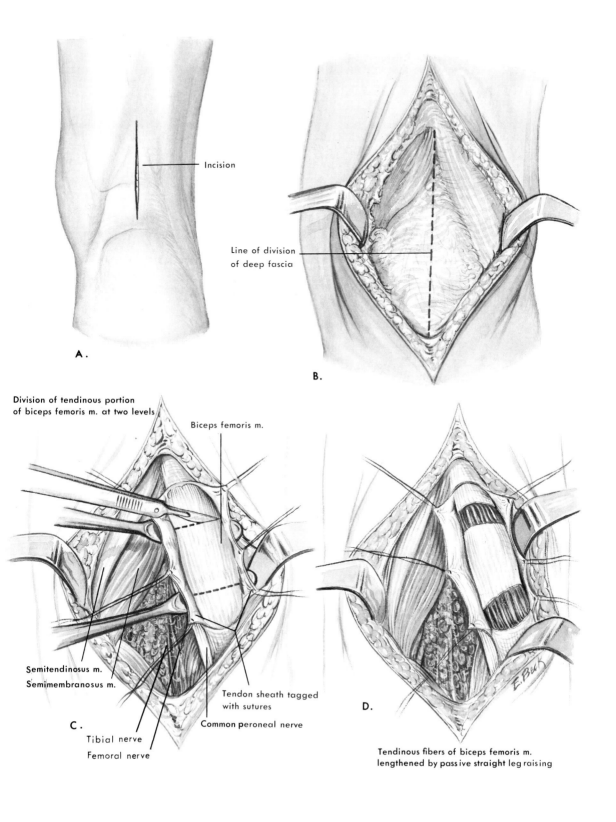

A.

Incision

B.

Line of division
of deep fascia

C.

Division of tendinous portion
of biceps femoris m. at two levels

Biceps femoris m.

Semitendinosus m.
Semimembranosus m.

Tibial nerve

Femoral nerve

Tendon sheath tagged
with sutures

Common peroneal nerve

D.

Tendinous fibers of biceps femoris m.
lengthened by passive straight leg raising

Fractional Lengthening of Hamstrings (Continued)

E. The semimembranosus tendon is then isolated in the medial compartment of the wound. The tendinous portion lies on its deep surface; to expose it the muscle is everted. The tendinous fibers are divided at two levels (similar to the biceps tendon), leaving the muscle fibers in continuity. Again, by extending the knee and flexing the hip, a sliding lengthening of the semimembranosus is performed.

F. Next, the semitendinosus is exposed. The tendinous portion is divided proximal to the musculotendinous junction.

G. If inadvertently the semitendinosus tendon ruptures, a Z-plasty is performed.

H. The tendon sheath of each tendon is meticulously closed. The deep fascia is not sutured. The subcutaneous tissue and skin are closed in routine manner and bilateral long leg casts are applied with the knees in full extension.

POSTOPERATIVE CARE

While the patient is in the solid cast, straight leg raising exercises are performed 15 times, once a day, for further stretching of the hamstrings. At the end of three to four weeks the casts are removed and new above-knee bivalved casts are made. Active and passive exercises are performed to develop knee flexion, first side-lying with gravity eliminated and then against gravity. The motor strength of the quadriceps is developed. Whenever functional range of motion of the knees is present, the patient is allowed to be ambulatory with appropriate support.

Plate 66. Fractional Lengthening of Hamstrings

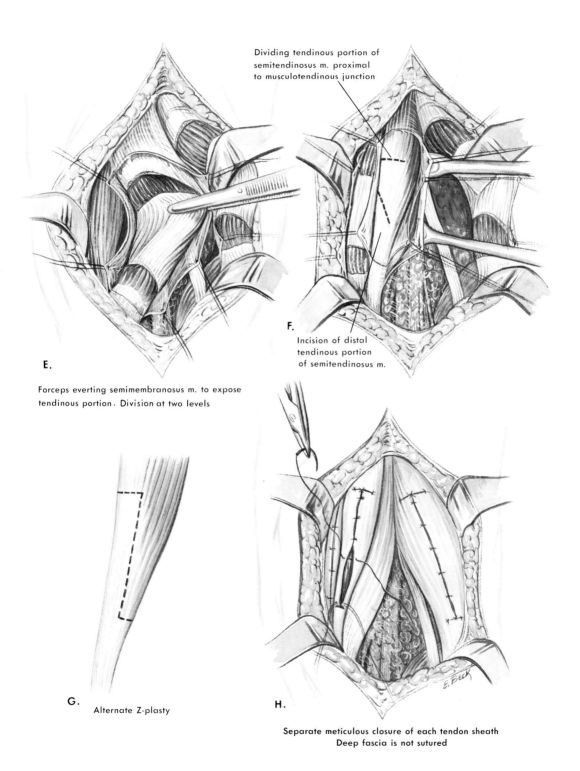

Dividing tendinous portion of
semitendinosus m. proximal
to musculotendinous junction

F.

Incision of distal
tendinous portion
of semitendinosus m.

E.

Forceps everting semimembranosus m. to expose
tendinous portion. Division at two levels

G. Alternate Z-plasty

H.

Separate meticulous closure of each tendon sheath
Deep fascia is not sutured

and hip flexion deformity. These deformities should be corrected first.

This author strongly recommends not performing multilevel surgery, i.e., lengthening the hamstrings simultaneously with hip flexor lengthening and adductor myotomy and heel cord lengthening. This is discouraged because only one tenth, if not less, of the patients will require fractional lengthening of the hamstrings at a later date. Furthermore, after multilevel surgery, postoperative training is made very difficult. As a rule, hip adductor myotomy and iliopsoas lengthening is performed first; at this time the gracilis is routinely lengthened. In the postoperative period the hamstrings are passively elongated by exercises, splinting, and prone posturing. Next, equinus deformity is corrected. If, at 6 to 12 months following a thorough trial period of conservative treatment, the child still walks with the knees flexed with a crouched posture and the hamstrings grab at 20 to 30 degrees on straight leg raising, or a flexion deformity of the knee persists, surgical lengthening of the hamstrings is indicated.

In the literature, three methods of surgical correction of hamstring spasticity and contracture are described: (1) distal hamstring lengthening,[196] (2) transfer of the hamstrings to the femoral condyles (Eggers' procedure),[150] and (3) proximal hamstring release at their origins.[491]

This author recommends a distal hamstring fractional lengthening as described by Green.[196] The biceps femoris, the semimembranosus, and the semitendinosus are all lengthened. The operative procedure is presented in Plate 66. Lengthening of the hamstrings preserves some degree of their motor function, thereby providing antagonist muscle balance against the quadriceps femoris. Transfer of the hamstrings to the femoral condyles or total release of the hamstrings proximally at their origin takes away the antagonistic action of the hamstrings against the quadriceps. Knee extension contracture because of imbalanced overactivity of the quadriceps may develop postoperatively. It is essential to maintain knee flexion against gravity. Reciprocal hip and knee flexion and dorsiflexion of the ankle are essential for a normal gait pattern. Distal fractional lengthening of the hamstrings is technically much simpler than transfer of hamstrings to the femoral condyles and proximal release of hamstrings; the risk of inadvertent injury to sciatic nerve is much less. In contrast to proximal hamstring release, the incision in distal hamstring lengthening is away from the perineum and affords less chance of infection; the procedure can be performed un-

der tourniquet ischemia, minimizing blood loss and postoperative hematoma. Distal lengthening corrects flexion deformity of the knee much more effectively than does proximal release, and it does not diminish the posterior stabilizing dynamic force provided by the hamstrings near their origin.

Eggers' transfer of the hamstring tendons to the femoral condyles is not recommended by this author (Fig. 5–57).[150] In a certain percentage of cases, the Eggers hamstring transfer will cause varying degrees of genu recurvatum, decreased posterior pelvic support, increase in lumbar lordosis, and weakening or loss of active knee flexion power.

Because of these problems, various authors have modified the original Eggers procedure. Pollock and English, for example, preserve at least one hamstring, either the semitendinosus

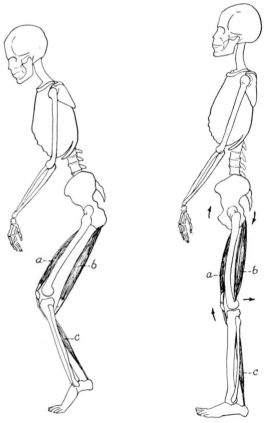

FIGURE 5–57. *Egger's transfer of hamstrings to femoral condyles.*

a. Quadriceps femoris muscle; *b.* hamstring muscles; *c.* soleus muscle. (From Eggers, G. N. M.: Transplantation of hamstring tendons to femoral condyles in order to improve hip extension and to decrease knee flexion in cerebral spastic paralysis. J. Bone Joint Surg., *34-A*:827, 1952. Reprinted by permission.)

or the semimembranosus.[423, 424] Keats and Kambin perform a Z-lengthening of the biceps femoris and transfer the medial hamstring to the femoral condyle.[286] Evans tenotomizes the gracilis, lengthens the biceps femoris and semimembranosus in their aponeurotic portion, and transfers only the semitendinosus to the ipsilateral femoral condyle.[156]

Mortens performs the same modification as Evans.[359] Masse and Audie, in assessing their results of hamstring transplantation to the femoral condyles, did not find any improvement in the strength or degree of active hip extension.[342]

Proximal Release of Hamstrings. Release of hamstrings from their origin on the ischial tuberosity was originally described by Seymour and Sharrard.[491] Subsequently, several other authors have reported the results of proximal hamstring release with modifications of operative technique and surgical approach.[38, 142, 436, 492]

Seymour and Sharrard and Drummond et al. performed the operation with the patient in prone position. Originally, Seymour and Sharrard described a vertical incision but later, because of the keloid formation, preferred a transverse incision. A 5- to 7-cm. transverse incision is made in the gluteal crease centered over the ischial tuberosity. Subcutaneous tissue and deep fascia are incised in line with the skin incision. With blunt and sharp dissection of deep fibrous septa the lower border of gluteus maximus is identified and retracted laterally and upward. Caution! Do not injure the posterior femoral cutaneous nerve. The sciatic nerve is identified and gently retracted laterally. The hamstrings are exposed by blunt dissection. They have a common tendon of origin. Flex the knee to relax the hamstrings and insert a blunt elevator-retractor deep to the tendons. The long heads of the biceps femoris and semitendinosus are superficial, and the semimembranosus is deep. The short head of biceps does not originate from the ischial tuberosity. With a nerve stimulator, ensure that the sciatic nerve is not mistaken for the semimembranosus.

Initially all the hamstrings were released by a transverse division using an electrocautery knife. Later, Drummond et al. performed a more limited recession, dividing the superficial biceps and semitendinosus, but leaving the deep semimembranosus intact.[142] Often, it is difficult to differentiate these muscles proximally because of their common origins. Later, Sharrard recommended an oblique incision from above downward and medially. The distal segments are resutured in an oblique position; they should not be allowed to retract freely without reattachment. Sharrard warned that

complete division without resuturing weakens the hamstrings excessively, with consequent serious functional complications of disabling genu recurvatum and lumbar hyperlordosis.[499]

The wound is closed after careful hemostasis. An above-knee cast is applied for a period of four to six weeks. The patient is allowed to walk when able to do so.

Sharps, Clancy, and Steel performed proximal hamstring release with the patient supine in lithotomy position with the hips and knees flexed 90 degrees.[492] The gluteus maximus tendon was identified and retracted laterally. The origin of hamstrings was exposed at the ischial tuberosity and released *extraperiosteally* by electrocautery. The sciatic nerve was identified with a nerve stimulator in some cases, whereas in others the nerve was protected by a retractor without actual visualization. An assistant held the hip flexed 90 degrees and gradually extended the knee during the sectioning of the hamstrings. The release was continued until the knee extended 5 degrees minus full extension with the hip flexed 90 degrees; often the total origin of the hamstrings was released. The hamstring release was *dynamic*. Sectioning continued until complete correction was obtained. The postoperative care of Sharps et al. differs from that of Drummond et al. Above-knee casts are applied with the knee in maximal extension for a period of six weeks; during this postoperative period if the knee could not extend fully at surgery, the flexion contracture was corrected by serial wedging casts. Following removal of the cast the patient was fitted in knee-ankle-foot orthosis for six months.

Bell developed an anterior approach to release the hamstrings proximally. The procedure is performed with the patient supine; this posture allows straight-leg raising, making determination of adequacy of lengthening simple. With the patient prone, straight-leg raising is difficult. The anteromedial approach allows proximal hamstring release to be combined with adductor myotomy and iliopsoas lengthening. A 5- to 7-cm. transverse incision is made in the upper adductor region of the thigh, in line with the inguinal crease, beginning 1 cm. anterior to the adductor longus tendon and extending posteriorly to the ischial tuberosity. The gracilis muscle is identified and sectioned with electrocautery. The plane between the hip adductors and medial hamstring is developed by blunt dissection. The sciatic nerve is identified; use electrical stimulation if necessary. The sciatic nerve should not be mistaken for the semimembranosus (which is tendinous proximally). With the use of electrocautery all the hamstrings are sectioned near their origins. Straight-leg raising is tested to ensure adequacy of correction. The wound is closed after hemostasis. Bell utilizes a removable splint, permitting walking several days postoperatively as soon as the patient is comfortable and is able to do so.[38]

There is controversy in the literature as to whether hamstring lengthening should be performed proximally or distally. Drummond et al. presented the results of total proximal release of the hamstrings in 25 patients (50 knees). In most instances the crouch posture was corrected, the gait was improved, and longer strides were possible. However, in seven patients (14 knees) genu recurvatum of 20 to 30 degrees developed; five of these patients did not have equinus deformity, whereas two patients did. In four patients a new disabling deformity of excessive lumbar lordosis developed, which was functionally disabling. One patient developed temporary sciatic nerve palsy; another, wound infection. Drummond et al. recommended that total proximal hamstring release no longer be performed. Sharps et al. retrospectively analyzed the results of proximal hamstrings in 32 patients (64 knees).[142] The average follow-up was nine years and five months. Straight-leg raising increased from 30 to 68 degrees, and knee flexion contracture decreased from 16 to 9 degrees. At follow-up only 4 of the 64 knees had mild (5 to 10 degrees) genu recurvatum, and the lumbar lordosis averaged 53 degrees. With their variation of postoperative care, i.e., supporting the knees in above-knee orthosis for a period of six weeks, devastating genu recurvatum and lumbar hyperlordosis were prevented.[492]

Reimers reported a prospective study of 112 operative procedures to correct hamstring contracture in 60 patients. Three different surgical techniques were utilized: (1) modified Eggers operation, (2) distal elongation of the hamstrings, and (3) proximal release of the hamstrings. He corrected flexion deformity of the hip and equinus of the ankle prior to hamstring release or lengthening. In the 27 patients treated by proximal hamstring release there was no genu recurvatum. Reimers recommends proximal hamstring release if the knee flexion contracture is less than 5 degrees, and distal elongation of the hamstrings if the knee flexion contracture exceeds 5 degrees.[436]

This author does not recommend proximal release of hamstrings in ambulatory patients. The potential of postoperative functionally disabling deformities of excessive lumbar lordosis and genu recurvatum dictates that the operation

not be performed in walkers. The only possible indication for proximal hamstring release is in nonambulators who are having difficulty sitting in a wheelchair; the extensor torque of the hamstrings restricts hip flexion, and the patient slides off the chair. In these patients the proximal hamstring release is performed through the anteromedial approach, as described by Bell, if the procedure is combined with adductor myotomy, which is often indicated. If adductor myotomy–flexion release is not indicated, the operation can be performed with the patient supine in the lithotomy position—somewhat cumbersome but allowing straight-leg raising to test the adequacy of hamstring lengthening.

It should be remembered that Sharrard's indication for proximal hamstring release is the spastic child with marked hamstring tautness (straight-leg raising 30 degrees or less) with a strong quadriceps femoris. The deforming effect of hamstrings is exerted at the hip: The child is unable to sit with the knees extended, sits with difficulty with the knees flexed and the pelvis rotated excessively.

EXTENSION CONTRACTURE OF THE KNEE

This is caused by spasticity of the quadriceps femoris muscle. The child walks with a stiff extended knee with loss of normal reciprocal hip and knee flexion. When the patient is seated with the knees over the edge of the table, the knees will not flex fully. In prone position with the hips in extension, the quadriceps muscle grabs on passive flexion of the knee. Upon further passive flexion of the knee, the pelvis will be elevated off the table because of the pelvic origin of the direct head of the rectus femoris (positive Ely test) (Fig. 5–58).

Treatment consists of passive stretching exercises of the spastic rectus femoris and active exercises to develop simultaneous knee and hip flexion in gait with dorsiflexion of the ankle. On occasion, the direct portion of the rectus femoris has to be released. This is particularly indicated when the extension contracture of the knee is moderate and is associated with flexion contracture of the hip. The operative technique is as follows:

A 3- to 5-cm. longitudinal incision is made directly over the origin of the rectus femoris. Subcutaneous tissue and deep fascia are divided. The medial and lateral borders of the rectus femoris are identified and, with a blunt instrument, dissected free of adjacent tissues. A curved Kocher hemostat is inserted under

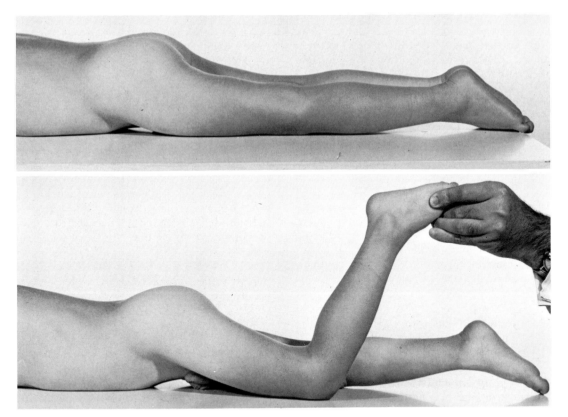

FIGURE 5–58. Positive Ely test.

In prone position, the quadriceps muscle will grab on passive flexion of the knee with the hips in extension. Upon further passive flexion of the knee, the pelvis will be elevated off the table because of the pelvic origin of the direct head of the rectus femoris muscle.

the origin of the rectus femoris, and the muscle is sharply divided. The wound is closed in the usual manner.

Postoperatively, the lower limbs are immobilized with the knees in 60 to 90 degrees of flexion for a period of two or three weeks. Active and passive exercises are performed to develop balance of motor strength between the extensors and flexors of the knee and reciprocal knee-hip flexion in gait. To maintain the lengthened position of the rectus femoris, the patient sleeps in a bivalved night cast or splint for several months with the hips in extension and the knees in 20 to 30 degrees of flexion.

Release of the rectus femoris is performed distally. When the extension contracture of the knee is severe, the patient walks with a stiff-knee gait, and there is no associated rotational malalignment in gait (in-toeing and out-toeing).

The operative technique of distal femoral recession is as follows: A 4-cm. long transverse incision centered 1 cm. above the superior pole of the patella is made. The wound edges are undermined, and the fascia is incised longitudinally. The insertion of the rectus femoris tendon to the patella is identified and sharply divided. The knee is flexed and the margins of the rectus femoris tendon are divided and released from the adjacent vastus medialis and vastus lateralis muscle fibers. The knee is acutely flexed so that the rectus tendon slides proximally for a distance of 2.5 cm. The recessed rectus tendon is sutured to the adjoining vastus muscles by several sutures. The wounds are closed in layers in the usual fashion. A knee immobilizer is applied for support, with the knee in extension for three to four weeks. The patient is allowed to ambulate and bear weight fully as soon as comfortable, several days postoperatively. Physical therapy in the form of knee flexion-extension exercises and gait training is performed several times a day.

Transfer of Distal Insertion of Rectus Femoris Tendon. When there is cospasticity and contracture of both quadriceps femoris and hamstring muscles, the gait will be "stiff-knee" (or "stiff-legged"). This may occur primarily or secondarily after hamstring lengthening. Perry proposed that inadequate initial knee flexion in gait in spasticity may be due to inadequate function of the sartorius, gracilis, and short head of biceps femoris; therefore, Gage et al. transferred the distal tendon of rectus femoris to the sartorius, with the result of improved knee flexion in swing phase of gait.[178b] Transfer of the rectus femoris tendon to sartorius did not change the foot progression angle to lateral rotation. It seems that the problem was inadequacy of anchoring the rectus femoris tendon to the soft, pliable sartorius muscle fibers; the rectus femoris tendon transfer functioned more as a distal rectus femoris release. By transferring the rectus femoris tendon to semitendinosus-semimembranosus or to the biceps tendon, rotational malalignment in gait can be corrected.

Indications for rectus femoris tendon transfer are: (1) stiff-knee gait with cospasticity of the quadriceps femoris and hamstring muscles; (2) 0 to 15 degrees of knee flexion on swing phase (short stride length); (3) prolonged and out-of-phase abnormal potentials of both quadriceps and hamstring muscles on dynamic gait electromyography; (4) good or normal motor strength of quadriceps femoris muscle; and (5) in-toeing or out-toeing gait.

When the stiff-knee gait is accompanied by lateral foot progression angle (out-toeing gait), the rectus femoris is transferred to the medial hamstring; when the foot progression angle is medial (in-toeing gait), it is transferred to the biceps femoris tendon.

The operative technique of distal rectus femoris transfer is as follows: A midline longitudinal incision is made over the lower thigh, beginning at the superior pole of the patella and extending proximally for a distance of 5 to 7 cm. The subcutaneous tissue and fasciae are divided in line with the skin incision. The wound edges are undermined. The rectus femoris tendon is identified and divided at its insertion to the patella. Longitudinal incisions are made over the medial and lateral borders of the rectus tendon. Then the tendon is dissected free from the underlying vastus intermedius and adjoining vastus medialis and lateralis muscles. The rectus tendon is mobilized and elevated proximally. The vastus lateralis and vastus medialis are sutured together. The rectus tendon is transferred subcutaneously and sutured either to the medial hamstrings or to biceps femoris tendon. The postoperative immobilization and physical therapy program is similar to that for distal release of rectus femoris.

The problem of distal release of rectus femoris or rectus femoris transfer is balancing forces between quadriceps femoris and hamstrings. There should be adequate quadriceps femoris motor strength to extend the knee fully against gravity and to maintain the knee extended at initial and midstance phases of gait; also, the quadriceps should be weak enough and the hamstrings strong enough to flex the knee in initial swing of 35 degrees and complete swing of 60 to 70 degrees. In the experience of this author, it is difficult to achieve such a "balancing act"; sometimes the quadriceps is weakened more than ideally, with the result of lack of full extension of the knee against gravity. Meticulous postoperative care is crucial for success.

Subtalar Extra-Articular Stabilization with Staples Without Arthrodesis. Crawford and associates performed this procedure in the young child (mean age three years) with spastic pes valgus and oblique or vertical talus that is flexible and can be fully corrected by plantar flexion and inversion of the foot-ankle.

The normal anatomic relationship of the subtalar joint was maintained by one or two laterally placed staples in the bodies of the talus and calcaneus. Originally, Crawford proposed this method of subtalar stabilization as a temporary procedure until the child is old enough (over six years of age) to have permanent subtalar extra-articular arthrodesis. However, the preliminary results in 28 feet with a follow-up of 3.5 years were good in 20, fair in 6, and poor in 2. Staple extrusion was not a problem after a mean follow-up of 3.5 years with most of the children over six years of age.

This author has had no personal experience with Crawford's staple stabilization of subtalar joint. Bone resorption around the staple prongs does occur, and arthrofibrosis because of cartilage degeneration due to immobilization is a definite problem. I recommend nonsurgical treatment in the young child with UCBL or supramalleolar foot orthosis. When flexible vertical talus cannot be corrected by orthotic devices, heel cord lengthening should be performed. If vertical talus persists despite correction of equinus deformity, soft-tissue repair (as described in the section on congenital convex pes valgus) should be considered. Stapling is a simpler procedure; however, will it provide permanent correction?

GENU RECURVATUM

In cerebral palsy, this is usually caused by spasticity of the quadriceps muscle or equinus deformity due to contracture of the triceps surae in the presence of weak hamstrings. Genu recurvatum is a definite complication of proximal hamstring release; however, it can be caused by distal hamstring lengthening if there is equinus deformity. It may also be produced by Eggers transfer of the hamstrings to the femoral condyles or recession of the heads of the gastrocnemius. Growth arrest of the anterior part of the proximal tibial apophysis by performing distal transplantation of the proximal tibial tubercle is another bony cause.

Treatment. Genu recurvatum is a very difficult problem to treat. Equinus deformity, if present, should be corrected by heel cord lengthening, followed by an aggressive regimen of physical therapy to develop simultaneous knee flexion with dorsiflexion of the ankle. An effective way to manage genu recurvatum is by use of a fixed ankle-foot orthosis with the ankle dorsiflexed.[460] If the patient is uncooperative, use of an above-knee orthosis may be indicated to prevent hyperextension of the knee. In the adolescent with marked genu recurvatum, flexion osteotomy of the proximal tibia and fibula or of the distal femur may be indicated (see section on poliomyelitis).

ELONGATED PATELLAR TENDON AND QUADRICEPS FEMORIS INSUFFICIENCY

When the patellar tendon is elongated and the patella is high-riding, there will be loss of full active extension of the knee joint. In such a case, the patellar tendon may be plicated or transferred distally to correct the deformity. However, it is imperative that knee flexion deformity and contracture of the hamstrings be corrected prior to advancing the patella distally. If, following fractional lengthening of the hamstrings, the patient is still unable to completely extend the knee and there is still quadriceps insufficiency that causes him to stumble or fall, a Chandler patellar advancement operation is indicated. This operative technique is described in Plate 67.

The Upper Limb

In spastic paralysis, the upper limb is usually characterized by the following deformities: thumb-in-palm, flexion of the fingers and wrist, pronation of the forearm, flexion of the elbow, and adduction and medial rotation of the shoulder.

The primary purpose of treatment of the upper limb in cerebral palsy is to improve function, i.e., reach, grasp, and release with the hand. Function in the upper limb is more complicated than that of the lower limb, demading finely coordinated motions and good muscle control. As a rule, surgical measures in the upper limb should be delayed until maturation of the central nervous system permits adequate functional training in the postoperative period. Astereognosis may hinder functional use of the hand. Coordination and cerebral control are not provided by surgical measures. In the hemiplegic child, the presence of a contralateral nonaffected hand is not a contraindication to surgery on the involved hand. The goals of surgery should be realistic, and the result of surgery should be compared with the previous disability rather than the function of the contralateral noninvolved limb.

Function of the upper limb in cerebral palsy has been graded by Mowery et al. as follows: (1) *excellent*—when there is good use of the hand with effective grasp and release and voluntary control; (2) *good*—when the involved hand is a helper with functional voluntary control and the grasp and release are effective; (3) *fair*—when the hand is primarily a helper with no effective use and grasp and release are moderate with fair control; and (4) *poor*—when there is no grasp and release and the hand is a "paperweight."[363]

In the preoperative assessment the following factors should be considered: adequacy of function of the entire upper limb, i.e., the shoulder, elbow, forearm, wrist, hand, and fingers. Are there mirror or mass movements indicating poor cerebral coordinated control of the upper limb? Is there cerebral control over individual muscles or muscle groups? Can the patient voluntarily activate an individual muscle on command? This determines the potential for active use of the hand if one restores balance of muscles, better functional position, and stability of the hand and wrist. What is the availability of muscles with good motor strength and cerebral control for transfers? The sensory status of the hand is important. Coordination, cerebral control, and epicritic sensation are not provided by surgical measures. Age and intelligence of the patient are other important considerations. The level of neurophysiologic maturation should be determined. Surgical measures should be designed to provide function commensurate with the level of neurophysiologic maturation.

Occasionally, cosmetic appearance becomes a consideration for surgical intervention. In an adolescent female, the acutely flexed wrist and clenched fingers in the palm may be very

Text continued on page 1722

Patellar Advancement by Plication of Patellar Tendon and Division of Patellar Retinacula

OPERATIVE TECHNIQUE

A. A transverse skin incision is made, centering over the knee joint and extending from the medial to the lateral condyle of the femur. Subcutaneous tissue and fascia are divided in line with the skin incision.

B. The wound flaps are retracted proximally and distally, exposing the high-riding patella, elongated patellar tendon, and patellar retinacula.

C. The wound flaps are approximated, and through separate stab wounds in the skin, a large threaded Steinmann pin is inserted transversely through the center of the patella and a similar pin is placed in the proximal tibia. The distal pin should be drilled from the lateral side and should be directed somewhat anteroposteriorly to prevent pressure irritation of the common peroneal nerve.

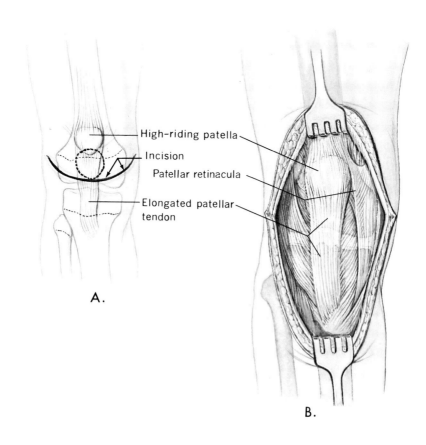

High-riding patella

Incision

Patellar retinacula

Elongated patellar tendon

A.

B.

C.

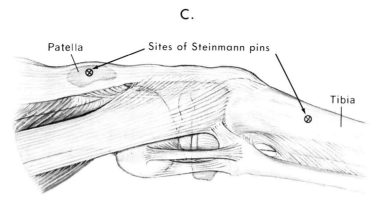

Patella

Sites of Steinmann pins

Tibia

Patellar Advancement by Plication of Patellar Tendon and Division of Patellar Retinacula (Continued)

D. The medial and lateral margins of the patellar tendon are identified. Longitudinal incisions are made on each side of the tendon, which is isolated and mobilized from subjacent and surrounding structures. Care should be taken not to open the capsule of the knee joint. Next, the patellar retinacula are divided medially and laterally.

E. The patella is pulled distally to its normal position in the intercondylar notch by traction on the proximal pin and manual pressure. The two pins are securely held together by a plate or external fixation apparatus. The patellar tendon is thoroughly freed from the underlying fat pad.

F. The patellar tendon is plicated, shortening it to the desired length. Its plicated ends are sutured together with 00 or 0 Tycron. Any bulky segment of the tendon is excised, if necessary. The wound is closed in layers and an above-knee cast is applied, which holds the knee in neutral position or 5 degrees of hyperextension. The pins are covered with petrolatum gauze to prevent skin slough from being incorporated in the cast. Adequate padding should be applied to prevent pressure sores.

POSTOPERATIVE CARE

About four to six weeks after surgery, the cast and pins are removed. Active and passive exercises are performed to regain muscle strength and range of motion. Weight-bearing is gradual and is protected with crutches. Full weight-bearing is allowed when the quadriceps is fair in motor strength.

Plate 67. Patellar Advancement by Plication of Patellar Tendon and Division of Patellar Retinacula

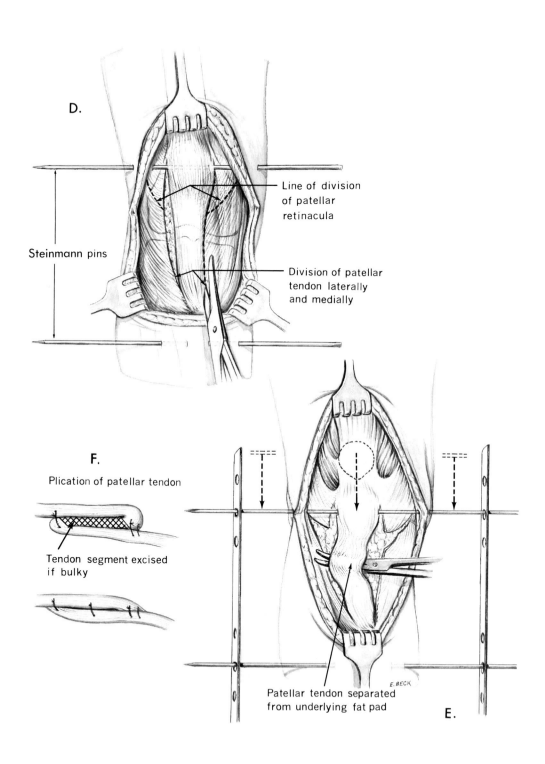

D.

Steinmann pins

Line of division
of patellar
retinacula

Division of patellar
tendon laterally
and medially

F.

Plication of patellar tendon

Tendon segment excised
if bulky

E. BECK

Patellar tendon separated
from underlying fat pad

E.

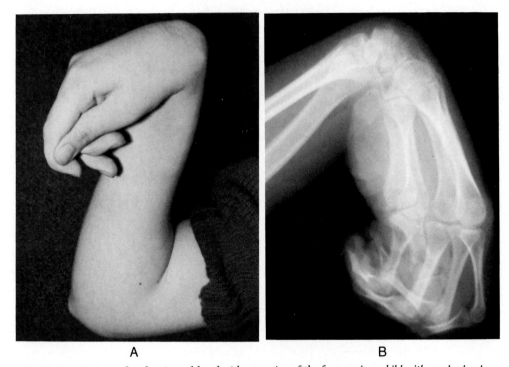

A   B

FIGURE 5–59. *Acute flexed wrist and hand with pronation of the forearm in a child with cerebral palsy.*

A. Photograph of patient's upper limb. **B.** Lateral radiogram showing the volar subluxation of the carpus.

disturbing psychologically (Fig. 5–59). Cosmetic improvement effected by placing the hand in a nearly normal position may be indicated despite poor functional potential. It will serve better as an assisting post.

The deformities of the upper limb are discussed individually.

THUMB-IN-PALM DEFORMITY

Thumb-in-palm deformity results from spasticity and contracture of the adductor pollicis or spasticity of the flexors of the thumb, or both. It is very disabling, as the thumb is in a poor position for effective function. Pulp-to-pulp action and lateral pinch are lost. Grasp is hindered, and entry of objects into the palm is blocked. In some patients, particularly those with tension athetosis, the thumb-in-palm position stimulates the so-called gripping reflex, in which the fingers are clenched in the palm over the thumb (Fig. 5–60A). Function of the thumb is intimately related to position and stability of the wrist. On hyperflexion of the wrist, the fingers and thumb extend out of the palm (Fig. 5–60B). When the wrist is dorsiflexed and placed in neutral position, the deformation of the thumb will be aggravated.

Stretching of the capsule may cause instability of the metacarpophalangeal joint of the thumb, resulting in hypermobility and subluxation, which interfere with complete extension of the thumb. Soft-tissue contracture in the web between the thumb and index metacarpals may develop in severe deformities; if left untreated, it will eventually cause subluxation of the carpometacarpal joint.

Deformities of the thumb in cerebral palsy may be classified as follows (according to House et al.[242]).

Type I—"Simple" metacarpal adduction contracture (Fig. 5–61A). In this form the first metacarpal is held in next to the second metacarpal owing to spasticity and myostatic contracture of the adductor pollicis and first dorsal interosseous muscle. There may be secondary contracture of the skin web between the thumb and index metacarpals. Metacarpophalangeal and interphalangeal joints of the thumb have normal range of motion, and the patient has varying degrees of voluntary cerebral control over the thumb extensors and flexors.

Type II—Metacarpal adduction contracture and metacarpophalangeal flexion deformity (Fig. 5–61B). In this form, in addition to the

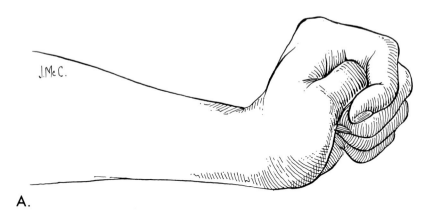

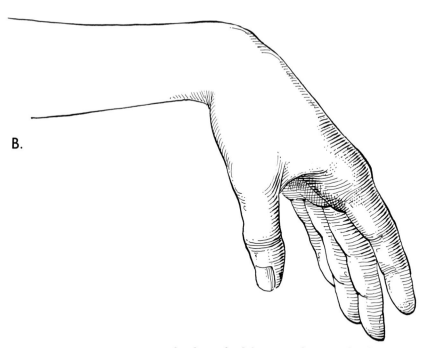

FIGURE 5–60. Thumb-in-palm deformity in the spastic hand.

A. Note the fingers are clenched in the palm over the thumb. **B.** On hyperflexion of the wrist, the fingers and thumb extend out of the palm.

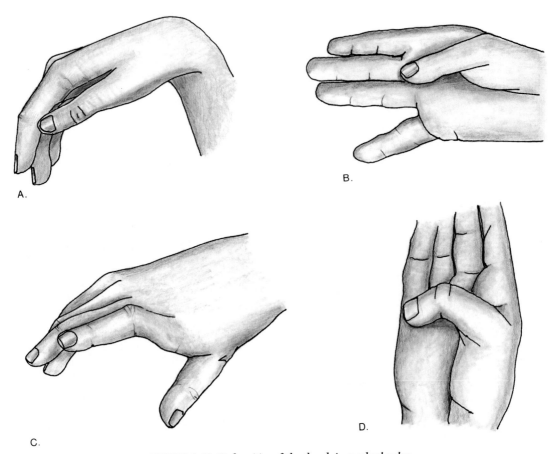

FIGURE 5–61. Deformities of the thumb in cerebral palsy.

A. Type I, simple metacarpal adduction contracture. **B.** Type II, metacarpal adduction contracture and metacarpophalangeal flexion deformity. **C.** Type III, metacarpal adduction contracture combined with a metacarpophalangeal hyperextension deformity or instability. **D.** Type IV, metacarpal adduction contracture combined with flexion deformity of the metacarpophalangeal and interphalangeal joints.

adduction contracture of the first metacarpal (as in Type I), there is flexion deformity of the thumb metacarpophalangeal joint due to spasticity and myostatic contracture of the flexor pollicis brevis muscle. There is normal mobility and relatively good function of the interphalangeal joint of the thumb.

Type III—Metacarpal adduction contracture combined with a metacarpophalangeal hyperextension deformity or instability (Fig. 5–61C). In this type of deformity the flexor pollicis longus is not spastic, the first metacarpal is adducted, and the thumb metacarpophalangeal joint is unstable and hyperextensible owing to compensatory overactivity of the extensor pollicis longus and brevis.

Type IV—Metacarpal adduction contracture combined with flexion deformity of the metacarpophalangeal and interphalangeal joints (Fig. 5–61D). This is caused by spasticity of the

flexor pollicis longus in association with spasticity and contracture of the intrinsic muscle of the thumb. The severity of the thumb-in-palm deformity is most marked in this type, and the disability is the greatest. The taut finger flexors trap the thumb under the flexed digits.

Treatment. Passive stretching exercises are performed several times a day to place the thumb metacarpal into abduction and the whole thumb into extension. Be sure not to subluxate the metacarpophalangeal joint. A persistent regimen of such therapy may prevent development of myostatic contracture and fixed deformity.

As soon as the child is old enough, normally by two or three years of age, a well-fitted opponens splint is used, which holds the thumb metacarpal in maximal abduction and the thumb phalanges in extension (Fig. 5–62). This opponens splint is worn as a night splint, which holds the wrist in dorsiflexion and the forearm

Text continued on page 1730

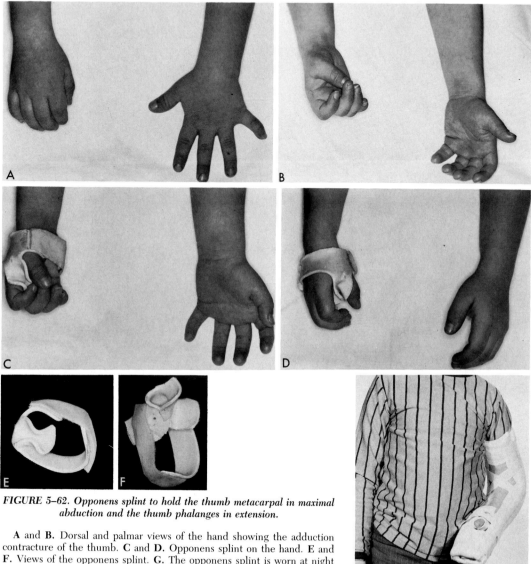

FIGURE 5–62. Opponens splint to hold the thumb metacarpal in maximal abduction and the thumb phalanges in extension.

A and **B.** Dorsal and palmar views of the hand showing the adduction contracture of the thumb. **C** and **D.** Opponens splint on the hand. **E** and **F.** Views of the opponens splint. **G.** The opponens splint is worn at night in a bivalved cast, which holds the wrist in dorsiflexion and the forearm in full supination.

Release of Adductor Pollicis Muscle in the Palm

OPERATIVE PROCEDURE

A. A skin incision is made in the palm beginning at the lateral border of the proximal palmar crease and extended proximally to the wrist. Subcutaneous tissue is divided in line with the skin incision.

B. The palmar aponeurosis is divided, taking due care not to injure the digital vessels and nerves.

C. The digital branches of the median nerve are visualized and kept out of harm's way. The second lumbrical muscle is retracted ulnarward, the flexor tendons of the index finger are retracted radially, and adductor pollicis muscle is visualized in the palm.

D. An incision is made at the origin of the adductor pollicis from the third metacarpal, and with periosteal elevators it is reflected radially and distally.

The tourniquet is released and after complete hemostasis a small Hemovac drain is used for closed suction. The subcutaneous tissue and the skin are closed in the usual fashion and a below-elbow cast is applied holding the thumb in maximal abduction.

Plate 68. Release of Adductor Pollicis Muscle in the Palm

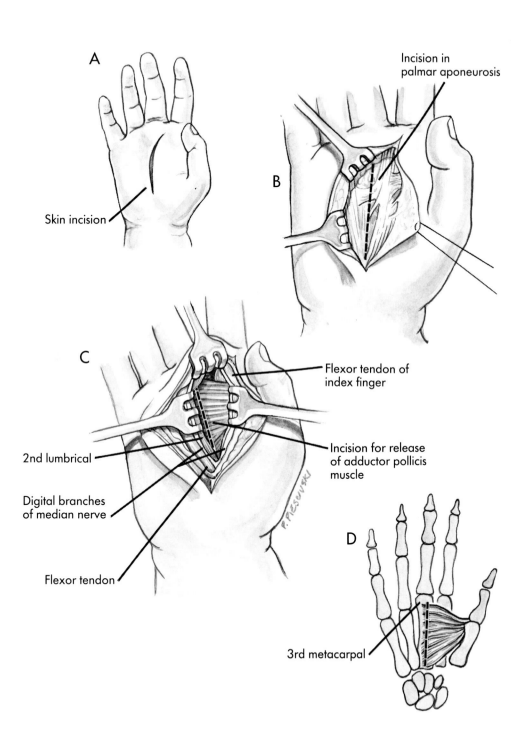

A

Skin incision

B

Incision in
palmar aponeurosis

C

Flexor tendon of
index finger

Incision for release
of adductor pollicis
muscle

2nd lumbrical

Digital branches
of median nerve

Flexor tendon

D

3rd metacarpal

Release of Adductor Pollicis Muscle in the Palm

OPERATIVE PROCEDURE

When adduction contracture of the thumb is not severe, this author prefers Z-lengthening of the adductor pollicis tendon through a dorsal incision.

E. A skin incision is made on the dorsum of the hand between the index and thumb metacarpals. The subcutaneous tissue is divided in line with the skin incision.

F. Adductor pollicis muscle is exposed and gently elevated from its underlying tendon. A Z-incision is made in the tendon.

G. The two ends of the tendon are closed with interrupted sutures elongating the adductor pollicis muscle.

The wound is closed in theusual fashion, and a below-elbow cast is applied holding the wrist in 20 degrees of dorsiflexion and the thumb in maximal abduction and leutral extension.

POSTOPERATIVE CARE

The cast is removed three weeks following surgery. A splint is manufactured for night use, holding the thumb in maximal abduction; another splint is made for day use. A physical therapy regimen consisting of active and passive exercises is prescribed.

Plate 68. Release of Adductor Pollicis Muscle in the Palm

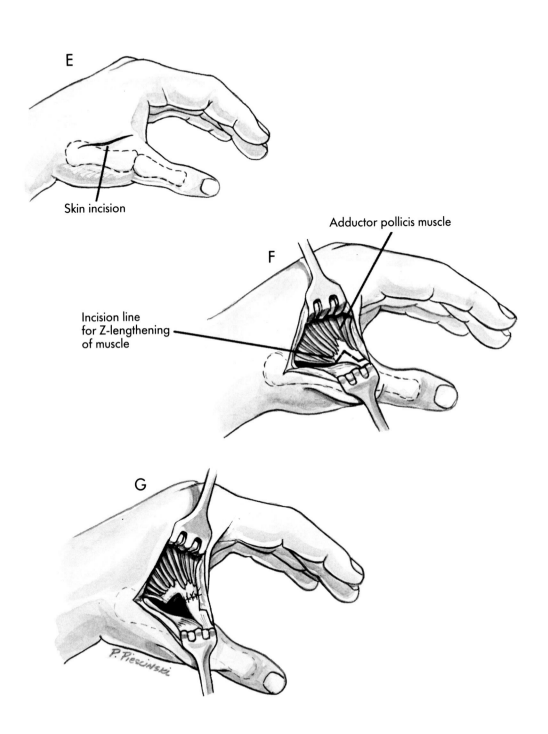

E

Skin incision

F

Adductor pollicis muscle

Incision line
for Z-lengthening
of muscle

G

P. Pieczinski

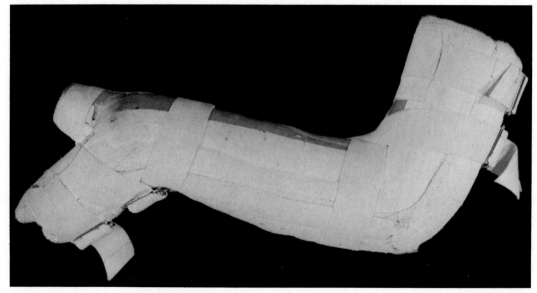

FIGURE 5–63. Bivalved above-elbow cast without opponens splint.

Often the thumb will slip proximally through the cast and cause subluxation of the metacarpophalangeal joint.

in full supination. Attempts to hold the thumb in corrected position in the bivalved long arm cast or plastic splint are usually unsuccessful and often result in deformity, as the thumb slips proximally through the cast and causes subluxation of the metacarpophalangeal joint (Fig. 5–63).

Surgical treatment is indicated when the thumb-in-palm is in the way of the fingers for grasp, or when the flexed-adducted thumb protrudes dorsally between the fingers, or when the thumb is unable to side pinch to the index finger.

The following modalities of treatment are available for operative correction of the thumb deformities in cerebral palsy: (1) muscle tendon lengthening or soft-tissue release (either at its origin or insertion); (2) muscle tendon transfers to enhance function of the weak muscles; and (3) stabilization of the unstable joints by capsulorrhaphy and volar plate plication in the young and arthrodesis in the skeletally mature hand.

Correction of Soft-Tissue Contractural Deformity. This should always be performed first. Adduction contracture of the thumb is best released in the palm at its origin from the metacarpals because this preserves some degree of function of thumb adduction. The operative technique is described and illustrated in Plate 68.

Release of thumb adductors at their insertion is technically much easier with fewer problems of surgical exposure and less risk of inadvertent division of nerves. The operative technique is described and illustrated in Plate 69. In moderately severe contracture, the adductor tendon can be lengthened by Z-plasty and its function preserved (see Plate 68, Steps **E** to **G**).

Neurectomy of the motor branches of the ulnar and median nerves to the adductor pollicis and intrinsic muscles of the thumb should not be performed because it causes muscle fibrosis and aggravates the contractural deformity.

If the flexor pollicis longus is very spastic and contracted, an attempt at passive stretching in a corrective cast is made; if unsuccessful, fractional lengthening of the flexor pollicis longus in the distal forearm is performed.

Muscle Tendon Transfers to Strengthen Motor Function of Thumb Abduction and Extension. After 6 to 12 months of aggressive therapy, if the thumb abductors and extensors continue to be cerebral zero in function and active voluntary motion does not develop, a tendon transfer to enhance their function should be considered. This should not be done simultaneously with adductor myotomy of the thumb, as release of the spastic adductor pollicis and flexor pollicis longus and proper postoperative training may be adequate to gain thumb abduction and extension.

Prior to tendon transfers to the abductor and extensor pollicis, there should be full passive abduction of the first metacarpal and full passive extension of the thumb. The metacarpophalangeal joint of the thumb should be stable.

The motor muscles usually available for transfer are the brachioradialis, the flexor digitorum sublimis of the ring or long finger, and the flexor carpi radialis. In spastic paralysis, the brachioradialis muscle is usually strong and under voluntary cerebral control. The amplitude of excursion of the divided tendon of the brachioradialis is approximately 1.5 cm. After thorough mobilization of the muscle from its surrounding fascia, its amplitude can be increased to 3 cm. The nerve and blood supply enters the brachioradialis muscle above the lateral epicondyle of the humerus; this allows thorough mobilization of the brachioradialis muscle without endangering its neurovascular supply. The surgical technique of brachioradialis transfer is illustrated in Plate 70.

If the flexor digitorum sublimis of the ring or long finger is used for a motor, the tendon is sectioned at the wrist and the distal end of the proximal segment sutured to the extensor pollicis longus and abductor pollicis brevis tendons in the same manner.

The flexor carpi radialis ordinarily should not be used as a motor if the flexor carpi ulnaris is transferred to the extensor carpi radialis or if there is the possibility of such a transfer in the future. Also, transfer of flexor carpi radialis will increase ulnar deviation of the wrist, which often is an already existing deformity of the spastic hand; also, it is best to maintain the action of a wrist flexor.

Rerouting of Extensor Pollicis Longus to Provide Thumb Abduction.[187–189] This is indicated when the patient hyperextends the interphalangeal joint of the thumb when attempting thumb abduction. It should be not be performed in the presence of instability and hyperextension of the metacarpophalangeal joint of the thumb, or when the interphalangeal joint of the thumb hyperextends but the metacarpophalangeal joint is in flexion. Prior to extensor pollicis longus rerouting it is imperative to stabilize the metacarpophalangeal joint of the thumb (if unstable) and fractionally lengthen (above the wrist) the flexor pollicis longus if it is spastic and contracted.

The operative technique of extensor pollicis longus rerouting is as follows: Make a lazy S-shaped incision beginning at the dorsoradial aspect of the interphalangeal joint of the thumb and terminating 3 to 4 cm. proximal to the radiocarpal joint. Caution! The scar should not be over the new course of the tendon. The extensor pollicis longus tendon is identified and

dissected free from the annular ligament and mobilized to its insertion. The thumb is fully abducted and medially rotated, and the extensor pollicis longus tendon is redirected to the volar and radial aspect of the thumb phalanges and the first metacarpal.

It can be held in place in several ways: Goldner recommends suturing the tendon into the subcutaneous tissue over an area of 4 to 5 cm.; this author recommends more secure fixation of the tendon in its position by providing a pulley through which the long extensor tendon traverses. This can be done by sectioning the extensor pollicis brevis tendon at the level of the radial styloid, pulling the distal end of the short extensor around the long extensor, and reattaching the short extensor tendon to its own muscle belly. An alternative method of reconstruction of a pulley above the radial styloid is by free tendon graft from the palmaris longus. Occasionally this author has rewound the extensor pollicis longus tendon through the abductor pollicis longus to enhance abductor pollicis longus muscle function. The wound is closed.

The hand, wrist, and forearm are immobilized for a period of three to four weeks in plaster of Paris cast with the thumb in full abduction and medial rotation. The extensor pollicis longus rerouting can be combined with flexor carpi ulnaris transfer; in such an instance the cast is above the elbow. This author has found the extensor pollicis longus rerouting to be a satisfactory way to provide thumb abduction; it is crucial, however, that the metacarpophalangeal joint be stable and that there be no flexed posture and contracture of the thumb metacarpal phalangeal joints.

In children, subluxation of the metacarpophalangeal joint of the thumb is treated by capsulorrhaphy ("capsulodesis"). The growth plate of the proximal phalanx of the thumb is proximal; this should not be disturbed. The deformity is usually one of hyperextension of the metacarpophalangeal joint. The whole width of the capsule on the volar surface is dissected free from the head of the first metacarpal (its growth plate is proximal) and, with the metacarpophalangeal joint in hyperflexion, is reattached proximally to the metacarpal head with 00 or 000 Mersilene suture through two drill holes. One or two smooth Kirschner wires may be inserted across the metacarpophalangeal joint to maintain its hyperflexed position securely. The thumb is immobilized in a below-elbow or above-elbow cast (length of the cast depending upon the associated deformities) for

Text continued on page 1738

Adductor Myotomy of the Thumb

OPERATIVE TECHNIQUE

A and **B**. A 2 to 3 cm. long oblique incision is made over the dorsum of the hand. It begins at the ulnar border of the first metacarpal head, extends proximally to the middle third of the metacarpal, and then swings ulnarward toward the base of the second metacarpal. One should avoid the distal margin of the thumb web, as the cicatrix may cause contracture of the web. This surgical approach permits stripping of the first dorsal interosseous muscle if necessary. When only an adductor tenotomy is to be done, an alternate approach is a 1.5 to 2 cm. long transverse incision immediately proximal to the flexor crease of the thumb. Again, the ulnar border of the incision should stop short of the distal margin of the thumb web. (When a Z-plasty of the contracted thumb web is indicated, a transverse skin incision is made at the distal border of the web, extending between the ulnar border of the proximal flexion crease of the thumb and the radial border of the proximal transverse crease of the palm, and two oblique cuts at a 45- to 60-degree angle are made for Z-lengthening.)

C. The subcutaneous tissue is divided. The first dorsal interosseous muscle is retracted proximally, and the tendon of the adductor pollicis is identified near its insertion.

D. With a staphylorrhaphy elevator, the adductor pollicis longus tendon is lifted dorsally and 1 cm. of the adductor tendon is excised near its insertion. Care should be exercised not to disturb the tendon mechanism of the extensors and the abductors of the thumb.

If the first dorsal interosseous muscle is contracted, it is stripped from the metacarpal with a periosteal elevator through the same incision.

The wound is closed in routine manner. A well-molded above-elbow cast is applied to hold the thumb metacarpal in maximal abduction, the metacarpophalangeal joint in neutral extension, and the interphalangeal joint in 10 degrees of flexion. The elbow should be in slight flexion with the forearm in full supination.

POSTOPERATIVE CARE

Three weeks after surgery the cast is bivalved and an opponens splint is made to hold the thumb in a position of maximal abduction and functional opposition. Active exercises are begun to develop active motion of the thumb in all directions—adduction, abduction, opposition, flexion, and extension. Passive exercises are also performed to maintain maximal range of motion. In the beginning two weeks, the opponens splint is worn continuously, except during the exercise periods; later the use of the splint is gradually decreased and an aggressive regimen of occupational therapy is instituted to develop function.

Plate 69. Adductor Myotomy of the Thumb

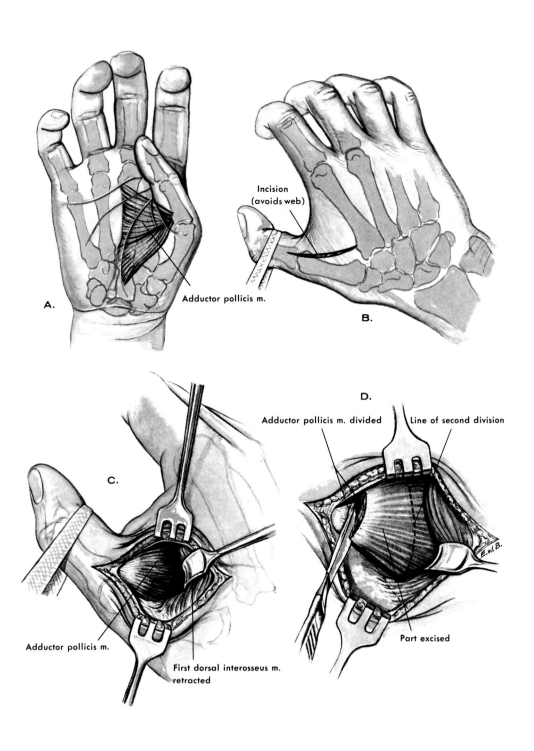

A.

Adductor pollicis m.

B.

Incision
(avoids web)

C.

Adductor pollicis m.

First dorsal interosseus m.
retracted

D.

Adductor pollicis m. divided

Line of second division

Part excised

Brachioradialis Transfer to Restore Thumb Abduction and Extension

OPERATIVE TECHNIQUE

A. A long dorsoradial incision is made, beginning at the radial styloid process and extending proximally to a point 2 cm. distal to the lateral epicondyle of the humerus. The subcutaneous tissue is divided and the wound edges are undermined and retracted.

B and **C.** The flat tendon of the brachioradialis is sectioned at its insertion into the base of the styloid process of the radius. The tendons of the abductor pollicis longus and extensor pollicis brevis are divided at their musculotendinous junction and marked with 00 silk whip sutures as they traverse from the dorsal to the volar aspect on the brachioradialis tendon. Injury to neurovascular structures should be avoided. The radial artery lies on the volar margin of the brachioradialis tendon, and on the ulnar side of the radial vessels is the flexor carpi radialis tendon. The radial nerve runs along the lateral aspect of the forearm deep to the brachioradialis muscle. In the upper third of the forearm, the nerve is radial to the radial artery; in the middle of the forearm it is immediately lateral to the artery, whereas in the lower third of the forearm the superficial branch of the nerve curves dorsally underneath the brachioradialis tendon to divide into the medial or lateral branches after penetrating the deep fascia on the dorsum of the wrist.

Plate 70. Brachioradialis Transfer to Restore Thumb Abduction and Extension

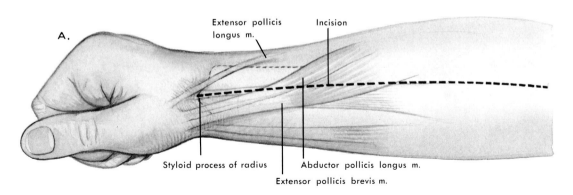

A.

Extensor pollicis longus m.

Incision

Styloid process of radius

Abductor pollicis longus m.

Extensor pollicis brevis m.

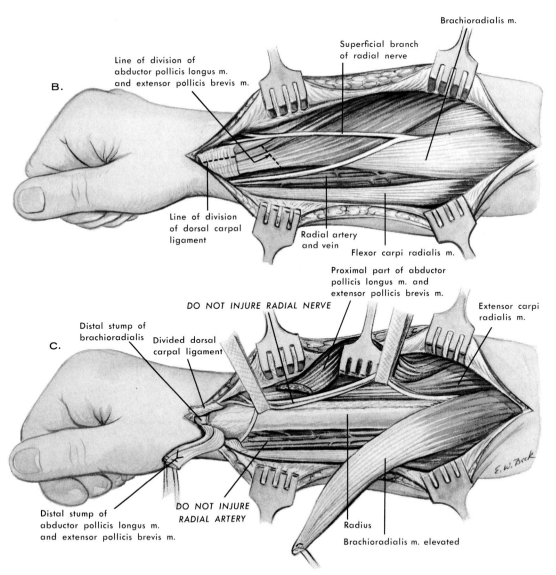

Brachioradialis m.

Superficial branch of radial nerve

B.

Line of division of abductor pollicis longus m. and extensor pollicis brevis m.

Line of division of dorsal carpal ligament

Radial artery and vein

Flexor carpi radialis m.

Proximal part of abductor pollicis longus m. and extensor pollicis brevis m.

DO NOT INJURE RADIAL NERVE

Extensor carpi radialis m.

C.

Distal stump of brachioradialis

Divided dorsal carpal ligament

Distal stump of abductor pollicis longus m. and extensor pollicis brevis m.

DO NOT INJURE RADIAL ARTERY

Radius

Brachioradialis m. elevated

E. W. Beck

Brachioradialis Transfer to Restore Thumb Abduction and Extension *(Continued)*

D. By sharp and dull dissection, the brachioradialis muscle is freed from the antebrachial fascia and the adjacent muscles (extensor carpi radialis dorsally and flexor carpi ulnaris anteriorly). It is imperative to mobilize the brachioradialis as proximally as possible (preferably immediately distal to the elbow joint) to gain maximal excursion of the muscle action and to have a straight line of muscle pull.

E. The extensor pollicis longus and abductor pollicis brevis tendons are sutured to the brachioradialis tendon by interrupted 00 silk sutures, and the tendon ends interwoven. The tension on the transferred tendon should be moderate, so that the first metacarpal can be passively adducted 1.5 cm. from the palm with the wrist in neutral position and passive pulp pinch is possible between the thumb and index finger. The wound is closed in layers and an above-elbow cast is applied with the elbow in 90 degrees of flexion, the wrist in neutral position, the first metacarpal in maximal abduction, and the thumb in neutral extension.

POSTOPERATIVE CARE

Three to four weeks following surgery, the cast is removed and active exercises are performed to develop function of the transferred brachioradialis muscle as an abductor and extensor of the thumb. Passive exercises are performed to maintain full range of motion of the joint. In the beginning a below-elbow splint is worn to maintain the thumb metacarpal in maximum abduction. Functional therapy is very important, such as holding water glasses of various sizes for thumb abduction and holding a pencil for thumb adduction.

Plate 70. Brachioradialis Transfer to Restore Thumb Abduction and Extension

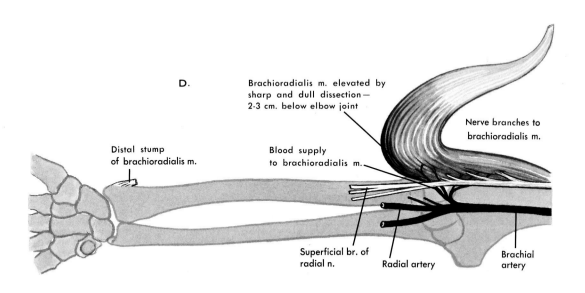

D.

Brachioradialis m. elevated by sharp and dull dissection — 2-3 cm. below elbow joint

Nerve branches to brachioradialis m.

Distal stump of brachioradialis m.

Blood supply to brachioradialis m.

Superficial br. of radial n.

Radial artery

Brachial artery

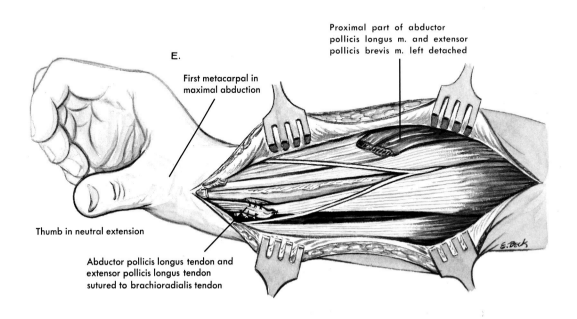

E.

Proximal part of abductor pollicis longus m. and extensor pollicis brevis m. left detached

First metacarpal in maximal abduction

Thumb in neutral extension

Abductor pollicis longus tendon and extensor pollicis longus tendon sutured to brachioradialis tendon

E. Beck

a period of four to six weeks. Then the cast and Kirschner wires are removed, and active exercises are performed. A splint is worn at night to maintain the flexed position of the metacarpophalangeal joint of the thumb and to prevent recurrence of deformity; the interphalangeal joint of the thumb should be in only 5 degrees of flexion in the splint.

In those of an older age group in whom growth is completed, arthrodesis of the metacarpophalangeal joint of the thumb is performed when there is marked hypermobility and gross subluxation. Fusion is achieved by excising the articular cartilage and utilizing the "peg" technique. Crisscross Kirschner wires or a small fragment AO or Herbert screws are inserted for secure internal fixation.

An intermetacarpal bone block between the first and second metacarpals or between the first and third metacarpals to place the thumb metacarpal rigidly in maximal abduction and opposition may be indicated. The procedure is performed when the thumb metacarpal is totally flail and when there is active voluntary flexion-extension of the thumb and index and long fingers. The stable thumb serves as an opposing post against which the index and long fingers pinch. (The operative technique is described and illustrated in Plate 88.) Parents and patient, however, should be forewarned that the rigid position of the stabilized thumb hinders fitting of gloves and makes it difficult for the patient to put his hand in his pocket.

FINGER DEFORMITIES

Flexion Deformity. Flexion at the metacarpophalangeal and interphalangeal joints is the most common deformity in the spastic hand. It is caused by spasticity and myostatic contracture of the flexor digitorum profundus and sublimis muscles. This is usually associated with flexion deformity of the wrist due to spasticity of the wrist flexors and pronation contracture of the forearm. Flexion deformity of the digits is increased by extension of the wrist, and it is diminished on hyperflexion of the wrist. With the wrist in maximal flexion, there will be a varying degree of active extension of the fingers out of the palm. Fixed joint contractures are usually not present.

Conservative methods of treatment should always be attempted prior to consideration of surgery. If flexion deformity is severe, it is best to apply a corrective above-elbow solid cast to stretch the flexion contracture of the digits and wrist and pronation contracture of the forearm.

The thumb is placed in abduction and extension. Caution! Do not dorsally subluxate the metacarpophalangeal joint of the thumb. The metacarpophalangeal and interphalangeal joints of the fingers are held in some flexion to prevent the disabling hyperextension deformity. Stretching of the finger flexors is accomplished by progressive extension of the wrist and by changing the cast weekly or biweekly. The deformity is corrected gradually, and the cast is well padded to prevent pressure sores. In about four to six weeks, a fair degree of correction can be obtained. Then a bivalved cast, or preferably a plastic splint, is made for night use, and passive stretching exercises are performed several times a day to maintain the correction. Active exercises are performed to develop voluntary finger control.

Surgical measures are indicated if the preceding conservative measures fail. The author prefers fractional lengthening of the finger and wrist flexors in the forearm at the distal musculotendinous junction. The procedure is simple and relatively safe and provides flexibility to obtain the desired degree of controlled lengthening. The operative technique is described and illustrated in Plate 71.

Release of the flexor-pronator origin for flexion deformities of the hand and wrist was originally described by Page.[382] Later, Inglis and Cooper evaluated their experience with 18 cases.[250] The procedure requires extensive soft-tissue and nerve dissection, creates antecubital and forearm dead space, and may cause supination contracture of the forearm due to loss of pronator power. Because of these possible complications, flexor-pronator origin release is not recommended by this author. Fractional lengthening of the flexors in the forearm is a much simpler and safer procedure. The surgical technique of flexor-pronator release at their origin is as follows:

The incision begins 5 cm. proximal to the medial epicondyle, curving radially at the elbow joint across the antecubital space and is extended distally on the volar surface of the ulna to end at the midpoint of the forearm. The subcutaneous tissue is divided, and the wound edges are retracted. Caution should be exercised not to injure the medial brachial cutaneous nerve and the medial antebrachial cutaneous nerve in the forearm. The ulnar nerve is identified, carefully dissected free, and elevated from its groove behind the medial epicondyle. The motor branches of the ulnar nerve to the flexor carpi ulnaris and to the two medial heads of the flexor digitorum profundus are exposed and gently dissected free to prevent traction injury to the nerve after release of the muscles.

Starting at the midpoint of the ulna, with a periosteal elevator, the flexor carpi ulnaris and flexor digitorum profundus are bluntly dissected free of their origins from the ulna and interosseous membrane. The release is continued proximally to the medial epicondyle. The ulnar nerve is retracted posteriorly, and the entire flexor-pronator muscle mass is sectioned at its origin from the medial epicondyle of the humerus. The median nerve is identified in the antecubital space as it passes through the pronator teres and is retracted forward. Next, the lacertus fibrosus is divided, and the remaining portions of the flexor muscle origin are elevated and released distally. The fascia of the brachialis is incised if there is any persistence of flexion deformity of the elbow. The ulnar nerve is then transplanted anteriorly from its groove. At this point, the fingers and wrist are passively extended and the flexor muscle mass origin is displaced 3 to 4 cm. distally from its original location. The distal displacement should not exceed 4 cm., as marked loss of pronation will occur and result in fixed supination contracture of the forearm. This retains some pronation power and helps to avoid such a postoperative supination contracture.

The wound is drained with closed suction catheters to prevent formation of a hematoma in the dead space, which can cause marked flexion contracture of the elbow with accompanying neuritis of the median and ulnar nerves. The wound is closed and the limb immobilized in an above-elbow cast, with the forearm in neutral rotation and the wrist and fingers in neutral position. Three weeks after surgery, the solid cast is removed and a bivalved cast is made to maintain the correction. Passive and active exercises are performed.

Swan-Neck Deformity. Swan-neck deformity of the fingers is caused by chronic overpull on the middle extensor band by the spastic intrinsic muscles and by the tenodesis effect of the extensor digitorum longus when the wrist is in flexion. The middle extensor band, as compared with the lateral extensor bands, is relatively short. Thus, the proximal interphalangeal joint hyperextends, and the distal interphalangeal joint goes into flexion. The volar capsule and retinacular ligaments become stretched and elongated. The lateral bands eventually are displaced dorsally, increasing the force that hyperextends the proximal interphalangeal joint.

The sublimis tenodesis of the proximal interphalangeal joint, as described by Swanson, will restrict extension of the proximal interphalangeal joint and will correct the swan-neck deformity.[541, 542] Prior to performing the Swanson procedure, the flexor carpi ulnaris should be transferred to the extensor carpi radialis longus to reinforce the power of the wrist dorsiflexors. By doing this at an early age in the pure spastic hand, the swan-neck deformity can be prevented or can be kept from being severe enough to warrant sublimis tenodesis. The swan-neck deformity in the mixed type of cerebral palsy (i.e., spastic and athetoid) or in pure tension athetosis presents a difficult and different problem; in these patients, Swanson's sublimis tenodesis should be performed with caution and only after thorough assessment of the pathomechanics and motor picture. It is best to tenodese only one slip of the flexor sublimis. The results in extrapyramidal involvement have not always been successful in this author's experience. In severe tension athetosis, sublimis tenodesis should not be performed.

The surgical technique of sublimis tenodesis of the proximal interphalangeal joint, as described by Swanson, is as follows:[541, 542]

A midlateral incision is made immediately dorsal to the flexion crease and extending from the distal end of the middle phalanx to the base of the proximal phalanx. The flexor sheath is incised, exposing the flexor tendons, which are retracted dorsally. The distal half of the volar surface of the proximal phalanx is subperiosteally exposed by resection of the periosteum, the palmar capsule, and the volar plate. Two small drill holes approximately 1 cm. apart are made through the neck of the proximal phalanx in the palmar to dorsal direction. With a curet, the two drill holes are connected on the palmar aspect, and the bone is roughened to give a raw surface of bone for attachment of the tendon. With a scalpel the sublimis tendon is scarified. Mersilene sutures are passed through these drill holes and through the sublimis tendon, firmly anchoring it to bone with the interphalangeal joint in 20 to 30 degrees of flexion. The flexed position of the proximal interphalangeal joint is further secured by placing a small Kirschner wire across it, which is cut off subcutaneously. The retinacular ligament and flexor sheath are closed with 0000 or 00000 plain catgut sutures and the skin with 0000 nylon. An above-elbow cast is applied; it should extend to the tip of the fingers with the wrist in neutral dorsiflexion, the forearm in full supination, and the elbow in 90 degrees of flexion.

Text continued on page 1744

Fractional Lengthening of Finger and Wrist Flexors in Forearm

OPERATIVE TECHNIQUE

A. A midline longitudinal incision is made in the middle three fourths of the volar surface of the forearm. The subcutaneous tissue and deep fascia are divided in line with the skin incision. The wound flaps are undermined, elevated, and retracted with four-prong rake retractors to expose the superficial groups of muscles. On the radial side of the flexor carpi ulnaris tendon, the ulnar vessels and nerves are identified and protected from injury; similarly, on the radial side of the flexor carpi radialis tendon, the radial vessels and nerve are isolated to protect them from inadvertent damage. Sliding lengthening of the flexor carpi radialis and flexor carpi ulnaris muscles is performed at the musculotendinous junction by making two incisions of their tendinous fibers, about 1.5 cm. apart, without disturbing underlying muscle tissue. The proximal incision is transverse and the distal one is oblique. The palmaris longus and flexor digitorum muscles are lengthened by only one transverse incision in each.

B. The wrist and the fingers are passively hyperextended. The tendinous parts will separate while the intact underlying muscle fibers will maintain continuity of the muscles.

Plate 71. Fractional Lengthening of Finger and Wrist Flexors in Forearm

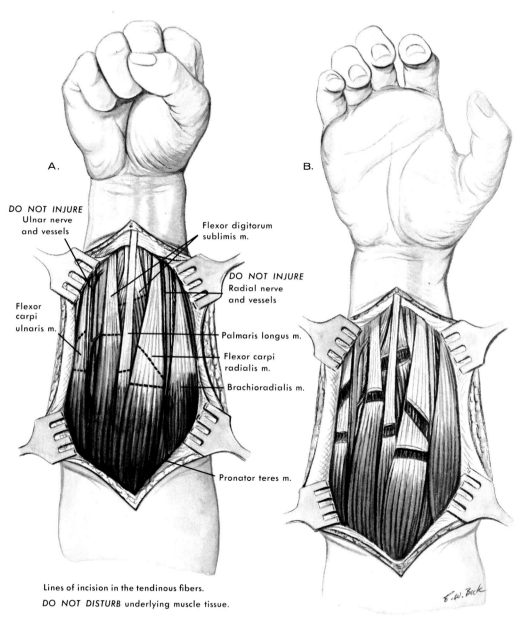

A.

DO NOT INJURE
Ulnar nerve
and vessels

Flexor digitorum
sublimis m.

DO NOT INJURE
Radial nerve
and vessels

Flexor
carpi
ulnaris m.

Palmaris longus m.

Flexor carpi
radialis m.

Brachioradialis m.

Pronator teres m.

B.

Lines of incision in the tendinous fibers.
DO NOT DISTURB underlying muscle tissue.

Separation of tendinous parts on extension
of wrist and digits

E. W. Beck

1741

Fractional Lengthening of Finger and Wrist Flexors in Forearm (Continued)

C and D. The deep volar muscles are exposed by retracting the brachioradialis muscle and radial vessels radially, and the flexor carpi radialis and flexor digitorum sublimis muscles ulnarward. The median nerve is identified and protected from injury by retracting it medially with the flexor carpi radialis muscle. The flexor pollicis longus and flexor digitorum profundus muscles are lengthened by making two incisions in their tendinous parts and sliding them in the same manner as that described for the superficial volar forearm muscles. Continuity of muscles is maintained by gentle handling of tissues and by taking care that there is adequate muscle substance underlying the divided tendinous parts. Sliding lengthening is achieved by separating the tendinous fibers by slow but firm extension of the thumb and four ulnar digits.

Next, the range of passive supination of the forearm is tested. If there is pronation contracture, the pronator teres muscle is lengthened by two oblique incisions, 1.5 cm. apart, of its tendinous fibers. Again, underlying muscle tissue should not be disturbed. The forearm is forcibly supinated; the tendinous segments will slide and separate, elongating the muscle.

The tourniquet is released and complete hemostasis is obtained. The deep fascia is not closed. The subcutaneous tissue and skin are approximated by interrupted sutures. An above-elbow cast that includes all the fingers and the thumb is applied to immobilize the forearm in full supination, the elbow in 90 degrees of flexion, the wrist in 50 degrees of extension, and the fingers and thumb in neutral extension.

POSTOPERATIVE CARE

Four weeks following surgery, the cast is removed and active exercises are started to develop motor power in the elongated muscle. Squeezing soft balls of varying sizes and other functional exercises are carried out several times a day. An aggressive occupational therapy program is essential. The corrected position is maintained in a bivalved cast. As motor function develops in the elongated muscle and its antagonists, the periods out of the cast are gradually increased.

Plate 71. Fractional Lengthening of Finger and Wrist Flexors in Forearm

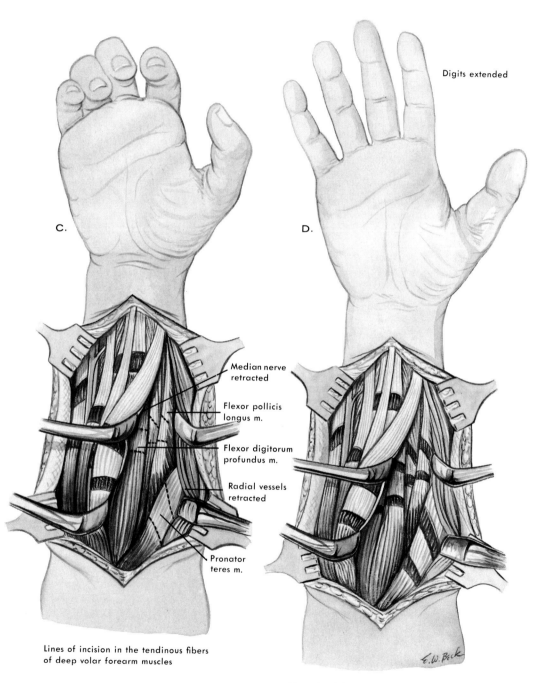

Digits extended

C.

D.

Median nerve retracted

Flexor pollicis longus m.

Flexor digitorum profundus m.

Radial vessels retracted

Pronator teres m.

E. W. Beck

Lines of incision in the tendinous fibers of deep volar forearm muscles

Note the sliding lengthening by separation of tendinous fibers

The cast and Kirschner wire are removed in four to six weeks. Passive and active exercises are performed under supervision of the therapist and the parents to develop functional range of motion. Extension of the proximal interphalangeal joints should be avoided. Splints that hold the proximal interphalangeal joints in flexion are utilized. These splints are worn during the day except for exercise periods for four to six weeks; then they are applied only at night, maintaining the fingers in flexion for another two to three months.

FLEXION DEFORMITY OF WRIST AND PRONATION CONTRACTURE OF FOREARM

This is a common deformity of spastic paralysis. Ability to extend the wrist and to supinate and pronate the forearm is fundamental to the effective use of the hand and fingers. The transfer of the flexor carpi ulnaris to the extensor carpi radialis longus or brevis was first described by Green in 1942. Thirty years' experience with 39 patients was reviewed by Green and Banks in 1962.[195] This transfer re-

moves the deforming force at the wrist, which pulls the hand into flexion and ulnar deviation; also, the rerouting of the tendon around the medial side of the ulna provides an active force that promotes supination of the forearm and dorsiflexion of the wrist (Fig. 5–64). It is indicated when the patient has adequate release but weak grasp; the wrist is in palmar flexion and ulnar deviation. In this deformed posture, the patient has difficulty in grasping objects, but when the wrist is passively dorsiflexed, the patient can extend his fingers and thumb fully, releasing the object. When the patient cannot extend his fingers with the wrist in dorsiflexed position, the flexor carpi ulnaris is transferred to extensor digitorum longus, provided there is full passive extension of all digits.

Prior to performing Green's flexor ulnaris transfer, the following essential prerequisites should be met: (1) The flexor carpi ulnaris should be normal or good in motor power. (2) There should be full range of passive supination of the forearm, dorsiflexion of the wrist, and extension of the fingers. If any fixed contractural deformity is present, it should be corrected by

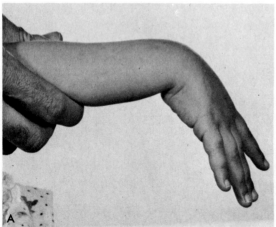

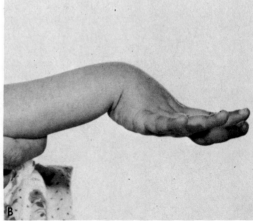

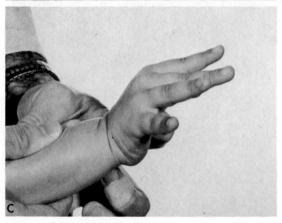

FIGURE 5–64. *Flexor carpi ulnaris transfer to extensor carpi radialis longus (Green procedure).*

A to C. Preoperative photographs.
Illustration continued on opposite page

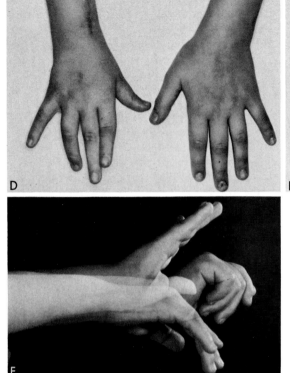

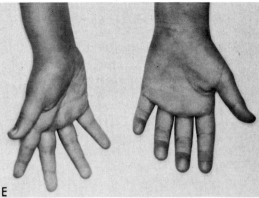

FIGURE 5–64 Continued. Flexor carpi ulnaris transfer to extensor carpi radialis longus (Green procedure).

D to F. Postoperative photographs.

successive stretching casts and an aggressive regimen of passive exercises. In severe and resistant cases, the pronator teres may have to be lengthened or reinserted to a wrist dorsi-flexor. Such procedures are usually indicated in neglected cases in which the patient has had no conservative therapy prior to surgery. (3) Motor control of the fingers is an equally important prerequisite for success of the operation. With the wrist in neutral extension, the patient should be able to extend the fingers actively (Fig. 5–65). If active finger action is not present, a passive stretching cast is applied, and in recalcitrant cases, fractional lengthening of the flexor digitorum profundus and sublimis is initially performed. (4) Voluntary control of the muscles of the hand-wrist, forearm, and elbow should be adequate to allow satisfactory function after the transplant. Diffuse hypotonia of the upper limb is a contraindication to flexor carpi ulnaris transfer. Hand placement test should be normal; if the patient cannot put his involved hand on an object on the examining table or on his knee, nose, or head, flexor carpi ulnaris transfer should not be performed; the operative procedure will not improve function. (5) Adequate sensory function in the hand is desirable; astereognosis is a great handicap to postoperative training but is not a contraindication to the procedure. It is true that function is propor-

tional to stereognosis and that best results are obtained in those with good stereognosis. However, significant improvement in function and

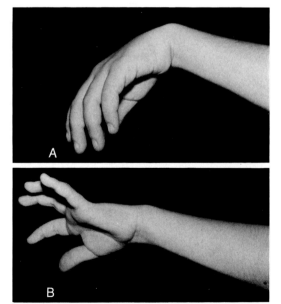

FIGURE 5–65. Prior to Green's flexor carpi ulnaris transfer the patient should be able to extend the fingers with the wrist in neutral extension.

A. Wrist in flexion. B. Note finger extension with wrist in extended position.

appearance can be obtained with surgery in those patients with "fair" stereognosis provided that they have satisfactory motor control of the upper limb. (6) The intellect of the child should be sufficient so that he cooperates with the postoperative habilitation. However, low IQ is not an absolute contraindication to surgery. A laborer with an IQ of 50 or 60 will benefit from the procedure because of improvement in the posture and strength of his hand. The grasp of the hand is weak when the wrist is palmar flexed. Placing the wrist in neutral or slightly dorsiflexed posture will strengthen the grasp. (7) The patient should be old enough to comply with the postoperative habilitation program. It is preferable to delay the flexor carpi ulnaris transfer until the patient is six or seven years of age. (8) Type of cerebral palsy. Any component of athetosis may lead to an undesirable hyperextension deformity of the wrist that may be more disabling than the original deformity.

The operative technique and postoperative care for Green's flexor carpi ulnaris transfer are described and illustrated in Plate 72.

Transfer of the flexor carpi ulnaris through the interosseous route is not indicated in spastic cerebral palsy.

Arthrodesis of the wrist in functional position is rarely performed in spastic paralysis. Wrist and forearm motions are important complements to effective use of the hand. In the experience of Green and Banks since the development of the flexor carpi ulnaris transfer, it has not been necessary to do a wrist fusion. The author recommends wrist fusion only in the athetoid patient in whom stabilization of the wrist in functional position enables active grasp and release and improves finger control. This can be done preoperatively by stabilizing the wrist with a plastic splint. Also, wrist fusion is indicated in the completely flail wrist-hand. In such an instance, stabilization of the wrist in neutral position will serve to improve function as an assisting post and provide a better hand cosmetically.

PRONATION CONTRACTURE OF THE FOREARM

Pronation contracture of the forearm may exist without flexion deformity of the wrist. The patient is able to extend the wrist, with normal muscle balance between the wrist flexors and extensors. In such an instance, lengthening of the pronator teres is performed, and later, reinforcement of active force of supination may be indicated by transfer of the flexor carpi ulnaris to the radius at the insertion of the brachioradialis tendon.

This is usually associated with flexion deformity of the wrist and elbow. It may be quite disabling and restrict function, preventing activities that require supination, such as turning a doorknob and receiving change. Fractional lengthening of the pronator teres at its insertion is a very simple procedure. It should be performed when the forearm cannot be supinated minus 45 to 30 degrees from neutral position. A 4 to 5 cm. longitudinal incision is made over the insertion of the pronator teres at the middle one third of the radius. Subcutaneous tissue and fasciae are divided in line with the incision. The brachioradialis is retracted medially, and the extensor carpi radialis longus is retracted dorsolaterally, exposing the tendon and muscles of the pronator teres. At its musculotendinous juncture, two transverse incisions are made 1 cm. apart, lengthening the pronator teres. The wound is closed over a closed Hemovac suction tube, and an above-elbow cast is applied, holding the forearm in full supination. This author has not found it necessary to transfer the pronator teres to the wrist extensors.[470]

This author has also found it unnecessary to transfer the pronator teres posteriorly to the anterolateral border of the radius, converting it from a pronator to a supinator. This operation was described by Sakellarides et al.[465] The results in their experience with 22 patients were good or excellent in 82 per cent. They felt that function of the upper limb was significantly improved by giving these patients the ability to supinate the forearm during activities requiring axial rotation of the forearm. In the experience of this author, flexor carpi ulnaris transfer is a more effective procedure to provide forearm supination.

In severe pronation contracture, the radial head may subluxate or dislocate posterolaterally. It is vital that during the examination of a child with cerebral palsy, the range of passive supination be tested and the radial head palpated to ensure that it is not subluxating. Dislocation of the radial head is a preventable deformity by simple lengthening of the pronator teres.

FLEXION DEFORMITY OF THE ELBOW

This is commonly present in cerebral palsy. The deformity is usually minimal or moderate and is effectively controlled by passive stretching exercises. Sometimes in neglected cases, it is very severe and presents a significant functional handicap. In such an instance, the biceps and brachialis muscles are lengthened in their musculotendinous portions. This author has found it unnecessary to perform a Z-lengthening of the biceps tendon or to divide the lacertus; however, in the very severe fixed flexion elbow deformity, this may be required.[354] Z-lengthening may cause weakening of supination of the forearm, and it is a calculated risk of the procedure. This author does not recommend neurectomy.

SHOULDER DEFORMITY

The usual shoulder deformity is one of medial rotation and adduction. Ordinarily, this is effectively managed by passive stretching exercises. Rarely, in neglected cases, lengthening of the pectoralis major and subscapularis muscles may be indicated.

Abduction contracture of the shoulder may develop in *acquired* cerebral palsy because of spasticity of the deltoid muscle. In the severe case it may be so disturbing cosmetically that a deltoid release at its insertion may be indicated (Fig. 5–66). This is performed through a longitudinal incision. The tendinous fibers of the anterior two thirds of the deltoid muscle are detached from their insertion to the tuberosity of the humerus, and the deltoid muscle is recessed (Fig. 5–67). The posterior one third of the deltoid should be avoided. Caution! Do not injure the radial nerve! The shoulder is immobilized for four weeks in a Velpeau bandage reinforced by a plaster of Paris cast.

Scoliosis

The incidence of structural scoliosis in adolescents and young adults with cerebral palsy is reported to be 15.2 per cent by Robson, and 21 per cent by Balmer and MacEwen. In 4 per cent of the cases of Robson, the scoliosis was considered to be moderately severe; in 6 per cent of the series of cases by Balmer and MacEwen, the curvature was more than 30 degrees.[16, 445]

Samilson and Bechard studied the incidence of scoliosis in 905 cerebral palsy patients who were institutionalized with severe involvement; of these, 232 (25 per cent) had scoliosis.[473]

Scoliosis may result from (1) *pelvic obliquity,*

Text continued on page 1755

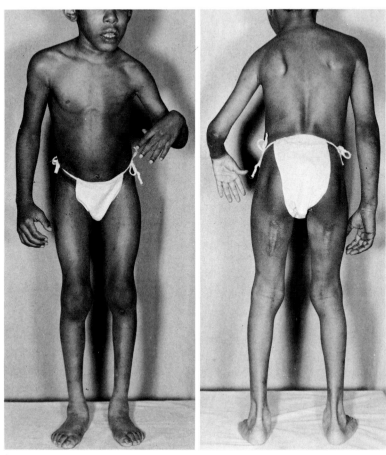

FIGURE 5–66. Abduction contracture of the shoulder in acquired cerebral palsy.

Flexor Carpi Ulnaris Transfer (Green Procedure)

OPERATIVE TECHNIQUE

The operation is usually performed with the patient in supine position; some surgeons, however, prefer the patient to be in prone position, as it facilitates manipulating the forearm and holding the wrist in dorsiflexed position. The author uses the prone position when there is pronation deformity of the forearm and medial rotation contracture of the shoulder.

A. An anteromedial incision is made over the flexor carpi ulnaris tendon. It starts at the flexor crease of the wrist and extends proximally and somewhat ulnarward over the belly of the muscle to the junction of the middle and upper thirds of the forearm (Green and Banks make two incisions, one distal and the other proximal).

B and **C.** The subcutaneous tissue is divided, and the tendon of the flexor carpi ulnaris is exposed. The ulnar nerve, lying immediately posterior to the tendon, is visualized and protected from injury. The tendon is detached at its insertion to the pisiform bone and mobilized proximally. The muscle fibers of the flexor carpi ulnaris take their origin from the ulna quite distally; they are stripped extraperiosteally from the underlying bone by sharp and dull dissection. The muscle is freed proximally as far as possible without disturbing its nerve supply from the ulnar nerve (which is the limiting factor of proximal dissection). The mobilization of the flexor carpi ulnaris should be high enough to allow its passage in a straight line from its origin to the dorsum of the wrist. The extensor compartment of the forearm is entered by excising a segment of the intermuscular septum at the medial margin of the ulna.

Plate 72. Flexor Carpi Ulnaris Transfer (Green Procedure)

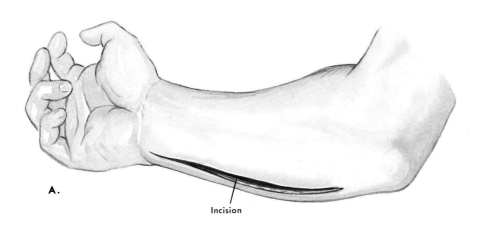

A.

Incision

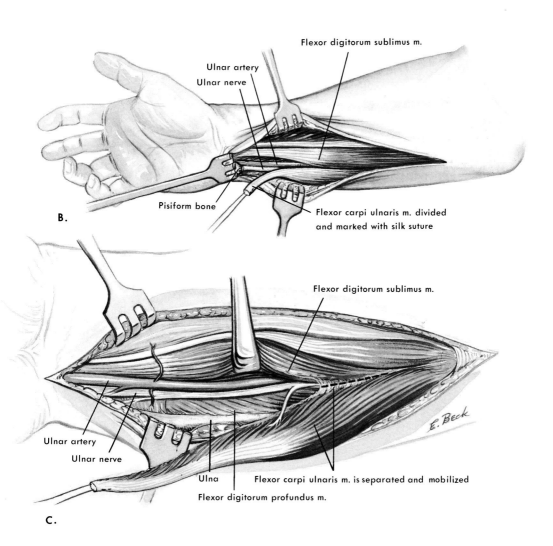

Flexor digitorum sublimus m.

Ulnar artery

Ulnar nerve

Pisiform bone

Flexor carpi ulnaris m. divided and marked with silk suture

B.

Flexor digitorum sublimus m.

E. Beck

Ulnar artery

Ulnar nerve

Ulna

Flexor carpi ulnaris m. is separated and mobilized

Flexor digitorum profundus m.

C.

Flexor Carpi Ulnaris Transfer (Green Procedure)
(Continued)

OPERATIVE TECHNIQUE

D. Next, a longitudinal incision is made on the dorsum of the wrist over the extensor carpi radialis longus and brevis tendons. It starts at the distal end of the radius immediately above the transverse crease and extends proximally for a distance of 3 cm.

E and **F.** The incision is carried through the subcutaneous tissue and fascia. The extensor carpi radialis longus (in line with the second metacarpal) and the extensor carpi radialis brevis (in line with the third metacarpal) tendons are identified and isolated.

An Ober tendon transfer is passed from the proximal portion of the ulnar incision to the wound on the dorsum of the wrist. The flexor carpi ulnaris tendon is passed around the ulna through the channel created by the Ober tendon transfer. The line of pull of the tendon should be as straight as possible. On the dorsum of the wrist and forearm the ulnaris tendon should be along the extensor communis tendons.

G and **H.** With a No. 11 blade knife a buttonhole is made in the extensor carpi radialis longus or brevis tendon. When there is ulnar deviation of the wrist, the ulnaris tendon is attached to the longus; when the wrist is in neutral posture, it is inserted into the radialis longus and brevis tendons. In the original description of Green, when there was ulnar deviation of the wrist the ulnaris tendon was attached to the longus.

With the forearm in full supination and the wrist in 25 degrees of dorsiflexion, the ulnaris tendon is sutured to the extensor tendon. The tension on the ulnaris tendon should be such that the wrist can be passively palmar flexed 40 degrees, but when the tension is released, it should resume a position of 35 to 45 degrees of dorsiflexion. The method of suturing is not important. The author prefers that the ulnaris tendon pass through the buttonhole and be sutured to itself. In addition, three interrupted sutures are used to transfix the ulnaris and radialis tendons securely.

I. The wound is closed in layers as an assistant holds the forearm in full supination and the wrist in marked dorsiflexion. An above-elbow cast is applied with the forearm in full supination, the wrist in 60 degrees of dorsiflexion, the thumb in abduction, the metacarpophalangeal joint in 15 degrees of flexion, and the interphalangeal joint in neutral extension.

POSTOPERATIVE CARE

About three to four weeks after operation, the cast is bivalved and physical therapy is started to develop function in the transferred muscle. In the beginning, it consists of guided active exercises, attempting ulnar deviation and dorsiflexion of the wrist and supination of the forearm. Exercises are performed three to four times a day under supervision of the therapist and later of the parents (after thorough instruction by the therapist). The limb is maintained in the bivalved cast or plastic splint in the desired position except for the exercise periods for the following three weeks. The time out of the cast is then gradually increased. When out of the cast and not exercising, the patient wears a light short arm orthosis or plastic splint, which holds the wrist in 30 degrees of dorsiflexion and the thumb in maximal abduction and opposition. The support is discontinued when the flexor carpi ulnaris muscle is fair in motor strength and the wrist can be maintained in dorsiflexed functional position. If there is a tendency for the wrist to drop into flexion, the support with the dorsiflexion orthosis is continued part time during the day. The use of a night splint is continued until good function has developed and there is no tendency for recurrence of the original deformity. This may take many months or even several years. During the growth period, exercises are continued, with emphasis on active exercises to improve function of the hand and passive stretching exercises to maintain range of motion and to prevent recurrence of contractural deformity.

Plate 72. Flexor Carpi Ulnaris Transfer (Green Procedure)

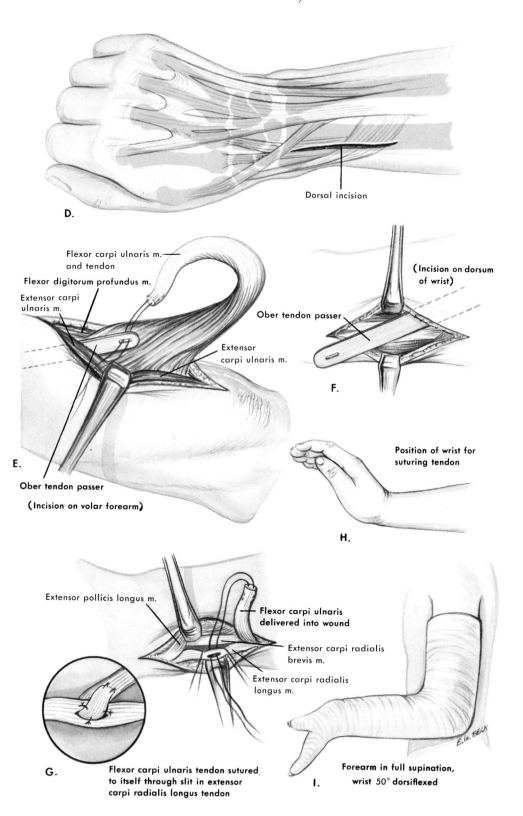

D.

Dorsal incision

Flexor carpi ulnaris m. and tendon

Flexor digitorum profundus m.

Extensor carpi ulnaris m.

Extensor carpi ulnaris m.

(Incision on dorsum of wrist)

Ober tendon passer

F.

E.

Ober tendon passer

(Incision on volar forearm)

Position of wrist for suturing tendon

H.

Extensor pollicis longus m.

Flexor carpi ulnaris delivered into wound

Extensor carpi radialis brevis m.

Extensor carpi radialis longus m.

G.

Flexor carpi ulnaris tendon sutured to itself through slit in extensor carpi radialis longus tendon

I.

Forearm in full supination, wrist 50° dorsiflexed

E.W. BECK

Flexor Carpi Ulnaris Transfer (Green Procedure) *(Continued)*

COMPLICATIONS

The reverse deformity of dorsiflexion contracture of the wrist may develop because of taut suturing of the flexor carpi ulnaris tendon with the wrist in 40 to 50 degrees of dorsiflexion. It is vital that the wrist be in only 25 degrees of dorsiflexion and that the wrist can be passively palmar flexed 40 degrees. Dorsiflexion deformity also may occur when the operation is performed in mixed cerebral palsy patients with spasticity and tension athetosis. The presence of extrapyramidal tract involvement is a contraindication to flexor carpi ulnaris transfer.

If dorsiflexion contracture of the wrist develops in the postoperative period, passive stretching casts are applied to correct, following which the wrist is supported part time in palmar flexed posture and exercises are performed to develop wrist flexion. If such nonoperative measures fail, the deformity is corrected by recessing the attachment of flexor carpi ulnaris near its insertion to extensor carpi radialis tendons.

Supination contracture is another complication that is often due to total release of the pronator teres performed simultaneously with flexor carpi ulnaris transfer. It is vital to lengthen and not totally release the pronator teres. Again, beware of the tension athetoid patient because reverse deformity may follow.

When there is flexion deformity of the wrist and pronation contracture of the forearm with good grasp by the weak extensors and release of the flexors, the flexor carpi ulnaris should be transferred to the extensor digitorum communis. The dynamic electromyographic studies of Hoffer et al. show that difficulty with a spastic hand is more that of weak release than that of weak grasp. Flexor carpi ulnaris is transferred to the finger extensors to improve finger extension, and flexor carpi ulnaris is transferred to extensor carpi radialis tendons to increase wrist extension alone. They recommend the following: Flexor carpi ulnaris is transferred to flexor digitorum communis when (1) release is weak; (2) grasp is adequate; and (3) EMG studies show that flexor carpi ulnaris is active. They recommend transfer of flexor carpi ulnaris to extensor carpi radialis tendons when (1) the grasp is weak with wrist flexion; (2) the release is adequate; (3) dynamic EMG studies show that the flexor carpi ulnaris is active with flexor digitorum pollicis. When deforming muscles are active throughout both phases of the grasp-release cycle, it is best to fractionally lengthen these muscles at the musculotendinous junction rather than transfer them.[227]

This author concurs with Hoffer et al.; however, when the finger and wrist flexors are lengthened fractionally at their musculotendinous juncture, he advises extensor tenodesis or shortening of the wrist extensors to provide some static support.

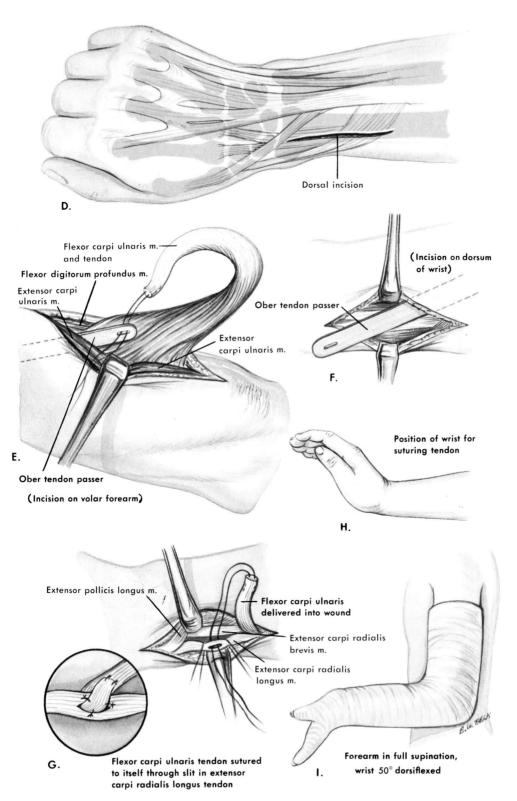

D.

Dorsal incision

Flexor carpi ulnaris m. and tendon

Flexor digitorum profundus m.

Extensor carpi ulnaris m.

Flexor carpi ulnaris m. and tendon

Extensor carpi ulnaris m.

Ober tendon passer

(Incision on dorsum of wrist)

F.

E.

Ober tendon passer

(Incision on volar forearm)

Position of wrist for suturing tendon

H.

Extensor pollicis longus m.

Flexor carpi ulnaris delivered into wound

Extensor carpi radialis brevis m.

Extensor carpi radialis longus m.

G.

Flexor carpi ulnaris tendon sutured to itself through slit in extensor carpi radialis longus tendon

I.

Forearm in full supination, wrist 50° dorsiflexed

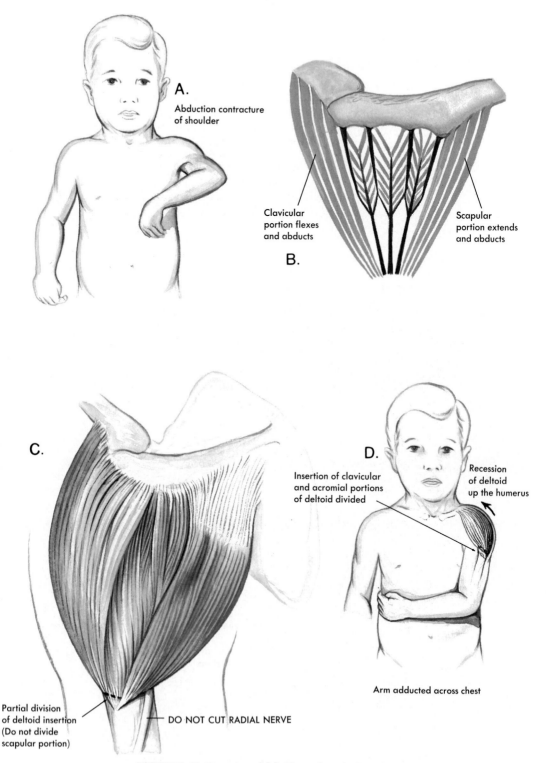

A.
Abduction contracture
of shoulder

Clavicular
portion flexes
and abducts

Scapular
portion extends
and abducts

B.

C.

D.

Insertion of clavicular
and acromial portions
of deltoid divided

Recession
of deltoid
up the humerus

Partial division
of deltoid insertion
(Do not divide
scapular portion)

DO NOT CUT RADIAL NERVE

Arm adducted across chest

FIGURE 5–67. Recession of deltoid muscle at its insertion.

which may be caused by asymmetrical involvement and contracture of the hip adductor or abductors, or by unilateral dislocation of the hip (Fig. 5–68); (2) *unilateral or asymmetrical spasticity or tension athetosis of the trunk musculature* (Fig. 5–69); (3) *congenital deformities of the vertebrae* such as hemivertebrae or unilateral bar; or (4) it may be *idiopathic.*

In cerebral palsy most of the curves are thoracolumbar or lumbar. Often there is exaggertion of dorsal roundback, which is postural and due to insufficiency of trunk extensor musculature.

TREATMENT

Ordinarily, orthotic devices are not well tolerated by the child with cerebral palsy. Cooperation is poor, and skin problems are frequent complications; however, early structural curves should be braced promptly and observed carfully for progression. Molded under-the-arm plastic body jackets are the orthosis of choice, especially for the common thoracolumbar and lumbar curves. High thoracic curves, however, require a Milwaukee brace.

Surgical intervention is indicated when there is curve progression and loss of function and when the curve is of high magnitude. Often, posterior fusion and internal instrumentation with Harrington rods or Luque intersegmental instrumentation is adequate; however, severe curves require combined anterior and posterior fusions. Preoperative traction is not effective in these patients.

The complication rate is very high, about 80 per cent; problems include pressure sores, wound healing problems, infection, instrumentation problems, pseudarthrosis, and death. Despite the great frequency of problems and complications, surgery is of definite benefit in the severely handicapped child with cerebral palsy. Stabilization of the spine significantly improves sitting balance and facilitates care of the patient.

Neurosurgical Modalities of Treatment

Rhizotomy of the Dorsal Nerve Roots. Experimentally in monkeys a flail limb results from cutting of the dorsal nerve roots. In time, some motor function returns. In the human, rhizotomy of the dorsal nerve roots has been performed; the initial results have been encouraging, with decrease in degree of spasticity.[39, 390] Data on long-term results are not available; at present, posterior rhizotomy for treatment of spasticity in cerebral palsy is considered investigational.

Stereotactic Surgery. Local destruction of selected areas of the brain by electric current or cryosurgery is reported to improve hyperkinesia and hypertonia.[77a, 77b, 191a, 379, 577a] Stereotactic surgery, however, has serious drawbacks: It

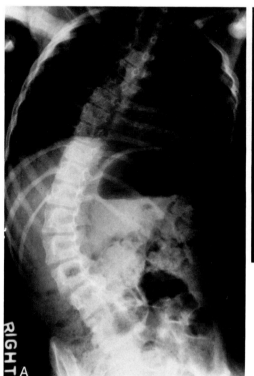

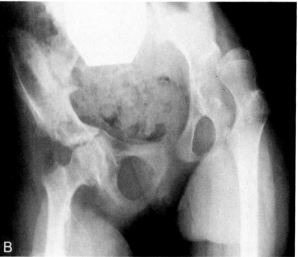

FIGURE 5–68. Severe cerebral palsy with dislocation of the left hip and severe thoracic lumbar scoliosis in a 12-year-old girl.

A. Anteroposterior radiogram of spine. **B.** Anteroposterior radiogram of hips.

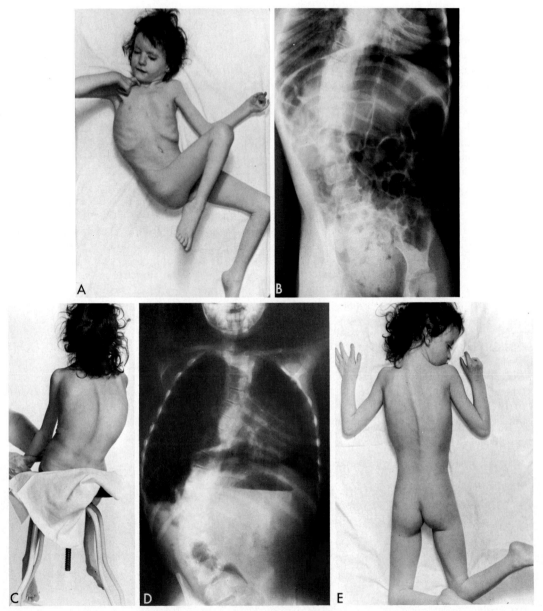

FIGURE 5–69. Scoliosis in a child with mixed type of cerebral palsy—spastic and tension athetoid.

A and B. Anteroposterior photograph and radiogram of patient. C and D. Posteroanterior photograph and radiogram with the patient sitting. E. When lying face down, the position is secure and tension athetosis is diminished. Note the decrease in the degree of curvature.

can cause autonomic and mental disturbance, motor dysfunction, and sensory impairment. Brain damage in cerebral palsy is diffuse, and interneuronal connections are complex. This author does not recommend stereotactic surgery because of its serious risks and gravity of complications.

Cerebellar Stimulation. Cooper introduced the "cerebellar pacemaker." A self-controlled stimulator was implanted on the surface of the cerebellum, and the tone of the spastic muscles decreased.[113] Davis et al. reported satisfactory results in a large series of 262 patients.[126] However, other investigators did not report any significant benefit from cerebellar stimulators.[41b, 259] At present the use of cerebellar pacemakers in the treatment of cerebral palsy patients is experimental; it is not recommended.

Drooling. Excessive salivation can be quite

disturbing to the parents and to the intellectually aware child, as the constant use of a bib is unsightly and inconvenient. Surgical treatment is not indicated in the infant and young child; however, in the older child and adolescent this author recommends plastic surgery. Excision of the salivary (submandibular) glands or transplantation of the salivary ducts to the tonsillar fossa is effective in decreasing excessive salivation.[347] Biofeedback methods have been tried and found to be successful in a small number of patients.[297]

References

1. Adler, N., Bleck, E. E., and Rinsky, L. A.: Decision-making in surgical treatment of paralytic deformities of the foot with gait electromyograms. Presented at the Annual Meeting of A.A.C.P.D.M., 1984. Dev. Med. Child Neurol., 27:106, 1985.
2. Albaugh, C. H.: Congenital anomalies following maternal rubella in early weeks of pregnancy with special emphasis on congenital cataract. J.A.M.A., 129:719, 1945.
3. Anderson, B.: Cerebral palsy. J. Oslo City Hosp., 4:65, 1954.
4. Angelini, L., Broggi, G., Nardocci, N., and Savoiardo, M.: Subacute cervical myelopathy in a child with cerebral palsy. Secondary to torsion dystonia? Childs Brain, 9:354, 1982.
5. Anthonsen, W.: Treatment of hip flexion contracture in cerebral palsy patients. Acta Orthop. Scand., 37:387, 1966.
6. Arvidsson, J., and Eksmyr, R.: Cerebral palsy and perinatal deaths in geographically defined populations with different perinatal services. Dev. Med. Child Neurol., 26:709, 1984.
7a. Ayres, A. J.: Characteristics of types of sensory integrative dysfunction. Am. J. Occup. Ther., 7:329, 1971.
7b. Ayres, A. J.: Effect of sensory integrative therapy on the coordination of children with choreoathetoid movements. Am. J. Occup. Ther., 31:291, 1977.
8. Badell-Ribera, A.: Cerebral palsy: Postural-locomotor prognosis in spastic diplegia. Arch. Phys. Med. Rehabil., 66:614, 1985.
9. Baker, L. D.: Triceps surae syndrome in cerebral palsy. Surgery, 68:216, 1954.
10. Baker, L. D.: Surgery in cerebral palsy. Arch. Phys. Med., 36:88, 1955.
11. Baker, L. D.: A rational approach to the surgical needs of the cerebral palsy patient. J. Bone Joint Surg., 38-A:313, 1956.
12. Baker, L. D., and Dodelin, R. A.: Extra-articular arthrodesis of the subtalar joint (Grice procedure): Results in seventeen patients with cerebral palsy. J.A.M.A., 168:1005, 1958.
13. Baker, L. D., Dodelin, R. A., and Bassett, F. H., III.: Pathological changes in the hip in cerebral palsy, incidence, pathogenesis, and treatment—preliminary report. J. Bone Joint Surg., 44-A:1331, 1962.
14. Baker, L. D., and Hill, L. M.: Foot alignment in the cerebral palsy patient. J. Bone Joint Surg., 46-A:1, 1964.
15. Balf, C. L., and Ingram, T. T. S.: Problems in the classification of cerebral palsy. Br. Med. J., 2:163, 1955.
16. Balmer, G. A., and MacEwen, G. D.: The incidence and treatment of scoliosis in cerebral palsy. J. Bone Joint Surg., 52-B:134, 1970.
17. Banks, H. H.: The foot and ankle in cerebral palsy. In Samilson, R. L. (ed.): Orthopedic Aspects of Cerebral Palsy. Philadelphia, J. B. Lippincott, 1975, pp. 212–215.
18. Banks, H. H.: The Grice procedure (letter). Clin. Orthop., 160:309, 1981.
18a. Banks, H. H.: Management of spastic deformities of the foot and ankle. Clin. Orthop., 122:70, 1972.
19. Banks, H. H., and Green, W. T.: The correction of equinus deformity in cerebral palsy. J. Bone Joint Surg., 40-A:1359, 1958.
20. Banks, H. H., and Green, W. T.: Adductor myotomy and obturator neurectomy for the correction of adduction contracture of the hip in cerebral palsy. J. Bone Joint Surg., 42-A:111, 1960.
21. Banks, H. H., and Panagakos, P.: Orthopaedic evaluation of the lower extremity in cerebral palsy. Clin. Orthop., 47:117, 1966.
22. Banks, H. H., and Panagakos, P.: The role of the orthopedic surgeon in cerebral palsy. Pediatr. Clin. North Am., 14:495, 1967.
23. Barbieri, E., and Garcia, M.: Observazioni sulla terapia chirurgica del piede spastico. Minerva Orthop., 21:639, 1970.
24. Barnett, H. E.: Orthopedic surgery in cerebral palsy. J.A.M.A., 150:1396, 1952.
25. Baron, M.: La chirurgie de l'infirmite motrice cerebrale chez l'enfant. Le pied. Rev. Chir. Orthop., 53:739, 1967.
26. Barr, J. S.: Muscle transplantation for combined flexion–internal rotation deformity of the thigh in spastic paralysis. Arch. Surg., 46:605, 1943.
27. Bassett, F. H.: The foot in cerebral palsy. In Giannestras, N. J.: Foot Disorders. Medical and Surgical Management. Philadelphia, Lea & Febiger, 1967, pp. 247–265.
28. Bassett, F. H., III: Cerebral palsy. Part II: Deformities of the feet due to cerebral palsy. A.A.O.S. Instr. Course Lect., 20:35, 1971.
29. Bassett, F. H., III, and Baker, D.: Equinus deformity in cerebral palsy. In Adams, J. P. (ed.): Current Practice in Orthopaedic Surgery. Vol. 3. St. Louis, C. V. Mosby, 1966, p. 59.
30. Batchelor, J. S.: Personal communication to Seymour, N. (#490).
31. Baumann, J. U.: 'Indication for Harrington's spine instrumentation for scoliosis in cerebral palsy. In Chapchal, G. (ed.): Operative Treatment of Scoliosis. Stuttgart, Georg Thieme Verlag, 1973, pp. 91–94.
32. Baumann, J. U., Meyer, E., and Schurmann, K.: Hip adductor transfer to the ischial tuberosity in spastic and paralytic hip disorders. Arch. Orthop. Trauma Surg., 92:107, 1978.
33. Bax, M.: Child abuse and cerebral palsy (editorial). Dev. Med. Child Neurol., 25:141, 1983.
34. Beals, R. K.: Spastic paraplegia and diplegia. An evaluation of non-surgical and surgical factors in influencing the prognosis for ambulation. J. Bone Joint Surg., 48-A:827, 1966.
35. Beals, R. K. J.: Developmental changes in the femur and acetabulum in spastic paraplegia and diplegia. Dev. Med. Child Neurol., 11:303, 1969.
36. Beaman, P.: Restriction, fatigue and motor activity in cerebral palsy. In Child Neurology and Cerebral Palsy. A report of an International Study Group, St. Edmund Hall, Oxford, 1960. Little Club Clinics in Developmental Medicine, No. 2, p. 82. London, Medical Advisory Committee of the National Spastics Society, 1961.
37. Beintema, D. J.: A Neurological Study of Newborn Infants. Clinics in Developmental Medicine No. 28. London, Spastics Society Medical Education and Information Unit in Association with William Heinemann Medical Books, 1968.

38. Bell, M.: Proximal hamstring release—anterior approach. Read at the 28th Annual Meeting of the Canadian Orthopaedic Association, Quebec City, Quebec, June 1972.

39. Benedetti, A., Colombo, F., Alexandre, A., and Pellegri, A.: Posterior rhizotomies for spasticity in children affected by cerebral palsy. J. Neurosurg. Sci., 26:179, 1982.

40a. Bennet, G. C., Rang, M., and Jones, D.: Varus and valgus deformities of the foot in cerebral palsy. Dev. Med. Child Neurol., 24:499, 1982.

40b. Bennett, J. T., Bunnell, W. P., and MacEwen, G. D.: Rotational osteotomy of the distal tibia and fibula. J. Pediatr. Orthop., 5:294, 1985.

41a. Bensahel, H., and Baum, C.: Le transfert des muscles adducteurs dans l'equilibration de la hanche chez l'enfant I.M.C. Ann. Chir. Infant., 15:179, 1974.

41b. Bensman, A. S., and Szegho, M.: Cerebellar electrical stimulation: a critique. Arch. Phys. Med. Rehab., 59:485, 1978.

42. Berenberg, W., and Ong, B. H.: Cerebral spastic paraplegia and prematurity. Pediatrics, 33:496, 1964.

43. Berger, W., Quintern, J., and Dietz, V.: Pathophysiology of gait in children with cerebral palsy. Electroencephalogr. Clin. Neurophysiol., 53:538, 1982.

44. Bertrand, P.: Correction du genu flexum chez les spastiques. Rev. Chir. Orthop., 45:416, 1959.

45. Bisla, R. S., Louis, H. J., and Albano, P.: Transfer of tibialis posterior tendon in cerebral palsy. J. Bone Joint Surg., 58-A:497, 1976.

46. Black, P. D.: Ocular defects in children with cerebral palsy. Br. Med. J., 281:487, 1980.

47. Black, P. D.: Visual disorders associated with cerebral palsy. Br. J. Ophthalmol., 66:46, 1982.

48. Blair, E., and Stanley, F. J.: An epidemiological study of cerebral palsy in Western Australia, 1956–1975. III. Postnatal aetiology. Dev. Med. Child Neurol., 24:575, 1982.

49. Blair, E., and Stanley, F.: Interobserver agreement in the classification of cerebral palsy. Dev. Med. Child Neurol., 27:615, 1985.

50. Blake, D. D., Andrasik, F., McCarran, M., and Quinn, S.: Validity of six measures for assessing social skills in cerebral palsied patients. Presented at the Annual Meeting of A.A.C.P.D.M., 1984. Dev. Med. Child Neurol., 27:98, 1985.

51. Bleck, E. E.: The management of hip deformities in cerebral palsy. In Adams, J. P. (ed.): Current Practice in Orthopaedic Surgery. Vol. 3. St. Louis, C. V. Mosby, 1966.

52. Bleck, E. E.: Spastic abductor hallucis. Dev. Med. Child Neurol., 9:602, 1967.

53. Bleck, E. E.: Postural and gait abnormalities caused by hip flexion deformity in spastic cerebral palsy. J. Bone Joint Surg., 53-A:1468, 1971.

54. Bleck, E. E.: Deformities of the spine and pelvis in cerebral palsy. In Samilson, R. L. (ed.): Orthopaedic Aspects of Cerebral Palsy. Philadelphia, J. B. Lippincott, 1975, pp. 124–144.

55. Bleck, E. E.: Locomotor prognosis in cerebral palsy. Dev. Med. Child Neurol., 17:18, 1975.

56. Bleck, E. E.: The hip in cerebral palsy. Orthop. Clin. North Am., 11:79, 1980.

57. Bleck, E. E.: Forefoot problems in cerebral palsy—diagnosis and management. Foot Ankle, 4:188, 1984.

58. Bleck, E. E.: Where have all the CP children gone?—The needs of adults. Dev. Med. Child Neurol., 26:675, 1984.

59. Bleck, E. E.: Orthopaedic Management of Cerebral Palsy. Philadelphia, J. B. Lippincott Co., 1987.

60. Bleck, E. E., and Holstein, A.: Iliopsoas tenotomy for spastic paralytic deformities of the hip. J. Bone Joint Surg., 46-A:375, 1964.

61. Blumel, J., Eggers, G. W. N., and Evans, E. B.: Genetic metabolic and clinical study on one hundred cerebral palsied patients. J.A.M.A., 174:860, 1960.

62. Bobath, B.: Treatment principles and planning in cerebral palsy. Physiotherapy, 49:122, 1963.

63. Bobath, B., and Finnie, N.: Re-education of movement patterns in everyday life in the treatment of cerebral palsy. Occup. Ther., 21:23, 1958.

64. Bobath, K.: The Motor Deficits in Patients with Cerebral Palsy. Clinics in Developmental Medicine No. 23. London, The Spastics Society Medical Education and Information Unit in Association with William Heinemann Medical Books, 1966.

65. Bobath, K., and Bobath, B.: Control of motor function in the treatment of cerebral palsy. Physiotherapy, 43:295, 1957.

66. Bobath, K., and Bobath, B.: An assessment of the motor handicap in children with cerebral palsy and of their response to treatment. Occup. Ther. J., 21:19, 1958.

67. Bobath, K., and Bobath, B.: The facilitation of normal postural reactions and movements in the treatment of cerebral palsy. Physiotherapy, 1:3, 1964.

68. Bobath, K., and Bobath, B.: The treatment of spastic paralysis by the use of reflex inhibition. Br. J. Phys. Med., 13:1, 1965.

69. Bohm, H., and Lippmann, J.: Care for cerebral palsied children and adolescents in a district. Z. Gesamte. Hyg., 27:160, 1981.

70. Bojarski, L.: Surgical treatment of clubfoot in spastic form of cerebral palsy by a modified Strayer's method with elongation of the Achilles tendon. Chir. Narzadow. Ruchu. Ortop. Pol., 47:77, 1982.

71. Bonnett, C., Brown, J. C., and Grow, T.: Thoracolumbar scoliosis in cerebral palsy. Results of surgical treatment. J. Bone Joint Surg., 58-A:328, 1976.

72. Bonnett, C., Brown, J. C., Perry, J., Nickel, V. L., Walinski, T., Brooks, L., Hoffer, M., Stiles, C., and Brooks, R.: Evolution of treatment of paralytic scoliosis at Rancho Los Amigos Hospital. J. Bone Joint Surg., 57-A:206, 1975.

73. Bowen, J. R., MacEwen, G. D., and Mathews, P. A.: Treatment of extension contracture of the hip in cerebral palsy. Dev. Med. Child Neurol., 23:23, 1981.

74. Bradford, E. H.: The surgical treatment of spastic paralysis in children. Trans. Am. Orthop. Assoc., 3:7, 1890. (Boston Med. Surg. J., 73:485, 1890.)

75. Braun, R. M., Mooney, V., and Nickel, V. L.: Flexor origin release for pronation-flexion deformity of the forearm and hand in the stroke patient. J. Bone Joint Surg., 52-B:907, 1970.

76. Braun, R. M., Vise, G. T., and Roper, B.: Preliminary experience with superficialis-to-profundus tendon transfer in the hemiplegic upper extremity. J. Bone Joint Surg., 56-A:466, 1974.

77a. Broggi, G., Angelini, L., and Giorgi, C.: Neurological and psychological side effects after stereotactic thalamotomy in patients with cerebral palsy. Neurosurgery, 7:127, 1980.

77b. Broggi, G., Bono, R., Giorgi, C., Nardocci, N., and Franzini, A.: Long term results of stereotactic thalamotomy for cerebral palsy. Neurosurgery, 12:195, 1983.

77c. Broms, J. D.: Sub-talar extra-articular arthrodesis—follow-up study. Clin. Orthop., 42:139, 1965.

78. Brooks, M., and Wardle, E. N.: Iliopsoas-muscle action and the shape of the femur. J. Bone Joint Surg., 44-B:398, 1962.

79. Brown, A.: A simple method of fusion of the subtalar joint in children. J. Bone Joint Surg., 50-B:369, 1968.

80. Brown, J. C., Swank, S. M., Matta, J., and Barras, D. M.: Late spinal deformity in quadriplegic children and adolescents. J. Pediatr. Orthop., 4:456, 1984.

81. Buchwald, E.: Physical Rehabilitation for Daily Living. New York, McGraw-Hill, 1952.

82. Buckley, E., and Seaber, J. H.: Dyskinetic strabismus as a sign of cerebral palsy. Am. J. Ophthalmol., 91:652, 1981.

83. Bunnell, W. P., and Goncalves, J.: Varus derotational osteotomy of the hip in cerebral palsy. Presented at the Annual Meeting of A.A.C.P.D.M., 1984. Dev. Med. Child Neurol., 27:102, 1985.

84. Bunnell, W. P., and MacEwen, G. D.: Non-operative treatment of scoliosis in cerebral palsy; preliminary report on the use of a plastic jacket. Dev. Med. Child Neurol., 19:45, 1977.

85. Burman, M. S.: Spastic intrinsic-muscle imbalance of the foot. J. Bone Joint Surg., 20:145, 1938.

86. Burygina, A. D., Nenko, A. M., and Muzyka, V. P.: Orthopedic treatment of children with diplegic form of infantile cerebral palsy. Ortop. Travmatol. Protez., 12:35, 1981.

87. Byers, R. K.: Evolution of hemiplegias in infancy. Am. J. Dis. Child., 6:915, 1941.

88. Cahuzac, M.: L'enfant infirme moteur d'origine cerebrale. Paris, Masson, 1977.

89. Cahuzac, M., Claverie, P., Olle, R., Mansat, C., Nichil, J., and Delpech, R.: Notre experience de la chirurgie du pied chez l'enfant infirme moteur cerebral. Chirurgie, 98:680, 1972.

90. Cahuzac, M., Nichil, J., Claverie, T., Mansat, M., and Delpech, R.: La main hemiplegique de l'enfant I.M.C. Rev. Chir. Orthop., 59:321, 1973.

91. Cain, R.: Drugs in paediatric rehabilitation. Int. Rehabil. Med., 5:181, 1983.

92. Campbell, J., and Ball, J.: Energetics of walking in cerebral palsy. Orthop. Clin. North Am., 9:374, 1978.

93. Carpenter, E. B.: Role of nerve blocks in the foot and ankle in cerebral palsy: Therapeutic and diagnostic. Foot Ankle, 4:164, 1983.

94. Carpenter, E. B., and Mikhail, M.: The use of intramuscular alcohol as a diagnostic and therapeutic aid in cerebral palsy (abstract). Dev. Med. Child Neurol., 14:113, 1972.

95. Carpenter, E. B., and Seitz, D. G.: Intramuscular alcohol as an aid in management of spastic cerebral palsy. Dev. Med. Child Neurol., 22:497, 1980.

96. Carroll, R. E.: The treatment of cerebral palsy in the upper extremity. Bull. N.Y. Orthop. Hosp., 3:1958.

97. Carroll, R. E., and Craig, F. S.: The surgical treatment of cerebral palsy—the upper extremity. Surg. Clin. North Am., 31:385, 1951.

98. Carruthers, D. G.: Congenital deaf mutism as sequela of rubella-like infection during pregnancy. Med. J. Aust., 1:315, 1945.

99. Castle, M. E., and Schneider, C.: Proximal femoral resection-interposition arthroplasty. J. Bone Joint Surg., 60-A:1051, 1978.

100. Chait, L. A., Kaplan, I., Stewart-Lord, B., and Goodman, M.: Early surgical correction in the cerebral palsied hand. J. Hand Surg., 5:122, 1980.

101. Chambers, E. F. S.: An operation for correction of flexible flat feet of adolescents. West. J. Surg., 54:77, 1946.

102. Chandler, F. A.: Re-establishment of normal leverage of patella in knee flexion deformity in spastic paralysis. Surg. Gynecol. Obstet., 57:523, 1933.

103. Chandler, F. A.: Patellar advancement operation. Revised technique. J. Int. Coll. Surg., 3:433, 1940.

104. Chigot, P. L., and Sananes, P.: Arthrodese de Grice; indications nouvelles et variant technique. Rev. Chir. Orthop., 51:53, 1965.

105. Chong, K. C., Vojnic, C. D., Quanbury, A. O., and Letts, R. M.: The assessment of the internal rotation gait in cerebral palsy. An electromyographic gait analysis. Clin. Orthop., 132:145, 1978.

106. Cigala, F., Marmo, C., and Misasi, M.: Baker's operation in correction of spastic equinus deformity of the foot. Chir. Organi Mov., 65:519, 1979.

107. Cohen, M. E., and Duffner, P. K.: Prognostic indicators in hemiparetic cerebral palsy. Ann. Neurol., 9:353, 1981.

108. Colton, C., Ransfor, A. E., and Lloyd-Roberts, G. C.: Transposition of the tendon of pronator teres in cerebral palsy. J. Bone Joint Surg., 58-B:220, 1976.

109. Conrad, J. A., and Frost, H. M.: Evaluation of subcutaneous heelcord lengthening. Clin. Orthop., 64:121, 1969.

110. Conrad, L., and Bleck, E. E.: Augmented auditory feed back in the treatment of equinus gait in children. Dev. Med. Child Neurol., 22:713, 1980.

111. Cooper, I. S.: Relief of juvenile involuntary movement disorders by chemopallidectomy. J.A.M.A., 164:1297, 1957.

112. Cooper, I. S.: Neurosurgical alleviation of intention tremor of multiple sclerosis and cerebellar disease. N. Engl. J. Med., 26:441, 1960.

113. Cooper, I. S.: Clinical and physiologic implications of thalamic surgery for dystonia and torticollis. Bull. N.Y. Acad. Med., 41:870, 1965.

114. Cooper, I. S., Riklan, M., Amin, I., Waltz, J. M., and Cullinan, T.: Chronic cerebellar stimulation in cerebral palsy. Neurology, 26:744, 1976.

115. Couch, W. H., DeRosa, G. P., and Throop, F. B.: Thigh adductor transfer for spastic cerebral palsy. Dev. Med. Child Neurol., 19:343, 1977.

116. Courville, C. B.: Cerebral Palsy. Los Angeles, San Lucas Press, 1954.

117. Courville, C. B.: Structural changes in the brain in cerebral palsy. *In* Illingworth, R. (ed.): Recent Advances in Cerebral Palsy. London, J. & A. Churchill, 1958.

118. Craig, C. L., Sosnoff, F., and Zimbler, S.: Seating in cerebral palsy—a possible advance. Presented at the Annual Meeting of A.A.C.P.D.M., 1984. Dev. Med. Child Neurol., 27:93, 1985.

119. Craig, J. J.: Cerebral palsy. *In* W. D. Graham (ed.): Modern Trends in Orthopaedics. London, Butterworths, 1967, p. 44.

120. Craig, J. J., and van Vuren, J.: The importance of gastrocnemius recession in the correction of equinus deformity in cerebral palsy. J. Bone Joint Surg., 58-B:84, 1976.

121. Crawford, A. H., Bilbo, J. T., and Schniegenberg, G.: Subtalar stabilization by staple arthrodesis in the young child. Orthop. Trans., 10:152, 1986.

122. Crothers, B., and Paine, R. S.: The Natural History of Cerebral Palsy. Cambridge, Harvard University Press, 1959.

123. Dale, A., and Stanley, F. J.: An epidemiological study of cerebral palsy in Western Australia, 1956–1975. II. Spastic cerebral palsy and perinatal factors. Dev. Med. Child neurol., 22:13, 1980.

124. Davidson, R. S., and Carroll, N. C.: Cerebral palsy associated with maple syrup urine disease. J. Pediatr. Orthop., 2:165, 1982.

125. Davis, G. T., and Hill, P. M.: Cerebral palsy. Nurs. Clin. North Am., 15:35, 1980.

126. Davis, R., Barolat-Romana, G., and Engle, H.: Chronic cerebellar stimulation for cerebral palsy—5 year study. Acta Neurochir. (Suppl. 30), 317, 1980.

127. Deaver, G. G.: Cerebral palsy: methods of treating the neuromuscular disabilities. Arch. Phys. Med., 37:363, 1956.

128. de Bruin, H., Russell, D. J., Latter, J. E., and Sadler, J. T.: Angle-angle diagrams in monitoring and quantification of gait patterns for children with cerebral palsy. Am. J. Phys. Med., 61:176, 1982.

129. Dekel, S., and Weissman, S. L.: Osteotomy of the

calcaneus and concomitant plantar stripping in children with talipes cavo-varus. J. Bone Joint Surg., 55-B:802, 1973.

130. Delpech, J. M.: Tenotomie due tendon d'Achille, Chirurgie Clinique de Montpellier, ou Observations et Reflexions Tirées des Travaux de Chirurgie Clinique de Cette Ecole. Paris, Gabon, 1823.

131. Denhoff, E.: Pre- and post-operative managment of the cerebral-palsied. *In* Samilson, R. L. (ed.): Orthopaedic Aspects of Cerebral Palsy. Clinics in Developmental Medicine, No. 52/53, p. 112. London, William Heinemann Medical Books, 1975.

132. Denhoff, E., and Robinault, I. P.: Cerebral Palsy and Related Disorders. A Developmental Approach to Dysfunction. New York, McGraw-Hill, 1960.

133. Denny-Brown, E.: The Basal Ganglia and Their Relation to Disorders of Movement. London, Oxford University Press, 1962.

134. Dennyson, W. G., and Fulford, G. E.: Subtalar arthrodesis by cancellous grafts and metallic internal fixation. J. Bone Joint Surg., 58-B:507, 1976.

135. Desbrosses, J., and Stagnara, P.: Grice's operation. Rev. Chir. Orthop., 54:791, 1968.

136. Diamond, L. J., and Jaudes, P. K.: Child abuse in a cerebral palsied population. Dev. Med. Child Neurol., 25:169, 1983.

137. Dimeglio, A., Pous, J. G., and Florensa, G.: La chirurgie du membre inferieur de l'infirme moteur cerebral. Du reeducateur au chirurgien. *In* Simon, L. (ed.): Actualites en Reeducation Fonctionelle et Readaptation. Paris, Masson, 1976, pp. 120–127.

138. Doman, R. J., Spitz, E. B., Zucman, E., Delacato, C. H., and Doman, G.: Children with severe brain injuries. Neurological organizations in terms of mobility. J.A.M.A., 174:257, 1960.

139. Dowd, C. N.: Tendon transfer for the correction of spastic hand deformity. Med. Rev., 78:175, 1910.

140. Drozda, I. U. A.: Cardiovascular and respiratory system indices in children with cerebral palsy. Pediatriia, 8:61, 1983.

141. Drummond, D. S., Rogala, E. J., Cruess, R., and Moreau, M.: The paralytic hip and pelvic obliquity in cerebral palsy and myelomeningocele. A.A.O.S. Instr. Course Lect., 28:7, 1979.

142. Drummond, D. S., Rogala, E. J., Templeton, J., and Cruess, R.: Proximal hamstring release for knee flexion and crouched posture in cerebral palsy. J. Bone Joint Surg., 56-A:1598, 1974.

143. Duncan, W. R.: Release of rectus femoris in spastic paralysis. Presented at the Meeting of the American Academy of Orthopaedic Surgeons, Los Angeles, 1955.

144a. Duncan, W. R.: Tonic reflexes of the foot. J. Bone Joint Surg., 42-A:859, 1960.

144b. Duncan, W., and Mott, D.: Foot reflexes and the use of the inhibitive cast. Foot Ankle, 4:145, 1983.

145. Durham, H. A.: A procedure for the correction of internal rotation of the thigh in spastic paralysis. J. Bone Joint Surg., 20:339, 1938.

146. Dwyer, F. C.: Osteotomy of the calcaneum in the treatment of grossly everted feet with special reference to cerebral palsy. *In* Huitième Congres International de Chirurgie Orthopedique, New York 1960. Societé Internationale de Chirurgie Orthopedique et de Traumatologie, p. 892. Brussells, Imprimerie Lielers, 1960.

147. Editorial: Child abuse and cerebral palsy. Lancet, 1:1143, 1983.

148. Egel, P.: Technique of Treatment for the Cerebral Palsied Child. St. Louis, C. V. Mosby, 1948.

149. Eggers, G. W. N.: Surgical division of the patellar retinacular to improve extension of the knee joint in cerebral spastic paralysis. J. Bone Joint Surg., 32-A:80, 1950.

150. Eggers, G. W. N.: Transplantation of hamstring tendons to femoral condyles in order to improve hip extension and to decrease knee flexion in cerebral palsy. J. Bone Joint Surg., 34-A:827, 1952.

151. Egger, G. W. N.: Selective surgery for the cerebral palsy patient. A.A.O.S. Instr. Course Lect., 12:221, 1955.

152. Eggers, G. W. N., and Evans, E. B.: Surgery in cerebral palsy. An instructional course lecture. J. Bone Joint Surg., 45-A:1275, 1963.

153. Eiben, R. M., and Crocker, A. C.: Cerebral palsy with the spectrum of developmental disabilities. *In* Thompson, G. H., Rubon, I. L., and Bilender, R. M. (eds.): Comprehensive Management of Cerebral Palsy. New York, Grune & Stratton, 1983, pp. 19–23.

154. Eilert, R. E., and MacEwen, G. D.: Varus derotation osteotomy of the femur in cerebral palsy. Clin. Orthop., 125:168, 1977.

155. Estève, R.: Un procede d'equilibration des pieds spastique. Vie Med., 1:51, 1970.

156. Evans, E. B.: The status of surgery of the lower extremities in cerebral palsy. Clin. Orthop., 47:127, 1966.

157. Evans, E. B.: The knee in cerebral palsy. *In* Samilson, R. L. (ed.): Orthopaedic Aspects of Cerebral Palsy. Clinics in Developmental Medicine No. 52/53, p. 173. London, William Heinemann Medical Books, 1975.

158. Evans, E. B., and Julian, J. D.: Modifications of the hamstring transfer. Dev. Med. Child Neurol., 8:539, 1966.

159. Evans, P. M., and Alberman, E.: Recording motor defects of children with cerebral palsy (letter). Dev. Med. Child Neurol., 27:404, 1985.

160. Eyring, E. J., Earl, W. C., and Brockmeyer, J. F.: Posterior tibial tendon transfers in neuromuscular conditions other than anterior poliomyelitis. Arch. Phys. Med., 55:124, 1974.

161. Fairbank, H. A. T.: Birth palsy: subluxation of the shoulder-joint in infants and young children. Lancet, 1:1217, 1913.

162. Fay, T.: Observations on the rehabilitation of movement in cerebral palsy problems. W.V. Med. J., 42:77, 1946.

163. Fay, T.: The use of pathological and unlocking reflexes in rehabilitation of spastics. Am. J. Phys. Med., 33:347, 1954.

164. Feldkamp, M.: Late results of hip and knee surgery in severely handicapped cerebral palsy patients. Arch. Orthop. Trauma Surg., 100:217, 1982.

165. Ferguson, R., and MacEwen, G. D.: Adductor tenotomies and obturator neurectomies in cerebral palsied children. Orthop. Trans., 2:51, 1978.

166. Ferreri, J. A.: Intensive stereognostic training. Am. J. Occup. Ther., 16:141, 1962.

167. Filler, B. C., Stark, H. H., and Boyes, J. H.: Capsulodesis of the metacarpophalangeal joint of the thumb in children with cerebral palsy. J. Bone Joint Surg., 58-A:667, 1976.

168. Fiorentino, M. R.: Reflex Testing Methods for Evaluating C.N.S. Development. Springfield, Charles C Thomas, 1973.

169. Fisher, R. L., and Shaffer, S. R.: An evaluation of calcaneal osteotomy in congenital clubfoot and other disorders. Clin. Orthop., 70:141, 1970.

170. Fleiss, O., Fleiss, H., and Pokorny, H.: Feedback therapy for improving heel contact and toe off motion during ambulation (author's transl.). Int. J. Rehabil. Res., 3:497, 1980.

171. Flodmark, A.: Augmented auditory feedback as an aid in gait training of the cerebral palsied child. Dev. Med. Child Neurol., 28:147, 1986.

172. Freud, S.: Infantile Cerebrallahmung. Nothnagel's

specielle Pathologie und Therapie 9. Volo. 2. Vienna, 1897.

173. Frost, H. M.: Surgical treatment of spastic equinus in cerebral palsy. Arch. Phys. Med. Rehabil., 52:270, 1971.

174. Fuldner, R. V.: Hamstring tenotomy in cerebral palsy. Results and rationale. J. Bone Joint Surg., 45-A:1545, 1963.

175. Fulford, G. E., and Brown, J. K.: Positions as a cause of deformity in children with cerebral palsy. Dev. Med. Child Neurol., 18:305, 1976.

176. Fulford, G. E., Cairns, T. P., and Sloan, Y.: Sitting problems of children with cerebral palsy. Dev. Med. Child Neurol., 24:48, 1982.

177. Gage, J. R.: Gait analysis for decision-making in cerebral palsy. Bull. Hosp. J. Dis. Orthop. Inst., 43:147, 1983.

178a. Gage, J. R., Fabian, D., Hicks, R., and Tashman, S.: Pre- and postoperative gait analysis in patients with spastic diplegia: A preliminary report. J. Pediatr. Orthop., 4:715, 1984.

178b. Gage, J. R., Perry, J., Hicks, R. R., Koop, S., and Wrentz, J. R.: Rectus femoris transfer as a means of improving knee function in cerebral palsy. Dev. Med. Child Neurol. In press.

179. Gaines, R. W., and Ford, T. B.: A systemic approach to the amount of Achilles tendon lengthening in cerebral palsy. J. Pediatr. Orthop., 4:448, 1984.

180. Galal, Z., and Said, M.: Anterior transposition of the tibialis posterior tendon in spastic equinus. A preliminary report. Egypt. Orthop. J., 6:209, 1971.

181. Gherlinzoni, G., and Pais, C.: Trattamento della lussazione patologica dell'anca: indicazione, tecnica e reultati lontani. Chir. Organi Mov., 34:335, 1950.

182. Girdlestone, G. R., and Somerville, E. W.: Tuberculosis of Bone and Joint. 2nd ed. New York, Oxford University Press, 1952.

183. Glynn, J. J., and Niebauer, J. J.: Flexion and extension contracture of the elbow. Surgical management. Clin. Orthop., 117:289, 1976.

184. Goldner, J. L.: Reconstructive surgery of the hand in cerebral palsy and spastic paralysis resulting from injury to the spinal cord. J. Bone Joint Surg., 37-A:1141, 1955.

185. Goldner, J. L.: Reconstructive surgery of the upper extremity affected by cerebral palsy or brain or spinal cord trauma. In Adams, J. P. (ed.): Current Practice in Orthopaedic Surgery. Vol. 3. St. Louis, C. V. Mosby, 1966.

186. Goldner, J. L.: Clinical management of the upper extremity in cerebral palsy. Dev. Med. Child Neurol., 10:250, 1968.

187. Goldner, J. L.: Upper extremity tendon transfers in cerebral palsy. Orthop. Clin. North Am., 5:389, 1974.

188. Goldner, J. L.: The upper extremity in cerebral palsy. In Samilson, R. L. (ed.): Orthopaedic Aspects of Cerebral Palsy. Clinic in Developmental Medicine No. 52/53, p. 221. London, William Heinemann Medical Books, 1975.

189. Goldner, J. L.: Upper extremity surgical procedures for patients with cerebral palsy. A.A.O.S. Instr. Course Lect. 28:37, 1979.

190. Goldner, J. L., and Fertic, D. C.: Upper extremity reconstructive surgery in cerebral palsy or similar conditions. A.A.O.S. Instr. Course Lect. 18:169, 1961.

191a. Gornall, P., Hitchcock, E., and Kirkland, I. S.: Stereotaxic neurosurgery in the management of cerebral palsy. Dev. Med. Child Neurol., 17:279, 1975.

191b. Grabe, R. P., and Thompson, P.: Lengthening of the Achilles tendon in cerebral paresis. S. Afr. Med. J., 56:993, 1979.

192. Grant, A. D., Feldman, R., and Lehman, W. B.: Equinus deformity in cerebral palsy: A retrospective

193. Green, N. E., Griffin, P. P., and Shiair, R.: Split posterior tibial transfer in cerebral palsy. J. Bone Joint Surg., 55-A:748, 1983.

194. Green, W. T.: Tendon transplantation of the flexor carpi ulnaris for pronation-flexion deformity of the wrist. Surg. Gynecol. Obstet., 75:337, 1942.

195. Green, W. T., and Banks, H. H.: Flexor carpi ulnaris transplant and its use in cerebral palsy. J. Bone Joint Surg., 44-A:1343, 1962.

196. Green, W. T., and McDermott, L. J.: Operative treatment of cerebral palsy of spastic type. J.A.M.A., 118:434, 1942.

197. Gregg, N.: Congenital cataract following German measles in the mother. Trans. Ophthalmol. Soc. Aust., 3:35, 1942.

198. Gregg, N.: Further observations on congenital defects in infants following maternal rubella. Trans. Ophthalmol. Soc. Aust., 4:119, 1946.

199. Grenier, A.: Early diagnosis of cerebral palsy . . . . Why do it? Ann. Pediatr. (Paris), 29:509, 1982.

200. Grice, D. S.: Extra-articular arthrodesis of the subastragalar joint for correction of paralytic flat feet in children. J. Bone Joint Surg., 34-A:927, 1952.

201. Grice, D. S.: Further experience with extra-articular arthrodesis of the subtalar joint. J. Bone Joint Surg., 37-A:246, 1955.

202. Griffin, P. P., Wheelhouse, W. W., and Shiavi, R.: Adductor transfer for adductor spasticity: Clinical and electromyographic gait analysis. Dev. Med. Child Neurol., 19:783, 1977.

203. Gritzka, T. L., Staheli, L. T., and Duncan, W. R.: Posterior tibial tendon transfer through the interosseous membrane to correct equinovarus deformity in cerebral palsy. An initial experience. Clin. Orthop., 89:201, 1972.

204. Gunsolus, P., Welsh, C., and Houser, C.: Equilibrium reactions in the feet of children with spastic cerebral palsy and of normal children. Dev. Med. Child Neurol., 17:580, 1975.

205. Hagberg, B., Hagberg, G., and Olow, I.: The changing panorama of cerebral-palsy in Sweden. Epidemiological trends 1959–78. Acta Paediatr. Scand., 73:433, 1984.

206. Hagberg, B., Lemperg, R., and Lundberg, A.: Transposition av gastrocnemius-muskulaturen vid spastiska former av cerebral pares nos barn. Nord. Med., 79:685, 1968.

207. Hagberg, B., Sanner, G., and Steen, M.: The dysequilibrium syndrome in cerebral palsy. Clinical aspects and treatment. Acta Paediatr. Scand. (Suppl.), 226:1, 1972.

208. Harris, M. M., and Dignam, P. F.: A non-surgical method of reducing drooling in cerebral-palsied children. Dev. Med. Child Neurol., 22:293, 1980.

209. Harris, S., and Riffle, K.: Effects of inhibitive ankle foot orthoses on standing balance in a child with cerebral palsy. Phys. Ther. J., 66:663, 1986.

210. Harris, S. R., Smith, L. H., and Krukowski, L.: Goniometric reliability for a child with spastic quadriplegia. J. Pediatr. Orthop., 5:348, 1985.

211. Haskin, M., Bream, J. A., and Erdman, W. J., II.: The Pennsylvania horseback riding program for cerebral palsy. Am. J. Phys. Med., 61:141, 1982.

212. Hellerbrandt, F. A.: Trends in the management of cerebral palsy (unpublished manuscript). Lectures in Medical College of Virginia, 1950–1951.

213. Henderson, J. L.: Cerebral Palsy in Childhood and Adolescence. A Medical, Psychological, and Social Study. Edinburgh, F. & S. Livingstone, 1961.

214. Hensey, O., Ilett, S. J., and Rosenbloom, L.: Child abuse and cerebral palsy (letter). Lancet, 2:400, 1983.

215. Hensinger, R. N.: Meeting highlights (1984 Annual

Meeting, American Academy for Cerebral Palsy and Developmental Medicine. Washington, D.C., October 24–27, 1984). J. Pediatr. Orthop., 5:372, 1985.

216. Heyman, C. H.: The surgical treatment of spastic paralysis. *In* Dean Lewis: Practice of Surgery. Vol. III. Hagerstown, Prior, 1945.

217. Hill, L. M., Bassett, F. H., and Baker, L. D.: Correction of adduction, flexion, and internal rotation deformities of the hip in cerebral palsy. Dev. Med. Child Neurol., 8:406, 1966.

218. Hodgen, J. T., and Frantz, C. H.: Subcutaneous tenotomy of the Achilles tendon. J. Bone Joint Surg., 20:419, 1938.

219a. Hoffer, M. M.: Basic considerations and classification of cerebral palsy. A.A.O.S. Instr. Course Lect., 25:96, 1976.

219b. Hoffer, M. M.: Current Concepts Review. Management of the hip in cerebral palsy. J. Bone Joint Surg., 68-A:629, 1986.

220. Hoffer, M. M., Abraham, E., and Nickel, V. L.: Salvage surgery at the hip to improve sitting posture of mentally retarded, severely disabled children with cerebral palsy. Dev. Med. Child Neurol., 14:51, 1972.

221. Hoffer, M. M., Barakat, G., and Koffman, M.: 10-year followup of split anterior tibial tendon transfer in cerebral palsied patients with spastic equinovarus deformity. J. Pediatr. Orthop., 5:432, 1985.

222. Hoffer, M. M., and Brink, J.: Orthopedic management of acquired cerebrospasticity in childhood. Clin. Orthop., 110:244, 1975.

223. Hoffer, M. M., and Bullock, M.: The functional and social significance of orthopedic rehabilitation of mentally retarded patients with cerebral palsy. Orthop. Clin. North Am., 12:185, 1981.

224. Hoffer, M. M., Garrett, A., Brink, J., Perry, J., Hale, W., and Nickel, V. L.: The orthopaedic management of brain-injured children. J. Bone Joint Surg., 53-A:567, 1971.

225a. Hoffer, M. M., and Holstein, A.: Hallux valgus—an acquired deformity of the foot in cerebral palsy. Foot Ankle, 1:33, 1980.

225b. Hoffer, M. M., and Koffman, M.: Cerebral palsy: The first three years. Clin. Orthop., 151:222, 1980.

226. Hoffer, M. M., Perry, J., Garcia, M., and Bullock, D.: Adduction contracture of the thumb in cerebral palsy. A preoperative electromyographic study. J. Bone Joint Surg., 65-A:755, 1983.

227. Hoffer, M. M., Perry, J., and Melkonian, G. J.: Dynamic electromyography and decision-making for surgery in the upper extremity of patients with cerebral palsy. J. Hand Surg., 4:424, 1979.

228. Hoffer, M. M., Reiswig, J. A., Garrett, A. M., and Perry, J.: The split anterior tibial tendon transfer in the treatment of spastic varus hindfoot of childhood. Orthop. Clin. North Am., 5:31, 1974.

229. Hoffer, M. M., Stein, G., Koffman, M., and Prietto, M.: Femoral varus-derotation osteotomy in spastic cerebral palsy. J. Bone Joint Surg., 67-A:1119, 1985.

230. Hohman, L. B.: Intelligence levels in cerebral palsied children. Am. J. Phys. Med., 32:282, 1953.

231. Hohman, L. B., Reed, R., and Baker, L. D.: Sensory disturbances in children with infantile hemiplegia, triplegia, and quadriplegia. Am. J. Phys. Med., 37:1, 1958.

232. Holm, V. A.: The cause of cerebral palsy. A contemporary perspective. J.A.M.A., 247:1473, 1982.

233. Holm, V. A., Harthun-Smith, L., and Tada, W. L.: Infant walkers and cerebral palsy. Am. J. Dis. Child., 137:1189, 1983.

234. Holt, K. S.: Deformity and disability in cerebral palsy. Dev. Med. Child Neurol., 5:629, 1963.

235. Holt, K. S.: Hand function in young cerebral palsied children. Dev. Med. Child Neurol., 5:635, 1963.

236. Holt, K. S.: Assessment of Cerebral Palsy. London, Lloyd Duke, 1965.

237. Holt, K. S.: Review: The assessment of walking in children with particular reference to cerebral palsy. Child Care Health Dev., 7:281, 1981.

238. Hood, P. N., and Perlstein, M. A.: Infantile spastic hemiplegia. V. Oral language and motor development. Pediatrics, 17:58, 1956.

239. Hoover, G. H., and Frost, H. M.: Dynamic correction of spastic rocker-bottom foot. Clin. Orthop., 65:175, 1969.

240. Horgan, J. S.: Reaction-time and movement-time of children with cerebral palsy: Under motivational reinforcement conditions. Am. J. Phys. Med., 59:22, 1980.

241. Houkom, J. A., Roach, J. W., Wenger, D. R., Speck, G., Herring, J. A., and Norris, E. N.: Treatment of acquired hip subluxation in cerebral palsy. J. Pediatr. Orthop., 6:285, 1986.

242. House, J. H., Gwathmey, F. W., and Fidler, M. O.: A dynamic approach to the thumb-in-palm deformity in cerebral palsy. J. Bone Joint Surg., 63-A:216, 1981.

243. Howard, C. B., McKibbin, B., Williams, L. A., and Mackie, I.: Factors affecting the incidence of hip dislocation in cerebral palsy. J. Bone Joint Surg., 67-B:530, 1985.

244. Hsu, L. C., Yau, A. C., O'Brien, J. P., and Hodgson, A. R.: Valgus deformity in the ankle resulting from fibular resection for a graft in subtalar fusion in children. J. Bone Joint Surg., 54-A:585, 1972.

245. Huang, S.-C., and Eilert, R. E.: Important radiographic signs for decision-making in surgery of the hip in cerebral palsy. Presented at the Annual Meeting of A.A.C.P.D.M., 1984. Dev. Med. Child Neurol., 27:100, 1985.

246. Hunt, J. C., and Brooks, A. L.: Subtalar extra-articular arthrodesis for correction of paralytic valgus deformity of the foot. J. Bone Joint Surg., 47-A:1310, 1965.

247. Hylton, N., and Uhri, B.: Inhibitive shoe inserts (paper). Inhibitive Foot Alignment Seminar. Kent, WA, April 14–15, 1984.

248. Illingworth, R.: Recent Advances in Cerebral Palsy. London, J. & A. Churchill, 1958.

249. Illingworth, R. S.: The Development of Infants and Young Children, Normal and Abnormal. 3rd Ed. Edinburgh, F. & S. Livingstone, Ltd., 1964.

250. Inglis, A. E., and Cooper, W.: Release of the flexor-pronator origin for flexion deformities of the hand and wrist in spastic paralysis. A study of eighteen cases. J. Bone Joint Surg., 48-A:847, 1966.

251. Inglis, A. E., Cooper, W., and Braton, W.: Surgical correction of thumb deformities in spastic paralysis. J. Bone Joint Surg., 52-A:253, 1970.

252. Ingraham, F. D., and Matson, D. D.: Subdural haematomas in infancy. Adv. Pediatr., 4:231, 1949.

253. Ingram, A. J.: Miscellaneous affections of the nervous system. *In* Edmonson, A. S., and Crenshaw, A. H. (eds.): Campbell's Operative Orthopaedics. 6th Ed. St. Louis, C. V. Mosby, 1980, pp. 1567–1641.

254. Ingram, A. J., Withers, E., and Speltz, E.: Role of intensive physical and occupational therapy in the treatment of cerebral palsy: Testing and results. Arch. Phys. Med., 40:429, 1959.

255. Ingram, T. T. S.: A study of cerebral palsy in the childhood population of Edinburgh. Arch. Dis. Child., 30:85, 1955.

256. Ingram, T. T. S.: Pediatric Aspects of Cerebral Palsy. Baltimore, Williams & Wilkins, 1964.

257. Ireland, M. L., and Hoffer, M.: Triple arthrodesis for children with spastic cerebral palsy. Dev. Med. Child Neurol., 27:623, 1985.

258. Ito, M., Okuno, T., Takao, T., Konish, Y., Yoshioka, M., and Mikawa, H.: Electroencephalographic and

cranial computed tomographic findings in children with hemiplegic cerebral palsy. Eur. Neurol., *20*:312, 1981.

259. Ivan, L. P., Ventureyra, E. C., Wiley, J., Doyle, D., Pressman, E., Knights, R., Guzman, C., and Utley, D.: Chronic cerebellar stimulation in cerebral palsy. Surg. Neurol., *15*:81, 1981.

260a. Ivey, A., McDaniel, C., Perkins, S., Roblyer, D. D., and Ruiz, J.: Supine stander for severely handicapped child. Phys. Ther., *61*:525, 1981.

260b. Ivey, A., and Roblyer, D. D.: Rollermobile for children with cerebral palsy. Phys. Ther., *60*:1162, 1980.

261. Jacobson, E.: Progressive Relaxation. 2nd Ed. Chicago, University of Chicago Press, 1938.

262. Jay, R. M., and Schoenhaus, H. D.: Further insights in the anterior advancement of tendo Achilles. J. Am. Podiatr. Assoc., *71*:73, 1981.

263. Jensen, G. D., and Alderman, M. E.: The prehensile grasp of spastic diplegia. Pediatrics, *31*:470, 1963.

264. Jones, A. R.: William John Little. J. Bone Joint Surg., *31-B*:123, 1949.

265. Jones, G. B.: Paralytic dislocation of the hip. J. Bone Joint Surg., *36-B*:375, 1954.

266. Jones, G. B.: Paralytic dislocation of the hip. J. Bone Joint Surg., *44-B*:573, 1962.

267. Jones, M. H.: Differential diagnosis and natural history of the cerebral palsied child. *In* Samilson, R. L. (ed.): Orthopaedic Aspects of Cerebral Palsy. Clinics in Developmental Medicine Vol. 52/53. Philadelphia, J. B. Lippincott, 1975, p. 5.

268. Jones, M. H., and Maschmeyer, J. E.: Childhood aims and adult accomplishments in cerebral palsy. Int. Rec. Med., *171*:219, 1958.

269. Jones, M. H., Sands, R., Hyman, C. B., Sturgeon, P., and Koch, F. P.: Study of the incidence of central nervous system damage following erythroblastosis foetalis. Pediatrics, *14*:346, 1954.

270. Jones, R., and Lovett, R. W.: Orthopedic Surgery. 2nd Ed. New York, William Wood & Co., 1929.

271a. Kabat, H.: Studies in neuromuscular dysfunction. XV. The role of central facilitation in restoration of motor function in paralysis. Arch. Phys. Med., *33*:532, 1952.

271b. Kabat, H.: Studies on neuromuscular dysfunction. *In* Payton, O. D., Hirt, S., and Newton, R. A. (eds.): Scientific Basis for Neurophysiologic Approaches to Therapeutic Exercise. Philadelphia, F. A. Davis, 1977, pp. 219–235.

272. Kabat, H., and Knott, M.: Principles of neuromuscular reeducation. Phys. Ther. Rev., *28*:107, 1948.

273. Kalen, V., and Bleck, E. E.: Prevention of spastic paralytic dislocation of the hip. Dev. Med. Child Neurol., *27*:17, 1985.

274. Kanda, T., Yuge, M., Yamori, Y., Suzuki, J., and Fukase, H.: Early physiotherapy in the treatment of spastic diplegia. Dev. Med. Child Neurol., *26*:438, 1984.

275. Karski, T., and Wosko, I.: Thom's surgical technic in the treatment of spastic contractures of the knee in children. Beitr. Orthop. Traumatol., *30*:90, 1983.

276. Kasser, J. R., and MacEwen, G. D.: Examination of the cerebral palsy patient with foot and ankle problems. Foot Ankle, *4*:135, 1983.

277. Keats, S.: Combined adductor-gracilis tenotomy and selective obturator nerve resection for correction of adduction deformity of the hip in children with cerebral palsy. J. Bone Joint Surg., *39-A*:1087, 1957.

278. Keats, S.: Surgery of the extremities in treatment of cerebral palsy. J.A.M.A., *174*:1266, 1960.

279. Keats, S.: An evaluation of surgery for the correction of knee-flexion contractures in children with cerebral spastic paralysis. J. Bone Joint Surg., *44*:1146, 1962.

280. Keats, S.: Surgical treatment of the hand in cerebral palsy: Correction of thumb-in-palm and other deformities. Report of nineteen cases. J. Bone Joint Surg., *47-A*:274, 1965.

281. Keats, S.: Cerebral Palsy. Springfield, Charles C Thomas, 1965.

282. Keats, S.: A simple anteromedial approach to the lesser trochanter of the femur for the release of the iliopsoas tendon. J. Bone Joint Surg., *49-A*:632, 1967.

283. Keats, S.: Excessive lumbar lordosis. Effect of iliopsoas tenotomy through an anteromedial approach to the lesser trochanter. Dev. Med. Child Neurol., *9*:115, 1967.

284. Keats, S.: Operative Orthopedics in Cerebral Palsy. Springfield, Charles C Thomas, 1970.

285. Keats, S.: Warning: Serious complications caused by the routine rerouting of the peroneus longus and brevis tendons in performing the Grice procedure in cerebral palsy (abstract). J. Bone Joint Surg., *56-A*:1304, 1974.

286. Keats, S., and Kambin, P.: An evaluation of surgery for the correction of knee flexion contracture in children with cerebral spastic paralysis. J. Bone Joint Surg., *44-A*:1146, 1962.

287. Keats, S., and Kouten, J.: Early surgical correction of the planovalgus foot in cerebral palsy. Extra-articular arthrodesis of the subtalar joint. Clin. Orthop., *61*:223, 1968.

288. Keats, S., and Morgese, A. N.: Excessive lumbar lordosis in ambulatory spastic children. Clin. Orthop., *65*:130, 1969.

289. Kendall, P. H., and Robson, P.: Lower limb bracing in cerebral palsy. Clin. Orthop., *47*:73, 1966.

290. Kennard, M. A.: Age and other factors in motor recovery from pre-central lesions in monkeys. Am. J. Physiol., *115*:138, 1936.

291. Kennard, M. A.: Re-organization of motor function in cerebral cortex of monkeys deprived of motor and pre-motor areas in infancy. J. Neurophysiol., *1*:477, 1938.

292. Khalili, A. A., and Benton, J. G.: A physiologic approach to the evaluation and management of spasticity with procaine and phenol nerve block. Clin. Orthop., *47*:97, 1966.

293. Kiessling, L. S., Denckla, M. B., and Carlton, M.: Evidence for differential hemispheric function in children with hemiplegic cerebral palsy. Dev. Med. Child Neurol., *25*:727, 1983.

294. King, H. A., and Staheli, L. T.: Torsional problems in cerebral palsy. Foot Ankle, *4*:180, 1984.

295. Kling, T. F., Kaufer, H., and Hensinger, R. N.: Split posterior tibial-tendon transfers in children with cerebral spastic paralysis and equinovarus deformity. J. Bone Joint Surg., *67-A*:186, 1985.

296. Knott, M., and Voss, D. E.: Proprioceptive Neuromuscular Facilitation. New York, Hoeber-Harper, 1956.

297. Koheil, R., Sochaniwskyj, A., Bablich, K., Kenny, D., and Milner, M.: Biofeedback techniques and behaviour modification in the conservative remediation of drooling in children with cerebral palsy. Scientific program, American Academy for Cerebral Palsy and Developmental Medicine, Seattle, 1985.

298. Koffman, M.: Proximal femoral resection of total hip replacement in severely disabled cerebral palsy patients. Orthop. Clin. North Am., *12*:91, 1981.

299. Kong, E.: Very early treatment of cerebral palsy. Dev. Med. Child Neurol., *8*:198, 1966.

300. Konig, F.: Osteoplastische Behandlung der Röntgenitalen Huftgelenksluxation (mit Demonstration eines Präparates). Verh. Dtsch. Gesellsch., *20*:75, 1891.

301. Kretzler, H. H., and Mooney, J. G.: Derotation osteotomy of the femur in cerebral palsy. J. Bone Joint Surg., *49-A*:196, 1967.

302. Kulakowski, S., and Larroche, J. C.: Cranial comput-

erized tomography in cerebral palsy. An attempt at anatomo-clinical and radiological correlation. Neuropediatrics, *11*:339, 1980.

303. Kyllerman, M.: Dyskinetic cerebral palsy. II. Pathogenetic risk factors and intra-uterine growth. Acta Paediatr. Scand., *71*:551, 1982.

304. Lagergren, J.: Prevalence rates for cerebral palsy (letter). Dev. Med. Child Neurol., *23*:818, 1981.

305. Lamb, D. W., and Pollack, G. A.: Hip deformities in cerebral palsy and their treatment. Dev. Med. Child Neurol., *4*:488, 1962.

306. Laseter, G. F.: Management of the stiff hand. Orthop. Clin. North Am., *14*:749, 1983.

307. Laskas, C. A., Muller, S. L., Nelson, D. L., and Wilson-Broyles, M.: Enhancement of two motor functions of the lower extremity in a child with spastic quadriplegia. Phys. Ther., *65*:11, 1985.

308. Lee, B. S., and Horstmann, H.: The brachioradialis for restoration of abduction and extension of spastic thumb in children. Orthopedics, 7:1445, 1984.

309a. Lee, C. L.: Role of lower extremity bracing in cerebral palsy. Dev. Med. Child Neurol., *24*:250, 1982.

309b. Lee, C. L., and Bleck, E. E.: Surgical correction of equinus deformity in cerebral palsy. Dev. Med. Child Neurol., *22*:287, 1980.

310. Legg, A. R.: Transplantation of tensor fasciae femoris in cases of weakened gluteus medius. J.A.M.A., *80*:242, 1923.

311. Legg, A. T.: Transplantation of tensor fasciae femoris in cases of weakened gluteus medius. N. Engl. J. Med., *209*:61, 1933.

312. Leiper, C. I., Miller, A., Lang, J., and Herman, R.: Sensory feedback for head control in cerebral palsy. Phys. Ther., *61*:512, 1981.

313. Lempberg, R., Hagberg, B., and Lundberg, A.: Achilles tenoplasty for correction of equinus deformity in spastic syndromes of cerebral palsy. Acta Orthop. Scand., *40*:507, 1969.

314. Letts, M., Shapiro, L., Mulder, K., and Klassen, O.: The windblown hip syndrome in total body cerebral palsy. J. Pediatr. Orthop., *4*:55, 1984.

315a. Levine, M. S.: Cerebral palsy diagnosis in children over age 1 year: Standard criteria. Arch. Phys. Med. Rehabil., *61*:385, 1980.

315b. Levine, M. S., and Kliebhan, L.: Communication between physician and physical and occupational therapists: a neurodevelopmentally based prescription. Pediatrics, *68*:208, 1981.

316. Levitt, S.: Physiotherapy in Cerebral Palsy. Springfield, Charles C Thomas, 1962.

317. Lewis, F. R., Samilson, R. R., and Lucas, D. B.: Femoral torsion and coxa valga in cerebral palsy. Dev. Med. Child Neurol., *6*:591, 1964.

318. Lindsley, D. B., Schreiner, L. H., and Magoun, H. W.: An electromyographic study of spasticity. *In* Payton, O. D., Hirst, S., and Newton, R. A. (eds.): Scientific Bases for Neurophysiologic Approaches to Therapeutic Exercises. Philadelphia, F. A. Davis, 1977, pp. 119–123.

319. Little, W. J.: The deformities of the human frame. Lancet, *1*:5, 1843.

320. Little, W. J.: On the Nature and Treatment of Deformities of the Human Frame (with Notes and Additions). London, Longmans, 1853.

321. Little, W. J.: On the influence of abnormal parturition, difficult labors, premature birth and asphyxia neonatorum on the mental and physical condition of the child, especially in relation to deformities. Lancet, *2*:378, 1861.

322. Lloyd-Roberts, G. C., Colton, C. L., and Ransford, A. O.: Transposition of the tendon of pronator teres in cerebral palsy. J. Bone Joint Surg., *58-B*:220, 1976.

323. Lloyd-Roberts, G. C., Jackson, A. M., and Albert, J. S.: Avulsion of the distal pole of the patella in cerebral palsy. J. Bone Joint Surg., *67-B*:252, 1985.

324. Lonstein, J. E.: Deformities of the spine in children with cerebral palsy. Orthop. Rev., *10*:33, 1981.

325. Lonstein, J. E., Winter, R. B., Moe, J. H., Bradford, D. S., and Akbarnia, B. A.: A combined anterior and posterior approach for the operative treatment of cerebral palsy spine deformity. Orthop. Trans., *2*:230, 1978.

326. Lord, J.: Cerebral palsy: A clinical approach. Arch. Phys. Med. Rehabil., *65*:542, 1984.

327a. McBride, R. D.: A conservative operation for bunions. J. Bone Joint Surg., *10*:735, 1928.

327b. McCall, R. E., Lillich, J. S., Harris, J. R., and Johnston, F. A.: The Grice extra-articular subtalar arthrodesis: a clinical review. J. Pediatr. Orthop., 5:442, 1985.

328. McCarroll, H. R.: Surgical treatment of spastic paralysis. *In* Instructional Course Lectures. The American Academy of Orthopedic Surgeons, Vol. 6. Ann Arbor, J. W. Edwards, 1949, pp. 134–151.

329. McCarroll, H. R., and Schwartzman, J. P.: Spastic paralysis and allied disorders. J. Bone Joint Surg., *25*:747, 1943.

330. McCue, F. C., Honner, R., and Chapman, W. C.: Transfer of the brachioradialis for hands deformed by cerebral palsy. J. Bone Joint Surg., *52-A*:1171, 1970.

331. McElroy, D. K.: Stabilization of the foot in cerebral palsy. Clin. Orthop., *34*:19, 1964.

332. MacEwen, G. D.: Operative treatment of scoliosis in cerebral palsy. Reconstr. Surg. Traumatol., *13*:58, 1972.

333. McIvor, W., and Samilson, R. L.: Fractures in patients with cerebral palsy. J. Bone Joint Surg., *48-A*:858, 1966.

334. MacKenzie, I. G.: Abnormalities of the hip in cerebral palsy. Dev. Med. Child Neurol., *17*:797, 1975.

335. Madigan, R. R., and Wallace, S. L.: Scoliosis in the institutionalized cerebral palsy population. Spine, *6*:583, 1981.

336. Majestro, T. C., Ruda, R., and Frost, H. M.: Intramuscular lengthening of the posterior tibialis muscle. Clin. Orthop., *79*:59, 1971.

337. Makin, M.: Tibiofibular relationship in paralyzed limbs. J. Bone Joint Surg., *47-B*:500, 1965.

338. Manley, M. T., and Gurtowski, J.: The vertical wheelchair: A device for ambulation in cerebral palsy. Arch. Phys. Med. Rehabil., *66*:717, 1985.

339. Marquis, P., Palmer, F. B., Mahoney, W. J., and Capute, A. J.: Extrapyramidal cerebral palsy: A changing view. J.D.B.P., *3*:65, 1982.

340. Martin, J. P.: Curvature of the spine in post-encephalitic Parkinsonism. J. Neurol. Neurosurg. Psychiatry, *28*:395, 1965.

341. Martz, C. D.: Talipes equinus correction in cerebral palsy. J. Bone Joint Surg., *42-A*:769, 1960.

342. Masse, P., and Audie, B.: Critical evaluation of Egger's procedure for the relief of knee flexion spasticity. Dev. Med. Child Neurol., *10*:159, 1968.

343. Masse, P., Baron, P., Cahuzac, M., Lacheretz, M., Martin, C. H., Quencau, P., and Roullet, J.: La chirurgie de l'infirmie mortice cerebrale chez l'enfant. Rev. Chir. Orthop., *53*:729, 1967.

344. Matev, I. B.: Surgical treatment of spastic "thumb-in-palm" deformity. J. Bone Joint Surg., *45-B*:703, 1963.

345. Matev, I. B.: Surgical treatment of flexion-adduction contracture of the thumb in cerebral palsy. Acta Orthop. Scand., *41*:439, 1970.

346. Mathews, S. M., Jones, M. H., and Sperling, S. C.: Hip derangements seen in cerebral palsied children. Am. J. Phys. Med., *32*:213, 1953.

347. Messingill, R.: Follow-up investigation of patients who

have had parotid duct transplantation surgery to control drooling. Ann. Plast. Surg., 2:205, 1978.

348. Michele, A. A.: Iliopsoas. Springfield, Charles C Thomas, 1962.

349. Milford, L.: The hand. *In* Edmonson, A. S., and Crenshaw, A. H. (eds.): Campbell's Operative Orthopaedics. 6th Ed. St. Louis, C. V. Mosby, 1980, pp. 110–417.

350. Miller, E., and Rosenfeld, G. B.: The psychologic evaluation of children with cerebral palsy and its implications in treatment. J. Pediatr., 41:613, 1952.

351. Mimran, R.: Transplantation du jambier posterieur sur le dos du pied. Rev. Chir. Orthop., 52:681, 1966.

352. Minear, W. L.: A classification of cerebral palsy. Pediatrics, 18:841, 1956.

353. Minns, R. A., Hazelwood, E., Brown, J. K., Fulford, G., and Elton, R. A.: Spina bifida and cerebral palsy. Z. Kinderchir., 34:370, 1981.

354. Mital, M. A.: Lengthening of the elbow flexors in cerebral palsy. J. Bone Joint Surg., 61-A:515, 1979.

355. Mital, M. A., and Sakellarides, H. T.: Surgery of the upper extremity in the retarded individual with spastic cerebral palsy. Orthop. Clin. North Am., 12:127, 1981.

356a. Molnar, G. E., and Gordon, S. V.: Predictive value of clinical signs for early prognostication of motor function in cerebral palsy. Arch. Phys. Med., 57:153, 1974.

356b. Monreal, F. J.: Consideration of genetic factors in cerebral palsy. Dev. Med. Child Neurol., 27:325, 1985.

357. Moreau, M., Drummond, D. S., Rogala, E., Ashworth, A., and Porter, T.: Natural history of the dislocated hip in spastic cerebral palsy. Dev. Med. Child Neurol., 21:749, 1979.

358a. Moreland, J. R., and Westin, G. W.: Further experience with Grice subtalar arthrodesis. Orthop. Trans., 1:109, 1977.

358b. Moreland, J. R., and Westin, G. W.: Further experience with Grice subtalar arthrodesis. Clin. Orthop., 207:113, 1986.

358c. Morgan, R. F., Hansen, F. C., Wells, J. H., and Hoopes, J. E.: The treatment of drooling in the child with cerebral palsy. Md. State Med. J., 30:79, 1981.

359. Mortens, J.: Orthopaedic operations in the treatment of children with cerebral palsy. Dan. Med. Bull., 12:22, 1965.

360. Mortens, J., Moller, H., and Salmonsen, L.: Early stabilizing operations for spastic talipes equino-valgus by Grice's extra-articular osteoplastic subtalar arthrodesis. Acta Orthop. Scand., 32:485, 1962.

361. Motonaga, M., Okahata, C., Kogure, K., Takeda, T., and Makino, C.: Nursing process: Nursing of children with cerebral palsy. Nursing of children with cerebral palsy: Case studies. Kurinikaru Sutadi., 2:1441, 1981.

362. Mott, D. M., and Yates, L.: An appraisal of inhibitive casting as an adjunct to the total management of the child with cerebral palsy. Proceedings of the A.A.C.P.D.M. meetings, Boston, 1980; Detroit, 1981.

363. Mowery, C. A., Gelberman, R. H., and Rhoades, C. E.: Upper extremity tendon transfers in cerebral palsy: Electromyographic and functional analysis. J. Pediatr. Orthop., 5:69, 1985.

364. Mullaferoze, P., and Vora, P. H.: Surgery in lower limbs in cerebral palsy. Dev. Med. Child Neurol., 14:45, 1972.

365. Murphy, D. P.: Ovarian irradiation and the health of the subsequent child: A review of more than 200 previously unreported pregnancies in women subjected to pelvic irradiation. Surg. Gynecol. Obstet., 48:766, 1929.

366. Murri, A.: Zur Adduktorenverlagerung nach Stephenson und Donovan unter besonderer Berucksichtigung der pathologischen Huftgelenkentwicklung beim zerebralbewegungsgestorten. Kind. Orthop. Prax., 13:178, 1977.

367. Murri, A., Fleiss, O., Fleiss, H., and Pokorny, H.: Biomechanical analysis after elongation of the Achilles tendon in patients with cerebral movement disorders. Wien. Med. Wochenschr., 132:507, 1982.

368. Mustard, W. T.: Iliopsoas transfer for weakness of the hip abductors. J. Bone Joint Surg., 34-A:647, 1952.

369. Nather, A., Fulford, G. E., and Stewart, K.: Treatment of valgus hindfoot in cerebral palsy by peroneus brevis lengthening. Dev. Med. Child Neurol., 26:335, 1984.

370. Nelson, K. B., and Ellenberg, J. H.: Children who "outgrew" cerebral palsy. Pediatrics, 69:529, 1982.

371. Nishihara, N., Tanabe, G., Nakahara, S., Imai, T., and Murakawa, H.: Surgical treatment of cervical spondylotic myelopathy complicating athetoid cerebral palsy. J. Bone Joint Surg., 66-B:504, 1984.

372. Norlin, R., and Tkaczuk, H.: One-session surgery for correction of lower extremity deformities in children with cerebral palsy. J. Pediatr. Orthop., 5:208, 1985.

373. Nuzzo, R. M.: Dynamic bracing: Elastics for patients with cerebral palsy. Clin. Orthop., 148:263, 1980.

374. Nwaobi, O. M.: Effects of body orientation in space on tonic muscle activity of patients with cerebral palsy. Dev. Med. Child Neurol., 28:41, 1986.

375. Nwaobi, O. M., Brubaker, C. E., Cusick, B., and Sussman, M. D.: Electromyographic investigation of extensor activity in cerebral palsied children in different seating positions. Dev. Med. Child Neurol., 25:175, 1983.

376. Ober, F. R.: Tendon transplantation in the lower extemity. N. Engl. J. Med., 209:52, 1933.

377. O'Brien, J. J., and Surkin, R. B.: The natural history of the dislocated hip in cerebral palsy. Dev. Med. Child Neurol., 20:241, 1978.

378. O'Brien, J. P., Dwyer, A. P., and Hodgson, A. R.: Paralytic pelvic obliquity. Its prognosis and management and the development of a technique for full correction of deformity. J. Bone Joint Surg., 57-A:626, 1975.

379. Ohye, C., Miyazaki, M., Hirai, T., Shibazaki, T., and Nagaseki, Y.: Stereotactic selective thalamotomy for the treatment of tremor type cerebral palsy in adolescence. Childs Brain, 10:157, 1983.

380. Okuno, T.: A radiological study of the hip in cerebral palsy in relation to pathogenesis of dislocation. J. Jpn. Orthop. Assoc., 59:55, 1985.

381. Osler, W.: The Cerebral Palsies of Children. A Clinical Study From the Infirmary of Nervous Diseases. London, Lewis, 1889.

382. Page, C. M.: An operation for the relief of flexion contracture in the forearm. J. Bone Joint Surg., 5:233, 1923.

383. Paine, R. S.: Neurological examination of infants and children. Pediatr. Clin. North Am., 7:471, 1960.

384. Paine, R. S.: Cerebral palsy: Symptoms and signs of diagnostic and prognostic significance. *In* Adams, J. P. (ed.): Current Practice in Orthopedic Surgery. Vol. 3. St. Louis, C. V. Mosby, 1966, p. 39.

385. Paine, R. S., and Oppe, T. E.: Neurological Examination of Children. Clinics in Developmental Medicine. Vol. 20/21. London, The Spastics Society Medical Education and Information Unit in Association with William Heinemann Medical Books, 1966.

386. Paluska, D. J., and Blount, W. P.: Ankle valgus after the Grice subtalar stabilization. Clin. Orthop., 59:137, 1968.

387a. Paneth, N., and Kiely, J.: The frequency of cerebral palsy: a review of population studies in industrialised nations since 1950. *In* Stanley, F., Alberman, E. (eds.): The epidemiology of the Cerebral Palsies.

Clinics in Developmental Medicine No. 87. London, S.I.M.P. with Blackwell Scientific; Philadelphia, J. B. Lippincott, 1984, pp. 46–56.

387b. Parsch, K.: Grice extra-articular arthrodesis (results, extensions in the range of indication). Z. Orthop., *111*:457, 1973.

388. Patella, V., and Martucci, G.: Transposition of the pronator radio-teres muscle to the radial extensors of the wrist, in infantile cerebral paralysis. An improved operative technique. Ital. J. Orthop. Traumatol., *6*:61, 1980.

389. Patella, V., Franchin, F., Moretti, B., and Mori, F.: Arthrodesis of the wrist with minifixators in infantile cerebral palsy. Ital. J. Orthop. Traumatol., *10*:75, 1984.

390. Peacock, W. J., and Arens, L. J.: Selective posterior rhizotomy for the relief of spasticity in cerebral palsy. S. Afr. Med. J., *62*:119, 1982.

391. Pedersen, H., Taudorf, K., and Melchior, J. C.: Computed tomography in spastic cerebral palsy. Neuroradiology, *23*:275, 1982.

392. Pendergast, J. J.: Congenital and other anomalies following rubella in mother during pregnancy. Med. J. Aust., *1*:315, 1945.

393. Perlstein, M. A.: Neurological sequelae of erythroblastosis fetalis. Am. J. Dis. Child., *79*:605, 1950.

394. Perlstein, M. A.: Infantile cerebral palsy. *In* Levine, S. Z., Anderson, J. A., et al. (eds.): Advances in Pediatrics. Vol. 7. Chicago, Year Book Medical Publishers, 1955.

395. Perlstein, M. A., and Barnett, H. E.: Nature and recognition of cerebral palsy in infancy. J.A.M.A., *148*:1389, 1952.

396. Perlstein, M. A., and Hood, P. N.: Infantile spastic hemiplegia. Pediatrics, *15*:676, 1955.

397. Perry, J.: Rehabilitation of the neurologically disabled patient—principles, practice and scientific basis. J. Neurosurg., *58*:779, 1958.

398. Perry, J.: Kinesiology of lower extremity bracing. Clin. Orthop., *102*:18, 1974.

399. Perry, J.: The cerebral palsy gait. *In* Samilson, R. L.: Orthopaedic Aspects of Cerebral Palsy. Clinics in Developmental Medicine No. 52/53. London, William Heinemann Medical Books, 1975, p. 71.

400. Perry, J., Antonelli, D., and Ford, W.: Analysis of knee joint forces during flexed-knee stance. J. Bone Joint Surg., *57-A*:961, 1975.

401. Perry, J., Easterday, C. S., and Antonelli, D. J.: Surface versus intramuscular electrodes for electromyography of superficial and deep muscles. Phys. Ther., *61*:7, 1981.

402. Perry, J., Giovan, P., Harris, L. J., Montgomery, I., and Azaria, M.: The determinants of muscle action in the hemiparetic lower extremity (and their effect on the examination procedure). Clin. Orthop., *131*:71, 1978.

403. Perry, J., and Hoffer, M. M.: Preoperative and postoperative dynamic electromyography as an aid in planning tendon transfers in children with cerebral palsy. J. Bone Joint Surg., *59-A*:531, 1977.

404. Perry, J., Hoffer, M. M., Giovan, P., Antonelli, D., and Greenberg, R.: Gait analysis of the triceps surae in cerebral palsy. A preoperative and postoperative clinical and electromyographic study. J. Bone Joint Surg., *56-A*:511, 1974.

405. Perry, J., Hoffer, M. M., Antonelli, D., Plut, J., Lewis, G., and Greenberg, R.: Electromyography before and after surgery for hip deformity in children with cerebral palsy. A comparison of clinical and electromyographic findings. J. Bone Joint Surg., *58-A*:201, 1976.

406. Peterson, L. T.: Tenotomy in the treatment of spastic paraplegia with special reference to the iliopsoas. J. Bone Joint Surg., *32-A*:875, 1950.

407. Pharoah, P. O.: Epidemiology of cerebral palsy: A review. J. R. Soc. Med., *74*:516, 1981.

408. Phelps, W. M.: Care and treatment of cerebral palsies. J.A.M.A., *111*:1, 1938.

409. Phelps, W. M.: Treatment of cerebral palsies. J. Bone Joint Surg., *22*:1004, 1940.

410. Phelps, W. M.: Treatment of cerebral palsies. Clinics, *2*:981, 1943.

411. Phelps, W. M.: The cerebral palsies. *In* Nelson, W. E. (ed.): Mitchell-Nelson Textbook of Pediatrics. Philadelphia, W. B. Saunders, 1950, p. 1361.

412. Phelps, W. M.: Braces—lower extremity—cerebral palsies. *In* American Academy of Orthopaedic Surgeons Instructional Course Lectures. Vol. 10. Ann Arbor, J. W. Edwards, 1953, p. 303.

413. Phelps, W. M.: Classification of athetosis with special reference to the motor classification. Am. J. Phys. Med., *35*:24, 1956.

414. Phelps, W. M.: Long-term results of orthopedic surgery in cerebral palsy. J. Bone Joint Surg., *39-A*:53, 1957.

415. Phelps, W. M.: The role of physical therapy in cerebral palsy. *In* Illingworth, R. S. (ed.): Recent Advances in Cerebral Palsy. London, J. & A. Churchill, 1958, p. 251.

416. Phelps, W. M.: Prevention of acquired dislocation of the hip in cerebral palsy. J. Bone Joint Surg., *41-A*:440, 1959.

417. Phelps, W. M.: Complications of orthopedic surgery in the treatment of cerebral palsy. Clin. Orthop., *53*:39, 1967.

418. Pierrot, A. H., and Murphy, O. B.: Heel cord advancement. Orthop. Clin. North Am., *5*:117, 1975.

419. Pinzur, M. S., and Sherman, R.: Modified Moberg opponensplasty in acquired spastic hemiplegia. Orthopedics, *8*:1151, 1985.

420. Pletcher, D. F., Hoffer, M. M., and Koffman, D. M.: Non-traumatic dislocation of the radial head in cerebral palsy. J. Bone Joint Surg., *58-A*:104, 1976.

421. Pollock, G. A.: Lengthening of the gastrocnemius tendons in cases of spastic equinus deformity. J. Bone Joint Surg., *35-B*:148, 1953.

422. Pollock, G. A.: Treatment of adductor paralysis by hamstring transfer. J. Bone Joint Surg., *40-B*:534, 1958.

423. Pollock, G. A.: Surgical treatment of cerebral palsy. J. Bone Joint Surg., *44-B*:68, 1962.

424. Pollock, G. A., and English, T. A.: Transplantation of the hamstring muscles in cerebral palsy. J. Bone Joint Surg., *49-B*:80, 1967.

425. Pollack, G. A., and Sharrard, W. J. W.: Orthopedic surgery in the treatment of cerebral palsy. *In* Illingworth, R. S. (ed.): Recent Advances in Cerebral Palsy. London, Churchill Livingstone, 1958, p. 286.

426. Pollock, J. H., and Carrell, B.: Subtalar extra-articular arthrodesis in the treatment of paralysis valgus deformities. A review of 112 procedures in 100 patients. J. Bone Joint Surg., *46-A*:533, 1964.

427. Polskoi, V. V.: Mechanism of development of abnormal hand postures in children with cerebral palsy. Zh. Nevropatol. Psikhiatr., *81*:357, 1981.

428. Preciso, G., Gallo, F., Matarazzo, E., and Novello, A.: Anesthesia problems in the orthopedic surgical management of children with infantile cerebral palsy. Minerva Anestesiol., *48*:319, 1982.

429. Prechtl, H., and Beintema, D.: The Neurological Examination of the Full Term Newborn Infant. Little Club Clinics in Developmental Medicine No. 12. London, Spastics Society Medical Education and Information Unit in Association with William Heinemann Medical Books, 1964.

430. Pritchett, J. W.: The untreated unstable hip in severe cerebral palsy. Clin. Orthop., *173*:169, 1983.

431. Rang, M., Douglas, G., Bennett, G. C., and Koreska,

J.: Seating for children with cerebral palsy. J. Pediatr. Orthop., *1*:279, 1981.

432. Ravelin, E. E.: Treatment of movement disorders in children with cerebral palsy by the method of programmed bioelectric stimulation. Pediatriia, *12*:41, 1980.

433. Ray, S. A., Bundy, A. C., and Nelson, D. L.: Decreasing drooling through techniques to facilitate mouth closure. Am. J. Occup. Ther., *37*:749, 1983.

434. Reimer, J.: A scoring system for the evaluation of ambulation in cerebral palsied patients. Dev. Med. Child Neurol., *14*:332, 1972.

435. Reimers, J.: Static and dynamic problems in spastic cerebral palsy. J. Bone Joint Surg., *55-B*:822, 1973.

436. Reimers, J.: Contracture of the hamstrings in spastic cerebral palsy. A study of three methods of operative correction. J. Bone Joint Surg., *56-B*:102, 1974.

437. Reimers, J.: The stability of the hip in children. A radiological study of the results of muscle surgery in cerebral palsy. Acta Orthop. Scand. (Suppl.), *184*:1, 1980.

438. Reimers, J.: Spastic paralytic dislocation of the hip (letter). Dev. Med. Child Neurol., *27*:401, 1985.

439. Reimers, J., and Bialik, V.: Influence of femoral rotation on the radiological coverage of the femoral head in children. Pediatr. Radiol., *10*:215, 1981.

440. Reimers, J., and Poulsen, S.: Adductor transfer versus tenotomy for stability of the hip in spastic cerebral palsy. J. Pediatr. Orthop., *4*:52, 1984.

441. Rembolt, R. R.: Emotional factors in residential care. Clin. Orthop., *47*:65, 1966.

442. Reynell, J. K.: Postoperative disturbance observed in children with cerebral palsy. Dev. Med. Child Neurol., 7:360, 1965.

443. Riordan, D. C.: Surgery of the paralytic hand. A.A.O.S. Instr. Course Lect. *16*:79, 1959.

444. Roberts, W. M., and Adams, J. P.: The patellar advancement operation in cerebral palsy. J. Bone Joint Surg., *35-A*:958, 1953.

445. Robson, P.: The prevalence of scoliosis in adolescents and young adults with cerebral palsy. Dev. Med. Child Neurol., *10*:447, 1968.

446. Robson, P.: Shuffling, hitching, scooting or sliding: Some observations in 30 otherwise normal children. Dev. Med. Child Neurol., *12*:608, 1970.

447. Rogers, M. H.: An operation for the correction of the deformity due to "obstetrical paralysis." Boston Med. Surg. J., *174*:163, 1916.

448. Rogtveit, A.: Extra-articular subtalar arthrodesis. According to Green-Grice in flat feet. Acta Orthop. Scand., *34*:367, 1964.

449. Rood, M. S.: Neurophysiologic reactions as a basis for physical therapy. Physiol. Rev., *34*:444, 1954.

450. Roosth, H. P.: The early release of spastic hip flexion deformity. Dev. Med. Child Neurol., 9:114, 1967.

451. Roosth, H. P.: Flexion deformity of the hip and knee in spastic cerebral palsy. J. Bone Joint Surg., *53-A*:1489, 1971.

452. Root, L.: Functional testing of the posterior tibial muscle in spastic paralysis. Dev. Med. Child Neurol., *12*:592, 1970.

453. Root, L.: Tendon surgery on the feet of children with cerebral palsy. Dev. Med. Child Neurol., *18*:671, 1976.

454. Root, L.: Varus and valgus foot in cerebral palsy and its management. Foot Ankle, *4*:174, 1984.

455. Root, L., Goss, J. R., and Mendes, J.: The treatment of the painful hip in cerebral palsy by total hip replacement or hip arthrodesis. J. Bone Joint Surg., *68-A*:590, 1986.

456. Root, L., and Spero, C. R.: Hip adductor transfer compared with adductor tenotomy in cerebral palsy. J. Bone Joint Surg., *63-A*:767, 1981.

457. Rose, J., Medeiros, J. M., and Parker, R.: Energy

cost index as an estimate of energy expenditure of cerebral-palsied children during assisted ambulation. Dev. Med. Child Neurol., *27*:485, 1985.

458. Rosenberg, B., Golan, J., Sternberg, N., and Ben-Hur, N.: A surgical treatment for drooling in cerebral palsy. Harefuah, *99*:156, 1980.

459. Rosenthal, R. K.: The use of orthotics in foot and ankle problems in cerebral palsy. Foot Ankle, *4*:195, 1984.

460. Rosenthal, R. K., Deutsch, S. D., Miller, W., Schuman, W., and Hall, J. E.: A fixed-ankle below-the-knee orthosis for the management of genu recurvatum in spastic cerebral palsy. J. Bone Joint Surg., *57-A*:545, 1975.

461. Rosenthal, R. K., Levine, D. B., and McCarver, C. L.: The occurrence of scoliosis in cerebral palsy. Dev. Med. Child Neurol., *16*:664, 1974.

462a. Ross, P. M., and Lyne, D.: The Grice procedure: indicators and evaluation of long term results. Clin. Orthop., *153*:195, 1980.

462b. Ruda, R., and Frost, H. M.: Cerebral palsy. Spastic varus and forefoot adductus, treated by intra-muscular posterior tibial tendon lengthening. Clin. Orthop., *79*:61, 1971.

463. Russ, J. D., and Soboloff, H. R.: A Primer of Cerebral Palsy. Springfield, Charles C Thomas, 1958.

464. Rutter, M., Graham, P., and Yule, W.: Neuropsychiatric Study in Childhood. Clinical in Developmental Medicine, No. 35/36. London, Spastics International Medical Publications with Heinemann Medical, 1970.

465. Sakellarides, H. T., Mital, M. A., and Lenzi, W. D.: Treatment of pronation contractures of the forearm in cerebral palsy by changing the insertion of the pronator radii teres. J. Bone Joint Surg., *63-A*:645, 1981.

466. Samilson, R. L.: Principles of assessment of the upper limb. Clin. Orthop., *47*:105, 1966.

467. Samilson, R. L.: Surgery of the upper limbs in cerebral palsy. Dev. Med. Child Neurol., 9:109, 1967.

468. Samilson, R. L.: Orthopaedic Aspects of Cerebral Palsy. Philadelphia, J. B. Lippincott, 1975.

469. Samilson, R. L.: Orthopaedic Aspects of Cerebral Palsy. Clinics in Developmental Medicine No. 52/53. London, William Heinemann Medical Books, 1975.

470. Samilson, R. L.: Tendon transfers in cerebral palsy (editorial). J. Bone Joint Surg., *58-B*:153, 1978.

471. Samilson, R. L.: Current concepts of surgical management of deformities of the lower extremities in cerebral palsy. Clin. Orthop., *158*:99, 1981.

472. Samilson, R. L.: Orthopedic surgery of the hips and spine in retarded cerebral palsy patients. Orthop. Clin. North Am., *12*:83, 1981.

473. Samilson, R., and Bechard, R.: Scoliosis in cerebral palsy: Incidence, distribution of curve patterns, natural history and thoughts on etiology. Curr. Pract. Orthop. Scand., *5*:183, 1973.

474. Samilson, R. L., Carson, J. J., James, P., and Raney, F. L., Jr.: Results and complications of adductor tenotomy and obturator neurectomy in cerebral palsy. Clin. Orthop., *54*:51, 1967.

475. Samilson, R. L., and Green, W. L.: Long-term results of upper limb surgery in cerebral palsy. Reconstr. Surg. Traumatol., *13*:43, 1972.

476. Samilson, R. L., and Hoffer, M. M.: Problems and complications in orthopaedic management of cerebral palsy. *In* Samilson, R. L. (ed.): Orthopaedic Aspects of Cerebral Palsy. Philadelphia, J. B. Lippincott, 1975, pp. 258–274.

477. Samilson, R. L., and Morris, J. M.: Surgical improvement of the cerebral palsied upper limb—electromyographic studies and results of 128 operations. J. Bone Joint Surg., *46-A*:1203, 1964.

478. Samilson, R. L., and Perry, J.: The orthopaedic assessment in cerebral palsy. *In* Samilson, R. L. (ed.):

Orthopaedic Aspects in Cerebral Palsy. Philadelphia, J. B. Lippincott, 1975, pp. 35–70.

479. Samilson, R. L., Tsou, P., Aamoth, G., and Green, W. M.: Dislocation and subluxation of the hip in cerebral palsy: pathogenesis, natural history and management. J. Bone Joint Surg., 54-A:863, 1972.

480. Sandifer, P. H.: Neurology in Orthopaedics. London, Butterworths, 1967.

481. Sanner, C., and Sundequist, U.: Acupuncture for the relief of painful muscle spasms in dystonic cerebral palsy. Dev. Med. Child Neurol., 23:544, 1981.

482. Schenectady County Study: Report of the New York State Joint Legislative Committee to study the problem of cerebral palsy. A Survey of Cerebral Palsy in Schenectady County. New York Legislation Document 55, Section 2, 1949.

483. Schneider, M., and Balon, K.: Deformity of the foot following anterior transfer of the posterior tibial tendon and lengthening of the Achilles tendon for spastic equinovarus. Clin. Orthop., 125:113, 1977.

484. Schultz, R. S., Chamberlain, S. E., and Stevens, P. M.: Radiographic comparison of adductor procedures in cerebral palsied hips. J. Pediatr. Orthop., 4:741, 1984.

485a. Scrutton, D. (ed.): The Management of Motor Disorders of Children with Cerebral Palsy. Clinics in Developmental Medicine, No. 90. London, S.I.M.P. with Blackwell Scientific; Philadelphia, J. B. Lippincott, 1984.

485b. Scrutton, D.: Aim-oriented management. In Scrutton, D. (ed.): The Management of Motor Disorders of Children with Cerebral Palsy. Clinics in Developmental Medicine. No. 90. London, S.I.M.P. with Blackwell Scientific; Philadelphia, J. B. Lippincott, 1984.

486. Seeger, B. R., and Caudry, D. J.: Biofeedback therapy to achieve symmetrical gait in children with hemiplegic cerebral palsy: Long term efficacy. Arch. Phys. Med. Rehabil., 64:160, 1983.

487. Seeger, B. R., Caudry, D. J., and O'Mara, N. A.: Hand-function in cerebral palsy: The effect of hip-flexion angle. Dev. Med. Child Neurol., 26:601, 1984.

488. Seeger, B. R., Caudrey, D. J., and Scholes, J. R.: Biofeedback therapy to achieve symmetrical gait in hemiplegic cerebral palsied children. Arch. Phys. Med. Rehabil., 62:364, 1981.

489. Sever, J. W.: Obstetric paralysis. Its etiology, pathology, clinical aspects and treatment, with a report of four hundred and seventy cases. Am. J. Dis. Child., 12:541, 1916.

490. Seymour, N., and Evans, D. K.: A modification of the Grice subtalar arthrodesis. J. Bone Joint Surg., 50-B:372, 1958.

491. Seymour, N., and Sharrard, W. J. W.: Bilateral proximal release of the hamstrings in cerebral palsy. J. Bone Joint Surg., 50-B:271, 1968.

492. Sharps, C. H., Clancy, M., and Steel, H. H.: A long-term retrospective study of proximal hamstring release for hamstring contracture in cerebral palsy. J. Pediatr. Orthop., 4:443, 1984.

493. Sharrard, W. J. W.: Muscle paralysis in poliomyelitis. Br. J. Surg., 44:471, 1957.

494. Sharrard, W. J. W.: The nature and management of spasticity. The peripheral surgery of spasticity. Proc. R. Soc. Med., 57:715, 1964.

495. Sharrard, W. J. W.: Posterior iliopsoas transplantation in the treatment of paralytic dislocation of the hip. J. Bone Joint Surg., 46-B:426, 1964.

496. Sharrard, W. J. W.: Paralytic deformity in the lower limb. J. Bone Joint Surg., 49-B:731, 1967.

497. Sharrard, W. J. W.: The orthopedic surgery of cerebral palsy and spina bifida. In Apley, A. G. (ed.): Recent Advances in Orthopaedics. London, J. & A. Churchill, 1969, p. 265.

498a. Sharrard, W. J. W.: The hip in cerebral palsy. In Tronzo, R. J. (ed.): Surgery of the Hip Joint. Philadelphia, Lea & Febiger, 1973, p. 145.

498b. Sharrard, W. J. W.: Indications for bracing in cerebral palsy. In Murdoch, G. (ed.): The Advance in Orthotics. London, Edward Arnold, 1976, pp. 453–461.

499. Sharrard, W. J. W.: Paediatric Orthopaedics and Fractures. 2nd Ed. Oxford, Blackwell Scientific Publications, 1979.

500. Sharrard, W. J. W., Allen, J. M. H., Heaney, S. H., and Prendiville, G. R. G.: Surgical prophylaxis of subluxation and dislocation of the hip in cerebral palsy. J. Bone Joint Surg., 57-B:160, 1975.

501. Sharrard, W. J. W., and Bernstein, S.: Equinus deformity in cerebral palsy. J. Bone Joint Surg., 54-B:272, 1972.

502. Sherk, H. H.: Treatment of severe rigid contractures of cerebral palsied upper limbs. Clin. Orthop., 125:151, 1977.

503. Sherk, H. H., Pasquariello, P. D., and Doherty, J.: Hip dislocation in cerebral palsy: Selection for treatment. Dev. Med. Child Neurol., 25:738, 1983.

504. Silfverskiold, N.: Reduction of the uncrossed two-joint muscles of the leg to one-joint muscles in spastic conditions. Acta Chir. Scand., 56:315, 1923–1924.

505. Silver, C. M., and Simon, S. D.: Gastrocnemius-muscle recession (Silfverskiold operation) for spastic equinus deformity in cerebral palsy. J. Bone Joint Surg., 41-A:1021, 1959.

506. Silver, C. M., Simon, S. D., and Lichtman, H. M.: Calcaneal osteotomy for valgus and varus deformities of the foot. Int. Surg., 58:24, 1973.

507. Silver, C. M., Simon, S. D., Lichtman, H. M., and Motamed, M.: Surgical correction of spastic thumb-in-palm deformity. Dev. Med. Child Neurol., 18:632, 1976.

508. Silver, C. M., Simon, S. D., Spindell, E., Lichtman, H. M., and Scala, M.: Calcaneal osteotomy for valgus and varus deformity of the foot in cerebral palsy. J. Bone Joint Surg., 49-A:232, 1967.

509. Silver, R. L., Rang, M., Chang, J., and de la Garza, J.: Adductor release in nonambulant children with cerebral palsy. J. Pediatr. Orthop., 5:672, 1985.

510. Simon, S. R., Deutsch, S. D., Nuzzo, R. M., Mansour, M. J., Jackson, J. L., Koskinen, M., and Rosenthal, R. K.: Genu recurvatum in spastic cerebral palsy. J. Bone Joint Surg., 60-A:882, 1978.

511a. Skinner, S. R., and Lester, D. K.: Dynamic EMG findings in valgus hindfoot deformity in spastic cerebral palsy. Orthop. Trans., 9:91, 1985.

511b. Skoff, H., and Woodbury, D. F.: Management of the upper extremity in cerebral palsy. J. Bone Joint Surg., 67-A:500, 1985.

512. Skrotzky, K.: Gait analysis in cerebral palsied and nonhandicapped children. Arch. Phys. Med. Rehabil., 64:291, 1983.

513. Smith, E. T.: Hip dislocation in cerebral palsy. Dev. Med. Child Neurol., 11:291, 1969.

514. Smith, J. B., and Westin, G. W.: Subtalar extra-articular arthrodesis. J. Bone Joint Surg., 50-A:1027, 1968.

515. Smith, R. J., and Hasting, H., II: Principles of tendon transfers to the hand. A.A.O.S. Instr. Course Lect. 29:129, 1980.

516. Smith, S. L., Gossman, M. R., and Canan, B. C.: Selected primitive reflexes in children with cerebral palsy: Consistency of response. Phys. Ther., 62:1115, 1982.

517. Staheli, L. T., Duncan, W. R., and Schaeffer, E.: Growth alterations in the hemiplegic child. A study of femoral anteversion neck-shaft angle, hip rotation, C. E. angle, limb length and circumference in 50 hemiplegic children. Clin. Orthop., 60:205, 1969.

518. Stahl, F.: Gastrocnemius recession. Acta Orthop. Scand., 32:466, 1962.
519. Stamp, W. G.: Bracing in cerebral palsy. J. Bone Joint Surg., 44-A:1457, 1962.
520. Stanley, F. J.: An epidemiological study of cerebral palsy in Western Australia, 1956–1975. Changes in total incidence of cerebral palsy and associated factors. Dev. Med. Child Neurol., 21:701, 1979.
521. Steel, H. H.: Triple osteotomy of the innominate bone. A procedure to accomplish coverage of the dislocated or subluxated femoral head in the older patient. Clin. Orthop., 122:116, 1977.
522. Steel, H. H.: Gluteus medius and minimus insertion advancement for correction of internal rotation gait in spastic cerebral palsy. J. Bone Joint Surg., 62-A:919, 1980.
523. Steindler, A.: Pathokenetics of cerebral palsy. A.A.O.S. Instructional Course Lectures. Vol. 9. Ann Arbor, J. W. Edwards, 1952, p. 118.
524. Stelling, F. H., and Meyer, L. C.: Cerebral palsy. The upper extremity. Clin. Orthop., 14:70, 1959.
525. Stephenson, Ch. T., and Donovan, M. M.: Transfer of hip adductor origins to the ischium in spastic cerebral palsy. J. Bone Joint Surg., 51-A:1050, 1969.
526. Stephenson, C. T., Griffith, B., Donovan, M. M., and Franklin, T.: The adductor transfer and iliopsoas release in the cerebral palsy hip. Orthop. Trans., 6:94, 1982.
527. Stephenson, T., and Donovan, M. M.: Transfer of the hip adductor origin to the ischium in spastic cerebral palsy. Dev. Med. Child Neurol., 13:247, 1971.
528. Stoffel, A.: The treatment of spastic contractures. Am. J. Orthop. Surg., 10:611, 1913.
529. Strayer, L. M., Jr.: Recession of the gastrocnemius, an operation to relieve spastic contracture of the calf muscles. J. Bone Joint Surg., 32-A:671, 1950.
530. Strayer, L. M., Jr.: Gastrocnemius recession. Five-year report of cases. J. Bone Joint Surg., 40-A:1019, 1958.
531. Stromeyer, G. F.: Beitragge zur operativen Orthopadik oder Erfahrungen uber die subcutane Durchschneidung verkurzter Muskein und deren Sehnen. Hanover, Helwing, 1838.
532. Sugita, H.: A study on the spinal deformity in cerebral palsy. Nippon Geka Hokan, 52:86, 1983.
533. Sussman, M. D.: Casting as an adjunct to neurodevelopmental therapy for cerebral palsy. Dev. Med. Child Neurol., 25:804, 1983.
534. Sutherland, D. H.: Gait Disorders in Childhood and Adolescents. Baltimore, Williams & Wilkins, 1984.
535. Sutherland, D. H., and Greenfield, R.: Double innominate osteotomy. J. Bone Joint Surg., 59-A:1082, 1977.
536. Sutherland, D. H., Larsen, L. J., and Mann, R.: Rectus femoris release in selected patients with cerebral palsy. A preliminary report. Dev. Med. Child Neurol., 17:26, 1975.
537. Sutherland, D. H., Schottstaedt, E. R., Larsen, L. J., Ashley, R. K., Callander, J. N., and James, P. M.: Clinical and electromyographic study of seven spastic children with internal rotation gait. J. Bone Joint Surg., 51-A:1070, 1969.
538. Sutherland, D. H., Olshen, R., Cooper, G., and Woo, S. K. Y.: The development of mature gait. J. Bone Joint Surg., 62-A:336, 1980.
539. Swanson, A. B.: Surgery of the hand in cerebral palsy and the swan-neck deformity. J. Bone Joint Surg., 42-A:951, 1960.
540. Swanson, A. B.: Surgery of the hand in cerebral palsy. Surg. Clin. North Am., 44:1061, 1964.
541. Swanson, A. B., Treatment of swan-neck deformity in cerebral palsied hand. Clin. Orthop., 48:167, 1966.
542. Swanson, A. B.: Surgery of the hand in cerebral palsy and muscle release procedures. Surg. Clin. North Am., 48:1129, 1968.
543. Swinyard, C. A.: Reflections about reflex therapy in cerebral palsy. Phys. Ther. Rev., 39:103, 1959.
544. Szalay, E. A., Roach, J. W., Houkom, J. A., Wenger, D. R., and Herring, A.: Extension-abduction contracture of the spastic hip. J. Pediatr. Orthop., 6:1, 1986.
545. Tabary, J.-C., Goldspink, G., Tardieu, C., Lombard, M., Tardieu, G., and Chigot, P.: Nature de la retraction des I.M.C. Mesure de l'allongement des sarcomeres du muscle etire. Rev. Chir. Orthop., 57:463, 1971.
546. Tachdjian, M. O., and Matson, D. D.: Orthopaedic aspects of intraspinal tumors in infants and children. J. Bone Joint Surg., 47-A:223, 1965.
547. Tachdjian, M. O., and Minear, W. C.: Hip dislocation in cerebral palsy. J. Bone Joint Surg., 38-A:1358, 1956.
548. Tachdjian, M. O., and Minear, W. C.: Sensory disturbances in the hands of children with cerebral palsy. J. Bone Joint Surg., 40-A:85, 1958.
549. Tardieu, C., Bret, M. D., Colbeau-Justin, P., and Huet de la Tour, E.: Relationship of triceps surae torques to photographed tibia-calcaneus angles in man. (II). Eur. J. Appl. Physiol., 37:153, 1977.
550. Tardieu, C., Colbeau-Justin, P., Bret, M. D., Lespargot, A., Huet de la Tour, E., and Tardieu, G.: An apparatus and a method for measuring the relationship of triceps surae torques to tibio-tarsal angles in man. Eur. J. Appl. Physiol., 35:11, 1976.
551. Tardieu, C., Huet de la Tour, E., Bret, M. D., and Tardieu, G.: Muscle hypoextensibility in children with cerebral palsy: I. Clinical and experimental observations. Arch. Phys. Med. Rehabil., 63:97, 1982.
552. Tardieu, G., Lespargot, A., and Tardieu, C.: To what extent is the tibia-calcaneum angle a reliable measurement of the triceps surae strength? Radiological correction of the torque-angle curve (III). Eur. J. Appl. Physiol., 37:163, 1977.
553. Tardieu, G., Tabary, J.-C., Tardieu, C., and Lombard, M.: Retraction, hyperextensibilite et "faiblesse" de l'I.M.C. expressions apparement opposees d'un meme trouble musculaire. Consequences therapeutiques. Rev. Chir. Orthop., 57:505, 1971.
554. Tardieu, G., Tardieu, C., Colbeau-Justin, P., and Bret, M. D.: Effects of muscle length on an increased stretch reflex in children with cerebral palsy. J. Neurol. Neurosurg. Psychiatry, 45:348, 1982.
555. Tardieu, G., Tardieu, C., Colbeau-Justin, P., and Lespargot, A.: Muscle hypoextensibility in children with cerebral palsy. II. Therapeutic implications. Arch. Phys. Med. Rehabil., 63:103, 1982.
556. Tardieu, G., Tardieu, C., Hariga, J., and Gagnard, L.: Treatment of spasticity by injection of dilute alcohol at the motor point or by epidural route. Clinical extension of an experiment on the decerebrate cat. Dev. Med. Child Neurol., 10:555, 1968.
557. Thibodeau, A. A., Wagner, L. C., and Carr, F. J.: Jun: The evaluation of surgical procedures on bones, muscles and peripheral nerves in spastic paralysis. Am. J. Surg., 43:822, 1939.
558. Thomas, A., Bax, M., Coombes, K., Goldson, E., Smyth, D., and Whitmore, K.: The health and social needs of physically handicapped young adults: Are they being met by the statutory services? Dev. Med. Child Neurol., 27(Suppl. 50), 1985.
559. Thometz, J. G., and Tachdjian, M. O.: Long-term follow-up of the flexor-carpi ulnaris transfer in spastic hemiplegia children. J. Pediatr. Orthop., 8:407, 1988.
560. Thompson, G. H., Likavec, M. J., Archibald, I., and Rush, T.: Atlantoaxial rotatory subluxation, congenital

absence of the posterior arch of the atlas, and cerebral palsy: An unusual triad. J. Pediatr. Orthop., 5:232, 1985.

561. Thompson, G. H., Rubin, I., and Bilenker, R.: Comprehensive management of cerebral palsy. J. Pediatr. Orthop., 5:610, 1985.

562. Thompson, S. B.: Indications for surgery in the lower limbs of the cerebral palsied child. Dev. Med. Child Neurol., 8:437, 1966.

563. Throop, F. B., DeRosa, G. P., Reeck, C., and Waterman, S.: Correction of equinus in cerebral palsy by the Murphy procedure of tendon calcaneus advancement: A preliminary communication. Dev. Med. Child Neurol., 17:182, 1975.

564. Thuilleux, G., and Tachdjian, M. O.: Traitement de la flexion pronation du poignet chez l'enfant hemiplegique. Rev. Chir. Orthop., 62:419, 1976.

565. Tizard, J. P. M.: Sensory defects in cerebral palsy. Cerebr. Palsy Bull., 2:40, 1960.

566. Tizard, J. P. M., Paine, R. S., and Crothers, B.: Disturbances of sensation in children with hemiplegia. J.A.M.A., 155:628, 1954.

567. Tohen, A. Z., Carmona, J. P., and Barrera, J. R.: The utilization of abnormal reflexes in the treatment of spastic foot deformities. Clin. Orthop., 47:77, 1966.

568. Tonnis, D., and Rauterberg, E.: Ergebnisse der orthopadisch-chirurgeschen Behandlung infantiler Cerebralparesen und die Indikation zur Operation. Arch. Orthop. Unfallchir., 62:29, 1967.

569. Townsend, W. R.: Tendon transplantation in the treatment of deformities of the hand. Medical News, 77, 2:41, 1900.

570. Truscelli, D., Lespargot, A., and Tardieu, G.: Variation in the long-term results of elongation of the tendo-Achilles in children with cerebral palsy. J. Bone Joint Surg., 61-A:466, 1979.

571. Turek, S. L.: Orthopaedics. Principles and Their Application. 4th Ed. Philadelphia, J. B. Lippincott, 1984, pp. 560–595.

572. Turner, J. W., and Cooper, R. R.: Anterior transfer of the tibialis posterior through the interosseous membrane. Clin. Orthop., 83:241, 1972.

573. Twitchell, T. E.: The neurologic examination in infantile cerebral palsy. Dev. Med. Child Neurol., 5:271, 1963.

574. Twitchell, T. E.: Sensation and the motor deficit in cerebral palsy. Clin. Orthop., 46:55, 1966.

575. Tylkowski, C. M., Rosenthal, R. K., and Simon, S. R.: Proximal femoral osteotomy in cerebral palsy. Clin. Orthop., 151:183, 1980.

576. Tylkowski, C. M., Simon, S. R., and Mansour, J. M.: The Frank Stinchfield Award Paper. Internal rotation gait in spastic cerebral palsy. In The Hip: Proceedings of the Tenth Open Scientific Meeting of the Hip Society. St. Louis, C. V. Mosby, 1982, pp. 89–125.

577a. Vasin, N. I., Nodvornik, P., Lesnov, N., Kadin, A. L., and Shramka, M.: Stereotaxic combined dentate-thalamotomy in the treatment of spastic-hyperkinetic forms of subcortical dyskinesias. Zhurnal Voprosy Neirokhirurgii Imeni N.N. Burdenko (Moskova), 6:23, 1979.

577b. Vidal, J., De Guillaume, P., and Vidal, M.: Balance of the pelvic girdle in cerebral palsy. Rev. Chir. Orthop., 70:297, 1984.

578a. Vojta, V.: Die zerebralen Bewegunstrorungen im Sauglingsalter, Frudiagnose und Frutherapie. 3rd ed. Stuttgart, F. Enke, 1981, pp. 183–189.

578b. Vojta, V.: The basic elements of treatment according to Vojta. In Scrutton, D. (ed.): The Management of the Motor Disorders of Children with Cerebral Palsy. Clinics in Developmental Medicine No. 90, London, S.I.M.P. with Blackwell Scientific; Philadelphia, J. B. Lippincott, 1984, pp. 75–85.

579. Vulpius, O., and Stoffel, A.: Orthopaedische Op-

erationslebre. 2nd Ed. Stuttgart, Ferdinand Enke, 1920.

580. Walshe, F. M. R.: On certain tonic or postural reflexes in hemiplegia with special reference to so-called "associated movements." Brain, 46:1, 1923.

581. Waters, R. L., Perry, J., McDaniels, J. M., and House, K.: The relative strength of the hamstrings during hip extension. J. Bone Joint Surg., 56-A:1592, 1974.

582. Watkins, M. B., Jones, R. B., Ryder, C. T., and Brown, T. H., Jr.: Transplantation of the posterior tibial tendon. J. Bone Joint Surg., 36-A:1181, 1954.

583. Watson-Jones, R.: Spontaneous dislocation of the hip. Br. J. Surg., 14:36, 1926.

584a. Watt, J., Sims, D., Harckham, F., Schmidt, L., McMillan, A., and Hamilton, J.: A prospective study of inhibitive casting as an adjunct to physiotherapy in the cerebral palsied child. Orthop. Trans., 8:110, 1984.

584b. Wesely, M. S., and Barenfeld, P. A.: Mechanism of the Dwyer calcaneal osteotomy. Clin. Orthop., 70:137, 1970.

585a. Westin, G. W., and Dye, S.: Conservative management of cerebral palsy in the growing child. Foot Ankle, 4:160, 1983.

585b. Wheeler, M. E., and Weinstein, S. L.: Adductor tenotomy-obturator neurectomy. J. Pediatr. Orthop., 4:48, 1984.

586. White, J. W.: Torsion of the Achilles tendon: Its surgical significance. Arch. Surg., 46:784, 1943.

587. White, W. F.: Flexor muscle slide in the spastic hand. The Max Page operation. J. Bone Joint Surg., 54-B:453, 1972.

588. Whitman, R.: A Treatise on Orthopaedic Surgery. 6th Ed. Philadelphia, Lea & Febiger, 1919.

589. Williams, P. F.: Restoration of muscle balance of the foot by transfer of the tibialis posterior. J. Bone Joint Surg., 58-B:217, 1976.

590. Woods, G.: Cerebral Palsy in Childhood. Bristol, John Wright & Sons, 1957.

591. Wright, T., and Nicholson, J.: Physiotherapy for the spastic child: An evaluation. Dev. Med. Child Neurol., 15:146, 1973.

592. Yu, W., and Schweigel, J. F.: Flexor digitorum sublimis to profundus tendon transfer for flexion deformities in spastic paralysis. Can. J. Surg., 17:225, 1974.

593. Yeates, H., and Mott, D. H.: Inhibitive casting. Paper read at the First William C. Duncan Seminar on Cerebral Palsy. Seattle, Children's Orthopaedic Hospital and Medical Center and the University of Washington, 1977.

593. Zachazewski, J., Eberle, E. D., and Jefferies, M.: Effect of tone-inhibitory casts and orthosis on gait. Phys. Ther., 62:145, 1983.

594. Zancolli, E.: The Structural and Dynamic Bases of Hand Surgery. Philadelphia, J. B. Lippincott, 1968.

595. Zancolli, E. A., Goldner, J. L., and Swanson, A. B.: Surgery of the spastic hand in cerebral palsy. Report of the Committee on Spastic Hand Evaluation. J. Hand Surg., 8:766, 1983.

596. Zancolli, E. A., and Zancolli, E. A., Jr.: Surgical management of the hemiplegic spastic hand in cerebral palsy. Surg. Clin. North Am., 61:395, 1981.

597. Zappert, J.: Ueber ein gehauftes Auftreten gutartiger Facialislamungen beim Kinde. Kinderheilk., 38:139, 1924.

598. Zausmer, E.: Locomotion in cerebral palsy. Clin. Orthop., 47:49, 1966.

599. Zervas, N. T., Horner, F. A., and Pickren, K. S.: The treatment of dyskinesia by stereotactic dentatectomy. Confin. Neurol., 29:93, 1967.

600. Zuckerman, J. D., Staheli, L. T., and McLaughlin, J. F.: Acetabular augmentation for progressive hip subluxation in cerebral palsy. J. Pediatr. Orthop., 4:436, 1984.

INTRACRANIAL TUMORS[1-33]

Intracranial tumors in childhood are common, being third in frequency to leukemia and neoplasms arising in the renal and suprarenal area. The highest incidence is in the age period from five to eight years. There is no significant sex predilection.

The orthopedic surgeon should keep in mind the possibility of an intracranial neoplasm when examining the child with an abnormality in gait, spasticity in the limbs, or torticollis. Also, since rehabilitation of the musculoskeletal system in the postoperative period is the concern of the orthopedist, he should be knowledgeable about the biology and prognosis of intracranial tumors.

Pathologic Considerations

Gliomas constitute a large proportion (about 75 per cent) of intracranial neoplasms found in children. Cerebellar astrocytomas, fourth ventricle medulloblastomas and ependymomas, and pontine gliomas are the common tumors, whereas the malignant glioblastoma multiforme (a common neoplasm in the cerebral hemisphere of adults) is relatively infrequent in children. Also, the benign lesions—meningiomas, acoustic neurinomas, and pituitary adenomas—which are the commoner types of adult tumors, are almost unknown in childhood. Other specific tumors encountered in childhood are craniopharyngioma, papilloma of the choroid plexus, glioma of the optic chiasm, and teratoma.

The anatomic location of intracranial neoplasms in children differs from that in adults. About two thirds of the tumors in children arise within the cerebellum, fourth ventricle, lower brain stem, cisterna magna, and cerebellopontine angle, whereas in the adult only one fourth of the tumors occur in these areas. In children, there is also a preponderance of tumors along the central neural axis. These account for the initial clinical manifestations being the result of increased intracranial pressure rather than a focal neurologic abnormality.

The common malignant intracranial tumors of childhood are medulloblastoma, pontine glioma, and third and fourth ventricular ependymomas, the prognoses for all of which are very poor. In the experience of Matson, 45 per cent of intracranial tumors should be considered benign; that is, they can be surgically excised with an 80 to 90 per cent cure rate. Figure 5–70 shows the incidence of various pathologic types of intracranial tumors in children under 12 years of age seen at the Children's Hospital Medical Center in Boston.[18] They are arbitrarily divided into benign and malignant, being so designated because of their histologic features and their anatomic accessibility for surgical excision.

Clinical Features

Often the initial manifestation of an intracranial tumor is increased intracranial pressure, the clinical features of which are headache, irritability, vomiting, somnolence, lethargy, papilledema, strabismus, diplopia, and increased head size. The pediatrician is ordinarily consulted for evaluation of these symptoms, and thus it is important that he keep in mind the possibility of an intracranial neoplasm when confronted with this complex of symptoms.

Neurologic manifestations depend upon the location of the tumor. When the lesion is located in the posterior fossa, neurologic symptoms and signs include ataxia (the child walks in a wide-based gait, develops a lurch, and falls frequently); dysmetria and adiadochokinesia; torticollis (the head is held tilted to one side with resistance to attempts to move it, and there is also palpable spasm of the cervical muscle); generalized muscular weakness, especially of the lower limbs, with hypotonia and hyporeflexia; nystagmus; cranial nerve paralysis (particularly the sixth); and tonic seizures. Tumors of the cerebral hemispheres cause disturbances of behavior, speech, or visual perception; motor, sensory, or reflex changes; and convulsive seizures. Suprasellar tumors (craniopharyngioma, optic pathway and hypothalamic gliomas, and epidermoid and teratoid tumors) produce visual disorders and disturbances of carbohydrate and water metabolism and of autonomic and pituitary function. Neoplasms in the brain stem are associated with pyramidal tract signs (spastic paralysis and hyporeflexia) and bilateral cranial nerve involvement.

Diagnostic Considerations

Radiograms of the skull will show changes in about 86 per cent of children with intracranial tumors. The increase in intracranial pressure causes the cranial sutures to separate—initially and most prominently, the coronal suture, followed by the sagittal and lambdoid, and rarely, the squamosal. The head of the infant generally enlarges from increased intracranial tension. Other abnormalities may include increased convolutional markings, localized thinning of one or more of the skull bones by erosion from the

BENIGN		MALIGNANT	
ASTROCYTOMA	87	MEDULLOBLASTOMA	63
Cerebellar	68	EPENDYMOMA	35
Cerebral	19	Sub-tentorial	20
EPENDYMOMA	7	Supra-tentorial	15
Sub-tentorial	2	GLIOMA of BRAIN STEM	39
Supra-tentorial	5	MIXED GLIOMA	15
GLIOMA of OPTIC PATHWAY	16	Cerebral	7
CRANIOPHARYNGIOMA	23	Cerebellar	8
DERMOID and EPIDERMOID CYST	12	GLIOBLASTOMA MULTIFORME	13
PAPILLOMA of CHOROID PLEXUS	12	GANGLIOGLIOMA	5
CAVERNOUS HEMANGIOMA	4	SARCOMA of MENINGES	4
MENINGIOMA	2	HAMARTOMA, III VENTRICLE	3
PARAPHYSIAL CYST	1	RETINOBLASTOMA	3
TUBERCULOMA	1	TERATOMA, MALIGNANT	2
CHORDOMA	1	METASTATIC WILMS TUMOR	1
NEUROFIBROMA	1	SPONGIOBLASTOMA	1
		MICROGLIOMA	1
		EMBRYONAL CELL CARCINOMA	1
		PINEALOMA	1
TOTAL	167(47%)	TOTAL	187(53%)

FIGURE 5–70. *Incidence of intracranial tumors in children.*

Three hundred and fifty-four consecutive intracranial tumors in children under 12 years of age were seen by the neurosurgical service, Children's Hospital Medical Center, Boston, between 1948 and 1961. Note that 47 per cent are considered benign. (From Matson, D. D., Intracranial tumors. *In*, Farmer, T. W., ed.: Pediatric Neurology. New York, Hoeber Medical Division, Harper and Row, Publishers, 1964, p. 475. Reprinted by permission.)

adjacent mass, and intracranial calcification (commonly seen with ependymomas and craniopharyngiomas).

Electroencephalography, computed axial tomography, and nuclear magnetic resonance imaging are invaluable in the diagnosis of brain tumor.[6, 15, 21, 30] The findings depend upon the location of the tumor. When the neoplasm is located in the cerebral hemisphere the electroencephalogram is almost always abnormal, whereas with tumors of the brain stem, ventricular system, and suprasellar area, the electroencephalogram may be normal. In the past, pneumoencephalography, contrast ventriculography, and arteriography were extremely important in the diagnosis and determination of the exact anatomic site of intracranial tumors. At present these studies are utilized occasionally; they have been replaced by the noninvasive CT and magnetic resonance imaging studies.

Caution should be exercised in performing lumbar puncture for cerebrospinal fluid examination in brain tumors in children, as a high percentage of these neoplasms are located in the posterior fossa, and a sudden reduction in pressure by lumbar puncture is very dangerous.

Treatment

Treatment is by surgical excision. When total excision of the tumor is impossible, however, and spinal fluid circulation is still disturbed, operative procedures are carried out to short-circuit the spinal fluid circulation around an area of obstruction. Radiation therapy and chemotherapy are indicated in malignant tumors.[9]

In the postoperative period, meticulous care should be given to the musculoskeletal system to prevent development of limb deformities and for functional rehabilitation. Often such care has been neglected because of the common misconception that all intracranial tumors in childhood have a poor prognosis for useful survival. In the modern era of neurosurgery and progress in anesthesia, temperature control, hemostasis, blood replacement, and endocrine and metabolic supportive treatment, the results of intracranial surgery of benign brain tumors are good. Details of orthopedic care depend upon the degree and distribution of neurologic deficit and paralysis. Active and passive exercises are performed and bivalved night casts are worn to prevent the development of deformities. Orthotic devices are used as indicated. In the residual stage, operative procedures are carried out, provided the lesion is stabilized and there is no change in the pattern of paralysis.

References

1. Bailey, P., Buchanan, D. N., and Bucy, P. C.: Intracranial Tumors of Infancy and Childhood. Chicago, University of Chicago Press, 1939.
2. Bloom, H. J.: Recent concepts in the conservative treatment of intracranial tumors in children. Acta Neurochir. (Wein), 50:103, 1979.
3. Bodian, M., and Lawson, D.: Intracranial neoplastic disease of childhood. Br. J. Surg., 40:368, 1953.
4. Cuneo, H. M., and Rand, C. W.: Brain Tumors of Childhood. Springfield, Charles C Thomas, 1952.
5. Danoff, B. F., Cowchock, F. S., Marquette, C., Mulgrew, L., and Kramer, S.: Assessment of the long-term effects of primary radiation therapy for brain tumors in children. Cancer, 49:1580, 1982.
6. Day, R. E., Thomson, J. L., and Schutt, W. H.: Computerised tomography and acute neurological problems of childhood. Arch. Dis. Child., 53:2, 1978.
7. Deen, H. G., Jr., Scheithauer, B. W., and Ebersold, M. J.: Clinical and pathological study of meningiomas of the first two decades of life. J. Neurosurg., 56:317, 1982.
8. Deutsch, M.: Radiotherapy for primary brain tumors in very young children. Cancer, 50:2785, 1982.
9. Deutsch, M., Albo, V., and Wollman, M. R.: Radiotherapy for cerebral metastases in children. Int. J. Radiat. Oncol. Biol. Phys., 8:1441, 1982.
10. Duffner, P. K., and Cohen, M. E.: Extraneural metastases in childhood brain tumors. Ann. Neurol., 10:261, 1981.
11. Farwell, J. R., Dohrmann, G. J., and Flannery, J. T.: Central nervous system tumors in children. Cancer, 40:3123, 1977.
12. Gjerris, F.: Clinical aspects and long-term prognosis of infratentorial intracranial tumors in infancy and childhood. Acta Neurol. Scand., 57:31, 1978.
13. Harrison, M. J.: The clinical presentation of intracranial abscesses. Q. J. Med., 51:461, 1982.
14. Heiskanen, O.: Intracranial tumors of children. Childs Brain, 3:69, 1977.
15. Kazner, E., Meese, W., and Kretzschmar, K.: The role of computed tomography in the diagnosis of brain tumors in infants and children. Neuroradiology, 16:10, 1978.
16. Kun, L. E., Mulhern, R. K., and Crisco, J. J.: Quality of life in children treated for brain tumors. Intellectual, emotional and academic function. J. Neurosurg., 58:1, 1983.
17. Matson, D. D.: Cerebellar astrocytoma in childhood. J. Pediatr., 18:150, 1956.
18. Matson, D. D.: Benign intracranial tumors of childhood. N. Engl. J. Med., 259:330, 1958.
19. Mayer, M., Ponsot, G., Kalifa, C., Lemerle, J., and Arthuis, M.: Thalamic tumors in children. A study of 38 cases (author's transl.). Arch. Fr. Pediatr., 39:91, 1982.
20. Mealy, J., Jr., and Hall, P. V.: Medulloblastoma in children. Survival and treatment. J. Neurosurg., 46:56, 1977.
21. Miller, J. H., Weinblatt, M. E., Smith, J. C., Fishman, L. S., Segall, H. D., and Ortega, J. A.: Combined computed tomographic and radionuclide imaging in the long-term follow-up of children with primary intra-axial intracranial neoplasms. Radiology, 146:681, 1983.
22. Papo, I., Caruselli, G., and Luongo, A.: External ventricular drainage in the management of posterior fossa tumors in children and adolescents. Neurosurgery, 10:13, 1982.
23. Pierre-Kahn, A., Hirsch, J. F., Renier, D., Sainte-Rose, C., Roux, F. X., and Pfister, A.: Intracranial ependymoma in children. Prognosis and therapeutic perspectives. Arch. Fr. Pediatr., 40:5, 1983.
24. Pierre-Kahn, A., Hirsch, J. F., Roux, F. X., Renier, D., and Sainte-Rose, C.: Intracranial ependymomas in childhood. Survival and functional results of 47 cases. Childs Brain, 10:145, 1983.
25. Raimondi, A. J., and Tomita, T.: Pineal tumors in childhood. Epidemiology, pathophysiology, and surgical approaches. Childs Brain, 9:239, 1982.
26. Russo, A., Delfini, R., Ciappetta, T., and Caroli, F.: Intracranial tumors during the first year of life: Clinicopathologic study of 24 cases. Ped. Med. Chir., 4:387, 1982.
27. Shillito, J.: An Atlas of Pediatric Neurosurgical Operations. Philadelphia, W. B. Saunders, 1982.
28. Stein, S. C.: Intracranial developmental cysts in children: treatment by cystoperitoneal shunting. Neurosurgery, 8:647, 1981.
29. Tadmor, R., Harwood-Nash, D. C., Scotti, G., Savoiardo, M., Musgrave, M. A., Fitz, C. R., Chuang, S., and Modan, M.: Intracranial neoplasms in children: the effect of computed tomography on age distribution. Radiology, 145:371, 1982.
30. Walker, A. E., and Hopple, J. L.: Brain tumors in children. General considerations. J. Pediatr., 35:671, 1949.
31. Weinblatt, M. E., Ortega, J. A., Miller, J. H., and Fishman, L. S.: The reliability of noninvasive diagnostic procedures in children with brain tumors. Am. J. Pediatr. Hematol. Oncol., 4:367, 1982.
32. Zimmerman, R. A., and Bilaniuk, L. T.: CT of primary and secondary craniocerebral neuroblastoma. A.J.R., 135:1239, 1980.

MYELOMENINGOCELE*

Myelomeningocele is a developmental defect of the vertebral arches and spinal cord characterized by a failure of fusion between the vertebral arches with dysplasia of the spinal cord and its membranes.

Spinal dysraphism and *myelodysplasia* are generic terms to encompass neural tube defects (NTD); however, under this general heading there are several specific entities that should be distinguished from each other.

Meningocele is an unfused condition of the vertebral arches with a visible meningeal sac along the spinal axis. The sac is filled with cerebrospinal fluid and composed of dura or

---

*Neurosurgical aspects written with David G. McClone, M.D., Ph.D., Professor and Head, Division of Neurosurgery, Children's Memorial Hospital, Chicago, Illinois.

dura and arachnoid, but no nerve tissue. There is no myelodysplasia of the spinal cord, nor is there any neurologic deficit; i.e., on neurologic examination there is no evidence of any sensory, motor, or reflex abnormality or sphincter disturbance.

In *myelomeningocele* the neural elements are abnormal and part of the sac. There is myelodysplasia of the spinal cord and neurologic deficit at and caudal to the level of the lesion.

The term *rachischisis* implies complete absence of all the covering structures so that the neural tissues themselves present on the surface of the body. The terms *myelocele, myelocystocele, hydromyelia,* and *myeloschisis* describe pathologic abnormalities of the spinal cord.

Incidence

The incidence of myelomeningocele varies in different parts of the world. The regional and national differences are possibly due to the different genetic compositions of the population and to environmental factors. The incidence of myelomeningocele is 2 per 1000 births in Birmingham[297] and North Hamptonshire, England;[340] 3 per 1000 in Liverpool;[550] and 4 per 1000 in South Wales.[308]

The incidence of myelomeningocele in the United States appears to be lower. O'Hare, in a survey of nearly a million and a half births at teaching centers in the United States, reported an incidence of 1.22 per 1000 births.[435] In community surveys, Alter reports a rate of 1.05 per 1000 live births in Charleston, South Carolina; a similar rate is given by Wallace et al. in New York.[6, 610] In Sweden, the incidence is 0.72 per 1000 live births.[228]

Myelomeningocele is slightly more common in females than in males. The sex ratio of male to female is reported as 1:1.15 by Doran and Guthkelch,[138] and 1:1.17 by Record and McKeown.[478]

Embryology

The central nervous system begins as a focal thickening caused by proliferation of ectodermal cells along the dorsum of the embryo. These cells increase in number and in height, ultimately forming a layer of pseudostratified epithelium. As the cells proliferate a groove forms in the sagittal plane of the cell mass. This groove deepens, bringing the lateral portions of the neural plate toward each other. Contractile proteins located within the superficial margin of these cells are felt to be responsible for the

actual contraction and drawing together of the neural folds. Progressive flexion brings the peripheral edges of the neural folds into contact. On about the twenty-first day, cell adhesion occurs at the point of contact, fusing the neural folds into the neural tube. Initially, fusion occurs near the center of the embryo at a point destined to become the craniovertebral junction. Fusion then proceeds longitudinally, in both caudal and cephalic directions simultaneously, forming the long neural tube. The cephalic (brain) end of the embryo closes first.

Just as the neural folds fuse together into the neural tube, the superficial ectoderm separates from the underlying (now fused) neural ectoderm and fuses with itself across the midline to close the back. The separation of superficial and neural ectoderm creates a plane into which mesenchymal cells migrate. This mesenchyme gives rise to the neural arch of the vertebrae and to paraspinal muscles. Closure of the neural ectoderm into a tubular structure and separation of the neural tube from the superficial ectoderm are critical events in the development of the central nervous system, and are completed by four weeks after fertilization.

Etiology

The cause of myelomeningocele remains obscure. It probably has multiple etiologies. *Genetic factors* are important; they are discussed under heredity. *Environment* plays a role in pathogenesis. *Nutritional factors* have also been postulated to play a role in myelomeningocele. At one time the potato was thought to be such a dietary factor.[108, 484] More recently, low folic acid intake by the mother prior to conception has been implicated. In a study from Britain, administration of preconceptual vitamins and folic acid supplements markedly reduced the expected recurrence rate of neural tube defects in families with prior births of children with myelomeningocele.[551] Analysis of the methods used in these studies casts doubt on the conclusion that vitamins and folic acid are effective in prevention of myelomeningocele. A larger, randomized study is needed.

Valproic acid, an anticonvulsant, is known to induce neural tube defects in at least some fetuses of mothers taking this medication.[96] Other teratogens can cause myelomeningocele in laboratory animals. Minor fluctuations in incubator temperature can prevent normal closure of the neural tube in chicks. Thus, a variety of environmental factors influence the occurrence of this congenital malformation. It is unlikely that there is one single cause.[315, 400]

Pathogenesis

Morgagni, in 1769, is often credited with developing the theory that myelomeningoceles result from rupture of the distal end of the neural tube.[409] According to the theory, when cerebral spinal fluid cannot escape from the ventricular pathways it flows instead into the central canal of the neural tube, distends the tube, and bursts it open at the distal end of the neural tube, creating the myelomeningocele. It is unlikely that Morgagni developed this theory, because the pathophysiology of cerebrospinal fluid flow was not understood at that time. Morgagni's real contribution was the association that he noted between hydrocephalus and spina bifida. It was von Recklinghausen who postulated that myelomeningocele resulted from a failure of closure of the neural tube.[476] This view was supported by Patten, who showed that overgrowth of the neural tube in myelomeningocele embryos implied lack of closure or interference with the closure of the neural tube.[451–453] More recently, Gardner and Paget postulated that intrauterine hydrocephalus causes the distal end of the neural tube to rupture, producing myelomeningocele.[196, 438] Refinements of this theory have been advanced to explain the development of the Chiari II, Dandy-Walker, and other malformations of the central nervous system as well as malformations of other organs of the body.

Myelomeningocele can be produced both by interfering with the closure of the neural tube and by causing rupture of the already closed neural tube.[363] In the chick embryo, simple alteration of the temperature of the incubator can result in neural tube defect. Closure of the neural tube can be prevented in mouse embryos, in vitro, by adding tunicamycin to the culture medium. Distention and rupture of the developing spinal cord in mouse embryos can be caused by poisoning the pregnant mouse with vitamin A.[363] Thus, primary failure of closure of the neural tube and secondary rupture of the once closed neural tube are both possible causes of myelomeningocele.

Heredity

There is a significantly greater incidence of myelomeningocele in the siblings of affected children than in the general population. The incidence of spina bifida and anencephaly is approximately the same, and the occurrence of either increases the risk for one or the other occurring in subsequent children.

Ingraham and Swam reported that 6 per cent of the families of 546 patients with spina bifida and cranium bifidum had a family history of similar malformations and that the expectancy of a second afflicted child being born was about 1 chance in 30.[272] The familial incidence in Doran and Guthkelch's series was 8.14 per cent;[139] in that of Smith, it was 7.8 per cent.[543]

Lorber studied the family histories of 722 infants born with spina bifida cystica. Of the 1256 siblings, 85 (6.8 per cent) had gross malformation of the central nervous system; spina bifida cystica was found in 54; anencephaly in 22; and uncomplicated hydrocephalus in 9. Eight per cent of the infants born after the index case were affected.[328] For a couple who already have an infant affected by myelomeningocele, the chance that any subsequent sibling will be affected by a major malformation of the central nervous system is approximately 1 in 14. Three fifths of any affected siblings are liveborn.

Lorber also reported a progressive increase in multiple cases in the family in accordance with increasing size. In sibships of five or more, mutiple cases occurred in 24.1 per cent. A positive family history among uncles, aunts, and cousins was obtained in 118 of the 722 families studied, with up to six cases in a single family.[328]

MacMahon et al. reported a 6.6 per cent incidence of major malfunctions of the central nervous system in siblings born after a child with spina bifida cystica.[362] Milham reported the incidence of malformation of the central nervous system in siblings of affected cases to be 16 times higher than in the general population.[396]

Yen and MacMahon, in a study of 1095 cases of anencephaly and spina bifida, reported a 4.6 per cent risk of recurrence in siblings born after the first index case.[639] Maternal age and parity seem to have relatively little effect. In 108 instances of affected twins, none of the co-twins was affected. Case reports of affected concordant twins have been published, but such instances are extremely rare.[172, 296, 289] Chromosomal abnormalities have not been demonstrated in myelomeningocele.

Inheritance pattern of myelomeningocele appears to be multifactorial, with modification by the environment.[90] The effect of environmental factors in prevalence of myelomeningocele is shown by the finding that Irish immigrants in Boston, Massachusetts, have a higher rate than other ethnic groups in Boston, but a lower rate than among the Irish in Ireland.[418] Japanese residing in Hawaii have a higher rate of involvement with myelomeningocele than those residing in Japan.[411]

In summary, the general population risk for a child to be born with myelomeningocele is 1 in 1000. The following should be stated to the family during genetic counseling; once a child is born with neural tube defect the risk for subsequent pregnancies increases to 50 per 1000 (a rise from 0.1 per cent to 5 per cent); after two children born with myelomeningocele, the risk increases to 100 per 1000 (or 0.1 per cent to 10 per cent—a 100 times greater risk than in the general population).[95, 309, 634]

Antenatal Diagnosis

At present there are two techniques utilized for antenatal diagnosis of myelomeningocele—ultrasound and determination of alpha-fetoprotein first by serum and then by amniocentesis. Following antenatal diagnosis, termination of pregnancy by abortion is an option that may not be acceptable to every parent or physician. Prenatal diagnosis also facilitates the early delivery and initial management of the child with a myelomeningocele. The parents have the right to their own choice, whereas physicians who object to possible abortion if antenatal diagnosis of myelomeningocele is made should refer the parents to physicians who do not have such personal constraints. The period of pregnancy when tests for antenatal diagnosis are performed is around 16 weeks of gestation. *Ultrasound* is performed first; it is an innocuous study. Longitudinal and transverse plane scanning of the fetal spine may show neural tube defects. Cranial anatomy is well demonstrated by ultrasound, making detection of anencephaly possible in almost all cases. Myelomeningocele, however, cannot be ruled out by ultrasound.

AMNIOCENTESIS

Alpha-fetoprotein (AFP) is a protein present in fetal tissues during development; from the sixth to the fourteenth weeks of gestation the presence of AFP in embryonic fluid is normal. As the embryo matures, closure of the abdominal wall anteriorly and the neural tube posteriorly prevents release of AFP into the amniotic fluid, so the level of amniotic AFP decreases to such low levels that it cannot be detected. Should the neural tube or the abdominal wall remain open, release of AFP into the amniotic fluid will continue and the concentration of amnionic AFP will remain high.[512] This allows for prenatal diagnosis of open neural tube defects by amniocentesis.[605] Increased levels of

AFP in amnionic fluid, and more recently in maternal blood samples, suggest the presence of an open neural tube defect.[56]

By combination of ultrasound and amniocentesis, antenatal diagnosis of anencephaly can be made in *all* fetuses and can be made in 80 to 90 per cent of cases of open neural tube.

Mothers with a previous history of a child with a neural tube defect or those with two serum samples showing elevated AFP should have fetal ultrasound and then amniocentesis. It should be remembered that amniocentesis is an invasive procedure and that there is a 0.5 per cent risk of producing a miscarriage. Acetylcholinesterase level determination in amniotic fluid by electrophoresis has diminished the number of false positive results.

Pathology

A masterful and thorough description of the pathologic findings of spina bifida cystica was given in 1888 by von Recklinghausen, who accurately dissected out both the spinal cord and the meninges in cases of myeloschisis and myelocystocele, and who first recognized every variety of spina bifida.[476]

The lesions may occur at any level along the spinal axis but are seen predominantly in the lumbosacral region. They are next most frequently found in the cervical spine area, and a smaller number of lesions are scattered along the thoracic region. The higher the level of the lesion, the less likelihood there is of severe neurologic involvement. In cervical lesions, for example, neurologic deficit is minimal because the majority are simple meningoceles with narrow necks to the sac. The converse is true for lesions below the first lumbar vertebra.

The great majority of the lesions are posterior, but in a very rare instance one may encounter an anterior or lateral meningocele, which should be considered in the differential diagnosis of atypical masses in the chest, retroperitoneal tissues, and pelvis. In these cases, myelography and, recently, magnetic resonance imaging will confirm the diagnosis. The anterior cysts protrude through the vertebral bodies, not through the vertebral arches.

The "different types" of myelomeningocele are best understood in terms of an archetypical anatomic deformity and variations on that archetype. The basic deformity consists of an open neural placode, which represents the embryologic form of the caudal end of the spinal cord. A narrow groove passes down the placode in the midline (Figs. 5–71 and 5–72). This represents the primitive neural groove and is directly

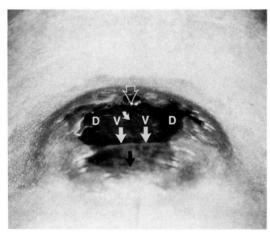

FIGURE 5–71.

A myelomeningocele demonstrates the ventral sulcus *(curved arrow)*, placode epithelial junction (↓ ↓), skin epithelial junction (↓), and the entrance to the central canal *(open arrow)*. Motor neurons (V) are medial and the dorsal root entry zones (D) are located laterally.

continuous with the central canal of the closed spinal cord above (and occasionally below) the neural placode. Cerebrospinal fluid passes down the central canal of the spinal cord and discharges from a small pit at the upper end of the placode to bathe the external surface of the neural tissue. This fluid does not indicate rupture of the myelomeningocele.

SKIN

Skin over a myelomeningocele sac is almost always incomplete. Normal skin surrounds the neural tissue but lies at a distance from it. Between the skin and the neural placode is a zone of thin epithelium. At points, skin may actually reach the edge of the neural placode. In the usual type of lesion, there is a raised mass on the back, covered laterally at its base by normal skin, but the apex of the mass is devoid of skin. It is covered by a tissue-paper-thin membrane (arachnoid) through which one may see nerve roots. Within a day or two, it presents the appearance of an ulcerated granulating surface. The lesion may heal over completely by epithelial growth from the periphery. Not infrequently, however, the mass will slough from secondary infection. If the infant does not die of meningitis, recurrent episodes of superficial infection and cellulitis will cause the mass to become puckered and crevassed. In the skin directly over the sac or surrounding it, one will often encounter pigmentary or hemangiomatous lesions.

MENINGES

Underlying the neural placode is the arachnoid sac and subarachnoid space. Since the superficial (dorsal) surface of the neural placode represents the everted interior of the neural tube, the deep (ventral) surface represents the entire outside of what should have been a closed neural tube. Thus the ventral nerve roots and the dorsal nerve roots arise from the deep (ventral) surface of the neural placode and pass through the subarachnoid space to their root sleeves. Because the placode is everted, the two dorsal roots (D) are lateral to the two ventral roots (V) in the order D VV D from left to right across the midline.

Underlying the skin, usually within a few millimeters of the edge of the skin, is the junction between skin and dura mater. Outside the dura mater is a true epidural space that

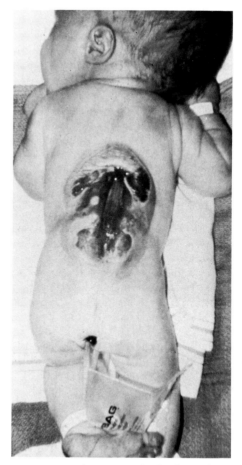

FIGURE 5–72. A large thoracolumbar lesion, but the basic anatomy remains the same.

Note that the legs and feet are well developed. The child had function through S1.

contains epidural fat. The underlying vertebral bodies are flattened and widened. The pedicles are everted and lie nearly horizontal in the coronal plane. The laminae are hypoplastic and often are also everted. The spinous processes are obviously absent. The paraspinal muscle masses are present but are everted with the pedicles and laminae. Thus, they lie anteriorly and often act as flexors and not extensors of the spine. The muscles can be markedly attenuated owing to the lack of innervation from the central nervous system.

The size of the sac on the child's back at the time of birth is dependent upon the amount of spinal fluid that is collected ventral to the neural placode. The majority of lesions will be flush with the child's back. A smaller number of placodes are raised far above the surface of the back by marked expansion of the subarachnoid space. These are properly designated *myelomeningoceles*. Generally, however, both types are grouped under the heading myelomeningocele.

SPINAL CORD

Myelodysplasia is always present. These variations in the dysplastic spinal cord may be classified into three types: (1) *Absent cord.* In extreme degrees of anencephaly with complete spina bifida, the cord may be totally absent. (2) *Split cord.* This may arise as a result of failure of fusion of the embryologic neural plates ("myeloschisis"), in which the cord is represented by only unformed strands of neural tissue with no central canal; or "schisis" of the cord may occur following its formation, a condition known as diastematomyelia. Diastematomyelia does occur without spina bifida as well. During surgery for myelomeningocele, or even in simple meningocele, a search must be made for a bony, cartilaginous, or fibrous spur that splits the cord. Its removal might prevent the possible subsequent increasing distortion of the cord and nerve roots with later growth of the vertebral column. (3) *Formed but dysplastic cord.* Commonly the cord is formed but dysplastic in the following ways. It may be cystic or cavitated; it may be solid, but degenerated and disorganized; or it may be grossly proliferated. Frequently all these features are found together in varying degrees.

Concurrent arteriovenous malformations and intraspinal lipomas also have been reported. Occasionally the neural placode is in a totally disorganized state. In these cases the neural placode appears to have undergone interuterine infarction, so portions of it are severely dysplastic and reduced to a simple membrane. This would support the concept that myelomeningocele is a progressive intrauterine disease.

PERIPHERAL ROOTS

Peripheral nerve development is not affected in myelomeningocele. At surgery and on dissection of the postmortem specimen, normal peripheral roots have been found in every case. However, inside the dura mater the roots appear to have tenuous connections with the cord itself and on occasion are hard to identify.

VERTEBRAE

The principal defect is the arrest of development of the laminae. It varies from one extreme of failure of the laminae and vertebral spines to fuse posteriorly, to the other extreme of total failure of formation of laminae, the pedicles alone being present. The intraspinal canal is widened as a result of lateral displacement of the pedicles on the vertebral bodies.

BRAIN

In myelomeningocele there may be associated anomalies of the cerebellum and brain stem, e.g., Chiari Type II deformity, in which the posterior lobe of the cerebellum, the medulla, and the fourth ventricle are herniated through the foramen magnum into the cervical spinal canal; in Chiari Type III, the more severe form, the entire cerebellum and lower brain stem are inferior to the foramen magnum. Hydrocephalus develops from obstruction of the flow of cerebrospinal fluid at the roof of the fourth ventricle by dislocation of the ventricle, by occlusion of the subarachnoid space at the site of herniation, by occlusion of the same space at the tentorial level by adhesive arachnoiditis, or by an associated aqueduct stenosis. Other causes of hydrocephalus in myelomeningocele are the Dandy-Walker malformation, which consists of marked distention of the fourth ventricle due to occlusion of the foramina of Luschka and Magendie; the "forking" of the aqueduct of Sylvius, in which the aqueduct is represented by two narrow channels situated in a sagittal plane; and aqueduct stenosis. Radiologic studies of cerebrospinal fluid dynamics in children with hydrocephalus have shown increased production of cerebrospinal fluid. Secondary changes in the brain develop as a result of increased pressure due to the hydrocephalus.

Clinical Features

The external appearance of the local lesion has been described previously. The size, location, and covering of the myelomeningocele sac

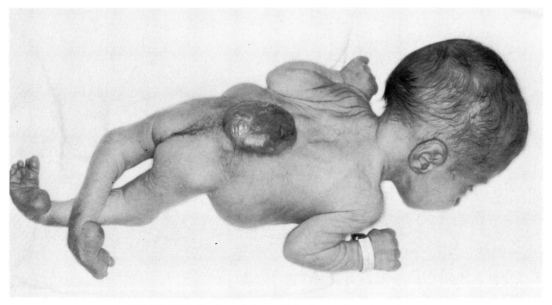

FIGURE 5–73. Newborn infant with lumbosacral myelomeningocele.

Note the severe equinovarus deformity of both feet.

are determined (Fig. 5–73). Any areas of ulceration or leakage of cerebrospinal fluid should be noted. The amount of neural tissue within the sac is determined by transillumination in a darkened room. The meningocele surface should be carefully inspected for the presence of any neural elements. The extent of bony defect in the vertebrae is noted by gentle palpation and confirmed by anteroposterior and lateral radiograms of the entire spine.

The adequacy of cerebrospinal fluid circulation is evaluated. One should look for any signs of hydrocephalus, such as dilatation of scalp veins, tension of the fontanelles, separation of cranial sutures, downward displacement of the eyes, and hollowness of the cranial percussion note. The occipitobregmatic circumference of the head is measured and compared with standard growth charts. It is important to record the rate of growth of the head by measuring its circumference at regular intervals. Radiograms of the skull are obtained.

The anus is inspected for rectal prolapse and eversion of anal skin. With loss of innervation of the rectal sphincter, there is lack of resistance and absence of reflex contraction as the examining finger is introduced into the rectum. The anal skin reflex is lost. Bladder sphincter control is checked by watching the infant pass urine. Intermittent dribbling of urine accentuated by suprapubic pressure indicates loss of vesical sphincter control. Suprapubic pressure has no effect on an infant with a normal bladder sphinc-

ter. Maceration of the perineal skin is another finding indicating lack of urinary control.

The degree and distribution of paralysis should be noted. A thorough neurologic evaluation of a newborn is difficult. The baby should be warm and hungry. By careful repeated examinations, a segmental level of neurologic deficit can be detected.

In lumbosacral lesions, paralysis of the lower limbs is flaccid, whereas in cervicothoracic lesions, it is of the spastic type because of partial cord involvement. Paralysis may be partial or complete below a certain neurosegmental level, with normal function above it.

The presence or absence of deep tendon and superficial skin reflexes is determined. In flaccid paralysis, there is total areflexia, whereas in spastic paralysis there will be hyperactive deep tendon reflexes, ankle clonus, and extensor plantar response. Sensory examination in a newborn is inadequate but should be attempted. The segmental innervation of cutaneous sensation in the lower limb is shown in Figure 5–74.

Motor strength of muscles is evaluated by observing the resting posture of the infant, by active motions of the limbs, and by the use of reflex stimulation techniques. Often it is difficult to accurately grade muscle strength; one determines whether the muscle strength is absent (zero), weak, or full-strength. Frequently the power of muscle groups (not individual muscles) is recorded, such as hip abductors, hip adductors, hip flexors, and knee extensors. The

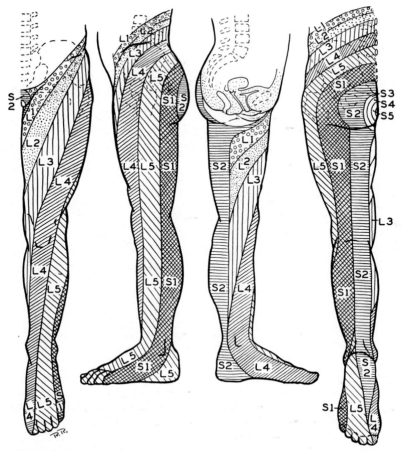

FIGURE 5–74. The segmental innervation of cutaneous sensation of the lower limb.

(From Keegan, J. J., and Garrett, F. D.: Segmental distribution of nerves in man. Anat. Rec., 102:409, 1948. Reprinted by permission.)

use of faradic current over nerve trunks and at motor points of muscles to stimulate muscle groups is recommended by Sharrard; Menelaus and this author have not been successful in this modality of investigation.[388, 528] The neurosegmental level of innervation of muscle groups is given in Figure 5–75; correlation between segmental innervation, reflexes, joint movement, and consequent deformities is shown in Figure 5–76.

The functional motor and sensory levels are related to, but not always consistent with, the anatomic level of the lesion. Often function is preserved below the anatomic segments involved. Asymmetry occurs and should raise the question of an additional lesion such as a diastematomyelia or hemimyelocele. It is important to establish as accurately as possible the functional level.

Deformities in myelomeningocele may be present at birth (congenital) or may develop postnatally (acquired). There may be coexisting congenital malformations. Deformities may be teratologic in origin, or they may result from dynamic muscle imbalance, from static forces of faulty posture, or from fibrotic contracture of muscles. Tethering of neural tissues may change the neurologic picture. Sensory, cerebellar, and cerebral abnormalities may affect posture and gait.

Most often, signs of deterioration will be subtle and insidiously progressive; only through close follow-up can such subtle deterioration be checkreined early. Somatosensory evoked potentials may be of some value in following patients for early signs of progressive paralysis.[480, 526]

Associated Congenital Anomalies

These may occur in any form and are present in about one third of the patients with myelo-

L1	L2	L3	L4	L5	S1	S2	S3

ILIO PSOAS
SARTORIUS
PECTINEUS
GRACILIS
ADD. LONGUS
ADD. BREVIS
ADDUCTOR MAGNUS
QUADRICEPS
OBT. EXT.
TIB. ANT.
TIB. POST.
TEN. FAS. LATA
GLUT. MED. & MIN.
SEMIMEMBRANOSUS
SEMITENDINOSUS
EXT. HALL. L.
EXT. DIG. L.
PER. TERT.
PER. BREVIS
PER. LONGUS
LAT. HIP. ROT.
GASTROCN.
SOLEUS & PLANT.
BICEPS FEMORIS
GLUTEUS MAX.
FLEX. HALL. L. & B.
FLEX. DIG. L. & B.
FOOT INTRINSICS

FIGURE 5–75. Neurosegmental innervation of muscles of lower limb.

(From Sharrard, W. J. W.: Posterior iliopsoas transplantation in the treatment of paralytic dislocation of the hip. J. Bone Joint Surg., *46-B*:427, 1964. Reprinted by permission.)

meningocele. A list, based on a study by Smith, of 170 anomalies in 101 children with spina bifida cystica is shown in Table 5–10.[543] The high incidence of congenital dislocation of the hip, talipes equinovarus, hemivertebrae, other anomalies of the spine, and abnormalities of the genitourinary system should be noted. An intravenous pyelogram and a thorough urologic evaluation is imperative in myelomeningocele patients. The possibility of congenital heart disease, malformations of the gastrointestinal tract, cleft palate, pilonidal sinus, or an imperforate rectum should be ruled out.

In the older child, the level of intelligence should be evaluated by a psychologist.

General Considerations and Principles of Treatment

An infant born with myelomeningocele poses complex medical, social, and ethical problems for the physicians, family, and society charged with his care.[377] Aristotle "resolved" the social problem by recommending infanticide.[17] Forestus (1610) first ligated the myelomeningocele sac.[186] Tulpius (1641) and de Ruysch and Morgagni (1806) recognized the association of the lesion with paralysis in the legs; they were aware of the concurrent hydrocephalus and attempted to improve the lives of these infants.[127, 594] Trowbridge (1828) claimed success-

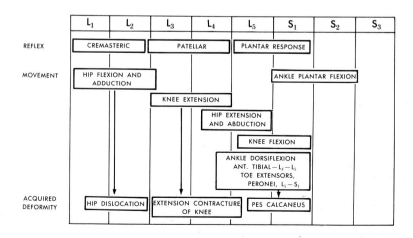

FIGURE 5–76. Segmental innervation of reflexes, joint movements, and consequent deformities.

Table 5–10. Associated Anomalies
in 101 Children with Spina Bifida Cystica*

System Involved		Number of Anomalies
Vertebral	Sacral agenesis and hemisacra	18
	Hemivertebrae, transitional vertebrae, fusion defects, fused ribs, etc. (including scoliosis and kyphosis)	18
Skeletal	Congenital talipes	37
	Congenital dislocation of hip	29
	Arthrogryposis	4
	Absent fibula	1
	Absent foot	1
	Extra rudimentary leg	1
	Syndactyly	2
Urinary	Megaureters and hydronephrosis	
	(a) with vesicoureteric reflux	22
	(b) without vesicoureteric reflux	4
	Vesicoureteric reflux in normal ureters	8
	Hypospadias	2
	Urethral diverticulum	1
	Posterior urethral valves	1
	Double ureters and kidneys	3
	Horseshoe kidney	1
	Exstrophy of bladder	1
Alimentary	Imperforate rectum	5
	Tracheo-oesophageal fistula	1
Cerebral	Encephalocele	1
	Congenital mental defect	5
Miscellaneous	Exomphalos	2
	Cleft palate	1
	Congenital cardiac lesions	3
	Sacral sinus	3
	Total	170

*From Smith, E. D.: Spina Bifida and the Total Care of Spinal Myelomeningocele. Springfield, Ill., Charles C Thomas, 1965, p. 49.

ful treatment of the sac, although his patients died with fever.[593] In the United States, use of Morton's Sclerosing Solutions (1875) and injections of iodine into the central nervous system led to violent convulsions and death.[410]

From the early 1900s onward, steady progress was made toward successful closure of the back without infection.[272] Individual patients began to survive, and the need to control hydrocephalus became paramount. As effective methods for dealing with hydrocephalus became available in the 1950s and 1960s, large numbers of patients survived longer, and centers began to advocate aggressive treatment of all children with myelomeningocele.[643] Unfortunately, the medical and surgical care of the period was not sufficiently advanced to deal with the new problems that arose as the chil-

dren survived longer, and opinion soon changed. Devastating shunt infection, poor intellectual development, urinary and fecal incontinence, impaired renal function, and serious musculoskeletal deformities led some surgeons to propose that the "quality of life" experienced by these patients was so poor, many of them would have been better off if allowed to die. Thus, Lorber in 1971 advocated the following "criteria" to predict which patients would have a good outcome and advocated use of these "criteria" to decide who should be treated and who should not be subjected to treatment and allowed to die: (1) hydrocephalus at birth with a grossly enlarged head with a maximum circumference of 2 cm. or more above the 90th percentile, related to birth weight; (2) level of paralysis of L2 and above; quadriceps femoris function was proposed to be "the passport to life"; (3) congenital rigid kyphosis or scoliosis; (4) infected sac and meningitis; (5) intracranial injuries and brain damage; and (6) multiple congenital anomalies and life-threatening diseases, such as of the heart or the kidneys. If these physical findings were present they were considered to be contraindications for early closure of the myelomeningocele sac.[330] With time, physicians treated fewer and fewer children with myelomeningocele despite beginning development of new and improved modalities of treatment for the secondary problems.

When an infant is born with myelomeningocele, a serious ethical question should be resolved, i.e., whether or not the child is to be treated. In the past there have been two possible avenues of approach: (1) The children were treated aggressively and given every opportunity to live, reducing their handicaps to a minimum; (2) infants were selected for treatment, and following the criteria set forth by Lorber, infants with poor prognosis were allowed to die, by neglecting treatment.

The validity of criteria used to determine whether or not to treat newborn children with myelomeningocele is best established by comparing the outcomes of patients in series that *do* and that *do not* select specific patients to treat. Series of unselected patients offer some insight into the impact of medical progress on the outcome of these children. Comparison between series of selected and unselected patients affords a type of "cost-benefit" analysis. Ethical considerations aside, it is important to determine (1) what percentage of those children selected for nontreatment who die would have been competitive in the community, and (2) what level of selection is "necessary" in order to obtain a significant improvement in overall functional level of the surviving population. Such information is critical to the decision-making process. Without such information, the physician cannot provide proper assistance to the parents of a newborn with myelomeningocele during the first critical days of the infant's life.

Between 1959 and 1984, four studies of unselected populations of newborns with myelomeningocele were carried out. Sufficiently long periods of follow-up provide accurate data on the success of treating myelomeningocele patients and the value of Lorber's criteria in predicting that success. These studies were those of Lorber (1971),[330] Ames and Schut (1972),[8] Soare and Raimondi (1977),[552] and McLone, Dias, Kaplan, and Sommers (1984)[356] (Graph 5–1). Review of this 25-year period (Graphs 5–2 and 5–3) documents a marked decrease in patient mortality, a marked decrease in the number of urinary diversions performed, a striking increase in urinary continence, and a gradual but significant improvement in ambulation and intelligence of the patient.

The long-term results in a *highly selected* population of presumably "best" patients with myelomeningocele have become available.[335] Graph 5–4 documents that the results of treatment of an *unselected* population of all patients with myelomeningocele compare favorably with groups of highly selected "best" patients. In the selected group, the overall mortality approaches 7 per cent, obviously because of the selection process itself. It is interesting to note that the mortality rate in that group selected to be the "best" patients is no different from the mortality rate in the group of McLone and associates of completely unselected patients. The only area in which the selected patients fared better than the unselected patients was in the percentage of children with an IQ greater than 80. Since no significant differences exist between (a) pop-

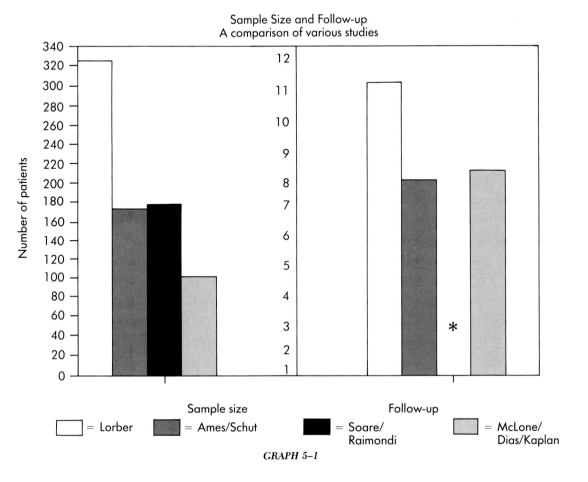

Sample Size and Follow-up
A comparison of various studies

Sample size

Follow-up

☐ = Lorber   ▨ = Ames/Schut   ■ = Soare/Raimondi   ▨ = McLone/Dias/Kaplan

GRAPH 5–1

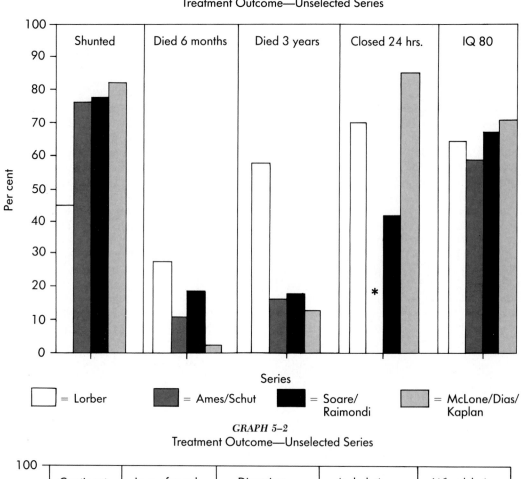

Treatment Outcome—Unselected Series

GRAPH 5–2

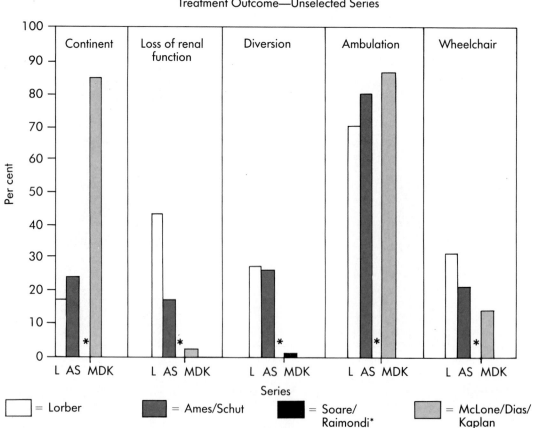

Treatment Outcome—Unselected Series

GRAPH 5–3

Selected Versus Unselected
Lorber 1981/McLone et al. 1984

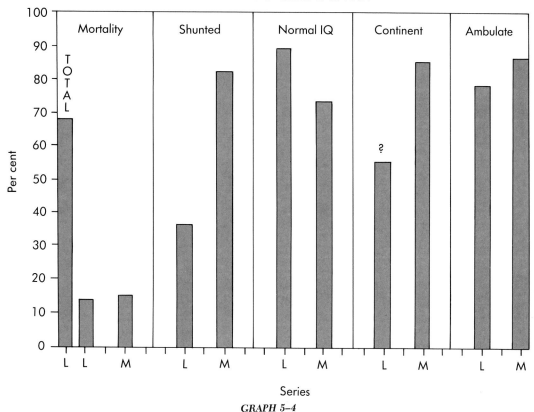

Series

GRAPH 5-4

ulations of children selected by criteria purported to be predictive of quality of survival and (b) populations in which all children were treated regardless of the extent of the problem at birth, most major centers currently treat nearly all newborn children with myelomeningocele. Full and aggressive treatment should be extended to all children, except those already agonal at birth.

Optimal care of the patient with myelomeningocele requires a comprehensive coordinated plan for the treatment of all lesions regardless of their level or extent. Past experience has taught that no valid criteria exist for selecting those newborns whose "quality of survival" would be so poor that it would be kinder to allow them to die. Because children with myelomeningocele require multidisciplinary care, a team composed of a pediatric neurosurgeon, a pediatric orthopedic surgeon, a urologic surgeon, and a neonatologist-pediatrician should be involved in the care of the infant from the beginning. The neurosurgeon and orthopedist should assess the patient within hours of birth to establish a baseline evaluation. The neuro-

surgeon should then discuss with the parents the likely prognosis for life and quality of life with and without surgical treatment. Because the parents are initially in a state of emotional shock and are ill informed or misinformed about spina bifida, the surgeon must make a special effort to bring to the parent the latest data on mortality, need for shunting, likelihood of normal intelligence, need for orthopedic procedures, likelihood of community ambulation, likelihood of continence, and possibility for ultimate self-support. If at all possible, the surgeon should make use of the spina bifida associations or another previously established network of parents of children with spina bifida. This will assist the parents of the child in question in speaking immediately with parents who faced similar problems and in joining a strong support group to help them withstand the stress of facing medical decisions.

In that context, the parents can gain as much "digested" information as possible to make an informed decision for their child and to give, or withhold, consent for immediate therapy and for subsequent management decisions.

The infant with myelomeningocele has multiple handicaps, each dysfunction and deformity requiring the frequent attention of many medical and surgical specialties. The cost of such care is prohibitive in terms of time as well as money for the average family who has to visit separate clinics. Also, the vision of a single physician can be myopic, his attention being directed primarily to one phase of therapy. To administer adequate total care to the child with myelomeningocele, it is imperative to have frequent interdisciplinary consultation. For these reasons, the child is best cared for in a special multidisciplinary clinic in a children's hospital, where the specialized services of the neurosurgeon, urologic surgeon, pediatric surgeon, orthopedic surgeon, neurologist, pediatrician, and physical and occupational therapists and orthotist are available.

Social and psychologic factors also have a tremendous impact on the lives of these multiply handicapped children, who are plagued by a pessimistic prognosis and inadequate motivation toward life and adjustment in the community. The roles of the special educator, vocational counselor, psychologist, and social worker are extremely important, as these workers enable the myelomeningocele child to compensate for his extreme physical disability by providing him with specialized education and vocational guidance. Finally, the total care of these children should be coordinated and supervised by an interested pediatrician who often functions as director of the team (Fig. 5–77).

A positive approach, beginning at birth, is important. Immediate steps toward total care and habilitation will prevent or minimize deformity and improve the emotional attitude of the family. It should be emphasized to the parents that with proper medical care most of these children *can* become useful members of the community.

Spina bifida parents' associations are extremely valuable for educating the parents, giving them the continued moral support so necessary for the adequate and proper care of these children. A stable and cooperative family is the most important part of the team in the total care of the child with myelomeningocele.

It is beyond the scope of this book to present detailed neurosurgical, urologic, and other aspects of medical treatment of the child with myelomeningocele; the neurosurgical management will be presented briefly because the orthopedic surgeon should be cognizant of the care of the central nervous system.

Neurosurgical Treatment*

The meningocele should be closed immediately as an emergency measure, since with such treatment there is greater preservation of innervation, and the eventual mortality rate is much lower than with delayed closure. Immediate repair of the meningocele combined with successful control of hydrocephalus by shunting procedures has decreased the mortality rate of myelomeningocele.

REPAIR OF MENINGOCELE

Several techniques for repair of the myelomeningocele have been described.[647] The technique described herein utilizes microneurosurgical principles and allows one to reconstruct the central canal of the spinal cord and the pia arachnoid–lined subarachnoid space.[355] This anatomic reconstruction allows the spinal cord to float freely in a cerebrospinal fluid compartment and establishes a microenvironment conducive to neuronal function.

The presence of function below the level of the myelomeningocele, postoperative recovery of motor function, and electrophysiologic studies indicate that the exposed neural tissue is viable and potentially capable of conducting motor and sensory impulses.[356, 480] Exposure of this tissue to trauma during birth and later drying of this tissue lead to a shocklike state of the spinal cord, which may be reversible with reconstruction of a more normal neural canal–meningeal environment.

In the surgical reconstruction, the following basic principles must be respected.

Early Closure. The myelomeningocele sac is closed as soon as possible, in order to prevent infection and a decrease in motor function. Our experience at Children's Memorial Hospital, Chicago, shows that the rate of ventriculitis in delayed closure is 37 per cent, as compared with an incidence of 7 per cent in patients with early closure.

The survival rate of unrepaired newborns who are fed but denied antibiotics is 40 to 60 per cent; many of these children have significant dysfunction of the central nervous system.[191] If antibiotics are added to the care of unrepaired children, the mortality and morbidity fall to a level similar to those of children repaired in the first 24 hours. Some children will require early

---
*Contributed by David G. McClone, M.D., Ph.D., Professor and Head, Division of Neurosurgery, Children's Memorial Hospital, Chicago, Illinois.

NEUROSURGEON

Meningocele
Myelomeningocele

C.F.S. LEAK   INFECTION

PARENTS

Hydrocephalus

MENINGITIC   NONABSORBPTION   ARNOLD-CHIARI

UROLOGIC SURGEON

INCONTINENCE
RETENTION
DIVERTICULA
PYELONEPHRITIS
RENAL FAILURE

PEDIATRIC SURGEON

ANORECTAL
INCONTINENCE
FECAL IMPACTION

ORTHOPEDIC SURGEON

SCOLIOSIS
LORDOSIS
DISLOCATION OF HIPS
EXT. CONTRACTURE-KNEE
FOOT DEFORMITIES
PARALYSIS

NEUROLOGIST-PEDIATRICIAN

PLASTIC SURGEON

ADMINISTRATIVE COORDINATOR

SOCIAL WORKER

PSYCHOLOGIST

VOCATIONAL COUNSELOR

SPECIAL EDUCATOR (S)

OCCUPATIONAL THERAPIST

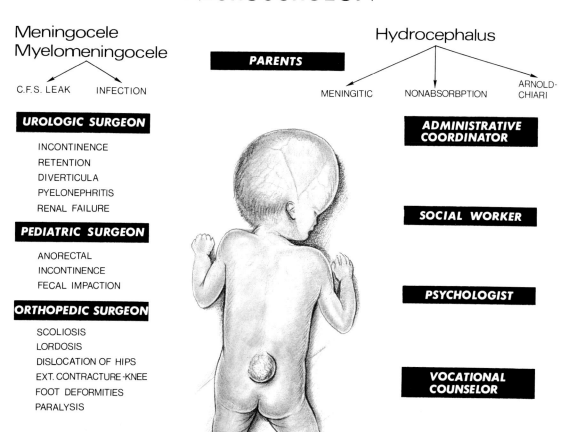

Myelomeningocele

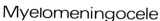

ORTHOTIST   **PHYSICAL THERAPIST**

FIGURE 5-77. *Total care of the infant with myelomeningocele—the team approach.*

shunt insertion because of severe progressive hydrocephalus or Chiari II hindbrain problems.

Delayed closure is purported to allow time for the physicians to educate and inform the family and to allow the parents to feel they are participating in the initial decision-making process. A review of 274 families from the myelomeningocele clinic at Children's Memorial Hospital, Chicago, showed that 52 per cent of the parents felt that they did not make an initial informed consent. Half the parents considered that at least six months was required before they knew 50 per cent or more of the problems involved with myelomeningocele. In this regard, it is noteworthy that 13 of the 274 families regretted their initial decision. In retrospect, 9 of the 13 felt that they would have preferred to delay early treatment. Three regretted agreeing to initial closure of the child's back. One regretted the decision to consent to the shunt procedure. There is no justification to delay neurosurgical treatment, as it will further complicate the future of these children.

Preservation of All Neural Tissue. It is often difficult to preserve all the neural tissue, because the mass of tissue may exceed the volume of the spinal canal. However, the neural tissue should be preserved even if it is necessary to construct a protruding sac to retain it.

Meticulous Care of the Exposed Tissue. The child should be kept on his abdomen to reduce mechanical trauma to the neural tissue. The exposed neural tissue must not be allowed to dry. For this purpose it must be kept covered with nonadherent dressings moistened with normal saline at body temperature. Scrubs or chemical antimicrobial agents should not be applied to the exposed neural tissue. During the subsequent surgical repair, great care must be taken to avoid drying, traction on neural elements, irrigation with hot saline, and cautery. With magnification and microinstrumentation, the inadvertent trauma to significant blood vessels can be avoided. Occasionally, the entire closure can be carried out without cautery. If cautery is used, only bipolar cautery should be employed.

Anatomic Reconstruction of the Neural Tissue and Coverings Under Magnification. The normal anatomic structures are almost always present, but are filleted open in the midsagittal plane, everted, and displaced laterally. They are often attenuated. The exposed neural surface is the ependymal surface of the neural placode and is continuous with the central canal of the spinal cord. The lateral edges of the neural tissue are developmentally the alar plate or the dorsal root entry zones. The medial portion of the placode is the basal plate or the ventral motor horn. Ventral to the placode, along either side of the midline, the motor roots exit from the placode. The sensory roots enter the cord at the periphery of the placode lateral to the motor roots. The ventral surface is covered with pia-arachnoid that is directly contiguous with the arachnoid membrane of the sac. The sac usually encloses an intact subarachnoid space. An understanding of this anatomy is essential to reconstituting the spinal cord and its coverings.

Cardiac and central temperature monitoring is essential. An intravenous canula is needed for fluid and blood replacement. Local or general anesthesia may be employed, but preexisting respiratory difficulties demand general anesthesia. General anesthesia makes the use of the operating microscope easier, while magnifying loupes are more convenient for local cases.

Dissection of the myelomeningocele begins at the junction of the abnormal covering epithelium and the normal skin.[355] This junction should be incised around the entire circumference of the myelomeningocele. Once this has been completed, the dissection is carried toward the neural placode. Dividing the epithelial junction from the neural tissue requires care because, on one hand, this is the region where dorsal roots and segmental vasculature enter the neural placode, and because, on the other hand, any residual skin elements may grow to become inclusion epidermoid tumors. When this has been completed, the neural tissue floats free on a sac of cerebrospinal fluid.

Reconstitution of the neural tube begins at the cephalic end; 7-0 to 10-0 suture is used in a running locked stitch to approximate the pia-arachnoid neural junction of one side with that of the other side. Care must be taken to pass the needle through pia-arachnoid and not through neural elements. The central canal should be closed throughout its entire length so that the neural placode becomes a neural tube. Because the arachnoid sac is directly continuous with the pia-arachnoid on the ventral surface of the placode, closing the neural placode into a neural tube simultaneously folds the arachnoid sac around the tube and encloses the cord within an envelope of cerebrospinal fluid. Suspending the closed neural tube in an intact cerebrospinal fluid compartment decreases the possibility of scarring and adherence of neural elements, which might later result in tethering of the spinal cord as the child grows.

The dissection now turns to the dura mater and the skin. The junction of dura mater and skin is usually located 1 to 2 cm. lateral to and beneath the point where the epithelium and skin were previously joined. This junction is incised, and the epidural fat layer is entered. The dural layer is freed medially only as far as is necessary to approximate the lateral edges in the midline, because the dura mater is often thin laterally where the nerve roots leave the canal. Once the dura mater is free, it is closed in the midline. This layer should be closed as "watertight" as possible. However, the dural closure must not constrict the underlying neural elements, nor should it interfere with the blood supply to the reconstructed cord. Potential recovery may be lost owing to ischemia or infarction if dura or fascial coverings constrict the underlying tissues. Such dural closure and, perhaps, interposition of a plastic dural substitute (Fig. 5–78) could further decrease the possibility of adhesions between the reconstructed spinal cord and the overlying closure.

Mobilization and midline approximation of lateral paraspinal muscle fascia is optional, depending on how substantial the dural closure is and how easy it is to obtain adequate lateral tissues.

Thoracic and upper lumbar myelomeningocele can be difficult to repair if associated with a kyphotic deformity. Reigel has described success with a procedure that has the benefits of making the closure easier, giving the child a flat back, and converting muscles from flexors of the spine to extensors, which prevents progression of the deformity.[481]

Closure of the skin should be carried out in the midsagittal plane, when possible. Future orthopedic procedures will be facilitated by a simple midline closure. Mobilization of the skin should also include the subcutaneous layer because the vascular supply to the skin comes from this layer. Blunt dissection in the plane between the muscle and subcutaneous fat is the best method to preserve the blood supply.

Some consideration of cosmesis should be taken here, but this is not a major factor if it poses any added stress to neural tissue.

Postoperative Care. In the past, great care was taken to prevent the child from lying on the recently repaired myelomeningocele. Special boards and slings were used to hold the child in the prone position. Not only did these means of immobilization prove to be unnecessary, but also they deprived the infant of the stimulation and human contact critical to early development.

At present, the child is given intravenous fluids with 10 per cent dextrose for the first 24 hours, and then the mother and nurses are allowed to feed the baby. Daily inspection of the closure is recommended for signs of infection, separation of the skin edges, or leakage of cerebrospinal fluid.

Careful Follow-Up of Patients and Aggressive Approach to Late Deterioration. Late deterioration of neurologic function is uncommon in patients with myelomeningocele. When pre-

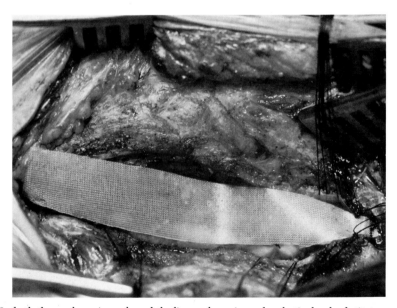

FIGURE 5–78. *In both the myelomeningocele and the lipomyelomeningocele, plastic dural substitutes prevent adhesions between the neural tissue and the closure.*

sent, it nearly always has a treatable cause. Late tethering of the spinal cord developed in only 1 of the initial 100 patients whose backs were closed by our reconstruction techniques.[248, 259, 360, 481] In two patients, a shunt revision was necessary to treat hydromyelia.[234] In two other children, inclusion dermoids necessitated reopening the lumbosacral incision. Detailed evaluation with ultrasound, CT, magnetic resonance imaging, and myelography are required to rule out remedial lesions in any patient with late deterioration in neurologic status, lest remediable causes go undiscovered.

HYDROCEPHALUS

The timing of the initial shunt would appear not to be critical to ultimate intellectual outcome. Stable ventriculomegaly is compatible with normal or even superior intellectual performance. On the other hand, delaying shunting until the cranial volume is fixed by closure of the fontanelle and approximation of the sutures increases the possibility of complicating postshunting subdural fluid collections. At present we believe that shunting is indicated whenever the patient suffers (1) rapidly progressive enlargement of the ventricular and/or head circumference; (2) hindbrain dysfunction related to Chiari II malfunction with stridor, apnea, and/or gastroesophageal reflux; (3) serious cosmetic deformity; and (4) developmental delay. Developmental delay may not be reversed by shunting. No predictive test is available at present to indicate when the shunt might be helpful. The shunt itself becomes the best test.

About 98 per cent of children born with myelomeningocele have or develop an enlarged ventricular system. In the last ten years the percentage of children requiring a shunt in our clinic has risen from 80 to 90 per cent. This increase is the result of the more liberal use of the CT scanner and ultrasound in the initial evaluation of the patient.

INTELLIGENCE

Intelligence Quotient. The majority of studies in the past decade have shown a significant reduction in intelligence quotient (IQ) when the myelomeningocele is associated with hydrocephalus severe enough to require a shunting procedure. In an earlier report by Soare and Raimondi, on 173 unselected children with myelomeningocele, the mean IQ of those with myelomeningocele alone was 102, whereas that of children with myelomeningocele associated with hydrocephalus was 87—a significant difference between the two groups.[552] Viewed an-

other way, 87 per cent of those with myelomeningocele alone had IQs greater than 80, whereas only 63 per cent of those with myelomeningocele and hydrocephalus had IQs above 80. Allowing for the heterogeneity of patient populations, differences in treatment regimens, and variations in intellectual testing batteries, it appeared sound to conclude that when hydrocephalus is associated with myelomeningocele, the IQ can be expected to be significantly lower.

In 1977, however, Hunt and Holmes reported that central nervous system (CNS) infection dramatically lowered the IQ of shunted hydrocephalic children with myelomeningocele as compared with children who either required no shunt or who required a shunt and remained infection free.[268] This then led us to reassess our previous data to see whether or not the presence of CNS infection would be an additional factor in intellectual outcome.[357]

A complete survey was made of the medical records of 167 of the original 173 patients in the Soare and Raimondi study. Specifically, information was obtained regarding the age of onset and duration of any infectious process as well as the causative organism and severity of the process as judged by CSF protein, glucose, and cell count. Accordingly, patients were placed into one of three categories: (1) not shunted, 39 patients; (2) shunted without CNS infection, 86 patients; and (3) shunted with infection, 42 patients. In this group, only shunted patients sustained a CNS infection.

As previously reported, the mean IQ of those not requiring a shunt was 102 with a standard deviation (S.D.) of 18, (the mean IQ for the normal population being 100 with a S.D. of 16). The mean IQ of those patients who were shunted but remained infection free was 95 with a S.D. of 19. This is not significantly different from the IQ of the nonshunted group. Those children who were shunted and then developed a CNS infection had a mean IQ of only 73 with a S.D. of 26. This is significantly different from the other two groups. Viewed another way, of those who did not require a shunt, 87 per cent had IQs greater than 80; of those shunted but infection free, 80 per cent had IQs over 80; and of those shunted with CNS infection, only 31 per cent had IQs over 80. Obviously, control of shunt infection must be a major concern of the neurosurgeon.[601]

Perceptual Motor Deficiency. Several reports indicate that children with myelomeningocele and hydrocephalus suffer significant perceptual motor deficiencies. In our patients the difference between chronologic age and perceptual motor age for those with hydrocephalus was two years, and for those without hydrocephalus was 1.5 years. Their differences are statistically significant as compared with the patients' normal siblings.

If central nervous system infection is taken into account, however, there is no difference between those patients without a shunt and those with an infection-free shunt; both groups still show greater perceptual motor difficulties than their normal siblings. Those children with CNS infection, however, show marked differences when compared with either their normal sibling or the other two groups.

In summary, then, it does not appear to us that hydrocephalus alone is a significant limiting factor in the ultimate intellectual development of children born with myelomeningocele. The result of infection upon the growing CNS, whether by direct neuronal destruction, by alteration of blood supply, or by a combination of these, is to reduce the IQ and to increase the perceptual motor deficits.

An IQ near 80 or greater makes it likely that one can be competitive in society. Seventy-three per cent of the 86 children who have survived from five to nine years in our recent series have an IQ of greater than 80.[356] These children are not problem free. Hand-eye coordination is diminished in many. Learning disabilities are now being identified in others.

Approximately 13 per cent of the children will survive in a noncompetitive condition. Mental retardation and problems with the Chiari II malformation are the major causes for the noncompetitive state. As stated previously, much of this mental retardation is acquired, or secondary, as a result of a complication of the treatment of hydrocephalus. However, primary retardation does occur, possibly because of rapidly progressive intrauterine hydrocephalus. These children are born with severe hydrocephalus and with portions of their cerebral mantle that do not thicken following shunting, leaving a porencephalic defect in the hemisphere.

URINARY INCONTINENCE

The single most significant medical advance in managing myelomeningocele patients is the establishment of urinary continence by clean intermittent catheterization (CIC) and pharmacotherapy.[240] Urinary continence now approaches 90 per cent in our five- to nine-year-old population. This single advance has had a profound impact on the author's ability to place these children into regular schools in the main-

stream of the education process. Urinary diversions are now rare and "undiversions" (reimplanting the ureters within the bladder) have been done in nearly 100 patients in the last nine years. A smaller number of select children have artificial urinary sphincters.[509]

HINDBRAIN DYSFUNCTION

The Chiari II hindbrain malformation continues to be the major cause of death in children with myelomeningocele.[82, 261] Almost all children with myelomeningocele have occasional problems referable to this hindbrain anomaly. In our initial series of 100 patients, 32 per cent had significant sequelae of hindbrain dysfunction. In 13 per cent the problems were severe and led to repeated hospitalization and surgical procedures to treat or manage the sequelae. One child was born with vocal cord paralysis. The other 12 developed problems in the neonatal period. Eleven of the 13 ultimately expired. Of the 32 children in our series, four had posterior fossa and cervical decompression because of progressive apnea. Two of the four died, one still requires a tracheostomy, and one has recovered. Of the remaining 28, nine died. Of the 19 survivors, one required a tracheostomy and 18 have recovered. The overall mortality rate in this group—34 per cent—is not significantly different from that reported in series in which all children have had cervical decompression. Rather, the natural history of hindbrain dysfunction would appear to be one of gradual improvement over time in those patients who survive the acute problems. Whether posterior fossa and cervical decompression in the neonate alters the course of this disease remains open to question. Neuroradiologic evaluation and brain stem evoked potentials may enable one to identify these children and anticipate their problems.[420–422]

MORTALITY

In this series operative mortality is defined as death prior to discharge from the hospital.[356] So defined, the operative mortality in the author's experience is 2 per cent. The overall mortality for the initial cohort of 100 patients, followed from five to nine years after closure of their backs, is 14 per cent. Survival curves for the last 100 children are identical to those for the first 100 children, indicating a stable death rate. No deaths have occurred after 48 months. Children with symptoms of hindbrain dysfunction contributed 11 of the 14 deaths in the first 100 patients. Thus the Chiari II dysfunction remains the principal cause of death.

It is obvious that significant progress has been

made in the understanding and management of myelomeningocele over the last 25 years; such progress continues today. In summary, the majority of mental retardation is acquired postnatally and is not intrinsic to the child with a myelomeningocele. Central nervous system infection is the principal cause of mental retardation in the myelomeningocele patient. Seventy-three per cent of surviving infants will have normal intelligence; however, the frequency of learning disabilities is likely to be high. The exact incidence of learning disability is only now being determined. Bladder and bowel control can be achieved by school age in almost 90 per cent of surviving children.

Greater than 80 per cent of patients with a myelomeningocele will be community ambulators by school age. This percentage will decrease by adulthood.

The Chiari II hindbrain malformation is the principal cause of mortality. Posterior fossa and/or cervical decompression is of questionable value in the treatment of patients with apnea, gastroesophageal reflux, and other symptoms normally attributed to hindbrain compression.

In an unselected population of patients with a myelomeningocele, 10 to 15 per cent of surviving children are likely *not* to be socially competitive and therefore will require some supportive care.

Our experience indicates that nearly all children born with a myelomeningocele should have the lesion repaired surgically, preferably within 24 hours, and should have their hydrocephalus treated. Purported "selection criteria" advocated in the past actually have little prognostic value. Their use has little effect on population outcome until more than 70 per cent of patients are selected for nontreatment. In fact, the ultimate outcome for patients in unselected series compares favorably with the outcome in series of patients managed in accordance with the "selection criteria" proposed. Deterioration in neurologic function is not regarded as a part of the natural history of myelomeningocele. Rather, myelomeningocele patients should have stable neurologic function as they grow. Any late deterioration in their condition signifies a complication that requires aggressive evaluation and treatment to return them to their steady state. Myelomeningocele is a chronic lifelong disease, requiring surveillance by knowledgeable physicians.

Orthopedic Management

The care of the musculoskeletal system of the infant with myelomeningocele begins from the day of birth. The orthopedist should be called in for consultation at the same time as the neurosurgeon, giving him an opportunity to evaluate the patient prior to closure of the lesion to determine the neurosegmental level of the lesion and the presence or absence of deformities of the limbs and spine.

All children with myelomeningocele are potentially capable of locomotion, provided they have normal function of their upper limbs, adequate stability of the spine, and motor strength of the trunk and hip musculature to enable them to elevate the pelvis and flex the hips. The goal of orthopedic treatment is to have these children walk with appropriate orthotic support by the age of 18 months. Upright posture opens new vistas with promise of a useful and satisfying life (Figs. 5–79 and 5–80), whereas recumbency will result in emaciation and large pressure sores that increase in size with malnutrition and infection; the bones become exposed; the debilitated child may expire within a few years.

The care of each patient is individualized, depending upon his unique problems. Several factors may act as deterrents to the achievement of a satisfactory level of functional performance; these may include problems of balance and posture resulting from hydrocephalus and brain damage, a poor attention span, and a lack of the necessary motivation to walk due to a low level of intelligence. Also, various behavioral aberrations and an unsatisfactory home environment may be detrimental to functional achievement.

AMBULATION

Walking ability in myelomeningocele patients may be subdivided into the following diminishing functional grades: (1) *Community walkers* are those who can walk and get around in the community with little or no restriction, managing public transport, stairs, and ramps. They may or may not require the support of orthoses or crutches. (2) *Household walkers* are those who can walk only on level terrain indoors or outdoors, transferring themselves in and out of a chair with minimal or no assistance. These patients require the support of orthoses and crutches. Community and household ambulators are classified as functional walkers. (3) *Nonfunctional walkers* are those who walk only during physiotherapy sessions; otherwise they are wheelchair bound. A nonfunctional walker often regresses in late childhood or adolescence to a nonwalker, but sometimes a motivated patient will progress to household ambulator. (4) *Nonwalkers* are those who use the wheel-

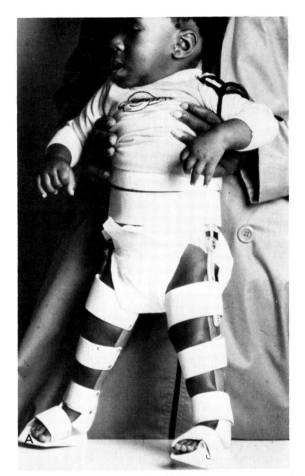

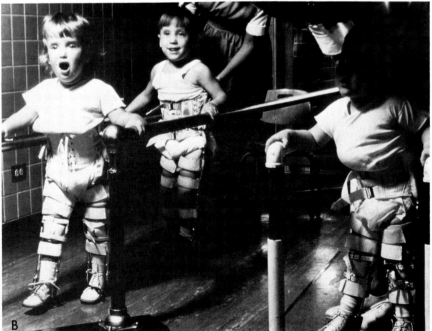

FIGURE 5–79. The goal of orthopedic management is ambulation at 16 to 18 months with the help of orthoses and crutches.

A. A 14-month-old infant with myelomeningocele held upright in braces. **B.** Gait training in parallel bars.

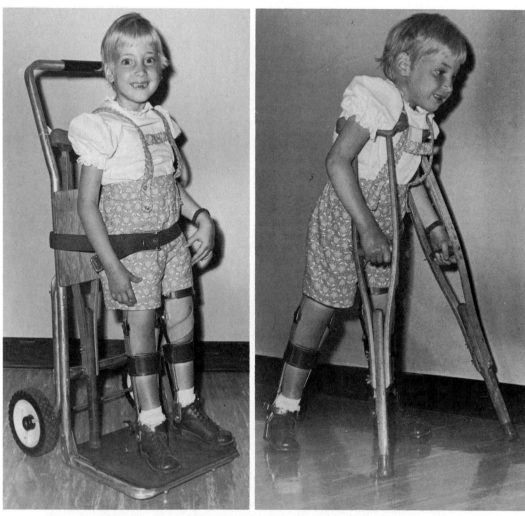

FIGURE 5–80. A child with myelomeningocele is capable of locomotion.

This child has been standing and walking since one and one half years of age. Upright posture opens new vistas with hope of a useful and satisfying life.

chair exclusively to get around, transferring themselves in and out of the wheelchair to their bed. One should make an attempt to predict the eventual ambulatory status of a child with myelomeningocele. Ambulatory status is related to energy expenditure necessary to walk. A number of factors that affect the long-term ambulatory potential of a patient with myelomeningocele are, in order of importance:

1. *The neurosegmental level of the lesion*– this is the most important factor. In the study by DeSouza and Carroll, in the group with sacral level lesions, over half were community ambulators; in the group with lower lumbar level lesions, a third; in the group with upper lumbar lesions, a tenth; and in the group with thoracic level lesions, none. Conversely, the relative numbers of nonwalkers and nonfunc-

tional walkers were least in the group with sacral level lesions and greatest in the group with thoracic lesions.[129] In the study by Asher and Olson, all the patients (with the exception of one) with sacral and fifth lumbar lesions were community walkers; patients with fourth lumbar lesions were usually functional ambulators whose ability to walk was markedly affected by musculoskeletal deformity; patients with upper lumbar and thoracic level lesions usually were not functional ambulators.[20]

2. *Motor power of the muscles in the limbs within a neurosegmental level.* The muscle strength of the limbs in the community and household ambulators is definitely superior to that of the nonfunctional ambulators and nonwalkers. Quadriceps femoris function is an important determinant of ambulatory function;

however, in addition to knee extensor motor strength, knee flexion is necessary for functional ambulation. Antigravity motor strength of hamstrings is important for stabilization of the pelvis and to decrease hip deformity. Hip abductor muscle power further stabilizes the pelvis. Patients with fourth lumbar level lesions have fair muscle strength of quadriceps and medial hamstrings (semimembranosus, semitendinosus, and gracilis); also in L4 level lesions there is usually poor strength of hip abductors.

3. *Extent and severity of musculoskeletal deformity.* Ambulatory function is adversely affected by hip deformity in third lumbar level lesions, by obesity and advancing age in first–second lumbar level lesions, and by knee-ankle-foot deformity in thoracic level lesions.[20]

4. *Obesity.* In general, more than one half of overweight children with myelomeningocele are nonfunctional ambulators. In part, obesity is the result of relative inactivity. The importance of controlling obesity cannot be overemphasized.

5. *Age of patient.* Ambulation usually deteriorates between 10 and 15 years of age, the patients tending to prefer a wheelchair to walking with orthotic devices. This appears to be related to weight gain, increased stature, and development of central nervous system lesions such as hydromyelia. Deterioration of ambulation is less in the male than in the female.

6. *Motivation* is vital in the ability to walk with braces.

7. The presence of *spasticity* tends to diminish ambulatory status, especially in association with spinal deformity, reduced muscle power, obesity, and marked retardation.

8. *Design and effectiveness of orthosis* is definitely a factor in determining ambulatory status. Operative procedures that prevent and correct musculoskeletal deformity and stabilize flail joints and collapsing spine will have a positive effect on ambulatory function.

In summary, neurosegmental level of paraplegia and motor strength of the muscles on the hip and lower limbs are the most important factors determining ambulatory function in patients with myelomeningocele. Patients with third lumbar level and higher lesions usually become nonambulatory with increasing age in adolescence; in patients with lesions at this level it is vital to control obesity and prevent musculoskeletal deformity. Stimulation of motivation and prevention of mental retardation by treating hydrocephalus are other factors. Patients with fourth lumbar or lower levels of paraplegia usually remain functional walkers.

Foot and Ankle

Deformities of the foot and ankle are very common in myelomeningocele. Some of them are congenital and others acquired postnatally. The causative factors are muscle imbalance, spasticity, fibrotic contracture of denervated muscles, intrauterine malposture assumed by a paralyzed foot, and habitual malposition of the limb adopted after birth; some deformities, however, may be of teratogenic origin.

Sharrard and Grosfield, in a study of 296 feet (148 patients with myelomeningocele), found 27 normal feet and 28 flail feet that were, however, not deformed.[531] At Children's Memorial Hospital in Chicago, 90 per cent of the patients with myelomeningocele had deformed feet; the distribution of deformities in 256 limbs in 123 children was as follows: (1) pes calcaneus, 89 feet; (2) talipes equinovarus, 83 feet; (3) pes equinus, 30 feet; (4) congenital convex pes valgus, 10 feet; and (5) miscellaneous, 18 feet. There was no deformity in 26 feet.[507] In analyzing the lower limbs of 350 patients with myelomeningocele, Lindseth found that 233 (or 63 per cent) had deformities of the feet (Table 5–11).[322]

Paralytic involvement of the lower limbs in myelomeningocele may be of two types. In the first, there is complete *flaccid* paralysis of the muscles below a certain segmental level with total loss of spinal cord function; in the second type, there is a reflex *spasticity* in isolated segments distal to the cord lesion.[564] Spastic and partial flaccid paralysis can cause muscle imbalance and result in deformities with skeletal growth. Sharrard and Grosfield observed no correlation between spontaneous motor activity and the type of deformity, but a strong correlation was noted between the deformity and the response of the lower limb muscles to faradic stimulation.[531]

Table 5–11. Foot Deformities in Patients with Myelomeningocele*

Level	Clubfoot	Calcaneo-valgus Deformity	Vertical Talus	No Deformity
Thoracic	40	8	0	38
L1, L2	22	4	1	13
L3	24	2	1	9
L4	50	4	0	14
L5	11	38	5	20
Sacral	19	4	0	41
Total	166	60	7	135

*In patients with asymmetrical paralysis, each foot was counted separately.

The type of paralytic foot deformity may be correlated with the neurosegmental level of the lesion. When it is *at or above the third lumbar segment*, the foot and ankle are flail; they may be in calcaneus, equinovarus, or valgus position as a result of intrauterine or postnatal malposture (Fig. 5–81). When these children are upright and begin to walk, valgus deformity will develop in response to the static forces of body weight.

When the lesion is *at the fourth lumbar segment*, the anterior tibial muscle will be active and strong, pulling the forefoot into dorsiflexion and inversion. The posture of the hindfoot is usually calcaneovalgus but occasionally may be equinus, with plantar flexion of the talus and dorsolateral subluxation or dislocation of the talocalcaneonavicular joint (paralytic vertical talus).

When involvement is *at the fifth lumbar level*, the long toe extensors, peroneus longus and brevis, and anterior tibial muscles are

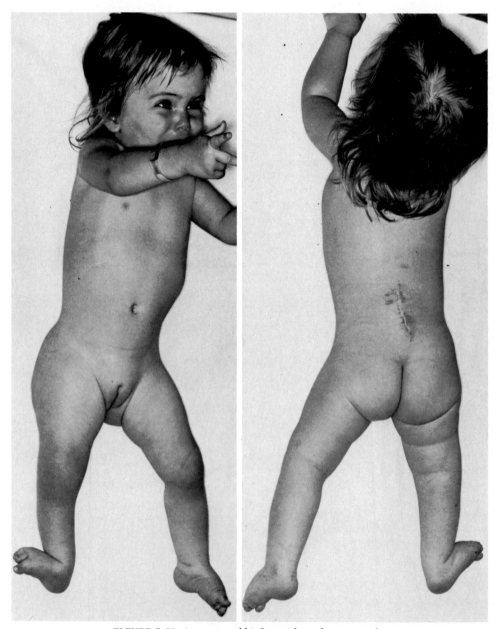

FIGURE 5–81. A one-year-old infant with myelomeningocele.

Note the calcaneovalgus deformity of the right foot caused by fibrosis of long toe extensors and peroneal muscles.

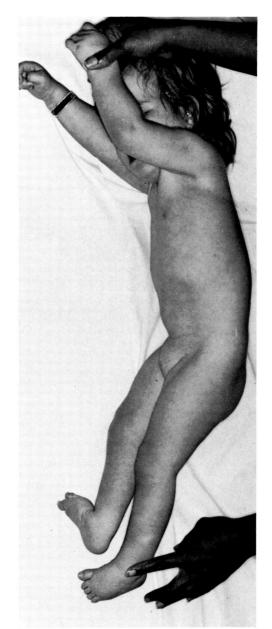

FIGURE 5–81 Continued. A one-year-old infant with myelomeningocele.

Note the calcaneovalgus deformity of the right foot caused by fibrosis of long toe extensors and peroneal muscles.

strong, whereas the triceps surae and long toe flexor muscles are paralyzed. A progressive calcaneus deformity will result if dynamic imbalance is not corrected (Fig. 5–82).

When the lesion is within the *first two sacral neurosegments* there is complete or partial paralysis of the long toe flexor and intrinsic muscles of the foot, with the long and short toe extensor muscles active; the resultant deformity is pes cavus with clawing of the toes.

Equinovarus deformity may result from a teratologic process at any level. Schafer and Dias report an equal distribution of talipes equinovarus (82 feet in 51 patients) between the thoracic, high lumbar, and low lumbar levels.[507]

The objective of treatment is to obtain a flexible, normally aligned plantigrade foot that can bear weight safely. Deformed feet will develop pressure sores, cellulitis, and osteomyelitis, which will eventually necessitate amputation. One cannot overemphasize the importance of diligent and persistent care of the feet of children with myelomeningocele. Management, however, does present certain difficult problems due to fibrosis of denervated

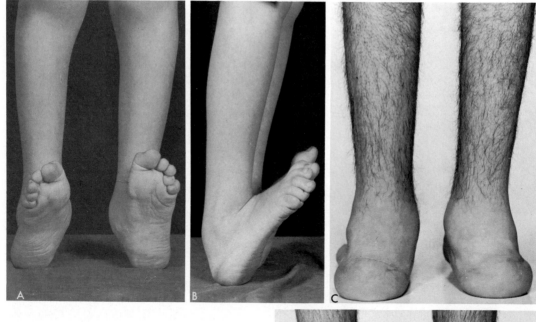

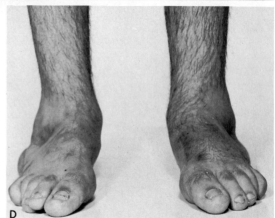

FIGURE 5–82. A myelomeningocele child with involvement at the fifth lumbar level.

The long toe extensor, peroneal, and anterior tibial muscles are normal in motor strength, whereas the triceps surae and long toe flexors are paralyzed. Severe calcaneus deformity of both feet has developed as a result of dynamic imbalance of muscles acting on the foot and ankle. A posterior transfer of the anterior tibial and peroneal muscles was performed to restore dynamic balance. **A** and **B.** Preoperative photographs at five years of age. **C** and **D.** Postoperative photographs when 14 years old.

muscles, sensory loss, and associated paralysis of the muscles controlling the hip and knee.

Treatment should begin at birth. There is no excuse for delay. A flexible deformity will become rigid with skeletal growth. The general tendency is to postpone the treatment of foot deformities because of the fear that it may interfere with nursing and surgical management of the spinal defect and hydrocephalus. The neurosurgeon should be requested to place the needles for intravenous administration of fluids in the upper limb when there is a deformity of the lower limb. Early soft-tissue surgery will prevent development of rigid structural bony deformities. Incomplete correction, muscle imbalance, and spasticity and fibrosis will cause a high rate of recurrence of foot deformity. It is vital to use night splints and day orthoses, to carry out an adequate physical therapy pro-

gram, and to balance muscle forces surgically to prevent recurrence of deformity. When muscle strength is inadequate and balancing of muscle forces is not feasible, it is best to section and excise tendons, making the foot-ankle flail and free of progressive deformity.

The specific deformities of the foot are discussed next.

PES CALCANEUS

Pes calcaneus is very common in myelomeningocele (see Figs. 5–81 and 5–82). On gross anatomic inspection the problem appears to be benign, but functionally it is very disabling. In calcaneus deformity the weight-bearing surface of the foot is shortened, and the stability of the base upon which the body is supported is diminished. In addition, excessive pressure is exerted on the posterior tuberosity of the dorsiflexed calcaneus and the plantar-flexed metatarsal heads. Pressure will lead to callosities and trophic ulcerations, which cause severe problems in insensitive feet.[178] Children with myelomeningocele have smaller feet than normal, and many of them put on excess weight as they get older. Hay and Walker found plantar pressures in children with myelomeningocele to be substantially higher than those in normal children of the same age.[243] This relative increase in perpendicular static pressure is partly due to the smaller feet in the child with spina bifida and, thereby, the greater pressure per unit of surface. Greater pressure is exerted on the hindfoot because of the vertical position of the os calcis in calcaneus deformity. In the normal limb, motion at the knee and ankle reduces the impact on foot-strike and in the stance phase in ambulation. In the braced, rigid knee and ankle of the child with myelomeningocele this compensatory mechanism is lacking, and the weight borne on the plantar aspect of the foot is increased.

The deformed calcaneus foot is difficult to fit with shoes. The prominent dorsum of the midfoot and interphalangeal joints of the clawed toes are rubbed and irritated by the shoe, and ulceration results. Because the posterior part of the heel is shortened or almost absent, it is difficult to keep the shoe on. Biomechanically, calcaneus posture of the ankle and instability in stance cause knee and hip flexion and increase the instability of an already precarious balance.[178]

The primary cause of calcaneus deformity is muscle imbalance between the active dorsiflexors of the ankle and the paralyzed plantar flexors. Being at the highest level of innervation, the tibialis anterior will function in fourth lumbar level lesions. The long toe extensors and peroneals will be strong in lesions at the fifth lumbar level.[531] Other deforming factors are fibrosis of the denervated muscles, spasticity, and malposture—intrauterine and postnatal. Greater motor strength of the lateral extensors (peroneus tertius, extensor digitorum communis, and peroneus brevis) over the tibialis anterior will cause calcaneovalgus deformity. Underdevelopment of the fibula in relation to the tibia will result in a high-riding lateral malleolus and lateral tilting of the ankle mortise.[73, 131, 369] Lateral tibial torsion is often associated with valgus foot and ankle. Calcaneovarus deformity is caused by the unbalanced action of the tibialis anterior; it is much less common than calcaneovalgus deformity.

In the newborn, treatment consists of passive manipulative exercises to elongate contracted soft-tissue structures on the dorsum of the ankle and leg. The rigid and severe calcaneus deformity may require the use of a plaster of Paris cast to retain the correction achieved by manipulation. As soon as the foot is brought to 10 to 20 degrees of plantar flexion, splints are used at night to maintain correction, and passive stretching exercises are continued.

If the calcaneus deformity cannot be prevented from progressing or recurring and the anterior tibial muscle is the deforming force, it is transferred posteriorly through the interosseous route. This procedure was originally described by Peabody for treatment of calcaneus deformity secondary to poliomyelitis.[457] Green and Grice have reported their technique and experience in the management of pes calcaneus.[210] The operative technique is described and illustrated in Plate 73.

This author recommends posterior transfer of the anterior tibial through the interosseous route, transfer of the peroneus longus to the os calcis, and suture of the distal stump of the peroneus longus to the peroneus brevis if the transferred muscles are good or normal in motor strength and the long toe extensors are strong. Additional important requisites are that the patient should have good hip flexors (and preferably knee flexors also) to clear the foot in gait as well as quadriceps femoris function. The patient should be between three and four years of age at the time of surgery. By then there will be a contracture of the anterior ankle capsule, and the foot will not go into equinus. With adequate postoperative care, the posterior transfer will be good on manual testing but poor when the patient rises on his toes. The objective of the posterior transfer is to halt progression of calcaneus deformity and to provide a plantigrade foot. If only the anterior tibial muscle is functioning and the long toe extensors are paralyzed, it is best to lengthen or simply section the anterior tibial tendon.

As reported in the literature, the results of posterior transfer of the tibialis anterior to the calcaneus have not been very encouraging. There were three failures in eight cases (37.5 per cent) reported by Hayes and colleagues, and 20 per cent of the series of 20 feet reported by Sharrard and Grosfield were failures.[246, 531] Menelaus recommends transfer of the anterior tibial tendon alone. When the toe extensors are functioning, Menelaus advises tenotomy of the extensor hallucis longus, extensor digitorum longus, and peroneus tertius.[388] Smith and Duckworth reported six poor results in nine

Text continued on page 1804

Posterior Tendon Transfer to Os Calcis for Correction of Calcaneus Deformity (Green and Grice)

OPERATIVE TECHNIQUE

It is best to place the patient in the prone position to facilitate the surgical exposure of the heel. The posterior tibial, and peroneus longus and brevis tendons are divided distally at their insertion and delivered into the proximal wound following the technique and steps described in Plate 40, page 982. When the flexor hallucis longus tendon is to be transferred, its distal portion is sutured to the flexor hallucis brevis muscle. The anterior tibial tendon is delivered into the calf and heel through the interosseous route.

A. A 5 cm. long posterior transverse incision is made around the heel along one of the skin creases in the part that neither presses the shoe nor touches the ground.

B. The skin and subcutaneous flaps are undercut and reflected, exposing the os calcis and the insertion of the tendo calcaneus. An L-shaped cut is made in the lateral two thirds of the insertion of the tendo calcaneus. The divided portion is reflected proximally, exposing the apophysis of the os calcis.

C. Next, with a %₆₄-inch drill, a hole is made through the calcaneus, beginning in the center of the apophysis and coming out laterally at its plantar aspect. With a diamond head hand drill and curet, the hole is enlarged to receive all the transferred tendons.

Plate 73. Posterior Tendon Transfer to Os Calcis for Correction of Calcaneus Deformity (Green and Grice)

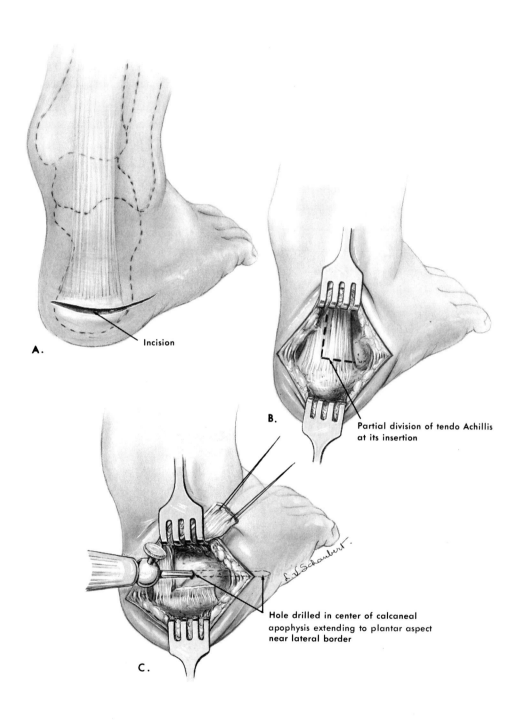

A.

Incision

B.

Partial division of tendo Achillis
at its insertion

C.

Hole drilled in center of calcaneal
apophysis extending to plantar aspect
near lateral border

Posterior Tendon Transfer to Os Calcis for Correction of Calcaneus Deformity (Green and Grice) (Continued)

D. Through a lateral incision, the intermuscular septum is widely divided between the lateral and posterior compartments. An Ober tendon transfer is inserted through the wound and directed anterior to the tendo calcaneus into the transverse incision over the os calcis. The threads of the whip sutures at the ends of the peroneal tendons are passed through the hole in the tendon passer and the tendons are delivered at the heel. The posterior tibial tendon is delivered at the heel by a similar route, through an incision in the intermuscular septum between the medial and posterior compartments and anterior to the tendo calcaneus. Next, with a twisted wire probe, the tendons are inserted in the hole and pulled through the tunnel in the calcaneus.

E. At their point of exit on the lateral aspect of the calcaneus the tendons are sutured to the periosteum and ligamentous tissues. The tendons are sutured under enough tension to hold the foot in 15 degrees of equinus when the remaining ankle dorsiflexors are fair in motor strength, and 30 degrees equinus if they are good or normal. The tendons are sutured to each other and to the periosteum of the apophysis of the calcaneus at the posterior end of the tunnel.

F and G. The divided portion of the tendo calcaneus is resutured in its original position posterior to the transferred tendons.

The wounds are closed and a long leg cast is applied, the knee in 45 to 60 degrees of flexion, the hindfoot 15 to 30 degrees equinus, but the forefoot neutral. Cavus deformity of the forefoot should be avoided.

POSTOPERATIVE CARE

Three to four weeks following surgery the solid cast is removed and a new above-knee bivalved cast is made to protect the limb at all times when exercises are not being performed. It is imperative to prevent forced dorsiflexion of the ankle and stretching of the transferred tendons.

Exercises are first performed side-lying and with gravity eliminated, and then in prone position against gravity (see Fig. 5–53 A and B). In order to teach the patient the new action of the transferred muscle, he is asked to move the foot in the direction of a component of the original action of the muscle and then to plantar-flex the foot. For example, when the peroneals are transferred, he is asked to evert and plantar-flex the foot; or when the anterior tibial is transferred, to invert and plantar-flex the foot. Soon, under supervision, guided dorsiflexion of the foot is performed along with plantar flexion. It is important to develop reciprocal motion and motor strength of agonists and antagonist muscles. Weight-bearing is not allowed. Ambulation is permitted in the above-knee bivalved cast with crutches.

In about four to six weeks when the transferred tendons are fair in motor strength the patient is allowed to stand on both feet. The heel of the foot that was operated on rests on a 3 cm. thick block to prevent stretching of the transferred tendons. Bearing partial weight on his foot, the patient should rise up on his tiptoes while holding on to a table with his hands or using two crutches.

When the transplant functions effectively on tiptoe standing, walking with crutches is begun with three-point gait and partial weight-bearing on the affected limb (Fig. 5–53 D). The heel of the shoe is elevated with a 1 to 1.5 cm. lift that tapers in front (toward the toes). Walking periods are gradually increased. When the transplant works effectively in gait and take-off has been developed in walking, standing tiptoe rising exercises are started without the support of crutches (Fig. 5–53 E). The knee should not be flexed and the patient should not lean forward while rising up on his toes at least three times (Fig. 5–53 F). This may take a long time (as much as a year or more), but it is a very important phase of postoperative management.

A plantar-flexion spring orthosis or an orthosis with a posterior elastic is worn when the patient is uncooperative in the use of crutches or when muscular control of the knee and hip is poor because of extensive paralysis. A stop at the ankle prevents dorsiflexion of the ankle beyond neutral position.

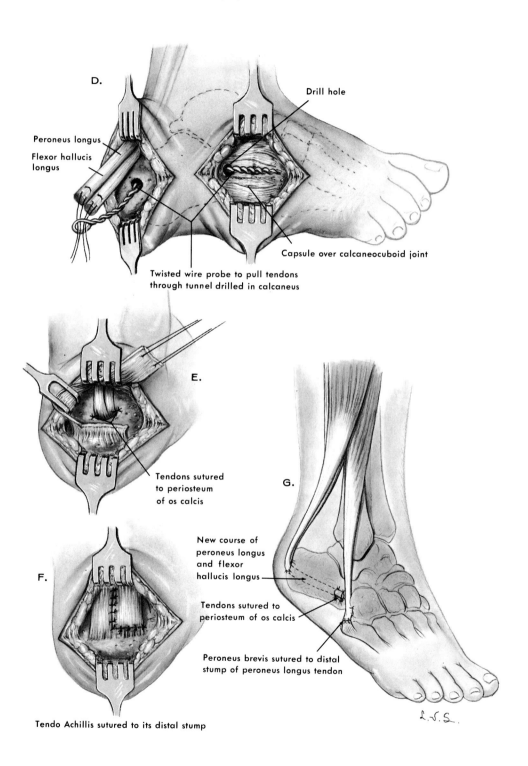

D.

Peroneus longus

Flexor hallucis longus

Drill hole

Capsule over calcaneocuboid joint

Twisted wire probe to pull tendons through tunnel drilled in calcaneus

E.

Tendons sutured to periosteum of os calcis

G.

New course of peroneus longus and flexor hallucis longus

Tendons sutured to periosteum of os calcis

Peroneus brevis sutured to distal stump of peroneus longus tendon

F.

Tendo Achillis sutured to its distal stump

L.S.S.

feet in which the extensor tendons were transferred to the heel, whereas in four calcaneus feet treated by extensor tenotomy there were no poor results.[549]

Posterior transfer of the anterior tibial tendon to the os calcis may be combined with tenodesis of the Achilles tendon to the tibia. Banta and co-workers reported the results in seven patients (14 feet). Following surgery, polypropylene ankle-foot orthoses were used to protect the transfers. Preoperative and postoperative gait analyses were performed. Results showed decreased knee flexion in stance and decreased ankle dorsiflexion in stance, with the achievement of a more upright posture. Prolongation of the firing time in both stance and swing phase was demonstrated by the EMG studies. Postoperatively, all patients showed improvement in step length, single limb support, and walking velocity. Force plate analysis showed reduction in the work required to ambulate. The progression of the calcaneus deformity was checked in all cases.[31] Equinus deformity did not develop as a consequence of the Achilles tenodesis. This author recommends a combination of Achilles tendon tenodesis to the tibia and posterior transfer of the anterior tibial tendon when the deformity is calcaneovarus. Often, however, the presenting deformity is a calcaneovalgus foot with an associated valgus ankle. In such a case, this author recommends a combination of posterior transfer of the anterior tibial tendon with calcaneofibular Achilles tendon tenodesis; this will stimulate distal growth of the fibula and prevent progression of the valgus inclination of the ankle.[131, 507]

Fibrosis and contracture of the denervated anterior crural muscles will cause calcaneus deformity. In severe cases there will be rigid contracture of the anterior capsule of the ankle joint. This type of pes calcaneus is treated by early radical excision of the tendons and tendon sheaths of the ankle dorsiflexors and anterior ankle capsulectomy. The skin may be very taut, preventing plantar flexion of the foot; in such a case, Z-plasty lengthening of the skin is performed.

Another type of calcaneus deformity is caused by spasticity of the ankle dorsiflexors and flaccid paralysis of the triceps surae. This type is treated by excision of the spastic tendons and their tendon sheaths.

In the older child with bony deformity, the calcaneocavus foot is corrected by posterior displacement osteotomy of the os calcis, by either Mitchell's oblique or Samilson's crescentic technique; it should be combined with plantar release as described in the section on pes cavus.[404, 504]

VALGUS ANKLE

Relative shortening of the fibula in relation to the tibia is common in the ankles of children with myelomeningocele. Makin described delay in ossification and shortening of the fibula in ten such patients.[369] Hollingsworth analyzed the radiograms of 39 children with myelomeningocele, of whom 32 showed slight to marked shortening of the fibula and a valgus ankle.[262] Dias studied the growth of the fibula and ankle mortise in 86 children with myelomeningocele who were between the ages of 18 months and 15 years.[131] The degree of fibular shortening was determined by comparing the radiograms of myelomeningocele children with radiograms showing the relationship between the distal fibular growth plate and the dome of the talus in 100 normal persons. During the first four years of life the normal distal physis of the fibula is slightly superior to the dome of the talus; at five years of age it is level with the talar dome; thereafter it gradually migrates inferiorly. At skeletal maturity it is situated approximately 3 mm. distal to the dome of the talus.

The degree of fibular shortening is determined by two factors: the severity of the paralysis of the triceps surae and the age of the patient. The fibula bears one sixth of the total body weight during stance and gait. Its longitudinal growth appears to be related to the strength of the posterior calf musculature, particularly of the soleus muscle. Weinert and associates have demonstrated with telephoto motion pictures and cineradiograms of weight-bearing and non-weight-bearing ankles that the fibula moves downward during the weight-bearing phase of gait; this serves to deepen the mortise and adds to the stability of the ankle.[616] The muscles taking origin from the fibula are the lateral head of the soleus and the flexor hallucis longus (both having innervations from the first and second sacral segments), and the tibialis posterior (innervated from the fifth lumbar segment). Growth of the fibula is stimulated by the dynamic force of muscle action and the static loading from body weight. When the soleus muscle is paralyzed, progressive shortening of the fibula takes place (Fig. 5–83). The age of the patient is another factor to consider; the older the patient, the greater the degree of shortening. According to Dias, the mean yearly increment of shortening is 1.3 mm.[131]

Relative shortening of the fibula and elevation

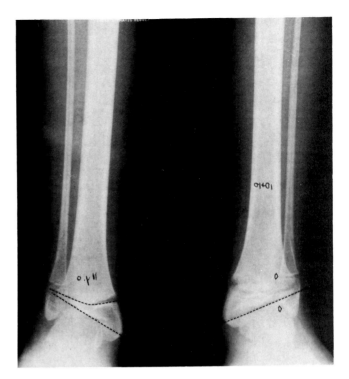

FIGURE 5–83. *Anteroposterior radiogram of both ankles in an eight-year-old child with myelomeningocele at the fourth lumbar level.*

Note the high-riding physis of the distal fibula and the valgus deformity of the ankle.

of the lateral malleolus result in instability of the ankle mortise and increasing lateral wedging of the distal tibial epiphysis (Fig. 5–84). Another pathogenic factor is uneven distribution of forces of body weight across the ankle mortise and distal tibial physis in the calcaneovalgus foot in stance and walking. The lateral epiphyseal growth of the distal tibia is retarded. The previously compressive forces across the medial aspect of the distal tibial physis become tensile; the traction effect may cause relative overgrowth of the medial malleolus. The prominent medial malleolus becomes irritated from the shoe and the medial upright of the orthosis; adventitious bursae may form, which may become infected. The short fibula will exert a tethering effect on the tibia and knee, causing progressively exaggerated lateral tibial torsion, genu valgum, and impairment of gait.

Treatment in the young child consists of calcaneofibular tenodesis. The technique is described and illustrated in Plate 74. The procedure was developed by Westin for correction of valgus ankle in poliomyelitis. Although not as effective in myelomeningocele, it does stimulate the growth of the fibula and prevents further progression of the valgus deviation of the ankle. In the active ambulatory patient, when the surgery is performed at four or five years of age, varying degrees of correction of the shortening of the fibula may be obtained. This author strongly recommends the procedure in children between four and six years of

dure in children between four and six years of age. In selected cases it may be combined with posterior transfer of the anterior tibial tendon to the os calcis.

In the child over eight years of age a supramalleolar tibial and fibular osteotomy is required to correct the valgus ankle. Sharrard and Webb perform a wedge resection osteotomy of the tibia.[533] This author, however, recommends a medial displacement and tilting osteotomy, which corrects the valgus ankle, elevates the medial malleolus, and lowers the fibular malleolus.[633] The technique of supramalleolar osteotomy of the tibia and fibula is described and illustrated in Figure 5–85.

Supramalleolar osteotomy may be combined with calcaneofibular tenodesis in the child between eight and ten years of age.

Stapling of the medial part of the distal tibial epiphysis is recommended by Burkus et al.[73] The procedure is indicated for patients whose physes will remain open for at least 18 months and whose progression of valgus deformity of the ankle is well documented. In a series of 25 ankles the valgus deformity was effectively controlled and adequately corrected. This author has had no personal experience with stapling of the medial part of the distal tibial physis in myelomeningocele.

TALIPES EQUINOVARUS

This common deformity of the foot in myelomeningocele is difficult to treat (Figs. 5–86 to

Calcaneofibular Tenodesis

OPERATIVE TECHNIQUE

The patient is placed in lateral position to facilitate the surgical exposure of the heel and lateral aspect of the ankle.

A. A longitudinal incision is made immediately posterior to the fibula; it begins at the tip of the lateral malleolus and extends proximally for a distance of 7 to 10 cm.

B. The subcutaneous tissue is divided, and the wound flaps are undercut and reflected, exposing the tendo calcaneus and the lateral surface of the fibula. The Achilles tendon is sectioned transversely at its musculotendinous junction, as proximally as possible. Obtain adequate length of the tendon.

C. Next, the distal physis of the fibula is identified and marked with a Keith needle. Radiograms are made with the Keith needle in place to verify the site of the growth plate, which should not be disturbed. With a dental drill a longitudinal slot about 3 cm. long and 0.5 to 0.75 cm. wide is made in the metaphyseal-diaphyseal area of the fibula. Its lower end should be 1 to 1.5 cm. proximal to the growth plate. The slot should be directed anteroposteriorly; do not break the lateral or medial cortex of the fibula.

D. The Achilles tendon is passed through the slot posteroanteriorly and sutured to itself under enough tension to hold the foot at an equinus angle of 15 to 20 degrees. The tendon is anchored to the periosteum of the fibula with additional sutures. Sometimes in the ankle of the child with myelomeningocele the fibula is so small and atrophied that it is safer to make a smaller slot, section the heel cord into halves, and pass only one half of the tendon through the slot and suture the other half to the fibular shaft through holes made with an electric drill. A calcaneofibular tenodesis may be combined with posterior transfer of the anterior tibial tendon to the os calcis through the interosseous route.

In calcaneus deformity secondary to overlengthening of the triceps surae in cerebral palsy, only the lateral half of the tendo calcaneus is attached to the fibula; its medial half is left continuous with the gastrocnemius-soleus muscle.

The tourniquet is released and, after complete hemostasis the wound is closed in the usual manner. An above-knee cast is applied with the ankle in 20 degrees of plantar flexion, but with the forefoot in neutral position. Avoid cavus deformity of the forefoot.

POSTOPERATIVE CARE

Four weeks following surgery the solid cast is removed and a new above-knee plastic splint is made to protect the limb, preventing forced dorsiflexion of the ankle and stretching of the tenodesis.

As soon as possible the child is fitted with an ankle-foot orthosis, in which a plantar flexion assist and stop at the ankle prevent dorsiflexion beyond minus 10 to 15 degrees. He is allowed to ambulate and bear weight with the support of crutches. The above-knee splint is worn at night. With the pull of the Achilles tendon the distal fibular epiphysis will grow, and gradually the lateral tilting of the ankle mortise will be corrected.

Plate 74. Calcaneofibular Tenodesis

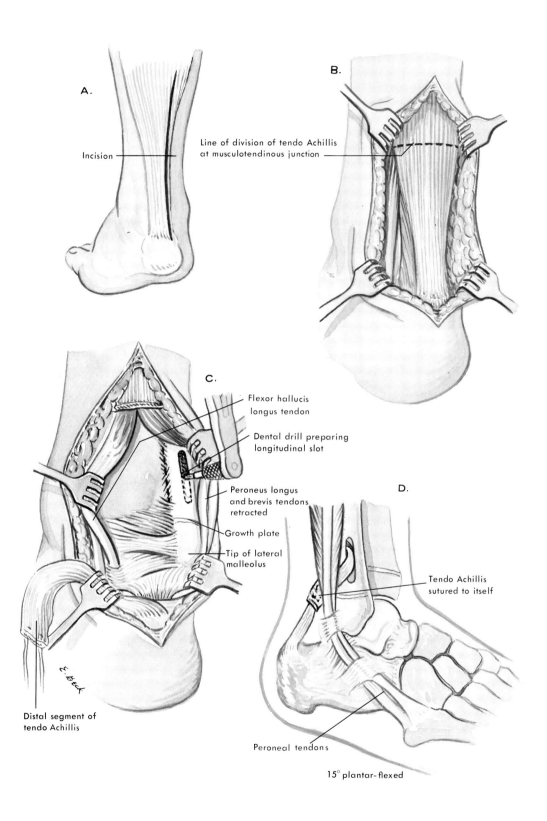

A.

Incision

B.

Line of division of tendo Achillis at musculotendinous junction

C.

Flexor hallucis longus tendon

Dental drill preparing longitudinal slot

Peroneus longus and brevis tendons retracted

Growth plate

Tip of lateral malleolus

Distal segment of tendo Achillis

D.

Tendo Achillis sutured to itself

Peroneal tendons

15° plantar-flexed

1807

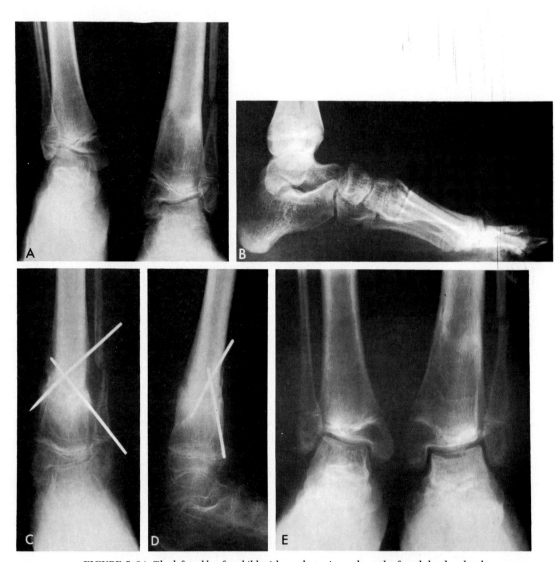

FIGURE 5–84. The left ankle of a child with myelomeningocele at the fourth lumbar level.

There are valgus ankle, high-riding fibular malleolus, and severe lateral wedging of the distal tibial epiphysis. **A.** Anteroposterior radiograms at six years old. Note the valgus ankle, especially on the left. **B.** Lateral view of the left foot, showing severe calcaneus deformity. **C** and **D.** Two-months-postoperative radiograms. The tendo Achillis is split and sutured to the distal fibular metaphyseal-diaphyseal junction. **E.** Two years postoperatively, radiograms of the left ankle show control and some correction of the valgus deviation of the ankle.

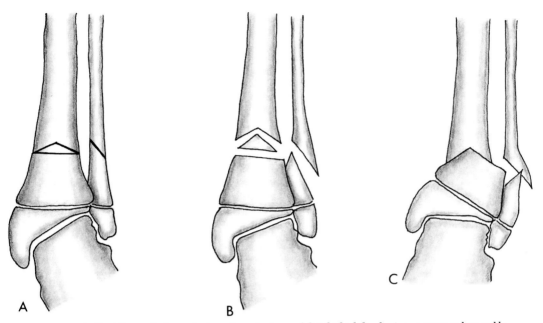

FIGURE 5–85. *Wiltse technique of triangular osteotomy of distal tibial diaphysis to correct valgus ankle.*

A. The lines of osteotomy. **B.** Triangular fragment of tibia excised. **C.** Medial rotation and lateral shift of the distal fragment will correct the valgus deformity without undesirable prominence of the medial malleolus; the shortening of the limb will be less than with a simple close-up osteotomy.

5–88). In the majority of the cases the deformity is very rigid and severe and has a high rate of recurrence despite adequate initial correction, behaving more like the clubfoot seen in arthrogryposis multiplex congenita. Talipes equinovarus in myelomeningocele is teratologic and paralytic, caused by lack of normal muscle forces in utero and arrest of development of the foot beyond the fetal stage of equinovarus posture. Often there is no muscle function of the limb below the knee. In about 10 per cent of the cases the equinovarus deformity is acquired and the result of muscle imbalance, spasticity, and fibrosis. The toe extensors, peroneals, and anterior tibial are paralyzed (sometimes the anterior tibial may be functioning); there is reflex activity and spasticity of the posterior tibial muscle; and there is fibrosis of the triceps surae, long toe extensors, and flexor hallucis longus.

Principles and details of management of talipes equinovarus are described in Chapter 7. Manipulative elongation of contracted soft tissues should be very gently performed to avoid

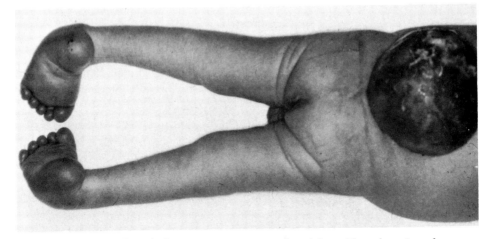

FIGURE 5–86. *Bilateral talipes equinovarus in a newborn infant with myelomeningocele.*

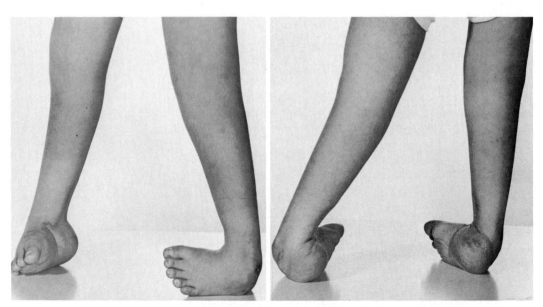

FIGURE 5–87. *A myelomeningocele child with severe bilateral talipes equinovarus.*

This is an example of deformity of the foot that is of teratologic origin.

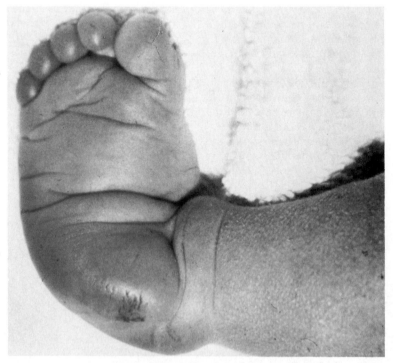

FIGURE 5–88. *Pressure sore on the heel of a child with myelomeningocele and talipes equinovarus.*

The cast should be applied not as a stretching device but as a retention apparatus to maintain the correction obtained by gentle manipulation.

fracture. Adhesive strapping or plaster of Paris casts should be properly padded and well molded. Sharrard and Grosfield report disastrous results from attempted conservative treatment of equinus and equinovarus deformities in children with myelomeningocele.[531] The same experience has *not* been shared by this author. It is strongly advocated that contractural deformities be corrected as much as possible by conservative methods. Partial correction of soft-tissue contractures will diminish the incidence of postoperative wound dehiscence. In the flail limb it is recommended that soft-tissue release (tenotomy of anterior tibial, posterior tibial, and Achilles tendons) be performed during the neonatal period at the time of sac closure or first shunt procedure. The mildly deformed foot can be corrected by nonsurgical means; in the great majority of cases, however, surgical correction is required. By three to six months of age, depending upon the size of the foot and general medical and neurosurgical status of the infant, an open reduction of the subluxated talocalcaneonavicular and calcaneocuboid joints is performed. The Cincinnati transverse incision is ideal, as it will allow complete subtalar release and correction of medial plantar subluxation of the talocalcaneonavicular and calcaneocuboid joints.

In the experience of Walker, V-Y plasty incision has been unsatisfactory. He recommends the rotation flap incision, as used by Holdsworth. The incision begins at the midpoint of the posterior aspect of the calf, extends distally to behind the medial malleolus, and then runs forward along the medial border of the foot. It then runs laterally across the dorsum at or just behind the metatarsal heads and turns proximally along the lateral border of the foot (Fig. 5–89A). The subcutaneous tissue is divided in line with the skin incision. The wound flap is raised, staying superficial to the venous arch (Fig. 5–89B and C). Posteromedial and plantar releases are performed to obtain full correction of the deformity. The tourniquet is released, and after complete hemostasis, the flap is rotated to close the defect on the medial aspect of the foot and ankle (Fig. 5–89D). Usually the return of circulation is adequate; occasionally there may be distal skin ischemia, which usually settles down during the period of cast immobilization. According to Walker, the rotation flap incision provides adequate skin cover at operation with the foot in plantigrade position, and scar contracture is not a problem.[606] This author has not found it necessary to utilize the flap incision.

During surgery one should excise the tendons of fibrosed muscles, the tendon sheaths, and the contracted joint capsules to prevent recurrence of deformity. It is crucial to provide meticulous postoperative care to prevent recurrence of deformity. Despite all efforts, recurrence of deformity is still high.[131, 388] Talectomy may be indicated between the ages of one and five years for the recurrent and rigid deformity.[535] Menelaus analyzed the outcome of talectomy in 41 feet (25 in patients with arthrogryposis multiplex congenita and 16 in those with spina bifida—among them, 14 with equinovarus deformity and 2 with vertical talus); the results were good in 32 feet (79 per cent); there was residual equinus deformity in 14 feet (14 per cent) and residual equinovarus deformity in 3 feet (7 per cent).[385] The technique of talectomy is described in Chapter 7. It should be combined with soft-tissue release and partial or complete resection of the cuboid bone. Menelaus states that during the past eight years the need for talectomy has been obviated by early soft-tissue release. Decancellation of the head and neck of the talus and cuboid bone (Verebelyi-Ogston procedure) is not recommended by this author.[191, 434]

PES EQUINUS

Varying degrees of pes equinus are quite common in myelomeningocele. It is caused by fibrosis and contracture of the triceps surae; if it is associated with contracture of the peronei the foot will be in equinovalgus position. Equinus deformity is very disabling, making it difficult to fit shoes and braces. Pressures sores on the heel become a chronic problem. In the flail limb, equinus deformity can be prevented by passive range of motion exercises and splinting the foot and ankle in neutral position at night. Moderate equinus deformity is corrected by section and excision of a segment of the Achilles tendon. Severe equinus deformity, as shown in Figure 5–90, requires radical excision of tendons and tendon sheaths, posterior capsulectomy of the ankle and subtalar joints, and sometimes sectioning of the inferior syndesmosis of the tibiofibular articulation to widen the ankle mortise. Postoperatively, it is essential to maintain the ankles and feet in corrected neutral position by splints at night and plastic orthoses in the shoes during the day.

PARALYTIC CONGENITAL CONVEX PES VALGUS

This is a rare congenital deformity, occurring in the feet of 5 to 10 per cent of children born

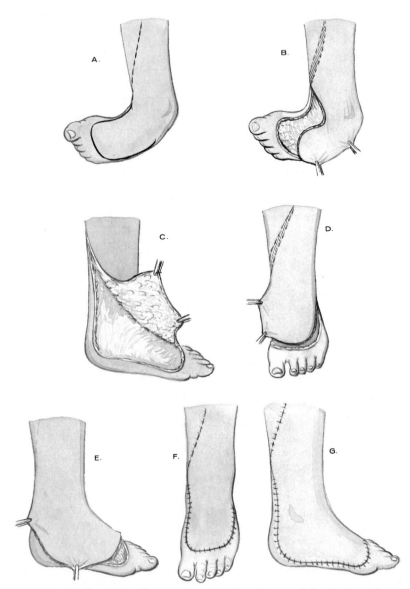

FIGURE 5–89. Rotation flap incision for correction of rigid equinovarus deformity in myelomeningocele.

A. The incision. **B** and **C.** Raising of the flap. **D.** Rotation of the flap. **E** to **G.** Resuturing of the flap with the foot in plantigrade position. (Redrawn after Walker, C.: The early management of varus feet in myelomeningocele. J. Bone Joint Surg., 53-*B*:465, 1977.)

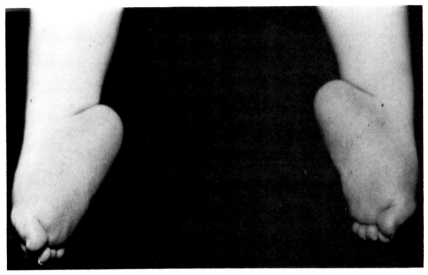

FIGURE 5–90. *Severe equinus deformity of both feet due to fibrosis and contracture of the triceps surae.*

with myelomeningocele. The talus is plantar flexed, and the talocalcaneonavicular and calcaneocuboid joints are partially or completely displaced dorsally and laterally. In clinical appearance, the paralytic and nonparalytic types are quite similar. The sole of the foot is convex, with the head of the talus prominent on the plantar and medial aspects of the foot; the hindfoot is everted and in equinus posture; and the forepart of the foot is abducted and dorsiflexed (Fig. 5–91).

The usual pattern of muscle imbalance found in association with paralytic vertical talus is normal strength in the anterior tibial, long toe extensor, and peroneal muscles; and paralysis of the triceps surae, tibialis posterior, long and short toe flexors, and intrinsic muscles of the foot, i.e., intact innervation down to the muscles supplied by the first sacral segment, with paralysis of the muscles supplied by the second and third sacral segments. Occasionally, congenital convex pes valgus is associated with complete paralysis of all muscles of the lower limb. The pathologic anatomy and radiographic features are discussed in the section on congenital convex pes valgus in Chapter 7. Usually the deformity is present at birth; occasionally it develops postnatally.[160]

The deformity is very rigid and does not respond to conservative therapy. It is strongly recommended that open reduction of the talocalcaneonavicular and calcaneocuboid joints be performed at three to six months of age, depending upon the general medical and neurosurgical status of the infant. The capsule of the talonavicular joint is reconstructed by plication

and tautening on its plantar and medial aspects, and the joint is fixed internally with a threaded Steinmann pin.

The details of the author's operative technique are described and illustrated in Chapter 7. The muscular forces acting on the foot are balanced by appropriate tendon transfers; commonly the anterior tibial tendon is transferred to the head-neck of the talus, and the peroneus brevis posteriorly to the os calcis. The peroneus longus is left to act as plantar flexor of the first metatarsal.

Duckworth and Smith, and Sharrard, recommend the following procedure: The operation is performed through three incisions, the first of which is made over the dorsum of the foot to the lateral aspect of the subtalar joint. A segment of the taut long toe extensor and peroneus tertius is excised (Sharrard recommends lengthening rather than sectioning of the toe extensors). The subtalar joint is opened laterally, and the interosseous talocalcaneal ligament is divided. The peroneus longus is lengthened by Z-plasty. The peroneus brevis is detached from the base of the fifth metatarsal. By this degree of soft-tissue release, a great deal of the dorsiflexion-abduction deformity of the forefoot and the valgus deformity of the hindfoot can be corrected. A separate longitudinal incision is made on the lateral side of the Achilles tendon. The peroneus brevis is delivered into the back of the ankle, and the tendo calcaneus is lengthened by Z-plasty. A third incision is made on the medial aspect of the foot, beginning below and behind the medial malleolus and extending distally to the base of

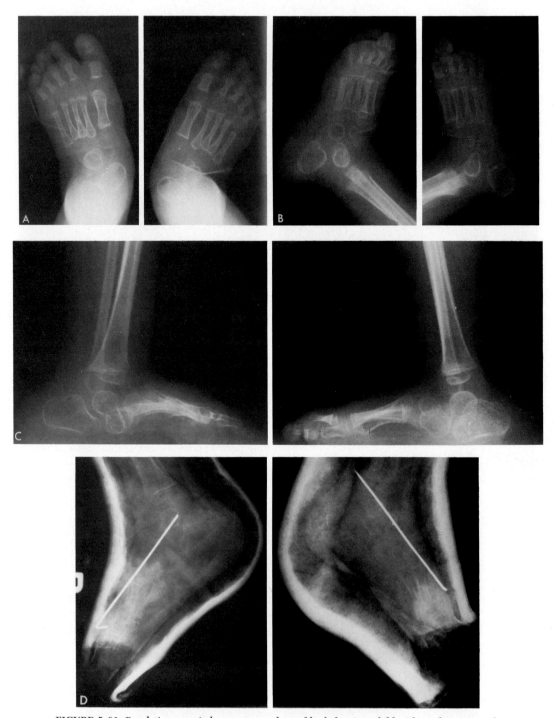

FIGURE 5–91. *Paralytic congenital convex pes valgus of both feet in a child with myelomeningocele.*

A and **B.** Radiograms of both feet at age of ten months. **C.** Lateral radiograms of the feet at two and one half years of age. Note the plantar-flexed talus with dislocation of the talonavicular joint. The os calcis is everted and somewhat equinus. The forefoot is abducted and slightly dorsiflexed. **D.** Postoperative lateral radiograms of both feet in cast. Open reduction of the talonavicular joint was performed. The Kirschner wire was introduced retrograde to maintain the reduction.

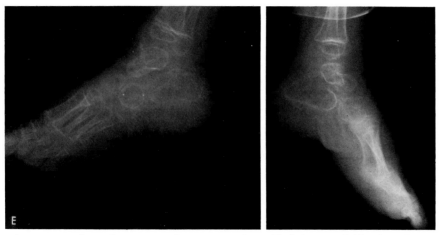

FIGURE 5–91 Continued. Paralytic congenital convex pes valgus of both feet in a child with myelomeningocele.

E. Six months after surgery. The radiograms of both feet show maintenance of reduction. The foot has normal alignment.

the first metatarsal. The dorsal capsule of the talonavicular joint and the tibionavicular ligament are sectioned, and the talonavicular joint is reduced. The tibialis posterior tendon is identified and isolated. The tibialis anterior tendon is detached from its insertion to the base of the first metatarsal. Next, the peroneus brevis tendon is passed across the back of the ankle joint deep to the neurovascular bundle, threaded down the tendon sheath of the tibialis posterior, and attached to the navicular bone. In case the peroneus brevis tendon is short and does not reach the navicular, it is sutured to

the tibialis posterior proximal to the level of the tendon sheath. The talonavicular joint is reduced and transfixed with a Kirschner wire, and the anterior tibial tendon is transferred to the neck of the talus (Fig. 5–92). The tourniquet is released, and after complete hemostasis, the wounds are closed and a below-knee cast is applied. The cast and Kirschner wire are removed in six weeks, at which time the limb is mobilized and walking with appropriate orthotic support is permitted.[160] Sharrard recommends simple division of the tendons in the flail limb with paralytic convex pes valgus.[527]

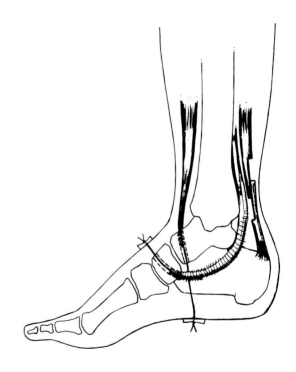

FIGURE 5–92. Composite diagram showing tendons transferred in operative correction of paralytic congenital convex pes valgus in myelomeningocele.

The tendo calcaneus is lengthened by Z-plasty. The anterior tibial tendon is transferred to the neck of the talus, and the peroneus brevis is detached from the base of the fifth metatarsal, passed behind the ankle joint deep to the neurovascular bundle, threaded down the sheath of the tibialis posterior tendon, and attached to the navicular. (From Duckworth, T., and Smith, T. W. D.: The treatment of paralytic convex pes valgus. J. Bone Joint Surg., 56-B:305, 1974. Reprinted by permission.)

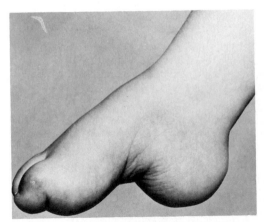

FIGURE 5–93. *Clawing of the hallux and pes cavus in myelomeningocele.*

This author advocates preservation of muscle function; i.e., do not section the tendons of the long toe extensors and peroneus tertius (if necessary, lengthen them). The peroneus brevis is transferred posteromedially to the navicular if the tibialis posterior is paralyzed; if the posterior tibial tendon is functioning, the posterior tibial tendon and plantar calcaneonavicular ligament are advanced distally to increase the support on the plantar aspect of the head of the talus. It is vital to plicate and tauten the capsule of the talonavicular joint on its medial and plantar aspects.

PES CAVUS AND CLAW TOES

With intact innervation down to the second sacral segment, there will be paralysis of the intrinsic muscles of the foot, but motor strength of the remaining muscles of the lower limbs will be normal. The dynamic muscle imbalance between the long toe extensors and flexors and the intrinsic muscles of the foot will gradually cause pes cavus and clawing of the toes (Figs. 5–93 and 5–94). Most of these children have quite adequate motor function in their lower limbs and are very active on their feet. Meticulous care should be given to the toe and forefoot deformities, however, to prevent the development of pressure sores on the toes or on the plantar surface of the metatarsal heads. The type of treatment varies with the severity of the deformity. In mild to moderate cases, treatment is by passive stretching exercises and a metatarsal pad. More severe deformity may require plantar fasciotomy and transfer of the long toe extensors to the metatarsal heads. In the older child, fusion of the proximal interphalangeal joint is indicated to correct hammertoe deformity.

For clawing of the great toe in the young child, Sharrard and Smith recommend tenodesis of the flexor hallucis longus. The hallux should be flexible; rigid deformity is a contraindication to the procedure.[532] The operation is performed under general anesthesia and tourniquet hemostasis. If cavus deformity is present, it is corrected by plantar release. A longitudinal incision is made over the medial aspect of the great toe and the distal third of the first metatarsal. The subcutaneous tissue is divided; the neurovascular bundle is identified and retracted dorsally. The flexor hallucis lon-

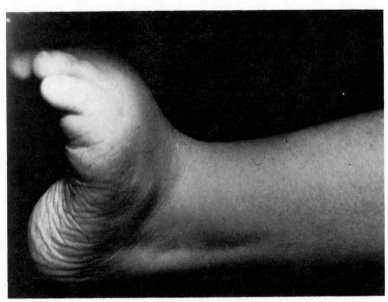

FIGURE 5–94. *Clawing of the hallux and the lesser toes in spina bifida.*

gus tendon is dissected free. If there is any contracture of the dorsal capsule of the metatarsophalangeal joint, it is released. In the middle half of the plantar surface of the proximal phalanx of the great toe, the periosteum and cortex are excised. Two 0 or 00 Tycron sutures are passed through the tendon of the flexor hallucis longus, and the tendon is secured to cancellous bone. The tension on the proximal part of the tendon maintains the metatarsophalangeal joint of the hallux in neutral extension. There should be no tension on the distal part of the tendon. A Kirschner wire is passed through both phalanges of the great toe at the first metatarsal. After closure of the wound, a below-knee walking cast is applied. The cast and pull-out wire are removed in six weeks. Sharrard has performed this operation in 17 feet and achieved good results in 15.[532] This author has had no experience with this operation. The treatment of pes cavus and pes calcaneovarus is discussed in Chapter 7; the same principles apply for treatment of pes cavus in myelomeningocele.

FLAIL ANKLE

This is best managed by ankle-foot orthosis. When the foot is plantigrade and free of deformity it may be stabilized by appropriate fusion, enabling the patient to discard orthotic support and use only crutches for walking. Be cautious! It is best to use AFO's until growth is completed. In the past, if the hip flexors and quadriceps femoris muscles were satisfactory, this author has performed a Chuinard type of ankle fusion when the child was eight or ten years of age. Delayed healing and development of Charcot-like changes were a problem, however, and therefore, at present, he does not recommend ankle fusion in myelomeningocele. It should never be combined with either a Green-Grice extra-articular arthrodesis or a triple arthrodesis (i.e., pantalar fusion) because of consequent trophic skin problems under the metatarsal heads. This is contrary to the report of Ruderman and associates.[500]

Torsional Deformities of the Tibia-Fibula

Lateral Tibiofibular Torsion. This is a common rotational deformity of the leg. Often it is associated with valgus deformity of the ankle. Contracture of the iliotibial band may be an etiologic factor—in such an instance there will be flexion-abduction–lateral rotation deformity at the hip. The gait pattern is lateral foot

progression angle—toeing-out. With lateral rotation of the tibia the medial malleolus is abnormally anterior in its position, causing problems with proper fitting of orthoses and pressure sores. Associated ankle valgus, high-riding fibular malleolus, and relative overgrowth of the medial malleolus aggravate the condition. Treatment consists of supramalleolar medial rotation osteotomy of the tibia and fibula; any associated valgus deformity of the ankle is corrected at the same time. Internal fixation is with AO plate and screws, or two staples, or crisscross threaded Steinmann pins. It is best to perform compression of osteotomized fragments, as delayed healing may be a problem. The distal level of the osteotomy minimizes the risk of compartment syndrome, which is a probable complication of proximal tibial osteotomy. With healing of the osteotomy, hypertrophic callus formation and bulkiness of the tibia may occur, possibly requiring adjustments of the orthosis.

Medial Torsion of the Tibia. This will cause medial foot progression—toeing-in gait. This is frequently seen in neurosegmental lesions of the fourth or fifth lumbar level with imbalance of muscle forces between medial hamstrings (which are strong) and biceps femoris (which is paralyzed). Initially, toeing-in is due to muscle imbalance; with time, however, structurally abnormal medial tibiofibular torsion develops. In some patients, excessive medial tibiofibular torsion can occur without muscle imbalance between the medial and lateral hamstrings.

Treatment. Lateral transfer of semitendinosus is performed in the young child (between two and four years of age), when the degree of medial tibiofibular torsion does not exceed 10 degrees. The operative procedure is Dias' modification of Golski and Menelaus.[134, 206] With the patient in prone position, an oblique longitudinal medial incision is made over the pes anserinus in line with the semitendinosus tendon. This author prefers to make a separate longitudinal incision over the posteromedial aspect of the distal thigh. The semitendinosus tendon is carefully identified, sectioned at its insertion, and freed proximally. It is delivered into the proximal wound. A third incision is then made posterolaterally over the biceps tendon, extending distally to the head of the fibula. Then the semitendinosus tendon is passed subcutaneously into the lateral wound. The common peroneal nerve is identified and protected from injury. The semitendinosus tendon is passed under the common peroneal nerve and woven through the biceps femoris tendon and sutured to the fibular head into the periosteum and biceps tendon with the leg held in maximal lateral rotation. The wounds are closed, and an above-knee cast is applied with the knee in 30 degrees of flexion for four to six weeks. Then the cast is removed, and the patient is allowed to walk with an ankle-foot orthosis.

When muscle imbalance between medial hamstrings and biceps femoris is associated with excessive structural medial tibiofibular torsion of greater than 10 degrees, lateral transfer of semitendinosus is combined with lateral rotation osteotomy of the tibia and fibula. Internal fixation is achieved with AO plate and screws.

Excessive medial tibiofibular torsion can occur without muscle imbalance; these cases are treated with simple lateral rotation osteotomy of the tibia and fibula. It should be emphasized that surgical procedures to correct rotational deformities of the lower limb in myelomeningocele should be performed only in patients who are community ambulators or have the potential to achieve such level of ambulatory function.

Knee

Deformities of the knee in myelomeningocele vary according to the level of paralysis. They are most common at lower thoracic and high lumbar neurosegmental levels; next in frequency are midlumbar and lower lumbar level lesions, with the least common being sacral level paralysis. The deformities may be one of four types: flexion, extension, valgus, or varus. Knee flexion deformity is the most common.

The following factors may cause knee deformity: (1) static forces of malposture, (2) fibrosis of muscles, (3) dynamic muscle imbalance, and (4) malunion of fractures. Functionally, knee deformities may be very disabling.

FLEXION DEFORMITY

In the neonate and the young infant, flexion contractures of the knee are normal, owing to intrauterine posture; they spontaneously correct by the age of three to four months of life.

Etiology. Fixed flexion deformity of the knee should be distinguished from functional secondary flexed posture of the knee assumed for compensation of calcaneus deformity of the ankle, caused by paralysis of the triceps surae muscle. In myelomeningocele children, the gluteus maximus is also paralyzed, further weakening antigravity muscle forces. The knee is flexed to provide plantigrade feet and ankles. In functional secondary knee flexion deformity,

there is no contracture of the hamstrings and no contracture of the posterior capsule of the knee joint.

Fixed flexion deformity of the knee is commonly found in high lumbar-thoracic neurosegmental level lesions. At this high level of paralysis the infant lies supine with the hips in abduction, flexion, and lateral rotation and the knees in flexion. Initially, contracture of the iliotibial band develops because of the malposture while recumbent and sitting. Later on, with persistence of malposture and skeletal growth, the fibrotic paralyzed hamstrings permanently shorten, and contracture of the posterior capsule and cruciate ligaments develops. It behooves the orthopedic surgeon to prevent these static soft-tissue contractural deformities by passive exercises, proper positioning, and appropriate splinting of the flexed lower limbs of the myelomeningocele infant.

Reflex spastic activity in the hamstring muscles is another factor in the pathogenesis of knee flexion deformity; spasticity of the hamstrings may be difficult to demonstrate in the infant but should be suspected and ruled out in every case of knee flexion deformity. Other causes include malunited distal metaphyseal-physeal injuries of the femur or upper tibia and prolonged immobilization of the knees in flexion in plaster of Paris casts or splints.

Clinical and Biomechanical Implications. A fixed knee flexion deformity of 15 degrees in a person with normal gluteus maximus and triceps surae muscle strength can be compensated for by postural adaptations of leaning forward and locking the hip joint, thereby diminishing the forces required by the quadriceps to stabilize the knee. In myelomeningocele with neurosegmental L4–L5 and higher level lesions, the gluteus maximus and triceps surae muscles are paralyzed and weak; therefore, such compensatory adaptation is not feasible. Another problem with myelomeningocele patients is the lack of proprioception, which impairs the ability of the patient to substitute stronger muscle groups for weak muscles. The energy demands necessary for walking in the child with a 20 degree fixed flexion deformity and L4–L5 neurosegmental level lesion are markedly increased. Perry et al. analyzed knee gait forces during flexed knee stance and found that the quadriceps force required to stabilize the knee is 75 per cent of the load of the femoral head at 15 degrees of knee flexion; 210 per cent at 30 degrees; and 410 per cent at 60 degrees.[462] Knee flexion deformity weakens the motor strength of the quadriceps. Whether a patient with myelomeningocele will be a community walker is often determined by the motor strength of the quadriceps. A myelomeningocele patient with a strong quadriceps will most probably walk. The importance of preventing and correcting knee flexion deformity is obvious.

Treatment. Progressive knee flexion deformity can be prevented by early splinting of the knees in extension, proper posturing, encouraging standing with appropriate orthotic support, and an adequate exercise regimen performed by the parents under the supervision of a physical therapist.

Fixed knee flexion contracture of 20 degrees or more requires surgical correction. The importance of early surgical release cannot be overemphasized. Stretching-wedging casts should not be applied because of the hazard of fractures and problems with pressure sores under the cast. Soft-tissue procedures should always be employed first. Posterior release of the knee should be thorough; *the objective is to correct the deformity fully and to hyperextend the knee.* One should not be satisfied with partial correction of flexion deformity. Both hip and knee flexion deformity, if present, should be corrected during the same period of anesthesia.

The operative technique to correct fixed knee flexion deformity by posterior soft-tissue release is as follows: The patient is placed in prone position (if hip flexion deformity requires correction, perform the hip surgery first with the patient supine, and then turn the patient prone and prepare and redrape for the posterior knee release). In order to minimize blood loss the knee surgery is performed under tourniquet ischemia. The surgical approach is preferably made through two 8 to 10 cm. long incisions, one posterolaterally and the other posteromedially. Other surgeons may prefer a transverse or a vertical longitudinal incision. Avoid injury to neurovascular structures. Identify and carefully isolate all major vessels and nerves! Through the lateral incision the common peroneal nerve is identified and gently retracted to prevent inadvertent injury. A portion of the tendon of biceps femoris and the iliotibial band are resected. Next, through the medial incision, the tendons of semitendinosus, semimembranosus, and gracilis are identified and isolated, and a 2 to 3 cm. portion of the tendons is resected. Function of sartorius should be preserved, if possible. Next, the popliteal vessels are retracted, and the musculotendinous origins of both heads of gastrocnemius are elevated extraperiosteally from the femoral condyles. The posterior capsule of the knee joint is exposed, and a capsulectomy (not capsulotomy) is performed through the posterior aspect of the knee joint. Caution! Do not injure the growth plate of the distal femur or proximal tibia. The knee joint is manipulated into extension; if it cannot be fully extended, the posterior part of the medial and lateral collateral ligaments and the posterior cruciate are divided. This author advises taking lateral radiograms of the knee in full extension in order to ensure and document that complete correction of the flexion deformity is achieved. The tourniquet is released, and after complete hemostasis, the wound is closed with Hemovac suction drainage. In the immediate postoperative period a compression dressing with a plaster posterior splint is applied with the knee in 10 to 30 degrees of flexion to prevent vascular compromise resulting from the postoperative development of hematoma and swelling in the popliteal region. Three to four days after surgery, an above-knee cast is applied, and the knee is maintained in complete extension for a period of two to three weeks. An above-knee posterior night orthosis is then made with the knee in full extension. The night splint is worn for several years.

Supracondylar Distal Femoral Extension Osteotomy. This is performed in the adolescent patient who is near skeletal maturity. Refrain from extension osteotomy in the child under ten years of age because of the great chance of recurrence of the flexion deformity! Soft-tissue release should be performed first, and then extension osteotomy, in order to minimize the degree of vertical tilting of the distal femoral articular plane.

The distal femoral metaphysis and shaft are exposed through a lateral approach. Caution! Do not injure the distal femoral physis! Use radiographic control to determine the proper level of osteotomy. An anteriorly based wedge of bone is removed with a posterior buttress on the lower end of the proximal segment (Fig. 5–95). A valgus or varus deformity can be simultaneously corrected by appropriate modification to the wedge. Internal fixation may be with a laterally placed AO blade plate or Cobra plate, or with an anteriorly placed prebent AO plate. Other less secure means of internal fixation are crisscross large threaded Steinmann pins or staples. More solid means of internal fixation are preferable because they allow early mobilization of the knee joint and weight bearing; disuse osteoporosis, stress fractures, and knee joint stiffness are thereby circumvented.

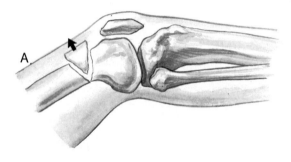

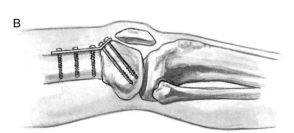

FIGURE 5–95. Extension osteotomy of the distal femur in the supracondylar region.

A. Note that the wedge of bone is based anteriorly. **B.** Internal fixation by plate and screws.

In the literature, results of surgical correction of knee flexion deformity are presented by Dupré and Walker,[162] Birch,[44] Menelaus,[388] Abraham et al.,[1] and Dias.[132] A critical analysis of the reported experiences of these authors highlights the following salient points: (1) Prevent knee flexion deformity by part-time splinting, posturing, and exercise regimen. (2) If flexion deformity develops and cannot be controlled by the foregoing conservative measures, operate early. (3) Correct hip flexion deformity first, knee flexion deformity second! Combine the two procedures under the same anesthesia. (4) Soft-tissue release should be thorough, and complete correction of the flexion deformity should be achieved on the operating table. Do not be satisfied with partial correction! Document the degree of correction by true lateral radiograms of the knee made on the operating table. (5) There is no place for anterior transfer of the hamstrings to the patella; the results are disappointing. (6) Perform supracondylar extension osteotomy of the femur in the adolescent patient who is skeletally mature, and not in the growing child. Internal fixation should be secure in order to provide early knee mobilization and weight bearing.

EXTENSION OR HYPEREXTENSION CONTRACTURE OF THE KNEE

This deformity may be caused by (1) dynamic imbalance of muscles resulting from normal strength of the quadriceps femoris muscle and paralyzed hamstrings (seen in lesions in which the level of involvement is distal to the third or fourth lumbar segment); (2) or it may be due to fibrosis of the quadriceps muscle (which usually occurs in higher levels of involvement with a flail lower limb); (3) or it may result from structural osseous deformity of the distal femur (such as that seen following malunited fractures).

Extension contracture of the knee is usually bilateral. The degree of deformity varies—the knee may be fixed in hyperextension with anterior subluxation of the knee joint, or it may be rigid in full extension with no subluxation. The degree of limitation of knee flexion range varies. Functionally the hyperextended knee and the knee fixed in full extension are very disabling. Ambulatory ability is markedly impaired. In the series of Lindseth, of 16 patients with extension contracture of the knee, only 3 were ambulatory; in 13 of these 16 patients, the neurosegmental level of the lesion was L-3.[322] Extension contracture of the knee makes sitting in a wheelchair and proper fitting of an orthotic device difficult. A stiff knee in extension will cause repeated fracture of the femur because of its levering action on the osteoporotic bone. The anesthetic aproprioceptive knee joint may develop arthrofibrotic and early degenerative changes under the abnormal stresses of body weight.

Extension deformity of the knee is commonly associated with other congenital deformities, particularly congenital dislocation of the hip (present in 95 per cent of the patients), talipes equinovarus (in 50 per cent), and lateral rotation deformity of the hip.

The pathologic anatomy varies according to the severity of the deformity. Often the quadriceps mechanism, particularly the rectus femoris, vastus intermedius, and lateralis, is fibrotic, and the entire extensor mechanism, including the patella, is laterally displaced. The anterior capsule is taut. In the rigid hyperextended knee the hamstring tendons are anterior to the axis of the knee joint motion, aggravating the hyperextension deformity. Ordinarily there are no abnormalities of the cruciate ligaments or the menisci.

Treatment. This depends upon the type of extension contracture of the knee. When the quadriceps femoris muscle is normal in motor strength and the extension contracture is due to dynamic imbalance between the knee flexors and extensors, a period of conservative management is employed. Genu recurvatum can usually be controlled by orthotic support, night splints, and gentle passive stretching exercises. In the older child posteromedial transfer of the rectus femoris to semitendinosus (when there is associated lateral rotation deformity of the hip) or posterolateral transfer to biceps femoris tendon at its insertion (when there is associated medial rotation deformity of the hip) with fractional lengthening of the vastus lateralis and intermedius may be employed. It should be emphasized that a split muscle is transferred across a weight-bearing joint; functionally it is not in phase. In the experience of this author, the results of posterior transfer of rectus femoris in myelomeningocele have not been satisfactory.

In quadriceps femoris fibrosis, conservative methods such as wedging casts, passive stretching exercises, and traction are not ordinarily tolerated by the myelomeningocele child. Often, conservative management proves to be unsuccessful, and when the child is about one year of age, open surgical lengthening of the fibrosed quadriceps femoris is performed. An inverted V incision in the quadriceps femoris in the suprapatellar region (Curtis-Fisher modification of the Bennett procedure) is recommended.[123] The taut anterior capsule of the knee joint is released; it is sectioned as far posteriorly as the anterior margin of the collateral ligaments. It is important that, on the operating table, 90 degrees of passive knee flexion be obtained. Then, with the knee bent 45 degrees, the quadriceps is resutured. Sometimes the patella may have to be excised in order to obtain relative length of the quadriceps mechanism and also to enable closure of the skin. An above-knee cast is applied with the knee flexed 45 degrees. The period of immobilization is about two to three weeks. Then the knee is supported part time during the day and all night in an above-knee splint with the knee in 45 degrees of flexion. Active and passive exercises to mobilize the knee are begun early in order to avoid joint stiffness, disuse atrophy of bone, and stress fractures.

GENU VALGUM

This is usually caused by contracture of the iliotibial band in lower thoracic and high lumbar neurosegmental level lesions. It may also be due to a malunited fracture of the distal femur or the proximal tibia. Occasionally, isolated spastic reflex activity of the biceps femoris may be a factor.[528] When the deformity is severe enough to interfere with fitting of an orthosis or to interfere with ambulation, sectioning of the iliotibial band is performed. A segment of the "spastic" biceps femoris is excised. If a malunited fracture is the cause of valgus deformity at the knee, it is corrected by osteotomy at the appropriate level.

VARUS DEFORMITY

Bony deformity due to malunited fractures may also cause genu varum. If it is severe enough, corrective osteotomy is indicated.

The Hip

Deformities of the hip in myelomeningocele may be subdivided into two general categories: first, contractural, and second, subluxation or dislocation. The *contractural deformities* are due to static forces of malposture, fibrosis, or muscle imbalance; they are flexion, lateral rotation-abduction, and adduction contractures of the hip. Involvement may be asymmetrical, depending upon the pattern of paralysis.

HIP SUBLUXATION-DISLOCATION

Hip dislocation in myelomeningocele may be categorized as *prenatal* (developing in utero), *perinatal* (occurring at birth), or *postnatal* (occurring later on in infancy and childhood.) It may be congenital or acquired secondary to muscle imbalance between hip flexors-extensors and hip adductors-abductors. Hip subluxation may be secondary to pelvic obliquity with the hip on the high side gradually displacing out of the acetabulum.

Sharrard has classified the patterns of muscle paralysis into six groups, correlating them with resultant acquired paralytic deformity of the hip (Fig. 5–96). *Group I* is characterized by total

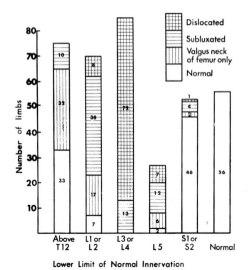

FIGURE 5–96. Hip disorders in 183 children with lumbar
myelomeningocele.

Radiographic status of the hip joint at 12 months of age,
related to the neurosegmental level of the lesion. (From
Sharrard, W. J. W.: Posterior iliopsoas transplantation in
the treatment of paralytic dislocation of the hip. J. Bone
Joint Surg., 46-B:427, 1964. Reprinted by permission.)

flail lower limbs due to complete paralysis below the level of the twelfth thoracic root. Mal-
positional or static deformities of the limbs
result from faulty posture in utero or in supine
or prone position in postnatal life (Fig. 5–97).
When these children begin to stand with support, coxa valga may develop with subsequent
subluxation of the hips. Complete dislocation
usually does not occur.

In *Group II* there is flaccid paralysis of the
muscles that are innervated distal to the first
and second lumbar nerve roots. Thus, the hip
flexors are good or fair in motor strength, and
the hip adductors are fair or poor; all other
muscles are paralyzed. Flexion deformity of the
hip is found in all patients at birth. During the
first year of life all patients develop progressively increasing flexion-adduction hip deformity with valgus deformity of the femoral neck.
Moderate or marked subluxation of the hips
will occur in four fifths of these children. If left
untreated, some of the subluxated hips will
become dislocated (about 10 per cent).

In *Group III* the upper three or four lumbar
nerve roots are intact, with paralysis distal to
this level. Motor strength is as follows: normal
hip flexors, good hip adductors, good quadriceps femoris, and fair sartorius and tensor fasciae latae; the hip abductors and extensors are
completely paralyzed; the anterior tibial muscle
is fair or good. At birth, marked flexion-adduc-

tion deformity of the hips is commonly present.
Extension contracture of the knee and pes varus
are common associated deformities. During the
first two years of life, frank dislocation of the
hip will develop in 80 per cent of the patients;
in the remaining 20 per cent, the hips are
subluxated, and if left untreated, they will become dislocated. Coxa valga is uniformly found
in all patients. The acetabulum appears normal
or will develop normally during the first year
of postnatal life.

In *Group IV*, all the lumbar nerve roots are
normal and the sacral segments are paralyzed.
In these patients the hip abductors are poor or
fair and the hamstrings are fair in motor
strength, while the hip extensors are paralyzed.
Progressively increasing flexion deformity of the
hip occurs in all, and coxa valga develops in 30
per cent of the patients. In *Group V*, characterized by paralysis distal to the first sacral root,
the gluteus maximus is the only hip muscle that
is weak. Mild flexion is the only acquired deformity in these patients. Paralytic subluxation
or dislocation does not take place. *Group VI* is
characterized by normal musculature in the
lower limbs with no acquired hip deformity.[515]

Dislocation of the hip in myelomeningocele,
when present at birth, is either prenatal or
perinatal; perinatal dislocation is easily reduced.
Prenatal dislocation cannot be reduced by the
Ortolani maneuver.

Diagnosis of hip dislocation in the newborn
with myelomeningocele is not difficult. Often,
however, the hips are examined inadequately
because the infant is in prone position to protect
the delicate posterior sac. It is difficult to perform the Barlow and Ortolani tests with the
infant lying face down on the Bradford frame.
He should be turned supine and gently supported by the nurse for thorough examination
of the hips. Ultrasound studies and radiographs
of the hips should always be obtained.

Ordinarily, a congenitally dislocated hip with
associated complete or partial paralysis is much
easier to reduce than if the limb had normal
musculature.

Treatment varies according to the type of
dislocation. In general, *prenatal rigid dislocation* of the hip in myelomeningocele should not
be treated. An attempt at closed reduction may
be made. If the hips are irreducible by closed
methods, open reduction should not be carried
out, as the result will often be a stiff, "frozen"
hip, which will prove to be a greater handicap
that will make sitting almost impossible. A
mobile dislocated hip with level pelvis is preferred over a reduced stiff hip with pelvic

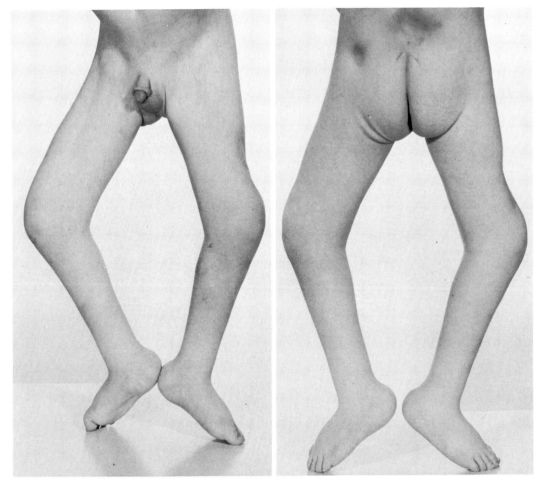

FIGURE 5–97. *A two-year-old child with myelomeningocele with paralysis below the twelfth thoracic level of innervation.*

Note the flexion, abduction, and lateral rotation contracture of both hips, flexion contracture of the knees, and bilateral pes equinus. These are static deformities produced by faulty posture in utero and in postnatal life. They can be prevented by positioning of the flail limbs of the paralyzed infant, by use of night splints, and by gentle passive stretching exercises.

Illustration continued on following page

obliquity. In low neurologic level lesions one may attempt open reduction of the hip with femoral shortening—particularly in unilateral dislocations. In the experience of this author the result may be satisfactory—a mobile, reduced, stable hip.

In *perinatal dislocation with partial or total paralysis* of the lower limbs, closed reduction in early infancy is a simple procedure. The femoral head can easily be lowered to the level of the acetabulum. Muscle forces across the hip joint are not severe enough to cause aseptic necrosis. Reduction with immobilization of the hips is often postponed until closure of the posterior defect is complete. Shunting procedures to control increasing hydrocephalus may be another cause of delay. During this period, however, the hips are maintained in abduction on the Bradford frame. *The Pavlik harness*

should not be used in treatment of paralytic hip dislocation in myelomeningocele. Following closed reduction, the exact position of immobilization of the hips in a plaster of Paris cast is an important consideration. Flexion-abduction–lateral rotation (the so-called frog-leg position) should be avoided; it will cause contracture of the iliotibial band. The hips should be placed in neutral or slight medial rotation and 40 to 50 degrees of abduction and only slight flexion of 20 to 30 degrees. The period of rigid immobilization in the cast is usually from six to eight weeks; then a bivalved hip spica cast or plastic splint (same position as above) is utilized to maintain the reduction; this is worn during sleeping hours.

The *unstable hip* that is dislocatable or subluxated is only splinted in the position as described above. The course of treatment follow-

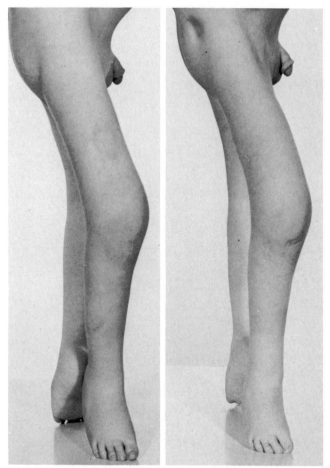

FIGURE 5–97 Continued. A two-year-old child with myelomeningocele with paralysis below the twelfth thoracic level of innervation.

ing this stage depends on the presence or absence of muscle imbalance. In involvement at *the higher levels,* i.e., the first lumbar level and above, with almost total paralysis of the lower limbs, the hips, once reduced, will usually remain so. Static deformities are usually prevented by proper splinting and by avoidance of faulty positions while lying or sitting. Coxa valga may develop as the child gets older, causing instability of the hip. In such an instance, varization osteotomy of the proximal femur is performed in selected cases.

With lower neurosegmental levels of involvement, i.e., the third lumbar level and below, stability of the hip joint depends entirely on the distribution of paralysis. The hip flexors and adductors are innervated by the upper three lumbar neurosegments, whereas the hip abductor-extensor muscle groups are innervated by the fourth and fifth lumbar and first sacral neurosegments. In the presence of muscle imbalance, e.g., strong hip flexor-adductors and

paralyzed hip extensor-abductors, the hips are at high risk for subsequent paralytic subluxation or dislocation.

Following reduction of the dislocated hip with muscle imbalance, the hip is maintained in a stable position in a bivalved hip spica cast or a plastic splint at night with the hips in 30 degrees of abduction, neutral extension, and medial rotation. The hips should not be immobilized in flexion because of the danger of development of troublesome flexion deformity. Splinting of the hips in abduction will delay and may even prevent eventual subluxation of the hip.[349, 350]

When progressive instability of the hip develops in the high-risk L3–L4 neurosegmental group, one should consider posterolateral transfer of the iliopsoas. With early surgical intervention and correlation of muscle imbalance, one may prevent eventual subluxation and dislocation of the hip and obviate the necessity of open reduction and capsular plication of the hip, thereby preventing the possible complication of postoperative stiffness of the hip joint.

Paralytic Subluxation or Dislocatable (Unstable) Hip in the Older Child. This is acquired as a result of muscle imbalance. Treatment of the hips should be carried out in patients who have potential for household or community ambulation, i.e., L3 or L4 neurosegmental level or better, and in children who are healthy. The presence of strong quadriceps femoris function is a reliable prognostic sign for walking. In general, a child who will walk will have done so by five to six years of age. If a patient is eight to ten years of age and still not walking, he should not be considered for major reconstructive surgery of the hip. These patients will function in life from a wheelchair; it is vital to keep their hips mobile.

The objectives of treatment of paralytic subluxation of the hip in the older child are (1) to correct pelvic obliquity; (2) to provide stability to the hip by correcting coxa valga and severe femoral antetorsion and by correcting acetabular dysplasia; and (3) to achieve muscle balance about the hip. These surgical procedures should be combined, preferably performed under one anesthesia or within one hospital admission. The period of total cast immobilization should be kept to the minimum. Multiple fractures following prolonged immobilization should be prevented.

Coxa valga and excessive femoral antetorsion are corrected by proximal femoral osteotomy performed at the intertrochanteric level with internal fixation by a pediatric hip screw plate (see section on congenital dislocation of the hip, Chapter 2, Plate 17, p. 402). If only femoral osteotomy is required, both hips can be operated on simultaneously. If femoral osteotomy is combined with innominate osteotomy or posterolateral iliopsoas or other muscle transfer, one side should be done, followed by the contralateral hip 10 to 14 days later.

Acetabular insufficiency in paralytic dislocation of the hip is posterior and superolateral; it is not anterior. Therefore, there is no place for the Salter or Pemberton pericapsular innominate osteotomy—these procedures are designed to provide anterolateral coverage, not posterolateral. The innominate osteotomy recommended by this author is the modified Albee shelf or (in the older child) Chiari's medial displacement osteotomy, which is extended inferiorly in its posterior part to provide posterior coverage.[80] In myelomeningocele, Chiari's osteotomy provides stability and increases acetabular capacity with minimal risk of postoperative stiffness of the hip (see Chiari's innominate osteotomy in the section on congenital hip dislocation).

Paralytic Dislocation of the Hip in the Older Child. In the past, the dislocated hips in the older age group were treated aggressively by open reduction, capsulorraphy, iliopsoas transfer, or proximal femoral and innominate osteotomy. The serious problem following surgery was stiffness of the hip because of lack of adequate motor power required to mobilize the hips. The stiff hips impeded sitting; the patients were even unable to stand effectively. It was noted that patients who were able to walk preoperatively did not walk well after surgery.[179] The long-term follow-up study of Barden et al. showed that the presence of hip dislocation did not prevent reasonable ambulatory function.[33] Feiwell et al. found that a level pelvis and good range of hip motion are requisites for maximal function; the presence of the femoral head in the acetabulum did not improve range of hip motion, did not increase ability to walk, did not decrease the extent of orthosis required for ambulation, and did not diminish pain or discomfort.[180]

In the analytic study of Asher and Olson it was demonstrated that in L3–L4 neurosegmental level lesions the most important factor affecting ambulation is hip deformity and not dislocation.[20] Therefore, in the older myelomeningocele child with frank dislocation of the hips, it is best to leave the hips dislocated; treatment efforts are directed toward the correction of pelvic obliquity and trunk balance. Surgery is performed to correct contractural hip deformities that are causing pelvic obliquity and interfering with bracing and ambulation.

This author recommends open reduction of the dislocated hip in an older patient with myelomeningocele when the patient is in excellent health with a good intellect, is a community ambulator (with neurosegmental level of L4–L5 or better), and has only unilateral dislocation. If all of these requisites are present, open reduction of the hip is combined with femoral osteotomy. Reduction should be concentric, and stability of reduction is enhanced by appropriate femoral and/or innominate osteotomy (Chiari). The operation should be performed by an experienced pediatric hip surgeon.

Specific Surgical Procedures on the Hip

Iliopsoas Transfer. Lateral transfer of iliopsoas was first described by Mustard primarily for treatment of paralytic hip instability and correction of gluteus medius lurch in poliomyelitis; 2 of the 50 cases of Mustard were in myelomeningocele hips.[415, 416] Further experience with the Mustard technique of iliopsoas showed that it is ineffective in preventing progressive hip subluxation. The procedure leaves the iliopsoas muscle anterior to the axis of flexion; hip abduction is improved to some degree, but the muscle imbalance between hip flexors and extensors persists.[121] The Mustard technique of anterolateral transfer of iliopsoas should not be performed in myelomeningocele.

Sharrard developed the posterior transfer of iliopsoas; the purpose of the operation was to remove the deforming force of iliopsoas and by the posterior transfer to act as an extensor and abductor of the hip. Hip flexion action was provided by the sartorius, rectus, and pectineus.[515] The popularity of the Sharrard posterior iliopsoas transfer waxed in the 1960s and waned in the 1970s. The results reported in the literature leave the reader confused. At present the primary *indication* for posterolateral transfer of iliopsoas is progressive instability of the hip in a young child with a L3–L4 neurosegmental level lesion. However, prior to transfer of the iliopsoas the following *requisites* should be met.

1. *Stable concentric reduction of the hip*—this is crucial! Anatomic factors causing hip instability should be corrected first. A lax capsule should be tautened by capsulorraphy. Coxa valga and excessive femoral antetorsion should be corrected by derotation varus osteotomy of the proximal femur at the intertrochanteric level. Superoposterolateral deficiency of the acetabulum is corrected by modified Albee shelf or Chiari's innominate osteotomy. In the experience of Carroll and Sharrard, only two hips became unstable after having been stabilized at the time of surgery.[89]

2. Prior to transfer of the iliopsoas the *passive range of hip abduction should be at least 45 to 50 degrees;* if the hip cannot be abducted, an adductor myotomy is performed to obtain adequate range of hip abduction. Should one posteriorly transfer the hip adductors (longus and brevis) instead of performing adductor myotomy? London and Nichols analyzed the results in two groups of patients. In the first group (25 procedures in 11 patients) the origins of the adductor longus, adductor brevis, and gracilis were transferred posteriorly to the ischial tuberosity; also, in the first group, iliopsoas was transferred to the greater trochanter in 15 hips. In the second group (39 procedures in 28 patients) only the iliopsoas was transferred. Comparison of the results showed that in the first group of patients (iliopsoas and hip adductor transfer) there was greater improvement in muscle balance, less severe flexion-

adduction contracture, and greater power in hip abduction-extension. There was a higher incidence of stable hips at follow-up of those in the first group as compared with the second group.[327] Benton et al. studied 31 subluxating or dislocated hips in 17 patients with myelomeningocele; all hips had posterior iliopsoas transfer, 13 hips had additional posterior transfer of hip adductors, and 11 hips had derotation varus osteotomy of the proximal femur. They found that the associated hip adductor transfer weakened the hip adductor strength, increased hip extensor strength, and enhanced action of the transferred iliopsoas. However, only 5 of the 13 hips in the associated adductor transfer group were located.[43] This author does not share the enthusiasm of Benton et al. and London and Nichols. Simple adductor myotomy is recommended by this author—the procedure is much simpler, with less risk of hematoma and postoperative wound infection.

3. Motor strength of the iliopsoas should be at least good and preferably normal. In the experience of this author the posterolaterally transferred iliopsoas rarely, if ever, functions as a hip extensor. As a hip abductor the transferred iliopsoas at its best is fair-minus or poor-plus in motor strength; seldom is it powerful enough to lift the lower limb against gravity. Often it functions as tenodesis.

4. Sartorius, pectineus, and rectus femoris muscles should be strong enough to flex the hip against gravity; otherwise, it is advisable not to weaken active flexion by iliopsoas transfer, as the patient will be unable to climb steps, such as to get on the school bus. When sartorius-pectineus muscles are weak, it is best to transfer the external oblique muscle.

5. The child should have a normal intelligence quotient, absent or controlled hydrocephalus, and good general health.

6. He should be a community ambulator or have the potential to be one.

7. Lastly, the operative procedure is technically demanding, and an important requisite is an experienced pediatric orthopedic hip surgeon.

The operative technique of posterolateral transfer of iliopsoas is described and illustrated in Plate 75. An illustrative case is shown in Figure 5–98. The following technical points and modifications from that of Sharrard are recommended: (1) It is best to detach the iliopsoas tendon from the lesser trochanter through a separate longitudinal adductor incision, immediately posterior to the adductor longus tendon. (2) Preserve lateral femoral cutaneous nerve.

Text continued on page 1836

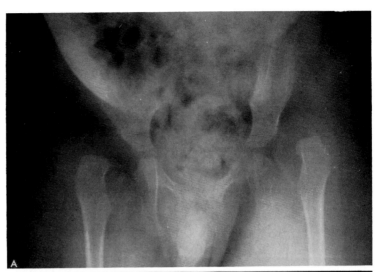

FIGURE 5–98. Bilateral congenital dislocation of the hip in a child with myelomeningocele.

The neurosegmental level of paralysis is distal to the third lumbar. The hip flexors and adductors are normal in motor strength, but the hip abductors and extensors are paralyzed. Bilateral open reduction, capsular plication, innominate osteotomy, and posterior iliopsoas transfer were performed in two stages. **A.** Preoperative radiogram. **B** and **C.** Postoperative radiograms. (The staples are used to fix the iliopsoas tendon to the subtrochanteric region of the femur.)

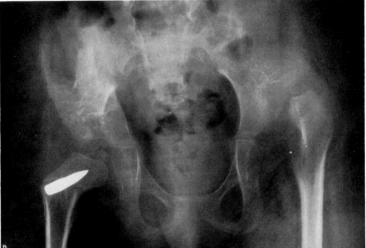

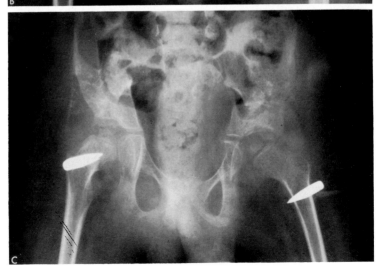

Iliopsoas Muscle Transfer for Paralysis of the Hip Abductors

OPERATIVE TECHNIQUE

The patient lies supine with a small sandbag under the sacrum and a larger sandbag under the ipsilateral scapula. The entire involved lower limb, the hip, the lower abdomen and chest, and the iliac and sacral regions are prepared sterile and draped so that the limb that is to be operated on can be freely manipulated and the incision extended to the posterior third of the iliac crest without contamination.

A. The skin incision extends forward from the junction of the posterior and middle thirds of the iliac crest to the anterior superior iliac spine; it is then carried distally into the thigh along the medial border of the sartorius muscle for a distance of 10 to 12 cm., ending 2 cm. distal to the lesser trochanter.

B. The deep fascia is incised over the iliac crest and the fascia lata is opened in line with the skin incision.

The lateral femoral cutaneous nerve is identified; it usually crosses the sartorius muscle 2.5 cm. distal to the anterior superior iliac spine and lies in close proximity to the lateral border of the sartorius. The nerve is mobilized by sharp dissection and protected by retracting it medially with a moist hernia tape. The wound flaps are undermined and retracted. The anterior medial margin of the tensor fasciae latae muscle is identified and, by blunt dissection, the groove between the sartorius and rectus femoris muscles medially and the tensor fasciae latae muscle laterally is opened. The dissection is carried deep through the loose areolar tissue that separates these structures, and the adipose tissue that covers the front of the capsule of the hip joint is exposed. The ascending branch of the lateral femoral circumflex artery and the accompanying vein cross the midportion of the wound; they are isolated, clamped, cut, and ligated.

The origin of the sartorius muscle from the anterior superior iliac spine is detached and the muscle is reflected distally and medially. The free end is marked with a silk whip suture for later reattachment. The origins of the two heads of the rectus femoris are divided and reflected distally. The femoral nerve and its branches to the sartorius and rectus femoris are identified. A moist hernia tape is passed around the femoral nerve for gentle handling. The femoral vessels and nerve are retracted medially.

C. The cartilaginous apophysis of the ilium is split and the dissection is deepened along the iliac crest down to bone. With a broad periosteal elevator the tensor fasciae latae and the gluteus medius and minimus muscles are stripped subperiosteally from the lateral surface of the ilium and reflected in one continuous mass laterally and distally to the superior margin of the acetabulum. Bleeding is controlled by packing the interval between the reflected muscles and ilium with laparotomy pads.

D. Then with a large periosteal elevator, the iliacus muscle is subperiosteally elevated and reflected medially, exposing the inner wall of the wing of the ilium from the greater sciatic notch to the anterior superior iliac spine.

By careful blunt dissection with a periosteal elevator, the iliacus muscle is freed, elevated, and mobilized from the inner wall of the ilium and the anterior capsule of the hip joint. It is important to stay lateral and deep to the iliacus muscle and work in a proximal to distal direction.

Plate 75. Iliopsoas Muscle Transfer for Paralysis of the Hip Abductors

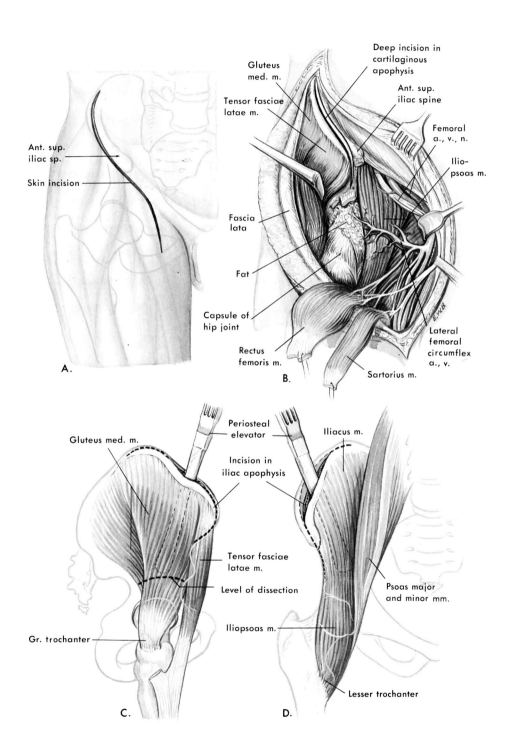

A.

Ant. sup. iliac sp.

Skin incision

B.

Gluteus med. m.

Tensor fasciae latae m.

Deep incision in cartilaginous apophysis

Ant. sup. iliac spine

Femoral a., v., n.

Ilio-psoas m.

Fascia lata

Fat

Capsule of hip joint

Rectus femoris m.

Sartorius m.

Lateral femoral circumflex a., v.

C.

Gluteus med. m.

Periosteal elevator

Incision in iliac apophysis

Tensor fasciae latae m.

Level of dissection

Iliopsoas m.

Gr. trochanter

D.

Iliacus m.

Psoas major and minor mm.

Lesser trochanter

Iliopsoas Muscle Transfer for Paralysis of the Hip Abductors (Continued)

E to G. Next, the hip is flexed, abducted, and laterally rotated, and with the index finger, the lesser trochanter is cleared of soft tissues proximally, posteriorly, and distally. The index finger is then placed on the posteromedial aspect of the lesser trochanter and is used to direct a curved osteotome to the superior and deep aspect of the base of the lesser trochanter.

The lesser trochanter is osteotomized and the distal insertion of the iliacus muscle on the linea aspera of the femur is freed with a periosteal elevator.

H. The iliacus and psoas muscles are reflected proximally by sharp and dull dissection. It is very essential not to injure the nerve to the iliacus, which at times enters the muscle belly quite distally; also, the femoral nerve should not be damaged. The author finds the use of a nerve stimulator of great help. Circumflex vessels are clamped, cut, and ligated as necessary.

I. In the middle third of the wing of the ilium a rectangular hole, usually 1½ to 2 inches, is cut with drill holes and osteotomes. The hole should be large enough to accommodate the transferred muscle. It should be located as far posteriorly as possible to allow a more direct line of muscle action. The limiting factor is the nerve supply to the iliacus, which should not be stretched.

Plate 75. Iliopsoas Muscle Transfer for Paralysis of the Hip Abductors

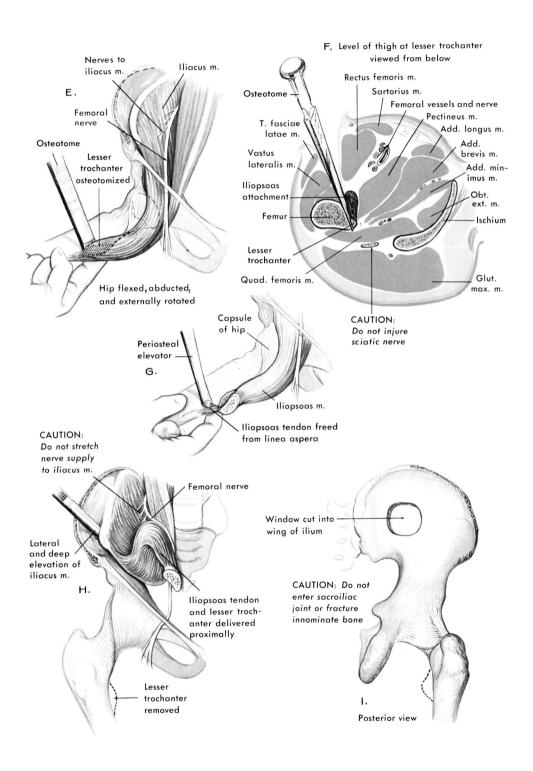

E.

Nerves to iliacus m.

Iliacus m.

Femoral nerve

Osteotome

Lesser trochanter osteotomized

Hip flexed, abducted, and externally rotated

F. Level of thigh at lesser trochanter viewed from below

Osteotome

Rectus femoris m.

Sartorius m.

Femoral vessels and nerve

Pectineus m.

Add. longus m.

Add. brevis m.

Add. minimus m.

Obt. ext. m.

Ischium

Glut. max. m.

T. fasciae latae m.

Vastus lateralis m.

Iliopsoas attachment

Femur

Lesser trochanter

Quad. femoris m.

CAUTION: *Do not injure sciatic nerve*

Capsule of hip

Periosteal elevator

G.

Iliopsoas m.

Iliopsoas tendon freed from linea aspera

CAUTION: *Do not stretch nerve supply to iliacus m.*

Femoral nerve

Lateral and deep elevation of iliacus m.

H.

Iliopsoas tendon and lesser trochanter delivered proximally

Lesser trochanter removed

Window cut into wing of ilium

CAUTION: *Do not enter sacroiliac joint or fracture innominate bone*

I.

Posterior view

1831

Iliopsoas Muscle Transfer for Paralysis of the Hip Abductors (Continued)

J. With the hip in extension and medial rotation, the greater trochanter is exposed by a longitudinal lateral incision. The vastus lateralis muscle is split and the lateral surface of the proximal 4 to 5 cm. of femoral shaft is subperiosteally exposed.

K. It is important not to damage the greater trochanteric apophyseal growth plate.

L. Next, a large Ober tendon passer is inserted through the hole in the wing of the ilium, directed deep to the glutei, and brought out in the greater trochanteric region by splitting the insertion of the fibers of the gluteus medius muscle.

M and **N.** The iliopsoas muscle is then transferred laterally by this route with the Ober tendon passer. The nerve supply to the iliacus is again checked to be sure it is not under great tension. Next, the hip is abducted at least 45 to 60 degrees and internally rotated 10 to 15 degrees. The site of insertion of the iliopsoas tendon on the femoral shaft is determined and is roughened with curved osteotomes. The muscle should be under proper tension.

Plate 75. Iliopsoas Muscle Transfer for Paralysis of the Hip Abductors

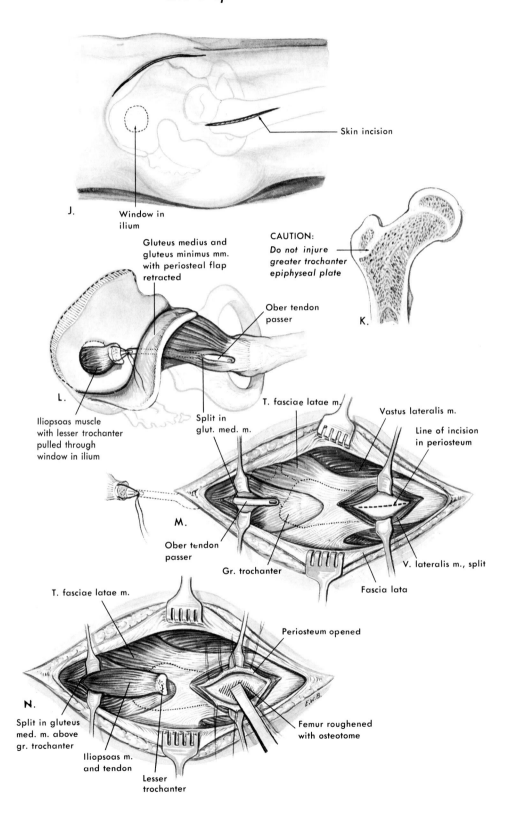

Skin incision

J.

Window in ilium

Gluteus medius and gluteus minimus mm. with periosteal flap retracted

CAUTION:
Do not injure greater trochanter epiphyseal plate

K.

Ober tendon passer

L.

Iliopsoas muscle with lesser trochanter pulled through window in ilium

Split in glut. med. m.

T. fasciae latae m.

Vastus lateralis m.

Line of incision in periosteum

M.

Ober tendon passer

Gr. trochanter

V. lateralis m., split

Fascia lata

T. fasciae latae m.

Periosteum opened

N.

Split in gluteus med. m. above gr. trochanter

Iliopsoas m. and tendon

Lesser trochanter

Femur roughened with osteotome

E.W.B.

Iliopsoas Muscle Transfer for Paralysis of the Hip Abductors (Continued)

O. The lesser trochanter is anchored to the proximal femur by one or two transversely placed small staples. Mustard recommends making a trap door in the femur into which the lesser trochanter is drawn and anchored by heavy wire sutures.

P. The periosteum and vastus lateralis muscle are sutured to the edges and over the iliopsoas tendon.

Q and **R.** The rectus femoris and sartorius muscles are sutured to the inferior and superior iliac spines, respectively. The tensor fasciae latae, the gluteus medius and minimus, and the abdominal muscles are sutured to the iliac crest. The wound is closed in layers in routine manner. A one and one half hip spica cast is applied, with the hip in 60 degrees of abduction, 10 to 15 degrees medial rotation, and slight flexion.

POSTOPERATIVE CARE

Four to six weeks following surgery, the patient is readmitted to the hospital and the cast is removed and a new bivalved hip spica cast made. This should be cut low on the lateral side so that hip abduction exercises can be performed in the posterior half of the cast. Radiograms of the hips are made to determine the stability of the hip joint. Great care should be exercised so that a pathologic fracture of the femur is not caused when the child is lifted out of the cast.

Training of the iliopsoas transfer follows the same general principles as those for training tendon transfers in poliomyelitis. In myelomeningocele, however, there is extensive paralysis of the lower limb, necessitating orthotic support, and the patient is much younger. Thus, as soon as the transferred iliopsoas has fair motor strength and the lower limbs can be adducted to neutral position, weight-bearing is permitted in bilateral above-knee orthoses. The butterfly pelvic band will keep the hips in 5 to 10 degrees of abduction during locomotion. At night, the hips and the transfer are protected in the bivalved hip spica cast or plastic hip-knee-ankle-foot orthosis (HKAFO).

Plate 75. Iliopsoas Muscle Transfer for Paralysis of the Hip Abductors

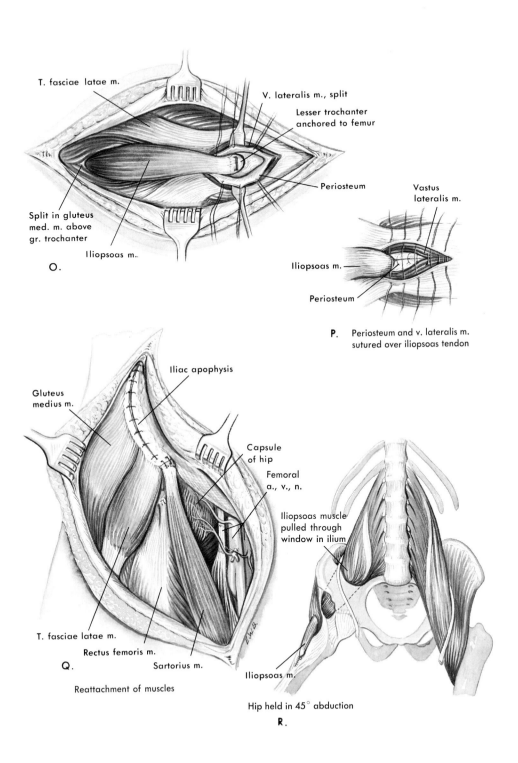

T. fasciae latae m.

V. lateralis m., split

Lesser trochanter anchored to femur

Periosteum

Vastus lateralis m.

Split in gluteus med. m. above gr. trochanter

Iliopsoas m.

O.

Iliopsoas m.

Periosteum

P.   Periosteum and v. lateralis m. sutured over iliopsoas tendon

Iliac apophysis

Gluteus medius m.

Capsule of hip

Femoral a., v., n.

Iliopsoas muscle pulled through window in ilium

T. fasciae latae m.

Rectus femoris m.

Q.

Sartorius m.

Reattachment of muscles

Iliopsoas m.

Hip held in 45° abduction

R.

(3) Dissect sartorius cautiously because its nerve supply should be preserved. (4) Instead of cutting a hole, one may cut a trough in the posterolateral region of the ilium. (5) Do not transfer the iliacus muscle external to the wall of the ilium because of increased danger of denervation of the muscle with consequent fibrosis, abduction contracture, and hip stiffness. (6) In the cast, do not force and immobilize the hips in marked abduction because this will cause avascular necrosis of the femoral head (25 per cent in the series of Carroll and Sharrard).[89]

Posterolateral transfer of iliopsoas is a difficult operation with inherent problems and complications. The parents and patient should be forewarned of the following: (1) The operative wounds are near the perineum; hence the risk of hematoma-infection is greater than ordinary. (2) The transferred tendon may pull off from the greater trochanter, necessitating reoperation and reattachment. (3) Following removal of the hip spica cast, multiple fractures may occur because of disuse osteoporosis. (4) The hip joint may become stiff because of fibrosis of the denervated muscle. (5) Avascular necrosis of the femoral head may develop. (6) Following transfer of iliopsoas, all patients have decreased power of active hip flexion. They may be unable to climb steps. Do not perform bilateral iliopsoas transfer until power of hip flexion against gravity on the operated hip is achieved!

External Oblique Transfer to the Greater Trochanter. The external oblique abdominal muscle may be transferred to the greater trochanter to restore hip abduction power. Originally it was developed by Lowman, who used part of the external oblique muscle and attached it to the greater trochanter with a strip of fascia lata.[338] Thomas, Thompson, and Straub transferred the entire muscle belly of the external oblique.[587] Following detachment of the insertion of the muscle, the entire muscle is mobilized to its origin; then the distal aponeurosis is attached to the greater trochanter. The external oblique transfer is definitely weaker than a strong iliopsoas transfer; however, it has the following advantages: (1) The external oblique muscle functions synergistically, while the iliopsoas functions antagonistically. (2) The transferred muscle is taken from the abdominal wall, leaving the remaining abdominal muscles (rectus abdominis, internal oblique, and transversus) to maintain integrity of the abdomen. Contrariwise, iliopsoas transfer weakens power of active hip flexion. The latter may be desirable in the presence of hip flexion deformity; however, if the sartorius-pectineus unit is not strong

enough to flex the hip against gravity, the patient loses ability to walk up steps. (3) When the external oblique is transferred, the ilium is not violated (no holes or trough in the bone), making future innominate osteotomy feasible, if necessary.

Isolated transfer of external oblique does *not* provide adequate hip abductor strength to stabilize the hip. Therefore, other muscles are added to increase the power of hip abduction. Tensor fasciae latae can be transferred posteriorly to the iliac crest to increase hip abductor strength. This operation was developed originally by Legg for poliomyelitis; later Barr used it for spastic cerebral palsy.[34] Lindseth used the posterior transfer of tensor fasciae latae in association with external oblique transfer. In the experience of Lindseth and also Dias, hip abductor strength is stronger, the hip muscles are better balanced, and the hips are more stable. Posterior transfer of hip adductors can be added to the external oblique transfer. Often these muscle transfers are combined with varus derotation osteotomy of the proximal femur at the intertrochanteric level. Isolated posterior transfer of tensor fasciae latae is ineffective in providing hip stability.[641] Finally, in order for any muscle-tendon transfer to function adequately, the hip should be concentrically reduced, be stable, and have full passive range of motion.

FLEXION DEFORMITY

This is more common in L3 and higher level lesions, developing when there is hip flexion power in the absence of hip extension strength. In the older child who is primarily a sitter, hip flexion deformity also results from static forces of malposture with a direct relation between the degree of flexion deformity and the time spent sitting.

Hip flexion deformity causes anterior pelvic tilt and compensatory excessive lumbar lordosis (Fig. 5–99 A and B). It may be associated with abduction–lateral rotation contracture of the hip. When involvement is unilateral or asymmetrical, infrapelvic pelvic obliquity may develop with secondary lumbosacral scoliosis. Often, hip flexion deformity is accompanied by knee flexion contracture. Both deformities impede walking, with or without orthosis.

Treatment. This varies according to the age of the patient and the severity of the deformity. In infancy, gentle passive stretching exercises are performed several times a day. Prone posturing during sleep and certain periods of the day will stretch out the hip flexors and prevent increase of the hip flexion deformity.

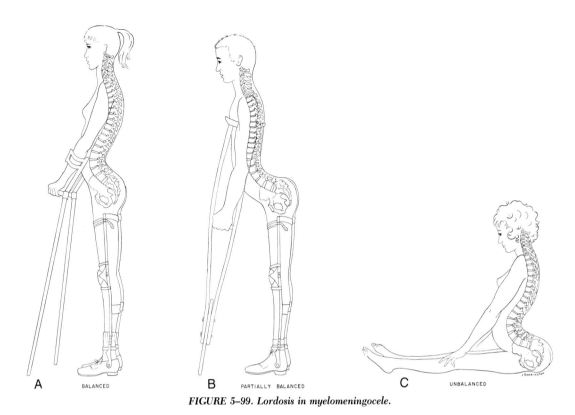

A. BALANCED B. PARTIALLY BALANCED C. UNBALANCED

FIGURE 5–99. Lordosis in myelomeningocele.

A. Balanced. B. Partially balanced. C. Unbalanced. (From Kilfoyle, R. M., Foley, J. J., and Norton, P. L.: The spine and pelvic deformity in childhood paraplegia. J. Bone Joint Surg., 47-A:661, 1965. Reprinted by permission.)

When a child is one year or older, a total-body orthosis (TLSHKAFO) with drop-lock hip and knee joints can be utilized to maintain the hip in neutral extension, 15 degrees of abduction, and neutral rotation. The drop-lock hip-knee joints will permit the child to sit and also, when locked in extension, to stand with support for short periods of time. Occasionally one may apply bilateral split Russel's skin traction to correct the hip flexion deformity; however, ulceration of the skin is a definite risk and meticulous nursing care is crucial when the patient is in traction.

Surgical measures are indicated to correct hip flexion deformity when the child is two years of age or older and the degree of fixed hip flexion deformity is 25 degrees or greater. Coexistent knee flexion deformity should be corrected simultaneously during the same anesthesia. The temptation is to procrastinate and delay surgical correction of hip flexion contracture. Operate early before the deformity becomes progressively fixed!

Soft-Tissue Release of the Hip Flexion Contracture. This is performed primarily in high-level lesions (L2 and higher) with poor motor strength of the lower limb musculature—patients who have a poor prognosis for functional walking. The goals of surgery are to provide full mobility of the hips and to correct anterior pelvic tilt and excessive lumbar lordosis. The operative procedure should be simple. The surgical exposure is through the anterior part of the incision utilized for Salter's innominate osteotomy. The iliopsoas tendon (about 1.5 to 2 cm.) and the reflected head of the rectus femoris are excised. In order to prevent recurrence of the deformity, *excision* is preferred over simple division. Fibrotic parts of the tensor fasciae latae and sartorius are divided. If possible, it is wise not to section the anterior capsule of the hip. Incomplete correction should be avoided. Perform a Thomas test on the operating table; continue anterior release until the hip hyperextends 20 degrees. Postoperative immobilization is in a bilateral above-knee hip spica cast with the hips in full extension, 10 to 15 degrees of abduction, and neutral rotation. The period of immobilization in spica cast should not exceed two weeks. When in the cast, the patient is placed upright in weight-bearing position several hours a day to minimize disuse atrophy and osteoporosis of the paralyzed limb bones and to prevent stress fractures. After removal of the cast the patient is fitted with a total-body orthosis, encouraging standing and walking several times a day. Hip extension and range-of-motion exercises are performed gently. The child should not sit for prolonged periods; instead he should be placed in prone position to maintain the hips and knees in extension.

Extension osteotomy of the proximal femur in the subtrochanteric region may be indicated in severe hip flexion deformity (exceeding 50 degrees) in an older child or adolescent. As a rule, bony procedures should be deferred until the patient is near skeletal maturity. Extension osteotomy should be performed after anterior soft-tissue release to decrease the degree of fixed flexion deformity. The two procedures can be combined. Correction of muscle imbalance prevents recurrence of the deformity. Surgical exposure may be through an anterolateral ap-

proach (if a bent AO plate for internal fixation is to be placed anteriorly), or through a posterior approach (as described by Root and Siegel,[494] if the internal fixation device is placed posteriorly). The anterior, lateral, and posterior aspects of the proximal femur are subperiosteally exposed from the level of the greater trochanteric apophyseal plate (which should not be disturbed) for a distance of 10 cm. inferior to the lesser trochanter. Next, with an electric drill, two threaded Steinmann pins are drilled into the upper and lower segments of the proposed osteotomy in an anteroposterior direction, at an angle determining the degree of flexion deformity to be corrected (Fig. 5–100). The wedge of bone to be resected is based posteriorly. There should be enough bone in the upper segment for screw insertion into the two holes of a pre-bent five-hole AO plate. The

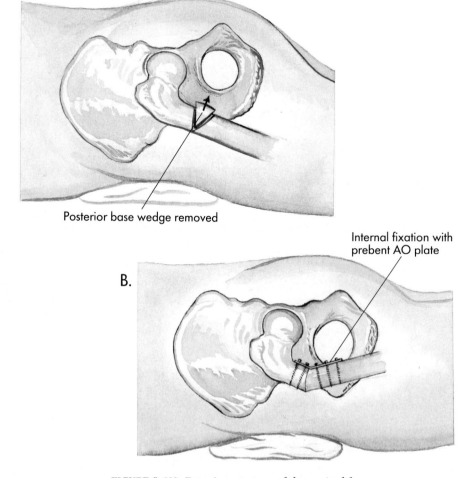

FIGURE 5–100. *Extension osteotomy of the proximal femur.*

A. Line of wedge osteotomy with its base anterior. **B.** Lateral view showing internal fixation with a pre-bent AO plate and five screws.

bone is then cut with an electric oscillating saw. The wedge of bone is removed. The two bone surfaces are apposed by extending the distal segment. Internal fixation is with a bent five-hole AO plate. The wounds are closed in routine fashion. A bilateral long leg hip spica cast is applied for external immobilization for four weeks. The child is allowed to stand several times a day in the cast, in order to prevent disuse atrophy, osteoporosis of the lower limb bones, and stress fractures. After cast removal, the child is fitted with appropriate orthosis for support and ambulation. In the older patient in whom secure internal fixation is achieved (a six- or seven-hole AO plate should be used), cast immobilization may be avoided. He is fitted with a hip-knee-ankle-foot orthosis (HKAFO) immediately after surgery. Splinting at night with the hips in extension and prone posturing are crucial to prevent recurrence of the hip flexion deformity.

A pitfall of extension osteotomy of the proximal femur is excessive extension; in such a case the combined fixed lumbar lordosis and restricted hip flexion will impede sitting posture.

There are two other procedures to increase hip extensor strength and prevent hip flexion deformity: (1) posterior transfer of the hip adductor origin to the ischial tuberosity, thus converting the flexor action of the deforming anterior hip adductors into extension; and (2) erector spinae transfer with fascia lata to the greater trochanter. The personal experience of the author with the preceding two procedures in patients with myelomeningocele has been disappointing. Hogshead and Ponseti reported results of fascia lata transfer to erector spinae in nine patients with myelomeningocele. The transfer provided a dynamic fasciodesis and relief of hip flexion contracture, stabilization of the hip, and relief of lumbar lordosis.[260]

ABDUCTION AND LATERAL ROTATION DEFORMITY OF THE HIP

Lateral rotation and abduction deformity of the hip usually occur together. They frequently occur in thoracic or upper lumbar level lesions with extensive paralysis of the muscles of the lower limbs. The infants lie with lateral rotation-abduction posture of the hips. Static forces of malposture are the pathogenic factor. In these infants, abduction-lateral rotation contracture of the hips can be prevented by proper posturing, splinting at night and certain periods of the day, and appropriate physical therapy consisting of range-of-motion exercises. Isolated lateral rotation deformity is very rare; it is caused by

the unbalanced muscle action of the iliopsoas. To demonstrate the role of the iliopsoas muscle, the range of medial rotation of the hip is determined with the hips in extension and in 90 degrees of flexion. If the range of medial rotation of the hip does not increase with flexing the hip, the iliopsoas is not the cause of the lateral rotation deformity of the hip.

Often, lateral rotation–abduction deformity of the hip is caused by contracture of the iliotibial band and tensor fasciae femoris. This is demonstrated by the Ober test (see Fig. 1–22, p. 30).

Tensor fasciae femoris is a flexor and abductor of the hip, and sartorius may also be contracted; therefore, the usual deformity is lateral rotation–abduction and varying degrees of flexion deformity—all three deformities occurring together. The short lateral rotators of the hip and posterior capsule of the hip joint may be contracted in severe deformity. A laterally transferred iliopsoas may contract and cause abduction contracture of the hip. Continuous lateral rotation posture of the hip will gradually decrease the degree of femoral antetorsion, and if untreated for a prolonged period, may even cause femoral retrotorsion. The hip should be carefully examined, assessing all pathogenic factors in lateral rotation–abduction contractures. Preoperatively it is desirable to perform a CT scan to determine the exact degree of femoral and acetabular torsion.

Bilateral abduction–lateral rotation contractures render orthotic fitting difficult, impairing ambulation and causing pressure ulcers at points of abnormal orthotic contact. Unilateral contracture of the iliotibial band will cause pelvic obliquity, with the contralateral femoral head gradually becoming displaced laterally and superiorly out of the acetabulum. Often the contracted iliotibial band causes flexion deformity of the knee and lateral tibiofibular torsion.

Treatment. This consists of soft-tissue release with Ober fasciotomy proximally and Yount fasciotomy distally (if a knee flexion deformity is present). The operative technique of the Ober-Yount procedure is described in the section on poliomyelitis. In unilateral involvement, especially if the contralateral hip is beginning subluxation, the hip with the release of the iliotibial band contracture is placed in the position of extension and neutral adduction-rotation, whereas the contralateral subluxating hip is immobilized in abduction and mild flexion in the hip spica cast (Fig. 5–101). In bilateral cases, the position of immobilization of the hips in the spica cast is neutral extension, 10 degrees

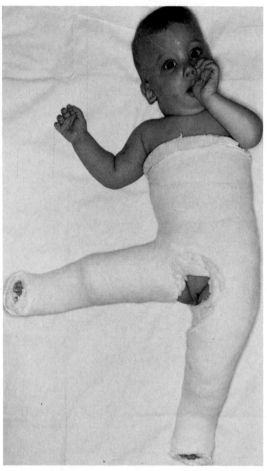

FIGURE 5–101. An infant with lumbosacral myelomeningocele and pelvic obliquity due to unilateral contracture of the iliotibial band on the left.

The right hip had become dislocated. The contracted iliotibial band on the left was released by the Ober-Yount procedure, and the right hip was reduced by closed manipulation. Note the position of immobilization of the hips in the hip spica cast—the left hip is in extension and neutral adduction, whereas the right hip is in wide abduction and in some flexion.

of abduction, and neutral rotation. The period of cast immobilization is only two weeks; it should not exceed three weeks. During the period of cast immobilization the child is placed upright for two to three hours a day. This position will assist in prevention of disuse osteoporosis and pathologic fractures. After removal of the cast the child is fitted with a total-body orthosis, with each hip in 10 degrees of abduction, neutral extension, and neutral rotation.

The severe fixed abduction–lateral rotation–flexion deformity of the hip requires radical soft-tissue release to correct rigid contractural

deformity of the lateral rotators of the hip and posterior part of the capsule of the hip joint. The operative technique is described by Menelaus.[388] It is usually required in children with high thoracolumbar lesions with no function below the first lumbar neurosegmented level. A lateral longitudinal incision is made extending from 4 to 5 cm. above to 4 to 6 cm. below the tip of the greater trochanter. The subcutaneous tissue and deep fascia are divided in line with the skin incision. By blunt dissection, the anterior, lateral, and posterior aspects of the hip joint are exposed. First, with the hip in minimal medial rotation and adduction the fibrotic gluteus medius and gluteus minimus are sectioned at their insertions. Next, the short lateral rotators and posterior hip joint capsule are divided. Then the fibrotic tensor fasciae latae and iliotibial band are released by excision of a 2 to 3 cm. segment. The iliopsoas tendon is sectioned at its insertion. The redundant anterior hip joint capsule is exposed, divided longitudinally near the acetabular rim, and plicated. Both hips are operated upon under one anesthesia. The blood loss is usually minimal. Postoperatively the child is placed in a bilateral long leg hip spica cast, with the hips in 10 degrees of abduction, minimal medial rotation, and neutral extension. The period of cast immobilization is three to four weeks, long enough for the reefed anterior capsule to heal.

Derotation osteotomy of the proximal femur, rotating the distal femoral segment medially, should not be performed when there is femoral retrotorsion. However, if there are no adaptive retrotorsional changes of the upper femur and there is femoral antetorsion as shown by CT scan, derotation osteotomy of the upper femur at the intertrochanteric or subtrochanteric level will achieve satisfactory result in correction of lateral rotation deformity of the hip. In the experience of Dias et al., in nine hips, the result was good in eight and fair in one.[134] Rigid internal fixation, such as with the AO plate, will obliterate the necessity of postoperative immobilization in a cast—permitting early standing and preventing osteoporosis of disuse.

HIP ADDUCTION DEFORMITY

This is common with high-level lesions when spasticity of the hip adductors leads to contractural deformity. It also occurs frequently in association with hip subluxation or dislocation. Unilateral hip adduction contracture can result in infrapelvic obliquity and scoliosis, impeding sitting and walking.

Treatment consists of surgical division of the

hip adductors—usually the longus and brevis (see cerebral palsy section, Plate 58, for operative technique). Because of incontinence there is a definite increased risk of fecal-urinary contamination of the operative wound. For this reason this author prefers a longitudinal incision instead of a transverse incision. Again, the period of immobilization in a hip spica cast should be short, usually about two weeks.

Posterior transfer of the anterior hip adductors to the ischium is *not* recommended by this author.

The Spine

Deformities of the spine are common, as the vertebral column is the primary site of involvement in myelomeningocele. With improved medical and surgical care, more and more of these children are surviving into adolescence, and the progressive deformities of the spine present serious and challenging problems to the orthopedic surgeon.

Scoliosis, kyphosis, and abnormal lordosis are the deformities frequently encountered. These may be present in pure form or in varying combinations. Spinal deformity may be present at birth or may develop in childhood or early adolescence. It is imperative that all patients with myelomeningocele have anteroposterior and lateral radiograms of the spine taken periodically for early detection of spinal deformities.

LORDOSIS

The most common of the spinal deformities in myelomeningocele is abnormal lordosis.

Etiology. Not present at birth, lordosis develops later on in childhood. It is often compensatory in origin for purposes of balance. In the presence of bilateral paralysis of the triceps surae and gluteus maximus muscles, but normal strength of the hip flexors and quadriceps femoris muscles, the patient stands with a characteristic calcaneus crouch posture; i.e., the hips and knees are flexed, the ankles are dorsiflexed, and the trunk is inclined forward. Stability is provided by the action of a strong quadriceps femoris muscle. Compensation and balance are provided by holding the lumbar spine in severe lordosis (see Fig. 5–99).

Hip flexion contracture will increase the pelvic inclination and force the lumbar spine into excessive lordosis. Muscle imbalance between hip flexors and extensors and contracture of the iliotibial band are common causes of flexion deformity of the hip. Posterior osseous defect of the lumbosacral spine, congenital spondylo-

listhesis, and posterior postsurgical scarring are other etiologic factors. Lordosis is usually present above the level of a lumbar kyphosis.

Types. Lordosis in myelomeningocele may be of two types: a *lower type*, in which the proximal end of the exaggerated anterior curve is at or below the third lumbar vertebra; and a *high type*, in which the lordotic curve extends from the second lumbar vertebra into the thoracic vertebrae, where lordosis is not normally present. The location and extent of lordosis usually correspond with the level of paralysis. Compensation of abnormal lordosis takes place by the development of a commensurate posterior curve in the spine (kyphosis) above and flexion of the hip below. In stance, when the center of gravity of the body falls immediately in front of the ankle joint, the lordosis is *balanced* and minimum external support is required for standing; when the center of gravity falls in front of the toes but the patient is able to stand with crutches, lordosis is *partially balanced*; and when crutch standing is impossible or impractical because of severity of lordosis, it is regarded as *off balance* (Figs. 5–101 and 5–102).

The functional performance of patients with low-type lordosis is better than that of those with high-type lordosis. Most patients with high-type lordosis are off balance or only partially balanced, whereas balance or partial balance of the spine is the rule in low-type lordosis.[296]

Treatment. Lordosis of the spine will progress with growth unless aggressive measures are taken to checkrein it. Knee-chest exercises are performed several times per day to maintain flexibility of the lumbosacral spine. Passive stretching exercises are carried out to correct hip flexion and iliotibial band contractures. Vigorous correction of hip flexion deformity is vital. A plastic TLSO, utilizing the Boston brace principle, may be used to support the trunk in sitting and in stance.

Surgical measures are directed toward elimination of deforming factors. If a strong iliopsoas muscle is causing the deformity, it is transferred posteriorly to the greater trochanter to function as a hip abductor and extensor, or if it is weak and spastic, it is lengthened. If iliotibial band contracture is present to a significant degree and does not respond to passive stretching exercises, it is surgically released by the Ober-Yount procedure. The first step is correction of fixed flexion deformity of the hips. Erector spinae transfer may improve trunk stability. Fascial transplants to reinforce abdominal mus-

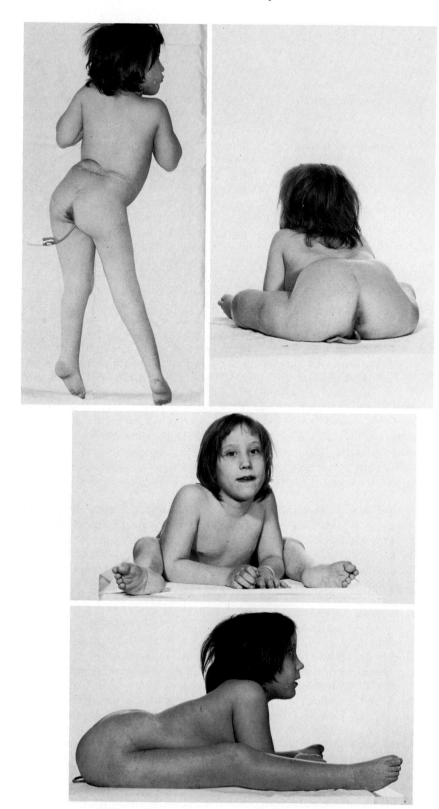

FIGURE 5–102. A seven-year-old girl with myelomeningocele.

Note the severe lordosis. The spine is decompensated and off-balance, making standing impossible. Sitting is assisted with support of hands.

culature may be considered.[296] In the experience of this author, erector spinae transfer and abdominal fascial transplants are ineffective to correct a fixed lumbar lordosis. These should not be employed.

Spinal fusion is indicated when the preceding measures fail to improve or arrest the increasing lordosis and there is progressive loss of balance. The sacrum should be included in the fusion area. Functional range of hip motion is a prerequisite for lumbosacral fusion; otherwise, the patient will be unable to sit. Anterior spinal fusion is performed first with Dwyer or Zielke instrumentation.[163, 644] Two weeks later, posterior spinal fusion is performed with internal instrumentation. The posterior fusion extends to include the sacrum. In the severe fixed lordosis, during the anterior approach, one may combine the disc excision with wedge resection of the vertebral bodies at the apex of the deformity.

SCOLIOSIS

Scoliosis in myelomeningocele may result from one or several of the following causes:

1. *Congenital bony anomalies*, such as hemivertebrae or failure of segmentation or unilateral segmental bar (Fig. 5–103). These congenital anomalies of the spine cause asymmetrical growth of the vertebral column and result in scoliosis (they are discussed in detail in Chapter 6).

2. *Local instability of the spine* due to absence of posterior elements and intervening ligaments, a pathogenic factor present in all children with myelomeningocele. A second factor is loss of stability provided by the muscles across the spinal segments as a result of paralysis (Figs. 5–104 and 5–105). In myelomeningocele, progressive neurologic dysfunction may occur secondary to hydromyelia or, later on in adolescence, because of tethering of the cord at the site of sac closure.

It is important to distinguish the congenital form from the paralytic spinal deformity in myelomeningocele. Paralytic deformities have no anomalies of the vertebrae, and the spine in infancy has no abnormal curvature. The curves usually develop between the ages of five and ten years. The paralytic curves are long and sweeping. They are associated with pelvic obliquity and decompensation of the torso.[475]

The natural history of untreated scoliosis in myelomeningocele is progression. If the cause of scoliosis, however, is hydromyelia and tethering of the cord, the degree of curvature may improve by shunting in hydromyelia and by release of the tethered cord. It is vital, therefore, to rule out hydromyelia and tethering of the cord in scoliosis in myelomeningocele. A neurosurgical consultation is obtained. First, dermatomal sensory evoked potentials are performed for screening and then high-resolution CT scanning, nuclear magnetic resonance imaging, or metrizamide myelography is carried out. Hydromyelia is diagnosed by alteration in the size of the spinal cord shadow between erect and supine postures and with delayed uptake of the metrizamide dye in the central canal (but visualized in the CT scan). Tethering of the spinal cord is detected by the presence of spinal cord below the third lumbar level and by ascending nerve roots.

Treatment. Management of hemivertebrae and unsegmented bar is discussed under congenital scoliosis in Chapter 6. The basic principle of treatment is to halt abnormal growth forces by early spinal fusion. The objective is prevention of progression of the curvature. In the presence of documented progression of the scoliosis, fusion should be performed early. Do not procrastinate and allow severe deformity to develop and then attempt to treat.

Scoliosis due to local instability of the spine (caused by muscle paralysis and absence of posterior elements—bony or ligamentous) may be managed nonoperatively initially, provided that the curve is flexible. In the wheelchair-bound child with myelomeningocele, provision of maximal possible trunk height is important. Delay of spinal fusion will allow further vertebral growth. Long spinal fusion in early childhood will cause substantial loss of trunk height. Another advantage of delaying surgery is to allow development of adequate bone stock for fusion.[68] It is important to closely follow the braced spine of these children—if progression of scoliosis cannot be controlled by orthosis, surgery should be performed.

Orthotic treatment of scoliosis in myelomeningocele is difficult and poses special problems. The first difficulty is skin tolerance: the support provided by the orthosis is passive; therefore, pressure on the skin should be minimized by increasing the area of contact pressure. This author uses the Boston brace; others may prefer the total extended support provided by a total body thoracolumbosacral orthosis (TLSO). The Milwaukee brace may be used; however, the pelvic girdle should be longer, extending proximally under the ribs to give some suspension. The thoracic and lumbar pads

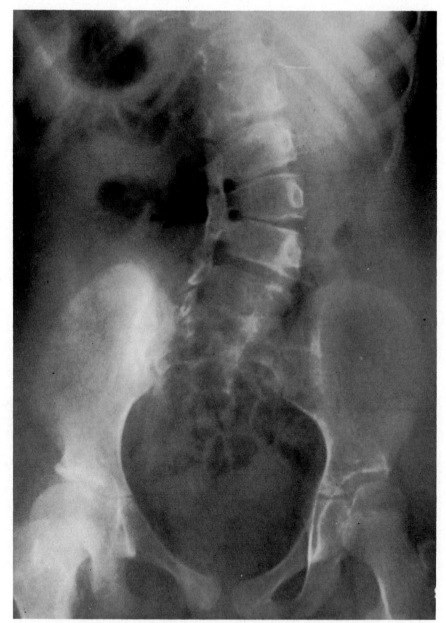

FIGURE 5–103. Congenital scoliosis in a child with myelomeningocele.

Note the unsegmented unilateral bar between the second and fourth lumbar vertebrae.

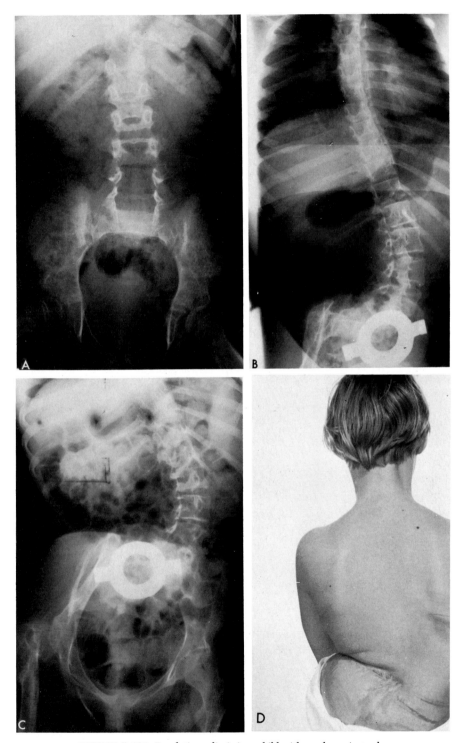

FIGURE 5-104. Paralytic scoliosis in a child with myelomeningocele.

Note the progression of the scoliosis and the fixed pelvic obliquity. Radiograms of the spine at three years of age (A); (B) at five years of age; and (C) at ten years of age. D. Clinical appearance of patient.

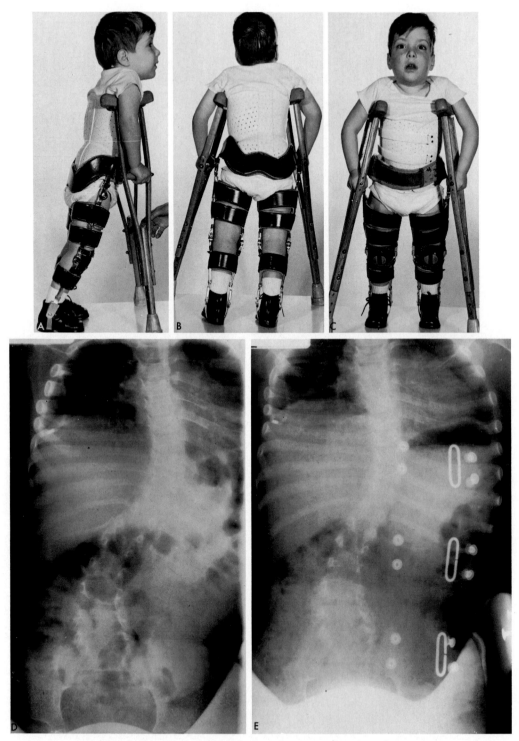

FIGURE 5–105. A five-year-old boy with myelomeningocele and paralytic scoliosis.

A plastic body jacket will support the trunk effectively; however, it will not prevent progression of the scoliosis. **A** to **C.** Clinical appearance of patient with the body jacket and orthosis. **D.** Standing radiogram of the spine without the body jacket support. **E.** Radiogram with the body jacket—note balancing of the trunk.

should be large. In all types of orthoses the pelvic girdle may be modified, if necessary, by an aperture for ilioconduits.

In the beginning, the periods in the brace are short, the wearing time slowly being increased until skin tolerance has developed. It may require four to six weeks, with frequent orthotic adjustments, before the child can wear the orthosis all day. It is best for the child not to sleep in the brace.

Operative correction of the curve and stabilization of the spine by instrumentation and fusion is indicated if the curve is not flexible; progression of the curve cannot be prevented by adequate wear of the orthosis, and fixed pelvic obliquity begins to develop.

The objectives of operative correction of scoliosis are to correct fixed pelvic obliquity, centralize the trunk, prevent decubitus ulcers, prevent respiratory dysfunction, improve ambulation, and improve self-image. Also, freeing a hand used for trunk support will enhance upper limb function.

Patients with myelomeningocele are frequently frail and tolerate the extensive spinal surgery poorly. The rate of complications is high, and there is a definite risk of operative mortality. Prior to surgery the patient should be assessed, analyzing the neurologic status, urinary tract function, cardiopulmonary status, and the various orthopedic deformities. The goals should be realistic. Major spinal surgery is contraindicated when life expectancy is short owing to systemic disease and also if there is uncontrolled hydrocephalus and severe mental retardation.

Active urinary tract infection should be treated before spinal surgery. If there is progressive neurologic loss, tethering of the spinal cord and hydrocephalus should be ruled out. In such an instance, appropriate neurosurgical treatment by release of tethered cord or shunting may arrest the progression of scoliosis and the degree of the curve may improve.

The hips are carefully examined to rule out infrapelvic (femoropelvic) obliquity. Prior to lumbosacral fusion, pelvic obliquity must be fully corrected by release of hip adduction and abduction contracture if they are the cause of fixed infrapelvic obliquity.

The skin over the lumbosacral spine is scarred by previous neurosurgical closure of the sac. Plastic surgical consultation is obtained if skin flaps will be required for wound closure.

Operative procedures should be planned in order to minimize the period of immobilization in cast. Prolonged cast immobilization causes severe osteoporosis and increases the risk of pathologic fractures.

Both anterior and posterior (circumferential) spinal fusions are almost always indicated. If posterior fusion alone is performed, the rate of pseudarthrosis is high and the correction obtained is lost. First, anterior fusion is performed, discs are excised, and the disc spaces are packed with autogenous rib, iliac, or bone-bank bone. Dwyer or Zielke instrumentation is centered at the apex of the deformity; it should span as long a segment of the thoracolumbar deformity as possible. Two weeks later, posterior spinal fusion and internal instrumentation are performed. The rods are contoured to restore a normal thoracic kyphosis and lumbar lordosis. They extend from the sacrum cephalad over the entire length of the deformity as seen on both the anteroposterior and the lateral radiograms. Alar hooks are used to transfix the rods to the sacrum.

Anterior instrumentation may block the degree of final correction. In general, in the child 12 years or under, anterior interbody fusion without instrumentation is performed; in the young patient the vertebral bodies are small and osteoporotic, making instrumentation insecure. Anterior instrumentation is usually utilized in the older adolescent.

Halo-femoral traction or halo-wheelchair traction is indicated only in curves greater than 100 degrees, with full comprehension of all possible problems and complications of such traction, especially cranial nerve palsy.[68]

Posterior fusion should be extended distally to the sacrum and proximally to one vertebra superior to the end of the curve. Facet fusion is performed whenever possible. The deficient posterior elements require long segments of bone graft—autogenous and homologous. Often, the bone grafts are layered on the concavity of the curve, where compression forces enhance rapid healing of the fusion mass. Bone grafts may be placed in gutter fashion beside the dysplastic vertebral bodies. In addition to Harrington rodding, one may use interlaminar wiring—this provides simultaneous segmental fixation with distraction transverse loading. The Luque rods have the serious problem of cutting through the thin iliac walls. Two weeks following surgery a pantaloon cast is applied, incorporating the thighs.

Complications of spinal surgery in myelomeningocele include pseudarthrosis, wound infection, decubitus ulcers, failure of internal fixation device with dislodging of hooks and rods protruding through the skin, and fractures due to osteoporosis of disuse in the cast. There is a definite risk of mortality.[69] These problems of extensive spinal surgery in myelomeningocele patients should be anticipated, and parents and patient should be forewarned.

The *pseudarthrosis* rate is high (about 25 per cent); this is because the vertebrae are dysplastic, the fusion area crosses the lumbosacral articulation, and the paralytic muscles provide poor support to the spine. Drummond et al. recommended routine exploration of the posterior spinal fusion five months postoperatively; the rods are removed without disturbing the hook purchase, the fusion mass is inspected, and sites of pseudarthrosis are repaired with fusion with autogenous bone from the fusion mass and bone-bank bone. The rods are replaced using the same hooks. Postoperatively another cast is applied for an additional four months. The total period of cast immobilization is nine months, during which time all pelvic obliquity, spinal deformity, and hip problems are corrected, adhering to the principle of planning all procedures within one cast period.[159]

Postoperative *wound infection* occurs in about 8 per cent of the cases. The relatively high infection rate is due to soaking of the wound dressing with feces and urine and poor skin coverage. If, at operation, there is any breach of the dural sac and leak of cerebrospinal fluid, it should be immediately repaired. Loss of neurologic function may occur following spinal fusion.

Despite all of these serious problems and complications of spinal surgery in myelomeningocele, it is recommended that the progressive fixed scoliosis be corrected and stabilized by fusion and instrumentation. Following surgery, new vistas are open to these disabled patients; with provision of spine stability and balance, they can sit and ambulate much more effectively, decubitus ulcers are prevented, and pulmonary function is improved.

KYPHOSIS

Kyphosis in myelomeningocele may be congenital or acquired.

Congenital lumbar kyphosis is uniquely found in myelomeningocele. It is characterized by a rigid posterior angulation of the spine limited to the area of the osseous defect. Its incidence is reported by Hoppenfeld to be 12.5 per cent.[263] The cause of congenital lumbar kyphosis in association with myelomeningocele is unknown. Sharrard believes that in such instances the lesional defect is very wide, the

erector spinae muscles are atrophic or absent, and the quadratus lumborum is displaced laterally, becoming a flexor of the lumbar spine. Thus the action of abdominal muscles is unopposed, and the lumbar kyphosis develops in utero.[530] An additional factor in progression of the kyphosis is the weakness or absence of function of the extensors of the lumbar spine in the presence of functioning psoas muscle and the crura of the diaphragm, which lie anterior to the kyphosis.[148]

The pathology of congenital lumbar kyphosis is well described by Hoppenfeld, and by Sharrard and Drennan.[263, 530]

The kyphotic deformity is evident at birth. The pedicles in the lesional area are spread widely apart and project posterolaterally, accentuating the kyphotic appearance and acting as pressure points over which the skin is blanched. The skin defect is extremely large, the open spinal cord being stretched over the kyphotic lumbar vertebrae.

The kyphosis is fixed—it cannot be reduced by passive manipulation and is not altered by changing the position of the infant from supine to prone. Upon sitting and standing the degree of kyphosis is increased by the incumbent body weight, and a compensatory thoracic lordosis develops above the kyphos. The pelvis will be markedly rotated, giving an apparent severe flexion deformity of the hips, with the plane of the lower limbs at right angles to the trunk (Fig. 5–106). This true congenital kyphosis should be distinguished from postural roundback, a condition characteristic of all infants who are placed in sitting posture. The postural kyphosis is flexible and can be corrected passively.

The deformity tends to increase with growth, and progressive neurologic deficit develops as a result of stretching of neural tissues over the kyphos. Skin necrosis and ulcers caused by pressure on the bony prominences (when the child is lying, sitting, or wearing an orthosis) are common. Mechanisms of compensation for abnormal kyphosis are the development of lordotic curves above and below the site of dorsal angulation, and hyperextension of the hip if the length of the spinal segment is not sufficient to form a lordosis. Kyphosis is *balanced* if the center of gravity of the body falls immediately anterior to the ankle joints; it is *partially balanced* when the center of gravity of the body falls behind the heels. Kyphosis is *unbalanced* when the patient is unable to stand or walk because of insufficient lordosis or hyperextension of the hip to compensate for the marked dorsal angulation of the spine (Figs. 5–106 and 5–107).

Radiograms demonstrate the characteristic findings. In the lesional area the spinous processes and laminae are absent and the interpedicular spaces markedly widened—these are common to all spina bifida cystica cases. In the lateral radiograms the localized kyphotic deformity is easily seen. The vertebral bodies are wedged anteriorly, mostly at the apex of the curve. The intervertebral disc interspaces are usually narrowed. The pelvic inclination is markedly increased, and the thighs seem to be elevated from their normal downward inclination to a more horizontal position (Fig. 5–108).

Treatment. Rigid kyphosis in myelomeningocele presents very difficult problems in management. Often the infants with congenital fixed lumbar kyphosis have a poor prognosis with marked hydrocephalus and extensive paralysis. Care of these children should be individualized. In the neonate, kyphosis will interfere with operative closure of the sac. Even with use of skin flaps and relaxing incisions, satisfactory skin closure without great tension is impossible. The skin closure breaks down, and secondary infection of the stretched neural tissues develops, causing complete paralysis of the lower limbs.

In the newborn, Sharrard has recommended correction of deformity by osteotomy of the spine with resection of one or more vertebral bodies at the apex of the kyphos. The vertebral bodies are removed laterally between the nerve roots to avoid injury to the large vessels traversing the posterior abdominal wall and to the neural tissues (Figs. 5–108 and 5–109). Postoperatively, the spine is held in extension by suspension-traction with adhesive straps on the abdomen and lower limbs, with the infant lying on a small Bradford frame. In the less severe deformity in the newborn, simple excision of the rudimentary laminae is performed in order to relieve the tension.[520]

Later on in childhood, the presence of severe rigid kyphosis impedes sitting, necessitating excision of the kyphosis and stabilization of the spine by fusion and internal fixation in order to provide stability. The height of the lumbar spine determines the vertical dimensions of the abdominal cavity; therefore, it is important to preserve the height of the lumbar spine as much as possible. It is best to excise the vertebral bodies between the apex of the kyphos and the apex of the lordosis, permitting approximation of the two adjacent vertebral bodies and allowing growth of the remaining lumbar vertebrae. Early fusion provides stability to the spine;

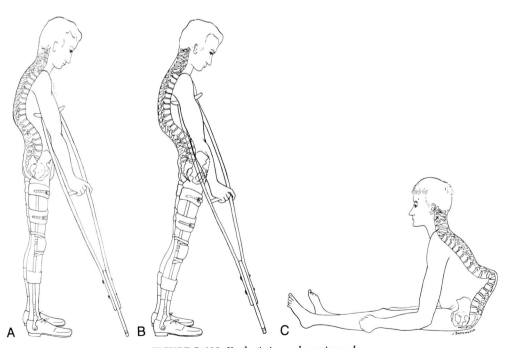

FIGURE 5–106. Kyphosis in myelomeningocele.

A. Balanced. **B.** Partially balanced. **C.** Unbalanced. (From Kilfoyle, R. M., Foley, J. J., and Norton, P. L.: The spine and pelvic deformity in childhood paraplegia. J. Bone Joint Surg., 47-A:668, 1965. Reprinted by permission.)

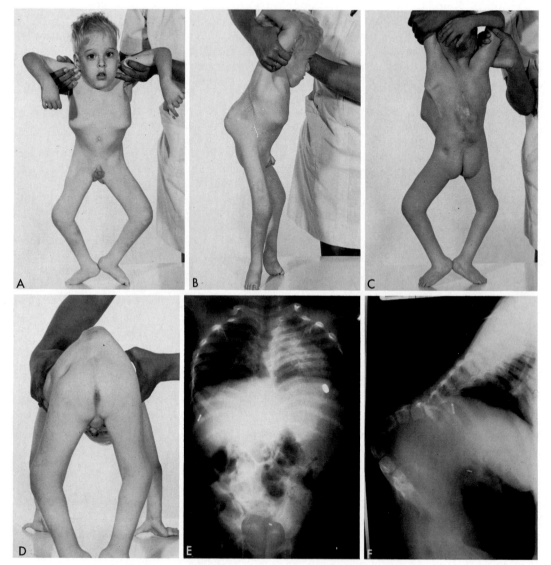

FIGURE 5–107. Congenital lumbar kyphosis in a two-year-old child with myelomeningocele.

A to D. Clinical appearance of patient. E and F. Radiograms of spine.

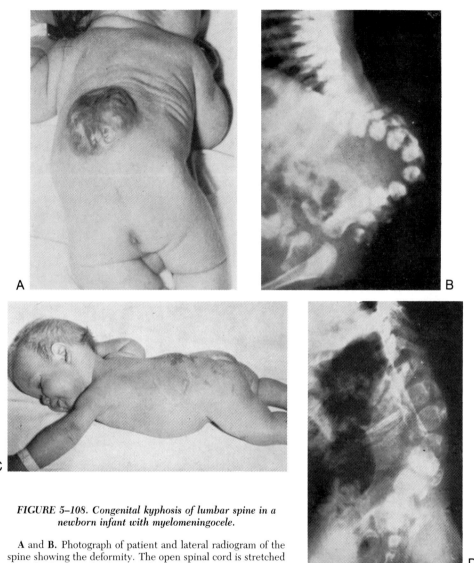

FIGURE 5-108. *Congenital kyphosis of lumbar spine in a newborn infant with myelomeningocele.*

A and **B.** Photograph of patient and lateral radiogram of the spine showing the deformity. The open spinal cord is stretched over the kyphotic lumbar vertebrae. **C** and **D.** Postoperative photograph and radiogram following neonatal osteotomy resection. Note improvement in the kyphotic deformity and the skin covering the spine. (From Sharrard, W. J. W.: Spinal osteotomy for congenital kyphosis in myelomeningocele. J. Bone Joint Surg., 50-B:466, 469, 1968. Reprinted by permission.)

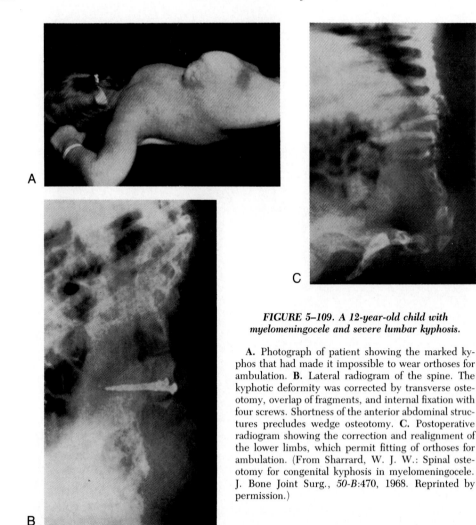

FIGURE 5–109. A 12-year-old child with myelomeningocele and severe lumbar kyphosis.

A. Photograph of patient showing the marked kyphos that had made it impossible to wear orthoses for ambulation. **B.** Lateral radiogram of the spine. The kyphotic deformity was corrected by transverse osteotomy, overlap of fragments, and internal fixation with four screws. Shortness of the anterior abdominal structures precludes wedge osteotomy. **C.** Postoperative radiogram showing the correction and realignment of the lower limbs, which permit fitting of orthoses for ambulation. (From Sharrard, W. J. W.: Spinal osteotomy for congenital kyphosis in myelomeningocele. J. Bone Joint Surg., *50-B*:470, 1968. Reprinted by permission.)

however, it shortens the height of the abdomen and trunk. The drawbacks of a shortened trunk should be carefully weighed against the advantages of spinal stability.

Duncan et al. described a technique of stretching of the apex by pulling the kyphosis anteriorly onto a rigid plate. The fixation device is attached to the vertebral bodies by a transverse screw with a ring plate in the bodies.[161] McKay had previously described a similar plate for correction of the kyphosis and stable internal fixation.[343]

Fractures

Fractures of the lower limbs are common in myelomeningocele, occurring in about 20 per cent of the patients.[388] The fracture may involve the metaphysis, diaphysis, or physis. The bone most commonly involved is the femur; next in frequency is the tibia.

ETIOLOGY

Several underlying abnormalities and other factors are responsible for the high incidence of pathologic fractures in myelomeningocele. The bone is osteoporotic, owing to muscular paralysis and disuse atrophy. The incidence of fractures tends to decrease as the child begins weight bearing and ambulation because the degree of osteoporosis diminishes. Fractures are more common in the flail limbs. In a survey of 122 children with myelomeningocele, James found 44 fractures in 28 limbs; the incidence of lower limb fractures was 7.5 per cent in children with strong quadriceps and 19 per cent in children with lower thoracic–high lumbar neurosegmental level lesions.[279] Fixed deformities of the knee, particularly extension contracture or stiffness of the hip, increase susceptibility to undue stress on the atrophic bones during application of the orthoses or night support.

The necessity for prolonged immobilization of the lower limbs in plaster of Paris casts following correction of hip dislocation—subluxation or scoliosis-kyphosis of the spine—increases the already existing paralytic bone atrophy and risk of fractures. Drummond et al. reported this high incidence of fractures in 40 myelomeningocele patients who had prolonged cast immobilization subsequent to major reconstructive surgery on the hips or spine. There were 18 fractures (9 in the supracondylar region of the femur, 4 in the diaphysis of the femur, 4 in the proximal metaphysis of the tibia, and 1 in the subtrochanteric region of the femur). The fractures occurred within one month of cast removal in 16 of the 18 fractures.[158]

Sensation is diminished or absent in patients with myelomeningocele, with the result that these children are oblivious to the pain of trauma and do not have protective reflex mechanisms. Also, the loss of sensation explains the secondary breakdown on attempted arthrodesis in patients with myelomeningocele. The physes and epiphyses of the long bones of the lower limbs in myelomeningocele can be repeatedly injured during daily walking activities. Gyepes et al. reported on six myelomeningocele patients (between the ages of 11 and 13 years) with physeal injuries in the region of the knee and ankle—none of these six patients used orthotic support for walking.[226] Another cause of physeal injury is passive joint movement or forced manipulation, such as during treatment of clubfoot or extension deformity of the knee.

The structural quality of bone in children with myelomeningocele is an additional factor. Ralis et al. compared 17 tibiae (dissected post mortem) of myelomeningocele infants with those of 14 normal controls. In the tibiae from myelomeningocele children with paralysis, the total area of cortical bone, its thickness, number of haversian systems, and number of large remodeling cavities were diminished. The total amount of osteoid tissue in the paralyzed limb bones of myelomeningocele is increased. This is especially noted in the subepiphyseal and metaphyseal regions. The new bone matrix is softened because of delay in mineralization of newly laid-down bone matrix. The remodeling of long bones is disturbed in myelomeningocele. Ralis et al. noted the tibiae in myelomeningocele children to be circular, as compared with the triangular shape of tibiae in normal children.[474]

CLINICAL FEATURES

The presence of fracture is usually discovered by the parents, the nurse, or the physical therapist, who will usually first note the increased local heat, swelling, gross deformity, and crepitation. Bruising and subcutaneous hematoma are characteristically absent. A healing fracture is occasionally found in radiographs taken for other reasons. It is often difficult to ascertain exactly when these fractures occurred. Ordinarily there is no history of acute trauma, such as a fall. They may also result from removal of a hip spica cast, or may occur during manipulation of the knee while a heavy patient is being turned, or may take place when the foot becomes entangled in the rails on the side of the bed. Passive manipulation of a joint for range-of-motion exercises may cause the fracture.

Systemic reactions of elevation of white blood cells and erythrocyte sedimentation rate may occur in fractures in myelomeningocele. Occasionally, systemic dysfunction may be severe with tachypnea or tachycardia resembling fat embolism syndrome; however, immediate improvement following administration of fluid and immobilization of the fracture indicates that the acute systemic reaction noted in these children is most probably related to problems of blood volume loss.[15]

Radiographic Findings. These vary according to the location of the fracture and stage of repair. Diaphyseal fractures of the femur are usually of the spiral or greenstick type. Metaphyseal fractures are usually minimally displaced in the flail limb. Physeal fracture-separation may manifest in its early stages in the form of widening of the physis, but later on there will be exuberant subperiosteal new bone formation. These radiographic changes represent responses to multiple minute fractures and subsequent healing in the metaphyseal-physeal junctions in insensitive limbs that are subjected to the stresses of weight-bearing. They should not be mistaken for osteomyelitis or a malignant bone tumor. The associated temperature and white blood cell elevation makes differential diagnosis from osteomyelitis difficult. There are reports of fractures in myelomeningocele children who were treated with antibiotics because of the misdiagnosis of infection.[591] Traumatic destruction of the distal femoral epiphysis in its posterolateral portion with sclerosis and bone fragmentation has been reported by Wolverson.[635] CT scan and linear tomography are of great value in establishing diagnosis in these difficult cases.

Neurotrophic joints usually do not develop in myelomeningocele, as weight-bearing is a prerequisite for the progressive changes of excessive bone production as well as the joint disintegration commonly seen in Charcot joints.

TREATMENT

Definite steps should be taken to prevent fractures. Parents, nurses, and attendant personnel should be informed of the danger of fracture and should exercise gentle care in the application of shoes, orthoses, or bivalved night casts, handling the child cautiously while performing passive exercises or while turning him, in routine bed care, and in daily activities. Stiff and rigid deformity of joints should be avoided; if present, the joints should be mobilized to functional range as a safeguard against fractures. As bone atrophy is an important factor and increases susceptibility to fractures, the limbs should be immobilized as briefly as possible. A bilateral above-knee, rather than a one and one half, hip spica cast should be applied when a hip joint is immobilized. Weight-bearing should be encouraged several hours a day to stimulate osteogenesis.

When a fracture occurs, pre-existing deformities should be carefully assessed. If the site of the fracture is convenient and is discovered early enough, it can be utilized as an osteotomy to correct a rotational or angular deformity. For example, a supracondylar fracture of the femur is commonly associated with hyperextension contracture of the knee; in such an instance, the distal femoral fragment is tilted posteriorly to correct the genu recurvatum. With subtrochanteric fractures of the femur, the status of the hip should be analyzed. Is there an indication for derotation or varization osteotomy of the proximal femur?

Fractures in myelomeningocele heal quite rapidly despite the absence of muscle tone. Treatment should be by nonoperative methods. Skeletal traction in femoral fractures is not tolerated. The Kirschner wire in the osteoporotic bone will often migrate distally and cause injury to the physis. It is simpler and more effective to manipulate the fracture into the desired position and to maintain reduction in a well-padded, snug bilateral above-knee hip spica cast. This also allows early weight-bearing with the support of the cast, minimizing disuse bone atrophy. Fractures of the tibia do not present any particular problem. Shortening due to overriding of fragments is not significant and not a problem. The objective is to achieve functional alignment and proper rotation in order to enable the child to stand and walk with orthotic appliances. Night bivalved casts or splints are not recommended, as such methods provide inadequate immobilization and frequently cause rotational and angular deformities or shortening. Two to three weeks of immobilization is all the duration required to achieve stability for removal of the cast and fitting with appropriate orthotic support. Pressure sores are a problem; the importance of adequate padding of the cast cannot be overemphasized. Delayed union or nonunion is not a problem; however, remodeling of long bone fracture in myelomeningocele is very poor. Remodeling usually does not occur because of lack of muscle forces across the fracture site and inadequate stresses of static forces of weight-bearing.

Physeal injuries can be complicated by growth arrest. Prolonged immobilization does not prevent growth disturbance; instead, it may initiate a vicious circle of multiple fractures. It is recommended that after an initial period of immobilization and protection of the part for three weeks, the cast be removed and the limb supported in an orthosis allowing weight-bearing and function.

Orthotic Management and Habilitation

The principal objective of orthopedic treatment of myelomeningocele is to achieve a stable posture with spine, hips, and lower limbs free of deformity, allowing the child to function at the maximal level of performance consistent with his neurologic level of involvement and intelligence.

To stand and walk, the myelomeningocele child will require the support of orthotic devices. Prerequisites for orthotic support in myelomeningocele are normal control of the head and neck, good sitting balance, and functionally adequate upper limbs for the handling of crutches. The children should possess sufficient intelligence and motivation to walk, and the parents should be cooperative. Ordinarily, any myelomeningocele child who meets these requirements is capable of some form of ambulation with an orthotic device. The purpose of the orthotic device is to compensate for the functional deficiency of the musculoskeletal system. The type of orthosis used depends upon the distribution and extent of paralysis and the need to prevent development of contractural deformities. Motor and neurophysiologic level of development and age of the patient are other determinants.

The orthosis should restrict the child's mobility as minimally as possible. The energy consumption needed for ambulation is increased with immobilization of each joint segment by an orthosis for support; therefore, the extent of orthosis prescribed should be kept to a minimum. It should be lightweight, durable, and adjustable for growth; the device should assist and not impede the activities of daily living of the child. It should be easy to apply and remove, comfortable, and cosmetically acceptable. An effective physical therapy program is vital. The orthotist should be an integral member of the team of a multidisciplinary myelomeningocele clinic. The neurosurgeon and urologist may have to be consulted in the design of the orthosis. The cost of the orthoses is usually high—requiring financial assistance from appropriate agencies and help from social workers in indigent cases.

During the first few months of life, the orthoses utilized are essentially to prevent development of contractural deformities. They primarily consist of an ankle-foot orthosis (AFO)—posterior splint—to maintain a flexible calcaneovalgus or supinated foot or an equinus ankle-foot in neutral position. Such an orthotic device does not correct a fixed deformity. The splint should be well padded to prevent pressure sores. The parents or nurses should be diligently instructed on how to place the orthosis on the child. Constant vigilance and meticulous skin care are vital.

In the infant with thoracolumbar level lesions, with flaccid paralysis of the lower limbs, it is important to place the child in a "total-body splint." This is a posterior thoracolumbosacral hip-knee-ankle-foot orthosis (TLSHKAFO), which holds each hip in 15 to 20 degrees of abduction, neutral rotation, and mild flexion (10 to 20 degrees) in the infant of three to six months; in the older infant the hips are in neutral extension-flexion and the knee-ankle-foot in neutral position. The objective of a "total-body splint" is to prevent the development of flexion–abduction–lateral rotation contracture of the hips, flexion deformity of the knees, and equinus and calcaneovarus deformities of the ankles. The "total-body splint" is used part-time only—at night and nap periods—and in conjunction with *gentle* range of motion of the joints.

The 9- to 12-month-old infant with good head, neck, and trunk control and normal function of the upper limbs is placed, for several hours a day, in the caster cart (or some other similar device). The caster cart, developed at the Ontario Crippled Children's Center, is a simple mobility aid, enabling the child with paralysis of the lower limbs to move around by turning the wheels of the cart (Fig. 5–110). It enhances motor strength of the upper limbs and development of head-trunk control. The child explores his environment and plays with his peers. The caster cart may be modified by adding a small table on the cart, under which the child extends his lower limbs and plays with toys placed on the table. When the child attempts to pull himself up, showing an interest in standing, he is fitted with a standing orthosis, such as an A-Frame or the parapodium. Upright posture opens new vistas with provision of a useful and satisfactory life, whereas recumbency will result in emaciation. In stance, bladder drainage and bowel function are better. The abdominal viscera are not pushing against the diaphragm. Breathing capacity is increased, and cardiovascular function is stimulated. Osteopenia in the lower limb bones and flexion contractural deformity of the hips and knees are prevented. Standing orthoses are particularly useful in high lumbar and thoracic level lesions. The patient can stand without crutches, liberating his upper limbs for functional activities.

The A-Frame (Fig. 5–111) is a simple standing device, made with a tubular frame in which the child with flail lower limbs can stand without crutches; however, it does not allow ambulation. The A-Frame is primarily utilized in high lumbar–low thoracic level lesions in children who have adequate control of the head, neck, and upper trunk. In cases with severe nervous system involvement and hydrocephalus, a head–neck–upper trunk extension device may be used for support.

The parapodium (Fig. 5–112) is designed to allow the child to stand without crutches and provides a limited degree of mobility. With a pivot gait pattern these children can move around without crutches. With crutches they ambulate with a swing-to or swing-through gait. Initially, the parapodium is used for brief peri-

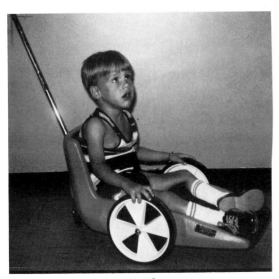

FIGURE 5–110. The caster cart.

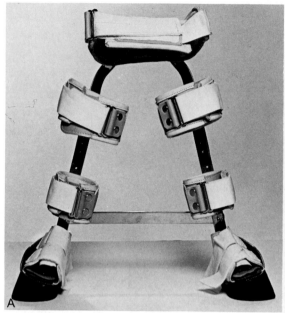

FIGURE 5–111. The A-Frame.

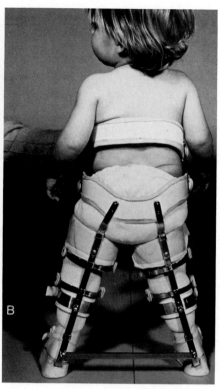

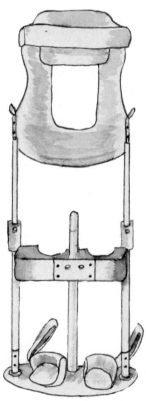

FIGURE 5–112. The parapodium.

ods, the anesthetic skin of the child being inspected for pressure sores. By unlocking the knees the child in the parapodium can sit.

The child with poor upper limb function but good head, neck, and trunk control may be fitted with the Shrewbury Swivel Walker.[388, 495] This rigid device allows rotation of the upper trunk with arm movement, achieving swivel ambulation with minimal energy requirements.

When the child is about two years of age and has been in the standing orthosis for a period of three to six months, his support needs by orthosis are reassessed. With growth and development the child gains balance, increases the motor strength of his upper limbs and trunk extensors, and achieves stable sitting balance. At this time the type of orthosis prescribed depends upon his neurosegmental level of involvement.

The child with a *thoracic level lesion* is unable to sit without support because of weak trunk musculature. A spine support is required for sitting. These children will be sitters and not walkers. It is crucial that the management plan be realistic. Upright posture can be provided, and during childhood these patients can achieve short periods of household ambulation with assistance and encouragement. Psychologic and physiologic benefits derived from upright posture and nonfunctional ambulation dictate a positive approach during the early developmental years of the child. This should be carried out with the understanding that in adolescence these patients will be wheelchair bound. The orthosis prescribed in thoracic level lesions should be a thoracolumbosacral–hip-knee-ankle-foot orthosis (TLSHKAFO) with a butterfly pelvic band, drop-lock hip and knee joints, and rigid ankles. By unlocking the hips and knees, these patients can sit.

In *upper lumbar level lesions* the hip flexors are present but hip extensors are absent. These patients with hip flexion power are fitted with a reciprocating gait orthosis (Fig. 5–113). In this device a cable extends from the thigh upright to the pelvic portion, crossing posteriorly to the hip joint axis; thereby, an extensor moment is provided, check reining hip flexion in stance. With loss of hip extensor control due to paralysis of the gluteus maximus the hips go into hyperflexion and the lumbar spine into lordosis, unless such an extensor force is provided by the orthosis. The orthosis is so designed that active flexion of one hip obligatorily extends the contralateral hip by the tension on the cable mechanism. The pelvis and thorax are stabilized and prevented from falling forward about the hip joint axis. The reciprocating gait orthosis is a flexion-driven hip extension orthosis. With crutches the patient walks with a reciprocating gait pattern by flexing one hip at a time. Activation of both hip flexors allows for a swing-through gait. Release of the cable allows bilateral hip flexion for sitting. The design of the orthosis allows stance with crutches. Accurate fit is essential. Adequate balance is critical; tall and obese patients have more difficulty in walking than do short, thin patients. A double-cable system is available for patients whose hips are hyperextensible.

In *low lumbar level lesions* the quadriceps femoris, hip flexors, and hamstrings are usually fair or better in motor strength. When the child is three to four years of age or older an ankle-foot orthosis (AFO) is prescribed for ambulation. In the younger child one often has to begin with a hip-knee-ankle-foot orthosis (HKAFO) and then remove the components of the orthosis cephalocaudally. Control of rotation of the lower limbs is often a problem following removal of the pelvic band. This is controlled by rotational straps or twister cables. The type of ankle joint of the orthosis depends upon the motor picture: For example, when the leg is totally flail a rigid ankle is given, whereas if the

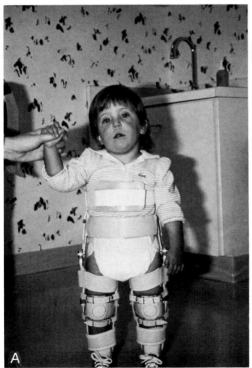 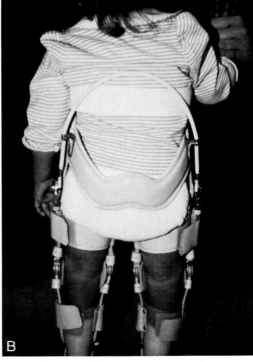

FIGURE 5–113. The reciprocating gait orthosis.

A and **B**. Anterior and posterior views of orthosis.

toe extensors and anterior tibial are normal, but the triceps surae is paralyzed, a plantar flexion assist ankle joint is prescribed.

In neurosegmental level lesions L5 or distal, patients may ambulate without crutches or external support; however, for long-distance walking crutches or canes are advisable.

In first sacral level involvement, triceps surae motor strength is weak, causing the patient to walk with a knee-hip flexion "crouched" posture. In this situation an AFO can block dorsiflexion of the ankle and improve the posture.

Obesity will present a formidable handicap to the myelomeningocele child, as it increases the amount of effort required for physical activity. It should be avoided by strict dietary control.

The use of wheelchairs should be discouraged for routine activities of daily living. However, when long distances beyond the functional competence of the patient are to be traveled, the use of a wheelchair is indicated. A wheelchair is a practical necessity when the level of paralysis is at the twelfth thoracic or first lumbar neurosegmental level.

The type of wheelchair provided should meet the individual requirements of the patient. Its size should be carefully measured. The seat is an important consideration in the design of the wheelchair utilized. Abnormal pressure on the trochanters, ischium, and sacrum should be avoided by the use of special cushions. The backrest should provide adequate trunk support. In patients with poor head and neck control, special head supports are given. The armrests should be detachable. Electric-powered wheelchairs are preferred over those that are manually propelled. The patient should have adequate intellect to understand the proper operation of the wheelchair.

The shuttlebug, hand cycles, and walkers are other mobility aids that are used as indicated.

References

1. Abraham, E., Verinder, D. G. R., and Sharrard, W. J. W.: The treatment of flexion contracture of the knee in myelomeningocele. J. Bone Joint Surg., 59-B:433, 1977.
2. Adams, M. M., Greenberg, F., Khoury, M. J., Marks, J., and Oakley, G. P., Jr.: Trends in clinical characteristics of infants with spina bifida—Atlanta, 1972–1979. Am. J. Dis. Child., 139:514, 1985.
3. Adams, M. M., Greenberg, F., Khoury, M. J., Marks, J., and Oakley, G. P., Jr.: Survival of infants with spina bifida—Atlanta, 1972–1979. Am. J. Dis. Child., 139:518, 1985.
4. Allen, B. L., Jr., and Ferguson, R. L.: The operative treatment of myelomeningocele spinal deformity—1979. Orthop. Clin. North Am., 10:845, 1979.
5. Alliaume, A.: Fractures des os longs dans les myelomeningoceles. Arch. Fr. Pediatr., 7:294, 1950.
6. Alter, M.: Anencephalus, hydrocephalus, and spina bifida. Arch. Neurol., 7:411, 1962.
7. Altman, B.: Care of children with spina bifida (letter). Am. J. Dis. Child., 136:280, 1982.
8. Ames, M. D., and Schut, L.: Results of treatment of 171 consecutive myelomeningoceles—1963 to 1968. Pediatrics, 50:466, 1970.
9. Anderson, E. M.: Cognitive deficits in children with spina bifida and hydrocephalus: A review of the literature. Br. J. Educ. Psychol., 43:257, 1973.
10. Anderson, E. M. P.: Impairment of a motor skill in children with spina bifida cystica and hydrocephalus. An exploratory study. Br. J. Psychol., 68:61, 1977.
11. Anderson, E.: The psychological and social adjustment of adolescents with cerebral palsy or spina bifida and hydrocephalus. Int. J. Rehabil. Res., 2:245, 1979.
12. Anderson, E. M., and Spain, B.: The Child with Spina Bifida. London, Methuen, 1977.
13. Anderson, T. E., Drummond, D. S., Breed, A. L., and Taylor, C. A.: Malignant hyperthermia in myelomeningocele: A previously unreported association. J. Pediatr. Orthop., 1:401, 1981.
14. Angle, C. R., Trembath, E. J., and Strond, W. L.: The myelodysplasia and hydrocephalus program in Nebraska: A 15 year review of costs and benefits. Nebr. Med. J., 62:391, 1977.
15. Anschuetz, R. H., Freehafer, A. A., Shaffer, J. W., and Dixon, M. S., Jr.: Severe fracture complications in myelodysplasia. J. Pediatr. Orthop., 4:22, 1984.
16. Aprin, H., and Kilfoye, R. M.: Extension contracture of the knee in patients with myelomeningocele. Clin. Orthop., 144:260, 1979.
17. Aristotle: Politics. In McKeon, R. (ed.): The Basic Works of Aristotle. New York, Random House, 1941.
18. Arregui, J., Cannon, B., Murray, J., and O'Leary, J. J.: Long-term evaluation of ischiectomy in the treatment of pressure ulcers. Plast. Reconstr. Surg., 36:583, 1965.
19. Arvidsson, J.: Children with myelomeningocele in a Swedish county. Current status after 15 years' treatment and future prospects. Lakartidningen, 76:4625, 1979.
20. Asher, M., and Olson, J.: Factors affecting the ambulatory status of patients with spina bifida cystica. J. Bone Joint Surg., 65-A:350, 1983.
21. Babbitt, A., and Dias, L. S.: Surgical treatment of talipes equino-varus in spina bifida. Myelomeningocele Seminar, Chicago, 1981.
22. Balog, B., and Skinner, S. R.: Unilateral duplication of the femur associated with myelomeningocele. J. Pediatr. Orthop., 4:488, 1984.
23. de Backer, E.: Spina bifida. Viewpoint of the urologist. Acta Orthop. Belg., 43:271, 1977.
24. Badell-Ribera, A., Shulman, K., and Paddock, N.: The relationship of non-progressive hydrocephalus to intellectual functioning in children with spina bifida cystica. Arch. Phys. Med., 45:443, 1964.
25. Bahnson, D. H.: Myelomeningocele and its problems. Pediatr. Annu., 11:528, 1982.
26. Bailey, B. N.: Bedsores, London, E. Arnold, 1967.
27. Baker, R. H., and Sharrard, W. J. W.: Correction of lordoscoliosis in spina bifida by multiple spinal osteotomy and fusion with Dwyer fixation: A preliminary report. Dev. Med. Child Neurol. (Suppl.), 29:12, 1973.
28. Banta, J. V., and Hamada, J. S.: Natural history of the kyphotic deformity in myelomeningocele. Proceedings of the Western Orthopedic Association. J. Bone Joint Surg., 58-A:279, 1976.
29. Banta, J. V., and Nichols, O.: Autogenous fibular subtalar arthrodesis in myelodysplasia. J. Bone Joint Surg., 55:1317, 1973.

30. Banta, J. V., and Park, S. M.: Improvement in pulmonary function in patients having combined anterior and posterior spinal fusion for myelomeningocele scoliosis. Spine, 8:765, 1983.

31. Banta, J. V., Sutherland, D. H., and Wyatt, M.: Anterior tibial transfer to the os calcis with Achilles tenodesis for calcaneal deformity in myelomeningocele. J. Pediatr. Orthop., 1:125, 1981.

32. Banta, J. V., Whiteman, S., Dyck, P. M., Hartleip, D. L., and Gilbert, D.: Fifteen year review of myelodysplasia. J. Bone Joint Surg., 58-A:726, 1976.

33. Barden, G. A., Meyer, L. C., and Stelling, F. H.: Myelodysplastics: Fate of those followed for twenty years or more. J. Bone Joint Surg., 57-A:643, 1975.

34. Barr, J. S.: Poliomyelitic hip deformity and the erector spinae transplant. J.A.M.A., 144:813, 1950.

35. Barson, A. J.: Spina bifida: The significance of the level and extent of the defect to the morphogenesis. Dev. Med. Child Neurol., 12:129, 1970.

36. Bassett, G. S., Weinstein, S. L., and Cooper, R. R.: Long-term follow-up of the fascia lata transfer for paralytic hip in myelodysplasia. Detroit, American Academy of Cerebral Palsy and Developmental Medicine, 1981.

37. Bauer, H., and Vojta, V.: Rehabilitation in the meningomyelodysplasias. Monatsschr. Kinderheilkd., 127:351, 1979.

38. Bauer, S. B., Labib, K. B., Dieppa, R. A., and Retik, A. B.: Urodynamic evaluation of boy with myelodysplasia and incontinence. Urology, 10:354, 1977.

39. Bauer, S. B., Colodny, A. H., and Retik, A. B.: The management of vesicoureteral reflux in children with myelodysplasia. J. Urol., 128:102, 1982.

40. Baumann, J. U., and Gross, R. H.: The treatment of the feet in meningomyelocele. Helv. Paediatr. Acta, 33:217, 1978.

41. Bazih, J., and Gross, R. H.: Hip surgery in the lumbar level myelomeningocele patient. J. Pediatr. Orthop., 1:405, 1981.

42. Beal, S.: The occurrence of spina bifida cystica in South Australia. Med. J. Aust., 2:597, 1967.

43. Benton, I. J., Salvati, E. A., and Root, L.: Reconstructive surgery in the myelomeningocele hip. Clin. Orthop. Rel. Res., 110:261, 1975.

44. Birch, R.: Surgery of the knee in children with spina bifida. Dev. Med. Child Neurol. (Suppl. 37), 18:111, 1976.

45. Blockey, N. J.: Aids for crippled children. Dev. Med. Child Neurol., 13:216, 1971.

46. Bluestone, S. S., and Deaver, G. G.: Habilitation of the child with spina bifida and myelomeningocele. J.A.M.A., 161:1248, 1956.

47. Blum, R. W.: The adolescent with spina bifida. Clin. Pediatr. (Phil.), 22:331, 1983.

48. Bodeker, J., and Nagel, R.: Intravesical and intraurethral pressure studies: Significance for the prognosis and the treatment of children with myelomeningocele. Urologe, 16:258, 1977.

49. Bonde, J., Mitrofanoff, P., and Lefort, J.: Treatment of myelomeningocele. A reassessment. Arch. Fr. Pediatr., 34:820, 1977.

50. Bonnett, C., Brown, J. C., Perry, J., et al.: Evolution of treatment of paralytic scoliosis at Rancho Los Amigos Hospital. J. Bone Joint Surg., 57:206, 1975.

51. Boothman, R.: Some observations on the management of the child with a spina bifida. Br. Med. J., 1:145, 1975.

52. Boris, M.: Increased incidence of meningomyelocele. J.A.M.A., 84:768, 1963.

53. Borjeson, M. C., Kornfalt, R., Lagergren, J., and Mortensson, W.: Children with spina bifida—report on a 10 year series. Lakartidningen, 75:3895, 1978.

54. Breed, A. L., and Healy, P. M.: The midlumbar myelomeningocele hip: mechanism of dislocation and treatment. J. Pediatr. Orthop., 2:15, 1982.

55. Breed, A. L., Ibler, I., and Etlanger, P.: The motorized wheelchair: New freedom, new responsibility, new problems in transportation. Dev. Med. Child Neurol., 23:113, 1981.

56. Brock, D. J., and Sutcliffe, R. G.: Alphafetoprotein in the antenatal diagnosis of anencephaly and spina bifida. Lancet, 2:197, 1972.

57. Brocklehurst, G.: Spina bifida for the clinician. Clin. Dev. Med., No. 57. London, Heinemann, 1976.

58. Brocklehurst, G., Gleave, J. R. W., and Lewin, W. S.: Early closure of myelomeningocele with special reference to leg movement. Dev. Med. Child Neurol., 13:51, 1967.

59. Brookes, M., and Wardle, E. N.: Muscle action and the shape of the femur. J. Bone Joint Surg., 44-B:398, 1962.

60. Brooks, A. L., and Saunders, E. A.: Fusion of the ankle in denervated extremities. South. Med. J., 60:30, 1967.

61. Broome, H. L., and Basmajian, J. V.: Survival of iliopsoas muscle after Sharrard procedure. An electromyographic study. Am. J. Phys. Med., 50:301, 1971.

62. Brown, H. P.: Management of spinal deformity in myelomeningocele. Orthop. Clin. North Am., 9:391, 1978.

63. Brunt, D.: Characteristics of upper limb movements in a sample of meningomyelocele children. Percept. Mot. Skills, 51:431, 1980.

64. Brunt, D.: Predictive factors of perceptual motor ability in children with meningomyelocele. Am. Correct. Ther. J., 35:42, 1981.

65. Buisson, J. S., and Hamblen, D. L.: Electromyographic activity of the transplanted iliopsoas in spina bifida cystica. J. Bone Joint Surg., 54-A:752, 1972.

66. Bunch, W. H.: The Milwaukee brace in paralytic scoliosis. Clin. Orthop., 110:63, 1975.

67. Bunch, W. H.: Treatment of the myelomeningocele spine. A.A.O.S. Instr. Course Lect., 25:93, 1976.

68. Bunch, W. H.: Myelomeningocele. In Lovell, W. W., and Winter, R. B. (eds.): Pediatric Orthopedics. Philadelphia, J. B. Lippincott, 1978, p. 381.

69. Bunch, W. M., Cas, A. S., Bensman, A. S., and Long, D. M. (eds.): Modern Management of Meningomyelocele. St. Louis, Warren H. Green, 1972.

70. Bunch, W. M., Cas, A. S., and Long, D. M.: Habilitation of the child with myelomeningocele. In Bunch, W. M., Cas, A. S., Bensman, A. S., and Long, D. M. (eds.): Modern Management of Myelomeningocele. St. Louis, Warren H. Green, 1972.

71. Bunch, W. M., and Hakala, M. W.: Iliopsoas transfers in children with myelomeningocele. J. Bone Joint Surg., 66:224, 1984.

72. Bunch, W. M., Scarff, T. B., and Dvonch, V.: Progressive neurological loss in myelomeningocele patients. Orthop. Trans., 5:32, 1981.

73. Burkus, J. K., Moore, D. W., and Raycroft, J. F.: Valgus deformity of the ankle in myelodysplastic patients. Correction by stapling of the medial part of the distal tibial physis. J. Bone Joint Surg., 65-A:1157, 1983.

74. Burney, D. W., and Hasma, W. R.: Spina bifida with myelomeningocele. Clin. Orthop., 30:167, 1963.

75. Butler-Smythe, A. C.: Spina bifida and hydrocephalus occurring in the same family. Lancet, 1:272, 1889.

76. Byrne, R. R., and Larson, L. J.: Hip instability in myelodysplasia. Clin. Orthop., 127:150, 1977.

77. Cameron, A. H.: The spinal cord lesion in spina bifida cystica. Lancet, 2:171, 1956.

78. Cameron, A. H.: Arnold-Chiari and other neuroanatomical malformations associated with spina bifida. J. Pathol. Bacteriol., 73:195, 1957.

79. Campbell, J. B.: Congenital anomalies of the neural axis. Surgical management based on embryological considerations. Am. J. Surg., 75:231, 1948.

80. Canale, S. T., Hammond, N. L., Cotler, J. M., and

Sneddon, H. E.: Pelvic displacement osteotomy for chronic hip dislocation in myelodysplasia. J. Bone Joint Surg., 57-A:177, 1975.

81. Carlioz, H., de la Caffiniere, J. Y., and Queneau, P.: 22 psoas transplantations by Sharrard's method. Rev. Chir. Orthop. (Suppl. 1), 57:187, 1971.

82. Carmel, P. W.: The Arnold-Chiari malformation. *In* McLaurin, R. L., and Epstein, F. (eds.): Pediatric Neurosurgery: Surgery of the Developing Nervous System. New York, Grune & Stratton, 1982, pp. 61–77.

83. Carr, J., Halliwell, M. D., and Pearson, A. M.: Educational attainments of spina bifida children attending ordinary or special schools. Spec. Educ. Forward Trends, 10:22, 1983.

84. Carr, T. L.: Orthopaedic aspects of one hundred cases of spina bifida. Postgrad. Med. J., 32:201, 1956.

85. Carroll, N.: The orthotic management of the spina bifida child. Clin. Orthop., 102:108, 1974.

86. Carroll, N. C.: The orthotic management of spina bifida children. Present status—future goals. Prosthet. Orthot. Int., 1:39, 1977.

87. Carroll, N. C.: Hip instability in children with myelomeningocele. Orthop. Clin. North Am., 9:403, 1978.

88. Carroll, N. C., Jones, D., Maschuich, W., Milner, M., and White, C.: Evaluation pertinent to the gait of children with myelomeningocele. Prosthet. Orthot. Int., 6:27, 1982.

89. Carroll, N. C., and Sharrard, W. J.: Long-term followup of posterior iliopsoas transplantation for paralytic dislocation of the hip. J. Bone Joint Surg., 54-A:551, 1972.

90. Carter, C. O.: Spina bifida and anencephaly: A problem in genetic-environmental interaction. J. Biol. Sci., 1:71, 1969.

91. Carter, C. O.: Genetics of common simple malformations. Br. Med. Bull., 32:21, 1976.

92. Carter, C. O., and Evans, K.: Children of adult survivors with spina bifida cystica. Lancet, 2:924, 1973.

93. Carter, C. O., and Evans, K.: Spina bifida and anencephalus in Greater London. J. Med. Genet., 10:209, 1973.

94. Carter, C. O., Evans, K. A., and Till, K.: Spinal dysraphism: A genetic relation to neural tube malformation. J. Med. Genet., 13:343, 1976.

95. Carter, C. O., and Fraser Roberts, J. A.: The risk of recurrence after two children with central nervous system malformation. Lancet, 1:306, 1967.

96. Center for Disease Control, Valproic Acid and Spina Bifida: A preliminary report—France. M.M.W.R., 31(42):565, 1982.

97. Chakour, K.: Deformities of the lower extremities and prosthetic devices in children with myelodysplasia. Arch. Orthop. Unfall-Chir., 70:101, 1971.

98. Channon, G. M., and Jenkins, D. H.: Aggressive surgical treatment of secondary spinal deformity in spina bifida children—Is it worthwhile? Z. Kinderchir., 34:395, 1981.

99. Charney, E. B., Rosenblum, M., and Finegold, D.: Linear growth in a population of children with myelomeningocele. Z. Kinderchir., 34:415, 1981.

100. Charney, E. B., Weller, S. C., Sutton, L. N., Bruce, D. A., and Schut, L. B.: Management of the newborn with myelomeningocele: Time for decision-making process. Pediatrics, 75:58, 1985.

101. Chiari, K.: Medial displacement osteotomy of the pelvis. Clin. Orthop., 98:55, 1974.

102. Childs, V.: Physiotherapy for spina bifida. Physiotherapy, 63:281, 1977.

103. Cholmeley, J. A.: Elmslie's operation for the calcaneus foot. J. Bone Joint Surg., 35-B:46, 1953.

104. Chrystal, M., and Hershey, L. S.: Total rehabilitation in relation to spina bifida. Phys. Ther. Rev., 31:357, 1951.

105. Chuinard, E. G., and Peterson, R. E.: Distraction-compression bone-graft arthrodesis of the ankle: A method especially applicable in children. J. Bone Joint Surg., 45-A:481, 1963.

106. Clairbois, J.: Orthopedic deformations of the hips in a child with myelomeningocele. Acta Orthop. Belg., 43:289, 1977.

107. Clairbois, J.: Surgical treatment of deformations of the hip in children with myelomeningocele. Acta Orthop. Belg., 43:317, 1977.

108. Clarke, C. A., McKendrick, O. M., and Sheppard, P. M.: Spina bifida and potatoes. Br. Med. J., 3:251, 1973.

109. Clark, J. A., Hsu, L. C. S., and Yau, A. C. M. C.: Viscoelastic behaviour of deformed spines under correction with halo pelvic distraction. Clin. Orthop., 110:90, 1975.

110. Clark, M. W., D'Ambrosia, R. D., and Ferguson, A. B., Jr.: Congenital vertical talus. Treatment by open reduction and navicular excision. J. Bone Joint Surg., 59-A:816, 1977.

111. Clarkson, J. D.: Self-catheterization training of a child with myelomeningocele (toileting independence, incontinent children). Am. J. Occup. Ther., 36:95, 1982.

112. Claussen, C. D., Lohkamp, F. W., and von Bazan, U. B.: The diagnosis of congenital spinal disorders in computed tomography (CT). Neuropaediatrie, 8:405, 1977.

113. Colgan, M. T.: The child with spinal bifida. Role of the pediatrician. Am. J. Dis. Child., 135:854, 1981.

114. Colonna, P. C.: An arthroplastic operation for congenital dislocation of the hip. A two-stage procedure. Surg. Gynecol. Obstet., 63:777, 1936.

115. Colonna, P. C.: Capsular arthroplasty for congenital dislocation of the hip: Indications and technique, some long-term results. J. Bone Joint Surg., 47-A:437, 1965.

116. Committee on Prosthetics Research and Development. The Child with an Orthopedic Disability, His Orthotic Needs and How to Meet Them. Washington, D.C., National Academy of Sciences, 1973.

117. Corcoran, P. J., Jebsen, R. H., Brengelmann, G. I., and Simons, B. C.: Effects of plastic and metal braces on speed and energy cost of hemiparetic ambulation. Arch. Phys. Med. Rehabil., 51:69, 1970.

118. Cotta, H., Parsch, K., and Schulitz, K. P.: The treatment of lumbar kyphosis in spina bifida cystica. Z. Orthop., 108:567, 1971.

119. Crooks, K. K., and Enrile, B. G.: Comparison of the ileal conduit and clean intermittent catheterization for myelomeningocele. Pediatrics, 72:203, 1983.

120. Crooks, K. K., Enrile, B. G., and Wise, H. A.: The results of clean intermittent catheterization on the abnormal upper urinary tracts of children with myelomeningocele. Ohio State Med. J., 77:377, 1981.

121. Cruess, R. L., and Turner, N. S.: Paralysis of hip abductor muscles in spina bifida. Results of treatment by the Mustard procedure. J. Bone Joint Surg., 52-A:1364, 1970.

122. Curtis, B. H.: The hip in the myelomeningocele child. Clin. Orthop., 90:11, 1973.

123. Curtis, P. E., and Fisher, R. L.: Congenital hyperextension with anterior subluxation of the knee. J. Bone Joint Surg., 51-A:255, 1969.

124. Darling, R. B.: Parents, physicians, and spina bifida. Hastings Cent. Rep., 7:10, 1977.

125. Davidson, R. G., and Sheffield, L. J.: Hazards of perinatal detection of neural tube defects by screening material serum for alpha fetoprotein. Can. Med. Assoc., 118:1186, 1978.

126. DeBruyere, M., Kulakowski, S., Malchaire, J., Delire, M., and Sokal, G.: HLA gene and haplotype frequencies in spina bifida. Population and family studies. Tissue Antigens, 10:399, 1977.

127. de Ruysch, F., and Morgani, G. B.: Anatomic and path-theories, terms. Considerations generales et ob-

servations particulaires sur le spina bifida. J. Med., 27:162, 1806.

128. DeSouza, L. J., and Carroll, N. C.: Paralysis of hip abductor muscles in spina bifida: Results of treatment by the Mustard procedure. J. Bone Joint Surg., 52:1364, 1970.

129. DeSouza, L. J., and Carroll, N. C.: Ambulation of the braced myelomeningocele patient. J. Bone Joint Surg., 58-A:1112, 1976.

130. DeVries, E.: Spina bifida occulta and myelo-dysplasia with unilateral clubfoot beginning in adult life. Am. J. Med. Sci., 175:365, 1928.

131. Dias, L. S.: Ankle valgus in children with myelomeningocele. Dev. Med. Child Neurol., 20:627, 1978.

132. Dias, L. S.: Surgical management of knee contractures in myelomeningocele. J. Pediatr. Orthop., 2:127, 1982.

133. Dias, L. S., and Hill, J. A.: Evaluation of treatment of hip subluxation in myelomeningocele by intertrochanteric varus derotation femoral osteotomy. Orthop. Clin. North Am., 11:31, 1980.

134. Dias, L. S., Jasty, M. J., and Collins, P.: Rotational deformities of the lower limbs in myelomeningocele. J. Bone Joint Surg., 66-A:215, 1984.

135. Dibbell, D. G., McCraw, J. B., and Edstrom, L. E.: Providing useful and protective sensibility to the sitting area in patients with meningomyelocele. Plast. Reconstr. Surg., 64:796, 1979.

136. Dippe, K., and Parsch, K.: Treatment of knee joint deformities in spina bifida. Helv. Paediatr. Acta, 33:205, 1978.

137. Donaldson, W. F.: Hip problems in the child with myelomeningocele. American Academy of Orthopedic Surgeons Symposium on Myelomeningocele. St. Louis, C. V. Mosby Co., 1972, p. 176.

138. Doran, P. A., and Guthkelch, A. N.: Studies in spina bifida cystica. I. General survey and reassessment of the problem. J. Neurol. Neurosurg. Psychiatry, 24:331, 1961.

139. Doran, P. A., and Guthkelch, A. N.: Studies on spina bifida. IV. The frequency and extent of the paralysis. J. Neurol. Neurosurg. Psychiatry, 26:545, 1963.

140. Dorner, S.: The relationship of physical handicap to stress in families with an adolescent with spina bifida. Dev. Med. Child Neurol., 17:765, 1975.

141. Dorner, S.: Adolescents with spina bifida. How they see their situation. Arch. Dis. Child., 51:439, 1976.

142. Dorner, S., and Atwell, J. D.: Family adjustment to the early loss of a baby born with spina bifida. Dev. Med. Child Neurol., 27:461, 1985.

143. Dowrick, P. W., and Dove, C.: The use of self-modeling to improve the swimming performance of spina bifida children. J. Appl. Behav. Anal., 13:51, 1980.

144. Drabu, J., and Walker, G.: Stiffness after fractures around the knee in spina bifida. J. Bone Joint Surg., 67-B:266, 1985.

145. Drago, J. R., Wellner, L., Sanford, E. J., and Rohner, T. J., Jr.: The role of intermittent catheterization in the management of children with myelomeningocele. J. Urol., 118:92, 1977.

146. Dransey, J., and Lindseth, R. E.: The polypropylene solid ankle orthosis. Orthot. Prosthet., 26:14, 1972.

147. Draycott, V.: The Draycott-Oswestry spina bifida splint. Physiotherapy, 68:154, 1982.

148. Drennan, J. C.: The role of muscles in the development of human lumbar kyphosis. Dev. Med. Child Neurol. (Suppl.), 22:33, 1970.

149. Drennan, J. C.: The hip in myelomeningocele. *In* Katz, J., and Siffert, R. (eds.): Disease of the Hip in Children. Philadelphia, J. B. Lippincott, 1973.

150. Drennan, J. C.: Management of myelomeningocele foot deformities in infancy and early childhood. A.A.O.S. Instr. Course Lect., 25:82, 1976.

151. Drennan, J. C.: Management of neonatal myelomeningocele. A.A.O.S. Instr. Course Lect., 25:65, 1976.

152. Drennan, J. C.: Orthotic management of the myelomeningocele spine. Dev. Med. Child Neurol. (Suppl. 37), 18:97, 1976.

153. Drennan, J. C.: Myelomeningocele. *In* Orthopedic Management of Neuromuscular Disorders. Philadelphia, J. B. Lippincott, 1983.

154. Drennan, J. C., and Freehafer, A. A.: Fractures of the lower extremities in paraplegic children. Clin. Orthop., 77:211, 1971.

155. Drennan, J. C., Renshaw, T. S., and Curtis, B. H.: The thoracic suspension orthosis. Clin. Orthop., 139:33, 1979.

156. Drennan, J. C., and Sharrard, W. J.: The pathological anatomy of convex pes valgus. J. Bone Joint Surg., 53-B:455, 1971.

157. Drummond, D. S., Moreau, M., and Cruess, R. L.: The results and complications of surgery for the paralytic hip and spine in myelomeningocele. J. Bone Joint Surg., 62-B:49, 1980.

158. Drummond, D. S., Moreau, M., and Cruess, R. L.: Post-operative neuropathic fractures in patients with myelomeningocele. Dev. Med. Child Neurol., 23:147, 1981.

159. Drummond, D. S., Rogala, E. J., Cruess, R., and Moreau, M.: The paralytic hip and pelvic obliquity in cerebral palsy and myelomeningocele. A.A.O.S. Instr. Course Lect., 29:7, 1979.

160. Duckworth, T., and Smith, T. W.: The treatment of paralytic convex pes valgus. J. Bone Joint Surg., 56-B:305, 1974.

161. Duncan, J. W., Lovell, W. W., Bailey, S. C., and Ransom, D.: Surgical treatment of kyphosis in myelomeningocele. J. Bone Joint Surg., 58-A:155, 1976.

162. Dupré, P. H., and Walker, G. L.: Knee problems associated with spina bifida. Dev. Med. Child Neurol. (Suppl.), 27:152, 1972.

163. Dwyer, A. F., Newton, N. C., and Sherwood, A. A.: An anterior approach to scoliosis. A preliminary report. Clin. Orthop., 62:192, 1969.

164. Dwyer, A. P.: A fatal complication of paravertebral infection and traumatic aneurysm following Dwyer instrumentation. Proceedings of the Australian Orthopedic Association. J. Bone Joint Surg., 61-B:239, 1979.

165. Dwyer, F. C.: Osteotomy of the calcaneum for pes cavus. J. Bone Joint Surg., 41-B:80, 1959.

166. Eckstein, H. B., and Vora, R. M.: Spinal osteotomy for severe kyphosis in children with myelomeningocele. J. Bone Joint Surg., 54-B:328, 1972.

167. Edvardsen, P.: Physeo-epiphyseal injuries of lower extremities in myelomeningocele. Acta Orthop. Scand., 43:550, 1972.

168. Edwards, J. H.: Congenital malformations of the central nervous system in Scotland. Br. J. Prev. Soc. Med., 12:115, 1958.

169. Eichenholtz, S. N.: Management of long bone fractures in paraplegic patients. J. Bone Joint Surg., 45-A:299, 1963.

170. Ekvall, S., Chen, I. W., and Bozian, R.: The effect of supplemental ascorbic acid on serum vitamin B12 levels in myelomeningocele patients. Am. J. Clin. Nutr., 34:1356, 1981.

171. Enrile, B. G., and Crooks, K. K.: Clean intermittent catheterization for home management in children with myelomeningocele. Clin. Pediatr., 19:743, 1980.

172. Eskelund, V., and Bartels, E. D.: Spina bifida umbalis in uniovular twins. Nord. Med., 11:2075, 1941.

173. Ette, S. I., and Adeloye, A.: Low levels of vitamins A, C, and E in Nigerian children with spina bifida cystica. Cent. Afr. J. Med., 28:116, 1982.

174. Evans, D.: Relapsed club foot. J. Bone Joint Surg., 43-B:722, 1961.

175. Evans, E. P., and Tew, B.: The energy expenditure of spina bifida children during walking and wheelchair ambulation. Z. Kinderchir., *34*:425, 1981.

176. Eyring, E. J., Wanken, J. J., and Sayers, M. P.: Spine osteotomy for kyphosis in myelomeningocele. Clin. Orthop., *88*:24, 1972.

177. Faber, L. A., and Ericksen, L. G.: Prenatal diagnosis of spina bifida. J. Iowa Med. Soc., *26*:359, 1936.

178. Feiwell, E.: Paralytic calcaneus in myelomeningocele. *In* McLaurin, R. L. (ed.): Myelomeningocele. New York, Grune & Stratton, 1977, pp. 447–460.

179. Feiwell, E.: Surgery of the hip in myelomeningocele as related to adult goals. Clin. Orthop., *148*:87, 1980.

180. Feiwell, E., Sakai, D., and Baltt, T.: The effect of hip reduction on function in patients with myelomeningocele. J. Bone Joint Surg., *60-A*:169, 1978.

181. Fisher, R. G., Uihlein, A., and Keith, H. M.: Spina bifida and cranium bifidum: Study of 530 cases. Proc. Staff Meet. Mayo Clin., *27*:33, 1952.

182. Fisher, R. L., and Schaffer, S. R.: An evaluation of calcaneal osteotomy in congenital clubfoot and other disorders. Clin. Orthop., *70*:141, 1970.

183. Fitzpatrick, W. F.: Sexual function in the paraplegic patient. Arch. Phys. Med. Rehabil., *55*:221, 1974.

184. Floyd, W., Lovell, W., and King, R. E.: The neuropathic joint. South. Med. J., *52*:563, 1959.

185. Forrest, D. M.: President's address. Spina bifida: Some problems in management. Proc. R. Soc. Med., *70*:233, 1977.

186. Forestus: Obs. Chir. Libri V, Lib. III, Obs. VII, 1610.

187. Fowler, I.: Responses of the chick neural tube in mechanically produced spina bifida. J. Exp. Zool., *123*:115, 1953.

188. Fraser, F. C.: Genetic counselling. Am. J. Hum. Genet., *26*:636, 1974.

189. Freehafer, A. A.: The treatment of myelomeningocele patients with paralytic hip deformities by iliopsoas transfer. Paraplegia, *11*:295, 1974.

190. Freehafer, A. A., Vessely, J. C., and Mack, R. P.: Iliopsoas muscle transfer in the treatment of myelomeningocele patients with paralytic hip deformities. J. Bone Joint Surg., *54-A*:1715, 1972.

191. Freeman, J. M.: Practical Management of Meningomyelocele. Baltimore, University Park Press, 1974.

192. Fry, A.: Spina bifida in binovular twins. Br. Med. J., *1*:131, 1943.

193. Fulford, G. E., and Cairns, T. P.: The problems associated with flail feet in children and treatment with orthoses. J. Bone Joint Surg., *60-B*:93, 1978.

194. Gardner, W. J.: Myelomeningocele, the results of rupture of the embryonic neural tube. Cleve. Clin. Q., *27*:88, 1960.

195. Gardner, W. J.: Myelocele: Rupture of the neural tube? Clin. Neurol. Neurosurg., *15*:57, 1968.

196. Gardner, W. J.: Etiology and pathogenesis of the development of myelomeningocele. *In* McLaurin, R. L. (ed.): Myelomeningocele. New York, Grune & Stratton, 1977, pp. 3–30.

197. Gardner, W. J.: Hydrodynamic factors in Dandy-Walker and Arnold Chiari malformation. Childs Brain, *3*:200, 1977.

198. Ger, R., and Levine, S. A.: The management of decubitus ulcers by muscle transposition. Plast. Reconstr. Surg., *58*:419, 1976.

199. Gillespie, R. B., and Wedge, J. H.: The problems of scoliosis in paraplegic children. J. Bone Joint Surg., *56-A*:1767, 1974.

200. Gillies, C. L., and Hartung, W.: Fracture of tibia in spina bifida vera. Radiology, *31*:621, 1938.

201. Gillman, J., Gilbert, C., and Gillman, T.: A preliminary report on hydrocephalus, spina bifida and other anomalies in the rat produced by trypan blue. Significance of these results in interpretation of congenital malformations following maternal rubella. S. Afr. J. Med. Sci., *13*:47, 1948.

202. Glancy, J.: A dynamic orthotic system for young meningomyeloceles: A preliminary report. Orthot. Prosthet., *30*:3, 1976.

203. Gluckman, S., and Barling, J.: Effects of a remedial program on visual-motor perception in spina bifida children. J. Genet. Psychol., *136*:195, 1980.

204. Goessens, H., and Parsch, K.: Surgical treatment of knee and foot deformities in spina bifida. Acta Orthop. Belg., *37*:216, 1971.

205. Golding, C.: Spina bifida and epiphyseal displacement. J. Bone Joint Surg., *42-B*:387, 1960.

206. Golski, A., and Menelaus, M. B.: The treatment of intoed gait in spina bifida patients by lateral transfer of the medial hamstrings. Aust. N.Z. J. Surg., *46*:157, 1976.

207. Gordon, Y. B., Kitau, M. J., Letchworth, A. T., Grudzinfkas, J. H., Usherwood, M. McD., and Chard, T.: Fetal wastage as a result of an alpha-fetoprotein screening program. Lancet, *1*:677, 1978.

208. Grace, H. J.: Prenatal screening for neural tube defects in South Africa. An assessment. S. Afr. Med. J., *22*:324, 1981.

209. Green, W. T.: Tendon transplantation in rehabilitation. J.A.M.A., *163*:1235, 1957.

210. Green, W. T., and Grice, D. S.: The management of calcaneus deformity. A.A.O.S. Instr. Course Lect., *13*:135, 1959.

211. Greene, S. A., Frank, M., Zachmann, M., and Prader, A.: Growth and sexual development in children with myelomeningocele. Eur. J. Pediatr., *144*:146, 1985.

212. Gressang, J.: Perceptual processes of children with myelomeningocele and hydrocephalus. Am. J. Occup. Ther., *28*:226, 1974.

213. Grice, D. S.: An extra-articular arthrodesis of the subastragalar joint for the correction of paralytic flat feet in children. J. Bone Joint Surg., *37*:246, 1952.

214. Griffiths, J. C., and Taylor, A. G.: The production of spinal jackets for children with spina bifida. J. Med. Eng. Technol., *4*:20, 1980.

215. Grimm, R.: Hand function and tactile perception in a sample of children with myelomeningocele. Am. J. Occup. Ther., *30*:234, 1976.

216. Gross, H. P.: Myelomeningocele in one identical twin. J. Neurosurg., *20*:439, 1963.

217. Gross, P. M., and Lyne, D.: The Grice procedure: Indications and evaluation of long-term results. Clin. Orthop., *153*:194, 1980.

218. Gross, R. H., Cox, A., Tatyrek, R., Pollay, M., and Barnes, W. A.: Early management and decision-making for the treatment of myelomeningocele. Pediatrics, *72*:450, 1983.

219. Gucker, T., III: The role of orthopaedic surgery in the long-term management of the child with spina bifida. Arch. Phys. Med. Rehabil., *45*:82, 1964.

220. Guess, R. L., and Turner, N. S.: Paralysis of hip abductor muscles in spina bifida. Results of treatment by the Mustard procedure. J. Bone Joint Surg., *52-A*:1364, 1975.

221. Gufgenheim, J. J., Gerson, L. P., Sadler, C., and Tullos, H. S.: Pathologic morphology of the acetabulum in paralytic and congenital hip instability. J. Pediatr. Orthop., *2*:397, 1982.

222. Gunberg, D. L.: Spina bifida and the Arnold-Chiari malformation in the progeny of trypan blue injected rats. Anat. Rec., *126*:343, 1956.

223. Guthkelch, A. N.: Studies in spina bifida cystica. II. When to repair the spinal defect. J. Neurol. Neurosurg. Psychiatry, *25*:137, 1962.

224. Guthkelch, A. N.: Studies in spina bifida cystica. IV. Anomalous reflexes in congenital spinal palsy. Dev. Med. Child Neurol., *6*:264, 1964.

225. Guttman, L.: Problems of treatment of pressure sores in spinal paraplegia. Br. J. Plast. Surg., 8:196, 1955.
226. Gyepes, M.: Metaphyseal and physeal injuries in children with spina bifida and myelomeningocele. A.J.R., 95:168, 1965.
227. Haddad, F. S.: Anterior sacral meningocele. Report of two cases and review of the literature. Can. J. Surg., 1:230, 1958.
228. Hagberg, B., Sjogren, I., Bensch, K., and Hadenius, A. M.: The incidence of infantile hydrocephalus in Sweden. Acta Paediatr. (Stockh.), 52:588, 1963.
229. Hall, J. E.: The anterior approach to spinal deformities. Orthop. Clin. North Am., 3:81, 1972.
230. Hall, J. E.: Current concepts review. Dwyer instrumentation in anterior fusion of the spine. J. Bone Joint Surg., 63-B:1188, 1981.
231. Hall, J. E., and Bobechko, W. P.: Advances in the management of spinal deformities in myelodysplasia. Clin. Neurol. Neurosurg., 20:164, 1973.
232. Hall, J. E., and Poitras, B.: The management of kyphosis in patients with myelomeningocele. Clin. Orthop., 128:33, 1977.
233. Hall, P. F.: Abortion of fetuses with spina bifida? (Letter). Can. Med. Assoc. J., 121:846, 1979.
234. Hall, P. V., Campbell, R. L., and Kalsbeck, J. E.: Meningomyelocele and progressive hydromyelia. J. Neurosurg., 43:457, 1975.
235. Hall, P. V., Lindseth, R. E., Campbell, R. K., and Kalsbeck, J. E.: Myelodysplasia and developmental scoliosis: A manifestation of syringomyelia. Spine, 1:50, 1976.
236. Hallock, H.: Surgical stabilization of dislocated paralytic hips: An end-result study. Surg. Gynecol. Obstet., 75:721, 1942.
237. Hamburgh, M.: The embryology of trypan blue induced abnormalities in mice. Anat. Rec., 119:409, 1954.
238. Hammock, M. K., Milhorat, T. H., and Brallier, D. R.: Computed tomography in the evaluation and management of patients with spina bifida. Z. Kinderchir., 34:334, 1981.
239. Handelsman, J. E.: Orthopaedic aspects of spina bifida cystica. South Afr. J. Surg., 9:183, 1971.
240. Hannigan, K. F.: Teaching intermittent self-catheterization to young children with myelodysplasia. Dev. Med. Child Neurol., 21:365, 1979.
241. Harris, J.: Ethical problems in the management of some severely handicapped children. J. Med. Ethics, 7:117, 1981.
242. Harrold, A. J.: Congenital vertical talus in infancy. J. Bone Joint Surg., 49-B:634, 1967.
243. Hay, M. C., and Walker, G.: Plantar pressures in healthy children and in children with myelomeningocele. J. Bone Joint Surg., 55-B:828, 1973.
244. Hayden, P. W., Davenport, S. L. H., and Campbell, M. H.: Adolescent with myelodysplasia: Impact of physical disability on emotional maturation. Pediatrics, 64:53, 1979.
245. Hayes, J. T., and Gross, H. P.: Orthopedic implications of myelodysplasias. J.A.M.A., 184:762, 1963.
246. Hayes, J. T., Gross, H. P., and Dow, S.: Surgery for paralytic defects secondary to myelomeningocele and myelodysplasia. J. Bone Joint Surg., 46-A:1577, 1964.
247. Hayes-Allen, M. C.: Obesity and short stature in children with myelomeningocele. Dev. Med. Child Neurol. (Suppl. 27), 14:59, 1972.
248. Heinz, E. R., Rosenbaum, A. E., Scarff, T. B., Reigel, D. H., and Drayer, B. P.: Tethered spinal cord following meningomyelocele repair. Radiology, 131:153, 1979.
249. Heizer, D.: Long-leg brace design for traumatic paraplegia. Phys. Ther., 47:824, 1967.
250. Herndon, C. H., and Heyman, C. H.: Problems in the recognition and treatment of congenital convex pes valgus. J. Bone Joint Surg., 45-A:413, 1963.
251. Herndon, C. H., Strong, J. M., and Heyman, C. H.: Transposition of the tibialis anterior in the treatment of paralytic talipes calcaneus. J. Bone Joint Surg., 38-A:751, 1956.
252. Herskowitz, J., and Marks, A. N.: The spina bifida patient as a person. Dev. Med. Child Neurol., 19:413, 1977.
253. Herzog, E. G., and Sharrard, W. J. W.: Calipers and braces with double hip locks. Clin. Orthop., 46:239, 1966.
254. Hewitt, D.: Geographical variations in the mortality attributed to spina bifida and other congenital malformations. Br. J. Prev. Soc. Med., 17:13, 1963.
255. Hewson, J. E.: Basic physiotherapy of spina bifida. Dev. Med. Child Neurol., 37:117, 1976.
256. Hide, D. W., Williams, H. P., and Ellis, H. L.: The outlook for the child with a myelomeningocele for whom early surgery was considered inadvisable. Dev. Med. Child Neurol., 14:304, 1972.
257. Hight, B., Redelman, K., and Hall, P. V.: Myelodysplasia: A progressive paraplegia and scoliosis. J. Neurosurg. Nurs., 8:28, 1976.
258. Hoffer, M. M., Feiwell, E., Perry, J., and Bonnett, C.: Functional ambulation in patients with myelomeningocele. J. Bone Joint Surg., 55-A:137, 1973.
259. Hoffman, H. J., Hendrick, E. B., and Humphreys, R. P.: The tethered spinal cord: Its protean manifestations, diagnosis and surgical correction. Childs Brain, 2:145, 1976.
260. Hogshead, H. P., and Ponseti, I. V.: Fascia lata transfer to the erector spinae for the treatment of flexion abductor contractures of the hip in patient with poliomyelitis and myelomeningocele. J. Bone Joint Surg., 46-A:1389, 1964.
261. Holinger, P. C., Holinger, L. D., Reichert, T. J., and Holinger, P. H.: Respiratory obstruction and apnea in infants with bilateral abductor vocal cord paralysis, myelomeningocele, hydrocephalus and Arnold-Chiari malformation. J. Pediatr., 92:368, 1978.
262. Hollingsworth, R. P.: An x-ray study of valgus ankles in spina bifida children with valgus flat foot deformity. Proc. R. Soc. Med., 68:481, 1975.
263. Hoppenfeld, S.: Congenital kyphosis in myelomeningocele. J. Bone Joint Surg., 49-B:276, 1967.
264. Huff, C. W., and Ramsey, P. L.: Myelodysplasia: The influence of the quadriceps and hip abductor muscles for ambulatory function and stability of the hips. J. Bone Joint Surg., 60-A:432, 1978.
265. Hull, W., Moe, J. H., and Winter, R. B.: Spinal deformity in myelomeningocele: Natural history, evaluation and treatment. J. Bone Joint Surg., 56-A:1767, 1974.
266. Hunt, G. M.: Spina bifida: Implications for 100 children at school. Dev. Med. Child Neurol., 23:160, 1981.
267. Hunt, G. M., and Holmes, A. E.: Factors relating to intelligence in treated cases of spina bifida cystica. Am. J. Dis. Child., 130:823, 1976.
268. Hunt, G. M., and Holmes, A. E.: Some factors relating to intelligence in treated children with spina bifida cystica. Dev. Med. Child Neurol. (Suppl. 35), 17:65, 1977.
269. Hunt, G. M., Walpole, L., Gleave, J., and Gairdner, D.: Predictive factors in open myelomeningocele with special reference to sensory level. Br. Med. J., 4:197, 1973.
270. Ingraham, F. D., and Fowler, F.: Lumbar myelomeningocele. Surg. Clin. North Am., 36:6, 1956.
271. Ingraham, F. D., and Hamlin, H.: Spina bifida and cranium bifidum. Surgical treatment. N. Engl. J. Med., 228:361, 1943.
272. Ingraham, F. D., and Swam, H.: Spina bifida and cranium bifida. I: A survey of five hundred forty-six cases. N. Engl. J. Med., 228:559, 1943.

273. Irwin, C. E.: The calcaneus foot. South. Med. J., 44:191, 1951.

274. Jackman, K. V., Nitschke, R. O., Haake, P. W., and Brown, J. A.: Variable abduction HKAFO in spina bifida patients. Orthot. Prosthet., 34:2, 329, 1980.

275. Jackson, R. D., Padgett, T. S., and Donovan, M. M.: Iliopsoas muscle transfer in myelodysplasia. J. Bone Joint Surg., 61-A:40, 1969.

276. Jackson, R. D., Padgett, T. S., and Donovan, M. M.: Posterior iliopsoas transfer in myelodysplasia. J. Bone Joint Surg., 56-A:198, 1974.

277. Jackson, R. W.: Correction of spinal curvature in paraplegics by the method of Harrington fusion. Med. Serv. J. Can., 22:486, 1966.

278. Jaeger, R.: Congenital spinal meningocele. J.A.M.A., 153:792, 1953.

279. James, C. C. M.: Fractures of the lower limb in spina bifida cystica: A survey of 44 fractures in 122 children. Dev. Med. Child Neurol., 22:88, 1970.

280. Jansen, J.: Spina bifida: Epidemiological data from a pilot study. Acta Neurol. Scand., 57:193, 1978.

281. Japas, L. M.: Surgical treatment of pes cavus by tarsal V osteotomy: Preliminary report. J. Bone Joint Surg., 58-A:927, 1968.

282. Jeffries, J. S., Killam, P. E., and Varni, J. W.: Behavioral management of fecal incontinence in a child with myelomeningocele. Pediatr. Nurs., 8:267, 1982.

283. Johnson, J. T. H., and Robinson, R. A.: Anterior strut grafts for severe kyphosis: Results of three cases with a preceding progressive paraplegia. Clin. Orthop., 56:25, 1968.

284. Jones, C. C. M., and Lassman, L. P.: Spinal Dysraphism. London, Butterworth, 1972.

285. Jones, G. B.: Paralytic dislocation of the hip. J. Bone Joint Surg, 36-B:375, 1954.

286. Jones, G. B.: Paralytic dislocation of the hip. J. Bone Joint Surg, 44-B:573, 1962.

287. Jones, J. D. L., and Evans, T. G.: Anterior sacral meningocele. J. Obstet. Gynaecol., 66:477, 1959.

288. Jones, T.: Spina bifida occulta: No paralytic symptoms until 17 years of age—spine trephined to relieve pressure on the cauda equina: Recovery. Br. Med. J., 1:173, 1891.

289. Josephson, J. F., and Waller, K. B.: Anencephaly in identical twin. Can. Med. Assoc. J., 29:34, 1933.

290. Kahanovitz, N., and Suncan, J. W.: The role of scoliosis and pelvic obliquity on functional disability in myelomeningocele. Spine, 6:494, 1981.

291. Kaplan, W. E., and Firlit, C. F.: Management of reflux in the myelodysplastic child. J. Urol., 129:1195, 1983.

292. Kaufmann, J.: Orthopedic aspects in the care of children with spina bifida. Padiatr. Grenzgeb., 14:115, 1975.

293. Katsen, M., Handelsman, J. E., Costas, S., and Schneier, N.: Experience in a spinal defects clinic. S. Afr. Med. J., 47:1912, 1973.

294. Kazak, A. E., and Clark, M. W.: Stress in families of children with myelomeningocele. Dev. Med. Child Neurol., 28:220, 1986.

295. Keats, S., and Morgese, A. N.: A simple anteromedial approach to the lesser trochanter of the femur for the release of the iliopsoas tendon. J. Bone Joint Surg., 49-A:632, 1967.

296. Kilfoyle, R. M., Foley, J. J., and Norton, P. L.: The spine and pelvic deformity in childhood and adolescent paraplegia. J. Bone Joint Surg., 47-A:659, 1965.

297. Knox, E. G.: Spina bifida in Birmingham. Dev. Med. Child Neurol., 13:14, 1967.

298. Kopits, S.: Orthopedic aspects of myelomeningocele. In Freeman, J. M. (ed.): Practical Management of Myelomeningocele. Baltimore, University Park Press, 1974, pp. 105–106.

299. Kowalski, M.: The place of orthopedic surgery in early rehabilitation of children with spina bifida. Acta Orthop. Belg., 43:297, 1977.

300. Kumar, S. J., Cowell, H. R., and Townsend, P.: Physeal, metaphyseal, and diaphyseal injuries of the lower extremities in children with myelomeningocele. J. Pediatr. Orthop., 4:25, 1984.

301. Kumar, S. J., and Townsend, P.: Posterolateral spinal fusion for the treatment of scoliosis in myelodysplasia. J. Pediatr. Orthop., 2:514, 1982.

302. Kupka, J., Rey, O. T., Geddes, N., and Carroll, N. C.: Developmental landmarks in spina bifida. Orthop. Clin. North Am., 9:97, 1978.

303. Langenskiöld, A.: Supination deformity of the forefoot. Acta Orthop. Scand., 48:325, 1977.

304. Laurence, E. R., Tew, B. J., and Jenkins, D. H.: Family reactions to surgical correction for kyphoscoliosis in spina bifida children: A preliminary report. Z. Kinderchir., 34:398, 1981.

305. Laurence, K. M.: The natural history of spina bifida cystica. Proc. R. Soc. Med., 53:1055, 1960.

306. Laurence, K. M.: New thoughts on spina bifida and hydrocephalus. Dev. Med. Child Neurol., 5:68, 1963.

307. Laurence, K. M.: The natural history of spina bifida cystica: Detailed analysis of 407 cases. Arch. Dis. Child., 39:41, 1964.

308. Laurence, K. M.: The survival of untreated spina bifida cystica. Dev. Med. Child Neurol. (Suppl. 11), 8:10, 1966.

309. Laurence, K. M.: The recurrence risk in spina bifida cystica and anencephaly. Dev. Med. Child Neurol., 20:23, 1969.

310. Laurence, K. M.: Vertebral abnormalities in first degree relatives of cases of spina bifida and of anencephaly. Arch. Dis. Child., 45:274, 1970.

311. Laurence, K. M.: Impact of antenatal diagnosis for central nervous system malformation in high-risk pregnancies and pregnancy screening in a high-risk community. Z. Kinderchir. Grenzgb., 22:383, 1977.

312. Laurence, K. M., Carter, C. O., and David, P. A.: Major central nervous system malformations in South Wales. Br. J. Prevent. Soc. Med., 22:146, 212, 1968.

313. Laurence, K. M., and Tew, B.: Follow-up of 65 survivors from the 425 cases of spina bifida born in South Wales between 1956 and 1962. Dev. Med. Child Neurol., 13:1, 1968.

314. Laurence, K. M., and Tew, B. J.: Natural history of spina bifida cystica and cranium bifida cysticum. Major central nervous system malformations in South Wales. Arch. Dis. Child., 46:127, 1971.

315. Layde, P. M., Edmonds, L. D., and Erickson, J. D.: Maternal fever and neural tube defects. Teratology, 21:105, 1980.

316. Leatherman, K. D., and Dickson, R. A.: Congenital kyphosis in myelomeningocele. Vertebral body resection and posterior spine fusion. Spine, 3:222, 1978.

317. Lee, E. H., and Carroll, N. C.: Hip stability and ambulatory status in myelomeningocele. J. Pediatr. Orthop., 5:522, 1985.

318. Letts, R. M., Fulford, R., and Hobson, D. A.: Mobility aids for the paraplegic child. J. Bone Joint Surg., 58-A:38, 1976.

319. Levitt, R. L., Canale, S. T., and Gartland, J. J.: Surgical correction of foot deformity in the older patient with myelomeningocele. Orthop. Clin. North Am., 5:19, 1974.

320. Lichtblau, S.: A medial and lateral release operation for a clubfoot. J. Bone Joint Surg., 55-A:1377, 1973.

321. Light, K., and van Blerk, P. J.: Causes of renal deterioration in patients with myelomeningocele. Br. J. Urol., 49:257, 1977.

322. Lindseth, R. E.: Treatment of the lower extremity in children paralyzed by myelomeningocele. A.A.O.S. Instr. Course Lect., 25:76, 1976.

323. Lindseth, R. E.: Posterior iliac osteotomy for fixed pelvic obliquity. J. Bone Joint Surg., 60-A:17, 1978.

324. Lindseth, R. E., and Glancy, J.: Polypropylene lower-extremity braces for paraplegia due to myelomeningocele. J. Bone Joint Surg., 56-A:556, 1974.

325. Lindseth, R. E., Hall, P., and DeSousa, C. R.: The effects of ventricular shunting on developmental scoliosis in myelomeningocele patients. Presented at Scoliosis Research Society, Seattle, 1979.

326. Lindseth, R. E., and Stelzer, L., Jr.: Vertebral excision for kyphosis in children with myelomeningocele. J. Bone Joint Surg., 61-A:699, 1979.

327. London, J. T., and Nichols, O.: Paralytic dislocation of the hip in myelodysplasia. J. Bone Joint Surg., 57-A:501, 1975.

328. Lorber, J.: Incidence and epidemiology of myelomeningocele. Clin. Orthop., 45:81, 1966.

329. Lorber, J.: Neurologic assessment of neonates with spina bifida. Clin. Pediatr., 7:676, 1968.

330. Lorber, J.: Results of treatment of myelomeningocele. Dev. Med. Child Neurol., 13:279, 1971.

331. Lorber, J.: Spina bifida cystica. Arch. Dis. Child., 47:854, 1972.

332. Lorber, J.: Selective treatment of myelomeningocele: To treat or not to treat. Pediatrics, 53:307, 1974.

333. Lorber, J.: Spina bifida: To treat or not to treat? Selection—the best policy available. Nurs. Mirror, 147:14, 1978.

334. Lorber, J., and Levick, K.: Spina bifida cystica: Incidence of spina bifida occulta in parents and in controls. Arch. Dis. Child., 42:171, 1967.

335. Lorber, J., and Salfiedl, S.: Results of selective treatment of spina bifida cystica. Arch. Dis. Child., 56:822, 1981.

336. Lorber, J., and Schloss, A. L.: The adolescent with myelomeningocele. Dev. Med. Child Neurol., 29:113, 1973.

337. Lowe, G. P., and Menelaus, M. B.: The surgical management of kyphosis in older children with myelomeningocele. J. Bone Joint Surg., 60-B:40, 1978.

338. Lowman, C. L.: Lateral fascial transplant for controlling a gluteus medius limp. Physiother. Rev., 27:355, 1947.

339. Luque, E. R., and Cardoso, A.: Segmental correction of scoliosis with rigid internal fixation. Preliminary report. Orthop. Trans., 1:136, 1977.

340. McAndrew, I.: Adolescents and Young People with Spina Bifida. Melbourne, Ability Press, 1977.

341. McCall, R. E., and Schmidt, W. T.: Clinical experience with the reciprocal gait orthosis in myelodysplasia. J. Pediatr. Orthop., 6:157, 1986.

342. McCormick, M. C., Charney, E. B., and Stemmler, M. M.: Assessing the impact of a child with spina bifida on the family. Dev. Med. Child Neurol., 28:53, 1986.

343. McKay, D. W.: The McKay plate for kyphosis of the spine. Presented at the Scoliosis Research Society, Louisville, September 1975.

344. McKay, D. W., Jackman, K. V., Nason, S. S., and Eng, G. E.: McKay stabilization in myelomeningocele. Dev. Med. Child Neurol. (Suppl.), 37:18, 1976.

345. McKeown, T., and Record, R. G.: Seasonal incidence of congenital malformations of the central nervous system. Lancet, 1:192, 1951.

346. McKibbin, B.: The action of the iliopsoas muscle in the newborn. J. Bone Joint Surg., 50-B:161, 1968.

347. McKibbin, B.: Conservative management of paralytic dislocations of the hip in myelomeningocele. J. Bone Joint Surg., 53-B:758, 1971.

348. McKibbin, B.: The use of splintage in the management of paralytic dislocation of the hip in spina bifida cystica. J. Bone Joint Surg., 55-B:163, 1973.

349. McKibbin, B., and Porter, R. W.: The incidence of vitamin-C deficiency in meningomyelocele. Dev. Med. Child Neurol., 9:338, 1967.

350. McKibbin, B., and Ralis, Z.: The effect of skeletal changes in hip joint stability in spina bifida. Dev. Med. Child Neurol. (Suppl.), 29:112, 1973.

351. McKibbin, B., Roseland, P. A., and Duckwith, T.: Abnormalities in vitamin-C metabolism in spina bifida. Dev. Med. Child Neurol. (Suppl.), 15:55, 1968.

352. McLaughlin, T. P., Banta, J. V., Gahm, N. H., and Raycroft, J. F.: Intraspinal rhizotomy and distal cordectomy in patients with myelomeningocele. J. Bone Joint Surg., 68-A:88, 1986.

353. McLone, D. G.: Technique for closure of myelomeningocele. Childs Brain, 6:65, 1980.

354. McLone, D. G.: Results of treatment of children born with a myelomeningocele. In Weiss, M. H. (ed.): Clinical Neurosurgery. Baltimore, Williams & Wilkins, 1983, pp. 407–412.

355. McLone, D. G., Czyzewski, D., Raimondi, A., and Sommers, R.: Central nervous system infections as a limiting factor in the intelligence of children with myelomeningocele. Pediatrics, 70:338, 1982.

356. McLone, D. G., Dias, L., Kaplan, W., and Sommers, M.: Concepts in the management of spina bifida. Proceedings of the American Society for Pediatric Neurosurgery. Concepts in Pediatric Neurosurgery. Basel, S. Karger, 1984.

357. McLone, D. G., Mutluer, S., and Naidich, T. P.: Lipomeningoceles of the conus medullaris. Concepts Pediatr. Neurosurg., 3:170, 1983.

358. McLone, D. G., and Naidich, T. P.: Spinal dysraphism: clinical and experimental. In Holtzman, R.N.N., and Stein, B.M. (eds.): The Tethered Spinal Cord. New York, Thieme Stratton, 1985, pp. 14–28.

359. McLone, D. G., and Naidich, T. P.: Terminal myelocystocele. Neurosurgery, 16:36, 1985.

360. McLone, D. G., Raimondi, A. J., and Sommers, R.: The results of early treatment of 100 consecutive newborns with myelomeningocele. Z. Kinderchir., 34:115, 1981.

361. McLone, D. G., Suwa, J., Collins, J. A., Poznanski, S., and Knepper, P. A.: Neurulation: Biochemical and morphological studies on primary and secondary neural tube defects. Proceedings of the American Society for Pediatric Neurosurgery. Concepts in Pediatric Neurosurgery 4. Basel, S. Karger, 1983, pp. 15–29.

362. MacMahon, B., Record, R. G., and McKeown, T.: Secular changes in the incidence of malformation of the central nervous system. Br. J. Soc. Med., 5:254, 1951.

363. MacMahon, B., Pugh, T. F., and Ingalls, T. D.: Anencephalus, spina bifida, and hydrocephalus. Br. J. Prev. Soc. Med., 7:211, 1953.

364. McMaster, W. C., and Silber, I.: An urological complication of Dwyer instrumentation. J. Bone Joint Surg., 57-A:710, 1975.

365. Mackel, J. C., and Lindseth, R. E.: Scoliosis in myelodysplasia. J. Bone Joint Surg., 57-A:1031, 1975.

366. Madden, B. K.: Orthopaedic aspects of spina bifida. Physiotherapy, 63:186, 1977.

367. Madigan, R. R., and Worrall, V. T.: Paralytic instability of the hip in myelomeningocele. Clin. Orthop., 125:57, 1977.

368. Maguire, C. D., Winter, R. B., Mayfield, J. K., and Erickson, D. L.: Hemimyelodysplasia: A report of 10 cases. J. Pediatr. Orthop., 2:9, 1982.

369. Makin, M.: Tibio-fibular relationship in paralyzed limbs. J. Bone Joint Surg., 47-B:500, 1965.

370. Manella, K. J., and Varni, J. W.: Behavior therapy in a gait-training program for a child with myelomeningocele. A case report. Phys. Ther., 61:1284, 1981.

371. Martin, M. C.: Physiotherapy in relation to myelomeningocele. Physiotherapy, 50:50, 1964.

372. Martin, M. C.: Spina bifida. Physiotherapy, 53:299, 1967.

373. Martin, P.: Marital breakdown in families of patients with spina bifida cystica. Dev. Med. Child Neurol., 17:757, 1975.

374. Master, C. L.: Pathogenesis of the Arnold-Chiari malformation: The significance of hydrocephalus and aqueduct stenosis. J. Neuropathol. Exp. Neurol., 37:56, 1978.

375. Matson, D. D.: Congenital spinal defects. Clin. Neurosurg., 8:185, 1962.

376. Matson, D. D.: Surgical repair of myelomeningocele. J. Neurosurg., 27:180, 1967.

377. Matson, D. D.: Commentaries. Surgical treatment of myelomeningocele. Pediatrics, 42:225, 1968.

378. Matson, D. D.: Neurosurgery of Infancy and Childhood. 2nd Ed. Springfield, Ill., Charles C Thomas, 1969.

379. Mayer, L.: Further studies of fixed pelvic obliquity. J. Bone Joint Surg., 18:87, 1936.

380. Mayer, L.: Tendon transplantation on the lower extremities. A.A.O.S. Instr. Course Lect., 6:189, 1949.

381. Mayfield, J. K.: Severe spine deformity in myelodysplasia and sacral agenesis: An aggressive surgical approach. Spine, 6:498, 1981.

382. Mazur, J. M., Stillwell, A., and Menelaus, M.: The significance of spasticity in the upper and lower limbs in myelomeningocele. J. Bone Joint Surg., 68-B:211, 1986.

383. Menelaus, M. B.: Posterior iliopsoas transfer. J. Bone Joint Surg., 48-B:592, 1966.

384. Menelaus, M. B.: Dislocation and deformity of the hip in children with spina bifida cystica. J. Bone Joint Surg., 51-B:238, 1969.

385. Menelaus, M. B.: Talectomy for equinovarus deformity in arthrogryposis and spina bifida. J. Bone Joint Surg., 53-B:468, 1971.

386. Menelaus, M. B.: Orthopaedic management of children with myelomeningocele. A plea for realistic goals. Dev. Med. Child Neurol. (Suppl.), 37:18, 1976.

387. Menelaus, M. B.: The hip in myelomeningocele—management directed towards a minimum number of operations and a minimum period of immobilization. J. Bone Joint Surg., 58-B:448, 1976.

388. Menelaus, M. B.: The Orthopedic Management of Spina Bifida Cystica. 2nd Ed. Edinburgh, Churchill-Livingstone, 1980.

389. Menelaus, M. B.: Progress in the management of the paralytic hip in myelomeningocele. Orthop. Clin. North Am., 11:17, 1980.

390. Menzies, R. G., Parkin, J. M., and Hey, E. N.: Prognosis for babies with meningomyelocele and high lumbar paraplegia at birth. Lancet, 2:993, 1985.

391. Meyer, P. R.: Lower limb orthotics. Clin. Orthop. Rel. Res., 102:58, 1974.

392. Meyer, S., and Landau, H.: Precocious puberty in myelomeningocele patients. J. Pediatr. Orthop., 4:28, 1984.

393. Michael, J. C. C.: Fractures in lower limbs in spina bifida cystica—a survey of 4 fractures in 122 children. Dev. Med. Child Neurol., 12:88, 1970.

394. Middleton, R. W. D.: Ankle valgus due to fibular growth abnormality. J. Bone Joint Surg., 57-B:118, 1975.

395. Milani-Comparetti, A., and Gidoni, E. A.: Routine developmental examination in normal and retarded children. Dev. Med. Child Neurol., 9:631, 1967.

396. Milham, S.: Increased incidence of anencephalus and spina bifida in siblings of affected cases. Science, 138:593, 1962.

397. Milhorat, T. H.: Hydrocephalus and the Cerebrospinal Fluid. Baltimore, Williams & Wilkins, 1972.

398. Miller, E., and Sethi, L.: The effect of hydrocephalus on perception. Dev. Med. Child Neurol. (Suppl.), 25:77, 1971.

399. Miller, J. H., Reid, B. S., and Kemberling, C. R.: Utilization of ultrasound in the evaluation of spinal dysraphism in children. Radiology, 143:737, 1982.

400. Miller, P., Smith, D. W., and Shepart, T. H.: Maternal hyperthermia as a possible cause of anencephaly. Lancet, 1:519, 1978.

401. Milunsky, A., and Alpert, E.: Prenatal diagnosis of neural tube defects I and II. J. Obstet. Gynecol. Neonatal Nurs., 48:1, 1976.

402. Minns, R. A., Hazelwood, E., Brown, J. K., Fulford, G., and Elton, R. A.: Spina bifida and cerebral palsy. Z. Kinderchir., 34:370, 1981.

403. Minns, R. A., Sobkowiak, C. A., Skardoutsou, A., Dick, K., Elton, R. A., Brown, J. K., and Forfar, J. O.: Upper limb function in spina bifida. Z. Kinderchir. Grenzgeb., 22:493, 1977.

404. Mitchell, G. P.: Posterior displacement osteotomy of the calcaneus. J. Bone Joint Surg., 59-B:233, 1977.

405. Moe, J. H., Winter, R. B., Bradford, D. S., and Lonstein, J. E.: Scoliosis and Other Spinal Deformities. Philadelphia, W. B. Saunders, 1978.

406. Molnar, G. E., and Taft, L. T.: Pediatric rehabilitation. Part II. Spina bifida and limb deficiencies. Curr. Probl. Pediatr., 7:2, 1977.

407. Moore, D. W., Raycroft, J. F., Loyer, R. E., and Paul, S. W.: The treatment of disabling foot and ankle valgus in myelodysplastic children. Presented at the 45th Annual Meeting of the American Academy of Orthopedic Surgeons, Dallas, February 1978.

408. Moore, T. S., Dreyer, T. M., and Bevin, A. G.: Closure of large spina bifida cystica defects with bilateral bipedicled musculocutaneous flaps. Plast. Reconstr. Surg., 73:288, 1984.

409. Morgagni, J. B.: The Seats and Causes of Disease Investigated by Anatomy. London, A. Millar and J. Caldwell, 1979.

410. Morton, N.: Spina bifida operata, treatment by injection. Br. Med. J., 1:381, 1875.

411. Mortonne, C. S., and Mi, M. P.: Genetics of Interracial Crosses in Hawaii. Basel, S. Karger, 1967.

412. Motloch, W.: The parapodium: An orthotic device for neuromuscular disorders. Artif. Limbs, 15:36, 1971.

413. Motloch, W.: Device design in spina bifida. In Murdoch, G.: The Advance of Orthotics. Baltimore, Williams & Wilkins, 1976.

414. Murphy, E. A., and Chase, G. A.: Principles of Genetic Counselling. Chicago, Year Book Medical Publications, 1975.

415. Mustard, W. T.: Iliopsoas transfer for weakness of the hip abductors. J. Bone Joint Surg., 34-A:647, 1952.

416. Mustard, W. T.: A follow-up study of iliopsoas transfer for hip instability. J. Bone Joint Surg., 41-B:289, 1959.

417. Mustard, W. T., and McDonald, G.: The Gallie tenodesis. Can. Med. Assoc. J., 75:271, 1956.

418. Naggan, L., and MacMahon, B.: Ethnic differences in the prevalence of anencephaly and spina bifida. N. Engl. J. Med., 227:1119, 1967.

419. Naidich, T. P., McLone, D. G., Schkolnik, A., and Fernbach, S. K.: Sonographic evaluation of caudal spine anomalies in children. A.J.R., 4:661, 1983.

420. Naidich, T. P., Pudlowski, R. M., and Naidich, J. B.: Computed tomographic signs of Chiari II malformation. II. Midbrain and cerebellum. Radiology, 134:391, 1980.

421. Naidich, T. P., Pudlowski, R. M., and Naidich, J. B.: Computed tomographic signs of Chiari II malformation. III. Ventricles and cisterns. Radiology, 134:657, 1980.

422. Naidich, T. P., Pudlowski, R. M., Naidich, J. B., et al.: Computed tomographic signs of Chiari II malformation. Part I. Skull and dural partitions. Radiology, 134:65, 1980.

423. Naik, D. R., and Emery, J. L.: The position of the spinal cord segments related to the vertebral bodies

in children with meningomyelocele and hydrocephalus. Dev. Med. Child Neurol. (Suppl.), 16:62, 1968.

424. Nash, D. F. E.: Meningomyelocele. Proc. R. Soc. Med., 56:506, 1963.

425. Nathanson, L., and Lewitan, A.: Dislocation of the hip associated with spina bifida. A.J.R., 51:635, 1944.

426. Nevin, R. S., Easton, J. K., McCubbin, H. I., and Birkebak, R. R.: Parental coping in raising children with have spina bifida cystica. Z. Kinderchir. Grenzgeb., 28:417, 1979.

427. Nielsen, H. H.: A longitudinal study of the psychological aspects of myelomeningocele. Scand. J. Psychol., 21:45, 1980.

428. Nogami, H., and Ingalls, T. H.: Pathogenesis of spinal malformations induced in the embryos of mice. J. Bone Joint Surg., 49-A:1551, 1967.

429. Norton, P. L., and Foley, J. J.: Paraplegia in children. J. Bone Joint Surg., 41-A:1291, 1959.

430. Nuzzo, R.: Dynamic bracing: Elastics for patients with cerebral palsy, muscular dystrophy and myelodysplasia. Clin. Orthop., 148:263, 1980.

431. Ober, F. R.: An operation for the relief of paralysis of the gluteus maximus muscle. J.A.M.A., 88:1063, 1927.

432. O'Brien, J. P.: The surgical management of paralytic scoliosis. J. Bone Joint Surg., 56-B:566, 1974.

433. O'Brien, J. P., Dwyer, A. P., and Hodgson, A. R.: Paralytic pelvic obliquity. J. Bone Joint Surg., 57-A:626, 1975.

434. Ogston, A.: A new principle of curing clubfoot in severe cases in children a few years old. Br. Med. J., 1:1524, 1902.

435. O'Hare, J. M.: Progress report in the study of congenital paraplegics. Proceedings of the Annual Clinical Paraplegia Conference, 1958.

436. Osebold, W. R., Mayfield, J. K., Winter, R. B., and Moe, J. H.: Surgical treatment of paralytic scoliosis associated with myelomeningocele. J. Bone Joint Surg., 64-A:841, 1982.

437. Oyewole, A., Adeloye, A., and Adeyokunnu, A. A.: Psychosocial and cultural factors associated with the management of spina bifida cystica in Nigeria. Dev. Med. Child Neurol., 27:498, 1985.

438. Paget, D. H.: Spina bifida and embryonic neuroschisis—A causal relationship: Definition of postnatal confirmations involving a bifid spine. Johns Hopkins Med. J., 128:233, 1968.

439. Paluska, D. J., and Blount, W. P.: Ankle valgus after Grice subtalar stabilization. Clin. Orthop. Rel. Res., 59:137, 1968.

440. Park, W. M., and Watt, I.: The preoperative aortographic assessment of children with spina bifida cystica and severe kyphosis. J. Bone Joint Surg., 57-B:112, 1975.

441. Parker, B., and Walker, G.: Posterior psoas transfer and hip instability in lumbar myelomeningocele. J. Bone Joint Surg., 57-B:53, 1975.

442. Parsch, K.: Grice extra-articular arthrodesis (results, extensions in the range of indication.) Z. Orthop., 109:458, 1973.

443. Parsch, K., and Goessens, H.: Surgical treatment of spinal column and hip deformities in spina bifida. Acta Orthop. Belg., 37:230, 1971.

444. Parsch, K., and Manner, G.: Prevention and treatment of knee problems in children with spina bifida. Dev. Med. Child Neurol. (Suppl. 37), 18:114, 1976.

445. Parsch, K., and Manner, G.: Surgical interventions for correction of deformations of the hip in children with spina bifida. Acta Orthop. Belg., 43:359, 1977.

446. Parsch, K., Rosska, K., and Goessens, H.: Does hip dislocation in meningomyelocele require a special treatment? A propos of 30 transplantations of the psoas by Sharrard's technic. Rev. Chir. Orthop., 56:683, 1970.

447. Parsch, K., and Schulitz, K. P.: Early orthopedic therapy of the child with cystic spina bifida. Z. Orthop., 109:458, 1971.

448. Parsons, J. G.: Assessment of aptitudes in young people of school-leaving age handicapped by hydrocephalus or spina bifida cystica. Dev. Med. Child Neurol. (Suppl.), 27:101, 1972.

449. Passo, S. D.: Positioning infants with myelomeningocele. Am. J. Nurs., 74:1658, 1974.

450. Passo, S. D.: Parents' perception, attitudes and needs regarding sex education for the child with myelomeningocele. Res. Nurs. Health, 1:53, 1978.

451. Patten, B. M.: Embryological stages in the development of spina bifida and myeloschisis. Anat. Rec., 94:487, 1946.

452. Patten, B. M.: Overgrowth of the neural tube in young embryos. Anat. Rec., 113:381, 1952.

453. Patten, B. M.: Embryological stages in the establishing of myeloschisis with spina bifida. Am. J. Anat., 93:365, 1953.

454. Patterson, W. R., Fitz, D. A., and Smith, W. S.: The pathologic anatomy of congenital convex pes valgus. J. Bone Joint Surg., 50-A:458, 1968.

455. Paul, S. W.: Spinal problems in myelomeningocele—orthotic principles. Prosthet. Orthot. Int., 1:30, 1977.

456. Paulos, L., Coleman, S., and Samuelson, K. M.: Pes cavovarus. J. Bone Joint Surg., 62-A:942, 1980.

457. Peabody, C. W.: Tendon transplantation in the lower extremity. A.A.O.S. Instr. Course Lect., 6:178, 1949.

458. Pemberton, P. A.: Pericapsular osteotomy of the ilium for treatment of congenital subluxation and dislocation of the hip. J. Bone Joint Surg., 47-A:65, 1965.

459. Perez-Marrero, R., Dimmock, W., Churchill, B. M., and Hardy, B. E.: Clean intermittent catheterization in myelomeningocele children less than 3 years old. J. Urol., 128:779, 1982.

460. Perricone, G., Granata, C., and Piazzini, D.: Electric stimulation test in myelomeningocele. Chir. Organi Mov., 65:303, 1979.

461. Perry, J.: The halo in spinal abnormalities. Orthop. Clin. North Am., 3:69, 1972.

462. Perry, J., Antonelli, D., and Ford, W.: Analysis of knee joint forces during flexed knee stance. J. Bone Joint Surg., 57-A:961, 1975.

463. Perry, J., and Nickel, V. L.: Total cervical-spine fusion for neck paralysis. J. Bone Joint Surg., 41-A:37, 1959.

464. Perspectives in spina bifida (Letter). Br. Med. J., 2:1368, 1978.

465. Piggott, H.: The natural history of scoliosis in myelodysplasia. J. Bone Joint Surg., 62-B:54, 1980.

466. Pilliard, D., Massy, P., and Taussig, G.: The hip in myelomeningocele. Orthop. Trans., 5:61, 1981.

467. Pinyerd, B. J.: Siblings of children with myelomeningocele: Examining their perceptions. Matern. Child Nurs. J., 12:61, 1983.

468. Poitras, B., and Hall, J. E.: Excision of kyphosis in myelomeningocele. J. Bone Joint Surg., 56-A:1767, 1974.

469. Poulton, M.: Walking aid for young paraplegics. Physiotherapy, 61:275, 1975.

470. Pouw, R.: Assessment of pre-school abilities based on spina bifida children. Br. J. Occup. Ther., 40:61, 1977.

471. Pressman, S. D.: Myelomeningocele: A multidisciplinary problem. J. Neurosurg. Nurs., 13:333, 1981.

472. Purath, W., Hellinger, J., and Schottmann, R.: Results of the surgical treatment of myelodysplastic paralytic luxation of the hip joint. Padiatr. Grenzgeb., 20:301, 1981.

473. Quilis, N. A.: Fractures in children with myelomeningocele. Report of 15 cases and review of the literature. Acta Orthop. Scand., 45:883, 1974.

474. Ralis, L. A., Ralis, H. M., Randall, M., Watkins, G.,

and Blake, P. D.: Changes in shape, ossification and quality of bones in children with spina bifida. Dev. Med. Child Neurol., 37:29, 1976.

475. Raycroft, J. F., and Curtis, B. H.: Spinal curvature in myelomeningocele. A.A.O.S. Symposium on Myelomeningocele. St. Louis, C. V. Mosby, 1972.

476. von Recklinghausen, F.: Untersuchungen uber der Spina bifida. Arch. Pathol. Anat., 105:243, 1886.

477. Record, R. G., and McKeown, T.: Congenital malformations of the central nervous system. I. A survey of 930 cases. Br. J. Soc. Med., 3:183, 1949.

478. Record, R. G., and McKeown, T.: Congenital malformations of the central nervous system. III. Risk of malformation in siblings of malformed individuals. Br. J. Soc. Med., 4:217, 1950.

479. Reigel, D. H.: Kyphectomy and meylomeningocele repair: Modern techniques in surgery. Neurosurgery, 13:1, 1979.

480. Reigel, D. H., Dallman, D. E., and Scarff, T. B.: Intra-operative evoked potential studies of newborn infants with myelomeningocele. Dev. Med. Child Neurol., 18:42, 1977.

481. Reigel, D. H., Scarff, T. B., and Woodford, J. E.: Surgery for tethered spinal cord in myelomeningocele patients. American Association of Neurological Surgeons, April 1976. Dev. Med. Child Neurol. (Suppl. 37), 18:165, 1977.

482. Reikeras, O., and Hellum, C.: Fractures in children with myelomeningocele. Arch. Orthop. Trauma Surg., 98:25, 1981.

483. Renoirte, P., and Bellen, P.: Place of orthosis in the treatment of sequelae of meningomyelocele. Acta Orthop. Belg., 43:345, 1977.

484. Renwick, J. H.: Hypothesis: Anencephaly and spina bifida are usually preventable by avoidance of a specific but unidentified substance present in certain potato tubers. Br. J. Prev. Soc. Med., 26:67, 1972.

485. Richards, I. D. G., Roberts, C. J., and Lloyd, S.: Area differences in prevalence of neural tube malformations in South Wales. Br. J. Prev. Soc. Med., 26:89, 1972.

486. Rickard, K., Brady, M. S., and Gresham, E. L.: Nutritional management of the chronically ill child. Congenital heart disease and myelomeningocele. Pediatr. Clin. North Am., 24:157, 1977.

487. Rickham, P. P.: Problems in the treatment of children with myelomeningocele. Changes in the indications for surgery during the last 30 years (Editorial). Helv. Paediatr. Acta, 33:187, 1978.

488. Ritter, M. A., and Wilson, P. D.: Colonna capsular arthroplasty. A long-term follow-up of forty hips. J. Bone Joint Surg., 50-A:1305, 1968.

489. Robin, G.: Fractures in childhood. Paraplegia, 3:165, 1966.

490. Robin, G.: Scoliosis of spina bifida and infantile paraplegia. Isr. J. Med. Sci., 8:1823, 1972.

491. Robin, G. C.: Scoliosis and neurological disease. Isr. J. Med. Sci., 9:578, 1973.

492. Robinson, J., Hewson, E., and Parker, P.: The walking ability of fourteen to seventeen year old teenagers with spina bifida. A physiotherapy study. Z. Kinderchir., 31:4, 1980.

493. Root, L.: Surgical treatment of mild hip dysplasia in spina bifida cystica. Orthop. Trans., 5:4, 1981.

494. Root, L., and Siegel, T.: Osteotomy of the hip in children: Posterior approach. J. Bone Joint Surg., 62-A:571, 1980.

495. Rose, G. K., and Henshaw, J. T.: A swivel walker for paraplegics: Medical and technical considerations. Biomed. Engin., 7:420, 1972.

496. Rose, G. K., Sankarankutty, M., and Stallard, J.: A clinical review of the orthotic treatment of myelomeningocele patients. J. Bone Joint Surg., 65-A:242, 1983.

497. Rose, G. K., Stallard, J., and Sankarankutty, M.: Clinical evaluation of spina bifida patients using hip guidance orthosis. Dev. Med. Child Neurol., 23:30, 1981.

498. Rosenblum, M. F., Finegold, D. N., and Charney, E. B.: Assessment of stature of children with myelomeningocele and usefulness of arm-span measurement. Dev. Med. Child Neurol., 25:338, 1983.

499. Rossak, K., Parsch, K., and Schulitz, K. P.: Treatment of hip joint luxations in myelomeningocele. Arch. Orthop. Unfall-Chir., 67:199, 1970.

500. Ruderman, R. J., Goldner, J. L., and Hardaker, W. T.: Pantalar fusion in myelodysplasia: A procedure too hastily rejected? Orthop. Trans., 4:152, 1980.

501. Rueda, J., and Carroll, N. C.: Hip instability in patients with myelomeningocele. J. Bone Joint Surg., 54-B:422, 1972.

502. Russell, D. S., and Donald, C.: Mechanism of internal hydrocephalus in spina bifida. Brain, 58:203, 1935.

503. Salter, R. B.: Innominate osteotomy in the treatment of congenital dislocation and subluxation of the hip. J. Bone Joint Surg., 43-B:518, 1961.

504. Samilson, R. L.: Crescentic osteotomy of the os calcis for calcaneovalgus feet. In Bateman, J. E. (ed.): Foot Science. Philadelphia, W. B. Saunders, 1976, p. 18.

505. Sand, P. L., Taylor, N., Hill, M., Kosky, N., and Rawlings, M.: Hand function in children with myelomeningocele. Am. J. Occup. Ther., 28:87, 1974.

506. Scarff, T. B., Toleikis, J. R., Bunch, W. H., and Parrish, S.: Dermatomal somatosensory evoked potentials in children with myelomeningocele. Z. Kinderchir., 28:384, 1979.

507. Schafer, M. F., and Dias, L. S.: Myelomeningocele. Orthopaedic Treatment. Baltimore, Williams & Wilkins, 1983.

508. Schwidde, J. T.: Spina bifida. Survey of two hundred twenty-five encephoceles, meningoceles and myelomeningoceles. Am. J. Dis. Child., 84:35, 1952.

509. Scott, F. B., Bradley, W. E., and Timm, G. W.: Treatment of urinary incontinence by an implantation prosthetic sphincter. Urology, 1:252, 1973.

510. Scouter, E. E.: Spina bifida and epiphyseal displacement. Report of 2 cases. J. Bone Joint Surg., 44-B:106, 1962.

511. Scranton, P. E., McMaster, J. H., and Kelly, E.: Dynamic fibular function. Clin. Orthop., 118:76, 1976.

512. Seppala, M., Ruoslahti, E.: Alpha-fetoprotein: Physiology and pathology during pregnancy and application to antenatal diagnosis. J. Perinat. Med., 1:104, 1973.

513. Sharrard, W. J. W.: Congenital paralytic dislocation of the hip in children with myelomeningocele. J. Bone Joint Surg., 41-B:622, 1959.

514. Sharrard, W. J. W.: The mechanism of paralytic deformity in spina bifida. Dev. Med. Child Neurol., 4:310, 1962.

515. Sharrard, W. J. W.: Posterior iliopsoas transplantation in the treatment of paralytic dislocation of the hip. J. Bone Joint Surg., 46-B:426, 1964.

516. Sharrard, W. J. W.: Spina bifida. Physiotherapy, 50:44, 1964.

517. Sharrard, W. J. W.: The segmental innervation of the lower limb muscles in man. Ann. R. Coll. Surg., 35:106, 1964.

518. Sharrard, W. J. W.: Modern trends in the treatment of spina bifida: Methods of assessment and their relation to treatment by early closure. Proc. R. Soc. Med., 60:767, 1967.

519. Sharrard, W. J. W.: Paralytic deformity in the lower limb. J. Bone Joint Surg., 49-B:731, 1967.

520. Sharrard, W. J. W.: Spinal osteotomy for congenital kyphosis in myelomeningocele. J. Bone Joint Surg., 50-B:466, 1968.

521. Sharrard, W. J. W.: Long-term follow-up of posterior

transplant for paralytic dislocation of the hip. J. Bone Joint Surg., 52-B:779, 1970.

522. Sharrard, W. J. W.: Neuromotor evaluation of the newborn. In A.A.O.S. Symposium on Myelomeningocele. St. Louis, C. V. Mosby, 1972.
523. Sharrard, W. J. W.: The orthopaedic surgery of spina bifida. Clin. Orthop. Rel. Res., 92:195, 1973.
524. Sharrard, W. J. W.: Supramalleolar wedge osteotomy of the tibia in children with myelomeningocele. J. Bone Joint Surg., 56-B:458, 1974.
525. Sharrard, W. J. W.: The orthopaedic management of spina bifida. Acta Orthop. Scand., 46:356, 1975.
526. Sharrard, W. J. W.: Orthopedic surgery of spina bifida. Acta Orthop. Belg., 43:330, 1977.
527. Sharrard, W. J. W.: Paralytic convex pes valgus (paralytic vertical talus). In McLaurin, R. L. (ed.): Myelomeningocele. New York, Grune & Stratton, 1977, pp. 461–467.
528. Sharrard, W. J. W.: Paediatric Orthopaedics and Fractures. 3rd Ed. Oxford, Blackwell Scientific Publications, 1980.
529. Sharrard, W. J. W., and Carroll, N. C.: Long-term follow-up of posterior iliopsoas transplant for paralytic dislocation of the hip. J. Bone Joint Surg., 52-B:779, 1970.
530. Sharrard, W. J. W., and Drennan, J. C.: Osteotomy-excision of the spine for lumbar kyphosis in older children with myelomeningocele. J. Bone Joint Surg., 54-B:50, 1972.
531. Sharrard, W. J. W., and Grosfield, I.: The management of deformity and paralysis of the foot in myelomeningocele. J. Bone Joint Surg., 50-B:456, 1968.
532. Sharrard, W. J. W., and Smith, T. W.: Tenodesis of flexor hallucis longus for paralytic clawing of the hallux in childhood. J. Bone Joint Surg., 58-B:458, 1974.
533. Sharrard, W. J. W., and Webb, J.: Supra-malleolar wedge osteotomy of the tibia in children with myelomeningocele. J. Bone Joint Surg., 56-B:458, 1974.
534. Sharrard, W. J. W., Zachary, R. B., Lorber, J., and Bruce, A. M.: A controlled trial of immediate and delayed closure of spina bifida cystica. Arch. Dis. Child., 38:18, 1963.
535. Sherk, H. H., and Ames, M. D.: Talectomy in the treatment of the myelomeningocele patient. Clin. Orthop. Rel. Res., 110:218, 1975.
536. Sherk, H. H., and Ames, M. D.: Functional results of iliopsoas transfer in myelomeningocele hip dislocation. Clin. Orthop. Rel. Res., 137:181, 1978.
537. Shulman, B. H.: Spina bifida with meningocele. Occurrence in two children of the same family. Arch. Neurol. Psychiatry, 47:474, 1942.
538. Shulman, B. H., and Ames, M.: Intensive treatment of fifty children born with myelomeningocele. N.Y. J. Med., 68:265, 1969.
539. Shurtleff, D. B.: Myelodysplasia: Management and treatment. Curr. Probl. Pediatr., 10:1, 1980.
540. Shurtleff, D. B., Goiney, R., Fordon, L. H., and Livermore, N.: Myelodysplasia: The natural history of kyphosis and scoliosis. A preliminary report. Dev. Med. Child Neurol. (Suppl. 37), 18:6, 1976.
541. Simmons, E. H.: Observations on the technique and indications for wedge resection of the spine. J. Bone Joint Surg., 50-A:847, 1968.
542. Singh, C. V.: Anaesthetic management of meningomyelocele and meningocele. J. Indian Med. Assoc., 75:130, 1980.
543. Smith, E. D.: Spina Bifida and the Total Care of Spinal Myelomeningocele. Springfield, Ill., Charles C Thomas, 1965.
544. Smith, E. T., Pevey, J. K., and Shindler, T. O.: The erector spinae transplant—a misnomer. Clin. Orthop., 30:144, 1963.
545. Smith, G. K.: Total care in spina bifida cystica. In Industrial Society and Rehabilitation—Problems and Solutions. Proceedings of the 10th World Congress of the International Society for Rehabilitation of the Disabled. Wiesbaden, 1966, p. 75. Heidelberg, I.S.R.D.

546. Smith, G. K.: Spina bifida. In Clinical Paediatric Surgery, 2nd Ed. London, Blackwell, 1976, p. 100.
547. Smith, G. K., and Smith, E. D.: Selection for treatment in spina bifida cystica. Br. Med. J., 4:189, 1973.
548. Smith, R. S.: Orthopedic considerations in the treatment of spina bifida. Surg. Gynecol. Obstet., 62:218, 1936.
549. Smith, T. W. D., and Duckworth, T.: The management of deformities of the foot in children with spina bifida. Dev. Med. Child Neurol. (Suppl.), 37:104, 1976.
550. Smithells, R. W., and Chin, E. R.: Spina bifida in Liverpool. Dev. Med. Child Neurol., 7:258, 1965.
551. Smithells, R. W., Sheppard, S., and Schorah, C. J.: Possible prevention of neural tube defects by periconceptional vitamin supplementation. Lancet, 1:647, 1980.
552. Soare, P. L., and Raimondi, A. J.: Intellectual and perceptual-motor characteristics of treated myelomeningocele children. Am. J. Dis. Child., 131:199, 1977.
553. Somerville, E. W.: Paralytic dislocation of the hip. J. Bone Joint Surg., 41-B:279, 1959.
554. Soutter, F. E.: Spina bifida and epiphyseal displacement: Report of two cases. J. Bone Joint Surg., 44-B:106, 1962.
555. Soutter, R.: A new operation for hip contracture in poliomyelitis. Boston Med. Surg. J., 170:380, 1914.
556. Spain, B.: Verbal and performance ability in preschool children with spina bifida. Dev. Med. Child Neurol., 16:773, 1974.
557. Specht, E. E.: Congenital paralytic vertical talus. An anatomical study. J. Bone Joint Surg., 57-A:842, 1975.
558. Spielrein, R. E.: An engineering approach to ambulation without the use of external power sources, of severely handicapped individuals. J. Aust. Inst. Engineers, 35:321, 1963.
559. Sriram, K., Bobechko, W. P., and Hall, J. E.: Surgical management of spinal deformities in spina bifida. J. Bone Joint Surg., 54-B:666, 1972.
560. Staheli, L. L.: Acetabular augmentation: A review of 50 cases. Orthop. Trans., 5:8, 1981.
561. Stark, G. D.: Neonatal assessment of the child with a myelomeningocele. Arch. Dis. Child., 46:539, 1971.
562. Stark, G. D.: Myelomeningocele: The changing approach to treatment. In Recent Advances in Paediatric Surgery, No. 3. London, Churchill Livingstone, 1975, p. 73.
563. Stark, G. D.: Spina Bifida. Problems and Management. London, Blackwell, 1977.
564. Stark, G. D., and Baker, G. C. W.: The neurological involvement of the lower limbs in myelomeningocele. Dev. Med. Child Neurol., 9:732, 1967.
565. Stark, G. D., and Drummond, M.: The spinal cord lesion in myelomeningocele. Dev. Med. Child Neurol. (Suppl. 25), 13:1, 1971.
566. Stark, G. D., and Drummond, M.: Results of selective early operation in myelomeningocele. Arch. Dis. Child. 48:676, 1973.
567. Stauffer, E. S., Hoffer, M., and Nickel, V. L.: Ambulation in thoracic paraplegia (Abstract). J. Bone Joint Surg., 54-A:1336, 1972.
568. Steel, H. H.: Triple osteotomy of the innominate bone. J. Bone Joint Surg., 55-A:343, 1973.
569. Steel, H. H., and Adams, D. J.: Hyperlordosis caused by the lumboperitoneal shunt procedure for hydrocephalus. J. Bone Joint Surg., 54-A:1537, 1972.
570. Stein, S. C., and Schut, L.: Hydrocephalus in myelomeningocele. Childs Brain, 5:413, 1979.
571. Steindler, A.: Stripping of the os calcis. J. Orthop. Surg., 2:8, 1920.

572. Steindler, A.: The treatment of pes cavus (hollow claw foot). Arch. Surg., 2:325, 1921.

573. Stephen, J. P., and Bodel, J. G.: Luque rod fixation in meningomyelocele kyphosis: A preliminary report. Aust. N.Z. J. Surg., 53:473, 1983.

574. Stern, M. B., Grant, S. S., and Isaacson, A. S.: Bilateral distal tibial and fibular epiphyseal separation associated with spina bifida: A case report. Clin. Orthop., 50:191, 1967.

575. Stillwell, A., and Menelaus, M. B.: Walking ability in mature patients with spina bifida. J. Pediatr. Orthop., 3:184, 1983.

576. Stoyle, T. F.: Prognosis for paralysis in myelomeningocele. Dev. Med. Child Neurol., 8:755, 1966.

577. Strach, E. H.: Orthopedic care of children with myelomeningocele. A modern programme of rehabilitation. Br. Med. J., 3:791, 1967.

578. Strach, E. H., and Orth, M. C.: Methods of bracing in the rehabilitation of the paraplegic child. Paraplegia, 11:137, 1973.

579. Sugar, M., and Kennedy, C. M.: The use of electrodiagnostic techniques in the evaluation of the neurological deficit in infants with meningomyelocele. Neurology, 15:787, 1965.

580. Sutow, W. W., and Pryde, A. W.: Incidence of spina bifida occulta in relation to age. Am. J. Dis. Child., 91:211, 1956.

581. Swinyard, C. A.: Comprehensive care of the child with spina bifida manifesta. Rehabilitation Monograph No. 31. New York, Institute of Rehabilitation Medicine, 1966.

582. Symposium on Spina Bifida, London, 1965. Proceedings. London, National Fund for Research into Poliomyelitis and Other Crippling Diseases. (Action for the Crippled Child Monograph.)

583. Taylor, L. J.: Excision of the proximal end of the femur for hip stiffness in myelomeningocele. J. Bone Joint Surg., 68-B:75, 1986.

584. Tew, B.: The "cocktail party syndrome" in children with hydrocephalus and spina bifida. Br. J. Disord. Commun., 14:89, 1979.

585. Tew, B., Evans, R., Thomas, M., and Ford, J.: The results of a selective surgical policy on the cognitive abilities of children with spina bifida. Dev. Med. Child Neurol., 27:606, 1985.

586. Tew, B. J., and Laurence, K. M.: The effects of admission to hospital and surgery in children with spina bifida. Dev. Med. Child Neurol. (Suppl 37), 18:6, 1976.

587. Thomas, L. I., Thompson, T. C., and Straub, L. R.: Transplantation of the external oblique muscle for abductor paralysis. J. Bone Joint Surg., 32-A:207, 1950.

588. Thomas, A., Bax, M., Coombes, K., Goldson, E., Smyth, D., and Whitmore, K.: The health and social needs of physically handicapped young adults: Are they being met by the statutory services? Dev. Med. Child Neurol. (Suppl. 50), 27:1, 1985.

589. Thompson, M. S., Cavin, E., and Phippen, W. G.: Fractures of the femora associated with spina bifida. Milit. Med., 129:841, 1964.

590. Thompson, T. C.: Astragalectomy and treatment of calcaneovalgus. J. Bone Joint Surg., 21:627, 1939.

591. Townsend, P. F., Cowell, H. R., and Steg, N. L.: Lower extremity fractures simulating infection in spina bifida. Clin. Orthop. Rel. Res., 144:255, 1979.

592. Trieshmann, H., Millis, M., Hall, J., and Watts, H.: Sliding calcaneal osteotomy for treatment of hindfoot deformity. Orthop. Trans., 4:305, 1980.

593. Trowbridge, A.: Three cases of spina bifida successfully treated. Boston Med. Surg. J., 1:753, 1828.

594. Tulpius, N.: Obs. Med. Lib. III Cap. XXIX, XXX. 229, 1641.

595. Turner, A.: Hand function in children with myelomeningocele. J. Bone Joint Surg., 67-B:268, 1985.

596. Turner, J. W., and Cooper, R. R.: Posterior transposition of tibialis anterior through the interosseous membrane. Clin. Orthop. Rel. Res., 79:71, 1971.

597. Tzimas, N., and Badell-Ribera, A.: Orthopedic and habilitation management of patients with spina bifida and myelomeningocele. Med. Clin. North Am., 53:502, 1969.

598. Uehling, D. T., Smith, J., Meyer, J., and Bruskewitz, R.: Impact of an intermittent catheterization program in children with myelomeningocele. Pediatrics, 76:892, 1985.

599. Vanderick, L. P.: Pathology and treatment of feet and knees in myelomeningocele. Acta Orthop. Belg., 43:306, 1977.

600. Variend, S., and Emery, J. L.: The pathology of the central lobes of the cerebellum in children with myelomeningocele. Dev. Med. Child Neurol., 32:99, 1974.

601. Venes, J. L.: Control of shunt infections. J. Neurosurg., 45:311, 1976.

602. Vigliarolo, D.: Managing bowel incontinence in children with meningomyelocele. Am. J. Nurs., 80:105, 1980.

603. Wagner, H.: Femoral osteotomies for congenital hip dislocation. Prog. Orthop. Surg., 2:85, 1978.

604. Wald, A.: Use of biofeedback in treatment of fecal incontinence in patients with meningomyelocele. Pediatrics, 68:45, 1981.

605. Wald, N. J., Cuckle, H., and Brock, D. J.: Maternal serum alpha fetoprotein measurement in antenatal screening for anencephaly and spina bifida in early pregnancy. Reports of a collaborative study of alpha fetoprotein in relation to neural tube defect. Lancet, 1:1323, 1977.

606. Walker, G.: The early management of varus feet in myelomeningocele. J. Bone Joint Surg., 53-B:462, 1971.

607. Walker, G., and Cheong-Leen, P.: Surgical management of paralytic vertical talus in myelomeningocele. Dev. Med. Child Neurol. (Suppl. 29), 15:112, 1973.

608. Walker, G. F., and Cheong-Leen, P.: The surgical management of paralytic vertical talus in myelomeningocele. J. Bone Joint Surg., 55-B:876, 1973.

609. Walker, J. H., Thomas, M., and Russell, I. T.: Spina bifida—the parents. Dev. Med. Child Neurol., 13:462, 1971.

610. Wallace, H. M., Baumgartner, L., and Rich, H.: Congenital malformations and birth injuries in New York City. Pediatrics, 12:525, 1953.

611. Wallace, S. J.: The effect of upper-limb function on mobility of children with myelomeningocele. Dev. Med. Child Neurol. (Suppl.), 29:84, 1973.

612. Warkany, J.: Morphogenesis of spina bifida. In McLaurin, R. L. (ed.): Myelomeningocele. New York, Grune & Stratton, 1977, pp. 31–39.

613. Warkany, J., Wilson, J. G., and Geiger, J. F.: Myeloschisis and myelomeningocele produced experimentally in the rat. J. Comp. Neurol., 109:35, 1958.

614. Watson, D., Pow, M., Ellam, A., and Costeloe, K.: Prevention of neural tube defects in an urban health district. J. Epidemiol. Community Health, 37:221, 1983.

615. Watson-Jones, R.: Spontaneous dislocations of the hip. Br. J. Surg., 14:36, 1926.

616. Weinert, C. R., McMaster, J. H., Scranton, P. E., Jr., and Ferguson, R. J.: Human fibular dynamics. In Bateman, J. E. (ed.): Foot Science. Philadelphia, W. B. Saunders, 1976. p. 1.

617. Weisl, H., and Matthews, J. P.: Posterior ilio-psoas transfer in the management of the hip in spina bifida: a review of 34 operations. Dev. Med. Child Neurol. (Suppl.), 29:100, 1973.

618. Weissman, S. L.: Capsular arthroplasty in paralytic dislocation of the hip: a preliminary report. J. Bone Joint Surg., 41-A:429, 1959.

619. Welbourn, H.: Spina bifida children attending ordinary schools. Br. Med. J., *1*:142, 1975.
620. Wenger, D. R., Jeffcoat, B. T., and Herring, J. A.: The guarded prognosis of physeal injury in paraplegic children. J. Bone Joint Surg., *62-A*:241, 1980.
621. Westin, G. W.: Tendon transfers about the foot, ankle and hip in the paralysed lower extremity. J. Bone Joint Surg., *47-A*:1430, 1975.
622. Westin, G. W., and DiFore, R. J.: Tenodesis of the tendo Achillis to the fibula for paralytic calcaneus deformity. J. Bone Joint Surg., *56-A*:1541, 1974.
623. Westin, G. W., and Marafioti, L. R.: Factors influencing the results of acetabuloplasty in children. J. Bone Joint Surg., *62-A*:765, 1980.
624. Wheatley, J. K., Woodard, J. R., and Parrott, T. S.: Electronic bladder stimulation of the management of children with myelomeningocele. J. Urol., *127*:283, 1982.
625. Whitehead, W. E., Parker, L. H., Masek, B. J., Cataldo, M. F., and Freeman, J. M.: Biofeedback treatment of fecal incontinence in patients with myelomeningocele. Dev. Med. Child Neurol., *23*:313, 1981.
626. Whitman, R.: Further observations on the treatment of paralytic talipes calcaneus by astragalectomy and backward displacement of the foot. Ann. Surg., *47*:264, 1908.
627. Wiener, A. S.: Pathogenesis of spina bifida and related congenital malformations. N.Y. J. Med., *47*:985, 1947.
628. Williams, P. F.: Surgical advances in the management of deformities of the spine and lower limbs in spina bifida. Aust. N.Z. J. Surg., *34*:250, 1965.
629. Williams, P. F.: Restoration of muscle balance of the foot by transfer of the tibialis posterior. J. Bone Joint Surg., *58-B*:217, 1976.
630. Williams, P. F., and Menelaus, M. B.: Triple arthrodesis by inlay grafting: a method suitable for the undeformed or valgus foot. J. Bone Joint Surg., *59-B*:333, 1977.
631. Willson, M. A.: Multidisciplinary problems of myelomeningocele and hydrocephalus. Phys. Ther. Rev., *45*:1139, 1965.
632. Wilner, I. A.: Familial repetition of myelomeningocele. J. Mich. Med. Soc., *48*:727, 1949.
633. Wiltse, L. L.: Valgus deformity of the ankle. J. Bone Joint Surg., *54-A*:595, 1972.
634. Wissinger, H. A., Tumer, Y., and Donaldson, W. F.: Posterior iliopsoas transfer: a treatment for some myelodysplastic hips. Orthopedics, *3*:865, 1980.
635. Wolverson, M. K., Sundaram, M., and Graviss, E. R.: Spina bifida and unilateral focal destruction of the distal femoral epiphysis. Skeletal Radiol., *6*:119, 1981.
636. Woodridge, C. P.: Purpose-designated vehicles. *In* Murdoch, G.: The Advance in Orthotics. Baltimore, Williams & Wilkins, 1976.
637. Wynne-Davies, R.: Congenital vertebral anomalies: aetiology and relationship to spina bifida cystica. J. Med. Genet., *12*:280, 1975.
638. Yates, G.: Molded plastic in bracing. Clin. Orthop. Rel. Res., *102*:46, 1974.
639. Yen, S., and MacMahon, B.: Genetics of anencephaly and spina bifida. Lancet, *2*:623, 1968.
640. Yngve, D. A., Douglas, R., and Roberts, J. M.: The reciprocating gait orthosis in myelomeningocele. J. Pediatr. Orthop., *4*:304, 1984.
641. Yngve, D. A., and Lindseth, R. E.: Effectiveness of muscle transfer in myelomeningocele hips measured by radiographic indices. J. Pediatr. Orthop., *2*:121, 1982.
642. Yount, C. C.: The role of the tensor fasciae femoris in certain deformities of the lower extremities. J. Bone Joint Surg., *8*:171, 1926.
643. Zachary, R. B.: The improving prognosis in spina bifida. Clin. Pediatr., *11*:11, 1972.
644. Zielke, K.: Ventrale Derotations-spondylodese, Behandlungsergenbnisse bei idiopathischen Lumbal-Skoliosen. Z. Orthop., *120*:320, 1982.
645. Ziller, R.: Neuropathic osteolysis following arthrodesis of the ankle joint in myelodysplasia. Beitr. Orthop. Traumatol., *21*:401, 1974.
646. Zippel, H.: Iliopsoas transposition in myelodysplastic paralytic luxation of the hip joints. Padiatr. Granzgeb., *20*:189, 1981.
647. Zook, E. G., Dzenitis, A. J., and Bennett, J. E.: Repair of large myelomeningoceles. Arch. Surg., *98*:41, 1969.

SPINAL DYSRAPHISM[1-57]*

Spinal dysraphism is a term used to refer to a complex group of developmental abnormalities of the spine and neural axis in which there is nerve tissue anomaly combined with bony anomalies of the vertebral column. This category of developmental affection encompasses a wide spectrum of conditions; at the severe extreme is myelomeningocele, and at the other end is a fibrous band in the spinal canal. In this section, lipomeningocele, lipomas of the filum terminale, and myelocystocele will be presented. Myelomeningocele and diastematomyelia are discussed separately. Dermal sinus, dermal and epidermal cysts, sacral agenesis, anomalous fibrous bands, tethered filum terminale, abnormal nerve roots, intradural angiomas and lipomas are other forms of spinal dysraphism; they will not be considered in this section.

Lipomyelomeningocele and Lipomas of the Filum Terminale

Lipomyelomeningocele is a dysraphic condition of the spine characterized by incorporation of subcutaneous fat in the distal part of the spinal cord. The lesion is often skin-covered, but the posterior elements of the vertebral column frequently are defective. The neuropathways are often intact; the neurologic deficit is caused primarily by tethering of the spinal cord to the surrounding fixed structures.

EMBRYOLOGY AND PATHOLOGY

Lipomyelomeningocele appears to be due to a single initial error in embryogenesis: focal premature separation of cutaneous ectoderm from neural ectoderm. In the normal state (Fig. 5–114), mesenchyme is always excluded from the dorsal surface of the neural plate and the

*Written with David G. McClone, M.D., Ph.D., Professor and Head, Children's Memorial Hospital, Northwestern University Medical School, Chicago, Illinois.

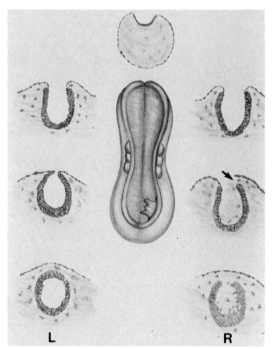

FIGURE 5–114. Spinal dysraphism.

A drawing of, on the left (L), normal sequence of closure, on the right (R), premature dysjunction (arrow) with mesenchyme entering the neural tube. In the center is a dorsal view with mesenchyme entering from the right side.

neural folds because (1) the cutaneous ectoderm is directly continuous with the neural ectoderm, and (2) the neural tube closes prior to dysjunction of cutaneous ectoderm from neural ectoderm. After normal dysjunction, the mesenchyme that streams in between the neural tube and the now separate cutaneous ectoderm gains contact with the *outer* surface of the neural tube only. The mesenchyme is induced to form meninges and bone by interaction with the outer surface of the neural tube.

Should the cutaneous ectoderm separate from neural ectoderm prematurely, before the neural tube closes, mesenchyme could gain access to the dorsal surface of the closing neural folds, the surface of which should form the interior or ependymal surface of the neural tube (Fig. 5–114). In such location, the mesenchyme might well prevent the neural folds from closing into the neural tube, creating a dorsal myeloschisis. Since the human neural tube closes progressively from cephalic end to caudal end, the cord segments above the pathologic segment would already have closed normally. The mesenchyme could then extend cephalad along the neural folds into the central canal of the normally fused

neural tube above. The cutaneous ectoderm would be expected to heal over in the dorsal midline.

If the development of normal meninges depends on a mutually interactive induction of surrounding mesenchyme by the *outer* surfaces of the cells that should have formed the neural tube, then that induction will be distorted secondarily. The neural ectodermal cells are splayed open by the dorsal myeloschisis. The meningeal cavity formed would be similarly splayed open. The meninges would be expected to stop exactly at the edge of the inducing cell surface, i.e., at the ventrolateral edge of the neural ectodermal plate (the future cleft spinal cord). Similarly, the dura would form only in relationship to the ventral surface of the neural plate. The dura would pass along the inner surface of the spinal canal ventrally and then would reflect back to the lateral edge of the neural tissue just where the outer surface of the neural ectoderm stopped. No dura would form in relationship to the dorsal "inner" surface of the neural ectoderm, so no dura would pass behind the cord. In effect, this would create a dorsal dural deficiency along the dorsal (inner) surface of the cord.

The dorsal surface of the cleft cord represents the cell surfaces that should have formed the central canal of the closed cord. It is postulated that these surfaces are capable only of inducing mesenchyme to form fat, some smooth muscle, and a little striated muscle. The fat formed would have the exact contour of the dorsal surface of the cleft cord, would fill the entire cleft, and would terminate laterally exactly at the edge of the inner surface of the neural tissue. In fact, the fat induced by the inner surface would stop just where the meninges induced by the outer surface began. The mesenchyme that extended cephalad within the central canal would also be induced to form fat and would be directly continuous with the fat within the dorsal cleft. Since the fat within the cleft lies along the dorsal dural defect, it is anatomically extradural and would, in turn, be directly continuous with the extracanalicular subcutaneous fat. If the premature dysjunction occurred unilaterally, the neural plate might well be rotated and the spinal and subcutaneous lipoma might well extend asymmetrically to one side of the midline.

Since the nerve roots develop from the neural plate itself, and since that plate was splayed open, the dorsal and ventral nerve roots would be expected to arise from the ventral surface of the neural plate (cleft cord) and grow outward through the subarachnoid space to their root sleeves. They would not be expected to traverse fat.

Spina bifida was induced by McLone and Naidich in the chick embryo over the normal avian glycogen body, a structure of uncertain function.[36] The glycogen body normally occupies a midline position in what closely resembles a dorsal myeloschisis. Its relationships are remarkably similar to those expected from the embryologic theory and to those observed in human lipomyeloschisis at surgery. It serves, therefore, as a paradigm for human lipomyeloschisis. Many features of this model have been reported previously by McLone and Naidich.[36]

In summary, the ventral surface of the neural plate can induce mesenchyme to form the meninges, whereas the dorsal surface of the neural plate can induce only the formation of fat. If the cutaneous ectoderm detaches from the neural crest prior to closure of the neural tube, mesenchyme streams into the neural groove. The mesenchyme is induced to form fat that prevents closure of the neural tube; thus a lipomyelomeningocele is formed.

Lipomas of the Filum Terminale. These are fatty masses located within the filum terminale (Figs. 5–115 and 5–116). These are anatomically and embryologically distinct from lipomyeloschisis. Filar lipomas result from defective development of the tail end of the spinal cord, perhaps because the caudal cell mass is not well organized and is still in a state of evolution or regression. What seems to happen is that the caudal cell mass (termed Hensen's node) will pinch off a series of beads—little cellular beads—composed of multipotential cells. Mesenchyme is initially interposed between these

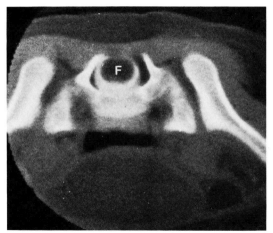

FIGURE 5–116. Spinal dysraphism.

A water contrast CT scan shows the large fat-filled filum (F) in the sacral sac.

beads. These beads will cavitate, link up with each other, and then cavitate into each other to create a tubular structure that ultimately forms everything in the tail end of the embryo, including the skeletal structure and filum terminale.

If one examines lipomas of the filum terminale in humans, they appear more likely to contain disparate elements such as striated muscle and a variety of other elements, whereas lipomas that occur higher up on the spinal cord at the thoracolumbar junction are almost pure lipomas. Presumably, the complex composition of the more distal level results from the less orderly sequence of development of the filum.

In the *subcutaneous lipoma with intradural stalk,* the fibrofatty stalk pierces the dura in an area of spina bifida occulta to attach to the filum terminale or conus medullaris; this anomaly probably develops during the stage of secondary neural tube formation by a disorganization of the process of retrogressive differentiation.

CLINICAL FEATURES OF SPINAL DYSRAPHISM

Most cases of lipomeningocele and lipoma of the filum terminale are asymptomatic during infancy. The only physical finding may be the lumbosacral *soft-tissue lump* (Fig. 5–117), which is regarded as a cosmetic deformity.

Cutaneous lesions may be present; it is vital to closely scrutinize the skin to detect abnormalities. The local increase in hair (hypertrichosis) may be minimal or abundant in the form of a fawn's tail (Fig. 5–118). The hypertrichosis may be associated with hemangiomata or telangiectasia. Sacral dimples in spinal dysraphism

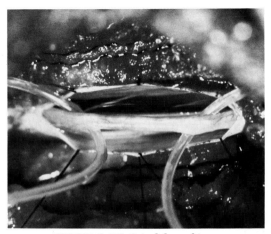

FIGURE 5–115. Spinal dysraphism.

A thickened filum terminale, containing fat, tethers the spinal cord. Normal nerves can be seen in the lumbar sac.

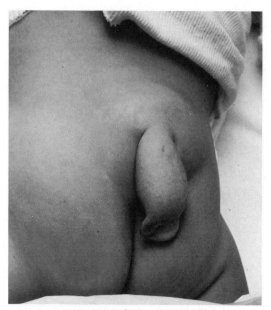

FIGURE 5–117. Spinal dysraphism.

A lipomyelomeningocele located at the lumbosacral level above the intergluteal fold. This appendage is present in a small number of cases.

are always in the midline; these dimples may be connected to a sinus tract (dermal sinus) or a fibrous band leading to bone or dura. One should be highly suspicious of skin dimples proximal to the fifth lumbar level, particularly when associated with spina bifida occulta. The location of the cutaneous lesion does not always correlate with the level of intraspinal lesion.

In spinal dysraphism, *musculoskeletal deformity* may be present at birth; it may manifest

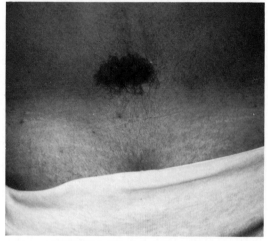

FIGURE 5–118. Spinal dysraphism.

Hypertrichosis in the lumbosacral area in a patient with spinal dysraphism.

as talipes equinovarus, congenital convex pes valgus, cavus, or simple equinus. There may be shortening or atrophy of the lower limb or congenital hip subluxation or dislocation. When an infant presents with a deformity of the lower limb, it is essential to examine the spine in order to rule out spinal dysraphism.

Neurologic deficit usually manifests during the second year of life. The child may have difficulty in learning to walk owing to muscle weakness or spasticity, or a child who was walking normally may develop a gait abnormality. On careful examination, one foot may be smaller than the opposite side, or a calf or thigh atrophy may be noted. One should suspect spinal dysraphism when a child who was previously functioning normally later develops progressive limp, muscle weakness, deformity of a foot or lower limb, scoliosis, or kyphosis. There may be a small ilium as a result of hypoplasia or absence of sacral nerve roots.

Sensory dysfunction is difficult to detect in an infant or young child. Loss of sensation usually manifests as skin ulceration or pressure areas. In spinal dysraphism there may be loss of tactile, hot-cold, vibratory, and position sense.

Bladder dysfunction is another manifestation of spinal dysraphism. Is there any abnormality of urination such as incontinence or enuresis? What is the level of bladder control? Is there a history of repeated episodes of cystitis?

In summary, clinical features that should make the orthopedic surgeon highly suspicious of spinal dysraphism are the presence of (1) a lumbosacral soft tissue mass; (2) deformity of the lower limbs and feet, especially if progressive; and (3) urologic disturbance such as incontinence and dribbling urine.

DIAGNOSIS

Often the initial physician fails to make the correct diagnosis, resulting in a delay of up to two to eight years. The diagnostic evaluation of the patient suspected of spinal dysraphism should include the following: (1) a thorough clinical examination of the musculoskeletal system, including muscle testing; (2) neurologic assessment; (3) ultrasound examination of the spine, especially in the infant (Fig. 5–119); (4) plain radiograms of the entire spine; (5) electromyography, which may show denervation potential and fibrillation; (6) dermatomal somatosensory evoked potentials (asymmetry of these SSE potentials is very suggestive of spinal dysraphism); (7) myelography with metrizamide (Fig. 5–120); and (8) computerized axial tomog-

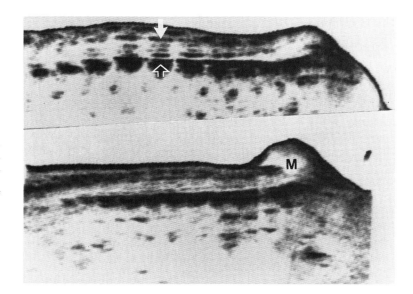

FIGURE 5–119. Spinal dysraphism.

An ultrasound of an infant shows the lamina (closed arrow), spinal cord (triple echoes), and vertebral bodies (open arrow). Note the meningocele (M) at the end of the cerebrospinal fluid space.

raphy and nuclear magnetic resonance imaging studies of the spine.

NEUROSURGICAL MANAGEMENT

The natural history of the neonatal lipomyelomeningocele is not well documented. In the literature, controlled studies are not available

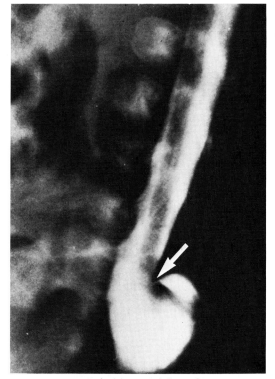

FIGURE 5–120. Spinal dysraphism.

A water contrast myelogram demonstrates the straight spinal cord and the sharp angulation (arrow) as the cord passes under the fibrous band of the bifid lamina.

to confirm the results of operated and untreated cases. Nonetheless, in our experience, one child, normal at birth, returned at six weeks of age with a flail lower limb and dribbling urine. This convinced us that neurologic deterioration could occur in these children early and over a very short period of time. We then decided that any child born with a lipomyelomeningocele should undergo surgery as soon as the proper neuroradiologic studies are completed.

The operative technique (Figs. 5–121 to 5–124) of resection of lipomyelomeningocele is as follows: A midline skin incision is made with the knife, followed by laser dissection thereafter. The knife is used for the skin incision because the laser sometimes interferes with skin healing. The skin is then undermined laterally, care being taken to leave intact a substantial layer of subcutaneous fat to provide the skin with vascular support. The most cephalic intact neural arch is then identified by palpation. One to two levels inferior to this palpation identifies the most cephalic, widely bifid laminae and a distinct, tough fibrous band that stretches across the midline to connect the club-shaped medial ends of the bifid laminae. This band appears to be a remnant of the tissue that should have formed the neural arch at that level. The band lies at the cephalic end of the fibrous defect in the spinal canal and tethers and kinks the dural tube, cord, and meningocele, which herniates dorsally through the fibrous defect. One of the most important parts of the surgical procedure is section and release of this "tethering" band. In fact, when the band is cut, the dural tube and lipoma almost jump out of the canal. Somatosensory evoked potentials (SSEPs) have shown increased amplitude and decreased la-

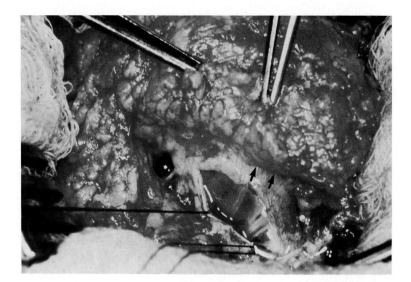

FIGURE 5–121. Spinal dysraphism.

An incision is made in the dura mater anterior and lateral to the lipoma-dura junction (arrows). Note the dorsal roots through the arachnoid as they pass to enter the cord at the junction of lipoma and dura mater.

tency immediately following section of the band. Although we have used SSEPs extensively in the past, it is not certain that SSEPs are truly of value intraoperatively. SSEPs stimulated at diverse points on the lower limbs can be used to determine the lowest functional dermatome. SSEPs will indicate that an error has been made but will not prevent the error in this type of complex operative procedure. This is not to minimize the need for SSEPs in other spinal procedures, especially in scoliosis surgery.

The next step in the surgical procedure is incision of the dura (1) on the side of the widest subarachnoid space and (2) away from the entry zones of the dorsal nerve roots. The widest

subarachnoid space typically lies on the side opposite the lipoma and can be identified readily by preoperative sonography, myelography, and/or intraoperative sonography through the intact dura. It is important to appreciate that the dura, the dorsal root entry zone of the placode, and the lipoma all come together at the same point. One is tempted to enter the subarachnoid space along the line at which the dura meets lipoma. This is the worst possible place to do so, since the dorsal roots and dorsal root entry zone lie immediately subjacent to this line of junction. One can inadvertently section the dorsal roots if the dura is not opened properly. In this author's opinion, the best way to avoid this risk is to make the initial dural incision (1) well lateral to the line of junction of lipoma and dura and (2) at a more

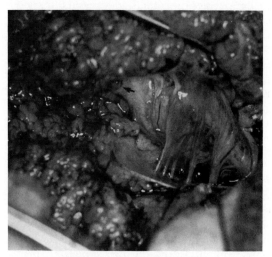

FIGURE 5–122. Spinal dysraphism.

The dura and arachnoid are now entirely open and the filum (arrow) has been cut. Note the caudal spinal cord and lipoma are only tethered by the nerve roots.

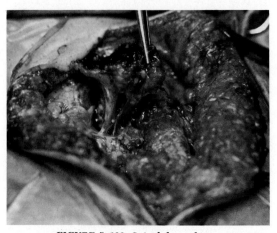

FIGURE 5–123. Spinal dysraphism.

The laser has been used to nearly totally remove the lipoma.

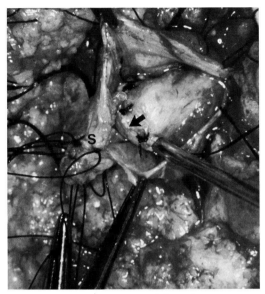

FIGURE 5–124. Spinal dysraphism.

The dural-arachnoid flaps are closed (arrow) over the caudal spinal cord and the distal cerebrospinal fluid sac is being constructed.

cephalic level where the anatomy is more nearly normal. Intraoperative sonography can be utilized at this point to delineate the structures beneath the point of initial dural incision.

The laminectomy is performed as high as is necessary to reach an area of dura that looks normal. Begin the incision laterally where the dura appears nearly normal! One can then see the intact arachnoid and, through the arachnoid, the dorsal nerve roots, which pass toward their entry zone just beneath the lipodural junction. The arachnoid is then opened and the dural/arachnoid incision is carried completely around the distal spinal cord under direct vision to preserve the nerve roots. This circumferential incision leaves a small circumferential flap of dura and subjacent pia-arachnoid attached to the placode at the lipodural junction. This flap will be used later in the closure.

The problem of visualizing the nerve roots and of getting lost chasing them through the fat is a real one. If one were to trace nerve roots beyond the lipomatous mass, one would be chasing them into the extradural location where nerve roots are supposed to be surrounded by fat in the normal state. This is an example of pursuing nerve roots into a fatty environment that does not represent a pathologic situation. The important anatomic structure to locate is the posterior margin of the dura. At that point, the operation is essentially over. One need not go any further.

Remove the lipomatous mass. This is adherent to the spinal cord; when it is excised, the spinal cord will be freed. The simplest and most rapid way to debulk the lipoma is with the laser. By playing it over the surface of the lipoma, one can virtually wipe away the fat and areolar tissue with only infrequent interruptions to cauterize larger bleeders with bipolar cautery. With a little experience, it is possible to reduce the lipoma to proper proportion by laser (see Fig. 5–123).

Great care must be taken not to attempt total removal of the lipoma. It is dangerous to remove the final few cell layers of lipoma because they extend down into the matrix of the cord. Therefore, stop the dissection at this point and begin closure by inverting the circumferential dural flap and subjacent pia-arachnoid over the distal cord and remaining lipoma! Because of the inversion, the smooth pia-arachnoid now lies superficial to the dura. The dura/pia-arachnoid flaps along each side are pulled together and overlapped to cover the distal end of the spinal cord (Fig. 5–124) with a smooth pial surface which, it is hoped, will reduce the incidence of retethering by scar. The residual portions of lipoma attached to the cord are incorporated beneath the closure. We used to reconstitute the dural sac with fascia, but now use Silastic or lyophilized dura to create a space that will distend with cerebrospinal fluid and provide an environment in which subsequent tethering is unlikely. In reviewing our cases, we have had three children in whom retethering occurred. On re-exploration, everything seemed intact, yet there was tethering of the spinal cord to the fascia. Because of this, we reverted to the use of plastics and lyophilized dura instead of paraspinous muscle fascia.

Two other technical points merit discussion. First, the tilted placode: When a placode is tilted over on its side, the dorsal and ventral nerve roots on the deep side are unusually short. One will have difficulty untethering the cord in this situation. At least we have never been able to untether it to our satisfaction. The superficial side can be untethered without difficulty. The cord then flops back and forth and moves up and down a little bit, but it remains tethered ventrolaterally by the short nerve roots of the deep side. The objective is to allow nerve roots to grow with time, thereby relieving the tethering effect. In this case, we simply do the remainder of the operation, remove the lipoma, and reconstitute the tube, leaving the placode tipped over and tied down in that corner.

The second problem is the concurrent skin appendage. Some children who have skin appendages associated with the lipoma present a problem because of a dermal sinus within the appendage. In this group untethering is difficult to accomplish. The sinus passes into the dorsum of the cord for some distance. Upon entering the spinal cord, it may merge with a lipoma that extends deep into the central canal of the cord.

The statistics of our patients are interesting. Postoperatively, the major improvements are in motor strength and (less commonly) in urologic function. One child who had never been continent in the five years of her life voided in the recovery room. For the first time she was able to feel herself urinate and, before discharge, she was continent of urine. Another child who began walking at 14 months came to us at 3 years of age unable to walk. The lipoma was removed, recovery began in the hospital, and the child was discharged walking. Obviously, some very dramatic results can be achieved by neurosurgical intervention. Motor improvement occurred in 50 per cent, and urologic improvement was seen in 7 per cent of the cases. However, half of the patients do not show motor improvement—rather, the function stabilizes.

The neurologic status in some children deteriorates. There appear to be three reasons for this:

First, mass effect: The lipomatous mass acts as an expansile tumor within the central canal, compressing the conus. The available evidence indicates that the lipoma is stable in cell number but increases in cell volume by progressive fat deposition. Such a mechanism would explain satisfactorily the observed deterioration in the early infantile period and during periods of rapid weight gain.

Second, tethering: Tethering of the spinal cord is caused by (1) the lipoma's attachment to subcutaneous fat, (2) the dura mater's being attached to the fascia of the paraspinal musculature, and (3) kinking at the fibrous band between the uppermost widely bifid laminae. Normal developmental growth spurts are usually associated with the onset or progression of symptoms.

Third, tethering of the cord by scarring into prior surgical closure: The goals of surgical repair, then, are decompression of neural elements by debulking sufficient lipoma to allow the conus to return to the canal, release of all fibrous bands tethering the cord, and prevention of retethering by reconstructing a neural tube and dorsal subarachnoid space lined with tissues that make retethering unlikely. Incomplete repairs of lipomyelomeningocele fail to achieve these goals and leave the child at increased risk of later neurologic deterioration.

Operative mortality has been 0 per cent in the series at the Children's Memorial Medical Center in Chicago. One child with purely orthopedic problems prior to surgery developed urinary incontinence in the postoperative period. Wound infections occurred in 9 per cent of the cases and meningitis in one child. These infections responded to routine measures, without increased deficits. Patients who were normal prior to surgery have remained intact during a follow-up period of several months to ten years. All the children are in regular school or (if less than school age) are expected to enter regular school. Repeat operation necessitated by retethering of the cord was done in six patients, although duraplasty was done at the time of the initial surgery in four of those children. In these four, the residual lipoma was adherent to the dural graft, which in turn was incorporated into the closure scar. Duraplasty alone apparently does not prevent retethering. It is still too early to tell whether terminal cord reconstitution will prevent such retethering.

Any child with a myelomeningocele or a lipomyelomeningocele who shows signs of neurologic deterioration should have thorough neurologic and neuroradiologic assessment for the possibility of retethering. Deterioration indicates that something has gone wrong. A complication has developed. Secondary deterioration is not the natural postoperative history of the disease. If the child with a dysraphic state deteriorates after surgery, then one of three things is likely to be taking place: The spinal cord may have become tethered, there is an inclusion dermoid, or there is hydromyelia. In our experience, these are all correctable lesions.

In addition to the lipoma, there are several congenital tumors that involve the distal spinal cord and cauda equina. This group of tumors may have cutaneous manifestations that betray their presence within the spinal canal. In presentation and course they are very similar to the other congenital lesions of the spinal cord. Some are lesions, such as a dermoid, a lipoma, a tethered cord, and an anterior meningocele, all occurring in the same child. We have also seen a diastematomyelia with a large bony spur and an associated intrathecal Wilms tumor. Other tumors include the dermoid, the teratomas, and glial series tumors, most often the ependymoma.

ORTHOPEDIC MANAGEMENT

The care of the musculoskeletal deformity depends upon its type. The basic principles of treatment of each deformity are discussed in the section on myelomeningocele. It is vital, however, to untether the spinal cord and nerve roots prior to orthopedic treatment in order to prevent recurrence of the deformity.

Postoperative care of children with lipomyelomeningocele or spinal dysraphism is best carried out in a multidisciplinary clinic that cares for children with myelomeningocele. The medical/surgical problems are similar, and the expertise required from the various subspecialties is the same.

Myelocystocele

Another entity that must be considered in the differential diagnosis of skin-covered lumbosacral masses is the terminal myelocystocele, which must be differentiated from sacral teratomas.

The myelocystocele and the teratoma differ from the lipomyelomeningocele by usually extending into the intergluteal fold. The myelocystocele is an accumulation of cerebrospinal fluid in the terminal ventricle of the spinal cord and therefore is really not a dysraphic condition. The consequences of this disease are very similar to those of the dysraphic states. Early treatment is indicated to prevent progressive loss of neuromuscular function.

The teratoma has quite a different prognosis and represents a neoplasm with the potential for malignant deterioration. The single best test for differentiating the teratoma from the myelocystocele is the ultrasound study. The teratoma usually contains solid tumor and extends into the presacral space, whereas the myelocystocele usually shows a two-compartment cystic structure posterior to the sacrum. Myelocystoceles are often associated with exstrophy of the bladder.

Tethered Cord

Limitation of movement of the distal end of the spinal cord can produce a variety of symptoms due to deterioration of cord function. The fixation or tethering of the end of the spinal cord allows intermittent bowstringing of the spinal cord between the normal cephalic attachment and the point of the tether.

In the past it was postulated that the symptoms of tethered cord are due to inability of the conus to ascend to its normal level of the first or second lumbar vertebra during growth. However, Barson demonstrated that the conus completes its ascent by two months of age.[4] It is now established that the symptoms of tethered

cord are caused by impaired mobility of the spinal cord. With flexion and extension of the trunk, repetitive forces of stretch are exerted on the spinal cord. When the spinal cord stretches under tension, the vasculature is attenuated and the spinal cord suffers intermittent ischemia. Stretching of the spinal cord impairs mitochondrial oxidation metabolism. Prolonged neuronal dysfunction will cause permanent damage to the perikarya and axon. Untethering of the spinal cord will improve the oxidation metabolism. The younger the age of the patient at the time of untethering, the greater is the degree of postoperative improvement.

The most common cause of tethered spinal cord is the lipomyelomeningocele. Second is retethering of the spinal cord after repair of myelomeningocele or a lipomyelomeningocele. The third cause is the lipoma of the filum terminale. Other causes are diastematomyelia, taut filum terminale, anomalous fibrous bands, and anomalous roots of spinal nerves.

CLINICAL FEATURES

The most frequent symptoms are subtle atrophy and orthopedic foot deformities. Pain radiating into the legs, especially with exercise, is common. Lordosis and flexed posture of the knees due to hamstring spasm on standing are common physical findings. Bladder and bowel symptoms may be present, signaling an urgent situation requiring immediate attention.

Prior to the onset of neurologic deficits, many of the spine and spinal cord anomalies can be suspected because of cutaneous hallmarks. Besides the obvious open lesions of myelomeningocele and the lumps of the lipoma, there are a series of diseases that place the apparently healthy child at risk of insidious or precipitous deterioration. Any skin lesion located over the spine should make one suspect an underlying process. Hemangiomas, pigmented spots, dimples, pits, and tufts of hair are some of the common indicators of occult disease.

Often the child with a short filum or lipomyelomeningocele will be asymptomatic, only to deteriorate during a phase of rapid growth in height. Recently it has become evident that adults who have tethered spinal cords who escaped deficits during the growth years and have done well may deteriorate in their fifth and sixth decades with the onset of kyphosis with aging.

In the myelomeningocele population, any of the aforementioned symptoms may occur. More often, however, subtle changes in tone, usually spasticity, muscle function loss, or the onset of scoliosis above the level of the lesion, are found. These changes are often insidious and will be picked up only by a scheduled routine of close observation. Periodic muscle examinations are vital.

In myelomeningocele, hydromyelia must be ruled out and differentiated from tethered cord. Hydromyelia may be treated simply by shunt revision. In our experience, shunt revision may relieve symptoms. The scoliotic curve usually corrects by several degrees.

TREATMENT

Tethered cord is released by the experienced neurosurgeon.

References

1. Al-Mefty, O., Kandzari, S., and Fox, J. L.: Neurogenic bladder and the tethered spinal cord syndrome. J. Urol., *122*:112, 1979.
2. Anderson, F. M.: Occult spinal dysraphism: diagnosis and management. J. Pediatr., *73*:163, 1968.
3. Anderson, F. M.: Occult spinal dysraphism: A series of 73 cases. Pediatrics, *55*:826, 1975.
4. Barson, A. J.: The vertebral level of termination of the spinal cord during normal and abnormal development. J. Anat., *106*:489, 1970.
5. Barson, A. J., and Sands, J.: Physical and biochemical characteristics of the human dysraphic spinal cord. Dev. Med. Child Neurol. (Suppl. 35)*17*:11, 1975.
6. Bassett, R. C.: The neurologic deficit associated with lipomas of the cauda equina. Ann. Surg., *131*:109, 1950.
7. Braun, I. F., Raghavendra, B. N., and Kricheff, I. I.: Spinal cord imaging using real-time high-resolution ultrasound. Radiology, *147*:459, 1983.
8. Bruce, D. A., and Schut, L.: Spinal lipomas in infancy and childhood. Childs Brain, *5*:192, 1979.
9. Cameron, A. H.: Malformation of the neural spinal axis, urogenital tract and foregut in spina bifida attributable to disturbances of the blastopore. J. Pathol., *73*:215, 1957.
10. Chapman, P. H.: Congenital intraspinal lipomas: anatomic considerations and surgical treatment. Childs Brain, *9*:37, 1982.
11. Chapman, P. H., and Davis, K. R.: Surgical treatment of spinal lipomas in childhood. *In* Raimondi, A. J. (ed.): Concepts in Pediatric Neurosurgery. Vol. 3. Basel, S. Karger, 1983, pp. 178–190.
12. Ehni, G., and Love, J. G.: Intraspinal lipomas. Report of a case; review of the literature and clinical and pathologic study. Arch. Neurol. Psychiatry, *53*:1, 1945.
13. Emery, J. L., and Lendon, R. B.: Lipomas of the cauda equina and other fatty tumors related to neurospinal dysraphism. Dev. Med. Child Neurol., (Suppl.)*20*:62, 1969.
14. Feingold, M.: Picture of the month. Lipomeningocele. Am. J. Dis. Child., *138*:89, 1984.
15. Finlay, D., Stockdale, H. R., and Lewin, E.: An appraisal of the use of diagnostic ultrasound to quantify the lumbar spinal canal. Br. J. Radiol., *54*:870, 1981.
16. Fitz, C. R., and Harwood-Nash, D. C.: The tethered conus. A.J.R., *125*:515, 1975.
17. Fukui, J., and Kakizaki, T.: Urodynamic evaluation of tethered cord syndrome including tight filum terminale. Urology, *16*:539, 1980.
18. Gardner, J. W.: The Dysraphic States. Amsterdam, Excerpta Medica, 1973.
19. Gillespie, R., Faithful, D., Roth, H., and Hall, J. E.: Intraspinal anomalies in congenital scoliosis. Clin. Orthop., *93*:103, 1973.
20. Hall, D. E., Udvarhelyi, G. B., and Altman, J.: Lumbosacral skin lesions as markers of occult spinal dysraphism. J.A.M.A., *246*:2606, 1981.
21. Harris, H. W., and Miller, O. F.: Midline cutaneous and spinal defects. Midline cutaneous abnormalities associated with occult spinal disorders. Arch. Dermatol., *112*:1724, 1976.
22. Hibbert, C. S., Delaygue, C., McGlen, B., and Porter, R. W.: Measurement of the lumbar spinal canal by diagnostic ultrasound. Br. J. Radiol., *54*:905, 1981.
23. Higginbottom, M. C., Jones, K. L., James, H. E., Bruce, D. A., and Schut, L.: Aplasia cutis congenita: a cutaneous marker of occult spinal dysraphism. J. Pediatr., *96*:687, 1980.
24. Hoffman, H. J., Hendrick, E. B., and Humphreys, R. P.: The tethered spinal cord: its protean manifestations, diagnosis and surgical correction. Childs Brain, *2*:145, 1976.
25. Hoffman, H. J., Taecholarn, C., and Hendrick, E. B.: Management of lipomyelomeningoceles. Experience at the Hospital for Sick Children, Toronto. J. Neurosurg., *62*:1, 1985.
26. James, C. C. M., and Lassman, L. P.: Spinal dysraphism: The diagnosis and treatment of progressive lesion in spina bifida occulta. J. Bone Joint Surg., *44-B*:828, 1962.
27. James, H. E., and Walsh, J. W.: Spinal dysraphism. Curr. Probl. Pediatr., *11*:1, 1980–81.
28. Johnson, A.: Fatty tumour from the sacrum of a child, connected with the spinal membranes. Trans. Pathol. Soc. Lond., *8*:16, 1857.
29. Johnson, A.: Sacrum of a child containing a fatty tumor connected with the interior of the spinal canal. Lancet, *7*:35, 1957.
30. Kadziolka, R., Asztely, M., Hansson, T., and Nachemson, A.: Ultrasonic measurement of the lumbar spinal canal. The origin and precision of the recorded echoes. J. Bone Joint Surg., *63-B*:504, 1981.
31. Lassman, L. P., and James, C. C. M.: Lumbosacral lipomas: critical survey of 26 cases submitted to laminectomy. J. Neurol. Neurosurg. Psychiatry, *30*:174, 1967.
32. Lemire, R. J., Graham, C. B., and Beckwith, J. B.: Skin-covered sacrococcygeal masses in infants and children. J. Pediatr., *79*:948, 1971.
33. Lichtenstein, B. W.: Spinal dysraphism, spina bifida and myelodysplasia. Arch. Neurol. Psychiatry, *44*:792, 1940.
34. Linder, M., Rosenstein, J., and Sklar, F. H.: Functional improvement after spinal surgery for the dysraphic malformation. Neurosurgery, *11*:622, 1982.
35. McLone, D. G., Mutluer, S., and Naidich, T. P.: Lipomeningoceles of the conus medullaris. *In* Raimondi, A. J. (ed.): Concepts in Pediatric Neurosurgery. Vol. 3. Basel, S. Karger, 1983, pp. 170–177.
36. McLone, D. G., and Naidich, T. P.: Spinal dysraphism: Clinical and experimental. *In* Holtzman, R. N. N., and Stein, B. M. (eds.): The Tethered Spinal Cord. New York, Thieme Stratton, 1985, pp. 14–28.
37. McLone, D. G., and Naidich, T. P.: Terminal myelocystocele. Neurosurgery, *16*:36, 1985.
38. Matson, D. D.: Neurosurgery of Infancy and Childhood. 2nd ed. Springfield, Ill., Charles C Thomas, 1969, p. 46.
39. Miller, J. H., Reid, B. S., and Kemberling, C. R.: Utilization of ultrasound in the evaluation of spinal dysraphism in children. Radiology, *143*:737, 1982.
40. Naidich, T. P., Fernbach, S. K., and McLone, D. G.: John Caffey Award. Sonography of the caudal spine and back: congenital anomalies in children. A.J.R., *142*:1229, 1984.

41. Naidich, T. P., McLone, D. G., and Mutluer, S.: A new understanding of dorsal dysraphism with lipoma (lipomyeloschisis): radiologic evaluation and surgical correction. A.J.R., *4*:103, 1983.
42. Padget, D. H.: Spina bifida and embryonic neuroschises—a causal relationship. Johns Hopkins Med. J., *123*:223, 1968.
43. Padget, D. H.: Neuroschisis and human embryonic maldevelopment. J. Neuropathol. Exp. Neurol., *29*:192, 1970.
44. Pang, D., and Wilberger, J. E.: Tethered cord syndrome in adults. J. Neurosurg., *57*:32, 1982.
45. Patten, B. M.: Embryological stages in the establishment of myeloschises with spina bifida. Am. J. Anat., *93*:385, 1953.
46. Pierre-Kahn, A., Lacombe, J., and Pichon, J.: Intraspinal lipoma with spina bifida. Prognosis and treatment in 73 cases. J. Neurosurg., *65*:756, 1986.
47. Raghavendra, B. N., Epstein, F. J., and Pinto, R. S.: The tethered spinal cord: diagnosis by high-resolution real-time ultrasound. Radiology, *149*:123, 1983.
48. Rogers, H. M., Long, D. M., Chou, S. N., et al.: Lipomas of the spinal cord and cauda equina. J. Neurosurg., *34*:349, 1971.
49. Roller, G. J., and Pribram, H. F. W.: Lumbosacral intradural lipoma and sacral agenesis. Radiology, *84*:507, 1965.
50. Scheible, W., James, H. E., Leopold, G. R., et al.: Occult spinal dysraphism in infants: screening with high-resolution real-time ultrasound. Radiology, *146*:743, 1983.
51. Schut, L., Bruce, D. A., and Sutton, L. N.: The management of the child with a lipomyelomeningocele. Clin. Neurosurg., *30*:446, 1983.
52. Streeter, G. L.: Factors involved in the formation of the filum terminale. Am. J. Anat., *25*:1, 1919.
53. Tavafoghi, V., Ghandcyi, A., Hambrick, G. W., et al.: Cutaneous signs of spinal dysraphism. Arch. Dermatol., *114*:573, 1978.
54. Thompson, W. F., and McKay, M.: Occult spinal dysraphism. Case Report and review of the literature. Orthopedics, *9*:402, 1986.
55. Till, K.: Spinal dysraphism—a study of congenital malformation of the lower back. J. Bone Joint Surg., *51-B*:415, 1969.
56. Udvarhelyi, G. B.: Mild forms of spinal dysraphism and associated conditions. *In* Freeman, J. M. (ed.): Practical Management of Meningomyelocele. Baltimore, University Park Press, 1974.
57. Yamada, S., Sinke, D., and Sanders, D.: Pathophysiology of "tethered cord syndromes." J. Neurosurg., *54*:494, 1981.

DIASTEMATOMYELIA[1-43]

Diastematomyelia is a congenital malformation of the neural axis in which there is a sagittal division of the spinal cord or its intraspinal derivatives; often it is associated with a projection of an osseous, fibrocartilaginous, or fibrous spur that is attached anteriorly to one or more vertebral bodies and posteriorly to the dura (Fig. 5–125). When a spur is present, the spinal cord is usually tethered by the spur and a thickened filum terminale. This entity should be distinguished from *diplomyelia*, a very rare anomaly in which the spinal cord is duplicated but not tethered (Fig. 5–126).

The pathogenesis of diastematomyelia is un-

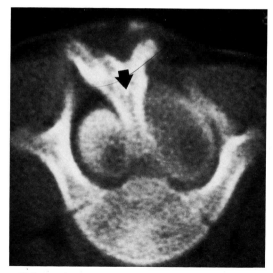

FIGURE 5–125. Diastematomyelia with a bone spur (arrow).

This case also had a tethered filum terminale and a Wilms tumor attached to the dorsum of the filum.

known. It appears that during the organization of the neural tube from the primitive neuroectoderm, aberrant mesodermal cells protrude into the neural tissue on its anterior surface instead of becoming arranged entirely around its periphery. They persist in this location, developing into a bony and dural septum. Associated multiple congenital anomalies of the vertebrae with some degree of incomplete spinal fusion are often present.

The bony or fibrocartilaginous spicule is usually located in the lumbar region, though it may be seen at a segmental level as high as the fifth thoracic vertebra. The osseous septum transfixes the spinal cord or cauda equina at a low anatomic level, checkreining its normal ascent during growth of the vertebral column, which terminates at the first two months of age. Later it impedes the normal mobility of the spinal cord during flexion-extension of the trunk with stretching of the spinal cord and roots. Progressive neurologic deficit distal to the level of the lesion develops.

The condition is more common in the female, accounting for about 75 per cent of the cases.

Clinical Picture

Abnormalities of motor function in the lower limbs are not ordinarily detected at birth. Hallmarks of the condition are the various types of skin defects that are found near the midline at the level of the lesion. The cutaneous abnormalities include abnormal tufts of hair (Fig. 5–

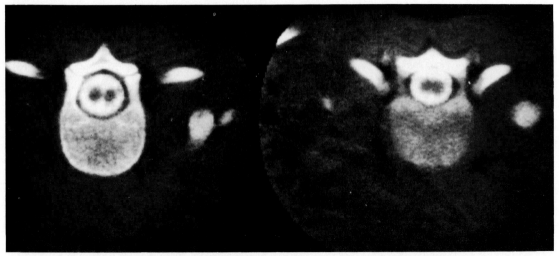

FIGURE 5–126. Diastematomyelia (diplomyelia) seen in a water-contrast CT scan.

The split cord was not tethered.

127), dimpling of the skin, ill-defined subcutaneous fatty tumors, and cutaneous vascular malformations. Localized scoliosis due to congenital anomalies of the vertebrae is not uncommon.

During the first two years of life, increasing disturbance of function of the lower limbs develops. The child may fail to walk at the expected normal time, or some abnormality of

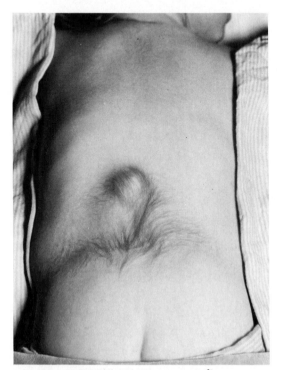

FIGURE 5–127. Diastematomyelia.

A hairy patch on the back of a child with a diastematomyelia.

gait may develop after the child has learned to walk properly. Muscle paralysis is often present, and it may be spastic or flaccid, depending upon the level of the lesion. The anterior tibial and peroneal muscles are often paralyzed. The type of limp depends upon the muscles involved. Atrophy of one or both lower limbs is a common finding. A varus, valgus, or cavus deformity of the foot is frequent. In thoracic lesions, the deep tendon reflexes are hyperactive with a positive ankle clonus and dorsiflexion response to the Babinski stimulus. In lumbar lesions the deep tendon reflexes may be diminished or absent. Poor rectal sphincter tone and urinary incontinence are frequent findings. Sensory examination may demonstrate a definite deficit, particularly in the saddle area.

Radiographic Findings

Radiograms of the spine will disclose widening of the spinal canal and interpedicular distance that is maximal at the level of the lesion but may extend over several adjacent segments (Fig. 5–128). It should be noted, however, that interpedicular widening is not diagnostic of diastematomyelia. The absence of thinning of the pedicles and lack of erosion of the posterior aspect of the vertebral bodies suggest a congenital origin for widening of the spinal canal rather than an expanding intraspinal mass, which would cause pressure erosion.

The bony spicule is best visualized in the anteroposterior projection as an irregular fragment of increased density, lying in the midline of the spinal canal. It is approximately 1 cm. in length (Fig. 5–129). In the lateral projection,

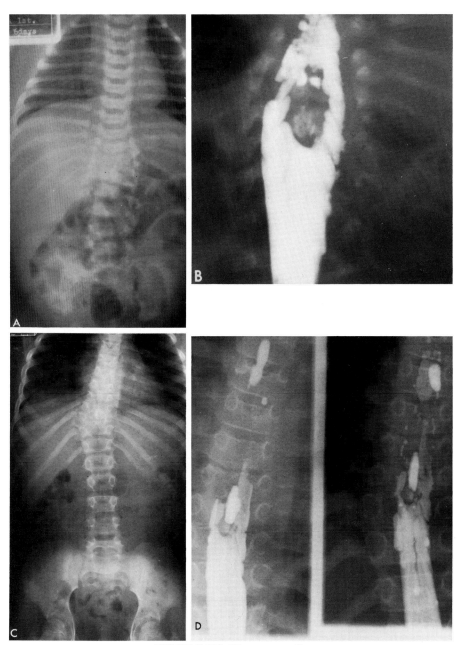

FIGURE 5–128. Diastematomyelia.

A and B. Diastematomyelia in a six-day-old infant. In the plain radiogram of the spine, note the widening of the interpediculate distance and hemivertebra, and in the myelogram, the midline bony spicule around which the opaque medium is divided into two columns. C and D. Diastematomyelia in an eight-year-old boy. Note the bony spicule and widening of the intraspinal canal.

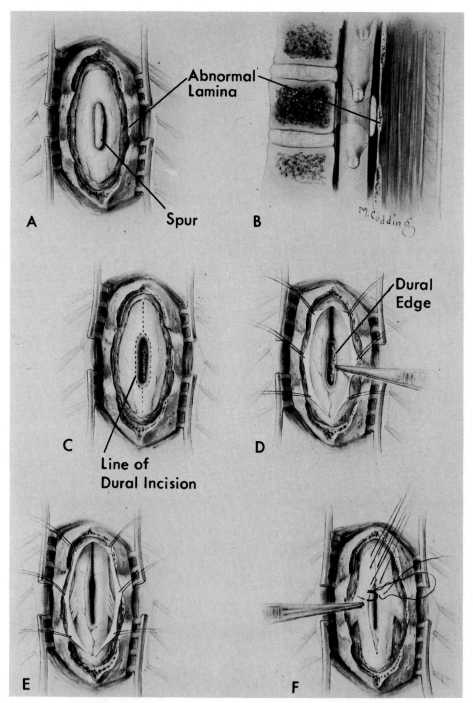

FIGURE 5–129. *Operative technique of excision of diastematomyelia.*

(From Matson, D. D., Woods, R., Campbell, J., and Ingraham, F. D.: Diastematomyelia (congenital clefts of the spinal cord): Diagnosis and surgical treatment. Pediatrics, 6:98, 1950. Reprinted by permission.)

the bony spicule may be seen as a radiopaque septum arising from the posterior surface of the vertebral body. In plain radiograms, bony septa was found in 16 of 41 patients in the series of James and Lassman, and in 16 of 25 patients by Sheptak and Susen.[19, 39]

Various other anomalies of the vertebrae are also present. These include decrease in the anteroposterior diameter of the vertebral bodies, hemivertebrae, failure of segmentation of vertebrae, and incomplete or absent fusion of laminae resulting in spina bifida. The level of the septum is best correlated with anomalies of the lamina—particularly the combination of intersegmental laminar fusion with spina bifida.

Myelography with metrizamide will usually visualize the pathologic changes and help to determine the exact level and extent of diastematomyelia. A characteristic finding is the division of the opaque medium into two columns that flow readily around the midline bony spicule and dural septum. It should be noted, however, that the spur is not always midline; the split of the spinal cord may be into symmetrical or asymmetrical segments. Myelography is of significant help in surgery; it is often combined with computerized axial tomography of the spine. In addition to identification of a cartilaginous or fibrous septum, myelography and CT scanning will detect the presence of other dysraphic lesions that may tether the cord. In 16 of the 21 cases of known diastematomyelia, Scottie et al. found other causes of tethering of the spinal cord.[37] It is wise to study the entire spine (prone and supine) in order to rule out the presence of multiple lesions. Recently, magnetic resonance imaging has replaced myelography, as it is noninvasive.

In the assessment of patients with suspected diastematomyelia, electromyographic studies will show denervation potential and fibrillation as a result of motor weakness of the affected muscle. In addition, dermatomal somatosensory evoked potentials are performed; the presence of asymmetry of these potentials is suggestive of diastematomyelia.

Treatment

The purpose of surgery in diastematomyelia is the prevention of progressive neurologic deficit. It is prophylactic rather than curative. In diastematomyelia, the spinal cord and cauda equina are transfixed by the midline bony spicule and the normal mobility of the cord is impaired, producing progressive neurologic deficit. The aim of surgery is not so much to attempt to reverse changes that are already present, but to prevent further neurologic deficit by allowing normal mobility of the spinal cord. This is especially true if correction of scoliosis or kyphosis is to be performed, as during correction of spinal curvature the tethered spinal cord is stretched, which can cause catastrophic deterioration in hindbrain and spinal cord function.

Neurosurgical excision of the septum is also recommended when there is progressive neurologic deficit or a recent development of neurologic dysfunction.

Patients with asymptomatic diastematomyelia or those with long-standing stable nonprogressive neurologic deficit are observed by thorough neurologic and musculoskeletal evaluations at periodic intervals—unless spinal surgery is contemplated.

The operation is a neurosurgical procedure (Fig. 5–129). A local laminectomy is performed, and most of the bony spicule is subperiosteally resected. Next, the dura is incised, arachnoidal adhesions to medial dural reflections are divided, and the remaining portion of the bony spicule and dural septa are excised. The taut filum terminale is cut, to release the cord. Thus the separate halves of the cord are freely movable and approximate each other. The dura is not closed anteriorly; posteriorly, however, it is approximated in a linear manner. Hydrocephalus or other clinical evidence of the Arnold-Chiari malformation is not a postoperative complication.

The role of the orthopedic surgeon is the care of muscle paralysis and deformities affecting the lower limbs. Treatment follows the same principles discussed in the section on poliomyelitis.

References

1. Anand, A. K., Kuchner, E., and James, R.: Cervical diastematomyelia: uncommon presentation of a rare congenital disorder. Comput. Radiol., 9:45, 1985.
2. Arredondo, F., Haughton, V. M., Hemmy, D. C., Zelaya, B., and Williams, A. L.: The computed tomographic appearance of the spinal cord in diastematomyelia. Radiology, 136:685, 1980.
3. Banniza von Bazan, U.: The association between congenital elevation of the scapula and diastematomyelia: a preliminary report. J. Bone Joint Surg., 61:59, 1979.
4. Barson, A. J.: The vertebral level of termination of the spinal cord during normal and abnormal development. J. Anat., 106:489, 1970.
5. Basauri, L., Palma, A., Zuleta, A., Holzer, F., and Poblete, R.: Diastematomyelia. Report of 10 cases. Acta Neurochir., 51:91, 1979.
6. Bremer, J. L.: Dorsal intestinal fistula: accessory neurenteric canal; diastematomyelia. Arch. Pathol., 54:132, 1952.
7. Cohen, J., and Sledge, C. B.: Diastematomyelia. Embryologic interpretation. Am. J. Dis. Child., 100:257, 1960.

8. Cowie, T. N.: Diastematomyelia with vertebral column defects. Br. J. Radiol., 24:156, 1951.
9. Cowie, T. N.: Diastematomyelia: Tomography in diagnosis. Br. J. Radiol., 25:263, 1952.
10. Eid, K., Hochberg, J., and Saunders, D. E.: Skin abnormalities of the back in diastematomyelia. Plast. Reconstr. Surg., 63:534, 1979.
11. Frerebeau, P., Dimeglio, A., Gras, M., and Harbi, H.: Diastematomyelia: report of 21 cases surgically treated by a neurosurgical and orthopedic team. Childs Brain, 10:328, 1983.
12. Gardner, J. W.: The Dysraphic States. Amsterdam, Excerpta Medica, 1973.
13. Giordano, G. B., and Cerisoli, M.: Diastematomyelia and scoliosis. Usefulness of CT examination. Spine, 8:111, 1983.
14. Goldberg, C., Fenelon, G., Blake, N. S., Dowling, F., and Regan, B. F.: Diastematomyelia: a critical review of the natural history and treatment. Spine, 9:367, 1984.
15. Han, J. S., Benson, J. E., Kaufman, B., Rekate, H. L., Alfidi, R. J., Bohlman, H. H., and Kaufman, B.: Demonstration of diastematomyelia and associated abnormalities with MR imaging. A.J.N.R., 6:215, 1985.
16. Hilal, S., Marton, D., and Pollack, E.: Diastematomyelia in children: Radiographic study of 34 cases. Radiology, 112:609, 1974.
17. Hulser, P. J., Schroth, G., and Petersen, D.: Magnetic resonance and CT imaging of diastematomyelia. Eur. Arch. Psychiatr. Neurol. Sci., 235:107, 1985.
18. Humphreys, R. P., Hendrick, E. B., and Hoffman, H. J.: Diastematomyelia. Clin. Neurosurg., 30:436, 1983.
19. James, C. C. M., and Lassman, L. P.: Diastematomyelia. Arch. Dis. Child., 35:315, 1960.
20. Jequier, S., Cramer, B., and O'Gorman, A. M.: Ultrasound of the spinal cord in neonates and infants. Ann. Radiol., 28:225, 1985.
21. Kennedy, P. R.: New data on diastematomyelia. J. Neurosurg., 51:355, 1979.
22. Lassale, B., Rigault, P., Pouliquen, J. C., Padovani, J. P., and Guyonvarch, G.: Diastematomyelia. Rev. Chir. Orthop., 66:123, 1980.
23. Martin, K., Krastel, A., Hamer, J., and Banniza, U. K.: Symptomatology and diagnosis of diastematomyelia of children. Neuroradiology, 16:89, 1978.
24. Mathieu, J. P., Decarie, M., Dube, J., and Marton, D.: Diastematomyelia. Study of 69 cases. Chir. Pediatr., 23:29, 1982.
25. Matson, D. D., Woods, R., Campbell, J., and Ingraham, F. D.: Diastematomyelia (congenital clefts of the spinal cord): Diagnosis and surgical treatment. Pediatrics, 6:98, 1950.
26. Maxwell, H., and Bucy, P.: Diastematomyelia. J. Neuropathol. Exp. Neurol., 5:165, 1946.
27. Naidich, T. P., Fernbach, S. K., McLone, D. G., and Shkolnik, A.: John Caffey Award: Sonography of the caudal spine and back: congenital anomalies in children. A.J.R., 142:1229, 1984.
28. Naidich, T. P., and Harwood-Nash, D. C.: Diastematomyelia: hemicord and meningeal sheaths; single and double arachnoid and dural tubes. A.J.N.R., 4:633, 1983.
29. Neuhauser, E. B. D., Wittenborg, M. H., and Dehlinger, K.: Diastematomyelia. Radiology, 54:659, 1950.
30. Pang, D., and Parrish, R. G.: Regrowth of diastematomyelic bone spur after extradural resection. Case report. J. Neurosurg., 59:887, 1983.
31. Perret, G.: Diagnosis and treatment of diastematomyelia. Surg. Gynecol. Obstet., 105:69, 1957.
32. Perret, G.: Symptoms and diagnosis of diastematomyelia. Neurology, 10:51, 1960.
33. Quaknine, G. E., Gadoth, N., Matz, S., and Shalit, M.: Congenital vascular malformation of spinal cord simulating diastematomyelia. Childs Brain, 5:513, 1979.
34. Sands, W. W., and Clark, W. K.: Diastematomyelia. Am. J. Roentgenol., 72:64, 1954.
35. Scatliff, J., Till, K., and Hoare, R.: Incomplete false and true diastematomyelia: Radiological evaluations by air myelography and tomography. Radiology, 116:349, 1975.
36. Schlesinger, A. E., Naidich, T. P., and Quencer, R. M.: Concurrent hydromyelia and diastematomyelia. A.J.N.R., 7:473, 1986.
37. Scotti, G., Musgrave, M. A., Harwood-Nash, D. C., Fitz, C. R., and Chuang, S. H.: Diastematomyelia in children: metrizamide and CT metrizamide myelography. A.J.R., 135:1225, 1980.
38. Sheptak, P. E.: Diastematomyelia-diplomyelia. In Handbook of Clinical Neurology. Amsterdam, North Holland, 1978, pp. 239–254.
39. Sheptak, P. R., and Susen, A. F.: Diatematomyelia. Am. J. Dis. Child., 113:210, 1967.
40. Weinstein, M. A., Rothner, A. D., Duchesneau, P., and Dohn, D. F.: Computed tomography in diastematomyelia. Radiology, 118:609, 1975.
41. Williams, R. A., and Barth, R. A.: In utero sonographic recognition of diastematomyelia. A.J.R., 144:87, 1985.
42. Winter, R. B., Haven, J. J., Moe, J. H., and LaGaard, S.: Diastematomyelia and congenital spine deformities. J. Bone Joint Surg., 56-A:27, 1974.
43. Yamada, S., Zinke, D., and Sanders, D.: Pathophysiology of "tethered cord syndromes." J. Neurosurg., 54:494, 1981.

SPINA BIFIDA OCCULTA

Failure of fusion of one or more of the vertebral arches is perhaps among the most common congenital anomalies. It is so frequent that it is often regarded as a normal variation.

Fusion of the vertebral arches does not take place until the first year of life and is not complete until adolescence. This fact accounts for the higher incidence of spina bifida occulta in the radiograms of the spine in children than in adults. One fourth of all infants and young children show some minor defect of the vertebral arches in radiographic examination.

The most common sites of spina bifida occulta are the fifth lumbar, first sacral, and cervical axis vertebrae. Much less frequently, the last two segments of the sacrum, the twelfth thoracic vertebra, and the first lumbar vertebra are affected.

Clinical Features

The majority of spina bifida occulta cases are of no clinical significance and show no evidence of neurologic deficit or musculoskeletal abnormality. Diagnosis is made incidentally on x-ray films of the spine obtained for some other purpose. There is, however, a small percentage of cases in which the central neural axis is involved as well as the bone, and in which surgical intervention may be indicated. Early recognition of these patients is desirable.

The skin over the lesion is usually normal

but may show various types of abnormalities, such as: (1) abnormal growth of a patch of hair, which may be coarse and several inches in length or may be silky and limited to a definite area; (2) a dimple that manifests itself as a depression in the skin in the midline with fixation of the epithelium to underlying layers (such dimples may mark either the level of an underlying spina bifida or the outlet of a continuous fibrous or fistulous tract extending directly into the spinal canal); the dimples may be minute or may present as open sinus tracts; (3) subcutaneous lipomas that are soft, nontender, and poorly circumscribed; and (4) hemangiomas in the midline along the spine, particularly in the lumbosacral level. In the suboccipital area, cutaneous port-wine stains are frequent but are of no clinical significance.

Even though the diagnosis of spina bifida occulta is established on radiologic examination, there is still much controversy over whether it is the cause of neurologic deficit, deformities of the lower limbs, or disturbances of bladder or bowel control. The vast majority of clinicians believe that it has no etiologic bearing. Myelography, CT scan, and magnetic resonance imaging are indicated whenever there is objective evidence of motor loss, sensory deficit, changes in reflexes, regression of bladder or bowel control, actual demonstration of urinary dribbling on pressure of the suprapubic region of the abdomen, palpable relaxation of the anal sphincter, or the presence of musculoskeletal deformity of the lower limb (such as atrophy or pes varus or pes cavus). Myelography and CT scan are performed to assess the significance of the spina bifida and to rule out intraspinal tumors. These will detect and localize filling defects caused by lesions such as intraspinal lipomatous masses, fibrous defects, bony spicules, dermoid cysts, or intraspinal meningoceles.

Treatment

Most individuals with spina bifida occulta do not require treatment. Surgery is performed in a very few selected patients for specific indications, which are as follows: (1) objective evidence of neurologic deficit, especially if it is increasing; (2) filling defect (demonstrated by metrizamide myelography) in the region of spina bifida in a patient with impaired neurologic function; or (3) aesthetic reasons—the presence of a large hairy patch or skin nevus that can be removed. During this purely cosmetic procedure for removal of large deforming cutaneous defects, one should observe whether

there are any connecting tracts from the skin to the spinal canal.

INTRASPINAL TUMORS[1-36]

Intraspinal tumors in children are rare, occurring about one-fifth as frequently as intracranial tumors in the same age group. Intraspinal gliomas (astrocytoma, ependymoma, and medulloblastoma) are the most common; next, in decreasing order of frequency, are neuroblastoma, extradural sarcomas arising in paraspinal lymphoid tissue, dermoid cyst, teratoma, lipoma, and intramedullary cysts. Neurofibroma and meningioma, which are so common in adults, are rarely encountered in children. Intraspinal tumors are twice as common in males as in females and are frequently found during the first four years of life (about half the tumors).

Clinical Picture

The initial symptoms of intraspinal tumors are usually manifested in the musculoskeletal system, and diagnosis is often not readily made. The presenting complaints and physical findings in 115 children with intraspinal tumors treated at the Children's Hospital Medical Center in Boston are shown in Figures 5–130 and 5–131.

Persistent or intermittent pain in the back, neck, trunk, or limbs not readily explained by local injury or some other disease process should suggest the possibility of an intraspinal tumor. The pain is usually ill-defined and poorly described; it is accentuated by physical activity, sneezing, coughing, straining, flexing the neck or back, or straight leg-raising.

The most common physical sign is motor weakness, which may be either flaccid or spastic, depending upon the level of the lesion. The parents may note that the child is unable to run or climb stairs as well as usual, or a limp may be the initial manifestation of motor weakness. An infant may tend to use one hand to the exclusion of the other when playing with toys. Muscle atrophy usually accompanies motor weakness.

Muscle spasm is a common finding, particularly in the paravertebral muscles. When the lesion is located in the cervical spine, it causes torticollis (Fig. 5–132).[17] Scoliosis may be the initial deformity (Fig. 5–133). The presence of pathologic reflexes is an important neurologic sign; an unequivocal upturning of the toe elicited by plantar stimulation at any time after infancy suggests the presence of a cervical or thoracic spinal cord lesion. Diminution or ab-

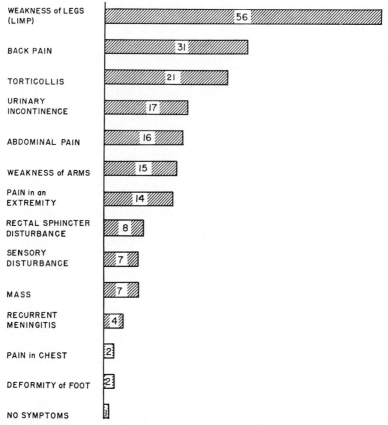

FIGURE 5-130. *Initial complaints of intraspinal tumors of childhood of 115 patients treated at the Children's Medical Center in Boston.*

(From Tachdjian, M. O., and Matson, D. D.: Orthopaedic aspects of intraspinal tumors in infants and children. J. Bone Joint Surg., 47-A:230, 1965. Reprinted by permission.)

sence of deep tendon reflexes in the upper or lower limbs is another valuable sign.

A change in bladder or bowel habits, such as incontinence, enuresis, urgency, dribbling, or increasingly severe constipation, may be the presenting complaint. A lax anal sphincter may be noted on rectal examination. Deformities of the foot—cavus, varus, or equinus—may be seen. A definite sensory level may be elicited in about one third of the patients. This usually consists of diminished awareness of pinprick or anesthesia caudal to a given dermatome. Other occasional physical findings with intraspinal tumors are visible or palpable paraspinal soft-tissue mass, local tenderness over the affected area of the spine, and vasomotor changes.

Radiographic Findings

On the initial plain radiogram, pathologic changes are often visible to make one suspicious of an intracranial neoplasm.

Widening of the spinal canal is a frequent finding. With the slowly growing intraspinal tumors of childhood, vertebral growth becomes altered in such a way that for long periods an expanding intraspinal mass is accommodated without visible evidence of bone erosion. With diligent measurements of the interpediculate spaces and sagittal diameter of the spinal canal, a local lesion may often be diagnosed early. The upper and lower limits of normal interpediculate measurements in infants and children were published by Simril and Thurston.[31] A simple, rapid, and accurate method of using drawings on transparencies to compare the interpediculate spaces in infants, children, and adults in a group of average normal persons of similar age and height was described by Haworth and Keillor.[12] Normal values for the sagittal diameter of the cervical spinal canal in children and young adults between the ages of 3 and 18 years of age have been published by Hinck and associates.[13] The sagittal diameter is measured from the middle of the posterior surface of the vertebral body to the nearest point on the ventral

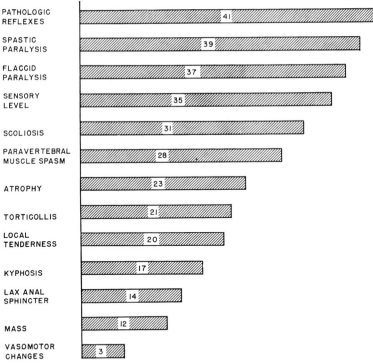

FIGURE 5–131. *Physical findings of intraspinal tumors of childhood of 115 patients treated at the Children's Medical Center in Boston.*

(From Tachdjian, M. O., and Matson, D. D.: Orthopaedic aspects of intraspinal tumors in infants and children. J. Bone Joint Surg., 47-A:231, 1965. Reprinted by permission.)

line of the cortex at the junction of the spinous process and laminae. Meticulous measurements made of both the interpediculate spaces on anteroposterior radiograms and the sagittal diameters on lateral projections may disclose minute localized increases that may be of diagnostic value.[10]

Naidich et al. retrospectively studied plain radiograms from 31 patients with pathologically proven intraspinal tumors to assess the reliability of radiographic signs commonly used to detect spinal cord tumors. Interpediculate distance was graphed onto standard curves. No single radiographic criteria allowed greater than 40 per cent true positive diagnosis. Use of multiple radiographic signs result in 55 per cent true positive diagnosis. This study stressed the importance of computed tomography scan and nuclear magnetic resonance imaging when intraspinal tumor is suspected in children.[24]

Other radiographic changes that may be seen in intraspinal tumors are thinning or erosion of the pedicles, erosion of the vertebral bodies or laminae, erosion of rib ends, paravertebral soft-tissue masses, calcification in the tumor, kyphoscoliosis, loss of cervical or lumbar lordosis, and often, in the case of intraspinal dermoid cysts, spina bifida or another congenital vertebral abnormality.

The radiographic examination should include the entire spine whenever an intraspinal tumor is suspected. A common error is failure to make radiograms at sufficiently high levels; in other words, radiograms may be obtained of only the lumbosacral spine because the presenting complaint is related to the feet or to sphincter disturbance, although intraspinal lesions at the cervical or thoracic level may cause symptoms and signs limited to the lower lumbar and sacral segments for a considerable time. It is also easy, particularly in a young child, to overlook minor sensory and motor disturbances involving the trunk. Obviously, the presence of hyperactive deep tendon reflexes in the lower limbs, toes upturned on plantar stimulation, ankle clonus, or spasm indicates an upper motor neuron deficit and, therefore, a lesion located cephalad to the first lumbar skeletal level.

Spinal cord tumors can be detected by imaging with high-resolution ultrasound, computed tomography, and nuclear magnetic resonance imaging (Fig. 5–134).[3, 19, 22, 31]

Myelography with metrizamide has particular value in a child in accurate determination of

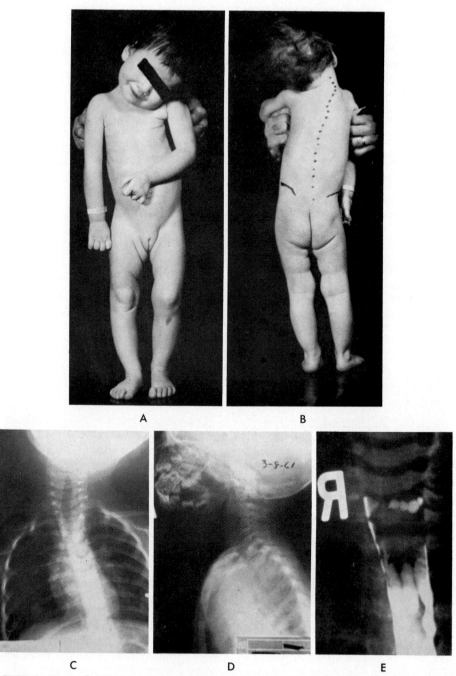

FIGURE 5–132. *Grade III-IV astrocytoma of the cervical spinal cord in a one-and-one-half-year-old girl.*

A and **B.** The initial symptom was left torticollis, as shown in these photographs of the patient. During the six months prior to admission she had been treated for left congenital torticollis by passive stretching exercises. **C** and **D.** Anteroposterior and lateral radiograms of the spine. Note the widening of the spinal canal without evidence of bone destruction. **E.** Myelogram shows the complete block at the second thoracic level. (From Tachdjian, M. O., and Matson, D. D.: Orthopaedic aspects of intraspinal tumors in infants and children. J. Bone Joint Surg., 47-A:227, 1965. Reprinted by permission.)

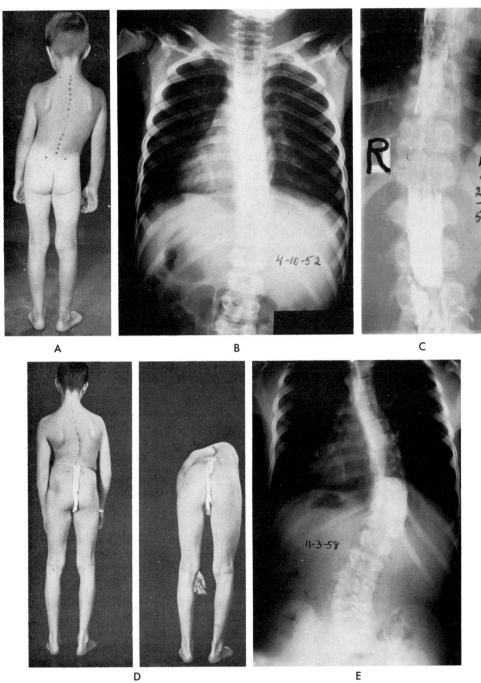

A   B   C

D   E

FIGURE 5–133. *Scoliosis as the initial manifestation of a cystic astrocytoma of the spinal cord in a five-and-one-half-year-old boy.*

A and **B.** Photograph and radiogram of the spine showing the right thoracolumbar scoliosis. Paravertebral muscle spasm and hyperactive deep tendon reflexes were found on careful neurologic examination. The total cerebrospinal fluid protein on lumbar puncture was 159 mg. per 100 ml. **C.** Myelogram showing block at the interspace between the twelfth thoracic and first lumbar vertebrae with fusiform expansion of the cord from this level to the tenth thoracic level. **D** and **E.** Photographs and anteroposterior radiogram of the spine four years after laminectomy and aspiration of the intraspinal cyst. The scoliosis has markedly increased. (From Tachdjian, M. O., and Matson, D. D.: Orthopaedic aspects of intraspinal tumors in infants and children. J. Bone Joint Surg., 47-A:241, 1965. Reprinted by permission.)

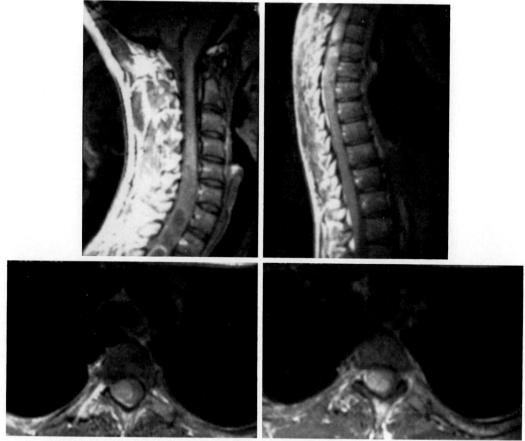

FIGURE 5–134. *Nuclear magnetic resonance image of the spine showing a tumor in the cervical and upper dorsal regions.*

A and **B.** Sagittal views of the cervical and dorsal regions. Note the increased radiopacity indicating the tumor (glioma). **C** and **D.** Transverse sections of the lower cervical and upper dorsal regions showing the tumor.

the level of the intraspinal tumor. The level of sensory and motor loss demonstrated by neurologic examinations alone may be inaccurate and mislead the surgeon in placing the laminectomy incision. The caudal extent of the intraspinal mass may be determined accurately by myelography, and the cephalic pole may be located, if necessary, by noting the descent of a small amount of opaque medium instilled into the cisterna magna. At present, with clear demonstration of intraspinal pathology by magnetic resonance imaging, myelography is performed less often.

Cerebrospinal Fluid Findings

It is imperative to perform lumbar puncture and analysis of cerebrospinal fluid, though it should be done cautiously when a spinal cord tumor is suspected, and only after critical examination of plain radiograms and magnetic resonance imaging of the entire spine. When-

ever the presence of a block is suggested by the finding of xanthochromia and the results of the Queckenstedt test, metrizamide myelography is performed at the same time, eliminating the need for an additional lumbar puncture. If neurologic signs suggest the presence of a tumor, myelography should be performed to detect the presence of tumor cells; this is of particular importance in the case of medulloblastoma and epidermoid and dermoid cysts.

The total protein content will be elevated whenever an intraspinal lesion encroaches upon the cerebrospinal fluid pathways below the level of the foramen magnum. The normal level in cerebrospinal fluid is 20 to 35 mg. per 100 ml.; when an intraspinal tumor is present, it may be elevated from 50 to 4000 mg. per 100 ml.

Differential Diagnosis

The possibility of an intraspinal tumor should always be considered when evaluating an abnormality of the musculoskeletal system. One cannot overemphasize this. Often an erroneous diagnosis is entertained initially, and needless treatment is carried out for prolonged periods before the lesion is identified. Such a delay in diagnosis will result in permanent damage to the cord (Fig. 5–135). Torticollis, idiopathic scoliosis, spastic cerebral palsy, traumatic subluxation of the cervical spine, acute back strain, spondylitis, poliomyelitis, muscular dystrophy, and infectious polyneuritis are some of the common orthopedic conditions for which intraspinal neoplasms are mistaken. Figure 5–136 illustrates a case of cystic astrocytoma of the cervical spinal cord that was erroneously diagnosed and treated as traumatic subluxation of the cervical spine.

Appendicitis is another diagnosis mistakenly made when the tumors involve the lower thoracic spinal cord and nerve roots. In the workup of a child with otherwise unexplored persistent abdominal pain, a thorough neurologic examination should be made and radiograms of the spine taken. A lumbar puncture should not be neglected.

Treatment

The treatment of intraspinal tumors is by surgical removal of the lesion. Benign lesions may be completely excised by a competent neurosurgeon. Infiltrating intramedullary lesions are ordinarily removed in two stages to prevent surgical damage to the cord. Surgery is supplemented by irradiation for malignant infiltrating gliomas and for extradural extensions of such tumors of paraspinal origin as neuroblastoma, reticulum cell sarcoma, and lymphoma. Urologic care in the form of constant bladder drainage is indicated in the immediate postoperative period. When cystometrograms indicate that urination is voluntary, the catheter is removed to facilitate skin care and to minimize the possibilities of urinary infection.

Postoperative care of the musculoskeletal system is very important. It is preferable, whenever possible, for the orthopedic surgeon to examine the patient preoperatively to assess the musculoskeletal deformities that may have been present for some time. Complete and thorough muscle examination should be carried out to record the degree of preoperative motor weakness. This measurement will serve as a baseline during the postoperative period. At operation, every effort should be made to preserve the integrity of the pedicles and the posterior joints, meticulous attention being paid to all anatomic structures that give stability to the spine. When

possible, the posterior spinal arch is reconstructed.[26] In childhood, when laminectomy extends over three or four vertebral segments, as is frequently the case, the spine should always be supported postoperatively by a cervical or cervicothoracic lumbosacral (CTLSO) orthosis or a plaster-of-Paris body jacket, depending upon the level of the laminectomy. Such support is particularly important when there is already associated muscle weakness, when there is existing deformity of the spine, or when the spine has been irradiated. All appliances should be carefully fitted and well padded to prevent pressure sores in anesthetic areas.

Postoperatively, if there is weakness of motor function in the lower limbs, its extent and any improvement or worsening should be assessed and recorded by periodic muscle examinations. Fundamental measures of orthopedic care include active exercises directed toward improving voluntary function in weak muscles; passive exercises to preserve the maximum range of motion in joints, with emphasis on correcting existing deformity; and the use of such supports as plastic splints or bivalved casts to prevent the development of additional deformity. When motor recovery takes place, the patient is permitted to walk under supervision with the aid of any necessary crutches and orthotic devices.

Orthopedic operative procedures are indicated in some patients to correct severe musculoskeletal deformities. Before performing any such surgery, it is imperative that one be sure that the disease process is stable and that the pattern of paralysis or deformity is not changing. The neurologic status of each patient should be thoroughly evaluated; when progressive neurologic deficit exists, examination of the spinal fluid and myelography should be performed. If there is any doubt, it is best to wait and observe the patient and re-evaluate the neurologic picture at intervals, especially when the intraspinal tumor is an astrocytoma, teratoma, intramedullary cyst, or ependymoma.

Progressive scoliosis and kyphosis are deformities that should be closely observed following surgery (Figs. 5–137 to 5–140).[4, 15, 25, 30, 33, 34] They occur in about one third of the patients as a result of postoperative irradiation, associated muscle weakness, or instability of the spine after extensive laminectomy. Other factors involved are the level of the lesion, the age of the patient, recurrence of the tumor with progressive increase of the intraspinal mass, and lack of postoperative support for the spine. A Milwaukee brace is used to prevent or improve an increasing kyphoscoliosis. When it is felt that

Text continued on page 1902

A

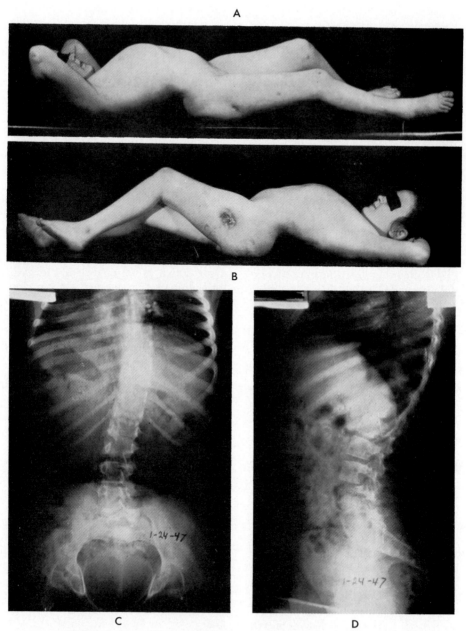

B

C   D

FIGURE 5–135. *A girl, 11 years old, with cystic teratoma of the spinal cord.*

Teratoma extends from the fifth thoracic to the second lumbar level. The lesion is a benign, slowly growing neoplasm. With early diagnosis and immediate surgical treatment, persistent injury to the spinal cord could have been prevented. **A** and **B.** Photographs of patient showing the flexion deformities of the hips and knees, the severe lumbar lordosis, and the deep ulcers over both greater trochanters. A diagnosis of chronic poliomyelitis had been made because of motor weakness in the lower limbs. This erroneous diagnosis could have been prevented by neurologic examination, which disclosed spasticity, hyperactive reflexes, and sensory disturbances. **C** and **D.** Anteroposterior and lateral radiograms of the spine. Note the marked widening of the spinal cord extending from the fifth thoracic to the second lumbar level, with thinning of the pedicles and erosion of the posterior aspect of the vertebral bodies, indicating an extensive, intraspinal mass of very long duration. The total spinal fluid protein was 3,900 mg. per 100 ml. (From Tachdjian, M. O., and Matson, D. D.: Orthopaedic aspects of intraspinal tumors in infants and children. J. Bone Joint Surg., 47-A:224, 1965. Reprinted by permission.)

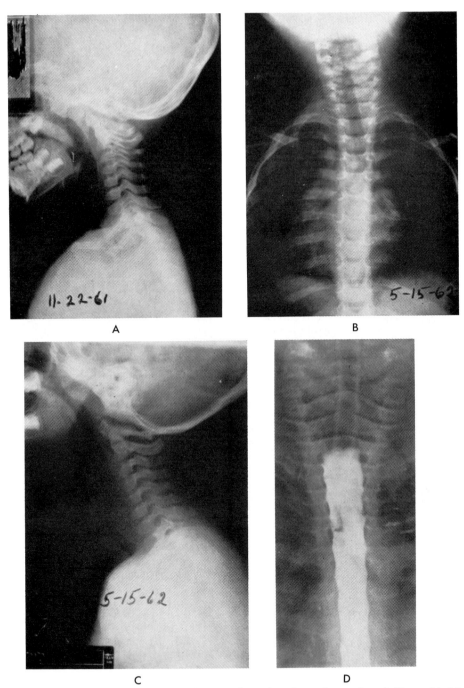

FIGURE 5–136. *Cystic astrocytoma of the cervical spinal cord in a three-and-one-half-year-old girl.*

The initial manifestations were torticollis on the right and paralysis of the right upper limb, precipitated by a fall from a kitchen stool. For six months after diagnosis of traumatic subluxation of the second or the third cervical vertebra she was treated by traction, first with head halter and then with Crutchfield tongs. **A.** Lateral radiogram of the cervical spine made at the time of injury. This was erroneously interpreted as showing subluxation of the second or the third cervical vertebra. The widening of the sagittal diameter of the spinal canal was missed. **B** and **C.** Anteroposterior and lateral radiograms of the cervical spine made six months later. Note the absence of bone erosion or destruction. There is no true subluxation or dislocation. The marked widening of both anteroposterior and sagittal diameters of the cervical spinal canal is evident. **D.** Myelogram shows almost complete block with greatly widened spinal canal above it. (From Matson, D. D., and Tachdjian, M. O.: Intraspinal tumors in infants and children. Postgrad. Med., *34:*282, 1963. Reprinted by permission.)

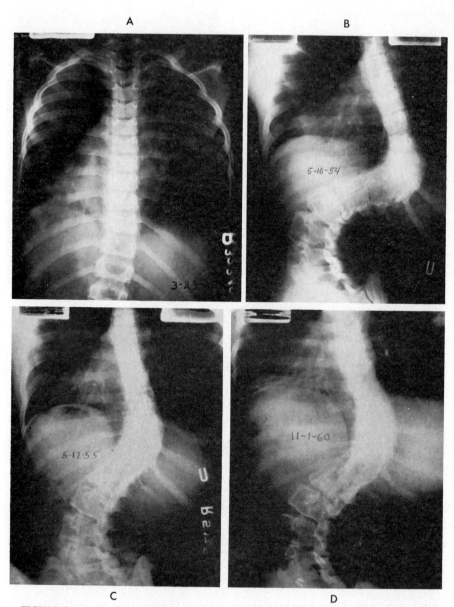

FIGURE 5–137. *Cystic intramedullary astrocytoma of the spinal cord in an 11-year-old boy.*

A. Initial radiogram of the spine. Note the minimal right thoracic curve and the widened interpediculate spaces of the tenth and eleventh thoracic vertebrae. **B.** Anteroposterior radiogram of the spine six years after operation, showing marked progression of the scoliosis. **C.** Anteroposterior radiogram of the spine made one year after spinal fusion from the fifth thoracic to the first lumbar vertebra. **D.** Anteroposterior radiogram of the spine made six years after fusion. The patient had increasing paraplegia in both lower limbs with complete block at the twelfth thoracic level, as shown by the myelogram. The area was surgically explored and the cyst aspirated through a burr hole. (From Tachdjian, M. O., and Matson, D. D.: Orthopaedic aspects of intraspinal tumors in infants and children. J. Bone Joint Surg., *47-A:239*, 1965. Reprinted by permission.)

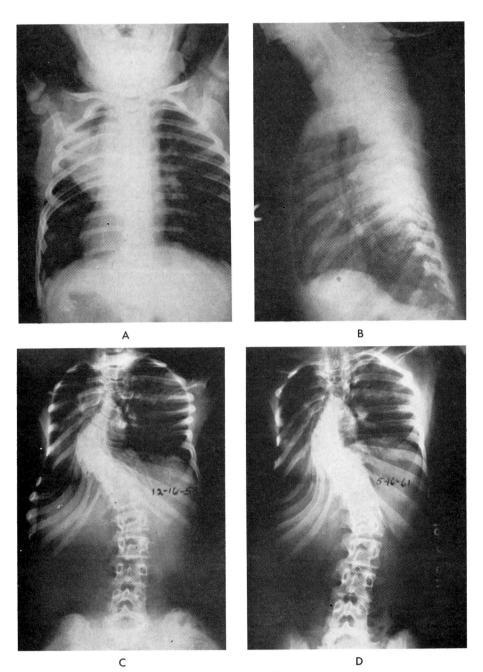

FIGURE 5–138. Extradural neuroblastoma in an infant.

A and **B.** Anteroposterior and lateral radiograms of the chest. Note the soft-tissue mass in the left paravertebral region with erosion of the ribs and thinning of the pedicles at the fourth and fifth thoracic vertebrae. On laminectomy an extradural neuroblastoma was found and was completely removed. The large retropleural tumor was excised two weeks later. Postoperatively she received 4,300 r of irradiation. **C.** Anteroposterior radiogram of the spine made nine years after laminectomy and irradiation. Note the severe left thoracic scoliosis. Spinal fusion was performed from the fourth to the eleventh thoracic vertebra. **D.** Anteroposterior radiogram of the spine made two years following fusion. (From Tachdjian, M. O., and Matson, D. D.: Orthopaedic aspects of intraspinal tumors in infants and children. J. Bone Joint Surg., 47-A:242, 1965. Reprinted by permission.)

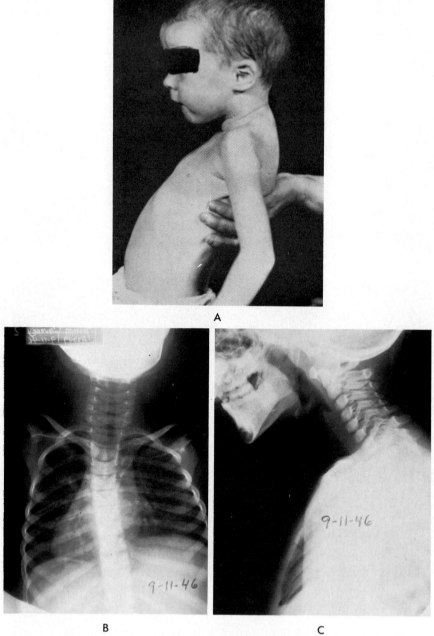

A

B   C

FIGURE 5–139. Glioma of the cervical spinal cord in a four-year-old girl.

A to C. Preoperative photograph and radiograms. Note the kyphosis and widening of the spinal canal in both anteroposterior and sagittal diameters with no evidence of bone erosion or destruction. (From Tachdjian, M. O., and Matson, D. D.: Orthopaedic aspects of intraspinal tumors in infants and children. J. Bone Joint Surg., *47-A*:243, 1965. Reprinted by permission.)

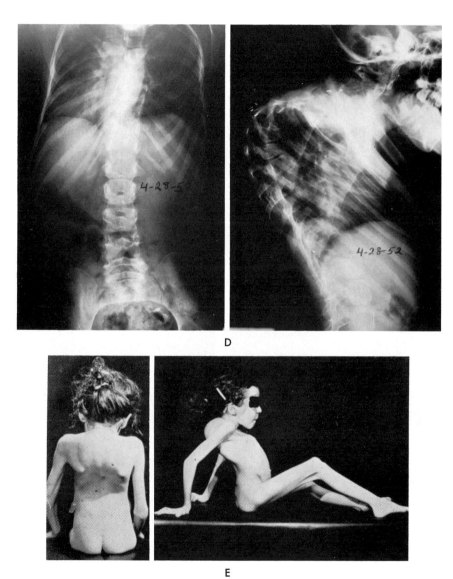

D

E

FIGURE 5–139 Continued. Glioma of the cervical spinal cord in a four-year-old girl.

D and **E**. Radiograms and photographs of patient six years after operation. Note the severe kyphosis. (From Tachdjian, M. O., and Matson, D. D.: Orthopaedic aspects of intraspinal tumors in infants and children. J. Bone Joint Surg., *47-A*:243, 1965. Lateral views in **D** and **E** from Matson, D. D., and Tachdjian, M. O.: Intraspinal tumors in infants and children. Postgrad. Med., *34*:283, 1963. Reprinted by permission.)

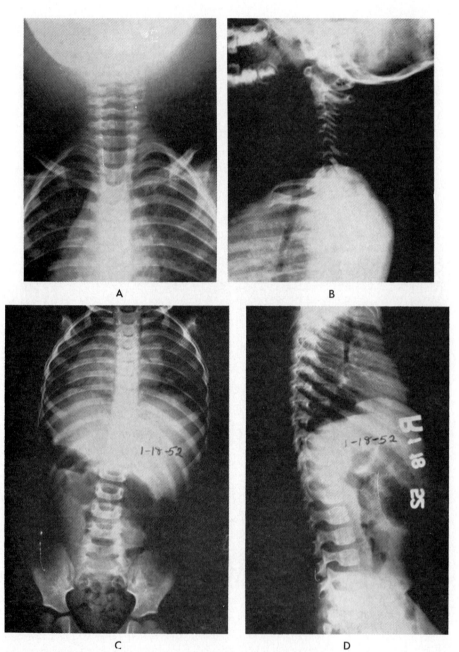

A

B

C

D

FIGURE 5–140. *Intramedullary Grade II astrocytoma of the lower cervical and upper thoracic spinal cord in a one-year-and-eight-month-old girl.*

A to **D.** Preoperative radiograms of the spine showing the widening of the spinal canal in the cervicothoracic region.

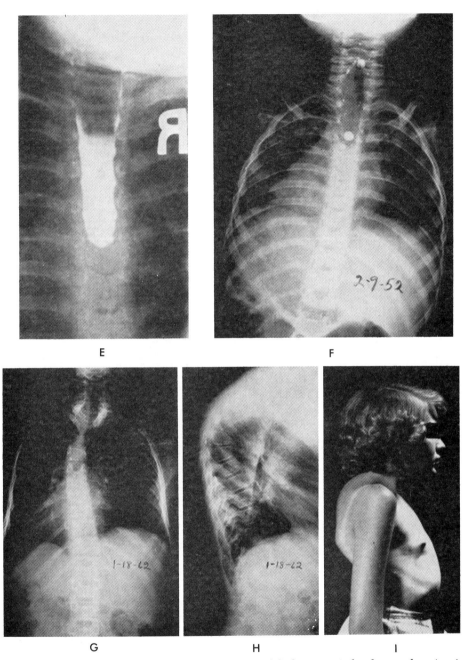

E   F

G   H   I

FIGURE 5–140 Continued. Intramedullary Grade II astrocytoma of the lower cervical and upper thoracic spinal cord in a one-year-and-eight-month-old girl.

E. Myelogram. Note the block with fusiform dilation of the spinal canal above the block. F. Immediate postoperative radiogram of the spine showing the extent of laminectomy. G to I. Radiograms and photograph of the patient ten years after the original operation. Note the severe kyphosis. (From Tachdjian, M. O., and Matson, D. D.: Orthopaedic aspects of intraspinal tumors in infants and children. J. Bone Joint Surg., 47-A:245, 1965. Reprinted by permission.)

a checkrein on progression is necessary, spinal fusion is indicated—but only when the tumor or neurologic disease process is reasonably stable and not obviously progressing. If in doubt, it is preferable to fuse only one side to facilitate subsequent laminectomy.

References

1. Armstrong, E. A., Harwood-Nash, D. C., Ritz, C. R., Chuang, S. H., Pettersson, H., and Martin, D. J.: CT of neuroblastomas and ganglioneuromas in children. A.J.R., 139:571, 1982.
2. Batnitzky, S., Keucher, T. R., Mealey, J., Jr., and Campbell, R. L.: Iatrogenic intraspinal epidermoid tumors. J.A.M.A., 237:148, 1977.
3. Braun, I. F., Raghavendra, B. N., and Kricheff, I. I.: Spinal cord imaging using real-time high-resolution ultrasound. Radiology, 147:459, 1983.
4. Catell, H. S., and Clark, G. L., Jr.: Cervical kyphosis and instability following multiple laminectomies in children. J. Bone Joint Surg., 49-A:713, 1967.
5. Chapman, P. H.: Congenital intraspinal lipomas: anatomic considerations and surgical treatment. Childs Brain, 9:37, 1982.
6. Cohen, J. Y., Lebatard-Sartre, R., Lajat, Y., Mitard, D., and David, A.: Sacral intraspinal lipoma associated with congenital iliac anomaly. Childs Brain, 8:181, 1981.
7. Conti, P., Conti, R., and Lo Re, F.: Two rare cases of intraspinal meningioma in childhood. Rev. Neurobiol., 27:536, 1981.
8. DeSousa, A. L., Kalsbeck, J. E., Mealey, J., Jr., Campbell, R. L., and Hockey, A.: Intraspinal tumors in children. A review of 81 cases. J. Neurosurg., 51:437, 1979.
9. DiRocco, C., Caldarelli, M., Puca, A., and Colosimo, C., Jr.: Multiple spinal meningiomas in children. Neurochirurgia, 27:25, 1984.
10. Elsberg, C. A., and Dyke, C. G.: The diagnosis and localization of tumors of the spinal cord by means of measurements made on the x-ray films of the vertebrae, and the correlation of clinical and x-ray findings. Bull. Neurol. Inst., 3:359, 1934.
11. Hagan, H., III, and Meyer, L. C.: Dermoid cyst of the spine in childhood. Orthopedics, 9:107, 1986.
12. Haworth, J. B., and Keillor, G. W.: Use of transparencies in evaluation of the width of the spinal canal in infants, children and adults. Radiology, 79:109, 1962.
13. Hinck, V. C., Hopkins, C. E., and Savara, B. S.: Sagittal diameter of the cervical spinal canal in children. Radiology, 79:97, 1962.
14. Holgersen, L. O., Santulli, T. V., Schullinger, J. N., and Berdon, W. E.: Neuroblastoma with intraspinal (dumbbell) extension. J. Pediatr. Surg., 18:406, 1983.
15. Johnston, E. C., II: Post laminectomy kyphoscoliosis following surgical treatment for spinal cord astrocytoma. Orthopedics, 9:587, 1986.
16. Kantrowitz, L. R., Pais, M. J., Burnett, K., Choi, B., and Pritz, M. B.: Intraspinal neurenteric cyst containing gastric mucosa: CT and MRI findings. Pediatr. Radiol., 16:324, 1986.
17. Kiwak, K. J., Deray, M. J., and Shields, W. D.: Torticollis in three children with syringomyelia and spinal cord tumor. Neurology, 33:946, 1983.
18. Kopelson, G.: Radiation tolerance of the spinal cord previously damaged by tumor and operation: long term neurological improvement and time-dose-volume relationships after irradiation of intraspinal gliomas. Int. J. Radiat. Oncol. Biol. Phys., 8:925, 1982.
19. Kucharczyk, W., Brant-Zawadzki, M., Sobel, D., Edwards, M. B., Kelly, W. M., Norman, D., and Newton, T. H.: Central nervous system tumors in children: detection by magnetic resonance imaging. Radiology, 155:131, 1985.
20. Latchaw, R. E., L'Heureux, P. R., Young, G., and Priest, J. R.: Neuroblastoma presenting as central nervous system disease. A.J.N.R., 3:623, 1982.
21. Matson, D. D., and Tachdjian, M. O.: Intraspinal tumors in infants and children. Postgrad. Med., 34:279, 1963.
22. Mikhael, M. A., Paige, M. L., and Thayer, C.: Computerized tomography of malignant pleural mesothelioma with spinal canal invasion. Comput. Radiol., 6:11, 1982.
23. Mirkin, L. D., and Azzarelli, B.: Spinal malignant schwannoma in a 5-year-old boy: Ultrastructural evidence of its perineural origin. Pediatr. Pathol., 1:211, 1983.
24. Naidich, T. P., Doundoulakis, S. H., and Poznanski, A. K.: Intraspinal masses: Efficacy of plain spine radiography. Pediatr. Neurosci., 12:10, 1985.
25. Packer, R. J., Zimmerman, R. A., Bilaniuk, L. T., Leurssen, T. G., Sutton, L. N., Bruce, D. A., and Schut, L.: Magnetic resonance imaging of lesions of the posterior fossa and upper cervical cord in childhood. Pediatrics, 76:84, 1985.
26. Peterson, H.: Spinal deformity secondary to tumor, irradiation and laminectomy. In Bradford, D., and Hensinger, R. (eds.): The Pediatric Spine. New York, Theime, 1985, p. 273.
27. Raimondi, A. J., Gutierrez, F. A., and DiRocco, C.: Laminectomy and total reconstruction of the posterior spinal arch for spinal cord surgery in childhood. J. Neurosurg., 45:555, 1976.
28. Rand, R. W., and Rand, C. W.: Intraspinal Tumors of Childhood. Springfield, Ill., Charles C Thomas, 1960, pp. 330–339.
29. Reimer, R., and Onofrio, B. M.: Astrocytomas of the spinal cord in children and adolescents. J. Neurosurg., 63:669, 1985.
30. Roberson, F. C., Ghatak, N. R., and Young, H. F.: Myelopathy presenting as an intrinsic spinal cord tumor. Surg. Neurol., 9:317, 1978.
31. Simril, W. A., and Thurston, D.: The normal interpediculate space in the spines of infants and children. Radiology, 64:340, 1955.
32. Tachdjian, M. O., and Matson, D. D.: Orthopaedic aspects of intraspinal tumors in infants and children. J. Bone Joint Surg., 47-A:223, 1965.
33. Tadmor, R., Cacayorin, E. D., and Kieffer, S. A.: Advantages of supplementary CT in myelography of intraspinal masses. A.J.N.R., 4:618, 1983.
34. Winter, R. B., and McBride, G. G.: Severe postlaminectomy kyphosis treatment by total vertebrectomy (plus late recurrence of childhood spinal cord astrocytoma). Spine, 9:690, 1984.
35. Yasuoka, S., Peterson, H. A., Laws, E. R., Jr., and MacCarty, C. S.: Pathogenesis and prophylaxis of postlaminectomy deformity of the spine after multiple level laminectomy. Difference between children and adults. Neurosurgery, 9:145, 1981.
36. Yasuoka, S., Peterson, H. A., and MacCarty, C. S.: Incidence of spinal column deformity after multilevel laminectomy in children and adults. J. Neurosurg., 57:441, 1982.

SPINAL MUSCULAR ATROPHY

This is a rare hereditary degenerative disease of the anterior horn cells of the spinal cord and occasionally of the motor neurons of the cranial nerves (fifth to twelfth, inclusive). It is characterized by progressive hypotonia and symmetrical paralysis of voluntary muscles. Involvement is greater in the lower than in the upper limbs, and the proximal muscle groups are more severely affected than the distal. There is no sensory disturbance. Pyramidal long-tract signs are absent. There is considerable variation in the age of onset of muscular atrophy, severity of weakness, and life span.

The condition was first described by Werdnig, in 1891, in two brothers.[74] A family of four affected children was reported by Hoffmann in 1893.[37] In the reported cases of Werdnig and Hoffmann the progressive muscle atrophy was noted at 6 to 12 months of age, with demise by the age of 6 years. The presence of spinal neural atrophy was recognized by Beevor.[3] A less severe variety of spinal muscular atrophy was described by Kukelberg and Welander in 1956.[41] A milder variety of the disease with a protracted course was also described by Wohlfart et al. in 1955.[78] The presentation of spinal muscular atrophy in the adult was described by Richter and McMasters.[54]

The condition is transmitted by an autosomal recessive gene, affecting both sexes equally. The affection appears to be more severe in the male. The etiology is unknown. The incidence is one in 15,000 live births. Carrier prevalence is 1 in 80.

Pathology

The anterior horn cells of the spinal cord and the motor cells of the cranial nerves undergo degenerative changes, with diminution in their number, pyknosis, central chromatolysis, neuronophagia, and gliosis. The condition begins and is most marked at the caudal end of the spinal cord and extends proximally to affect the motor nuclei of the cranial nerves. Involvement is always symmetrical. Secondary wallerian degeneration takes place in the anterior roots and nerves, which become pale and thin; the medullated fibers disappear and are replaced by fibrous tissue. The skeletal muscles develop denervation atrophy characterized by smallness and narrowness of the muscle fibers, an increase in the sarcolemmal nuclei, and preservation of the longitudinal and transverse striations and their internal architecture. The bundles of atrophic muscle fibers are separated by fat and fibrous tissue.

At autopsy, the diaphragm is normal in all cases, and the involuntary musculature of the intestine, bladder, heart and sphincters is not affected.

Clinical Features

The degree of muscular atrophy and weakness varies. As a rule, the age of onset can be correlated with the extent of the disease and the length of the period of survival. Byers and Banker, in a review of their personal experience with 52 cases, separated the patients into three types. The first group, *acute infantile variety* (Type I), has the onset in utero or in the first months of life, the weakness is generalized, and death occurs early owing to respiratory failure. The second category, *the chronic infantile variety* (Type II), comprises those cases with onset somewhere between the second and twelfth postnatal months, usually during the middle of the first year. The muscle weakness is more localized; after initial progression of atrophy the disease remains static for long periods, and there is a longer life expectancy. The *juvenile variety* (Type III) is the third group. The symptoms begin in the second year of life or later. Muscle weakness has gradual onset and is localized. The disease pursues a slowly progressive course with a survival period of many years.[9]

It is vital to recognize the three varieties, particularly to distinguish the benign chronic types from the acute infantile type in order to give an accurate prognosis and provide appropriate orthopedic care.

The patients of the *first group (acute infantile variety)* are the most severely involved. Some abnormality of the fetus is reported by most mothers, who usually state that in late pregnancy fetal movements were unusually diminished and then became totally absent. At birth or within the first few weeks of life, inactivity and "flopping" of the baby are noted. There is conspicuous generalized weakness of the voluntary muscles, the limb girdle and trunk muscles being most severely affected. The degree of paralysis is less severe distally, with persistence of function of the muscles controlling the fingers and toes until late in the disease. Extraocular movements are usually normal.

These infants are unable to move their limbs; they lie in a characteristic posture with the hips flexed, abducted, and laterally rotated; the shoulders abducted and laterally rotated; the knees and elbows flexed; the forearms pronated; and the hands elevated above the head. The infant is so limp and flaccid that he can be manipulated into any posture. The head control is poor or absent. The patients cannot raise their head. They do not turn over and never develop sitting balance. Respiratory movements are paradoxical because of the coexistence of intercostal paralysis and a well-functioning diaphragm. The chest is compressed anteroposteriorly and the lower ribs are often flared in a bell shape.

The deep tendon reflexes are absent. Sensation, sphincter function, and intelligence are normal. Corticospinal tract signs are absent. Dysphagia is present in some. Paralysis of the facial muscles gives a "bland" facial expression. Fasciculations of the tongue are frequently seen. The sucking and gag reflexes are eventually lost.

Bulbar muscle weakness and respiratory insufficiency result in recurrent pneumonia and atelectasis. The heart tends to be unaffected. The course of the disease is rapidly progressive, and the infant usually dies of respiratory infection at the average age of ten months. Patients who survive beyond two years of age with aggressive medical care usually die before ten years of age.

In the *second group (chronic infantile variety)*, in which muscular weakness is first detected between 2 and 12 months, the lower limbs are more severely affected than the arms. The patellar tendon reflex is absent, but the biceps and triceps reflexes are retained for some time. The deep tendon reflexes are gradually lost centrifugally. On attempting active motions, the infant commonly exhibits a fine tremor in the arms and hands owing to inequality of weakness of antagonistic muscles. Fasciculations may be noted in the tongue, the deltoid muscle, and the intrinsic muscles of the hand. About three fourths of these children develop sitting balance, and a few are able to crawl or stand up by holding onto furniture. The course of the disease is less rapidly progressive, the average age of death being 42 months (i.e., four times the longevity of Group I). With intensive medical and orthopedic care these children can survive into late adolescence or early adult life.

The *third group (chronic juvenile variety)* constitutes a small percentage of cases of spinal muscular atrophy. In these children, symptoms begin from 12 months on. The gluteus maximus and thigh muscles are principally affected. Tremor and muscular fasciculations are usually

present. The biceps and triceps tendon reflexes are normal. The ankle jerk may be depressed. These children are usually able to sit up at 6 months of age and to stand and walk between 12 and 24 months. The clinical course is quite benign. In the past, the average length of survival was seven years; however, with adequate medical care patients live to the age of 20 to 30 years.

Kugelberg-Welander disease is the most benign form of spinal muscular atrophy; it has an insidious onset, usually between 2 and 15 years of age.[41] The presenting manifestation is weakness of the hip extensor and abductor muscles. These cases have been mistaken for Duchenne type of muscular dystrophy, as in both conditions the patients have a waddling gait, positive Gower's sign, and difficulty in climbing stairs. On occasion the patient with Kugelberg-Welander disease will have hypertrophy of the calves. As the disease progresses the shoulder girdle muscles are involved. Late in the course of the disease the hands become affected with tremor and muscle weakness. Facial musculature weakness is rare. Prognosis for life is almost normal in these patients; however, functionally most of these patients are wheelchair bound by the fourth decade of life.

Functional classification of spinal muscular atrophy was given by Evans, Drennan, and Russman. They noted the actual degree of involvement as the important guide to prognosis.[20] *Group I* patients never develop the strength to sit independently; their head control is poor and delayed. *Group II* patients develop head control. They develop sitting balance but cannot assume sitting posture actively from a supine posture. They cannot walk even with orthotic support. *Group III* patients pull themselves up to stand and walk in a limited fashion with or without orthotic support. *Group IV* patients develop the ability to walk, run, and climb stairs without holding onto the rail before the onset of weakness.[20] This functional classification has definite advantages: It is easy to apply, correlates with the development of secondary deformity, and assists with the planning of long-term care of the musculoskeletal system.

Laboratory Findings

Serum creatine phosphokinase (CPK) and serum aldolase are elevated in Kugelberg-Welander disease and the juvenile variety of spinal muscular atrophy, whereas in the acute and chronic infantile varieties (Groups I and II), in which there is paucity of muscle mass, serum CPK is normal.

Motor nerve conduction velocities are normal. Electromyography will show denervation atrophy with some evidence of reinnervation; there are fibrillation potentials at rest with high-amplitude long-duration polyphasic potentials. Muscle biopsy will show evidence of neural atrophy, with the atrophic fibers having a unique round outline.

Differential Diagnosis

Infantile muscular atrophy must be distinguished from a number of conditions. Cerebral palsy, particularly the extrapyramidal type, is initially manifested by a stage of hypotonia and flaccid paralysis prior to the development of athetosis and rigidity. Hypotonia may also be a prominent symptom of glycogen storage disease with involvement of the anterior horn cells. Traumatic transverse myelitis may result from obstetrical injury and may produce flaccid paralysis of the limbs and trunk. Muscular dystrophy in infancy is rare but can occur. Peripheral neuropathy, such as acute infectious polyneuritis and chronic hypertrophic neuritis, may have its onset in early infancy and cause flaccid paralysis. Benign congenital hypotonia is distinguished from Werdnig-Hoffmann disease by the preservation of tendon reflexes and lack of progression of paralysis. The differential diagnosis of hypotonia in infants and children is given in Table 5–12.

Treatment

There is no specific therapy. The majority of infantile-type patients with spinal muscular atrophy survive into adolescence or early adulthood, and patients with the juvenile type live to be adults. These patients require long-term planning for care and support. Each case is individually assessed as to potential of future locomotion. Functional grouping of cases serves as a practical guide for planning of future orthopedic care.

In infancy the goals of therapy are to prevent the development of contractural deformity of the hips, knees, ankles, and feet. Passive exercises are performed several times a day in order to prevent flexion-abduction lateral rotation deformity of the hips, flexion deformity of the knees, and equinovarus or equinovalgus deformity of the feet. Sleeping in prone posture is encouraged. When the infant is 6 to 12 months of age, appropriate light plastic splints are manufactured to maintain the joints in functional position. These splints are worn during the night and at naptime.

In infantile muscular atrophy the patients are usually confined to a wheelchair from infancy; these children develop flexion contractures of the hips and knees. Flexion deformities up to 30 to 45 degrees are treated by night splints, exercise, and serial stretching casts as indicated. The flexion deformities, however, tend to be progressive, and by the age of eight to ten years they may be as much as 80 to 90 degrees. Severe flexion deformity of the hips causes excessive lumbar lordosis and makes sleeping and sitting posture uncomfortable; also, it tends to predispose to hip dislocation and pain. Therefore, when flexion deformity of the hips exceeds 45 to 60 degrees and cannot be controlled by appropriate orthotic support and physical therapy, radical soft-tissue release of the hip and knee flexors is performed. The hips and knees are operated on at the same time. In Group III (functional classification) patients, 20 to 30 degree flexion deformities of the knees and hips weaken further biomechanically the already weakened hip and knee extensors, interfering with independent stance and walking. In these patients, moderate flexion deformities are treated aggressively by cast or, if necessary, by surgical release; postoperatively, above-knee orthotic support and crutches are provided for locomotion. By such orthopedic measures, walking can be prolonged for up to an additional five years (Fig. 5–141).

Unilateral hip dislocation causes pelvic obliquity and secondary scoliosis; the hip should be relocated, when possible. The care of bilateral hip dislocation is individualized. This author favors reduction, as dislocated hips tend to aggravate lumbar lordosis. When the hip is painful and irreducible, resection of the proximal femoral neck and head may be performed. Subtrochanteric abduction Schanz femoral osteotomy may relieve pain in selected cases. In functional Group I and Group II patients, soft-tissue release to correct equinovarus or equinovalgus deformities of the foot-ankle is indicated to allow application of shoes and to relieve pressures causing skin ulceration. In functional Group III and Group IV patients, paralytic and static deformities of the foot-ankle are corrected by cast and/or surgery to provide a plantigrade foot for locomotion. Orthotic devices are provided for support. Occasionally, triple arthrodesis is indicated in these patients. This procedure corrects deformity and provides stability to the paralytic deformed feet.

Table 5–12. *Clinico-Anatomic Classification and Differential Diagnosis of the Hypotonic Child Syndrome**

	Cerebral Hypotonic Diplegia	Infantile Muscular Atrophy	Acute Infective Polyneuritis	Juvenile Myasthenia Gravis	Progressive Muscular Dystrophy	Polymyositis	Benign Congenital Hypotonia
Site of lesion	Cerebrum	Anterior horn cells	Peripheral nerves	Myoneural junction	Skeletal muscle	Skeletal muscle	Skeletal muscle
Inheritance	None	Recessive	None	Not defined	Sex-linked	None	None
Sex preponderance	None	None	None	Females	Males	Females	None
Limb musculature involved	Distal more than proximal	Generalized	Distal more than proximal	Generalized	Proximal	Proximal	Generalized
Cranial muscle pareses	Facial and pseudo-bulbar	Bulbar in late stages	Facial often, bulbar less often	Eyelids very often, ocular, facial, bulbar	None	Pharyngeal 50%	None
Respiratory paralysis	None	Common	Less common	Common 43%	Late	Occasional	Mild
Muscle fasciculations	None	Common	Less common	None	None	None	None
Muscle atrophy	Moderate	Severe	Moderate to severe	Mild	Severe	Mild (with tenderness)	Moderate
Pseudohypertrophy	None	None	None	None	Characteristic	Occasional	None
Deep tendon reflexes	Brisk or normal	Absent	Absent	Normal	Variable, usually depressed	Variable, usually depressed	Normal or depressed
Sensory defect	Cortical	None	Frequent	None	None	Usually none	None
Mental defect	Severe	None	None	None	Moderate	None	None or moderate
Muscle biopsy	Normal	Grouped atrophy	Atrophy	Lymphorrhages	Degeneration, variation in fiber size	Degeneration, and inflammatory cells	Small fibers
Electromyography	Normal	Fibrillations; sparse, giant action potentials	Fibrillations; sparse action potentials	Decline in amplitude of potentials	Short, low amplitude potentials	Fibrillations; short, low amplitude potentials	Normal or low amplitude potentials
Serum creatinine kinase, SGOT, aldolase	Normal	Normal	Normal	Normal	Increased	Increased	Normal
Spinal fluid protein	Normal	Normal	Often high	Normal	Normal	Usually normal	Normal
Specific therapy	None	None	Steroids (?)	Rest and anticholinesterase drugs	None	Steroids	None
Course	Nonprogressive	Rapid	Acute or subacute	Prolonged, remittent	Chronic	Acute, subacute, or chronic	Nonprogressive
Prognosis	Severe chronic disability	Fatal, usually within 2 yr. (4 wk. to 20 yr.)	Recovery in 80%	Complete remission in 25% within 6 yr.; fatal in 5%	Fatal within 20 to 30 yr.	Remission in 80%	Gradual improvement

*From Millichap, J. G.: The hypotonic child. Reproduced by special permission from *Brennemann's Practice of Pediatrics*, Vol. IV, Chapter 16. Hagerstown, Md., Medical Department, Harper & Row, Publishers, Inc., 1966.

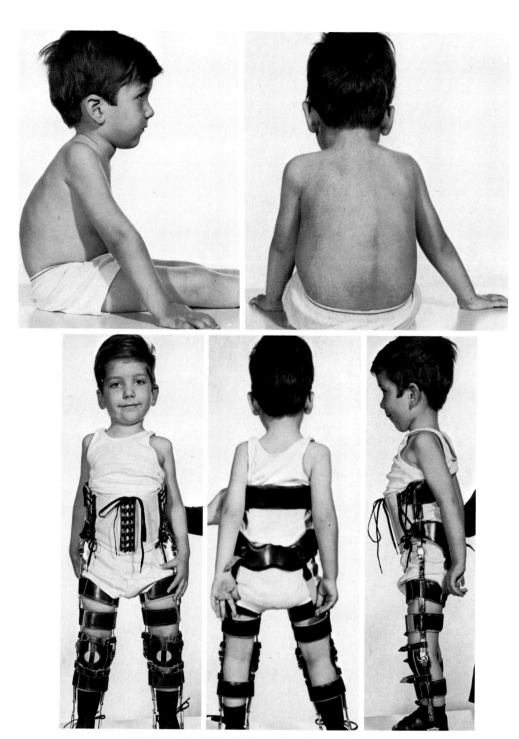

FIGURE 5–141. Child with Werdnig-Hoffmann disease.

With orthotic support and crutches he is able to ambulate.

Spinal deformity is the most serious orthopedic problem in spinal muscular atrophy, particularly in functional Groups I and II patients. The scoliosis appears early in life and progresses rapidly. In functional Group III patients a mild scoliosis develops early but does not progress rapidly until the age of 10 to 12 years. It seems that once the patient is confined to a wheelchair, the scoliosis progresses rapidly and relentlessly. Scoliosis is relatively less of a problem in functional Group IV patients who retain their walking ability. The goals of treatment of spinal deformity are to prevent or decrease the rate of progression of the scoliosis by the application of appropriate spinal orthosis, and then at appropriate skeletal age to stabilize the paralytic spine by spinal fusion and internal instrumentation. It should be emphasized that orthosis is a temporary measure, borrowing time for skeletal growth. It does not usually prevent progression of the scoliosis. The following program for management of scoliosis is recommended[12, 20]

Group I patients are managed by a sitting spinal orthosis, which may be built into a wheelchair. Thoracic suspension orthosis may be tried but usually is not well tolerated. These infants suffer from repeated respiratory infections. They are very poor surgical risks; the mortality rate is high. *Group II* patients are treated with total contact spinal orthosis when the scoliosis progresses to 15 to 20 degrees, which is usually by the age of three years. Several years later a thoracic suspension orthosis is prescribed. When the degree of scoliosis progresses to 50 degrees or more, posterior spinal fusion is performed with segmental instrumentation. Postoperatively, external support to the spine is not required. *Group III* patients are treated with spinal orthotics when the curvature progresses to 20 degrees. In these patients, thoracic suspension orthosis is usually not required and a Milwaukee brace is poorly tolerated.[36] Ordinarily, the scoliosis in Group III patients is progressive, requiring stabilization of the spine in early adolescence. In *Group IV* patients one should examine the spine carefully, as 50 per cent of these patients develop scoliosis. Orthotic support is provided as indicated. Spinal fusion is required occasionally.

When performing spinal fusion and internal fixation with segmental instrumentation in spinal muscular atrophy, it is vital to stabilize the trunk over a level pelvis.

References

1. Aprin, H., Bowen, J. R., MacEwen, G. D., and Hall, J. E.: Spine fusion in patients with spinal muscular atrophy. J. Bone Joint Surg., *64-A*:1179, 1982.
2. Batten, F. E.: Progressive spinal muscular atrophy of infants and young children. Brain, *33*:433, 1911.
3. Beevor, C. E.: A case of congenital spinal muscular atrophy (family type), and a case of haemorrhage into the spinal cord at birth, giving similar symptoms. Brain, *25*:85, 1902.
4. Benady, S. G.: Spinal muscular atrophy in childhood: review of 50 cases. Dev. Med. Child Neurol., *20*:746, 1978.
5. Bonnett, C., Brown, J. C., Perry, J., Nickel, V. L., Walinski, T., Brooks, L., Hoffer, M., Stiles, C., and Brooks, R.: Evaluation of treatment of paralytic scoliosis at Ranchos Los Amigos Hospital. J. Bone Joint Surg., *57-A*:206, 1975.
6. Brandt, S.: Werdnig-Hoffmann's Infantile Progressive Muscular Atrophy. Copenhagen, E. Munksgaard, 1950.
7. Buchthal, F., and Olsen, P. Z.: Electromyography and muscle biopsy in infantile spinal muscular atrophy. Brain, *93*:15, 1970.
8. Burke, S. W., Jameson, V. P., Roberts, J. M., Johnston, C. E., and Willis, J.: Birth fractures in spinal muscular atrophy. J. Pediatr. Orthop., *6*:34, 1986.
9. Byers, R. K., and Banker, B. Q.: Infantile muscular atrophy. Arch. Neurol., *5*:140, 1961.
10. Daher, Y. H., Lonstein, J. E., Winter, R. B., and Bradford, D. S.: Spinal surgery in spinal muscular atrophy. J. Pediatr. Orthop., *5*:391, 1985.
11. Dorr, J. R., Brown, J. C., and Perry, J.: Results of posterior fusion in patients with spinal muscular atrophy. A review of 25 cases. J. Bone Joint Surg., *55-A*:436, 1973.
12. Drennan, J. C.: Orthopaedic Management of Neuromuscular Disorders. Philadelphia, J.B. Lippincott, 1983, 137–154.
13. Dubowitz, V.: Infantile spinal muscle atrophy: a progressive study with particular reference to a slowly progressive variety. Brain, *57*:767, 1964.
14. Dubowitz, V.: The Floppy Infant. London, William Heineman, 1969.
15. Dubowitz, V.: Benign infantile spinal muscular atrophy. Dev. Med. Child Neurol., *16*:672, 1974.
16. Duval-Beaupère, G., Barois, A., Quinet, I., and Estournet, B.: Respiratory, spinal and thoracic problems in children with prolonged spinal muscular atrophy. Arch. Fr. Pediatr., *42*:625, 1985.
17. Dyken, P., and Krawiecki, N.: Neurodegenerative diseases of infancy and childhood. Ann. Neurol., *13*:351, 1983.
18. Echenne, B., Georgesco, M., and Dapres, G.: Motor nerve conduction velocity in infantile spinal muscular atrophy. Diagnostic problems. Rev. Electroencephalogr. Neurophysiol. Clin., *13*:329, 1984.
19. Eng, G. D., Binder, H., and Koch, B.: Spinal muscular atrophy: experience in diagnosis and rehabilitation management of 60 patients. Arch. Phys. Med. Rehabil., *65*:549, 1984.
20. Evans, G. A., Drennan, J. C., and Russman, B. S.: Functional classification and orthopaedic management of spinal muscular atrophy. J. Bone Joint Surg., *73-B*:516, 1981.
21. Fishman, M. A., and Finegold, M.: Progressive neurologic deterioration in a hypotonic infant. J. Pediatr., *107*:634, 1985.
22. Fredericks, E. J., and Russman, B. S.: Bedside eval-

uation of large motor units in childhood spinal muscular atrophy. Neurology, 29:398, 1979.

23. Gardner-Medwin, D., Hudgson, P., and Walton, J. N.: Benign spinal muscular atrophy arising in childhood and adolescence. J. Neurol. Sci., 5:121, 1967.

24. Gobernado, J. M., Riva, C., Gimeno, A., Garcia-Albea, E., and Anaya, A.: Juvenile proximal spinal muscular atrophy with early hypertrophy of calves. Postgrad. Med., 59:327, 1983.

25. Gotz, E., and Bogosyan, S.: Anaesthesia in juvenile muscular atrophy (Kugelberg-Welander syndrome). Anaesth. Intensivther. Notfallmed., 15:360, 1980.

26. Granata, C., Cornelia, F., Bonfiglioli, S., Mattutini, P., and Merlini, L.: Promotion of ambulation of patients with spinal muscular atrophy by early fitting of knee-ankle-foot orthosis. Dev. Med. Child Neurol., 29:221, 1987.

27. Greenfield, J. G., Cornman, T., and Shy, G. M.: The prognostic value of the muscle biopsy in the "floppy infant." Brain, 81:461, 1958.

28. Greenfield, J. G., and Stern, R. O.: The anatomical identity of the Werdnig-Hoffmann and Oppenheim forms of infantile muscular atrophy. Brain, 50:652, 1927.

29. Grinker, R. R.: The pathology of amyotonia congenita. A discussion of its relation to infantile progressive muscular atrophy. Arch. Neurol. Psychiatry, 18:982, 1927.

30. Grunebaum, M., Nutman, J., and Nitzan, M.: The pharyngolaryngeal deficit in the acute form of infantile spinal muscular atrophy (Werdnig-Hoffman disease). Pediatr. Radiol., 1:67, 1981.

31. Gui, L., Savini, R., Merlini, L., Granata, C., Bonfiglioli, S., and Mattutini, P.: Il trattamento chirurgico della scoliosi nella atrofia muscolare spinale: primi risultati. Arch. Ortop. Rheum., 97:21, 1984.

32. Hardman, R.: The floppy infant. Am. J. Dis. Child., 101:145, 1961.

33. Hausmanowa-Petrusewicz, I., Borkowska, J., and Zaremba, J.: Juvenile motor neuron diseases—the sex influence in benign juvenile pseudodystrophic spinal muscular atrophy. Adv. Neurol., 36:131, 1982.

34. Hausmanowa-Petrusewicz, I., Zaremba, J., and Borkowska, J.: Chronic spinal muscular atrophy of childhood and adolescence: problems of classification and genetic counselling. J. Med. Genet., 22:350, 1985.

35. Hausmanowa-Petrusewicz, I., Zaremba, J., Borkowska, J., and Szirkowiec, W.: Chronic spinal muscular atrophy of childhood and adolescence—sex influence. J. Med. Genet., 21:447, 1984.

36. Hensinger, R. N., and MacEwen, G. D.: Spinal deformity associated with heritable neurological conditions: spinal muscular atrophy, Friedreich's ataxia, familial dysautonomia and Charcot-Marie-Tooth disease. J. Bone Joint Surg., 58-A:13, 1976.

37. Hoffmann, J.: Ueber chronische spinale Muskelatrophie im Kindsalter, auf familiarer Basis. Dtsch. Z. Nervenheilk., 3:427, 1893.

38. Hsu, J. D.: Extremity fracture in children with neuromuscular disease. Johns Hopkins Med. J., 145:89, 1979.

39. Isenberg, D. A., and Kahn, P. A.: The distal form of spinal muscular atrophy: an unusual case demonstrating the intermediate variety. Postgrad. Med. J., 58:554, 1982.

40. Kon, T. H. H. G.: "Do you shake hands with mothers of floppy babies?" Br. Med. J., 289:485, 1984.

41. Kugelberg, E., and Welander, L.: Heredo-familial juvenile muscular atrophy simulating muscular dystrophy. A.M.A. Arch. Neurol. Psychiatry, 75:500, 1956.

42. Levesque, J., LePage, F., Boeswillwald, M., and Gruner, J.: Congenital familial muscular dystrophy simu-

lating Werdnig-Hoffmann-Oppenheim disease. Arch. Fr. Pediatr., 13:202, 1956.

43. Linson, M., Bresnan, M., Eraklis, A., and Shapiro, F.: Acute gastric volvulus following Harrington rod instrumentation in a patient with Werdnig-Hoffmann disease. Spine, 6:522, 1981.

44. Meadows, J. C., Marsden, D. C., and Harriman, D. G. F.: Chronic spinal muscular atrophy in adults. Part I. The Kugelberg-Welander syndrome. J. Neurol. Sci., 9:527, 1969.

45. Miike, T., Tamari, H., Ohtani, Y., Nakamura, H., Matsuda, I., and Miyoshino, S.: A fluorescent microscopy study of biopsied muscles from infantile neuromuscular disorders. Acta Neuropathol., 59:48, 1983.

46. Moosz, A., and Dubowitz, V.: Spinal muscular atrophy in childhood. Two clues to clinical diagnosis. Arch. Dis. Child., 48:386, 1973.

47. Munsat, T. L., Woods, R., Fowler, W., and Pearson, C. M.: Neurogenic muscular atrophy of infancy with prolonged survival. The variable course of Werdnig-Hoffmann disease. Brain, 92:9, 1969.

48. Neame, W.: Case study—Werdnig Hoffmann disease. Master G. B.: The story of a remarkable child, his family, and community. N.Z. Nurs. J., 73:27, 1980.

49. Nesterov, L. N., Suscheva, G. P., Bjatkina, S. K., and Novikova, N. P.: The clinical pictures, pathogenesis and geneology of hereditary spinal progressive muscular atrophies. Zh. Nevropatol. Psikhiatr., 84:321, 1984.

50. Pearn, J.: Autosomal dominant spinal muscle atrophy. A clinical and genetic study. J. Neurol. Sci., 38:263, 1978.

51. Pearn, J. H., Gardner, D., and Wilson, J.: A clinical study of chronic childhood spinal muscular dystrophy. A review of 141 cases. J. Neurol. Sci., 38:23, 1978.

52. Piasecki, J. O., Mahinpour, S., and Levine, D. B.: Long-term follow-up of spinal fusion in spinal muscular atrophy. Clin. Orthop., 207:44, 1986.

53. Renault, F., Raimbault, J., Praud, J. P., and Laget, P.: Electromyographic findings in 50 cases of severe infantile spinal muscular atrophy (Werdnig-Hoffmann disease). Rev. Electroencephalogr. Neurophysiol. Clin., 13:301, 1984.

54. Richter, P. L., and McMasters, R. E.: Spinal muscular atrophy in the adult: contemporary views of a classical problem. South. Med. J., 65:317, 1972.

55. Riddick, M. F., Winter, R. B., and Lutter, L. D.: Spinal deformities in patients with spinal muscle atrophy. A review of 36 patients. Spine, 7:476, 1982.

56. Sandifer, P. H.: The differential diagnosis of flaccid paralysis. Proc. R. Soc. Med., 48:186, 1955.

57. Savini, R., Cervellati, S., Granata, C., and Merlini, L.: La scoliosi nelle atrofie muscolari prossimali infantili. *In* Progressi in Patologia Vertebrale. Bologna, Gaggi, 1980.

58. Schwentker, E. P., and Gibson, D. A.: The orthopedic aspects of spinal muscular atrophy. J. Bone Joint Surg., 58-A:32, 1976.

59. Shapira, Y., Amit, R., and Rachmilewitz, E.: Vitamin E deficiency in Werdnig-Hoffmann disease. Ann. Neurol., 10:266, 1981.

60. Shapiro, F., and Bresnan, M. J.: Orthopaedic management of childhood neuromuscular disease. Part I: Spinal muscular atrophy. J. Bone Joint Surg., 64-A:785, 1982.

61. Shy, G. M., and Magee, K. R.: A new congenital nonprogressive myopathy. Brain, 79:610, 1956.

62. Siegel, I. M., and Silverman, M.: Upright mobility system for spinal muscular atrophy patients. Arch. Phys. Med. Rehabil., 65:418, 1984.

63. Skouteli, H., and Dubowitz, V.: Fasciculation of the eyelids: an additional clue to clinical diagnosis in spinal muscular atrophy. Neuropediatrics, 15:145, 1984.

64. Schwentker, E. P., and Gibson, D. A.: The orthopaedic

aspects of spinal muscular atrophy. J. Bone Joint Surg., 58-A:32, 1976.

65. Tadonio, R. F.: Segmental spinal instrumentation in the management of neuromuscular spinal deformity. Spine, 7:305, 1982.

66. Thieffry, S., Arthus, M., and Bargeton, E.: Werdnig-Hoffmann: 40 cases with 11 autopsies. Rev. Neurol., 93:621, 1955.

67. Towfighi, J., Young, R. S. K., and Ward, R. M.: Is Werdnig-Hoffmann disease a pure lower motor neuron disorder? Acta Neuropathol., 65:270, 1985.

68. Turner, J. W. A.: On amyotonia congenita. Brain, 72:25, 1949.

69. Virmani, V., and Mohna, P. K.: Non-familial spinal segmental muscular atrophy in juvenile and young subjects. Acta Neurol. Scand., 72:336, 1985.

70. Walsh, F. S., and Moore, S. E.: Expression of muscle cell surface antigen 5.1H11 in infantile or juvenile spinal muscular atrophy. Neurology, 36:1140, 1986.

71. Walton, J.: Amyotonia congenita. Lancet, 1:1023, 1956.

72. Walton, J.: The "floppy" infant. Cerebral Palsy Bull., 2:10, 1960.

73. Welander, L.: Myopathia distalis tarda hereditaria. Acta Med. Scand. (Suppl.), 265:1, 1951.

74. Werdnig, G.: Zwei fruhim famile hereditare fall von progressiver muskelatrophie unter dem bild der dystrophie, aber auf neurotischer grundlage. Arch. Psychiatr. Nervenkr., 22:237, 1891.

75. Whelan, T. B.: Neuropsychological performance of children with Duchenne muscular dystrophy and spinal muscular atrophy. Dev. Med. Child Neurol., 29:212, 1987.

76. Wijngaarden, G. K. van, and Bethlem, J.: Benign infantile spinal muscular atrophy. A prospective study. Brain, 96:163, 1973.

77. Winson, E. J., Murphy, E. G., Thompson, M. W., and Reed, T. E.: Genetics of childhood spinal muscular atrophy. J. Med. Genet., 8:143, 1971.

78. Wohlfart, G., Fex, J., and Eliasson, S.: Hereditary proximal muscle atrophy: a clinical entity simulating progressive muscular dystrophy. Acta Psychiatr. Scand., 39:395, 1955.

79. Woolf, A. L.: Muscle biopsy in the diagnosis of the "floppy baby": infantile hypotonia. Cerebral Palsy Bull., 2:19, 1960.

80. Zellweger, H., Simpson, J., McCormick, W. F., and Ionasescu, V.: Spinal muscular atrophy with autosomal dominant inheritance. Neurology, 22:957, 1972.

POLIOMYELITIS

Poliomyelitis is an acute infectious disease caused by a group of neurotrophic viruses that initially invade the gastrointestinal and respiratory tracts and subsequently spread to the central nervous system through the hematogenous route. The poliomyelitis virus has a special affinity for the anterior horn cells of the spinal cord and for certain motor nuclei of the brain stem. These cells undergo necrosis with loss of innervation of the motor units that they supply.

The first description of paralytic poliomyelitis was given by Underwood, in 1789.[322]

Infection may be caused by Type I, II, or III poliomyelitis virus. There is no cross immunity between the various types of polio virus; thus infection may recur in the same individual.[210, 269]

Polio virus is a member of the enterovirus group that includes the Coxsackie and the ECHO viruses. Paralytic disease that is clinically and pathologically indistinguishable from poliomyelitis can be produced by various other members of the enterovirus group. These viruses may be isolated on tissue culture.

In the past, poliomyelitis was an epidemic disease in the summer and fall months, with sporadic cases occurring throughout winter and spring. The development and widespread use of prophylactic vaccine has greatly reduced the incidence of poliomyelitis; however, sporadic cases still do occur and the continued rehabilitation of patients who have had the disease is still a concern of the orthopedic surgeon.[210, 270, 273, 277, 302]

This textbook deals with general principles of management of paralytic deformities of the musculoskeletal system resulting from poliomyelitis. These principles not only are applicable to treatment of poliomyelitis but also are fundamental to management of similar problems of flaccid paralysis due to other causes. For a detailed account of the disease and its medical aspects of management, the reader is referred to the voluminous literature on the subject.

Pathology

The polio virus has a definite predilection for the anterior horn cells of the spinal cord as well as for certain motor nuclei in the brain stem. The lumbar and cervical enlargements of the cord are the most commonly affected. The damaging action upon the motor neurons may be *direct*, i.e., by the toxic effects of the virus, or *indirect*, by ischemia, edema, and hemorrhage in their supportive glial tissue.[29]

The motor neurons swell and the Nissl substance in their cytoplasm undergoes chromatolysis. An inflammatory reaction ensues, with infiltration of polymorphonuclear and mononuclear cells into the gray matter, particularly in the perivascular areas. The necrotic bodies are subsequently replaced by scar tissue.

Involvement of the anterior horn cells varies from minimal injury with temporary inhibition of metabolic activity with rapid recovery to complete and irrevocable destruction.

Paralysis is of the flaccid type, with the individual motor units following the "all or none" law, because the virus affects the anterior horn cells rather than the muscle. The percentage of motor units destroyed varies, and the resultant muscle weakness is proportionate to the number of motor units that are lost: for example, a muscle with "poor" muscle strength will have 20 per cent of its motor units functioning, whereas a muscle with "good" motor strength will have 80 per cent of its motor units functioning. These remaining functional motor units are called *guiding neuromuscular units* and are of particular importance in retaining the patterns of motion of the individual muscles or muscle groups during the recovery stage. The recovery in muscle power is primarily dependent upon restitution of the anterior horn cells of the spinal cord that have been damaged but not destroyed.

Immediately following onset, it is difficult to give an accurate prognosis as to the rate and extent of spontaneous recovery. It is best to assume that the involved muscles will recover until that time when the subsequent course of the disease demonstrates otherwise. Muscle recovery is most marked in the first three to six months, with this potential ceasing at approximately 16 to 18 months after the onset.

The two primary factors to consider in the prognosis are the severity of initial paralysis and the diffuseness of its regional distribution. If total paralysis of a muscle persists beyond the second month, severe motor cell destruction is indicated, and the likelihood of any significant return of function is poor. If the initial paralysis is partial, the prognosis is better.

The condition of the neighboring muscles is another consideration. A weakened muscle surrounded by completely paralyzed muscles has less chance of recovery than a muscle of corresponding power that is surrounded by muscles that are strong. Muscle spasm, contracture of antagonist muscle groups, deformity, and inadequate early treatment are other factors that may interfere with recovery of muscle function.

The course of the disease is subdivided into the following stages:

The *acute phase* (lasting from five to ten days) is the period of acute illness when paralysis may occur. It is further subdivided into the *preparalytic phase* and the *paralytic phase*. The acute phase is ordinarily considered to terminate 48 hours following the return to normal temperature.

The *convalescent phase* encompasses the 16-month period following the acute phase; during this time a varying degree of spontaneous recovery in muscle power takes place. This phase is also further subdivided into the *sensitive phase* (lasting from two weeks to several months) characterized by hypersensitivity of muscles, which are tender and "in spasm," and the *insensitive phase*, in which the muscles are

no longer sensitive but are still in the period of recovery.

The *chronic* or *residual phase* is the final stage of the disease after the recovery of muscle power has taken place. It encompasses the rest of the patient's life span following termination of the convalescent period.[201]

Treatment

The management of poliomyelitis varies with the stage of the disease and the severity and extent of paralysis.[117, 118] Treatment in the acute febrile stage is primarily the domain of the pediatrician or internist, with the patients being admitted to the services in infectious disease hospitals or isolation units of general hospitals. Care of the musculoskeletal system, however, is important from the first day of the disease. It is imperative that the orthopedic surgeon be called in consultation to examine a suspected case prior to performance of lumbar puncture. He should be responsible for all orders concerning the management of the musculoskeletal system. The pediatrician is responsible for general care of the patient, especially any problems of respiratory and bulbar involvement, should they develop. Once the patient has been afebrile for 18 hours (i.e., termination of the acute stage), he should be transferred to the service of the orthopedic surgeon, who assumes the dominant role. Such delineation and continuity of supervision is mandatory, as it stimulates early attention to deforming tendencies and prevents their development.

ACUTE PHASE

During this initial febrile phase of the disease, the primary concern of the orthopedic surgeon is the comfort of the patient and prevention of deformity. It is best to place the patient at complete bed rest and restrict his physical activities to a minimum. The patient is irritable and apprehensive. It is important to reassure him and allay his fears.

General medical measures consist of administration of a varied diet with a relatively high fluid intake, attention to urinary retention and bladder paralysis, prevention of constipation and fecal impaction, and analgesia for pain. Opiates and other medications that have a depressing action on the central nervous system should not be given in the presence of impending paralysis of the muscles of respiration.

A detailed determination of the severity and extent of muscle paralysis is not warranted during this febrile period. By gentle handling of the limbs and trunk, however, an approximate assessment of the degree and distribution of motor weakness can be made without much distress to the patient. This initial muscle examination has its diagnostic and therapeutic implications. It will also provide the necessary information to prevent the development of potential deformities consequent to paralysis.

Ordinarily, paralysis develops two or three days after onset of fever and increases in severity for several days. Progressive involvement will cease only after return of elevated temperature to normal. Characteristically paralysis in poliomyelitis is asymmetrical. In the presence of symmetrical paralysis of the limbs and trunk, a paralytic disease other than poliomyelitis should be considered. In a large epidemic the care of patients will be much simplified if those with paralysis are separated from those without paralysis.

Patients with bulbar and respiratory involvement require specialized intensive care. An early appraisal of the distribution and extent of paralysis will help to detect muscle weakness in certain areas, which should alert the clinician to the possible development of such distressing complications. For example, a patient who cannot lift his head because of paralysis of anterior neck muscles or one who has a nasal intonation to his voice, difficulty in swallowing, and weakness of facial muscles should be watched carefully for bulbar involvement. Prompt diagnosis and treatment are essential to keep the patient's airways open, since the condition may be fatal. Aspiration of unswallowed secretions is a definite danger. The foot of the bed is elevated and the patient is placed in prone or lateral position. Frequent suction or postural drainage is usually required. Occasionally tracheostomy may be necessary.

Another anatomic area that should be observed for muscle weakness is the shoulder girdle. The nerve supply of the deltoid muscle is the fifth cervical root, which is adjacent to the fourth cervical root innervating the diaphragm. Consequently, progressive paralysis of the deltoid muscle is usually followed by paralysis of the intercostal muscles and the diaphragm. Is there an increased rate of breathing? Is the patient using accessory muscles of respiration? Is he restless, anxious, and disoriented? These are signs that should alert the physician to the possible need for a mechanical respirator. Paralysis of the diaphragm is easily detected on fluoroscopy. Abdominal muscle weakness is determined by asking the patient to lift his head and shoulder or the lower limbs. Asymmetry of

power is shown by the Beevor's sign, which is the shift of the umbilicus toward the stronger muscles.

The patient should be positioned to provide correct anatomic alignment of the limbs and proper posture of the trunk. The aim is to prevent development of deformities. The bed should give adequate support and should not sag. A firm foam rubber mattress is preferable. Bedboards should be placed beneath the mattress and should be hinged to permit sitting in the later convalescent period. A padded footboard is used to maintain the ankles and feet in neutral position when the patient is lying supine or prone. By pulling the end of the mattress away from the footboard about 10 cm., an interspace is provided in which the heels are allowed to fall. Periods in the supine position should be alternated with periods of prone posture, the latter position being important for maintenance of good muscle tone of the gluteus maximus and erector spinae muscles.

When the patient is lying on his back, the knees should be held in slight flexion with padded rolls under them and behind the proximal ends of the tibiae in order to prevent genu recurvatum and posterior subluxation of the tibiae. A slightly flexed position of the knees will relax the sensitive hamstrings. Excessive flexion of the knees, however, should be avoided. Sandbags or rolled pads are placed on the lateral sides of the thighs and legs to prevent external rotation deformity of the lower limbs. Intermittent use of rolls between the scapulae will prevent hunching forward of the shoulders.

The limbs should not be maintained in rigidly fixed positions. Several times a day, the joints are carried passively through their range of motion; this will help to relieve muscle pain. Overstretching of muscles, however, should be avoided. The patient should be handled as gently as possible. Passive motion of the joints of a limb is imperative to prevent stiffness and myostatic contractures. At times, when there is severe spasm of the hip flexors, hamstrings, and gastrocnemius, the sensitivity and pain of muscles will be so great that anatomic alignment cannot be assumed without excessive discomfort.

Muscle Spasm. A principal manifestation of poliomyelitis in its early stages—the so-called muscle spasm—is characterized by protective contraction of the muscles to prevent a potentially painful movement. Muscle resistance to stretch is more descriptive of this reflex guarding action of the muscles, which resembles the muscle spasm associated with painful phenomena such as hamstring spasm in synovitis of the knee. True spasticity and signs of upper motor neuron involvement are absent. The exact cause of muscle pain and sensitivity is unknown. Most probably it is due to inflammatory changes in the posterior ganglia and meninges. Other possible causes are lesions in the reticular substance and lesions of the internuncial neurons in which inhibitory fibers to the anterior horn cells are affected.

The degree of muscle pain and sensitivity varies considerably. Some muscle discomfort is usually present in the preparalytic period. Nerve traction tests, such as those of Lasègue and Kernig, increase " muscle spasm" and pain. Spontaneous severe pain is rare, though it is occasionally seen in the adult patient. The important consideration is that the painful strong muscles tend to shorten during the sensitive phase; if they are maintained in their shortened position, myostatic contracture and fixed deformity will develop.

Moist Heat. In the acute and sensitive phase of convalescence, moist heat will serve to relieve sensitivity of the muscles and alleviate discomfort. Physiologically, heat will increase the local temperature and increase blood flow to the muscle. It has no specific therapeutic effect on the course of the paralysis and actual recovery of the involved nerve cells. Heat is more beneficial if applied for intermittent short periods.

In the acute phase, in order to minimize handling of the patient, a "lay-on wool pack" is used. It consists of three layers, one of wool blanket material (wrung out of boiling water by passing it twice through a wringer), and one of waterproof material that, in turn, is covered by an outer layer of wool blanket. The number and duration of the use of these packs is individualized, depending upon the intensity of pain and spasm. In general, two moist heat packs are applied during a 20-minute period. Continuous and overzealous use of heat should be avoided, as it can be tiring and harmful to the patient. It is best used prior to physiotherapeutic measures in order to assist in developing greater range of joint motion and to facilitate the performance of active exercises. Warm tub baths are substituted for the "lay-on packs" within a few days after the patient's temperature has returned to normal and when his general condition permits. The buoyant effect of the water makes execution of motion in the weakened muscles easier. Active exercises in water should be closely supervised so that the patient does not substitute stronger muscles for the weaker ones. Again, the patient's comfort is the primary consideration. The temperature of the tub baths should be about 100° F., and the total period of immersion in the tub should not exceed 20 minutes. In cases with extensive paralysis, overhead cranes may be used to lower the patient directly into the tub from the stretcher.

CONVALESCENT PHASE

The objectives of treatment during the convalescent stage are (1) the attainment of maximum recovery in individual muscles; (2) the restoration and maintenance of a normal range of joint motion; (3) the prevention of deformities and their correction if they occur; and (4) the achievement of as good a physiologic status of the neuromusculoskeletal system as is possible.[117]

In the early part of the convalescent stage, because muscle sensitivity and "spasm" are still present, the use of hot packs is continued for the comfort of the patient. Passive exercises are performed four to six times a day to prevent development of contractural deformity. When there is limitation of joint motion, gentle passive stretching exercises are added to the therapy program. This exercise regimen should not cause the patient discomfort; however, the threshold of pain may be very low in an apprehensive sensitive person. A firm but sympathetic attitude by the therapist is important, and the patient should be encouraged more each time to gain a greater degree of motion. Tendencies toward deformity should be observed, such as external rotation and abduction of the hips, plantar flexion of the feet, or adduction of the shoulders. Passive stretching exercises should be directed toward preventing and correcting deformity.

Several days after the onset of the convalescent stage, a complete muscle examination should be performed. Ordinarily it is done in stages in order not to fatigue or disturb the patient. This initial motor assessment provides a basis for comparison with subsequent examinations, and it also serves as a guide to the therapy regimen that is to be instituted. The rate and extent of muscle recovery is determined by repeating these muscle tests periodically, i.e., monthly during the first four months, bimonthly during the following eight months, and then quarterly during the second year of the disease. The prognostic value of the serial muscle tests is evident; when a muscle exhibits little or no improvement in power during a three-month period, it is unlikely that it will recover or gain strength of functional significance. In this case, the patient should be fitted with appropriate orthotic support and allowed greater activity. On the other hand, a muscle that shows steady improvement has a good possibility of recovery to a functional level; hence, it is unwise to apply an above-knee orthosis on this patient's weak limb and permit him to walk.

In the management of the convalescent stage of poliomyelitis, the following principles of neuromuscular function must be considered.[117]

Patterns of Motor Activity. Motions of a limb are complex and are not the result of isolated contraction of a single muscle. The functions of many muscles are integrated and coordinated in execution of a motion and are controlled by the automatic reflexes of the central nervous system. In dorsiflexion of the ankle, for example, the anterior tibial muscle, toe extensors, and the peroneus tertius are the prime movers that execute the desired movement, whereas the triceps surae and the toe flexors are the antagonist muscles that become relaxed because of the reciprocal innervation of the agonist and antagonist muscles. The synergist and fixation muscles also contract while the prime mover acts.

In the presence of muscle weakness, the tendency is to use a strong group of muscles that can perform the action more easily and readily, thus excluding the weaker muscles from the pattern of motor activity. A muscle that has been temporarily paralyzed will be left out of the pattern of motion permanently if other muscles substitute for its action during the period of its recovery. In the convalescent stage, these muscular substitutions and abnormal patterns of motor activity should be avoided.

Some neuromuscular units often remain intact in the paralyzed muscles; these act as "guiding contractile units," and in performance of active exercises, these functioning neuromuscular units should be utilized to guide the part in execution of normal motion.

For example, in re-education of a poor anterior tibial muscle, the ankle joint is first passively dorsiflexed through its full arc of motion, stretching any contracture of the triceps surae muscle that is present. The limb is then placed in a side-lying position to eliminate force of gravity, and the ankle joint is again passively dorsiflexed in some inversion through its full range, assisting the patient to localize the action of the anterior tibial muscle and emphasizing that substitution by the toe extensors and peroneus tertius muscle should be avoided.

Next the patient is asked to produce an active, sustained contraction of the anterior tibial throughout its full arc of motion, first with and then without assistance. As the muscle becomes stronger, the limb is placed in supine position to make the muscle work against gravity and gradually increasing manual resistance is applied. The active exercises are graduated on the basis of performance. Muscles that are overworked will lose strength.

In poliomyelitis, reciprocal innervation between agonist and antagonist muscles is often disturbed, with resultant loss of synergistic muscular action and normal pattern of motor activity.

Fatigue. A paralyzed muscle is easily fatigued. This is readily shown by its rapid loss of power and its inability to function following several effective contractions. Forcing such a weak muscle beyond its point of maximal action does not increase its strength: on the contrary, it will inhibit the recovery of the paralytic muscle. It is important to observe the level of functional activity of a weak muscle so that it is not forced to exceed its capability.

Contractural Deformity and Progressive Loss of Function. Flaccid paralysis is the chief cause of functional loss. Muscular action is also inhibited by pain, sensitivity, and "spasm." When a muscle is maintained in a shortened position for a prolonged period, it will develop myostatic contracture. Muscle imbalance and increased stress due to abnormal patterns of activity are other factors producing deformity. Growth is an important consideration in the management of poliomyelitis in children. The contour of bony structures is influenced by paralysis and dynamic muscle imbalance. For example, when the triceps surae muscle is weak, and the ankle dorsiflexors are of normal motor strength, progressive calcaneus deformity of the hindfoot will result. If the child is permitted to walk without support and protection, the loss of power of the triceps surae muscle will be greater, as it is working against gravity. Figure 5–142 presents the "vicious circle" of factors that cause progressive loss of function in poliomyelitis.

In the *asensitive stage*, proper alignment of the limbs and full range of joint motion must be restored and maintained. Passive stretching exercises are performed vigorously. In the presence of muscle imbalance and when there is a tendency to develop contracture, bivalved casts should be used at night to maintain the part in correct position. When a deformity is fixed, wedging casts or traction may be applied.

Active exercises are performed to integrate recovering motor units into the normal pattern

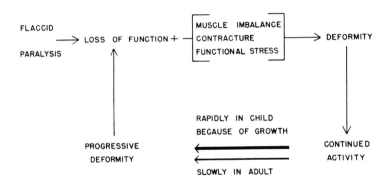

FIGURE 5–142. Diagram showing the principal factors concerned with progressive loss of function in the residual stage of poliomyelitis.

(From Green, W. T., and Grice, D. S.: The management of chronic poliomyelitis. American Academy of Orthopedic Surgeons Instructional Course Lectures, Vol. 9, p. 86. Ann Arbor, Mich., J. W. Edwards, 1952. Reprinted by permission.)

of motion; their primary objective is not to produce hypertrophy of muscles that are already functioning normally. Hydrotherapy and active exercises in a pool are utilized for patients with extensive paralysis. Motion of the hips, shoulders, and trunk is greatly facilitated in the pool, as the buoyant effect of the water facilitates the coordinated motion of the parts. Strict supervision by the therapist is mandatory, however, to prevent substitution of strong muscles for those that are weak. Excessive exercises and overwork should be avoided. Patients with extensive paralysis are initially instructed to ambulate in the pool; when there is adequate control of the trunk and lower limbs, this is no longer necessary. Standing balance should be developed first and then walking with the help of crutches. The gait pattern should be reciprocal four-point gait, the amount of body weight borne depending upon the degree of paralysis. The physical therapist assists in locomotion, so that abnormal mechanisms will not develop. During the convalescent period, use of an orthosis should be restricted to a minimum, as it increases the work load on the paralytic levels and tends to produce abnormal gait patterns. In severe paralysis of the lower limbs and trunk, however, locomotion may be impossible without the support of an adequate orthosis. General activities of the patient are gradually increased. During the first few minutes of locomotion the gait may be very effective, but with fatigue it may become very poor. Random, purposeless activity should be discouraged.

CHRONIC PHASE

The purposes of treatment in the residual stage are to enable the patient to attain maximal function and to obtain the greatest amount of productive activity in spite of residual weakness.[118] With continued growth and use of the limb, progressive deformities may develop, which will ultimately cause loss of function.

Hence, an equally important task during the chronic stage is to prevent deformities and to correct them, should they develop. The residual stage is a dynamic, not a static, period. Much can be done to improve the functional capacity of the patient. Aspects of treatment are discussed under the headings of Physical Therapy, Orthoses and Apparatus, and Surgery.

Physical Therapy. In the residual stage the physical therapy regimen is directed toward (1) prevention or correction of deformity by passive stretching exercises; (2) increase of motor strength of muscles by active or hypertrophy exercises; and (3) achievement of maximum functional activity.[194]

Active Hypertrophy Exercises. It is obvious there is little to be gained by exercising zero or trace muscles that remain so after 18 months, and the same is true of muscles that have a good or normal rating. Active hypertrophy exercises are performed primarily for the benefit of marginal muscles to elevate or maintain their functional level. For example, when the anterior tibial and toe extensor muscles are fair in motor strength and the triceps surae muscles are normal, it is important that active exercises of the ankle dorsiflexors be performed to maintain them at the antigravity functional level. The calf muscles should also be passively stretched to prevent the development of equinus deformity; this is implemented by the use of a night bivalved cast, which holds the foot out of equinus and in neutral position. Progressive resistance exercises utilize activity graded in proportion to the strength of the involved muscles; their use is recommended in the residual stage of poliomyelitis to increase the strength and improve the endurance of such individual muscles or groups of muscles as a fair quadriceps or triceps surae or a fair plus hip abductor muscle to the maximum capacity. Whether progressive resistive exercises are of any permanent value when the motor strength of a muscle is less than fair minus is doubtful; a poor quadriceps muscle cannot, by hypertrophy exercises, be improved to fair strength so that it can lift the leg against gravity. Correction of flexion deformity of the knee, however, may provide added strength by eliminating the need for the quadriceps muscle to work against deformity.

Passive Stretching Exercises. Prevention of contractural deformity is much simpler than its correction. When a limb is continuously maintained in one position, contracture and fixed deformity will develop as a result of the effects of gravity and dynamic imbalance of muscles. An ankle joint held in plantar flexion because of weak dorsiflexors and strong triceps surae will develop progressive equinus deformity if the ankle is not passively stretched into dorsiflexion every day. Passive stretching exercises should be performed gently, several times a day. In the presence of muscle imbalance, however, they are not adequate to prevent deformity and other measures should be employed, such as the use of a removable bivalved long leg night cast, which holds the foot in neutral position, and the wearing of a below-knee dorsiflexion-assist spring orthosis during the day. Later, during the chronic stage, muscle balance may be restored by transfer of muscles.

Functional Training. The purpose of such a therapy program is to enable the patient to overcome the handicaps imposed by his physical disability. The residual deficit in function varies, depending upon the extent and severity of paralysis. The needs of a growing child progressively change. In the residual stage the patient is taught how to use all the available muscles in order to accomplish a task successfully. This is in contrast to the convalescent stage, when he is not allowed to substitute stronger muscles for weaker ones. For example, when the anterior tibial is poor in motor strength in the convalescent stage, the child is not permitted to use his toe extensors to dorsiflex the foot when active exercises are performed with the anterior tibial. In the chronic stage, when anterior tibial function is still poor, he is taught how to dorsiflex his foot by using his toe extensors and peroneal muscles.

At times, the activity of stronger muscles is suppressed in order to prevent the development of deformity. For example, an individual with normal sartorius, biceps femoris, and peroneal muscles, but poor iliopsoas, medial hamstring, and anterior tibial muscles will walk with marked external rotation deformity of the foot and leg. It is important to supervise his gait,

teaching him to suppress the eversion power of the peroneals and the externally rotating power of the biceps femoris and the sartorius to prevent development of external rotation deformity of the lower limb.

To teach a child merely to walk with crutches and orthoses is not satisfactory. He should be instructed in activities of daily living, such as how to get in and out of chairs, to open doors, and to enter an automobile.

Orthoses and Other Apparatus. Use of an apparatus may be necessary during the asensitive period of the convalescent stage and the residual stage of poliomyelitis. The primary purposes of the orthosis are (1) to support the patient, enabling him to walk and increasing his functional activity; (2) to protect a weak muscle from overstretching; (3) to augment the action of weak muscles or to substitute for those completely lost; (4) to prevent deformity and malposition; and (5) to correct deformity by stretching certain groups of muscles that have been contracted. The elements of support, substitution, and correction may be combined in a single apparatus. In general, dynamic splinting

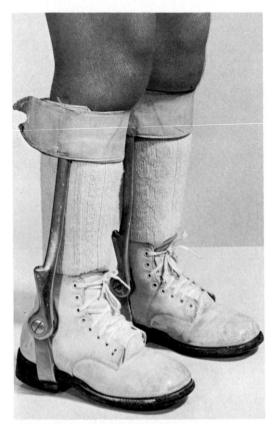

FIGURE 5–143. Plantar flexion assist below-knee orthosis with a dorsiflexion stop at neutral position.

is more desirable than static splinting. For example, when the toe extensor and anterior tibial muscles are paralyzed and the triceps surae muscle is normal, a dorsiflexion-assist spring orthosis (which acts as an active substitute for the weak ankle dorsiflexors) is preferable to a below-knee caliper orthosis with a posterior stop that prevents plantar flexion of the ankle beyond neutral position. In paralysis of the gastrocnemius and soleus muscles, a plantar flexion–assist spring below-knee orthosis with a dorsiflexion stop at neutral position is prescribed (Fig. 5–143). In the presence of a flail ankle and foot, a double-action ankle joint (both plantar flexion– and dorsiflexion-assist) is given, and a varus or valgus T-strap added to the shoe, as necessary. Also, inside or outside wedges to the shoe are given, depending upon the deformity of the foot (see Chapter 7).

When the muscles controlling the knee are paralyzed, an above-knee orthosis with a drop-lock knee joint is prescribed. This type of orthosis will provide knee stability for walking and can be unlocked during sitting. If genu recurvatum results from paralysis of the triceps surae in the presence of some strength of the quadriceps femoris, it can be controlled by an above-knee orthosis with a free knee joint so constructed as to prevent complete extension of the orthosis at the knee. Proper positioning of the thigh and calf bands will also check genu recurvatum. Genu varum or knock-knee pads are padded as necessary. When flexion deformity of the knee is present as a result of dynamic imbalance between the hamstrings and quadriceps femoris muslces, a well-padded anterior knee pad is given. An Engen extension knee orthosis is worn at night to correct flexion deformity of the knee.

When the muscles controlling the hip are weak, stability of the hip joint can be provided by an ischial weight-bearing thigh socket; crutches are used if necessary. Rotational alignment of the lower limbs is obtained by the addition of rotation straps or twisters. Ordinarily the patient does walk better without a pelvic band and drop-lock hips; however, in a young child with gluteus maximus paralysis, they may be used temporarily for balance. Often the spine will also require support. Upon resumption of upright posture, the abdominal muscles will overstretch, and severe lumbar lordosis and paralytic scoliosis will develop. Any asymmetrical involvement of the abdominal and trunk musculature should always be carefully noted. An abdominal corset support with metal stays often serves to control abdominal muscle paralysis. In the presence of weakness of the trunk extensors, a spinal orthosis with an abdominal corset is given. If the spine is unstable and collapsing, it may be supported by a molded plastic body jacket constructed from a plaster-of-Paris cast made with the patient standing with traction from a head sling. In paralytic scoliosis, usually a Milwaukee brace is worn, provided that the paralysis of the lower limbs is not very extensive and that the wearing of such an appliance does not prevent ambulation. In such instances, the Milwaukee brace is used intermittently during periods of recumbency or sitting, or both.

In the upper limb, the paralyzed shoulder muscles, particularly the deltoid, are best protected from the effects of gravity with a sling; this allows functional use of the forearm and hand. During the initial period of six to eight weeks, an abduction shoulder splint may be worn at night and during part of the day to prevent overstretching of the deltoid muscle; this is particularly indicated when there is associated paralytic subluxation or dislocation of the shoulder joint. A cock-up wrist splint is given when the wrist extensors are paralyzed, and an opponens splint when there is weakness of the opponens of the thumb. When there is paralysis of the intrinsic muscles of the hand, hyperextension of the metacarpophalangeal joints is prevented by a knuckle-bender dynamic splint.

Certain general principles should be followed in regard to use of an apparatus in poliomyelitis:

Whenever satisfactory recovery of function is expected, an orthosis should be used with caution in the lower limbs, since its use will tend to produce an abnormal gait pattern. Thus, during the early convalescent period, the use of an orthosis should be deferred until after maximum recovery of muscle function has taken place. Locomotion without an orthosis but with the support of crutches should be attempted, in order to stimulate active muscular function by the exercise derived from walking. Use of an orthosis should not, however, be postponed if deformities tend to develop incident to the stresses of weight-bearing. The needs of each patient are different, depending upon the severity of muscle weakness and the degree of dynamic imbalance of muscles. In the presence of extensive paralysis of the lower limbs, use of an orthosis may be the only means of stance and locomotion.

As a general principle, use of an orthosis should be as minimal as the condition permits. For example, when a patient with paralysis of both lower limbs is fitted with two above-knee orthoses, he will also require the use of two crutches to walk. If he is to use two crutches, he can do as well with an above-knee orthosis on one leg only, only minimal motor strength being required of the other leg to walk without an orthosis. During the stance phase on the leg without the orthotic support, the tripod base is completed by the two crutches; the knee is stabilized by locking it in hyperextension. Fair motor strength in the ankle dorsiflexors and hip flexor muscles will clear the lower limb in the swing phase. For prevention of fatigue, however, bilateral above-knee orthoses are used.

It is imperative to explain to the patient the reasons for the use of the orthosis. He should understand clearly that wearing the orthosis will help him at this stage of the disease, and that, at a later date, it may be discarded following training or reconstructive surgery. For example, the use of a dorsiflexion-assist below-knee orthosis may be unnecessary following a successful anterior transfer of the peroneal tendons, or an opponens splint may be discarded after a satisfactory opponens tendon transfer; or when the child becomes an adult, he may no longer require the above-knee orthosis used to prevent genu recurvatum.

It is always wise to question at intervals whether the continued use of the orthosis is necessary. Before advising that use of an orthosis be discontinued, one should be quite certain that there is no possibility for development of progressive deformities and that the level and quality of functional performance will not deteriorate.

Surgery. A multitude of operative procedures may be employed both in the correction of paralytic deformities and in the total physical rehabilitation of the child with poliomyelitis. These procedures may include fasciotomy, capsulotomy, tendon transfers, osteotomy, and arthrodesis. Leg length inequality commonly occurs in poliomyelitis as a result of shortening in the paralyzed leg. The various methods of equalizing leg lengths are presented in Chapter 7.

Principles of Tendon Transfer. Tendon transfer is the shifting of the insertion of a muscle from its normal attachment to another site to replace active muscular action that was lost by paralysis and to restore dynamic muscle balance. The procedure was originally described by Nicoladoni in 1882. Many surgeons have devised various types of tendon transfers and established their usefulness. Lange, Velpeau, Vulpius, Codivilla, Mayer, Biesalski, Gold-

thwait, Ober, Steindler, Bunnell, and Green are some who may be mentioned.* The term *tendon transplantation* should not be used interchangeably with the term *tendon transfer,* as the two are not synonymous. Tendon transplantation refers to the procedure of "excision of a tendon and its use as a free graft." In *muscle transplantation,* both the origin and the insertion of a muscle are detached, and the entire muscle with its intact neurovascular supply is transplanted to a completely new site.

Basic principles of tendon transfers have been outlined by Green:

1. The muscle to be transferred must have adequate motor strength to carry out the new function. As a rule, the motor rating of the muscle should be good or normal to warrant transfer. The function that the transferred muscle is intended to perform is another consideration. In the lower limb, for example, in the presence of drop foot, anterior transfer of the peroneus longus is adequate to produce effective ankle dorsiflexion, whereas in calcaneus limp, posterior transfer of the peroneus longus alone to the os calcis is not sufficient to substitute for the gastrocnemius-soleus action, and the additional action of two or three motors such as the flexor digitorum communis and anterior tibial muscles is required. Ordinarily one grade of motor power is lost after a muscle is transferred.

2. The range of motion of muscles on contraction is an important consideration. This range must be similar to that of the muscles for which they are being substituted; also, whenever muscles are transferred in combination, their range of contraction should not differ significantly. The transfer of antagonistic muscles ordinarily is not as effective as that of muscles having similar function or corollary activity. However, with meticulous postoperative care, antagonistic muscles may be transferred effectively with good results; the posterior transfer of the anterior tibial to the os calcis and of the hamstring muscles to the patella are common examples of such antagonistic transfers.

3. In choosing the muscles for transfer the loss of original function that will result from the tendon transfer must be balanced against the gains to be obtained. For example, in the presence of hip flexor weakness, the hamstring muscles should not be transferred to the patella for quadriceps paralysis, as loss of active knee

---

*See References 26, 41, 69, 113, 189, 215–217, 222, 242–246, 303–311, 328.

flexion added to lack of hip flexion will be a greater disability. Whenever possible, muscle balance must be restored. Ideally a deforming muscle force must be shifted so as to substitute for an essential weakness. In the foot and ankle, for example, the muscles of inversion and eversion and those of plantar flexion and dorsiflexion should be balanced. A common pitfall is transfer of the peroneus longus muscle posteriorly to the os calcis in the presence of a strong anterior tibial muscle. Normally, the anterior tibial muscle dorsiflexes the first metatarsal and the peroneus longus opposes this action. With posterior transfer of the peroneus longus, the unopposed anterior tibial gradually causes the first metatarsal to ride up, producing a dorsal bunion. Thus the peroneus longus should not be transferred to the os calcis unless the anterior tibial is shifted from its insertion on the first metatarsal to the midline of the foot.

4. The joints upon which the transferred muscle is to act should have functional range of motion. All contractural deformity should be corrected by wedging casts or soft-tissue release prior to tendon transfer. An anterior transfer for drop foot, for example, should not be performed in the presence of equinus deformity of the ankle.

5. A smooth gliding channel with adequate space must be provided for excursion of the tendon in its new location. The paratenon and synovial sheath are preserved over the tendon surface during dissection. It is preferable to pass the tendon beneath the deep fascia through tissues that permit free gliding rather than subcutaneously. A wide portion of the intermuscular septum is excised whenever muscles are passed from one muscle compartment to another. Sufficient space should be provided for the tendon so that adhesions will not form. An Ober tendon passer of appropriate size should be used to redirect the tendon to its new insertion: It spreads the tissues and prevents binding.

6. The neurovascular supply of the transferred muscle must not be damaged while transferring the tendon. One must be careful not to denervate the muscle while freeing it for redirection. When the tendon is pulled up from the distal wound into the proximal incision, traction should not be applied on the origin of the muscle. Stretching of the motor nerve is prevented by use of the double-hand technique; i.e., with a moist sponge, the proximal segment of the tendon is held steady while, with another sponge, traction is applied on its distal segment. Acute angulation or torsion of the neurovascular bundle is another cause of injury. Gentle handling is imperative for preservation of innervation and function of the transferred muscle.

7. In the rerouting of the tendon a *straight line* of contraction must be provided between the origin of the muscle and its new insertion. Angular courses and passages over pulley systems should be avoided. In order to allow adequate freeing of the muscle toward its origin, the incision over the belly of the muscle must be long and proximally located.

8. The tendon should be reattached to its new site under sufficient tension so that the transferred muscle will have a maximal range of contraction. The transferred muscle should be tested at surgery to ensure that it will hold the part in optimal position. Ordinarily, in the lower limb, where weight-bearing forces are involved, the tendon is attached to bone, whereas in the upper limb it is sutured to the tendon. An important technical detail is scarification of the distal segment of the tendon that is to be anchored to a bone or tendon; this is achieved by excision of the sheath and paratenon and "roughening" of the tendon by scraping and crosshatching it with a knife. The position of immobilization in a plaster-of-Paris cast should allow the transferred tendon to be in a relaxed attitude in order to diminish any tension on the tendon while healing. For example, when the flexor carpi ulnaris is transferred to the extensor carpi radialis longus, the tension on the tendon should be sufficient to hold the wrist in 30 degrees of dorsiflexion. Yet when the cast is applied, the wrist is immobilized in the overcorrected position of 45 to 50 degrees of dorsiflexion.[116]

Postoperative Care and Training. These are fundamental in obtaining a good result. The following principles, given by Green, should be followed meticulously.

First, the age of the patient at the time of tendon transfer is an important preoperative consideration. The child should be old enough, preferably over four years of age, to cooperate in the training of the transfer. A delay in tendon transfer in the presence of muscle imbalance will lead to progressive deformity. Usually, conservative measures should be undertaken to control deforming factors, but in certain instances, early surgery is indicated when such a delay of tendon transfer results in increasing structural deformity. A common example is the rapid development of progressive calcaneus deformity of the foot with paralysis of the gastrocnemius-soleus muscles and strong ankle dorsiflexors. An early posterior transfer will prevent the development of a deformed foot.

Support of the part in overcorrected position

should be continued until the muscle has assumed full function and until there is no tendency for the deformity to recur. Use of a bivalved cast will serve to hold the transferred tendon in a relaxed position.

It is best to teach the patient preoperatively to localize contracture in the muscle to be transferred. Active exercises are continued postoperatively as soon as the reaction to surgery and pain has subsided. The surgeon should assist the physical therapist during the initial exercises. When tendon transfer is combined with arthrodesis, muscle re-education is delayed until adequate bony union has taken place.

The patient is instructed to contract the transferred muscle voluntarily, moving the part through the arc of motion that was the original normal action of the muscle, while the therapist manually guides the part to move in the direction that is intended to be provided by the transfer. For example, when the peroneus longus muscle is transferred anteriorly to the base of the second metatarsal, the active motion called for is eversion in combination with guided dorsiflexion, or if the anterior tibial muscle has been transferred posteriorly to the os calcis, active inversion is combined with guided plantar flexion of the ankle; in anterior transfer of the hamstrings to the patella for quadriceps femoris paralysis, the patient is placed in side-lying position and is asked to extend the hip actively (using the hamstrings) as the knee is guided into extension; or when the flexor carpi ulnaris is transferred to the extensor carpi radialis longus, the wrist is gently guided into extension as the patient deviates it ulnarward. With one hand, the therapist should palpate the belly and tendon of the transferred muscle to ensure its contraction. In the beginning, the exercises are performed in the bivalved cast. Motion of the concerned joint is executed slowly, steadily, and smoothly through as full a range as possible. Soon the limb is taken out of the plaster cast and is properly positioned, and measures are taken to prevent stretching of the tendon out of its resting position.

Occasionally the patient is unable to contract the transferred muscle actively and has difficulty in "finding" it. To enable him to use the transfer actively and to assist him in acquiring the feeling desired, the therapist may exert gentle mild tension on the transferred tendon, have the patient shift positions during attempts at active contraction, or advise him in the use of corollary motions. If, after two weeks, such difficulty in "finding" the transfer persists, electrical stimulation may be employed to initiate contraction as the patient himself attempts to use the muscle. After a few sessions, the patient begins to "feel" the transfer and to contract it voluntarily.

As soon as the patient is able to contract the transferred muscle actively, exercises in the direction of the original action of the muscle are discontinued and only those motions in the new function provided by the transfer are performed.

When the transferred muscle develops poor motor strength, i.e., can carry the part through the full range of motion with gravity eliminated, the physical therapist instructs one of the parents to perform the exercises with the patient. The exercise regimen is supervised by the physical therapist and the surgeon, who check it at weekly or biweekly intervals.

In the beginning, the limb should be retained in the bivalved cast for support except during the exercise periods. As soon as the motor strength of the transfer becomes fair, the use of a bivalved cast during the day is gradually discontinued. Controlled activities are permitted to develop function. These are permitted sooner in the upper than in the lower limb. The age and dependability of the patient are other considerations. Resistive exercises to develop power are begun whenever the transfer has a normal range of action and is fair in strength. It is also important to exercise the antagonistic muscles to prevent disuse atrophy.

The next stage of training is the incorporation of the transfer into the new functional pattern. This is particularly important in the lower limb, in which the muscles are concerned with gait. For example, the action of the peroneus transfer may be good, dorsiflexing the ankle through full range and taking moderate resistance; yet, during locomotion, voluntary control over the transfer is "lost" and the patient walks with a drop-foot gait. The transition to walking requires diligent supervision. Of particular importance is the use of crutches—they serve to protect the limb from undue strain and at the same time allow the patient to be taught the use of the transfer and to become accustomed to it. First the patient is asked to take a single step, ensuring that the muscle contracts and dorsiflexes the ankle. As soon as the transfer functions throughout all the phases of a single step, the walking periods are gradually increased until the normal gait pattern becomes a conditioned reflex.

The use of orthoses in the postoperative

period should be judicious and for specific reasons. Orthotic support protects the part and allows early activity. This is indicated particularly when paralysis is extensive, as in myelomeningocele. In a posterior transfer to the os calcis, for example, a plantar flexion–assist orthosis with a dorsiflexion stop at right angles with crutches may be used to aid developing function in the transfers and prevent stretching. However, standing and walking exercises are also performed without the brace to stimulate function in the transfer.

Prolonged use of a bivalved night cast is very important to prevent development of contractural deformity that will oppose the action of the transfer, as for example, in the instance of anterior transfer for dorsiflexion, equinus deformity of the ankle. From the beginning, daily stretching exercises should be a part of the exercise regimen. Stretching and night support are continued over a long period of time, until the muscle has developed full strength and there is balanced function between the agonist and antagonist muscles with no tendency for recurrence of the original deformity. In fact, stretching and active exercises should be a simple rule of daily living.

Arthrodesis to provide stability and correct osseous deformity may be indicated, particularly in the foot. However, if dynamic balance is established prior to development of structural deformity, arthrodesis may be unnecessary. When it is necessary to combine arthrodesis with tendon transfer, muscle re-education must be delayed until adequate bony union has taken place.

The Hip

SOFT-TISSUE CONTRACTURE

The common deformity of the hip secondary to soft-tissue contracture is one of flexion, abduction, and external rotation. Several factors must be considered in its pathogenesis. During the acute and convalescent stages of poliomyelitis, the patient lies supine in the so-called frog-leg attitude with the hips flexed, abducted, and externally rotated; the knees flexed; and the feet in equinovarus posture. This position is assumed because of spasm of the hamstrings, hip flexors, tensor fasciae latae, and hip abductor muscles, and because of the forces of gravity acting on the flail lower limbs. Maintenance of the lower limbs in malposture results in permanent shortening of the soft tissues. Contracture of the intermuscular septa and enveloping fasciae takes place first. This fact can be easily

observed at surgery. Upon sectioning of the contracted fasciae that cover normal muscle fibers, and 2 to 3 cm. retraction of the cut edges of the fascia, the underlying muscle tissue will be found to be in relaxed condition when it is elevated with tissue forceps. Partially paralyzed muscle becomes shortened because of contracture of the involved fibrosed muscle fibers scattered throughout the normal muscle tissue. Adaptive shortening of normal muscle occurs later. Structural bony deformity develops with growth in the presence of soft-tissue contracture and dynamic muscle imbalance.

The iliotibial band (or tract) is the thickened lateral portion of the fascia lata located along the entire lateral aspect of the thigh and extending from the greater trochanteric region to below the knee. Superiorly, the iliotibial band is attached to the iliac crest by three prongs: a middle one through the aponeurosis over the gluteus medius, an anterior one through the tensor fasciae latae, and a posterior one through the gluteus maximus (Fig. 5–144).

Throughout its extent on the lateral aspect of the thigh, the iliotibial tract is continuous on its deep surface with the lateral intermuscular septum, through which it is firmly attached to the linea aspera on the posterior aspect of the femur. At the knee joint level, fascial expansions from the anterior border of the iliotibial tract join expansions that emanate from the quadriceps muscle to form the lateral patellar retinaculum. The lower end of the iliotibial band is attached to the lateral condyle of the tibia and the head of the fibula. Proximally the iliotibial band is located in a plane that is anterior and lateral to the axis of the hip joint, whereas distally, in a normal limb, the iliotibial tract inserts on the tibia in front of the axis of the knee joint. Irwin states, however, that the lower part of the iliotibial tract lies in a plane posterior and lateral to the axis of the knee joint.[172]

Contracture of the iliotibial band may contribute directly or indirectly to the development of the following deformities.[99, 103, 172, 175, 345]

The Lower Limb

Flexion, Abduction, and External Rotation Contracture of Hip. The shortened iliotibial band, which is in a plane anterior and lateral to the hip joint, will draw the femur into flexion and abduction at the hip with the pelvis as the fixed point. External rotation deformity is due to maintenance of the malposture of the "frog-leg" position. The related muscles, i.e., the tensor fasciae latae, reflected head of the rectus femoris, sartorius, and external rotators of the hip, undergo myostatic contracture if the fascial

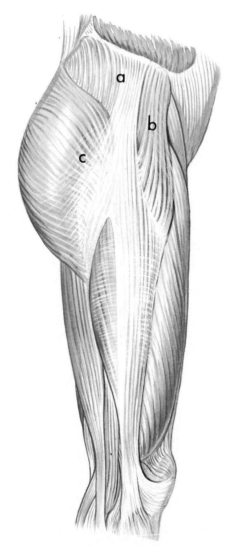

FIGURE 5–144. *The three-pronged attachment of the upper part of the iliotibial band to the iliac crest.*

There is a middle prong (a) through the aponeurosis over the gluteus medius, an anterior one (b) through the tensor fasciae latae, and a posterior one (c) through the gluteus maximus. Proximally, the location of the iliotibial tract is anterior and lateral to the axis of the hip, whereas inferiorly, in the normal knee, it inserts on the tibia well in front of the axis of the knee joint.

contracture is not corrected. The fixed soft-tissue contracture will cause anteversion of the proximal femur.

Flexion and Valgus Deformity of Knee and External Torsion of Tibia. The iliotibial band crosses lateral to the axis of the knee. When it is contracted a force is exerted on the lateral aspect of the joint and the tibia is gradually abducted on the femur. Its deforming action resembles that of a taut string on the concavity of an archer's bow. Irwin proposed that flexion

deformity of the knee developed as a result of the location of the band in a plane posterior to the axis of motion of the knee joint.[172] However, subsequent studies have not supported this observation. The short head of the biceps takes its origin in part from the intermuscular septum, which in turn is attached to the iliotibial band. Flexion deformity of the knee will develop as a result of spasm and subsequent myostatic contracture of the short head of the biceps. Prolonged maintenance of the knee in flexion will cause contracture of the patellar retinacula and soft tissues behind the knee.

External Torsion of the Tibia and Subluxation of the Knee Joint. The pull of the laterally located iliotibial band and the short head of the biceps femoris gradually rotates the tibia and fibula externally on the femur. When the contracture is not controlled, the deforming forces will cause posterolateral subluxation of the knee with displacement of the fibular head into the popliteal space.

Positional Pes Varus. This results from an ill-fitted orthosis that fails to compensate for the external tibial torsion. The axes of the knee and ankle joints do not occupy the same horizontal plane in external torsion of the tibia. When an above-knee orthosis manufactured with these joints in the same horizontal plane is fitted to a limb with external tibial torsion, the appliance will force the foot into varus position so that the ankle is in line with the knee joint. Initially the varus deformity is a purely functional one (the foot will assume normal alignment when the lateral upright of the orthosis is allowed to rotate externally on the thigh); it will later become fixed owing to permanent shortening of the soft tissues and adaptive osseous changes in the tarsal bones.

The Pelvis and Trunk

Pelvic Deformity, Lumbar Scoliosis, Subluxation of Contralateral Hip. In abduction deformity of the hip due to iliotibial band contracture, the pelvis is level or is at a right angle to the vertical axis of the trunk as long as the affected hip is maintained in abduction; however, when it is brought parallel to the vertical axis of the body in the weight-bearing position, the pelvis is forced to assume an oblique position. This pelvic obliquity is due to contracture below the iliac crest. A lumbosacral scoliosis, convex to the low side of the pelvis, simultaneously develops. The contralateral hip will subluxate.

Exaggerated Lumbar Lordosis. This is produced when there is bilateral flexion contracture of the hips. It is a compensatory response to the increased pelvic inclination when the trunk assumes an upright position.

Treatment. Static malpostural deformities of the lower limbs in the acute and subacute stages of poliomyelitis can be prevented by the use of bivalved casts, which maintain the joints in neutral position. A horizontal bar in the posterior half of the cast or a rotational strap will control malrotation at the hips. The knees should be in slight flexion to prevent genu recurvatum. Passive exercises are performed to maintain full range of joint motion.

Minimal contracture of the iliotibial band can be corrected by passive stretching exercises, which follow the same steps as in the Ober test (see Fig. 1–22). They can also be performed in the supine position, with the hip that is to be stretched overhanging the edge of the bed. In the older patient the iliotibial band can be stretched by the following exercise: The patient should stand sideways about 2 feet away from the wall with the hip that is to be stretched placed facing it. With the feet on the ground and the legs together, the hip is brought toward the wall to the count of 10 and is then returned to the original position. This exercise should be performed in sequences of 20 times, three times a day.

When the iliotibial band is contracted to such a degree that fixed deformity at the hip and knee with tilting of the pelvis has resulted, correction cannot be obtained by manipulative stretching or application of a series of plaster casts. The pelvis cannot be locked securely enough to permit stretching forces to be exerted on the shortened iliotibial band; instead, the pelvis will be tilted into an oblique and hyperextended position, stretching the lateral and anterior abdominal muscles on the side of the contracture.

Surgical intervention is the only way to correct the deformity. The shortened soft tissues must be sectioned proximally as well as distally by combining Ober's fasciotomy with Yount's procedure.[244, 345] As stated previously, the primary cause of the deformities is contracture of the intermuscular septa, the enveloping fascia, and the fibrosed muscular tissue in the partially involved muscles. Normal muscle tissue should not be divided.

Ober's and Yount's fasciotomies are performed as follows:

Both lower limbs and hips are prepared and draped sterile. *Ober's fasciotomy* is performed through an incision that starts at the junction of the posterior and middle thirds of the iliac crest and then extends distally to the anterior superior iliac spine, where it swings posterolaterally for a distance of 10 cm. The wound flaps are mobilized to expose the sartorius, rectus femoris, tensor fasciae femoris, and gluteus medius and minimus muscles. The enveloping fascia of these muscles, the intermuscular septa, the intervening fibrosed muscular tissue, and the iliotibial band are sectioned as far back as the greater trochanter. The Ober and Thomas tests are performed to determine by palpation the presence of any tight bands, which, if present, are divided. Normal muscle tissue and the anterior capsule of the hip joint should not be divided. The contracted fibers of the Bigelow ligament can be released without entering the hip joint. *Yount's procedure* consists of excision of a segment of the iliotibial band and of the lateral intermuscular septum in the distal thigh. A midlateral longitudinal incision is made beginning immediately above the knee joint line and extending cephalad for a distance of 10 cm. The subcutaneous tissue is divided and the wound flaps are mobilized by blunt dissection to expose the anterolateral aspect of the thigh in its distal one fourth. Next a 7 cm. block of the iliotibial band, the fascia lata covering the vastus lateralis muscle, and the lateral intermuscular septum are excised. It is important to divide the lateral intermuscular septum down to the femur. If it is contracted and contributes to flexion deformity of the knee, the lateral patellar retinaculum is also divided.

In severe cases with lateral rotatory subluxation of the knee, the biceps femoris muscle is lengthened by the fractional method, extreme care being taken not to injure the common peroneal nerve (see Plate 66). This can be performed through the same incision. Then an attempt at reduction is made by forcibly extending and internally rotating the knee. Often a Z-lengthening of the fibular collateral ligament will be necessary to achieve reduction.

Both the hip and the thigh wounds are closed routinely. Bilateral long leg casts are applied, holding the knees in full extension. Metal rings are anchored on the cast on both its anterior and its posterior aspects so that the patient can be placed in suspension traction. One set of rings is placed in the distal one fourth of the leg and another set of rings in the proximal one fourth of the leg. Rotational straps can be added to the plaster cast if necessary. The patient is placed on two or three half mattresses so that his lower limbs can hang free at the edge of the mattress and his hips can be hyperextended or flexed by suspension (Fig. 5–145). An infant or small child can be placed on a bent hyperex-

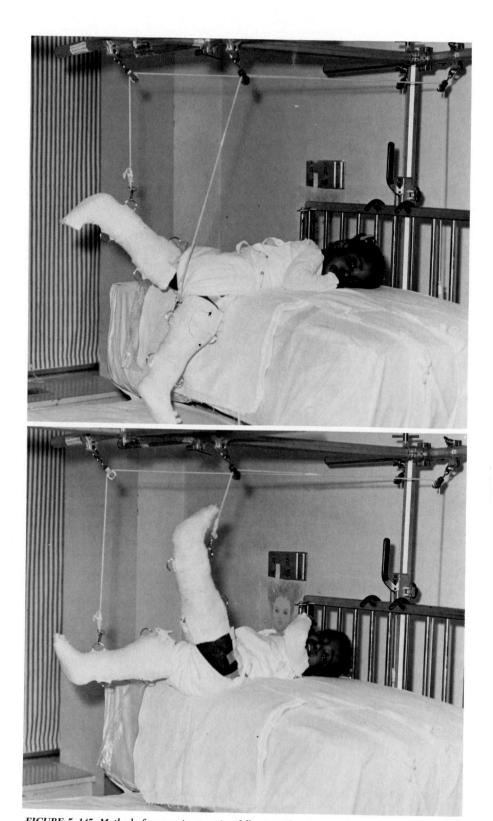

FIGURE 5–145. Method of suspension-traction following Ober-Yount release of the iliotibial band.

tended Bradford frame to achieve the same result. The opposite lower limb is flexed at the hip to obliterate the lumbar lordosis. The affected limb is gradually hyperextended, adducted, and internally rotated at the hip, stretching out all remaining contractural deformity. The same position of the hips can be accomplished with the patient prone or supine. In bilateral cases the hips are alternated several times a day. Manipulative stretching exercises are performed three times a day. Meticulous observation of circulation and sensation in the toes is imperative, especially if excessive shortening of neurovascular structures was observed at operation.

In myelomeningocele patients with impaired sensation, stretching by the method described may cause pressure sores. Atrophied bones of these children may also be fractured easily by vigorous manipulations or stretching procedures.

Passive stretching by the preceding suspension-traction method is continued for a period of three weeks.

With progressive longitudinal growth of the femur, contracture of the iliotibial band will recur unless passive stretching exercises and proper positioning of the joints in bivalved casts are continued during periods of growth.

GLUTEUS MEDIUS PARALYSIS

When the hip abductor muscles are paralyzed, the trunk will sway toward the affected side and the contralateral side of the pelvis will drop during the weight-bearing phase of gait. Lateral stability of the hip joint is best provided by transferring the *iliopsoas muscle* from the lesser trochanter to the greater trochanter (see Plate 75). The author commonly performs the Sharrard modification of the Mustard iliopsoas transfer, making the hole in the ilium as far posteriorly as the nerve supply to the iliacus will allow.[235, 236] One cannot overemphasize the importance of using a nerve stimulator while transferring the iliopsoas muscle. Details of postoperative care following iliopsoas transfer are described in the section on myelomeningocele. The hip should be protected with crutches until the transferred iliopsoas is fair plus or good in motor strength and the Trendelenburg test is negative. During this period the patient should sleep in a bivalved hip spica cast, which maintains the hip in 40 to 60 degrees of abduction. Active hip abduction exercises should be performed diligently—graduating from the supine position to side-lying against gravity, and then to standing Trendelenburg.

The *external oblique abdominal muscle* can be used to restore hip abduction power. Lowman used part of the external oblique muscle and attached it to the greater trochanter with a strip of fascia lata.[202-204] Thomas, Thompson, and Straub transferred the entire muscle belly of the external oblique.[315] The remaining abdominal muscles (rectus abdominis, internal oblique, and transversus muscles) will maintain integrity of the abdominal wall. The author has had no personal experience with external oblique muscle transfer for paralysis of hip abductors. Physiologically, the procedure is sound; for details of operative technique, the reader is referred to the original article.[315] Also, the tensor fasciae latae muscle may be transferred posteriorly on the iliac crest for increase of hip abduction strength.[192]

GLUTEUS MAXIMUS PARALYSIS

Instability of the hip and exaggerated lumbar lordosis result from paralysis of the gluteus maximus muscle. In gait, the trunk lurches backward when the body weight is borne on the affected side. When the hip flexor muscles are of normal strength, increasing flexion deformity of the hip will develop.

For motor evaluation of the gluteus maximus muscle, the patient is placed in prone position, with the lower limbs hanging off the examining table. The knee is in flexion to eliminate action of the hamstrings. The patient is asked to extend his hip against gravity and manual resistance. The position also serves to evaluate the degree of flexion deformity of the hip when it is extended passively. If the patient is unable to lift the thigh against gravity, he is placed in side-lying position to eliminate the force of gravity. Any abduction contracture is best determined by the Ober test, as the degree of hip abduction noted on maximal extension of the hip in prone position is not as accurate.

In gluteus maximus paralysis, stability of the pelvis may be provided by the addition of posterior gluteal crisscross straps between the pelvic band and the thigh band of the above-knee orthosis; an alternative method is to discard the pelvic band and fit an ischial weight-bearing quadrilateral socket to the upper thigh segment of the orthosis. Often, however, the additional support of one or two crutches is required.

Muscle transfers to restore gluteus maximus function are not always successful and should be undertaken only after considerable deliberation. Lange transferred the erector spinae muscle to the greater trochanter, using silk

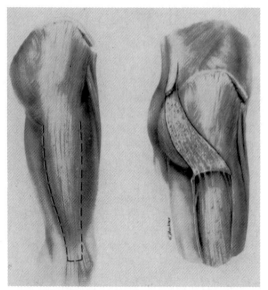

FIGURE 5–146. *Erector spinae transfer or fascia lata transfer to the greater trochanter.*

(From Hogshead, H. P., and Ponseti, I. V.: Fascia lata transfer to the erector spinae. J. Bone Joint Surg., 46-A:1390, 1964. Reprinted by permission.)

sutures to obtain length.[183, 189] Ober and Hey Groves used a strip of fascia lata to attach the erector spinae muscle to the greater trochanter.[127, 240]

The technique of Ober was further improved by Barr, who used a wide strip of fascia lata, including the iliotibial tract and tensor fasciae latae muscle (Fig. 5–146).[11] Contractures about the hip, such as fascia and tight intermuscular septa, are released, particularly those that are anterior and lateral to the hip joint. Complete mobilization of the iliotibial tract and shift of its pull laterally to the greater trochanter removes a major deforming force. Release of contracted investing fascia about the shortened erector spinae muscle permits rotation of the pelvis to nearly normal position and diminishes the severity of fixed lumbar lordosis.

Malrotation of the limb is prevented and corrected by transfer of the insertion of the tensor fasciae latae into the greater trochanter. Stability of hip is provided if there is power in the erector spinae and tensor fasciae latae muscles, which act in conjunction as a diagastric muscle transfer. The operation does not significantly improve the extensor or abductor power of the hip, but appears to produce a more dynamic fasciodesis. Stance and gait are improved by relief of hip flexion contracture, stabilization of the hip, and relief of lumbar lordosis.[293]

The operative technique, as advocated by Barr in 1964, is as follows:

Operative Technique [Barr]. The patient, under general anesthesia, is placed in the lateral position with both limbs flexed 90 degrees at the hip and knee; the affected limb is uppermost, abducted, and resting on pillows. The skin of the lumbar region, buttock, and limb is prepared from the ribs to the mid-calf. The operative field is draped so that the limb can be moved freely. The incision in the thigh begins just anterior to the head of the fibula and ends proximally just distal to the anterior superior iliac spine passing over the greater trochanter. The iliotibial band is exposed through its full length and breadth and is divided transversely at the level of the distal pole of the patella. A stout silk suture is passed through its free end and as wide a strip of fascia as it is possible to obtain is dissected upward and preserved as the tendon of insertion of the tensor fasciae latae muscle. Beginning at the trochanteric level, the dissection is carried toward the anterior iliac spine, mobilizing the distal half of the tensor fasciae latae muscle and preserving its neurovascular bundle. The intermuscular septa and other contracted fascial structures at the knee and anterior to the hip are divided as necessary while an assistant holds the hip and knee in as much extension as possible. The sartorius and rectus muscles are tenotomized if they are contracted and totally paralyzed. The iliopsoas tendon, if need be, may be divided at its insertion but should be transposed to a more proximal and anterior position in the intertrochanteric region. The anterior capsule of the hip may also be divided through the same incision if it prevents extension of the hip. The neurovascular bundle is preserved.

Subperiosteal anchorage of the fascial strip to the femur is accomplished by making two parallel longitudinal incisions, usually five to six centimeters long, through the origin of the vastus lateralis and the periosteum, one on the anterolateral, the other on the posterolateral aspect of the femur just below the greater trochanter and tunneling beneath the periosteum to join the two incisions. The strip of fascia is then passed through the tunnel and secured to the periosteum by silk sutures. This must be done with the hip held in as much extension as possible, without putting undue force on the tissues, and maintaining slight abduction and neutral position as regards rotation.

The lumbar incision is about 15 cm. long. It is made parallel to and 5 to 8 cm. lateral to the line of the spinous processes of the fourth and fifth lumbar and first sacral vertebrae. The inferior end of the incision is located medial to and about 5 cm. distal to the posterior superior iliac spine. The incision is deepened through the lumbodorsal fascia, which is reflected to expose the underlying erector spinae muscle. By blunt dissection along a vertical line, the lateral two-thirds of this muscle mass is mobilized and freed from the medial one-third, which is left attached to the adjacent spinous processes and laminae. The mobilized muscle is freed by sharp dissection from its origin to the ilium and sacrum. Since the nerve and blood supply to this muscle is segmental and enters from its ventral surface, it may be necessary to sacrifice one or two of the most distal neurovascular bundles in order to mobilize a 10 cm. length of muscle mass.

By means of a long tendon carrier, the free end of the fascia lata is passed within the gluteal muscle compartment entering the lumbar incision just medial to the posterior superior iliac spine. The tunnel at its point of emergence is carefully dilated by the surgeon's finger so that the fascia can glide freely. The gliding deep surface of the fascia should be placed as it lies ventrally. With the hip held in extension, the fascia is attached, under moderate tension, to the free end of the mobilized erector spinae muscle. This is best done by laying the ventral surface of the muscle on the subcutaneous surface of the fascial strip, passing the suture in the end of the fascia through the muscle, as far proximally as possible, and then fixing the edges of the fascia to the edges of the muscle flap by a series of interrupted sutures. The distal end of the muscle is thus covered on its deep surface by the fascia lata. The lumbar incision is closed in layers; it is usually possible to close the lumbodorsal fascia over the transplant partially. The thigh incision is closed in a routine manner. No attempt should be made to close the defect in the fascia of the thigh. After application of sterile dressings, the extremity is immobilized by elastic bandages and long plaster splints which extend from the ribs to the toes. The hip is immobilized in as much extension as can be obtained comfortably. No attempt is made to correct the hip-flexion contracture completely at this time.

Technique for Correction of Remaining Contractures in Poliomyelitic Deformities. After ten days to two weeks, when the incisions have healed, the remaining contractures are gradually stretched out. The lumbar spine and the opposite lower extremity are immobilized in a spica with that hip in sufficient flexion to obliterate the lumbar lordosis. A separate toe-to-groin cast is applied to the affected limb with the knee preferably in almost complete extension. With the patient supine the affected limb in its plaster cast is suspended from an overhead frame. The contracture can then be stretched gradually and completely by lowering the limb in day-to-day increments until the hip comes into hyperextension. During this procedure, the circulation and sensation in the toes should be watched carefully, especially if excessive shortening of the femoral vessels and nerves was observed at operation.

If a knee-flexion deformity is present it may be corrected simultaneously by wedging the cast.

As a rule the deformity is satisfactorily corrected in two to three weeks. The apparatus is then removed and assistive muscle re-education exercises are begun with the patient in recumbency. Underwater exercises are of value. A bivalved long spica to hold the hip in the corrected position should be worn at night for several months. Walking with crutches is permit-

ted as soon as the transplant functions satisfactorily, usually about six weeks postoperatively. Many patients require bilateral transplants and should undergo operation in two stages, four to six weeks apart. Careful gait training is essential if the best results are to be obtained.*

Hogshead and Ponseti found the formation of an erector spinae flap in myelomeningocele to be difficult. The procedure was bloody and the ramifications of the meningocele sac were inadvertently entered, with the result that there was troublesome drainage of cerebrospinal fluid through the wound. Since, in their experience, erector spinae transfer did not provide active power of hip extension or abduction, they recommended attachment of the distal end of the fascia lata band to the freed lumbodorsal fascia at the level of the third or fourth lumbar vertebra (Fig. 5–147). They term the operative procedure fascia lata transfer to the erector spinae.[157] The route of the transfer should be subfascial, and its direction from the greater trochanter to the region of the posterior superior iliac spine should be as far posterior as possible.

Caution should be exercised in the anterior release of soft-tissue contracture of the hip. Every effort should be made to preserve viable muscles and their nerve and blood supply. The anterior capsule of the hip should not be sectioned, in order to prevent anterior dislocation of the femoral head. When contracture of the anterior capsule is fixed and it limits extension of the hip, it is *lengthened.*

In the Sharrard modification of the Mustard operation a hole is made in the posterior part of the ilium and the iliacus muscle is sutured to the lateral surface of the ilium (see Plate 75). The operation was designed to provide power of hip extension as well as hip abduction. Unfortunately, the motor nerve supply of the iliacus muscle is frequently distal in its location, limiting the degree of posterior positioning of the iliac hole. In the author's experience, Sharrard iliopsoas transfer has not been successful in providing active power of hip extension against gravity in the presence of complete paralysis of the gluteus maximus muscle. When the hamstring muscles are normal in motor strength and the gluteus maximus is only partially paralyzed, it will restore functional strength of hip extension and give substantial improvement in gait.

*From Barr, J. S.: Discussion. J. Bone Joint Surg., 46–A:1402, 1964. Reprinted with permission.

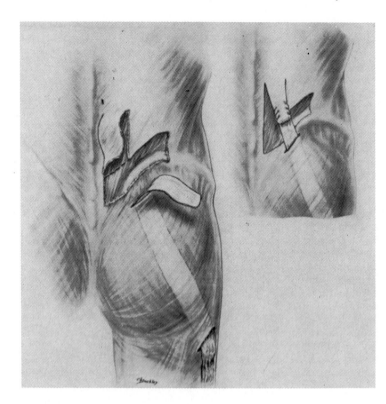

FIGURE 5–147. *Fascia lata transfer to lumbodorsal fascia to provide posterior stability to the hip joint.*

(From Hogshead, H. P., and Ponseti, I. V.: Fascia lata transfer to the erector spinae. J. Bone Joint Surg., 46-A:1404, 1964. Reprinted by permission.)

PARALYTIC DISLOCATION OF THE HIP

Hip dislocation in poliomyelitis is an acquired deformity caused by flaccid paralysis and the resulting muscular imbalance that develops. When, in a young child, the gluteus maximus and medius muscles are paralyzed and the hip flexors and adductors are of normal strength, eventual luxation of the hip is almost inevitable. Loss of hip abductor power causes retardation of growth from the greater trochanteric apophysis. Disparity of relative growth from the capital femoral epiphysis and the greater trochanteric apophysis causes increasing valgus deformity of the femoral neck. In severe cases, the angle between the neck and shaft of the femur increases to 180 degrees. Excessive anteversion of the femoral neck may also develop. When the angle between the femoral neck and the horizontal plane of the pelvis approaches 90 degrees, the hip joint becomes mechanically unstable. Gradually, under the forces of body weight, the capsule becomes lax and the femoral head rides out of the acetabulum. The empty acetabulum retains an adequate depth for several years following paralytic dislocation. With lack of concentric pressure of the femoral head in the acetabulum, however, progressive shal-lowness and obliquity of the acetabular roof develop. Thus, factors in the pathogenesis of true paralytic dislocation are muscle imbalance, coxa valga, and laxity of the capsule. In treatment, it is important to remember that coxa valga precedes subluxation and shallowness of the acetabulum.[176, 177, 295]

Acquired hip dislocation does not usually occur in a totally flail lower limb, particularly if the patient has been walking with the support of an orthosis. If inadequately treated, however, the flail hip may develop abduction–flexion–external rotation contracture due to shortening of the iliotibial band. When the lower limbs are aligned parallel to the vertical axis of the body in the weight-bearing position, the pelvis will be forced into an oblique position. The contralateral hip, i.e., the one on the high side of the pelvis, is in a markedly functional valgus position and will become dislocated eventually. Pelvic obliquity may result also from the foregoing factors; another cause may be severe structural scoliosis in the suprapelvic region. This type of scoliosis should be distinguished from positional scoliosis that is produced by pelvic obliquity due to contractural deformities below the pelvis.

Treatment. Dislocation of the hip in poliomyelitis may be prevented by restoration of dynamic balance about the hip; this is achieved by appropriate muscle transfers. If the age of onset of paralysis and muscle imbalance is less than two years, iliopsoas transfer to restore power of hip abduction is performed when the child is four or five years old. If the coxa valga deformity is less than 150 degrees, a preliminary varization osteotomy is unnecessary; the valgus deformity will correct itself with growth once hip abductor power is restored. If the coxa valga deformity is greater than 150 degrees, it is best to correct the deformity and obtain a femoral neck-shaft angle of 110 degrees prior to iliopsoas transfer.

If, at the time of paralysis, the patient is more than two years of age, iliopsoas transfer may be postponed and the stability of the hip followed by taking periodic radiograms. When the coxa valga exceeds 160 degrees and the femoral head starts to subluxate laterally, varization osteotomy is performed. In patients under six years of age, the femoral neck-shaft angle is reduced to 105 degrees; in older patients, the angle is corrected to 125 degrees. Often, if dynamic muscle imbalance persists, valgus deformity will recur with growth. The procedure should be followed in six months to a year with an iliopsoas transfer.

The operative technique of varization osteotomy follows the same principles as those of valgus osteotomy. First, if there is any adduction contracture of the hip, it should be passively stretched and corrected by split Russell traction, gradually bringing the hips into wide abduction. Adductor myotomy of the hip should be avoided whenever possible. The anterolateral surface of the subtrochanteric region of the femur is subperiosteally exposed, as described in Plate 17 on page 402. The line of osteotomy is shaped like a modified dome with a lateral buttress of cortical bone in the proximal segment to lock the upper end of the distal segment while the femoral shaft is adducted. This procedure is the reverse of valgus osteotomy. Rotational malalignment can be corrected at the same time. The author uses Crow pins or threaded Steinmann pins and Roger Anderson apparatus to fix the fragments together. Others may use a bone plate with four screws, a blade plate, or two staples. It is a matter of personal preference and depends upon past experience. Blundell Jones exposes the trochanteric region of the proximal femur posterolaterally with the patient in prone position and corrects the valgus deformity by excision of a wedge of bone with its base medially.[176, 177]

When the hip is completely dislocated, the hip joint capsule is stretched out and lax. Paralytic hip dislocation is very easily reduced. In the beginning the femoral head can be relocated into the acetabulum by simple abduction of the hip. Later on, however, soft-tissue contracture may develop and an initial period of skin or skeletal traction will then be indicated. Prolonged immobilization of the hip following reduction in a spica cast is not recommended. Following removal of the cast, the dislocation will recur. The use of a solid hip spica cast does not correct the etiologic factors; it has the additional disadvantage of causing disuse atrophy of muscles and bone. To stimulate normal growth of the proximal femur, weight-bearing should be restored as soon as possible.

Reefing and repair of the capsule is essential. It is described and illustrated in Plate 14, page 382. An iliopsoas transfer is performed at the same time to restore power of hip abduction and muscle balance about the hip. If the acetabulum is shallow and maldirected, the procedure may be combined with a Salter innominate osteotomy.

Arthrodesis of the Hip. Stabilization of the hip in poliomyelitis may result in increased ability to walk and eliminate the necessity for use of orthotic support. The procedure does have serious disadvantages, however, which should be carefully considered. Sharp et al. reported a series of 16 hip fusions performed in children for paralysis caused by poliomyelitis.[289] There was a high percentage of fractures (eight of the femur and one of the tibia). In addition, there were three cases of pseudarthrosis and one of slipped capital femoral epiphysis. In three patients, the hip was fused and subsequently required correction by femoral osteotomy. One patient had marked limitation of knee motion following prolonged immobilization in the cast; in another, amputation was indicated because of excessive shortening of the limb.

A stiff hip burdens the spine and knee with abnormal stress and strain. Thus, ligamentous instability of the knee, progressive lumbosacral scoliosis, and trunk instability due to extensive paralysis of abdominal muscles are absolute contraindications to hip fusion in poliomyelitis. A functional quadriceps femoris is desirable but not absolutely necessary, provided there is no flexion deformity of the knee, and stability of the foot and ankle is provided by a strong triceps surae muscle or by pantalar arthrodesis in a 15 degree equinus position. Stability of the flail knee is achieved as the body weight falls on the ball of the foot by forcing the heel on the ground and driving the knee into hyperextension (Fig. 5–148).

Hallock, in 1942, 1950, and 1958, reported

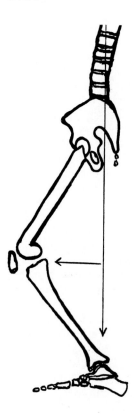
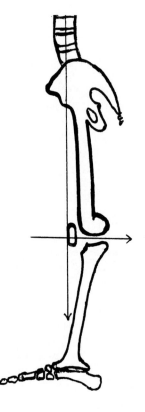

FIGURE 5–148. *The principle of dynamic knee stabilization when the hip is fused and the ankle is fixed in slightly equinus position.*

On the left is shown the collapsible knee when the hip and ankle are flail; on the right, stability of the knee is achieved when the body weight falls on the ball of the foot, forces the heel to the ground, and locks the knee, driving it into hyperextension. (From Sharp, N., Guhl, J. F., Sorenson, R. I., and Voshell, A. F.: Hip fusion in poliomyelitis children. J. Bone Joint Surg., *46-A*:122, 1964. Reprinted by permission.)

an enlarging series of hip fusions being performed in patients with flail lower limbs resulting from poliomyelitis.[135-137] In the beginning, the procedure was employed only in those instances in which there was painful arthritic subluxation or dislocation of the hip, or when previous reconstructive operations such as open reduction, shelf stabilization, or muscle transfers failed. Later, Hallock extended his indications to include several individuals with severe hip lurch from extensive hip muscle paralysis without dislocation. He found his results to be most gratifying: The arthrodesis relieved pain, achieved stability, and decreased the limp. Hallock recommended that the optimum position of fusion be 35 degrees of flexion, neutral rotation, and neutral abduction-adduction position, except in females or when considerable shortening is present, in which cases 10 or 15 degrees of abduction is advised for biologic reasons and to compensate in some measure for the inequality of leg length.[136]

When there is marked shortening of the flail limb, making equalization impractical, hip fusion should not be performed. The age of the patient is another consideration; it is imperative that he be mature enough to understand the disadvantages of a stiff hip. Hip fusion in a paralytic flail lower limb is controversial and should be considered only after thorough and meticulous assessment of the patient.

The Knee

QUADRICEPS FEMORIS PARALYSIS

The quadriceps is commonly affected by poliomyelitis. When there is slight genu recurvatum and adequate strength of the triceps surae and hamstring muscles, the knee is stabilized by locking it in hyperextension (Fig. 5–149). These patients are able to walk quite satisfactorily. During the stance phase of gait, quadriceps weakness is compensated by tilting the trunk and center of gravity of the body forward. The only functional disabilities are difficulty in climbing steps and running. In the presence of knee flexion deformity, however, the knee joint becomes unstable because it cannot be locked in hyperextension.

When the hamstring muscles are normal, they can be transferred anteriorly to the patella and the ligamentum patellae so as to provide extension and stability of the knee. This pro-

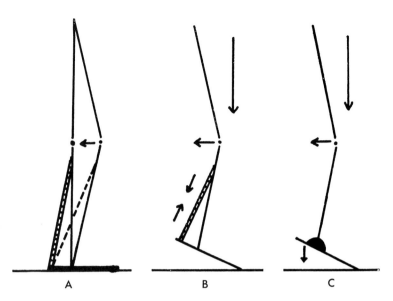

FIGURE 5-149. The effect of
muscle-controlled or fixed talipes
equinus upon extension of the knee.

A. Normal action of soleus as an extensor of the knee with the foot on the ground. B. Soleus as a fixator of the foot in equinus position. C. Rigid equinus foot, showing effect of body weight in extending the knee. (Vertical arrows represent body weight. Horizontal arrows indicate direction of movement of the knee joint.) (From Robins, R. H. C.: The ankle joint in relation to arthrodesis of the foot in poliomyelitis. J. Bone Joint Surg., 41-B:340, 1959; modified from Steindler, after von Baeyer. Reprinted by permission.)

cedure is advised when instability of the knee interferes with ordinary walking or when with such a transfer the patient will be able to dispense with his orthosis. Each case, however, must be individually considered. When the hip flexors are less than fair in motor strength, anterior transfer of hamstrings is absolutely contraindicated. Following surgery, the patient will be unable to clear his limb from the floor; consequently, his disability will be greater. The triceps surae muscle must be at least fair in strength; if not, with loss of all dynamic posterior knee support, marked genu recurvatum will develop. It is preferable to have adequate strength of the gluteus maximus and hip abductor muscles. Prior to tendon transfer, any flexion contracture of the knee and equinus deformity of the ankle should be fully corrected by wedging casts. The mechanics of patellofemoral articulation should be normal. Any significant malalignment of the lower limb, such as marked genu valgum, should also be corrected preoperatively.

A number of muscles have been transferred to restore knee extension power, namely, the biceps femoris, semitendinosus, sartorius, tensor fasciae latae, and adductor longus.*

The transfer of both the biceps femoris and the semitendinosus muscle is the procedure of choice. The strength of the tensor fasciae latae and sartorius muscles is not sufficient to substitute for the quadriceps. In an electromy-

ographic study of 21 patients with paralysis of the lower limb due to poliomyelitis, in whom 39 muscle transfers for quadriceps paralysis were performed, Sutherland, Bost, and Schottstaedt reported the following results: 10 to 14 hamstring transfers achieved conversion from swing phase to stance phase activity (roughly comparable to that of the normal quadriceps femoris); 2 of 11 sartorius transfers and 4 of 12 tensor fasciae latae transfers achieved stance phase activity.[314]

The operative technique of transfer of the biceps femoris and semitendinosus muscles, as described by Crego and Fischer, and Schwartzmann and Crego, is as follows (Fig. 5–150).[73, 285]

The patient is placed supine with a large sandbag under the ipsilateral hip so that he is tilted 45 degrees to the opposite side and the knee to be operated on is in semiflexion. A longitudinal incision is made over the posterolateral aspect of the thigh, starting immediately above the head of the fibula and extending proximally to terminate at the junction of the proximal and middle thirds of the thigh. The subcutaneous tissue and deep fascia are incised in line with the skin incision. The common peroneal nerve, located posteromedial to the biceps tendon, is identified and gently retracted posteriorly with a moist umbilical tape. The biceps femoris tendon is dissected free of its surrounding soft tissues and is retracted anterolaterally. At its point of attachment the lateral collateral ligament to the fibular head is quite adherent to the biceps tendon; great caution is exercised to protect it and not to divide it. Next, the biceps tendon is detached from its

*See References 36, 43, 73, 148, 182, 184, 252, 264, 285, 320.

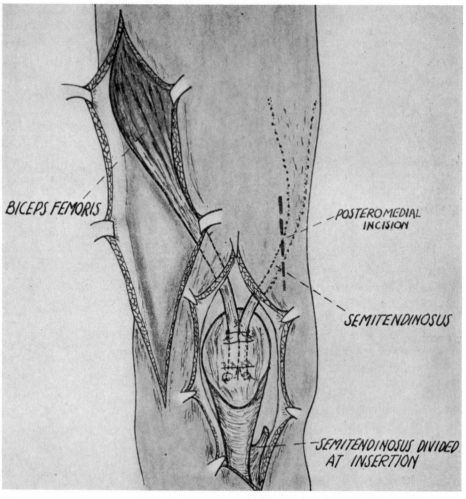

FIGURE 5–150. Transfer of semitendinosus and biceps femoris tendons to patella to restore knee extension.

(From Schwartzmann, J. R., and Crego, C. H.: Hamstring tendon transplantation for the relief of quadriceps femoris paralysis in residual poliomyelitis. J. Bone Joint Surg., 30-A:545, 1948. Reprinted by permission.)

insertion to the head of the fibula. By sharp and dull dissection, the muscle bodies of the short and long heads of the biceps muscle are freed proximally as high as possible, care being taken to preserve their nerve and blood supply. The new direction of the line of pull of the transfer must be as nearly vertical as possible; if they run horizontally, the muscles will pull the patella in a posterior direction.

Next, a transverse incision is made over the anterior aspect of the knee, centering over the distal third of the patella. The subcutaneous tissue and deep fascia are divided. The wound flaps are undermined to expose the patella and patellar tendon. With a large Ober tendon transfer, a wide subcutaneous tunnel is made, extending from the patella incision to the one on the lateral thigh. A 10 to 15 cm. long

segment of the intermuscular septum and the iliotibial band is excised to allow free gliding of the transferred muscle belly.

Next, the sandbag is removed and placed under the opposite hip so that the patient is positioned semilaterally, being turned to the ipsilateral side. A longitudinal incision is made over the posteromedial aspect of the thigh, beginning 3 cm. proximal to the popliteal crease and extending to the junction of the middle and proximal thirds of the thigh. The subcutaneous tissue and deep fascia are divided. The semitendinosus tendon is isolated and through a separate small incision over the anteromedial aspect of the proximal leg, it is detached from its insertion on the tibia. It is easy to identify the semitendinosus tendon in the distal leg wound by pulling on it in the proximal thigh wound; anatomically, at its insertion, the semitendinosus tendon is located posterior to the sartorius tendon and inferior to the tendon of the gracilis. Next, the semitendinosus tendon is delivered into the proximal wound and dissected free to the middle third of the thighs. Through a wide subcutaneous tunnel from the anterior transverse knee incision to the posteromedial thigh incision, the semitendinosus tendon is rerouted and delivered into the prepatellar area. Again, the deep fascia is widely incised to avoid angulation and to permit free gliding of the semitendinosus tendon.

Next, the prepatellar bursa is reflected and retracted to one side and an I-shaped incision is made through the quadriceps tendon and periosteum over the anterior surface of the patella. These tissues are stripped and reflected medially and laterally. With a %4-inch drill two oblique longitudinal tunnels are made through the patella, starting at the superolateral and superomedial poles of the patella and emerging at each side of the patellar tendon. The tunnels are enlarged with progressively increasing sizes of hand drills and curets. One should be cautious so that the articular surface of the patella is not damaged.

With braided silk whip sutures on their ends, the biceps femoris tendon and the semitendinosus tendon are each pulled through their respective tunnels in the patella and sutured to the patellar tendon under tension. Additional interrupted sutures are placed proximally and distally, fixing the biceps and semitendinosus tendons to the rectus femoris and patellar tendons. The soft tissues are sutured over the anterior aspect of the patella and the wounds are closed. A long leg cast is applied, which holds the knee in neutral position, but not in hyperextension.

Meticulous postoperative care is very important to obtain a satisfactory result. Tension on the transferred hamstring is prevented by avoiding flexion of the hip. The patient is kept supine in bed for a period of three weeks, and it should be strongly emphasized to personnel that he is not to sit.

Functional training of the transfer is begun three to five days following surgery, or as soon as the patient is comfortable. The patient is placed on his side to eliminate the force of gravity. The knee and hip are slightly flexed, and the patient is asked to extend his hip and knee. Active contraction of hamstrings as knee extensors is initiated by having them execute their former action of hip extension. Then active guided knee extension exercises are performed

from starting positions of greater knee flexion and decreasing hip flexion; the patient should soon be encouraged to divorce the two movements of knee and hip extension. The active exercise of knee extension is performed with the hip in the partially flexed position of the normal pattern of locomotion without, however, extending the hip.

The function of the antagonist muscles should not be ignored. Active knee flexion exercises are carried out (through a limited range initially), making sure that the transferred muscle is not used in both extensor and flexor functions.

As soon as the transferred muscle is fair minus in motor strength, the patient, while still supine in bed, is asked to go slowly through the motions of walking: namely, ankle-foot dorsiflexion and hip flexion, followed by knee extension (using the transfer), hip extension, and ankle plantar flexion. The same exercises are performed standing, first in parallel bars, and then in crutches. During the stance phase, hyperextension of the knee should be avoided. A night bivalved cast is worn for 8 to 12 months to prevent stretching of the transferred muscles. Orthotic devices to support the knee are not usually necessary, unless their use is indicated for control of the foot and ankle.

Genu recurvatum is a not infrequent complication; it occurs in 10 to 20 per cent of the reported cases, being a natural consequence of an operation in which the hamstring muscles that normally provide dynamic support to the knee posteriorly are removed and transferred anteriorly. Other contributory factors in its pathogenesis are (1) pes equinus, (2) selection of patients with inadequate (less than fair) strength in the triceps surae muscle, (3) immobilization of the knee in hyperextension in the postoperative period, (4) lack of an adequate and diligent postoperative exercise regimen with the resultant failure to develop active knee flexion against gravity, and (5) improper use of orthotic support following surgery. The development of genu recurvatum can be minimized if the preceding combination of factors is circumvented.

Lateral instability of the knee often results from inadvertent operative division of the tibial or fibular collateral ligaments while detaching the semitendinosus and biceps tendons from their insertion.

Lateral dislocation of the patella commonly occurs when the biceps femoris alone is transferred; this complication can be prevented by transfer of both the biceps and the semitendinosus muscles.

Failure of transfer may be due to denervation of the muscles during proximal dissection, to inadequate postoperative training, or to binding down of the transfer by adhesions in sharp angular pathways to the patella.

FLEXION DEFORMITY OF THE KNEE

Contracture of the iliotibial band due to static forces of malposture of a flail lower limb will cause flexion contracture of the knee along with flexion–abduction–external rotation deformity of the hip, genu valgum, and external tibial torsion. This deformity is preventable, and if minimal, it can be corrected by passive exercises and wedging casts.[72, 142] When it is marked, Ober-Yount open surgical release of the contracted iliotibial band will be required.

Flexion contracture of the knee may also result from a dynamic imbalance between the quadriceps femoris and hamstring muscles (Fig. 5–151). As stated previously, when there is flexion deformity of the knee, paralysis of the quadriceps muscle cannot be compensated by locking the knee in hyperextension, and the knee will then be unstable. Thus it is imperative that knee flexion deformity be fully corrected.

It is important to understand the pathomechanics of a knee that has become fixed in flexion. In the normal knee, the last 5 degrees of extension are accompanied by medial rotation of the femur on the tibia—a movement that tightens the collateral ligaments and oblique posterior ligament, thus locking the knee in extension. As the axis of knee motion does not pass through the joint line, but through the upper attachments of the collateral ligaments, the tibial plateau has to glide forward on the femoral condyles. In fixed flexion deformity of the knee this normal gliding movement does not take place; instead, a simple rocking motion occurs. When the knee is forced into extension, the tibia subluxates posteriorly, and the knee joint becomes incongruous and painful. In correction of fixed flexion deformity of the knee, it is important to preserve joint congruity by pulling the tibial plateau forward on the femoral condyles. This is accomplished by skeletal traction through a pin in the proximal tibia, following section of the contracted iliotibial band and patellar retinacular expansions that are usually adherent to the joint capsule and that obliterate the lateral recesses. Posterior capsulotomy of the knee is usually not required.

Supracondylar osteotomy may be indicated in cases in which fixed flexion deformity is very marked and there are structural bony changes in the femoral condyles. Osteotomy is also

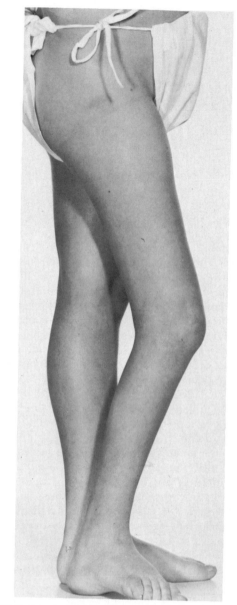

FIGURE 5–151. Flexion deformity of the right knee in poliomyelitis.

Dynamic imbalance between quadriceps femoris and hamstring muscles caused the deformity. Note also the calcaneovalgus deformity of the right foot.

indicated to align the lower limb when significant genu valgum persists following correction of soft-tissue contracture.[132]

GENU RECURVATUM

Hyperextension of the knee in poliomyelitis may develop as a result of stretching of the soft tissues in the back of the knee or may be due to structural bone changes with depression and

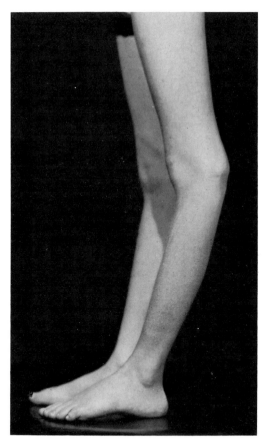

FIGURE 5-152. *Genu recurvatum in a patient with chronic poliomyelitis.*

to the epiphyseal plate of the upper end of the tibia, thus avoiding any injury to the epiphyseal plate. The tendons are firmly anchored with the knee in 30 degrees of flexion. An above-knee cast is worn for six weeks. The knee is then further protected for three months in an above-knee orthosis that limits extension of the knee at 5 degrees less than neutral. In a long-term follow-up note, Heyman reported complete and lasting correction in five cases, with extension of the knee limited to a point just short of neutral. In the experience of the author, however, under the forces of body weight, the tendons and shortened soft tissues eventually become stretched and the deformity recurs. The author recommends the Heyman tenodesis operation for genu recurvatum in a patient under ten years of age in whom osseous structural changes in the tibial plateau have not yet taken place. To prevent deformity from recurring until skeletal growth has been completed, the patient sleeps in a night bivalved cast, which holds the knee in 40 degrees of flexion. For walking, the knee is held in 5 to 10 degrees of flexion in an above-knee orthosis.

The second type of genu recurvatum develops when there is equinus deformity of the ankle with normal triceps surae and hamstring muscles but a weak quadriceps femoris muscle. The paralyzed quadriceps muscle is unable to lock the knee in neutral extension, and on heel-strike the proximal end of the tibia is forced into hyperextension with limited dorsiflexion of the ankle. With continued walking and stresses of weight-bearing, the anterior portion of the tibial plateau becomes depressed and is tilted inferiorly. The bony deformity is corrected either by open-up wedge osteotomy or by close-up wedge osteotomy of the proximal tibia.[170, 312] It is usually performed at the subcondylar level distal to the proximal tibial tubercle. It is best to delay surgery until completion of skeletal growth. The technique described by Irwin is simple and very satisfactory (Fig. 5-153 A and B).[170] A modified dome-shaped osteotomy will achieve the same result (Fig. 5-153 C and D).

The author, however, prefers an open-up wedge osteotomy (Fig. 5-153 E and F). The operative technique is as follows:

A curved transverse incision is made across the anterior aspect of the leg, centering 1.5 cm. distal to the proximal tibial tubercle. The lateral limb of the incision is continued proximally to terminate immediately superior and posterior to the upper end of the fibula. Subcutaneous tissue and fasciae are divided in line with the skin incision, and the wound flaps are mobilized

downward sloping of the anterior portion of the tibial plateau.

The first type occurs when there is extensive paralysis of the lower limb with marked weakness of the hamstrings, triceps surae, and quadriceps femoris muscles (Fig. 5-152). There is often calcaneus deformity of the foot. With continued weight-bearing, the hamstring and triceps surae muscles and the capsule and ligaments in the posterior aspect of the knee will stretch and elongate. The degree of genu recurvatum rapidly increases with loss of the support normally provided by the muscles and ligaments. Functional disability is usually great; an above-knee orthosis with a posterior knee strap is frequently required to support the knee. Heyman recommends the use of peroneal tendons to construct posterior check ligaments to prevent hyperextension of the knee.[152-154] When there is associated excessive lateral instability of the knee, the collateral ligaments are also reinforced. The tendons are passed through drill holes that are superior to the epiphyseal plate at the lower end of the femur, and interior

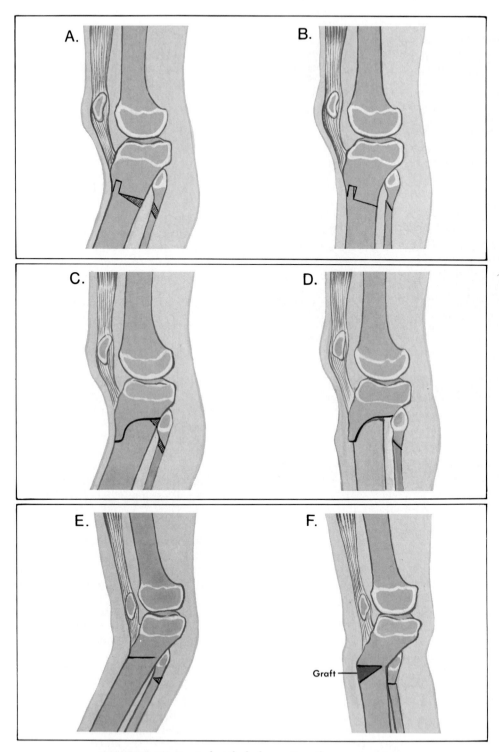

FIGURE 5–153. Surgical method of correction of genu recurvatum.

A and **B.** Irwin technique. **C** and **D.** Modified dome osteotomy. **E** and **F.** Open-up wedge osteotomy.

and retracted. First, the neck and 2 cm. of the proximal shaft of the fibula are extraperiosteally exposed. Meticulous attention must be paid to avoiding damage to the common peroneal nerve and proximal fibular epiphyseal plate (if open). With drill holes and a sharp thin osteotome, a simple short oblique osteotomy of the proximal shaft of the fibula is performed. Often it is desirable to excise a wedge of bone from the proximal fibula with its base posteriorly.

Next, a T-shaped incision is made in the periosteum over the anteromedial surface of the proximal tibia. The growing apophysis of the proximal tibial tubercle and the upper epiphyseal plate of the tibia should not be disturbed by stripping the periosteum. The level of osteotomy is immediately distal to the proximal tibial tubercle; its line is marked with a starter, and then drill holes are made through the anteromedial and lateral cortices, leaving the posterior cortex of the tibia intact.

Next, three large threaded Steinmann pins are chosen and their fit in the Roger Anderson apparatus is double-checked. Starting from the medial side, the first threaded Steinmann pin is placed transversely through the distal portion of the proximal fragment. The pin should just engage in the lateral cortex of the tibia (avoiding injury to the common peroneal nerve), and it should be more posterior in position away from the proximal tibial tubercle. The second and third Steinmann pins are placed transversely through the distal fragment of the tibia 5 and 10 cm., respectively, distal to the osteotomy site. Then the tibia is divided with an osteotome, leaving the posterior cortex intact. By keeping the proximal tibial fragment in maximal hyperextension by forward pull on the first Steinmann pin and by manual pressure on the anterior surface of the knee and distal thigh, the leg and the distal segment of the tibia are forced posteriorly, creating a wedge-shaped defect at the osteotomy site with its base anteriorly. A lamina spreader may be used effectively to open up the wedge.

Osteotomes of different widths are placed into the osteotomy site to determine the size of the iliac bone graft wedges, which are taken in routine manner with both cortices intact. It is best to take radiograms with the proper osteotome placed at the osteotomy site to double-check the correction. The degree of angulation at the osteotomy site should be approximately 10 degrees greater than that of the genu recurvatum, and the longitudinal axis of the distal fragment of the tibia should be parallel with that of the femur. The proximal tibial fragment should be in hyperextension.

Next, two iliac bone graft wedges are placed at the osteotomy site (one is medial, the other lateral to the tibial crest); these are locked in place with an impactor. The surrounding spaces are firmly packed with bone graft chips. The lateral bars of the Roger Anderson apparatus are tightened to provide additional stability to the osteotomy site. The correction obtained is then rechecked with radiograms. The wound is closed in the usual manner. The Roger Anderson apparatus is padded with petrolatum gauze in order to prevent its incorporation in the cast. An above-knee cast is applied with the knee in extension.

FLAIL KNEE

A flail knee is unstable (Fig. 5–154). For weight-bearing it requires the support of an above-knee orthosis with a drop-lock knee. With such an orthosis, the patient is able to flex his knee while sitting. Arthrodesis of the knee should not be performed in children; it is best postponed until adult life, when the patient is mature enough to understand and assess the advantages and disadvantages of a fused stiff knee. In unilateral involvement the author does not recommend arthrodesis of the knee, especially if there is associated muscle weakness of the hip and foot. When both lower limbs are paralyzed, however, one limb can be supported in an above-knee orthosis and the other knee stabilized by fusion, provided the hip has normal musculature and the foot is fixed in slightly equinus posture. For technical details of arthrodesis of the knee, the reader is referred to the References.[66, 228]

SPECIFIC DEFORMITIES OF THE FOOT AND ANKLE

Paralysis of the muscles acting on the foot may result in various deformities and functional disability of the foot, depending upon the particular muscle or muscles involved and the strength of the remaining musculature.

The stability of the foot is dependent on several factors: the contour of the bones and the articular surfaces, the integrity of the ligamentous and capsular support, and the motor strength of the muscles.

The combined mobility of the foot and ankle is equal to that of a universal joint. Motions of the ankle, subtalar, and midtarsal joints are related to each other. In inversion of the hindfoot, for example, the os calcis is displaced forward, producing adduction and inversion of the forefoot; when the hindfoot is everted, the os calcis moves backward and the forefoot is abducted and everted. When the ankle joint is

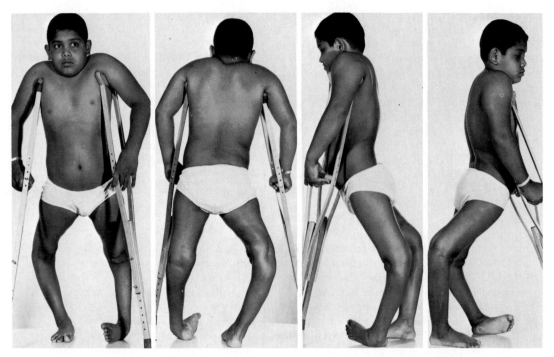

FIGURE 5–154. Bilateral unstable flail knees in a patient with chronic poliomyelitis.

plantar flexed, the hindfoot inverts, whereas in dorsiflexion of the ankle, the hindfoot everts. The foot is most stable in eversion and dorsiflexion and least stable in equinus position and inversion.

The muscles that produce *plantar flexion* are the gastrocnemius-soleus, flexor hallucis longus, flexor digitorum longus, peroneus longus, peroneus brevis, and posterior tibial. *Dorsiflexor muscles* are the anterior tibial, extensor hallucis longus, extensor digitorum communis, and peroneus tertius. The muscles that produce *inversion* are the posterior tibial, flexor hallucis longus, and anterior tibial; the *evertors* of the foot are the peroneus brevis, peroneus tertius, extensor digitorum communis, and extensor hallucis longus. The muscles that plantar flex the ankle and foot provide the force for forward propulsion of the body during locomotion. The dorsiflexor muscle group clears the foot during the swing phase of gait.

About two thirds of the total musculature of the leg is constituted by the triceps surae—one of the strongest muscles in the body. It acts on the foot as a first-class lever with the ankle joint as a fulcrum. The working capacity of the triceps surae is 6.5 kg.-m., whereas that of the dorsiflexors of the ankle joint is only 1.4 kg.-m., or a relative ratio of 4:1. This gross discrepancy of muscle mass betwen the plantar flexors and

dorsiflexors of the ankle is the result of developmental and mechanical factors. The strength of the calf muscles is a necessary antigravitational force against the elevated center of gravity of the body in the upright posture. Also, since the center of gravity of the human body falls anterior to the ankle joint, there is a strong rotatory component in ankle dorsiflexion that the triceps surae must counteract. The muscles that provide lateral stability to the foot in plantar flexion are the posterior tibial and peroneals, whereas in dorsiflexion it is provided by the action of the anterior tibial and extensor digitorum communis.

Muscle imbalance will produce progressive deformity. This is flexible in the beginning, but with skeletal growth, fixed soft-tissue and structural osseous deformity will develop. The deformities of the foot and loss of function produced by muscle imbalance are predictable. The *dynamic imbalance* from paralysis of the major muscle groups, the resultant deformity, and its treatment are presented in Table 5–13.

Paralysis of Peroneal Muscles. When the peroneus longus and brevis muscles are paralyzed, the os calcis is pulled into inversion by the strong posterior tibial muscle. The forefoot adducts following inversion of the hindfoot and also because of the unopposed action of the anterior tibial muscle. Gradually, a varus defor-

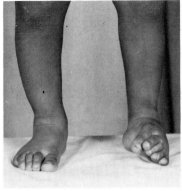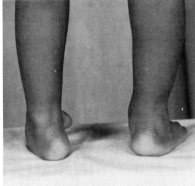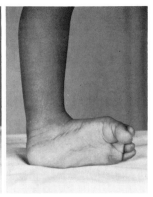

FIGURE 5–155. Paralytic pes varus.

The deformity is the result of paralysis of the peroneus longus and brevis muscles. The hindfoot is inverted by the pull of the strong posterior tibial muscle, and the forefoot is adducted and inverted by the unopposed action of the anterior tibial muscle. Note that the first metatarsal is dorsiflexed and a dorsal bunion is produced.

mity of the foot is produced (Fig. 5–155). Normally, the peroneus longus depresses the first metatarsal and the anterior tibial raises it. When the peroneus longus muscle is paralyzed, the first metatarsal becomes dorsiflexed by the unopposed action of the anterior tibial, and a dorsal bunion will result. The opposing actions of the peroneus longus and anterior tibial muscles on the first metatarsal should always be considered whenever there is a dynamic imbalance between the two.

Treatment consists of lateral transfer of the anterior tibial to the base of the second metatarsal bone. Lateral stability of the foot will then be adequate, and arthrodesis is not required.

Paralysis of Peroneals, Extensor Digitorum Longus, and Extensor Hallucis Longus. The deformity resulting from paralysis of these muscles will be moderately varus and somewhat equinus. Dynamic balance of the foot is restored by lateral transfer of the anterior tibial muscle to the base of the third metatarsal bone. Pes valgus may result if the anterior tibial is transferred to the fourth or fifth metatarsal bone. The operative technique of lateral transfer of the anterior tibial tendon is as follows:

A longitudinal incision is made over the medial aspect of the foot; it begins at the base of the first metatarsal bone and extends proximally parallel to the course of the anterior tibial tendon for a distance of 3 cm. The anterior tibial tendon is detached from its insertion into the base of the first metatarsal bone and the medial and under surface of the first cuneiform bone. A Mersilene or Dacron whip suture is inserted into the distal end of the tendon. By sharp dissection, the tendon is mobilized over

the dorsum of the foot. The dorsalis pedis artery, lying between the tendon of the extensor hallucis longus and the first tendon of the extensor digitorum longus, should not be divided.

Then a second 8- to 10-cm. longitudinal incision is made over the anterior tibial compartment in the distal third of the leg beginning at the upper border of the transverse crural ligament. The subcutaneous tissue and deep fascia are divided. The anterior tibial tendon is located immediately on the tibia. The anterior tibial vessels lie between the anterior tibial and extensor hallucis longus muscles in the middle third of the leg. At the ankle, the extensor hallucis longus tendon crosses the anterior tibial vessels from the lateral to the medial side. The deep peroneal nerve is located on the lateral side of the anterior tibial vessels in the upper third of the leg, in front of the artery in the middle third, and then again lateral in the distal third. Caution should be exercised in order not to injure the deep peroneal nerve and the anterior tibial vessels. The anterior tibial sheath is divided and by gentle traction, using the two-hand technique, the tendon is delivered into the proximal wound. Transfer of the anterior tibial tendon on the dorsum of the foot distal to the transverse crural ligament from the medial to the lateral side will not correct the varus action of the muscle.

Next, an incision 3 cm. long is made over the dorsum of the foot with its center over the base of the third metatarsal bone. With an Ober tendon passer, the anterior tibial tendon is delivered into the dorsum of the foot, passing deep to the transverse crural ligament to pro-

Table 5–13. *Tendon Transfers for Paralytic Deformities of the Foot and Ankle*

Dynamic Imbalance		Deformity of Foot	Tendon Transfer	Remarks
Paralyzed or Weak	*Normal or Strong*			

Peroneus longus
Peroneus brevis
	Anterior tibial
	Extensor hallucis
	  longus
	Extensor digit.
	  communis
	Posterior tibial
	Gastrocnemius-
	  soleus
	Flexor hallucis longus
	Flexor digit. longus
		Varus
		
		Dorsal bunion (first
		  metatarsal
		  dorsiflexed because
		  of unopposed action
		  or anterior tibial)
			Lateral transfer of
			  anterior tibial to
			  base of second
			  metatarsal
				Perform transfer before fixed deformity
				  develops
				Lateral stability will be retained
				Do not transfer more lateral than second
				  metatarsal in presence of strong extensor
				  digit. communis (will cause pes valgus)

Peroneus longus
Peroneus brevis
Extensor digit.
  communis
Extensor hallucis
  longus
	Anterior tibial
	Posterior tibial
	Gastrocnemius-
	  soleus
	Flexor hallucis longus
	Flexor digit. longus
		Varus, some equinus	Lateral transfer of
			  anterior tibial to
			  base of third
			  metatarsal
				Do not transfer further lateral than base of
				  third metatarsal (will cause pes valgus)

Peroneus longus
Peroneus brevis
Extensor digit.
  communis
Extensor hallucis
  longus
Anterior tibial
	Posterior tibial
	Gastrocnemius-
	  soleus
	Flexor hallucis longus
	Flexor digit. longus
		Equinovarus	Anterior transfer of
			  posterior tibial
			  tendon through
			  interosseous space
			  to base of third
			  metatarsal
				Postoperatively, equinovarus deformity
				  should be fully corrected by stretching
				  cast or soft-tissue surgery
				May consider reinforcing posterior tibial
				  transfer by adding flexor hallucis longus
				  or flexor digit. longus to anterior transfer
				  through interosseous space; anterior
				  tenodesis to prevent dropping down of
				  foot is another choice
				Postoperatively, support transfer by
				  dorsiflexion-assist below-knee orthosis

Anterior tibial	*Peroneus longus*
	Peroneus brevis
	Extensor hallucis
	  longus
	Extensor digit.
	  communis
	Gastrocnemius-
	  soleus
	Posterior tibial
	Flexor hallucis longus
	Flexor digit. longus
		Equinovalgus
		
		Cock-up deformity of
		  toes (overactivity of
		  toe extensors
		  displaces proximal
		  phalanges of toes
		  into hyperextension
		  and depresses
		  metatarsal heads)
		Occasionally cavovarus
		  deformity of foot
		  results (unopposed
		  peroneus longus acts
		  as depressor of first
		  metatarsal)
			Anterior transfer of
			  peroneus longus to
			  base of second
			  metatarsal (suture
			  peroneus brevis to
			  distal stump of
			  peroneus longus)
				Do not attach peroneus longus to first
				  metatarsal (will displace it upward and
				  cause dorsal bunion)
				Transfer long toe extensors to heads of
				  metatarsals if cock-up deformity of toes
				  is present
				If both peroneals are transferred, lateral
				  instability of foot will develop,
				  necessitating stabilization by subtalar
				  extraarticular or triple arthrodesis

Gastrocnemius-
  soleus (motor
  strength zero or
  trace)
	Peroneus longus
	Peroneus brevis
	Flexor hallucis longus
	Posterior tibial
	
	Flexor digit. longus
	Anterior tibial
	Extensor hallucis
	  longus
	Extensor digit.
	  communis
		Calcaneus or
		  calcaneocavus
			Posterior transfer (to
			  os calcis) of both
			  peroneals,
			  posterior tibial,
			  and flexor hallucis
			  longus
				Caution—Prevent development of dorsal
				  bunion by lateral transfer of anterior
				  tibial to base of second metatarsal within
				  a year
				In adolescent patient with fixed calcaneus
				  deformity, before tendon transfers,
				  perform triple arthrodesis with posterior
				  shift of os calcis to correct bony
				  deformity
				In young child, calcaneus deformity will
				  correct with subsequent growth;
				  however, subtalar extra-articular
				  arthrodesis may be required for lateral
				  stability

Gastrocnemius-
  soleus (motor
  strength poor)
	As above	Calcaneus or
		  calcaneocavus
			Posterior transfer (to
			  os calcis) of
			  posterior tibial and
			  peroneus longus
				Suture distal stump of peroneus longus to
				  peroneus brevis
				Watch closely for possible development of
				  dorsal bunion; lateral transfer of anterior
				  tibial to base of second metatarsal may
				  be indicated

Table 5–13. *Tendon Transfers for Paralytic Deformities of the Foot and Ankle* Continued

Dynamic Imbalance				
Paralyzed or Weak	*Normal or Strong*	*Deformity of Foot*	*Tendon Transfer*	*Remarks*
Gastrocnemius-soleus Posterior tibial Peroneus longus Peroneus brevis	*Anterior tibial* *Flexor hallucis longus* Extensor hallucis longus Extensor digit. communis Flexor digit. longus	Calcaneovarus	Posterior transfer (to os calcis) of anterior tibial and flexor hallucis longus	Suture distal stump of flexor hallucis longus to flexor hallucis brevis Interphalangeal joint fusion of great toe may be necessary
Anterior tibial Gastrocnemius-soleus	*Peroneus longus* *Peroneus brevis* *Posterior tibial* Flexor hallucis longus Flexor digit. longus Extensor hallucis longus Extensor digit. longus	Calcaneovarus	Posterior transfer (to os calcis) of both peroneals and posterior tibial	Perform triple arthrodesis in adolescence to provide lateral stability to hindfoot
Gastrocnemius-soleus Posterior tibial Peroneus longus Peroneus brevis Flexor hallucis longus Flexor digit. longus	*Anterior tibial* Extensor hallucis longus Extensor digit. communis	Calcaneovarus	Posterior transfer (to os calcis) of anterior tibial	Protect transfer with plantar flexion–assist orthosis until skeletal maturity Consider tendo Achillis tenodesis In adolescence, if adequate function exists in transferred anterior tibial, foot is stabilized by triple arthrodesis If anterior tibial function is inadequate, Chuinard type ankle fusion is performed (will provide stability and gait will improve considerably)
Gastrocnemius-soleus Posterior tibial Peroneus longus Peroneus brevis Flexor hallucis longus Flexor digit. longus Anterior tibial	Extensor hallucis longus Extensor digit. communis	Calcaneovalgus (minimal)	Ankle fusion (Chuinard type)	Stability and muscle control of knee should be adequate Full knee extension and functioning hamstrings are prerequisite
Flail ankle and foot (all muscles paralyzed)	None except short toe flexors and intrinsic muscles of foot	Flexion of toes and metatarsus varus Hindfoot neutral or valgus (may be in inversion due to contracture of plantar fascia)	Pantalar arthrodesis Resect motor branches of plantar nerves	As above
Anterior tibial Extensor hallucis longus Extensor digit. communis Peroneus longus Peroneus brevis Posterior tibial	Gastrocnemius-soleus Flexor digit. longus Flexor hallucis longus	Equinus	Anterior transfer of flexor digit. longus and flexor hallucis through interosseous space Anterior tenodesis	Do not lengthen tendo Achillis (will produce calcaneus deformity) Disability is little (patient must lift leg to clear toes) Stretch triceps surae, use night support to prevent fixed equinus deformity

duce straight dorsiflexion. It is securely fixed to the base of the third metatarsal bone with the ankle joint in neutral position or dorsiflexed 5 degrees. The muscle should be under physiologic tension. The wounds are closed in routine fashion and a long leg cast is applied, with the ankle in 5 degrees of dorsiflexion and the knee in 45 degrees of flexion.

Paralysis of Anterior Tibial Muscle. Dorsiflexor and inversion power of the foot is lost when the anterior tibial muscle is paralyzed, and equinovalgus deformity of the foot will

develop (Fig. 5–156). The toe extensors are overactive in an attempt to substitute for the action of the anterior tibial in dorsiflexion of the ankle. The proximal phalanges of the toes become hyperextended and depress the metatarsal heads, causing cock-up deformity of the toes. Equinus deformity of the ankle gradually results from contracture of the triceps surae. Occasionally cavovarus deformity of the foot may result because of the action of the peroneus longus muscle, which acts as a depressor of the first metatarsal. On active dorsiflexion of the ankle,

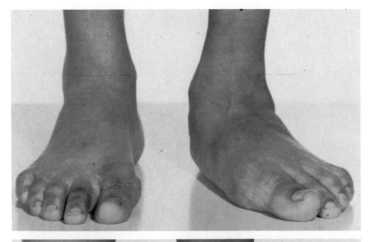

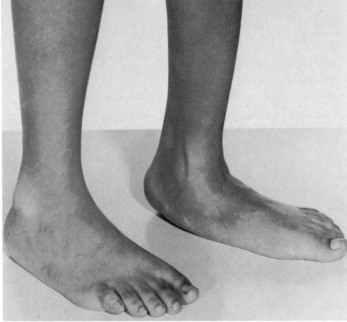

FIGURE 5-156. Equinovalgus deformity of the foot as a result of paralysis of the anterior tibial muscle.

the forefoot is everted, but on weight-bearing it goes into inversion to permit horizontal contact of all metatarsal heads with the ground. The heel will invert following the forefoot inversion.

During the convalescent phase of poliomyelitis, aggressive measures should be taken to retain passive range of dorsiflexion of the ankle joint. Passive heel cord stretching exercises are performed every day. At night, a bivalved cast or a plastic splint is used to hold the ankle in neutral position, and during the day an ankle-foot dorsiflexion-assist orthosis supports the ankle and foot.

If proper treatment is neglected, fixed equinus deformity may develop. In that event, the heel cord should not be lengthened, and every effort should be made to retain full function of the triceps surae muscle. Range of dorsiflexion of the ankle may be obtained with a wedging cast or a below-knee walking cast with an anterior heel. In severe fixed equinus deformity, posterior capsulotomy of the ankle and subtalar joints is performed and the heel cord is stretched with skeletal traction through a threaded Steinmann pin in the os calcis. Functional disability is great following loss of plantar flexion power.

Dorsiflexion power of the ankle is restored by anterior transfer of the peroneus longus tendon to the base of the second metatarsal bone. The peroneus brevis is sutured to the distal stump of the peroneus longus. The operative technique and postoperative care for

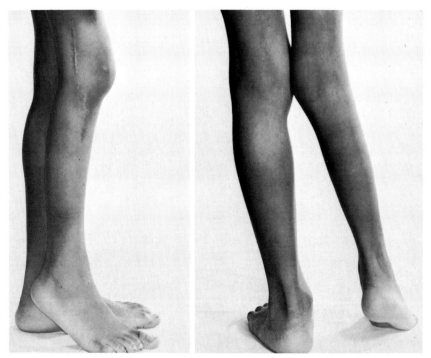

FIGURE 5-157. *Equinovarus deformity of right ankle and foot caused by unopposed action of the triceps surae and posterior tibial muscles.*

anterior transfer of the peroneus longus are described and illustrated in Appendix Plate A, following p. 2182. The peroneus longus tendon should not be attached to the base of the first metatarsal, since it will displace the bone upward and cause a dorsal bunion. If there is a cock-up deformity of the toes, the long toe extensors are transferred to the heads of the metatarsals. If both peroneals are transferred, lateral instability of the foot develops, requiring stabilization of the hindfoot by extra-articular subtalar arthrodesis or triple arthrodesis.

Paralysis of Anterior Tibial, Toe Extensors, and Peroneals. Equinovarus deformity of the foot will develop from the unopposed action of the posterior tibial and triceps surae muscles (Fig. 5-157). Treatment consists of anterior transfer of the posterior tibial tendon through the interosseous space to the base of the third metatarsal or second cuneiform (Appendix Plate B, following p. 2182). Preoperatively, equinovarus deformity should be fully corrected by a stretching cast. Soft-tissue release may be indicated for correction of the fixed pes varus.

The flexor digitorum longus or flexor hallucis longus may be transferred anteriorly through the interosseous route to reinforce the strength of dorsiflexion power of the posterior tibial transfer. Anterior tenodesis is another method of preventing the foot from dropping down in

plantar flexion. In the postoperative period, the anterior transfer and tenodesis should be supported in an ankle-foot dynamic dorsiflexion-assist orthosis during the day and a bivalved cast or plastic splint at night.

Paralysis of Triceps Surae Muscle. When the gastrocnemius and soleus muscles are weak or paralyzed, the patient walks with a calcaneus limp, i.e., there is weakness or lack of push-off. The tibia is displaced posteriorly on the talus by the forward thrust of the trunk, and the foot is forced into excessive dorsiflexion at the ankle joint.

The tendo Achillis inserts into the posterior aspect of the apophysis of the os calcis. Normally, the force exerted by the triceps surae muscle elevates the heel, depresses the anterior end of the os calcis, and pushes the body forward. The longitudinal arch is flattened as the head of the talus plantar flexes with the anterior end of the os calcis. In paralysis of the gastrocnemius and soleus muscles, the head of the talus and anterior end of the os calcis are displaced upward to a more vertical position. This results in the disappearance of the normal prominence of the heel and an increase in the range of dorsiflexion of the ankle (Fig. 5-158). When the accessory plantar flexor muscles (i.e., the posterior tibial, flexor hallucis longus, flexor digitorum longus, and peroneals) are strong,

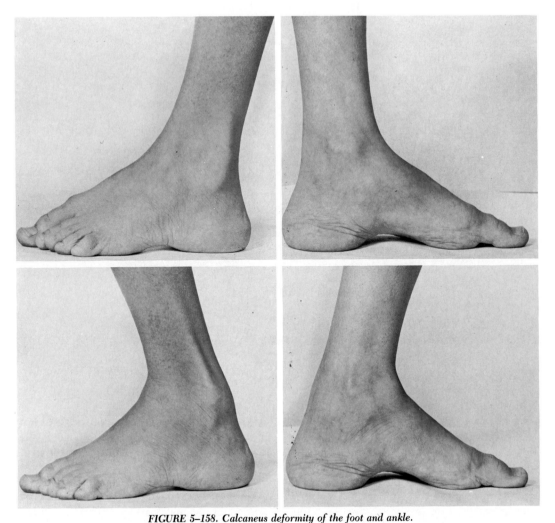

FIGURE 5–158. *Calcaneus deformity of the foot and ankle.*

Note the posterior shift of the tibia over the talus during push-off.

the forefoot is forced into equinus position, producing a calcaneocavus deformity. The foot is shortened by plantar flexion of the metatarsals and by rotation of the os calcis into a vertical position. Soon the plantar fascia and short flexors of the toes will contract and act as a bowstring, pulling together the metatarsal heads and the os calcis, and increasing the cavus deformity (Fig. 5–159). The calcaneocavus deformity progressively increases with every step. With paralysis of the triceps surae, growth of the apophysis of the os calcis is retarded. This is particularly important in a young child in whom, following an early and successful posterior tendon transfer to the os calcis, the calcaneus deformity of the heel may be restored to normal.

As stated previously, the triceps surae muscle is the strongest muscle of the foot. Therefore, it is desirable to transfer three or four muscles

posteriorly to the os calcis depending upon their availability and the degree of weakness of the triceps surae. Plantar flexion at the ankle is more important functionally than dorsiflexion.

When the motor strength of the triceps surae muscle is zero, both peroneus longus and brevis, the posterior tibial, and the flexor hallucis longus are transferred to the os calcis. The anterior tibial is transferred laterally to the base of the second metatarsal within a year to prevent formation of a dorsal bunion. In adolescents with fixed calcaneus deformity, the hindfoot is stabilized by triple arthrodesis, the bony deformity is corrected, and the os calcis is shifted posteriorly. In a young child, calcaneus deformity will be corrected by subsequent growth if the posterior transfer is successful; however, a subtalar extra-articular arthrodesis may be required later for lateral stability.

Only the peroneus longus and posterior tibial

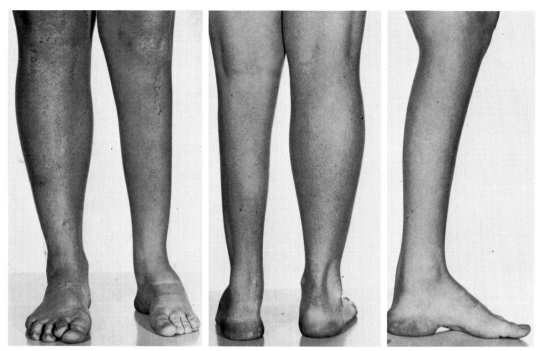

FIGURE 5-159. Calcaneocavus deformity of the left foot and ankle.

muscles are transferred when the gastrocne-mius-soleus muscles are poor in motor strength. The distal stump of the peroneus longus is sutured to the peroneus brevis. If a dorsal bunion tends to develop, lateral transfer of the anterior tibial to the base of the second meta-tarsal may again be indicated.

When the posterior tibial and peroneal mus-cles are paralyzed along with the triceps surae, the muscles available for posterior transfer are the anterior tibial and flexor hallucis longus. The flexor digitorum longus may be added if necessary. The interphalangeal joints, particu-larly that of the great toe, are fused.

When the anterior tibial muscle is paralyzed with the triceps surae, posterior transfer of both peroneals and the posterior tibial is performed; lateral stability of the hindfoot is provided by triple arthrodesis.

The anterior tibial muscle is transferred to the os calcis when all the plantar flexor muscles are paralyzed. The posterior transfer is pro-tected with a plantar flexion–assist ankle-foot orthosis until skeletal maturity. Tendo Achillis tenodesis may be performed to provide poste-rior stability to the ankle joint. In adolescence, if plantar flexion function of the transferred anterior tibial is adequate, the hindfoot is sta-bilized by triple arthrodesis.

When the anterior tibial function is inade-quate, Chuinard-type ankle fusion is per-

formed. When only the toe extensors are func-tioning, there will be no muscles available for posterior transfer. An ankle fusion is performed, provided there is adequate stability and muscle control of the knee.

The operative technique and postoperative care for posterior tendon transfer to the os calcis are presented in Plate 73.

Dorsal bunion is characterized by dorsiflexion of the first metatarsal and plantar flexion of the great toe (Fig. 5–160). It is caused by muscle imbalance—weakness or absence of the pero-neus longus muscle (plantar flexor of the first metatarsal) against normal strength of the an-terior tibial muscle (dorsiflexor of the first meta-tarsal) or flexor hallucis brevis and longus. There are two types of dorsal bunion—one in which there is primary dorsiflexion of the first metatarsal and secondary plantar flexion of the hallux, and another in which there is primary plantar flexion of the hallux with resultant up-ward displacement of the metatarsal head. The author has treated dorsal bunion successfully by open-up wedge osteotomy of the base of the first metatarsal and transfer of the flexor hallucis longus to the head of the first metatarsal. McKay transfers tendinous insertions of the flexor hallucis brevis and abductor and adductor hallucis to the neck of the first metatarsal (Fig. 5–161). He believes these muscles have better mechanical advantage after transfer than the

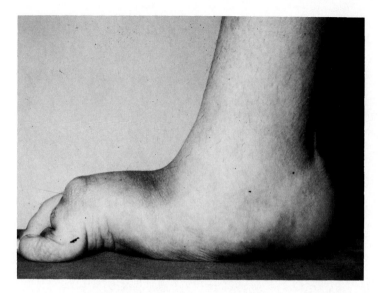

**FIGURE 5–160. Dorsal bunion
of left foot.**

Note the dorsiflexion of the first metatarsal and plantar flexion of the great toe.
(Courtesy of Dr. D. W. McKay.)

flexor hallucis longus; furthermore, the deforming action of the flexor hallucis brevis is also
removed. The operative technique is as follows:
A longitudinal incision is made on the medial
aspect of the foot, extending from the base of
the first metatarsal to the interphalangeal joint
of the great toe. The abductor hallucis and
medial part of the flexor hallucis brevis are
identified, detached from their insertion, and
dissected free; as much tendon as possible
should be preserved (Fig. 5–162A). Then the
lateral tendon of the flexor hallucis brevis and
the tendon of the adductor hallucis are sectioned from their insertion and dissected free.
The sesamoid bones in the tendinous part of
the flexor hallucis brevis are carefully removed.
If there is associated hallux valgus the abductor
hallucis is left intact; if hallux varus is present
the adductor hallucis is left attached to its
insertion. Next, a circumferential incision is
made in the periosteum of the first metatarsal
at its neck and elevated for a distance of 1 cm.
The abductor hallucis and medial part of the
flexor hallucis brevis are transferred medially
to the dorsal aspect of the metatarsal neck; the
adductor hallucis and lateral part of the flexor
hallucis brevis are transferred dorsally between
the first and second metatarsals (Fig. 5–162B).
All four tendons are sutured together, creating
a myotendinous ring around the neck of the
metatarsal (Figs. 5–161C and 5–162C). The
collar of periosteum is sutured to the tendon.
Next the interphalangeal joint of the great toe
is stabilized by tenodesis or arthrodesis. A below-knee walking cast is applied and worn for

three to four weeks. McKay reports complete
correction in ten feet (Figs. 5–163 and 5–164).

Arthrodesis of the Foot and Ankle

In the operative treatment of the paralyzed
foot, a multitude of surgical procedures have
been developed to provide stability, to correct
deformity, and to improve function.

The history of the evolution of stabilizing
operations of the foot and ankle is given in
Table 5–14. Detailed accounts of these procedures are to be found in the original contributions and in the comprehensive historical reviews by Hart, Hallgrimsson, and
Schwartz.[134, 143, 284]

In general, stabilizing operations on the foot
and ankle can be subdivided into the following:
(1) triple arthrodesis, (2) extra-articular subtalar
arthrodesis, (3) ankle fusion, and (4) anterior or
posterior bone blocks to limit motion at the
ankle joint. These procedures may be performed alone or in combination.

TRIPLE ARTHRODESIS

This procedure was devised by Ryerson in
1923 and consists of fusion of the subtalar,
calcaneocuboid, and talonavicular joints.[268] The
operation is designed to provide lateral stability,
and it will also correct deformity if the articular
surfaces are resected by pattern. In locomotion,
the essential motions of the foot and ankle are
plantar flexion and dorsiflexion. In the presence
of muscle weakness, triple arthrodesis will stabilize the hindfoot and diminish the functional

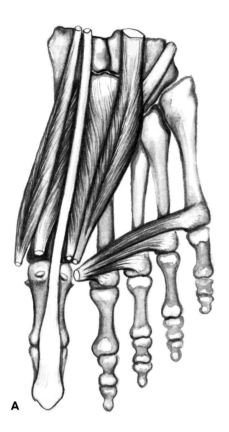

A

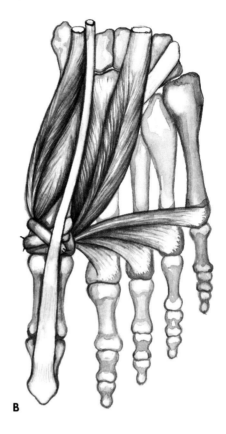

B

FIGURE 5–161. McKay's technique for correction of dorsal bunion.

A. Plantar view of right foot showing section of abductor hallucis, adductor hallucis, and flexor hallucis brevis from base of proximal phalanx. **B.** Tendinous portions of these muscles transferred to neck of first metatarsal as seen from plantar aspect. **C.** Dorsal view showing tendons transferred to the dorsum of the first metatarsal neck. (Courtesy of Dr. D. W. McKay.)

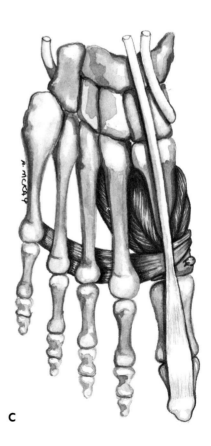

C

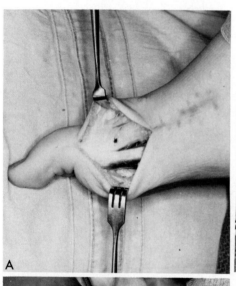

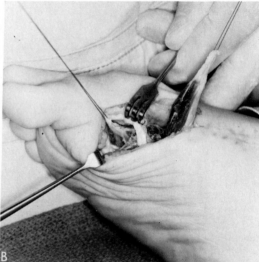

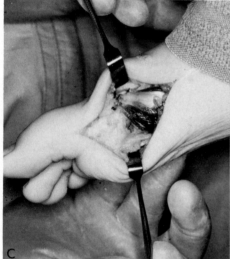

FIGURE 5–162. McKay's technique for correction of dorsal bunion as seen during surgery.

A. Note the abductor hallucis muscle. **B.** The suture on the right is attached to the abductor hallucis and the medial head of the flexor hallucis brevis; the other suture is attached to the adductor hallucis and the lateral head of the flexor hallucis brevis. The flexor hallucis longus tendon is in the middle of the wound. **C.** The four tendons are sutured over the dorsum of the neck of the first metatarsal and to the adjoining capsule and periosteum, providing a myotendinous ring. (Courtesy of Dr. D. W. McKay.)

Table 5–14. *History of Stabilizing Operations of the Foot and Ankle*

1879	Albert	Tibiotarsal or ankle joint arthrodesis
1879	Von Lesser	Tibiotarsal or ankle joint arthrodesis
1884	Samster	Ankle and subtalar joint arthrodesis
1901	Whitman	Talectomy and posterior displacement of the foot
1905	Nieny	Talocalcaneal and talocalcaneonavicular or subtalar arthrodesis
1908	Jones	Talocalcaneal and talocalcaneonavicular or subtalar arthrodesis
1908	Goldthwait	Supratalar and infratalar arthrodesis
1911	Lorthioir	Pantalar arthrodesis (temporary removal of the talus)
1911	Ombredanne	Surgical approach for exposure of the subtalar and midtarsal joints
1912	Soule	Talonavicular arthrodesis
1912	Soule	Talonavicular and subtalar arthrodesis
1913	Davis	Subtalar arthrodesis (transverse horizontal section of the tarsus) with posterior displacement of the foot
1915	Albee	Talonavicular arthrodesis with bone graft peg
1916	Davis	Subtalar or calcaneotalar and calcaneotalonavicular arthrodesis
1919	Dunn	Midtarsal tarsectomy and calcaneotalar arthrodesis
1920	Toupet	Posterior bone check
1921	Hoke	Calcaneotalonavicular arthrodesis resection, reshaping and reimplantation of head and neck of the talus, and posterior displacement of the foot.
1922	Dunn	Excision of navicular bone, calcaneotalocuneiform and calcaneocuboid arthrodesis with posterior displacement of the foot
1922	Putti	Anterior bone check
1922	Steindler	Pantalar arthrodesis (talus not temporarily removed)
1923	Ryerson	Triple (subtalar and calcaneocuboid) arthrodesis
1923	Ryerson	Lateral arthrodesis (cuneonavicular, first and fifth tarsometatarsal arthrodesis)
1923	Campbell	Posterior bone block
1925	Smith and von Lackum	Calcaneotalonavicular and calcaneocuboid arthrodesis, excision of head and neck of talus with posterior displacement of the foot
1927	Lambrinudi	Resection of wedge of bone from plantar aspect of head and neck of talus to lock the talus in equinus position at the ankle while the rest of the foot is in the desired degree of dorsiflexion
1933	Brewster	Calcaneonaviculocuneiform arthrodesis, excision of head and neck of the talus, posterior displacement of the foot and countersinking of the body of the talus in the os calcis
1935	Girard	Arthrodesis of subtalar and calcaneocuboid joints; shortening of the neck of the talus; posterior displacement of foot; construction of ankle joint mortise
1952	Grice	Extra-articular arthrodesis of subtalar joint
1963	Chuinard and Peterson	Distraction-compression bone graft arthrodesis of the ankle

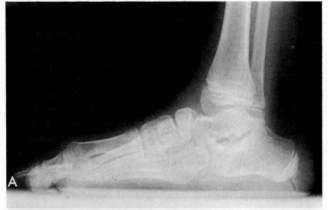

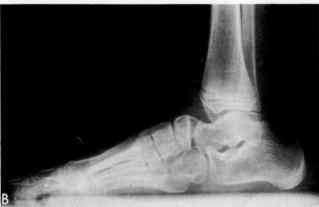

FIGURE 5–163. McKay's technique for correction of dorsal bunion.

A. Preoperative lateral radiogram of the foot, showing the deformity. **B.** Postoperative lateral x-ray of the foot. Note the excellent correction. (Courtesy of Dr. D. W. McKay.)

demand on the remaining active muscles by reducing the number of joints that they control.

Triple arthrodesis is described and illustrated in Appendix Plate C, following p. 2182.

The subtalar and midtarsal joint motions are particularly important for balance when an individual is walking upon rough or uneven terrain. The loss of lateral mobility of the hindfoot following triple arthrodesis may result in difficulty in locomotion on an irregular surface.

Triple arthrodesis may exert excessive ligamentous strain on the ankle joint. It is imperative to determine the stability of the body of the talus in the ankle mortise. This is done clinically by testing passive lateral motion of the ankle. If ankle stability is questionable, weight-bearing anteroposterior radiograms of the ankle with the hindfoot first in forced maximal eversion and abduction and then in forced inversion and adduction are taken. Normally, there is no lateral motion of the body of the talus in the ankle mortise except when the ankle is in marked plantar flexion; then it may be present in minimal amount. When there is marked instability of the ankle joint, varus or valgus deformity of the hindfoot may recur

following triple arthrodesis, and stabilization of the ankle joint may be indicated.

Anterior subluxation of the ankle joint may be present in severe equinus deformity; this should be ruled out by making lateral radiograms of the ankle with the foot in maximal plantar flexion and in forced dorsiflexion.

Alignment and weight-bearing lines of the lower limb should be carefully studied. The presence of bowleg, knock-knee, or any excessive medial or lateral tibial torsion should be noted. Lateral tibial torsion and genu valgum are common deformities in poliomyelitis. In stance, does the center of gravity of the body fall on the second metatarsal bone? Failure to recognize malalignment of the leg will result in improper positioning of the foot. During surgery, it is mandatory that the knee be draped sterile in the operative field. The foot should be aligned with the ankle mortise and not with the knee (Fig. 5–165). If there is significant torsional or angular deformity of the leg, it is corrected at a subsequent operation.

The growth of the foot in a young child should not be disturbed. The tarsal bones grow concentrically at their periphery, and resection of

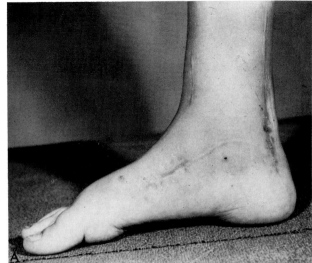

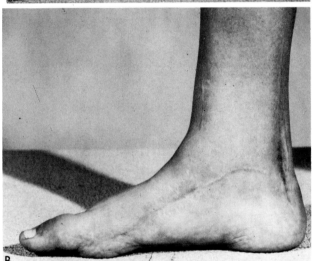

FIGURE 5–164. Dorsal bunion corrected by McKay's technique.

A. Preoperative photograph. Patient had developed dorsal bunion following cuneiform open wedge osteotomy (Fowler's procedure) for cavovarus foot. **B.** Postoperative lateral view of foot showing correction. (Courtesy of Dr. D. W. McKay.)

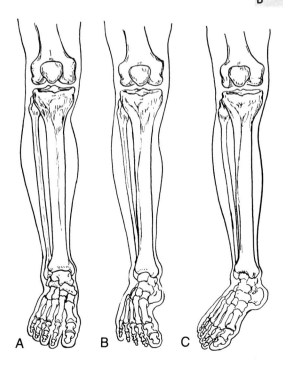

FIGURE 5–165. Alignment of the foot.

A. Normal foot, ankle, and knee alignment without tibial torsion. **B.** *Incorrect.* Foot is aligned with knee, not ankle, in the presence of external tibial torsion. **C.** *Correct.* Foot is aligned with ankle joint in the presence of external tibial torsion. (From Patterson, R. L., Parrish, F. F., and Hathaway, E. N.: Stabilizing operations on the foot. J. Bone Joint Surg., 32-A:3, 1950. Reprinted by permission.)

A   B   C

their articular surfaces will inhibit their growth. Triple arthrodesis should be deferred until the foot has achieved skeletal maturity, which in girls is 10 to 12 years, and in boys, 12 to 14 years.

The osseous deformity of the foot should be carefully analysed in the preoperative radiograms. These should include anteroposterior and mediolateral weight-bearing views of the foot and ankle. It is important to make the radiograms with the foot held in the positions of maximum correction. Tracings of the foot are made on x-ray negative films. The foot and ankle are divided into three segments, according to function: (1) the talus with the tibia and ankle joint; (2) the os calcis; and (3) the tarsal bones, the joints distal to the midtarsal joint, the metatarsals and phalanges. The talus is the only tarsal bone that transmits the entire body weight; thus, the importance of double-checking the stability of the body of the talus in the ankle mortise cannot be overemphasized.

The pattern of osteotomies and the plane of resection of the articular surfaces of each joint should be carefully and precisely planned. It is best to draw these lines on tracings of the preoperative lateral radiograms of the foot.

In the correction of varus deformity a wedge of bone with its base facing laterally is resected from the talonavicular and calcaneocuboid joints (Fig. 5–166). Lateral displacement of the forefoot is often prevented by the "beak" of the navicular bone, which projects posteriorly along the medial side of the head of the talus. It is important to excise this "beak" flush with the main body of the navicular—through a separate incision if necessary. The planes of osteotomies of the talonavicular and calcaneocuboid joints should be parallel to each other in the vertical axis in order to have close apposition of bones. To correct varus deformity of the heel, a laterally based wedge is resected from the subtalar joint. Most of the bone should be removed from the superior surface of the calcaneus. Only a minimal amount of bone should be excised from the talus. A slight valgus position of the heel will provide stability; however, the hindfoot should not be placed in more than 5 to 10 degrees of eversion, as it will cause difficulty in the proper wearing of shoes and is not cosmetically satisfactory. A varus position of the heel should not be accepted.

Valgus deformity of the foot is corrected by excision of a medially based wedge from the midtarsal area and another wedge, also based medially, from the subtalar region. The use of a laminectomy spreader in the subtalar joint will adequately expose the medial side of the hindfoot. Great care should be exercised not to injure the posterior tibial nerves and artery, which lie adjacent and superficial to the flexor hallucis longus tendon. In the valgus foot, the os calcis is everted and the head of the talus is plantar flexed over the medial aspect of the foot. The common tendency is to excise a large wedge in order to reduce the calcaneus medially beneath the talus. This should be avoided, as it will reduce the height of the hindfoot and lower the malleoli, resulting in a wide ankle contour and extreme difficulty in fitting shoes. When correcting severe valgus, varus, or calcaneus deformity of the foot, it is best to add bone graft wedges rather than to excise too much bone. Resection of excessive bone from the talus and navicular may also cause avascular necrosis of these tarsal bones with subsequent degenerative arthritis of the ankle and pseudarthrosis of the talonavicular joint.

For restoration of alignment of the calcaneus foot, a wedge of bone based posteriorly is resected from the subtalar joint (Fig. 5–167). Often there is associated cavus deformity, which is corrected by excising a wedge based dorsally from the talonavicular and calcaneocuboid joints. It is imperative to displace the os calcis posteriorly to provide a longer lever arm. When contracted, the anterior capsule of the ankle joint is stretched out preoperatively by passive manipulation and corrective casts. Release of soft-tissue contracture may be indicated when the contracture is very fixed. It is imperative to obtain normal range of plantar flexion of the ankle.

In severe talipes calcaneus, the bony deformity and soft-tissue contracture are rigid, fixing the talus and os calcis in marked dorsiflexion. The associated cavus deformity will be marked, with severe contracture of the plantar fascia and osseous changes in the midtarsal bones. Correction of deformity by wedge resections will result in appreciable reduction in the height and length of the foot.

Plantar fasciotomy is performed first. The anterior capsule of the ankle joint is released through an anterolateral approach. Next, the articular surfaces of the subtalar and talonavicular and calcaneocuboid joints are minimally resected, exposing raw cancellous bone. The calcaneus deformity is corrected by inserting an anteriorly based wedge of bone graft in the subtalar joint. Forefoot equinus deformity can be corrected by excising a wedge of bone based dorsally from the talonavicular and calcaneocuboid joints. Frequently, the author postpones

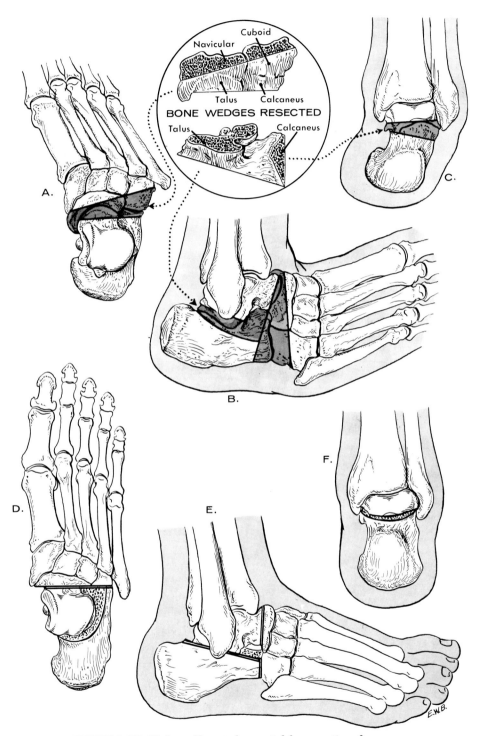

FIGURE 5–166. Wedges of bone to be resected for correction of pes varus.

A to **C**. Three views of the varus deformity. Shaded areas show amount of bone wedges to be resected. **D** to **F**. Corrected positions of the bones postoperatively.

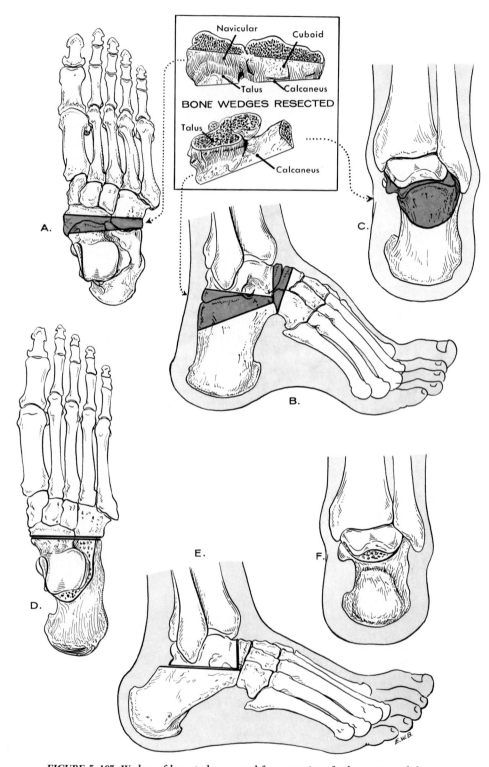

FIGURE 5–167. *Wedges of bone to be removed for correction of calcaneocavus deformity.*

A, B, and **C.** Dorsal, lateral, and posterior views show the deformity. Shaded areas indicate amount of bone removed. **D** to **F.** Positions of the bones after correction of deformity by triple arthrodesis. Note the posterior displacement of the hindfoot.

surgical correction of the cavus deformity until solid healing of the triple arthrodesis has taken place. During the application of the above-knee cast, however, it is important to immobilize the heel in moderate plantar flexion and the forefoot in maximal dorsiflexion. The common pitfall is to hold the forefoot in equinus position, permitting the cavus deformity to increase. The metatarsal heads should be well padded to prevent skin slough. Three to four months later, the metatarsals are osteotomized at their base and elevated into dorsiflexion, correcting the forefoot equinus deformity. In this way, some degree of mobility of the naviculocuneiform and cuneiform metatarsal joints is preserved.

Talectomy will correct the severe calcaneus deformity.[161, 206, 317, 335, 336] However, it reduces the height of the foot, lowers the malleoli, and causes great difficulty in fitting shoes. This is particularly disturbing to women. Fibroarthrosis and degenerative arthritis of the ankle joint will often develop in later years. For these reasons, astragalectomy is not recommended.

In classic triple arthrodesis, it is difficult to displace the os calcis backward. Dunn described a method of excising the navicular and part of the head and neck of the talus to permit posterior displacement of the calcaneus.[90, 91] Hoke had previously resected the navicular and head and neck of the talus; after subtalar joint resection and posterior displacement of the foot, he recommended reshaping and reimplanting the head and neck of the talus.[160] The Hoke and Dunn procedures, however, shorten the foot and increase the likelihood of pseudarthrosis of the talonavicular joint. For these reasons, the author prefers correction of calcaneus deformity by bone graft wedges.

In correction of pes equinus, fixed contracture of the posterior capsule of the ankle and subtalar joints and the triceps surae muscle must be corrected preoperatively. As stated previously, function of the gastrocnemius-soleus muscles should be maintained as much as possible. Wedging casts are tried first, followed by posterior capsulotomy and skeletal traction through the os calcis. In severe equinus deformity, limited heel cord lengthening may have to be performed, but it is preferable to leave some tightness of the triceps surae. It is imperative that the foot be dorsiflexed to neutral position; otherwise a rocker-bottom deformity will result. In patients with cerebral palsy, the author maintains reduction with a large Kirschner wire. One pin is placed through the os calcis into the talus and across the ankle joint into the tibia, while the other transfixes the

talonavicular joint. When equinus posture is due simply to drop foot and the foot can be passively dorsiflexed beyond neutral position, it is preferable to perform tendon transfer anteriorly to provide power of active dorsiflexion. If adequate muscles are not available for anterior transfer, the triple arthrodesis may be modified to prevent the foot from dropping down into plantar flexion. Lambrinudi, in 1927, described a method of triple arthrodesis in which a wedge of bone is excised from the plantar aspect of the head and neck of the talus and the distal sharp margin of the body of the talus is inserted into a prepared trough in the navicular. Thus the talus is locked in equinus position at the ankle joint, whereas the rest of the foot is maintained in the desired degree of dorsiflexion.[186]

The Lambrinudi operation is not recommended by the author, as his experience with it has been unsatisfactory. For adequate correction of equinus deformity, too much bone has to be resected from the talus, with consequent development of avascular necrosis of the talus, talonavicular pseudarthrosis, flattening of the superior surface of the talus, and painful arthritis of the ankle.[100, 144, 187, 208, 214, 250]

EXTRA-ARTICULAR SUBTALAR ARTHRODESIS

Grice, at the suggestion of William T. Green, developed a method of fusion of the subtalar joint by insertion of autogenous bone grafts in the sinus tarsi in the lateral aspect of the foot for correction of paralytic pes valgus and restoration of the height of the longitudinal arch.[121, 123] Any interference with subsequent normal growth of the foot is minimal, at most, because the procedure is extra-articular. The operative technique is described and illustrated in Plate 65. Pitfalls and complications are discussed in the section on cerebral palsy.

ANKLE FUSION AND PANTALAR ARTHRODESIS*

When surgical reconstruction is being considered for a flail foot and ankle, their relationship to the lower limb as a whole should be carefully assessed, since there is often associated paralysis of the muscles throughout the lower limb.

Pantalar arthrodesis is surgical fusion of the joints around the talus, i.e., the ankle, subtalar, and talonavicular joints; the calcaneocuboid joint (which is not an articulation of the talus)

---

*See References 4, 13, 27, 49, 56, 115, 138, 165, 181, 198, 250.

is also included in the stabilization, thus making the procedure a combination of triple arthrodesis and ankle fusion.

Lorthioir, as he originally reported the procedure in 1911, extirpated and replaced the talus as an autogenous bone graft.[200] In 1922, Steindler advised against the temporary removal of the talus from the wound because of the danger of avascular necrosis; he also included the calcaneocuboid joint in the fusion to provide stability and to maintain correction.[306]

When the muscles below the knee are paralyzed, pantalar arthrodesis will provide stability to the ankle and hindfoot, thus eliminating the need for orthotic support, provided the gluteus maximus is of adequate strength and the knee is stable. Extensor strength of the knee is desirable but not imperative. When the quadriceps muscle is paralyzed, stability of the knee joint is provided by shifting the center of gravity of the body forward anterior to the plane of the knee joint. To lock the knee in extension, the tibia should not be allowed to come forward through a dorsiflexion movement of the ankle, either by a strong triceps surae muscle or by a fixed equinus ankle joint. A good gluteus maximus muscle will transmit push-off power to the ball of the foot when the ankle is rigid and the knee is locked in extension.

Position of ankle fusion is an important consideration. In arthrodesis of the ankle, excessive plantar flexion to stabilize the knee in extension during the stance phase of gait or to compensate for a short limb will result in increased pressure on the metatarsal heads. Callosities will form and eventually the skin will ulcerate. Consequently, in later adult life, pain in the forefoot will be a constant complaint. Unequal heel heights are another cause of dissatisfaction; often patients would rather accept shortening and a full sole build-up. It is imperative that the position of ankle fusion be 5 to 10 degrees equinus. Lateral radiograms of the foot and ankle should be made at the time of surgery, and the position of stabilization of the ankle accurately measured with a goniometer.

Pronation or supination of the forefoot results in unequal pressure on its sides and may also cause painful callosities and ulceration. When the forefoot is in supination, callosities develop over the fifth metatarsal head, whereas in pronation they develop over the first and second metatarsal heads; and when in excessive equinus inclination, over the first and fifth metatarsal heads.

The plantar surface of the foot should be in the normal weight-bearing position, with no pronation or supination or uneven pressure under the metatarsal heads. The lateral border of the foot should be straight, with the heel in neutral or slightly valgus position and the ankle in less than 10 degrees of plantar flexion.

Waugh, Wagner, and Stinchfield reported the results of 116 pantalar arthrodeses in 97 patients with a mean follow-up of five years and an average follow-up of 6.9 years. In general, pantalar arthrodesis was found to be an effective and satisfying procedure. About 80 per cent of the patients had no complaints referable to their pantalar arthrodesis. Adequate compensatory motion developed in the forepart of the foot, so that rigidity of the feet was not a problem, despite fusion of the ankle and hindpart of the foot. Of the 52 patients who had used an orthosis preoperatively, 47 were able to discard it following fusion. Pseudarthrosis occurred in 14.7 per cent of the cases.[331]

When the foot has normal alignment and adequate bony and ligamentous stability, the author recommends ankle fusion only, using the distraction-compression bone graft arthrodesis described by Chuinard and Peterson (Appendix Plate D, following p. 2182).[63] In the paralyzed limb, there are no compressional forces to maintain the tibia and talus in close apposition, and the weight of the cast pressing on the dorsum of the foot may distract them.

ANTERIOR OR POSTERIOR BONE BLOCKS TO LIMIT MOTION AT ANKLE

In pes calcaneus, construction of a bone buttress anteriorly in the talus will limit dorsiflexion of the ankle by impinging upon the anterior lip of the distal tibia, whereas in equinus deformity of the foot, plantar flexion of the ankle may be restricted by bone block construction on the posterior aspect of the talus.[46, 47, 109, 110] These procedures were developed for use in cases of paralytic calcaneus or drop foot, when there is no musculature available for transfer to provide plantar flexion or dorsiflexion power. Long-term follow-up studies of bone block operations have disclosed a high incidence of recurrence of deformity and fibrous ankylosis or painful degenerative arthritis of the ankle joint. The author does not recommend bone blocks to limit motion at the ankle, as the procedure has all the disadvantages of arthrodesis of the ankle without providing the pain-free stability of the latter.

The only indication for a posterior bone block is in a female patient who desires to wear shoes with heels of varying height and who has fair strength of the triceps surae muscle but no dorsiflexor power. Following triple arthrodesis, small subarticular grafts are placed posteriorly to lift the articular surface of the posterior aspect of the talus and limit plantar flexion. Massive bone grafts that abut the posterior aspect of the tibia should not be used. The small blocks placed beneath the articular surface of the talus are just as effective, heal rapidly, can be performed in combination with triple arthrodesis, and are less likely to cause pain.[120]

The Trunk

The etiology and treatment of pelvic obliquity are discussed in the section on contracture of the iliotibial band. Pelvic obliquity may also be caused by unilateral paralysis of the quadratus lumborum muscle. Paralysis of the abdominal muscles will result in exaggeration of the anterior pelvic tilt and an increase in lumbar lordosis. Lowman has described fascial transplants to substitute for the paralyzed abdominal muscles. For indications and operative technique the reader is referred to Lowman, Dickson, Clark and Axer, Mayer, and Williamson, Moe, and Basom.[6, 65, 85, 202–204, 221, 339]

The treatment of postpolio paralytic scoliosis follows the same principles as that of idiopathic scoliosis (see Chapter 6.)

The Shoulder

The shoulder joint is a multiaxial one. On full abduction of the shoulder, the scapulothoracic motion contributes 60 degrees and the glenohumeral movements, 120 degrees, in a ratio of 1:2. When the arm is abducted to 90 degrees, the arm should rotate externally to allow full abduction. Full 180 degree forward flexion is permitted by internal rotation of the arm. Extension of the shoulder joint is limited to 80 degrees by the mechanical block of the acromion process and the adjacent spine of the scapula. Normal scapulohumeral rhythm is imperative for execution of graceful motions and strength of the shoulder joint.[274]

Functional classification of the muscles acting at the shoulder joint, as given by Saha, is as follows:[275, 276]

Prime Movers. These are the deltoid and clavicular head of the pectoralis major. They provide the greatest amount of active power in shoulder abduction, exerting force in three directions. Their insertion is most distal from the shoulder joint, at the juncture of the middle and upper thirds of the humeral diaphysis. When these prime movers are paralyzed, nat-

ural automatic substitution of function with adjacent motors is not feasible. To restore active shoulder abduction, muscle transfer is required.

Steering Group. This group consists of the subscapularis, supraspinatus, and infraspinatus muscles. Their force is exerted at the junction of the head-neck and shaft of the humerus, their primary function being to stabilize the humeral head in the glenoid cavity by steering, i.e., by rolling and gliding movement. Secondarily, they assist in shoulder abduction.

The infraspinatus muscle acts primarily as a posterior glider of the humeral head during the final stages of full abduction. The supraspinatus and subscapularis muscles are indispensable for shoulder abduction, steering the head of the humerus during abduction in different planes through an arc of 150 degrees. The scapula moves anteriorly and posteriorly and rotates vertically through the extremes of the arc (about 30 degrees on either side). In general, vertical gliding of the humeral head is accomplished by the muscle fibers acting in the plane of motion, whereas the muscle fibers that are anterior and posterior to these act to glide the humeral head in the horizontal plane at succeeding stages of shoulder abduction.

Depressor Group. This consists of the sternal head of the pectoralis major, the latissimus dorsi, and the teres major and teres minor. (Teres minor is included in this group, as electromyographic evidence has shown that it participates in this motion, though anatomically it is classified as belonging to the short rotator group.) The function of these muscles is to rotate the shaft of the humerus during abduction and to depress the humeral head, assisting in the last few degrees of full abduction. The steering action that they exert on the humeral head is minimal, however.

Scapular rotation takes place through its body in an anteroposterior axis and contributes about 60 degrees of total shoulder abduction. Fixation of the scapula is equally important during abduction provided by gravity and the lower fibers of the serratus.

When the deltoid and clavicular head of the pectoralis major are paralyzed, it is important to determine the action of the steering group of muscles when performing tendon transfers to restore shoulder abduction. If the latter are paralyzed, transfer of a single muscle (such as the trapezius) or several muscles to a common attachment to restore function will give at best only 90 degrees of shoulder abduction and scapulohumeral rhythm will still be disturbed. According to Saha, if there is paralysis of any

Table 5–15. *Possible Tendon Transfer to Restore Power at the Shoulder Joint**

Muscle Requiring Replacement or Reinforcement	Action	Choice of Muscles for Transfer (in Order of Preference)
Deltoid and clavicular head of pectoralis major	Prime mover (abduction)	1. Trapezius (as far down as possible on shaft)
Supraspinatus	Superior glider	1. Levator scapulae (first choice because of direction and length of its fibers) 2. Sternocleidomastoid 3. Scalenus anterior 4. Scalenus medius 5. Scalenus capitis (All act from above and are good substitutes)
Infraspinatus	Posterior glider (acting from behind)	1. Latissimus dorsi 2. Teres major
Subscapularis	Posterior glider	1. Upper two digitations of serratus anterior 2. Pectoralis minor 3. Pectoralis major (whole or part) (These muscles act in almost same direction as fibers of subscapularis)

*Modified from Saha, A. K.: Surgery of the paralyzed and flail shoulder. Acta Orthop. Scand., Suppl. 97, p. 40, 1967.

two of the steering group of muscles, appropriate tendon transfers should be performed to restore their function. This is as imperative as trapezius transfer for paralysis of the deltoid.

Table 5–15 gives Saha's recommendations for possible tendon transfers to restore power at the shoulder joint.

The Saha trapezius transfer for paralysis of the deltoid is shown in Figure 5–168. The upper and middle trapezius is completely mobilized from its insertion, providing an additional 5 cm.

of length without disturbing the nerve and blood supply to the muscle. The detached portion of the trapezius with the distal end of the clavicle, the capsule of the acromioclavicular joint, the acromion process, and the adjoining portion of the posterior border of the spine of the scapula are rerouted and attached by two screws to the humeral shaft as far distally as possible. The acromion is crushed to aid coaptation with the curve of the shaft of the humerus.

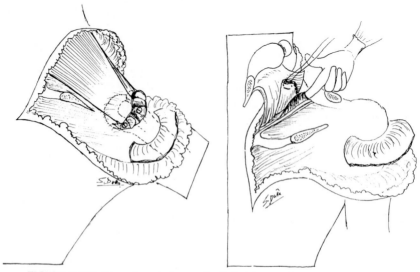

FIGURE 5–168. *Trapezius muscle transfer (Saha) for paralysis of deltoid muscle.*

(From Saha, A. K.: Surgery of the paralyzed and flail shoulder. Acta Orthop. Scand., Suppl. 97, p. 57, 1967. Reprinted by permission.)

Transfer of the upper two digitations of the serratus anterior for paralysis of the subscapularis is shown in Figure 5–169. Levator scapulae transfer for paralysis of the supraspinatus is shown in Figure 5–170; pectoralis minor transfer for paralysis of the subscapularis in Figure 5–171; sternocleidomastoid transfer for paralysis of the supraspinatus in Figure 5–172; and either latissimus dorsi or teres major transfer, or both, for paralysis of the subscapularis in Figure 5–173. For technical details the reader is referred to the original paper of Saha.[276]

ARTHRODESIS OF THE SHOULDER

This is indicated when there is paralytic subluxation or dislocation of the shoulder and extensive paralysis of the scapulohumeral muscles. Because scapulothoracic motion will serve as a substitute for that of the glenohumeral joint, it is important that the motor strength of the trapezius and serratus anterior be normal. The direct action of the scapula will move the arm. Normal function of the hand, however, is a primary requisite. It is best to delay shoulder arthrodesis until after epiphyseal closure has taken place.

The optimum position for shoulder fusion, as recommended by the Research Committee of the American Orthopedic Association, is 50 degrees of abduction, 20 degrees of flexion, and 25 degrees of internal rotation. This position is very functional, allowing the patient to reach his face and the top of his head with the elbow flexed.[15]

It is wise, however, to consider the sex and occupation of the patient, and the regional muscle power and functional status of the opposite limb. In general, office workers require more abduction than do laborers. In females, the degree of abduction should be less, since this permits the scapula a better resting position in relation to the trunk. For cosmetic reasons, females strongly object to the winging of the scapula. The lesser degree of abduction is functionally compensated by fusing it in greater internal rotation. The most acceptable position of shoulder arthrodesis in females is 30 degrees of glenohumeral abduction, 5 to 10 degrees of flexion, and 45 degrees of internal rotation. The shoulder should never be fused in external rotation, as the limb will be positioned in an awkward and functionally poor position. It should be explained to the patient that following surgery, extension and rotation of the shoulder will be limited and that he will have difficulty in lying on the side of the arthrodesis to sleep. Fusion of both shoulders should never be performed because of the loss in range of motion.

Arthrodesis of the shoulder will increase the power of both flexion and extension of the elbow and will provide adduction power to the shoulder, enabling the patient to grip an object between his arm and body.

For technical details of shoulder fusion, the reader is referred to the original papers in the references.* It should be emphasized, however, that the position of fusion should be calculated according to the angle between the humerus and scapula rather than that of the arms and thorax. Internal fixation is imperative; otherwise, the angle will be changed in the shoulder spica cast.

The Elbow

Loss of elbow flexion results from paralysis of the biceps brachii and the brachialis muscles. The resultant functional deficit is considerable, as the patient is unable to bring his hand to his head, mouth, or trunk.

A number of operative procedures have been devised to restore elbow flexion: (1) Steindler flexorplasty;[303] (2) transfer of the distal third of the pectoralis major muscle (Clark);[64] (3) transfer of the pectoralis major tendon (Brooks and Seddon);[38] (4) transfer of the sternocleidomastoid muscle (Bunnell);[41] (5) transfer of latissimus dorsi (Hovnanian);[162] (6) transfer of pectoralis minor (Spira);[299] (7) anterior transfer of the triceps brachii tendon to the biceps insertion on the radial tuberosity (Bunnell and Carroll).[41, 50]

Prior to the selection of a specific procedure, it is imperative to assess carefully the motor strength of the muscles of the entire upper limb and the functional status of the opposite limb. With paralysis of the elbow flexors, there is often a varying degree of paresis of the muscles of the scapulohumeral joint, forearm, and hand.

Function of the hand is of primary concern. Restoration of elbow flexion is only one step in total functional reconstruction of the upper limb, and procedures on the hand should precede those on the elbow. In the absence of a functional hand, flexorplasty of the elbow should not be performed.

STEINDLER FLEXORPLASTY

Steindler, in 1918, described a procedure in which the humeral origins of the flexor carpi radialis, the palmaris longus, the pronator teres, the flexor digitorum sublimis, and the flexor carpi ulnaris are transferred to a more proximal site on the humerus, thereby changing the leverage of these muscles across the elbow joint

---

*See References 15, 20, 34, 39, 40, 56–58, 108, 179, 330.

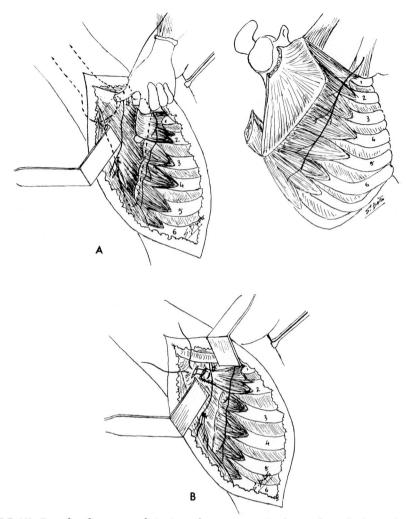

FIGURE 5–169. Transfer of upper two digitations of serratus anterior for paralysis of subscapularis muscle.

(From Saha, A. K.: Surgery of the paralyzed and flail shoulder. Acta Orthop. Scand., Suppl. 97, p. 59, 1967. Reprinted by permission.)

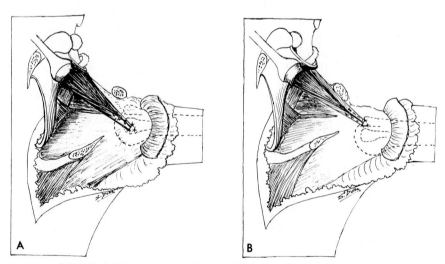

FIGURE 5–170. Levator scapulae transfer for paralysis of supraspinatus.

(From Saha, A. K.: Surgery of the paralyzed and flail shoulder. Acta Orthop. Scand., Suppl. 97, p. 60, 1967. Reprinted by permission.)

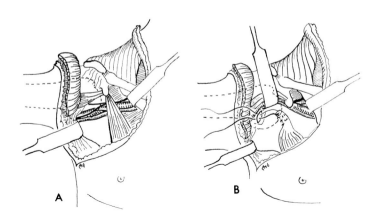

FIGURE 5–171. Pectoralis minor transfer for paralysis of subscapularis.

(From Saha, A. K.: Surgery of the paralyzed and flail shoulder. Acta Orthop. Scand., Suppl. 97, p. 61, 1967. Reprinted by permission.)

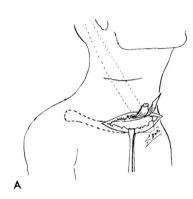

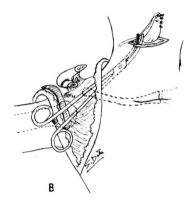

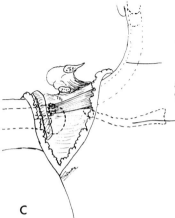

FIGURE 5–172. Sternocleidomastoid transfer for paralysis of supraspinatus muscle.

(From Saha, A. K.: Surgery of the paralyzed and flail shoulder. Acta Orthop. Scand., Suppl. 97, p. 62, 1967. Reprinted by permission.)

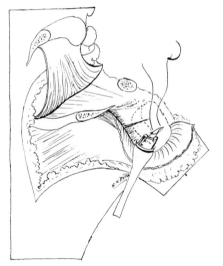

FIGURE 5–173. Latissimus dorsi or teres major transfer for paralysis of subscapularis muscle.

(From Saha, A. K.: Surgery of the paralyzed and flail shoulder. Acta Orthop. Scand., Suppl. 97, p. 64, 1967. Reprinted by permission.)

and enhancing their flexor action at the elbow.[303] Later, he reviewed the results of flexorplasties of the elbow and pointed out that the disadvantage of this transfer was an increase in the pronatory action of these muscles on the forearm.[307–309, 311]

Bunnell modified the Steindler flexorplasty by attaching the transferred muscles to the lateral border of the humerus to decrease their tendency to cause pronation. In order to reach the lateral border of the humerus, the common flexor muscles had to be elongated with a fascial graft (Fig. 5–174).[41] This method of fascial lengthening is technically difficult if one is to obtain secure fixation and maximum strength of the flexorplasty. Mayer and Green attached the transferred muscles on the anterior surface of the humerus through holes drilled in bone.[223] This direct fixation to bone ensured firm healing of the transferred muscle. The operative technique of Steindler flexorplasty as modified by Mayer and Green is described and illustrated in Appendix Plate E, following p. 2182.

Carroll and Gartland reported the results of Steindler flexorplasty in 27 patients.[52] Kettlekamp and Larson evaluated the results of Steindler flexorplasty in 15 patients, determining the maximum strength of the flexorplasty through a useful range of flexion. Nine of the fifteen patients were able to lift a weight of 1 pound or greater to 110 degrees of flexion. Upon correlating the strength of the flexorplasty with the degree of flexion contracture of the elbow, they found the average strength of the flexor-

plasty to be 2 pounds to 110 degrees of flexion when the degree of flexion contracture was between 30 and 60 degrees. The mechanical advantage and strength of the transfer were increased in the presence of flexion contracture of the elbow.[178] When there is marked paralysis of the opposite limb, the strength restored by flexorplasty is a greater consideration than is cosmetic appearance.

Mayer and Green, however, emphasize the importance of the appearance of the arm, preferring that the flexion position of the elbow not exceed 15 degrees. They recommend that a turnbuckle extension orthosis be worn at night to prevent the development of flexion contracture of the elbow. As soon as the strength of the transfer is fair or fair plus, a night splint is used and passive stretching exercises of the elbow flexors are performed.[223]

The motor strength of the triceps is another important factor in the development of flexion contracture of the elbow, as this contracture represents the residuum of flexorplasty and the end result of dynamic imbalance between elbow flexors and extensors over the years. A flexion deformity of the elbow greater than 30 degrees will usually develop when the triceps brachii is less than fair in motor strength. In the presence of a weakened triceps brachii, the period of postoperative immobilization should be short,

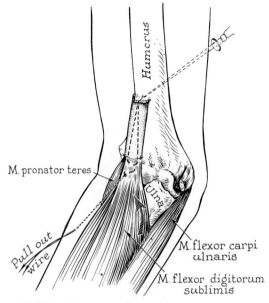

FIGURE 5–174. Bunnell's modification of Steindler flexorplasty of the elbow.

The common flexor muscles are elongated by a fascial graft. (From Bunnell, S.: Restoring flexion to the paralytic elbow. J. Bone Joint Surg., 33-A:566, 1951. Reprinted by permission.)

and assisted active exercises should be started on the fifth to seventh postoperative day, taking precautions to prevent the transfer from being stretched away from the bone. There should be an extensive period of postoperative splinting at night with the elbow in extension.

Loss of supination is an inherent complication of Steindler flexorplasty. The attachment of the transferred muscles as far laterally on the humerus as possible minimizes the severity of pronation contracture; however, even with this precaution a varying degree of pronation deformity of the forearm results in the presence of dynamic imbalance between a strong pronator teres and a paralyzed biceps brachii—its chief supinator opponent. The strength of the flexorplasty is not influenced by the degree of pronation contracture; however, it does impair the position of the hand and impedes its functional use. If the motor strength of the supinators of the forearm is poor, flexor carpi ulnaris transfer to the dorsum of the radius is performed to enhance supinator function and to prevent development of pronation contracture of the forearm.

In poliomyelitis, paralysis of the elbow without paralysis of the muscles that control the scapulohumeral joint is rarely seen. A flail shoulder will greatly impede the effectiveness of the flexorplasty. In the abducted position of the shoulder, the force of gravity assists elbow flexion and the amount of strength required to flex the elbow is decreased. Arthrodesis of the shoulder will markedly improve the results of flexorplasty.

Overestimation of the motor strength of the common flexor muscle group is a frequent pitfall, and accounts for poor results in some patients. For the transfer to function effectively, these muscles must rate at least good in motor strength. If they are weaker, other reconstructive methods must be employed. The flexor digitorum sublimis may be strong and the flexor carpi ulnaris and carpi radialis weak; in such an instance, following Steindler flexorplasty, flexion of the elbow is accomplished only by clenching the fingers, and any relaxation of the grip will allow the elbow to extend. This interferes with function of the hand, which is the primary interest of the patient.

PECTORALIS MAJOR TRANSFER TO RESTORE ELBOW FLEXION

A portion of the pectoralis major transfer was used by Clark to restore active elbow flexion.[64] The nerve supply of the distal third of the pectoralis major muscle (from branches of the medial thoracic nerve) is separate from that of its proximal part. This inferior strip of the pectoralis major muscle, which is 5 to 7 cm. in width, is freed from the chest wall and mobilized toward the axilla as far as its nerve and blood supply will allow. The muscle is then passed subcutaneously down the arm and sutured to the biceps tendon. The reader is referred to Clark's original description for the specific technical details.[64] Clark's operation is particularly indicated in patients with traction injury of the upper trunk of the brachial plexus, in whom the clavicular head of the pectoralis major is paralyzed but the sternal head is normal in motor strength. Seddon reported satisfactory results in 15 of 16 of Clark's pectoralis major transfers.[286] In a more recent report by Segal, Seddon, and Brooks, the results of Clark's operation in 17 patients were graded excellent or good in 47 per cent and fair or failure in 53 per cent.[287]

Brooks and Seddon devised a technique in which the entire pectoralis major muscle is transferred to restore elbow flexion.[38] The gap between the distal end of the pectoralis major tendon and the tuberosity of the radius is bridged by the long head of the biceps, which is detached from its origin and completely mobilized. Reducing the blood supply of the biceps brachii induced conversion of the muscle into tendon. The procedure was recommended by Brooks and Seddon in those patients in whom either the lower part of the pectoralis major is paralyzed (or too weak for the Clark transfer) but the clavicular head is strong, or the entire muscle is of such weakness that it is desirable to use all the active muscle. They reported the results as excellent or good in six; fair in two; and failure in two (one patient had arthrogryposis multiplex congenita, and the other poliomyelitis).

The operative technique of the Brooks-Seddon procedure is described and illustrated in Plate 90. The author recommends its use when the Steindler flexorplasty is not applicable; of course, it should be employed only when the biceps brachii is completely and permanently paralyzed. The procedure does restore some degree of active supination of the forearm and rarely limits passive extension of the elbow.

One disadvantage of the pectoralis major transfer is that in the presence of weak scapulohumeral muscles, active flexion of the elbow is often accompanied by shrugging, adduction, and internal rotation of the shoulder. These undesirable motions, with the hand hitting the chest wall, seriously impair the result of the operation. If there is appreciable paralysis of the shoulder muscle, the pectoralis major transfer must be followed by arthrodesis of the scapulohumeral joint.

PECTORALIS MINOR TRANSFER

Spira, in 1957, reported the successful use of the pectoralis minor as a motor to restore elbow flexion. The patient had complete paralysis of the pectoralis major, biceps brachii, and brachialis muscles. A tube of fascia lata was used to bridge the gap between the detached origin of the pectoralis minor and the paralyzed biceps tendon.[299]

STERNOCLEIDOMASTOID TRANSFER

Bunnell utilized the sternocleidomastoid muscle as a motor to restore active elbow flexion.[41] The sternoclavicular insertion of the sternocleidomastoid muscle is detached, and by gentle blunt dissection the distal half of the muscle is mobilized. A long tube of fascia lata is used to bridge the gap, extending from the distal end of the sternocleidomastoid muscle and then passing forward subcutaneously in the arm to the elbow where the graft is attached to the tuberosity of the radius (Fig. 5–175).

Carroll reported the results of 15 cases of sternocleidomastoid transfer with satisfactory results in 80 per cent. He stressed the importance of placing the transferred muscle under maximal tension at the time of operation.[51]

In the personal experience of the author with seven patients, the strength of elbow flexion following Bunnell's sternocleidomastoid transfer is excellent; however, the aesthetic appearance of the procedure is very grotesque and is objectionable, particularly in females. It should be used in cases in which it is the only method available, but must be limited to the male patient only, in whom function is the primary consideration and the resultant deformity can be hidden by the buttoned collar of a shirt.

ANTERIOR TRANSFER OF TRICEPS BRACHII

This was described by Bunnell in 1948 and in 1951, and later by Carroll, who showed the feasibility and effectiveness of the procedure without the use of the fascial graft that was recommended by Bunnell.[41, 150] In 1970 Carroll reported the results of triceps transfer in 15 patients (8 with arthrogryposis multiplex congenita, and 7 with post-traumatic and paralytic loss of elbow flexion). The criteria of success were the inability to flex the elbow against gravity and to bring the hand to the mouth before surgery and the ability to do so postoperatively. The results of Carroll were as follows: In the post-traumatic and paralytic group there were five successes, one limited result, and one failure; in the arthrogrypotic group, there were five successes, one limited result, and two failures.[53]

The operative technique described by Carroll is as follows:

The patient is placed in lateral position. A midline incision is made on the posterior aspect of the arm, beginning in its middle half and extending distally to a point lateral to the olecranon process; then the incision is carried over the subcutaneous surface of the shaft of the ulna for a distance of 5 cm. The subcutaneous tissue is divided, and the wound flaps are mobilized. The ulnar nerve is identified and mobilized medially to protect it from injury. The intermuscular septum is exposed laterally. The triceps tendon is detached from its insertion with a long tail of periosteum. Then the triceps muscle is freed and mobilized proximally as far as its nerve supply permits. The motor branches of the radial nerve to the triceps enter the muscle in the interval between the lateral and medial heads as the radial nerve enters the musculospiral groove. The distal portion of the detached triceps is then sutured to itself to form a tube. Through a curvilinear incision in the antecubital fossa, the interval between the brachioradialis and the pronator teres is developed. With an Ober tendon passer, the triceps tendon is passed into the anterior wound subcutaneously, superficial to the radial nerve. With the elbow in 90 degrees of flexion and the forearm in full supination, the triceps tendon is either sutured to the biceps tendon or anchored to the radial tuberosity by a suture passed through a drill hole (Fig. 5–176). The wound is closed in routine fashion. An above-elbow cast is applied with the elbow in 90 degrees of flexion and full supination for four weeks, at which time immobilization is discontinued and active exercises are begun. Gravity provides extension to the elbow.[53]

Loss of active extension against gravity is a definite disadvantage of anterior transfer of the triceps. The operation should be restricted to exceptional cases in which restoration of elbow flexion is imperative and in which no other tendon transfer is possible. Another indication for anterior transfer of the triceps is that of brachial plexus injuries, in which simultaneous contraction of the triceps (the antagonistic muscle) occurs on active flexion of the elbow, and

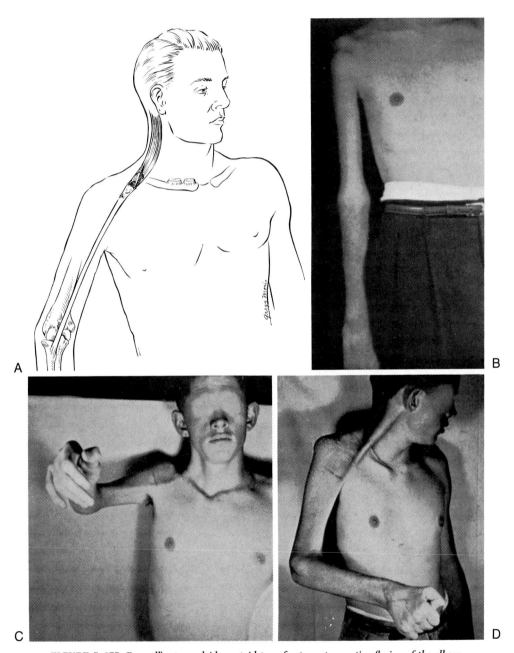

FIGURE 5–175. *Bunnell's sternocleidomastoid transfer to restore active flexion of the elbow.*

A. Drawing showing the sternocleidomastoid muscle transfer. **B.** Preoperative photograph of patient with flail shoulder and elbow and partially paralyzed hand. The shoulder was fused; the sternocleidomastoid muscle was transferred; the wrist was arthrodesed in functional position. **C** and **D.** Postoperative photographs show the result. Function of the useless right upper limb was greatly improved. (From Bunnell, S.: Restoring flexion to the paralytic elbow. J. Bone Joint Surg., *33-A*:569, 1951. Reprinted by permission.)

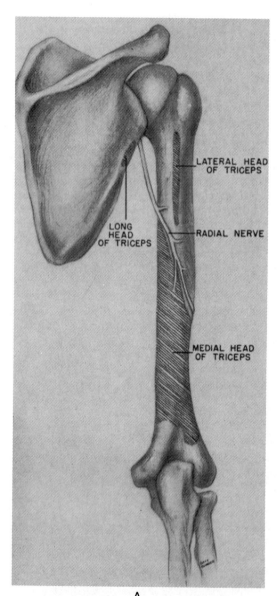

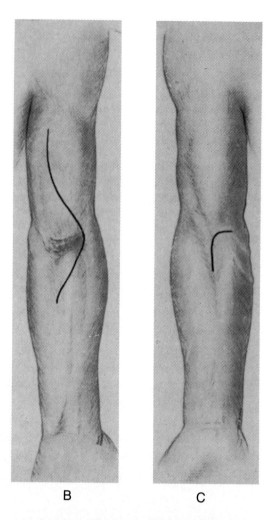

B   C

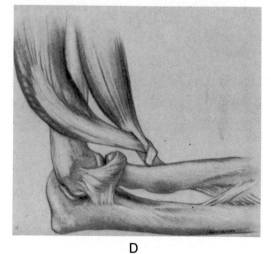

A

D

FIGURE 5–176. *Carroll's modification of Bunnell's anterior transfer of triceps for paralysis of biceps.*

A. The motor branches of the radial nerve are given off in the area between the medial and lateral heads of the triceps muscle. **B.** The long curvilinear incision avoids pressure points of the elbow and gives adequate exposure. **C.** Only a small incision is necessary to expose the ulnar aspect. **D.** The tendon of the mobilized triceps brachii is woven through the biceps tendon with the elbow in flexion. It may be anchored directly to the radial tuberosity. (From Carroll, R. E.: Restoration of flexor power to the flail elbow by transplantation of the triceps tendon. Surg. Gynec. Obstet., 95:686, 1952. Reprinted by permission.)

the action of the pectoralis major transfer is impaired. This simultaneous flexion-extension mass action can be successfully overcome by anterior transfer of the triceps into the flexor apparatus.

LATISSIMUS DORSI TRANSFER

Hovnanian described a method of transfer of the origin and belly of the latissimus dorsi muscle into the arm.[162] This is feasible because the nerve supply of the latissimus dorsi (the thoracodorsal nerve) is a long nerve (12 to 17 cm. in length) and is highly mobile and easily identified; also, the blood supply of the latissimus dorsi muscle enters from a wide zone in its proximal third. Thus the latissimus dorsi can be mobilized without denervating or devascularizing the muscle. Active elbow flexion is restored by anchoring the origin of the latissimus dorsi muscle into the biceps tendon near the radial tuberosity; active extension of the elbow is given by suturing it to the olecranon (Fig. 5–177).

PARALYSIS OF TRICEPS BRACHII MUSCLE

Loss of active extension of the elbow due to paralysis of the triceps muscle seldom causes significant disability because the elbow will extend passively under the force of gravity. A strong triceps is not essential for crutch walking, provided good shoulder depressors are present. A triceps strap or band is added to the crutch and with the elbow locked in slight hyperextension, the patient can ambulate quite well. If there is marked paralysis of both lower limbs and trunk, however, a functional triceps is desirable in order to lock the elbow in extension in daily activities such as arising from a bed or chair, or reaching for objects overhead.

Various operative procedures have been devised to restore active extension of the elbow. Trapezius muscle transfer was used in 1930 by Lange, who detached it from the acromion and joined it by long silk sutures to the olecranon.[189] Ober and Barr described a technique for transferring the brachioradialis muscle by rerouting it at the elbow to a more posterior position.[246] Extensor carpi radialis longus muscle was added to the brachioradialis muscle transfer if greater strength was necessary. The transfer of flexor carpi radialis and ulnaris muscles was proposed by Hohmann.[158, 159] Friedenberg transferred the biceps brachii for triceps paralysis.[106] The posterior part of the deltoid was proposed by d'Aubigné.[5] Latissimus dorsi was used for transfer to restore elbow extension by Hohmann; Lange; Harmon; Schottstaedt,

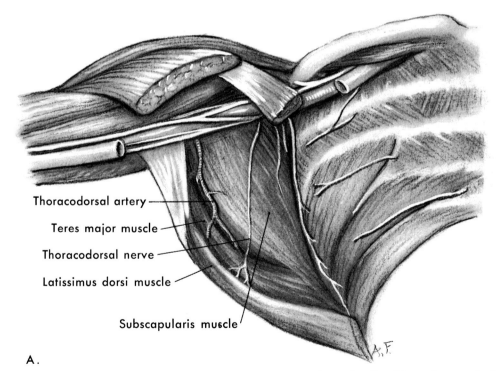

Thoracodorsal artery

Teres major muscle

Thoracodorsal nerve

Latissimus dorsi muscle

Subscapularis muscle

A.

FIGURE 5–177. Latissimus dorsi transfer to restore flexion or extension at the elbow (Hovnanian operation).

A. The anatomy of the axilla and the latissimus dorsi muscle. (From Hovnanian, A. P.: Latissimus dorsi transplantation at the elbow. Ann. Surg., *143*:493, 1956. Reprinted by permission.)

Illustration continued on following page

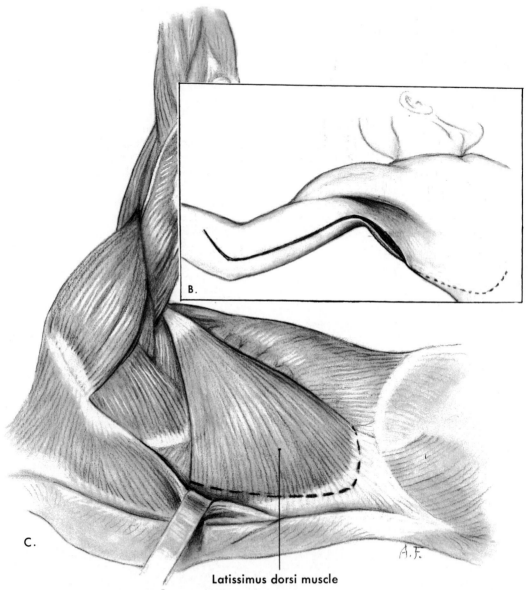

Latissimus dorsi muscle

FIGURE 5–177 Continued. Latissimus dorsi transfer to restore flexion or extension at the elbow (Hovnanian operation).

   B. Skin incision used to restore elbow flexion. The lumbar extension of the skin incision is shown by dotted lines. **C.** The line of section of latissimus dorsi muscle across its musculofascial portion inferiorly and its muscle fibers superiorly. (From Hovnanian, A. P.: Latissimus dorsi transplantation at the elbow. Ann. Surg., *143*:493, 1956. Reprinted by permission.)

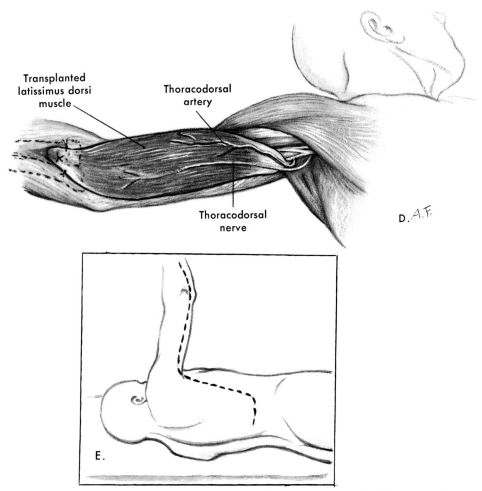

Transplanted
latissimus dorsi
muscle

Thoracodorsal
artery

Thoracodorsal
nerve

D. A.F.

E.

FIGURE 5–177 Continued. *Latissimus dorsi transfer to restore flexion or extension at the elbow (Hovnanian operation).*

D. To restore elbow flexion, the belly and origin of the latissimus dorsi is transferred into the anteromedial aspect of the arm, and its origin is anchored into the biceps tendon near the radial tuberosity. **E.** Skin incision used to restore elbow extension. (From Hovnanian, A. P.: Latissimus dorsi transplantation at the elbow. Ann. Surg., *143*:493, 1956. Reprinted by permission.)

Illustration continued on following page

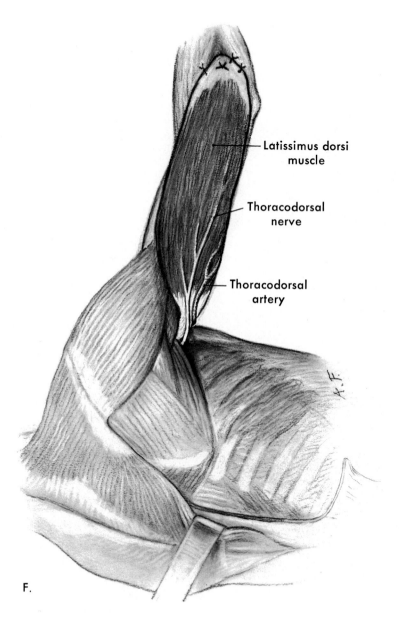

Latissimus dorsi
muscle

Thoracodorsal
nerve

Thoracodorsal
artery

F.

FIGURE 5–177 Continued.
Latissimus dorsi transfer to restore
flexion or extension at the elbow
(Hovnanian operation).

F. The latissimus dorsi muscle is
transferred to the posterior aspect of
the arm and anchored to the olecranon and triceps tendon. (From Hovnanian, A. P.: Latissimus dorsi transplantation at the elbow. Ann. Surg.,
143:493, 1956. Reprinted by permission.)

Larsen, and Bost; Hovnanian; and duToit and Levy.[88, 139, 158, 159, 162, 189, 283]

The relative merits and shortcomings of the various procedures are not discussed here as the author has had no personal experience with them. The Hovnanian transfer of the origin of the latissimus dorsi to the olecranon, leaving its insertion intact, is recommended, as the procedure is physiologically sound and has been successful in the author's experience.

The Forearm

Fixed supination and pronation contractures of the forearm are deformities in flaccid paralysis that require surgical treatment.

Supination contracture of the forearm is rare but disabling. It results from selective paralysis of the four muscles that originate from the medial epicondyle of the humerus (the pronator teres, flexor carpi ulnaris, palmaris longus, and flexor carpi radialis) in the presence of a strong biceps brachii muscle. Contracture of the interosseous membrane soon develops. With growth and under the influence of unopposed action of the biceps brachii muscle, osseous changes take place, causing the radius to become curved and spiral around the ulna. If deformity remains uncorrected and there is still muscle imbalance, progressive fixed deformity will develop, with permanent shortening of the soft tissues, primarily the interosseous membrane, biceps brachii, and supinator muscles. The radius becomes markedly bowed and the radioulnar joints may subluxate. In children under 12 years of age, closed osteoclasis of the middle third of both bones of the forearm is recommended by Blount.[28] Because of recurrence of deformity, which can occur with further growth, he advises overcorrection. In two of the nine reported cases, osteoclasis was later repeated because of recurrence of supination contracture.

Zaoussis corrected the fixed supination deformity by open osteotomy near the tuberosity of the radius.[349] He found more or less permanent "blocking" of the forearm rotation following surgery, but the synostosis of the proximal radius and ulna did not seem to impair the functional result. As internal fixation was not used by Zaoussis, angulation, displacement, and delayed union of the osteotomy occurred; however, these complications did not affect the cosmetic and functional result.

The transfer of the biceps brachii to the side of the radial tuberosity opposite its normal insertion was mentioned by Schottstaedt, Larsen, and Bost.[283] A year later Grilli described the operative technique of rerouting the biceps tendon insertion to the radial side of the neck of the radius to convert its function from a supinator to that of pronator.[124]

Zancolli included surgical release of the contracted soft tissues in biceps transfer, especially the interosseous membrane.[348] He reported satisfactory results in 14 patients with supination contracture of the forearm (eight patients had obstetrical brachial plexus paralysis, four patients had poliomyelitis, and two patients, traumatic quadriplegia). Correction was maintained in all 14 patients. Active pronation (measuring 10 to 60 degrees and using the transferred biceps brachii muscle) was achieved in eight patients. Active supination (measuring 20 to 80 degrees) was retained in eight patients. The procedure permits a more normal anatomic relationship of the radius and ulna to develop, resulting in nearly normal shape of the forearm. For details of operative technique, the reader is referred to the original paper of Zancolli.[348]

References

1. Abo, W., Chiba, S., Yamanaka, T., Nakao, T., Hara, M., and Tagaya, I.: Paralytic poliomyelitis in a child with agammaglobulinemia. Eur. J. Pediatr., *132*:11, 1979.
2. Anderson, J. G., and Brandsma, J. W.: Bilateral opponens replacement in post polio thenar paralysis, using different techniques. A case report. Hand, *15*:221, 1983.
3. André, F. E.: Control of poliomyelitis by vaccination in Belgium. Rev. Infect. Dis., *6*:(Suppl. 2), 419, 1984.
4. Ansart, M. B.: Pan-arthrodesis for paralytic flail foot. J. Bone Joint Surg., *33-B*:503, 1951.
5. d'Aubigné, R. M.: Chirurgia Orthopedique des Paralysis. Paris, Masson & Cie, 1959.
6. Axer, A.: Transposition of gluteus maximus, tensor fasciae latae and ilio-tibial band for paralysis of lateral abdominal muscles in children after poliomyelitis. A preliminary report. J. Bone Joint Surg., *40-B*:644, 1958.
7. Axer, A.: Intro-talus transposition of tendons for correction of paralytic valgus foot after poliomyelitis in children. J. Bone Joint Surg., *42-A*:1119, 1960.
8. Baptista Risi, J., Jr.: The control of poliomyelitis in Brazil. Rev. Infect. Dis., *6*:(Suppl. 2), 400, 1984.
9. Baker, A. B., and Cornwell, S.: Poliomyelitis: the spinal cord. A.M.A. Arch. Pathol., *61*:185, 1956.
10. Baker, L. D., and Dodelin, C. D.: Extra-articular arthrodesis of the subtalar joint (Grice procedure). J.A.M.A., *168*:1005, 1958.
11. Barr, J. S.: Poliomyelitic hip deformity and the erector spinae transplantation. J.A.M.A., *144*:813, 1950.
12. Barr, J. S.: Discussion. J. Bone Joint Surg., *46-A*:1402, 1964.
13. Barr, J. S., and Record, E. E.: Arthrodesis of the ankle for correction of foot deformity. Surg. Clin. North Am., *27*:1281, 1947.
14. Barr, J. S., Stinchfield, A. J., and Reidy, J. A.: Sympathetic ganglionectomy and limb length in poliomyelitis. J. Bone Joint Surg., *32-A*:793, 1950.
15. Barr, J. S., Freiberg, J. A., Colonna, P. C., and

Pemberton, P. A.: A survey of end-results on stabilization of the paralytic shoulder. Report of the research committee of the American Orthopaedic Association. J. Bone Joint Surg., 24:699, 1942.

16. Bass, J. W., Halstead, S. B., Fischer, G. W., Podgore, J. K., and Wiebe, R. A.: Oral polio vaccine. Effect of booster vaccination one to 14 years after primary series. J.A.M.A., 239:2252, 1978.

17. Basu, R. N., and Sokhey, J.: Prevalence of poliomyelitis in India. Indian J. Pediatr., 51:515, 1984.

18. Basu, S. N.: Paralytic poliomyelitis in children: some facts and figures from a hospital at Calcutta—Part I. Indian J. Public Health, 29:175, 1985.

19. Basu, S. N.: Paralytic poliomyelitis in children—Part II. Age, sex, and seasonal distribution. Indian J. Public Health, 29:183, 1985.

20. Bateman, J. E.: The Shoulder and Environs. St. Louis, C. V. Mosby, 1954.

21. Bellier, G., and Carlioz, H.: The prediction of growth in long bones in poliomyelitis (author's transl.). Rev. Chir. Orthop., 65:373, 1979.

22. Benyi, P.: A modified Lambrinudi operation for drop foot. J. Bone Joint Surg., 42-B:333, 1960.

23. Bergeisen, G. H., Bauman, R. J., and Gilmore, R. L.: Neonatal paralytic poliomyelitis. A case report. Arch. Neurol., 43:192, 1986.

24. Bernier, R. H.: Improved inactivated poliovirus vaccine: an update. Pediatr. Infect. Dis., 5:289, 1986.

25. Bickel, W. H.,and Moe, J. H.: Translocation of the peroneus longus tendon for paralytic calcaneus deformity of the foot. Surg. Gynec. Obstet., 78:627, 1944.

26. Biesalski, K., and Mayer, L.: Die Physiologische Sehnenverpflanzung. Vol. 14. Julius Springer, 1916.

27. Bingold, A. C.: Ankle and subtalar fusion by transarticular graft. J. Bone Joint Surg., 38-B:862, 1956.

28. Blount, W. P.: Osteoclasis for supination deformities in children. J. Bone Joint Surg., 22:300, 1940.

29. Bodian, D.: Poliomyelitis. Neuropathologic observations in relation to motor symptoms. J.A.M.A., 134:1148, 1947.

30. Bradford, E. H., and Lovett, R. W.: Treatise on Orthopedic Surgery. London, Bailliere, Tindall and Cox, 1915, p. 486.

31. Brewster, A. H.: Countersinking the astragalus in paralytic feet. N. Engl. J. Med., 209:71, 1933.

32. Britian, H. A.: Architectural Principles in Arthrodesis. 2nd. Ed. Edinburgh, E. & S. Livingstone, 1952.

33. Broca, J. S., Chaturvedi, S. K., and Mathur, G. M.: Prevalence of residual polio paralysis in children of 5–15 years age group in Ajmer City. Indian J. Public Health, 29:193, 1985.

34. Brockway, A.: An operation to improve abduction power of the shoulder in poliomyelitis. J. Bone Joint Surg., 21:451, 1939.

35. Broderick, T. F., Reidy, J. A., and Barr, J. S.: Tendon transplantation in the lower extremity. A review of end results in poliomyelitis. II. Tendon transplantation at the knee. J. Bone Joint Surg., 34-A:909, 1952.

36. Broms, J. D.: Subtalar extra-articular arthrodesis. Follow-up study. Clin. Orthop., 42:139, 1965.

37. Brooks, D. M.: Symposium on reconstructive surgery of paralyzed upper limb: tendon transplantation of the forearm and arthrodesis of the wrist. Proc. R. Soc. Med., 42:838, 1949.

38. Brooks, D. M., and Seddon, H. J.: Pectoral transplantation for paralysis of the flexors of the elbow. A new technique. J. Bone Joint Surg., 41-B:36, 1959.

39. Brooks, D. M., and Zaoussis, A.: Arthrodesis of the shoulder in reconstructive surgery of paralysis of the upper limb. J. Bone Joint Surg., 41-B:207, 1959.

40. Buck-Gramcko, H.: Zur technik der intrartikularen Schultergelenksarthrosese. Z. Orthop., 91:198, 1959.

41. Bunnell, S.: Restoring flexion to the paralytic elbow. J. Bone Joint Surg., 33-A:566, 1951.

42. Burman, M.: Paralytic supination of the forearm. J. Bone Joint Surg., 38-A:303, 1956.

43. Caldwell, G. D.: Transplantation of the biceps femoris to the patella by the medial route in poliomyelitic quadriceps paralysis. J. Bone Joint Surg., 37-A:347, 1955.

44. Caldwell, G. D.: Correction of paralytic footdrop by hemigastrosoleus transplant. Clin. Orthop., 11:81, 1958.

45. Calmes, S. H.: Memories of polio. Arch. Intern. Med., 144:1273, 1984.

46. Campbell, W. C.: An operation for the correction of "drop-foot." J. Bone Joint Surg., 5:815, 1923.

47. Campbell, W. C.: End results of operation for correction of drop-foot. J.A.M.A., 85:1927, 1925.

48. Carayon, A., Bourrel, P., Bourges, M., and Touze, M.: Dual transfer of the posterior tibial and flexor digitorum longus tendons for drop foot. Report of thirty-one cases. J. Bone Joint Surg., 49-A:144, 1967.

49. Carmack, J. C., and Hallock, H.: Tibiotarsal arthrodesis after astragalectomy, a report of eight cases. J. Bone Joint Surg., 29:476, 1947.

50. Carroll, R. E.: Restoration of flexor power to the flail elbow by transplantation of the triceps tendon. Surg. Gynecol. Obstet., 95:685, 1952.

51. Carroll, R. E.: Restoration of elbow flexion by transplantation of the sternocleidomastoid muscle. Proceedings of the American Society of Surgery of the Hand. J. Bone Joint Surg., 44-A:1039, 1962.

52. Carroll, R. E., and Gartland, J. J.: Flexorplasty of the elbow. An evaluation of a method. J. Bone Joint Surg., 35-A:706, 1953.

53. Carroll, R. E., and Hill, N. A.: Triceps transfer to restore elbow flexion. J. Bone Joint Surg., 52-A:239, 1970.

54. C.D.S.C. Report: Outbreak of poliomyelitis in Finland. Br. Med. J. (Clin. Res.), 291:41, 1985.

55. Chambers, E. F. S.: Operation for correction of flexible flat feet in adolescents. West. J. Surg., 54:77, 1946.

56. Charnley, J.: Compression arthrodesis of the ankle and shoulder. J. Bone Joint Surg., 33-B:180, 1951.

57. Charnley, J.: Compression Arthrodesis. London, E. & S. Livingstone, 1953.

58. Charnley, J., and Houston, J. K.: Compression arthrodesis of the shoulder. J. Bone Joint Surg., 46-B:614, 1964.

59. Chaves, J. P.: Pectoralis minor transplant for paralysis of the serratus anterior. J. Bone Joint Surg., 33-B:228, 1951.

60. Chen, C. J., Lin, T. M., and You, S. L.: Epidemiological aspects of a poliomyelitis outbreak in Taiwan, 1982. Ann. Acad. Med. Singapore, 13:149, 1984.

61. Chigot, P. L., and Sananes, P.: Arthrodese de Grice. Variente technique. Rev. Chir. Orthop., 51:53, 1965.

62. Cholmeley, J. A.: Elmslie's operation for the calcaneus foot. J. Bone Joint Surg., 33-B:228, 1951.

63. Chuinard, E. G., and Peterson, R. E.: Distraction-compression bone-graft arthrodesis of the ankle. A method especially applicable for children. J. Bone Joint Surg., 45-A:481, 1963.

64. Clark, J. M. P.: Reconstruction of biceps brachii by pectoral muscle transplantation. Br. J. Surg., 34:180, 1946.

65. Clark, J. M. P., and Axer, A.: A muscle-tendon transportation for paralysis of the lateral abdominal muscles in poliomyelitis. J. Bone Joint Surg., 38-B:475, 1956.

66. Cleveland, M.: Operative fusion of the unstable or flail knee due to anterior poliomyelitis. A study of late results. J. Bone Joint Surg., 14:525, 1932.

67. Clippinger, F. W., Jr., and Irwin, C. E.: The opponens transfer, analysis of end results. South. Med. J., 55:33, 1962.

68. Close, J. R., and Todd, F. N.: The phasic activity of the muscles of the lower extremity and the effects of tendon transfer. J. Bone Joint Surg., *41-A*:189, 1959.
69. Codivilla, A.: Meine Erfahrugen uber Schnenverpflanzungen. Z. Orthop. Chir., *12*:221, 1904.
70. Conner, A. N.: The treatment of flexion contractures of the knee in poliomyelitis. J. Bone Joint Surg., *52-B*:138, 1970.
71. Coonrad, R. W., Irwin, C. E., Gucker, T., III, and Wray, J. B.: The importance of plantar muscles in paralytic varus feet. The results of treatment by neurectomy and myotenotomy. J. Bone Joint Surg., *38-A*:563, 1956.
72. Cravener, E. K.: Device for overcoming non-bony flexion contractures of the knee. J. Bone Joint Surg., *12*:437, 1930.
73. Crego, C. H., Jr., and Fischer, F. J.: Transplantation of the biceps femoris for the relief of quadriceps femoris paralysis in residual poliomyelitis. J. Bone Joint Surg., *13*:515, 1931.
74. Crego, C. H., Jr., and McCarroll, H. R.: Recurrent deformities in stabilized paralytic feet. A report of 1100 consecutive stabilizations in poliomyelitis. J. Bone Joint Surg., *20*:609, 1938.
75. Cross, A. B.: Crawling patterns in neglected poliomyelitis in the Solomon Islands. J. Bone Joint Surg., *59-B*:428, 1977.
76. Dalakas, M. C., Elder, G., Hallett, M., Ravits, J., Baker, M., Papadopoulos, N., Albrecht, P., and Sever, J.: A long-term follow-up study of patients with post-poliomyelitis neuromuscular symptoms. N. Engl. J. Med., *314*:959, 1986.
77. Davidson, W. D.: Traumatic deltoid paralysis treated by muscle transplantation. J.A.M.A., *106*:2237, 1936.
78. Davis, G. G.: Wedge-shaped resection of the foot for the relief of old cases of varus. N.Y. J. Med., *56*:379, 1892.
79. Davis, G. G.: The treatment of hollow foot (pes cavus). Am. J. Orthop. Surg., *11*:231, 1913.
80. Davis, J. B., and Cotrell, G. W.: A technique for shoulder arthrodesis. J. Bone Joint Surg., *44-A*:657, 1962.
81. Dehne, E., and Hall, R. M.: Active shoulder motion in complete deltoid paralysis. J. Bone Joint Surg., *41-A*:745, 1959.
82. Dekking, F.: Poliomyelitis in the Netherlands. Ned. Tijdschr. Geneeskd., *122*:1142, 1978.
83. Den Hartog, J. G.: Hip and knee flexion contracture after poliomyelitis. South. Med. J., *73*:694, 1980.
84. Dickson, F. D.: An operation for stabilizing paralytic hips: a preliminary report. J. Bone Joint Surg., *9*:1, 1927.
85. Dickson, F. D.: Fascial transplants in paralytic and other conditions. J. Bone Joint Surg., *19*:405, 1937.
86. Dickson, F. D., and Diveley, R. L.: Operation for correction of mild claw foot, the results of infantile paralysis. J.A.M.A., *87*:1275, 1926.
87. Dunne, J. W., Harper, C. G., and Hilton, J. M.: Sudden infant death syndrome caused by poliomyelitis. Arch. Neurol., *41*:775, 1984.
88. duToit, G. T., and Levy, S. J.: Transposition of latissimus dorsi for paralysis of the triceps brachii. Report of a case. J. Bone Joint Surg., *49-B*:135, 1967.
89. Drew, A. J.: The late results of arthrodesis of the foot. J. Bone Joint Surg., *33-B*:496, 1951.
90. Dunn, N.: Stabilizing operations in the treatment of paralytic deformities of the foot. Proc. R. Soc. Med. (Section of Orthopaedics), *15*:15, 1922.
91. Dunn, N.: Suggestion based on ten years' experience of arthrodesis of the tarsus in the treatment of deformities of the foot. *In* Robert Jones Birthday Volume. London, Oxford University Press, 1928, p. 395.
92. Durman, D. C.: An operation for paralysis of the serratus anterior. J. Bone Joint Surg., *27*:380, 1945.
93. Eaton, G. O.: Results of abdominal stabilization. South. Med. J., *34*:443, 1941.
94. Eberle, C. F.: Pelvic obliquity and the unstable hip after poliomyelitis. J. Bone Joint Surg., *64-B*:300, 1982.
95. Elkins, E. C., Janes, J. M., Henderson, E. D., and McLeod, J. J., Jr.: Peroneal translocation for paralysis of plantar flexor muscles. Surg. Gynecol. Obstet., *102*:469, 1956.
96. Elmslie, R. L.: *In* Turner, G. G. (ed.): Modern Operative Surgery. 2nd Ed. London, Cassell & Co., 1934.
97. Emmel, H. E., and LeCoco, J. R.: Hamstring transplant for the prevention of calcaneocavus foot in poliomyelitis. J. Bone Joint Surg., *40-A*:911, 1958.
98. Fernandez de Castro, J.: Mass vaccination against poliomyelitis in Mexico. Rev. Infect. Dis., *6*:397, 1984.
99. Fitchet, S. M.: "Flexion deformity" of the hip and the lateral intermuscular septum. N. Engl. J. Med., *209*:74, 1933.
100. Fitzgerald, F. P., and Seddon, H. J.: Lambrinudi's operation for drop-foot. Br. J. Surg., *25*:283, 1937.
101. Flexner, S., and Lewis, P. A.: Transmission of acute poliomyelitis to monkeys. J.A.M.A., *53*:1639, 1909.
102. Flint, M. H., and MacKenzie, I. C.: Anterior laxity of the ankle. A cause of recurrent paralytic drop foot deformity. J. Bone Joint Surg., *44-B*:377, 1962.
103. Forbes, A. M.: The tensor fasciae femoris as a cause of deformity. J. Bone Joint Surg., *10*:579, 1928.
104. Fried, A., and Hendel, C.: Paralytic valgus deformity of the ankle. Replacement of the paralyzed tibialis posterior by the peroneus longus. J. Bone Joint Surg., *39-A*:921, 1957.
105. Friedenberg, Z. B.: Arthrodesis of the tarsal bones. A study of failure of fusion. Arch. Surg., *57*:162, 1948.
106. Friedenberg, Z. B.: Transposition of the biceps brachii for triceps weakness. J. Bone Joint Surg., *36-A*:656, 1954.
107. Gaebler, J. W., Kleiman, M. B., French, M. L., Chastain, G., Barrett, C., and Griffin, C.: Neurologic complications in oral polio vaccine recipients. J. Pediatr., *108*:878, 1986.
108. Gill, A. B.: A new operation for arthrodesis of the shoulder. J. Bone Joint Surg., *13*:287, 1931.
109. Gill, A. B.: An operation to make a posterior bone block at the ankle to limit foot-drop. J. Bone Joint Surg., *15*:166, 1933.
110. Girard, P. M.: Ankle joint stabilization with motion. J. Bone Joint Surg., *17*:802, 1935.
111. Goldner, J. L.: Paralytic equinovarus deformities of the foot. South. Med. J., *42*:83, 1949.
112. Goldner, J. L., and Irwin, C. E.: Paralytic deformities of the foot. *In* A.A.O.S. Instructional Course Lectures. Vol. 5. Ann Arbor, J. W. Edwards, 1948.
113. Goldthwait, J. E.: Tendon transplantation in the treatment of deformities resulting from infantile paralysis. Boston Med. Surg. J., *133*:447, 1895.
114. Goldthwait, J. E.: The direct transplantation of muscles in the treatment of paralytic deformities. Five cases of transplantation of the sartorius muscle. Boston Med. Surg. J., *137*:489, 1897.
115. Goldthwait, J. E.: An operation for the stiffening of the ankle joint in infantile paralysis. Am. J. Orthop. Surg., *5*:271, 1908.
116. Green, W. T.: Tendon transplantation in rehabilitation. J.A.M.A., *163*:1235, 1957.
117. Green, W. T., and Grice, D. S.: The treatment of poliomyelitis: Acute and convalescent stages. A.A.O.S. Instructional Course Lectures. Vol. 13. Ann Arbor, J. W. Edwards, 1951, p. 261.
118. Green, W. T., and Grice, D. S.: The management of chronic poliomyelitis. A.A.O.S. Instructional Course Lectures. Vol. 9. Ann Arbor, J. W. Edwards, 1952.

119. Green, W. T., and Grice, D. S.: The surgical correction of the paralytic foot. A.A.O.S. Instructional Course Lectures. Vol. 10. Ann Arbor, J. W. Edwards, 1953, pp. 343–363.

120. Green, W. T., and Grice, D. S.: The management of calcaneus deformity. A.A.O.S. Instructional Course Lectures. Vol. 13. Ann Arbor, J. W. Edwards, 1956, pp. 135–149.

121. Grice, D. S.: An extra-articular arthrodesis of the subastragalar joint for correction of paralytic flat feet in children. J. Bone Joint Surg., 34-A:927, 1952.

122. Grice, D. S.: Further experience with extra-articular arthrodesis of the subtalar joint. J. Bone Joint Surg., 36-A:246, 1955.

123. Grice, D. S.: The role of subtalar fusion in the treatment of valgus deformities of the feet. Instructional Course Lect., 16:127, 1959.

124. Grilli, F. P.: Il trapianto del bicipite brachiale in funzione pronatoria. Arch. Putti, 12:359, 1959.

125. Grist, N. R.: Poliomyelitis vaccine precautions (Editorial). Br. Med. J. (Clin. Res.), 287:1823, 1983.

126. Grist, N. R., and Bell, E. J.: Paralytic poliomyelitis and nonpolio enteroviruses: studies in Scotland. Rev. Infect. Dis. (Suppl.), 2:385, 1984.

127. Groves, E. W. H.: Some contributions to the reconstructive surgery of the hip. Br. J. Surg., 14:486, 1927.

128. Guidal, P., and Sodeman, T.: Results of 256 tri-articular arthrodeses of the foot in sequelae of infantile paralysis. Acta Orthop. Scand., 1:199, 1930–1931.

129. Guillozet, N.: Perthes disease after poliomyelitis. Recognition and management of aseptic capital femoral necrosis. Clin. Pediatr., 20:19, 1981.

130. Gunn, D R., and Molesworth, B. D.: The use of tibialis posterior as a dorsiflexor. J. Bone Joint Surg., 39-B:674, 1957.

131. Haas, S. L.: The treatment of permanent paralysis of the deltoid muscle. J.A.M.A., 104:99, 1935.

132. Haas, S. L.: Correction of extreme flexion contracture of the knee joint. J. Bone Joint Surg., 20:839, 1938.

133. Hajar, M. M., Zeid, A. S., Saif, M. A., Parvez, M. A., Steinglass, R. C., and Crain, S.: Prevalence, incidence, and epidemiological features of poliomyelitis in the Yemen Arab Republic. Bull. WHO, 61:353, 1983.

134. Hallgrimsson, S.: Studies on reconstructive and stabilizing operations on the skeleton of the foot, with special reference to subastragalar arthrodesis in treatment of foot deformities following infantile paralysis. Acta Chir. Scand. (Suppl. 78), 88:1, 1943.

135. Hallock, H.: Surgical stabilization of dislocated paralytic hips: end-results study. Surg. Gynecol. Obstet., 75:742, 1942.

136. Hallock, H.: Arthrodesis of the hip for instability and pain in poliomyelitis. J. Bone Joint Surg., 2-A:904, 1950.

137. Hallock, H.: Hip arthrodesis in poliomyelitis. Bull. N.Y. Hosp., 2:18, 1958.

138. Hamsa, W. R.: Panastragaloid arthrodesis. A study of end-results in eighty-five cases. J. Bone Joint Surg., 18:732, 1936.

139. Harmon, P. H.: Anterior transplantation of the posterior deltoid for shoulder palsy and dislocation in poliomyelitis. Surg. Gynecol. Obstet., 84:117, 1947.

140. Harmon, P. H.: Technic of utilizing latissimus dorsi muscle in transplantation for triceps palsy. J. Bone Joint Surg., 31-A:409, 1949.

141. Harmon, P. H.: Surgical reconstruction of the paralytic shoulder by multiple muscle transplantation. J. Bone Joint Surg., 32-A:583, 1950.

142. Hart, V. L.: Corrective cast for flexion-contracture deformity of the knee. J. Bone Joint Surg., 16:970, 1934.

143. Hart, V. L.: Arthrodesis of the foot in infantile paralysis. Surg. Gynecol. Obstet., 64:794, 1937.

144. Hart, V. L.: Lambrinudi operation for drop-foot. J. Bone Joint Surg., 22:937, 1940.

145. Henderson, M. S.: Reconstructive surgery in paralytic deformities of the lower leg. J. Bone Joint Surg., 11:810, 1929.

146. Henry, A. H.: An operation for slinging a dropped shoulder. Br. J. Surg., 15:95, 1927.

147. Henry, A. H.: Extensile Exposure Applied to Limb Surgery. 2nd. Ed. Baltimore, Williams & Wilkins, 1957.

148. Herndon, C. H.: Tendon transplantation at the knee and foot. A.A.O.S. Instructional Course Lectures. Vol. 18. St. Louis, C. V. Mosby, 1961.

149. Herndon, C. H., Strong, J. M., and Heyman, C. H.: Transposition of the tibialis anterior in the treatment of paralytic talipes calcaneus. J. Bone Joint Surg., 38-A:751, 1956.

150. Herzmark, M. H.: Traumatic paralysis of the serratus anterior relieved by transplantation of the rhomboidei. J. Bone Joint Surg., 33-A:235, 1951.

151. Heydarian, K., Akbarnia, B. A., Jabalameli, M., and Tabador, K.: Posterior capsulotomy for the treatment of severe flexion contracture of the knee. J. Pediatr. Orthop., 4:700, 1984.

152. Heyman, C. H.: A method for the correction of paralytic genu recurvatum. Report of a bilateral case. J. Bone Joint Surg., 6:689, 1924.

153. Heyman, C. H.: Operative treatment of paralytic genu recurvatum. J. Bone Joint Surg., 29:644, 1947.

154. Heyman, C. H.: Operative treatment of paralytic genu recurvatum. J. Bone Joint Surg., 44-A:1246, 1962.

155. Hildebrandt, A.: Uber eine neue Methode der Muskel-transplantation. Arch. Klin. Chir., 78:75, 1906.

156. Hipps, H. E.: Clinical significance of certain microscopic changes in muscles of anterior poliomyelitis. J. Bone Joint Surg., 24:68, 1942.

157. Hogshead, H. P., and Ponseti, I. V.: Fascia lata transfer to the erector spinae for the treatment of flexion-abduction contractures of the hip in patients with poliomyelitis and meningomyelocele. Evaluation of results. J. Bone Joint Surg., 46-A:1389, 1964.

158. Hohmann, G.: Eratz des gelahmten Biceps brachii durch den Pectoralis major. Munchen Med. Wochenschr., 65:1240, 1918.

159. Hohmann, G.: Operative Verwertung erhaltener Muskeln bei kinderlahmung. Munchen Med. Wochenschr., 92:249, 1950.

160. Hoke, M.: An operation for stabilizing paralytic feet. Am. J. Orthop. Surg., 3:494, 1921.

161. Holmdahl, H. C.: Astragalectomy as a stabilizing operation for foot paralysis following poliomyelitis; results of a follow-up investigation of 153 cases. Acta Orthop. Scand., 25:207, 1956.

162. Hovnanian, A. P.: Latissimus dorsi transplantation for loss of flexion or extension at the elbow. Ann. Surg., 143:493, 1956.

163. Hsu, L. C., O'Brien, J. P., Yau, A. C. M. C., and Hodgson, A. R.: Batchelor's extra-articular subtalar arthrodesis. A report on sixty-four procedures in patients with poliomyelitis deformities. J. Bone Joint Surg., 58-A:243, 1977.

164. Hunt, J. C., and Brooks, A. L.: Subtalar extra-articular arthrodesis for correction of paralytic valgus deformity of the foot. Evaluation of forty-four procedures with particular reference to associated tendon transference. J. Bone Joint Surg., 47-A:1310, 1965.

165. Hunt, W. S., Jr., and Thompson, H. A.: Pantalar arthrodesis. A one-stage operation. J. Bone Joint Surg., 36-A:349, 1954.

166. Inclan, A.: End results in physiological blocking of flail joints. J. Bone Joint Surg., 31-A:748, 1949.

167. Ingersoll, R. E.: Transplantation of peroneus longus to anterior tibial insertion in poliomyelitis. Surg. Gynecol. Obstet., 86:717, 1948.

168. Ingram, A. J., and Hundley, J. M.: Posterior bone block of the ankle for paralytic equinus. An end-result study. J. Bone Joint Surg., 33-A:679, 1951.

169. Irwin, C. E.: Transplants to the thumb to restore function of opposition. End results. South. Med. J., 35:257, 1942.

170. Irwin, C. E.: Genu recurvatum following poliomyelitis: controlled method of operative correction. J.A.M.A., 120:277, 1942.

171. Irwin, C. E.: Subtrochanteric osteotomy in poliomyelitis. J.A.M.A., 133:231, 1947.

172. Irwin, C. E.: The iliotibial band, its role in producing deformity in poliomyelitis. J. Bone Joint Surg., 31-A:141, 1949.

173. Irwin, C. E., and Eyler, D. L.: Surgical rehabilitation of the hand and forearm disabled by poliomyelitis. J. Bone Joint Surg., 33-A:679, 1951.

174. Johnson, E. W., Jr.: Results of modern methods of treatment of poliomyelitis. J. Bone Joint Surg., 27:223, 1945.

175. Johnson, E. W., Jr.: Contractures of the iliotibial band. Surg. Gynecol. Obstet., 96:509, 1953.

176. Jones, G. B.: Paralytic dislocation of the hip. J. Bone Joint Surg., 36-B:375, 1954.

177. Jones, G. B.: Paralytic dislocation of the hip. J. Bone Joint Surg., 44-B:573, 1962.

178. Kettelkamp, D. B., and Larson, C. B.: Evaluation of the Steindler flexorplasty. J. Bone Joint Surg., 45-A:513, 1963.

179. Key, J. A.: Arthrodesis of the shoulder by means of osteoperiosteal grafts. Surg. Gynecol. Obstet., 50:468, 1930.

180. Khuri Bulos, N., Melnick, J. L., Hatch, M. H., and Dawood, S. T.: The paralytic poliomyelitis epidemic of 1978 in Jordan: epidemiological implications. Bull. WHO, 62:83, 1984.

181. King, B. B.: Ankle fusion for the correction of paralytic drop foot and calcaneus deformity. Arch. Surg., 40:90, 1940.

182. Kleinberg, S.: The transplantation of the adductor longus in its entirety to supplement the quadriceps femoris. Bull. Hosp. Joint Dis., 18:117, 1957.

183. Kreuscher, P. H.: The substitution of the erector spinae for paralyzed gluteal muscles. Surg. Gynecol. Obstet., 40:593, 1925.

184. Kuhlmann, R. F., and Bell, J. F.: A clinical evaluation of tendon transplantation for poliomyelitis affecting the lower extremities. J. Bone Joint Surg., 34-A:915, 1952.

185. Kumar, K., and Kapahtia, N. K.: The pattern of muscle involvement in poliomyelitis of the upper limb. Int. Orthop., 10:11, 1986.

186. Lambrinudi, C.: New operation on drop-foot. Br. J. Surg., 15:193, 1927.

187. Lambrinudi, C.: A method of correcting equinus and calcaneus deformities at the sub-astragaloid joint. Proc. R. Soc. Med. (Section of Orthopaedics), 26:788, 1933.

188. Landsteiner, K., and Popper, E.: Uberstragung der Poliomyelitis acuta auf Affen. Z. Immunitatsforsch. Exp. Ther. Orig., 2:377, 1909.

189. Lange, F.: Die epidemische Kinderlahmung. Munich, J. F. Lehmann, 1930.

190. Leavitt, D. G.: Subastragaloid arthrodesis for the os calcis type of flat foot. Am. J. Surg., 59:501, 1943.

191. LeCoeur, P.: Procedes de restauration de la flexion du coude paralytique. Rev. Chir. Orthop., 39:655, 1953.

192. Legg, A. T.: Transplantation of tensor fasciae femoris in cases of weakened gluteus medius. J.A.M.A., 80:242, 1923.

193. Legg, A. T.: Tensor fasciae femoris transplantation in cases of weakened gluteus medius. N. Engl. J. Med., 209:61, 1933.

194. Legg, A. T., and Merrill, J. T.: Physical Therapy in Infantile Paralysis. Hagerstown, Md., W. F. Prior Co., 1932.

195. Leong, J. C., Alade, C. O., and Fang, D.: Supracondylar femoral osteotomy for knee flexion contracture resulting from poliomyelitis. J. Bone Joint Surg., 64-B:198, 1982.

196. Leong, J. C., Wilding, K., Mok, C. K., Ma, A., Chow, S. P., and Yau, A. C. M. C.: Surgical treatment of scoliosis following poliomyelitis. A review of one hundred and ten cases. J. Bone Joint Surg., 63-A:726, 1981.

197. Lewis, D. D.: Trapezius transplantation in the treatment of deltoid paralysis. J.A.M.A., 55:2211, 1910.

198. Liebolt, F. L.: Pantalar arthrodesis in poliomyelitis. Surgery, 6:31, 1939.

199. Lipscomb, P. R., and Sanchez, J. J.: Anterior transplantation of the posterior tibial tendon for persistent palsy of the common peroneal nerve. J. Bone Joint Surg., 43-A:60, 1961.

200. Lorthioir, J.: Huit cas d'arthrodese du pied avec extirpation temporaire de l'astragale. J. Chir. Ann. Soc. Belge Chir., 11:184, 1911.

201. Lovett, R. W.: The Treatment of Infantile Paralysis. Philadelphia, P. Blakiston's Son & Co., 1916.

202. Lowman, C. L.: Abdominal Fascial Transplants. Privately printed. Los Angeles, 1954.

203. Lowman, C. L.: Fascial transplants in paralysis of abdominal and shoulder girdle muscles. A.A.O.S. Instructional Course Lectures. Vol. 14. Ann Arbor, J. W. Edwards, 1957, p. 300.

204. Lowman, C. L.: Fascial transplants in relation to muscle function. J. Bone Joint Surg., 45-A:199, 1963.

205. Lundbeck, H.: International symposium of poliomyelitis control. Strategies for control: a discussion. Rev. Infect. Dis. (Suppl.), 2:483, 1984.

206. MacAusland, W. R., and MacAusland, A. R.: Astragalectomy (the Whitman operation) in paralytic deformities of the foot. Ann. Surg., 80:861, 1924.

207. McFarland, B.: Paralytic instability of the foot (Editorial). J. Bone Joint Surg., 33-B:493, 1951.

208. MacKenzie, I. G.: Lambrinudi's arthrodesis. J. Bone Joint Surg., 41-B:738, 1959.

209. Macnicol, M. F., and Catto, A. M.: Twenty-year review of tibial lengthening for poliomyelitis. J. Bone Joint Surg., 64-B:607, 1982.

210. Magoflin, R. L., Lennette, E. H., Hollister, A. C., Jr., and Schmidt, N. J.: An etiology study of clinical paralytic poliomyelitis. J.A.M.A., 175:269, 1961.

211. Makin, M.: Tibiofibular relationship in paralyzed limbs. J. Bone Joint Surg., 47-B:500, 1965.

212. Makin, M.., and Yossipovich, Z.: Translocation of the peroneus longus in the treatment of paralytic pes calcaneus. A follow-up study of thirty-three cases. J. Bone Joint Surg., 48-A:1541, 1966.

213. Malvarez, O.: Arthrodesis subastragalina extraarticular en el pie valgo pronado pavalitico. Arthrodesis minima. Estudio de 87 casos. Rev. Ortop. Traum. Lat. Am., 2:251, 1957.

214. Marek, F. M., and Schein, A. J.: Aseptic necrosis of the astragalus following arthrodesing procedures of the tarsus. J. Bone Joint Surg., 27:587, 1945.

215. Mayer, L.: The physiological method of tendon transplantation. I. Historical: anatomy and physiology of tendons. Surg. Gynecol. Obstet., 22:182, 1916.

216. Mayer, L.: The physiological method of tendon transplantation. II. Operative technique. Surg. Gynecol. Obstet., 22:298, 1916.

217. Mayer, L.: The physiological method of tendon transplantation. III. Experimental and clinical experiences. Surg. Gynecol. Obstet., 221:472, 1916.

218. Mayer, L.: Transplantation of the trapezius for paralysis of the abductors of the arm. J. Bone Joint Surg., 9:412, 1927.

219. Mayer, L.: Fixed paralytic obliquity of the pelvis. J. Bone Joint Surg., 13:1, 1931.

220. Mayer, L.: Operative reconstruction of the paralyzed upper extremity. J. Bone Joint Surg., 21:377, 1939.

221. Mayer, L.: The significance of the iliocostal fascial graft in the treatment of paralytic deformities of the trunk. J. Bone Joint Surg., 26:257, 1944.

222. Mayer, L.: The physiologic method of tendon transplants. Reviewed after forty years. A.A.O.S. Instructional Course Lectures. Vol. 13. Ann Arbor, J. W. Edwards, 1956, p. 116.

223. Mayer, L., and Green, W.: Experience with the Steindler flexorplasty at the elbow. J. Bone Joint Surg., 36-A:775, 1954.

224. Mayer, T. R.: Duration of vaccine-induced poliomyelitis immunity. J. Fam. Pract., 19:385, 1984.

225. Maynard, F. M.: Post-polio sequelae—differential diagnosis and management. Orthopedics, 8:857, 1985.

226. Medin, O.: L'état aigu de la paralysie infantile. Arch. Med. Enf., 1:257, 1898.

227. Mertens, T., Schurmann, W., Kruppenbacher, J. P., Eggers, H. J., Rheingans, K., Kellermann, K., and Leidel, J.: Two cases of vaccine-induced poliomyelitis. Acta Paediatr. Scand., 73:133, 1984.

228. Miller, O. L.: Paralytic knee fusions. South. Med. J., 20:782, 1927.

229. Miller, O. L.: Surgical management of pes calcaneus. J. Bone Joint Surg., 18:169, 1936.

230. Mitchell, G. P.: Posterior displacement of poliomyelitis scoliosis. J. Bone Joint Surg., 59-B:233, 1977.

231. de Morais, J. C., Eduardo, M. B., Camargo, M. C., Correa, M. V., Alves, M. C., and Adorno, R. C.: Epidemiological course of poliomyelitis 1970–1981, in Sao Paulo. Rev. Paul Med., 99:34, 1982.

232. Mortens, J., and Pilcher, M. F.: Tendon transplantation in the prevention of foot deformities after poliomyelitis in children. J. Bone Joint Surg., 38-B:633, 1956.

233. Mortens, J., Gregersey, P., and Zachariae, L.: Tendon transplantation in the foot after poliomyelitis in children. Acta Orthop. Scand., 27:153, 1957–1958.

234. Moses, P. D., Pereira, S. M., John, T. J., and Steinhoff, M.: Poliovirus infection and Bell's palsy in children. Ann. Trop. Paediatr., 5:195, 1985.

235. Mustard, W. T.: Iliopsoas transfer for weakness of the hip abductors: preliminary report. J. Bone Joint Surg., 34-A:647, 1952.

236. Mustard, W. T.: A follow-up study of iliopsoas transfer for hip instability. J. Bone Joint Surg., 41-B:289, 1959.

237. Nicoladoni, C.: Nachtrag zum Pes calcaneus und zur Transplantation der Peronealschnen. Arch. Klin. Chir., 27:660, 1881.

238. Nieny, K.: Behandlung der Fussdeformation bei ausgedehnten Lahmungen. Arch. Orthop. Unfallchir., 3:60, 1905.

239. Nyholm, K.: Elbow flexorplasty in tendon transposition (an analysis of the functional results in 26 patients). Acta Orthop. Scand., 33:30, 1963.

240. Ober, F. R.: An operation for relief of paralysis of the gluteal maximus muscle. J.A.M.A., 88:1063, 1927.

241. Ober, F. R.: Operative and postoperative treatment of infantile paralysis. N. Engl. J. Med., 205:300, 1931.

242. Ober, F. R.: An operation to relieve paralysis of the deltoid muscle. J.A.M.A., 99:2182, 1932.

243. Ober, F. R.: Tendon transplantation in the lower extremity. N. Engl. J. Med., 209:52, 1933.

244. Ober, F. R.: The role of the iliotibial band and fascia lata as a factor in the causation of low back disabilities and sciatica. J. Bone Joint Surg., 18:105, 1936.

245. Ober, F. R.: Transplantation to improve the function of the shoulder joint and extensor function of the elbow joint. A.A.O.S. Lectures on Reconstructive Surgery. Vol. 2. Ann Arbor, J. W. Edwards, 1944, p. 274.

246. Ober, F. R., and Barr, J. S.: Brachioradialis muscle transposition for triceps weakness. Surg. Gynecol. Obstet., 67:105, 1938.

247. Paluska, D. J., and Blount, W. P.: Ankle valgus after the Grice subtalar stabilization: the late evaluation of a personal series with a modified technic. Clin. Orthop., 59:137, 1968.

248. Parekh, P. K.: Flexion contractures of the knee following poliomyelitis. Int. Orthop., 7:165, 1983.

249. Parsons, D. W., and Seddon, H. J.: The results of operations for disorders of the hip caused by poliomyelitis. J. Bone Joint Surg., 50-B:266, 1968.

250. Patterson, R. L., Parrish, F. F., and Hathaway, E. N.: Stabilizing operation on the foot. A study of the indications, techniques used and end results. J. Bone Joint Surg., 32-A:1, 1950.

251. Pauker, E.: Correction of the outwardly rotated leg from poliomyelitis. J. Bone Joint Surg., 41-B:70, 1959.

252. Peabody, C. W.: Tendon transposition: an end-result study. J. Bone Joint Surg., 20:193, 1938.

253. Peabody, C. W.: Tendon transposition in the paralytic foot. A.A.O.S. Instructional Course Lectures. Vol. 6. Ann Arbor, J. W. Edwards, 1949, p. 178.

254. Peabody, C. W., Draper, G., and Dochez, A. R.: A clinical study of acute poliomyelitis. Monograph No. 4. New York, Rockefeller Institute of Medical Research, 1912.

255. Perry, J., and Fleming, C.: Polio: Long-term problems. Orthopedics, 8:877, 1985.

256. Pollock, J. H., and Carrell, B.: Subtalar extra-articular arthrodesis in the treatment of paralytic valgus deformities. A review of 112 procedures in 100 patients. J. Bone Joint Surg., 46-A:533, 1964.

257. Pollock, L. J.: Accessory muscle movement in deltoid paralysis. J.A.M.A., 79:526, 1922.

258. Putti, V.: Rapporti statici fra piede e ginocchio nell'arto paralitico. Chir. Organi Mov., 6:125, 1922.

259. Putti, V.: Due sindromi paralitiche del'arto superiore Note di fisiopatologia della rotazione antibrachiale. Chir. Organi Mov., 26:215, 1940.

260. Pyka, R. A., Coventry, M. B., and Moe, J. H.: Anterior subluxation of the talus following triple arthrodesis. J. Bone Joint Surg., 46-A:16, 1964.

261. Rapp, I. H.: Serratus anterior paralysis by transplantation of pectoralis minor. J. Bone Joint Surg., 36A:852, 1954.

262. Reidy, J. A., Broderick, T. F., Jr., and Barr, J. S.: Tendon transplantation in the lower extremity. A review of end results in poliomyelitis. I. Tendon transplantation about the foot and ankle. J. Bone Joint Surg., 34-A:900, 1952.

263. Riedel, G.: Zur Frage der Muskeltransplantation bei Deltoides lahmung. Ergeb. Inn. Chir. Orthop., 21:489, 1928.

264. Riska, E. B.: Transposition of the tractus iliotibialis to the patella as a treatment of quadriceps paralysis and certain deformities of the lower extremity after poliomyelitis. Acta Orthop. Scand., 32:140, 1962.

265. Rissler, J.: Kenntnis der Veranderungen des Nervensystems bei Poliomyelitis anterior acuta. Nord. Med. Ark., 11:22:1, 1888.

266. Roundtree, C. R., and Rockwood, C. A., Jr.: Arthrodesis of the shoulder in children following infantile paralysis. South. Med. J., 52:861, 1959.

267. Rugtveit, A.: Extra-articular arthrodesis according to Green-Grice, in flat feet. Acta Orthop. Scand., 34:367, 1964.

268. Ryerson, E. W.: Arthrodesing operations on the feet. J. Bone Joint Surg., 5:453, 1923.

269. Sabin, A. B.: Pathology and pathogenesis of human poliomyelitis. J.A.M.A., 120:506, 1942.

270. Sabin, A. B.: Oral poliovirus vaccine. History of its development and prospects. Eradication of poliomyelitis. J.A.M.A., *194*:872, 1965.

271. Sabin, A. B.: Oral poliovirus vaccine: history of its development and use and current challenge to eliminate poliomyelitis from the world. J. Infect. Dis., *151*:420, 1985.

272. Sabin, A. B.: Strategy for rapid elimination and continuing control of poliomyelitis and other vaccine preventable diseases of children in developing countries. Br. Med. J. (Clin. Res.), *292*:531, 1986.

273. Sabin, A. B., Michaels, R. H., Spigland, I., Pelon, W., Rhim, J. A., and Wahr, R. E.: Community-wide use of oral poliovirus vaccine. Am. J. Dis. Child., *101*:546, 1961.

274. Saha, A. K.: Theory of Shoulder Mechanism: Descriptive and Applied. Springfield, Ill., Charles C Thomas, 1961.

275. Saha, A. K.: Surgical rehabilitation of paralyzed shoulder following poliomyelitis in adults and children. J. Int. Coll. Surg., *42*:198, 1964.

276. Saha, A. K.: Surgery of the paralyzed and flail shoulder. Acta Orthop. Scand., Suppl. 97, 1967.

277. Salk, J. E.: Studies in human subjects on active immunization against poliomyelitis. J.A.M.A., *151*:1081, 1953.

278. Sammons, J. H.: Polio—out of sight, out of mind (Editorial). J.A.M.A., *238*:2403, 1977.

279. Scheer, G. E., and Crego, C. H., Jr.: A two-stage stabilization procedure for correction of calcaneocavus. J. Bone Joint Surg., *38-A*:1247, 1956.

280. Schnute, W. J., and Tachdjian, M. O.: Intermetacarpal bone block for thenar paralysis following poliomyelitis. J. Bone Joint Surg., *45-A*:1663, 1963.

281. Schonberger, L. B., Kaplan, J., Kim Farley, R., Moore, M., Eddins, D. L., and Hatch M.: Control of paralytic poliomyelitis in the United States. Rev. Infect. Dis. (Suppl.), *2*:424, 1984.

282. Schottsdaedt, E. R., Larsen, L. J., and Bost, F. C.: Complete muscle transposition. J. Bone Joint Surg., *37-A*:897, 1955.

283. Schottstaedt, E. R., Larsen, L. J., and Bost, F. C.: The surgical reconstruction of the upper extremity paralyzed by poliomyelitis. J. Bone Joint Surg., *40-A*:633, 1958.

284. Schwartz, R. P.: Arthrodesis of subtalus and midtarsal joint of the foot; historical review, preoperative determinations, and operative procedures. Surgery, *20*:619, 1946.

285. Schwartzmann, J. R., and Crego, C. H., Jr.: Hamstring-tendon transplantation for the relief of quadriceps femoris paralysis in residual poliomyelitis. A follow-up study of 134 cases. J. Bone Joint Surg., *30-A*:541, 1948.

286. Seddon, H. J.: Transplantation of pectoralis major for paralysis of the flexors of the elbow. Proc. R. Soc. Med., *42*:837, 1949.

287. Segal, A., Seddon, H. J., and Brooks, D. M.: Treatment of paralysis of the flexors of the elbow. J. Bone Joint Surg., *41-B*:44, 1959.

288. Seymour, N., and Evans, D. K.: A modification of the Grice subtalar arthrodesis. J. Bone Joint Surg., *50-B*:374, 1968.

289. Sharp, N. N., Guhl, J. F., Sorensen, R. I., and Voshell, A. F.: Hip fusion in poliomyelitis in children. A preliminary report. J. Bone Joint Surg., *46-A*:121, 1964.

290. Sharrard, W. J. W.: Muscle recovery in poliomyelitis. J. Bone Joint Surg., *37-B*:63, 1955.

291. Siffert, R. S., Forster, R. I., and Nachamie, B.: "Beak" triple arthrodesis for correction of severe cavus deformity. *In* DePalma, A. F. (ed.): Clinical Orthopedics and Related Research. Vol. 45. Philadelphia, J. B. Lippincott, 1966.

292. Smith, A. deF., and Lackum, H. L.: Subastragaloid arthrodesis. Surg. Gynecol. Obstet., *40*:836, 1925.

293. Smith, E. T., Pevey, J. K., and Shindler, T. O.: The erector spinae transplant—a misnomer. Clin. Orthop., *30*:144, 1963.

294. Smith, J. B., and Westin, G.: Subtalar extra-articular arthrodesis. J. Bone Joint Surg., *50-A*:1027, 1968.

295. Somerville, E. W.: Paralytic dislocation of the hip. J. Bone Joint Surg., *41-B*:279, 1959.

296. Soule, R. E.: Further considerations of arthrodesis in the treatment of lateral deformity of the foot. Am. J. Orthop. Surg., *12*:422, 1915.

297. Soutter, R.: A new operation for hip contractures in poliomyelitis. Boston Med. Surg. J., *170*:380, 1914.

298. Spira, E.: The treatment of dropped shoulder; a new operative technique. J. Bone Joint Surg., *30-A*:220, 1948.

299. Spira, E.: Replacement of biceps brachii by pectoralis minor transplant. Report of a case. J. Bone Joint Surg., *39-B*:126, 1957.

300. Staples, O. S.: Posterior arthrodesis of the ankle and subtalar joints. J. Bone Joint Surg., *38-A*:50, 1956.

301. Staples, O. S., and Watkins, A. L.: Full active abduction in traumatic paralysis of deltoid. J. Bone Joint Surg., *25*:85, 1943.

302. Steigman, A. J.: The control of poliomyelitis. J. Pediatr., *59*:163, 1961.

303. Steindler, A.: A muscle plasty for the relief of flail elbow in infantile paralysis. Interstate Med. J., *25*:235, 1918.

304. Steindler, A.: Orthopedic reconstruction work on hand and forearm. N.Y. Med. J., *108*:1117, 1918.

305. Steindler, A.: Operative treatment of paralytic conditions of the upper extremity. J. Orthop. Surg., *1*:608, 1919.

306. Steindler, A.: The treatment of the flail ankle; panastragaloid arthrodesis. J. Bone Joint Surg., *5*:284, 1923.

307. Steindler, A.: Reconstructive Surgery of the Upper Extremity. New York, D. Appleton & Co., 1923, p. 56.

308. Steindler, A.: Orthopedic Operations. Indications, Technique, and End Results. Springfield, Ill., Charles C Thomas, 1940, p. 129.

309. Steindler, A.: Muscle and tendon transplantation at the elbow. A.A.O.S. Instructional Course Lectures on Reconstruction Surgery. Ann Arbor, J. W. Edwards, 1944, p. 276.

310. Steindler, A.: Newer pathological and physiological concepts of anterior poliomyelitis and their clinical interpretation. J. Bone Joint Surg., *29*:59, 1947.

311. Steindler, A.: Reconstruction of poliomyelitis upper extremity. Bull. Hosp. Joint Dis., *15*:21, 1954.

312. Storen, G.: Genu recurvatum. Treatment by wedge osteotomy of tibia with use of compression. Acta Chir. Scand., *114*:40, 1957.

313. Straub, L. R., Harvey, J. P., Jr., and Fuerst, C. E.: A clinical evaluation of tendon transplantation in the paralytic foot. J. Bone Joint Surg., *39-A*:1, 1957.

314. Sutherland, D. H., Bost, F. C., and Schottstaedt, E. R.: Electromyographic study of transplanted muscles about the knee in poliomyelitic patients. J. Bone Joint Surg., *42-A*:919, 1960.

315. Thomas, C. I., Thompson, T. C., and Straub, C. R.: Transplantation of the external oblique muscle for abductor paralysis. J. Bone Joint Surg., *32-A*:207, 1950.

316. Thompson, C. E.: Fusion of the metacarpals of the thumb and index finger to maintain functional position of the thumb. J. Bone Joint Surg., *24*:907, 1942.

317. Thompson, T. C.: Astragalectomy and the treatment of calcaneovalgus. J. Bone Joint Surg., *21*:627, 1939.

318. Thompson, T. C.: A modified operation for opponens paralysis. J. Bone Joint Surg., *24*:632, 1942.

319. Toupet, R.: Technique d'enchevillement du tarse,

realisant l'arthrodese de torsion et la limitation des movements d'extension du pied. J. Chir. (Paris), 16:268, 1920.

320. Towsend, W. R.: Treatment of the paralytic clubfoot by arthrodesis. Am. J. Orthop. Surg., 3:378, 1905.

321. Tubby, A. H.: A case illustrating the operative treatment of paralysis of serratus magnus by muscle grafting. Br. Med. J., 2:1159, 1904.

322. Underwood, M.: Treatise on Diseases of Children with General Directions of Infants from Birth. London, J. Churchill, 1789.

323. Von Baeyer, H.: Translokation von Schuen. Z. Orthop. Chir., 56:552, 1932.

324. Von Heine, J.: Beobachtungen uber Lahmungszustande der unteren Extremitaten und deren Behandlung. Stuttgart, Kohler, 1810.

325. Von Lesser, L.: Ueber operative Behandlung des Pes varus paralyticus. Zbl. Chir., 6:497, 1879.

326. Wagner, L. C.: Modified bone block (Campbell) of ankle for paralytic foot drop with report of twenty-seven cases. J. Bone Joint Surg., 13:142, 1931.

327. Wagner, L. C., and Rizzo, P. C.: Stabilization of the hip by transplantation of the anterior thigh muscles. J. Bone Joint Surg., 18:180, 1936.

328. Waterman, J. H.: Tendon transplantation. Its history, indications and technic. Med. News, 81:54, 1902.

329. Watkins, M. B., Jones, J. B., Ryder, C. T., Jr., and Brown, T. H., Jr.: Transplantation of the posterior tibial tendon. J. Bone Joint Surg., 36-A:1181, 1954.

330. Watson-Jones, R.: Extra-articular arthrodesis of the shoulder. J. Bone Joint Surg., 15:862, 1933.

331. Waugh, T. R., Wagner, J., and Stinchfield, F. E.: An evaluation of pantalar arthrodesis. A follow-up study of one hundred and sixteen operations. J. Bone Joint Surg., 47-A:1315, 1965.

332. Weissman, S. L.: Capsular arthroplasty in paralytic dislocation of the hip. A preliminary report. J. Bone Joint Surg., 41-A:429, 1959.

333. Weissman, S. L., Torok, G., and Kharmosh, D.: L'arthrodese extraarticulaire avec transplantation tendineuse concomitante dans le traitement du pied plat valgue paralytique de jeune enfant. Rev. Chir. Orthop., 43:79, 1957.

334. Westin, G. W.: Tendon transfer about the foot, ankle, and hip in the paralyzed lower extremity. (Instructional Course Lecture). J. Bone Joint Surg., 42-A:1430, 1965.

335. Whitman, A.: Astragalectomy and backward displacement of the foot. An investigation of its practical results. J. Bone Joint Surg., 4:266, 1922.

336. Whitman, R.: The operative treatment of paralytic talipes of the calcaneus type. Am. J. Med. Sci., 122:593, 1901.

337. Wickman, O. L.: Studien uber Poliomyelitis acuta. Arb. Path. Inst. Univ. Helsingfors. Berl., 1:109, 1905.

338. Willard, DeF. P.: Subastragalar arthrodesis in lateral deformities of paralytic feet. Am. J. Orthop. Surg., 14:323, 1916.

339. Williamson, G. A., Moe, J. H., and Basom, W. C.: Results of the Lowman operation for paralysis of the abdominal muscles. Minn. Med., 25:117, 1942.

340. Wilson, F. C., Jr., Fay, G. F., Lamotte, P., and Williams, J. C.: Triple arthrodesis. A study of the factors affecting fusion after three hundred and one procedures. J. Bone Joint Surg., 11:40, 1929.

341. Wilson, P. D.: Posterior capsulotomy in certain flexion contractures of the knee. J. Bone Joint Surg., 11:40, 1929.

342. Wright, P. F., Hatch, M. H., Kasselberg, A. G., Lowry, S. P., Wadlington, W. B., and Karzon, D. T.: Vaccine-associated poliomyelitis in a child with sex-linked agammaglobulinemia. J. Pediatr., 91:408, 1977.

343. Yadav, S. S.: Complete rotation of the leg with associated deformities in poliomyelitis. Clin. Orthop., 76:287, 1976.

344. Yadav, S. S.: Muscle transfer for abduction paralysis of the shoulder in poliomyelitis. Clin. Orthop., 135:121, 1978.

345. Yount, C. C.: The role of the tensor fasciae femoris in certain deformities of the lower extremities. J. Bone Joint Surg., 8:171, 1926.

346. Yount, C. C.: An operation to improve function in quadriceps paralysis. J. Bone Joint Surg., 20:314, 1938.

347. Zachariae, L.: The Grice operation for paralysis flat feet in children. Acta Orthop. Scand., 33:80, 1963.

348. Zancolli, E. A.: Paralytic supination contracture of the forearm. J. Bone Joint Surg., 40-A:1275, 1967.

349. Zaoussis, A. L.: Osteotomy of the proximal end of the radius for paralytic supination deformity in children. J. Bone Joint Surg., 45-B:523, 1963.

FRIEDREICH'S ATAXIA (HEREDITARY SPINOCEREBELLAR ATAXIA)[1-57]

In Friedreich's ataxia, the most common of the hereditary cerebellar ataxias, both the cerebellar and the spinal cord pathways are involved. In the spinal cord, there are degenerative changes of the dorsal and ventral spinocerebellar tracts, the corticospinal tracts, and the posterior column. The anterior horn cells are usually normal. In the cerebellum there is atrophy of the Purkinje's cells and the dentate nuclei. Changes in the brain stem may occur. Degeneration of the corticospinal tract may occasionally extend above the level of the medulla to involve the cerebral cortex.

The etiology of the disease is unknown. Males and females are affected equally. It is definitely hereditary and is commonly transmitted by an autosomal recessive gene; however, there is an autosomal dominant form. Often it can be traced through a number of generations. In some members of a family, it may occur only in the mild and incomplete form.

Clinical Features

The onset of symptoms is usually in childhood, between the ages of seven and ten years, but often is so insidious that it is difficult to determine when the condition was first present.

An unsteady gait is almost always the first symptom to attract attention. The child has a tendency to stagger and fall, has difficulty in making sudden turns, and is unable to keep pace with his playmates in motor activities. The unsteady gait is more marked in the dark. The child is clumsy. Over a period of years, these symptoms progress and ataxia of the upper limbs develops. Parents notice that the child cannot handle a fork or spoon without spilling the food. He has difficulty in learning to write.

The gait is unsteady and has a wide base. Heel-to-toe walking is usually impossible. The patient sways and reels and places the feet irregularly. Stance is unsteady and Romberg's sign is present. The ataxia is both spinal and cerebellar in type. There is always a greater degree of ataxia in the legs than in the upper limbs. Heel-to-shin ataxia and later finger-to-nose ataxia may be demonstrated. There is slowness of the alternating movements of the hands. Certain characteristic musculoskeletal deformities are observed. A slowly progressive scoliosis, usually in the thoracic region, is most common and is present in approximately 80 to 90 per cent of patients. The feet, as a rule, show symmetrical cavus deformity with marked elevation of the longitudinal arch, equinus deformity of the forefoot, and claw toes. Pes cavus may be the initial deformity prior to the development of any neurologic signs. The plantar fascia is contracted in about half the cases. Varus deformity is present with the pes cavus and increases the disability. In the early phases the cavus deformity is flexible and can be passively corrected by elevation of the metatarsal heads. Later, however, the deformity increases with growth and becomes fixed.

Muscle imbalance is an important factor in the pathogenesis of pes cavus. On muscle examination of 43 patients with Friedreich's ataxia, Makin found definite muscle weakness in 27 cases. Ten patients had normal musculature, and in six the muscle picture was unrecorded. Peroneal muscle weakness was the most common finding, either in isolated form or in combination with paresis of the anterior tibial.

Later in the course of the disease, the patient may have difficulty with writing and eating with a fork or spoon. Speech is often explosive, slurred, and staccato. Head tremor may be seen. Cranial nerves are normal; eventually, however, a horizontal or rotatory nystagmus develops.

The deep tendon reflexes—the knee and ankle jerks—in the lower limbs are usually absent very early in the course of the disease. Subsequently, the biceps and triceps jerks in the arms disappear. The plantar response is extensor, but this sign may be delayed for a few years.

On sensory examination, position and vibration sense and two-point discrimination are lost, initially in the feet and later in the hands. Touch, pain, and temperature modalities of sensation are preserved.

Tachycardia and evidence of cardiac failure develop eventually. Occasionally, optic atrophy may develop. On rare occasions, mentation may deteriorate. Diabetes mellitus occurs more commonly in patients with Friedreich's ataxia than in the normal population.

Diagnosis

The diagnosis is suggested when a child presents with pes cavus, scoliosis, signs of involvement of the spinocerebellar tracts of the spinal cord, and a positive family history of similar disorders.

Nerve conduction studies show slight decrease in motor fiber conduction velocity but marked decrease in sensory action potential. This finding distinguishes Friedreich's ataxia from hereditary motor sensory neuropathies—in the latter there is marked decrease in motor nerve conduction. Cardiac manifestations will further substantiate the likelihood of Friedreich's ataxia. In the electrocardiogram, conduction defects with bundle branch block or complete heart block may be seen as a result of myocardial fibrosis; the T-waves are inverted.

Radiograms of the spine will reveal the structural scoliosis. The cerebrospinal fluid findings are within normal limits. Muscle biopsy shows denervation atrophy with the finding of small and large fiber group atrophy. The differential diagnosis of chronic progressive ataxia is presented in Table 5–16.

Prognosis

The course of classic Friedreich's ataxia is steadily progressive to complete disability. Remissions are uncommon in Friedreich's ataxia. An early onset is a poor prognostic sign. The history of the course of the disease in other members of the family will aid in estimating the rate of progression. Ordinarily the age of onset and rate of progression are similar in the siblings. The ataxia is severe by the age of 20 years, and usually the patient is confined to a wheelchair by the age of 30 years. Scoliosis steadily increases with progression of the disease.

Death usually results from myocardial failure due to interstitial myocarditis or from respiratory infection. The average duration of the disease from its onset until death is 25 years, with death generally occurring before the age of 40 years. Abortive cases are not uncommon; the disease may become arrested at almost any stage or may have such a slow course that the patient will have a normal life span.

*Table 5–16. Differential Diagnosis of Chronic Progressive Ataxia**

Clinical Disorder	Preceding History	Usual Year of Onset in Children	Examination	Usual Laboratory Examination	Usual Prognosis
Arnold-Chiari malformation	Headache, dysphagia		Palatal and tongue weakness, pyramidal signs, ataxia	May have hydrocephalus, spina bifida	Slowly progressive; stationary after surgery
Hereditary spinocerebellar ataxia	Stumbling, dizziness, familial incidence	7–10	Ataxia, loss of position sense, extensor plantar responses, kyphoscoliosis, pes cavus	Occasional associated EKG changes	Progressive with death usually by 30 years of age
Bassen-Kornzweig syndrome	Fatty diarrhea at 6 weeks to 2 years of age	2–17	Cerebellar ataxia, posterior column signs, retinitis pigmentosa, scoliosis, pes cavus	Acanthocytosis, lack of beta-lipoprotein in serum	Slowly progressive
Dentate cerebellar ataxia	Myoclonus, convulsions	7–17	Ataxia with severe intention tremor		Slowly progressive
Hereditary cerebellar ataxia	Familial incidence	3–17	Ataxia, optic atrophy, occasionally associated posterior column and pyramidal tract signs	Pneumoencephalogram: small cerebellar folia	Slowly progressive
Ataxia telangiectasia	Recurrent sinopulmonary infections in ⅔ of cases; familial incidence	1–3	Oculocutaneous telangiectasia at 4 to 6 years; ataxia, choreoathetosis, dysarthria	Chest x-ray may reveal bronchiectasis	Death before 25 years of age
Cerebellar tumors	Headache, vomiting		Papilledema, ataxia, nystagmus	Skull x-rays: separation of sutures	Progressive until operation
Multiple sclerosis	Preceding neurologic symptoms	14–17	Optic neuritis; brain stem, cerebellar, pyramidal or sensory signs	Spinal fluid may reveal increased cells, protein or gamma globulin	Exacerbations and remissions
Spinal cord tumor	May have numbness or bladder disorder		Ataxia with weakness or sensory loss	Defect on myelography	Progressive until operation

*From Farmer, T. W.: Pediatric Neurology. New York, Hoeber Medical Division, Harper & Row, 1964, p. 525.

Treatment

There is no specific treatment for the fundamental disease process. Prevention and adequate correction of the foot deformity will aid in prolonging the period of ambulation and delay the day that the patient will eventually become wheelchair bound. Pes cavus is the most frequent deformity; its management is discussed in Chapter 7. Tendon transfers are occasionally performed on the hand to improve function. Spinal fusion for progressive scoliosis is often indicated, especially when the scoliosis is progressive and hinders cardiopulmonary function. Orthosis is not tolerated by patients with Friedreich's ataxia, and progression of scoliosis cannot be controlled by bracing.

Makin, in a review of the end results of operative procedures on 34 patients with Friedreich's ataxia with an average follow-up of 7.2 years, emphasized that structural foot deformities and instability often contribute to abnormalities of gait and stance, and that the correction of these deformities has a markedly beneficial effect on the ataxia.[31]

References

1. Ackroyd, R. S., Finnegan, J. A., and Green, S. H.: Friedreich's ataxia. A clinical review with neurophysiological and echocardiographic findings. Arch. Dis. Child., 59:217, 1984.
2. Allard, P., Dansereau, J., Duhaime, M., and Geoffroy, G.: Scoliosis assessment in Friedreich's ataxia by means of intrinsic parameters. Can. J. Neurol. Sci., 11:582, 1984.
3. Barbeau, A.: The Quebec Cooperative study of Friedreich's ataxia: 1974–1984—10 years of research. Can. J. Neurol. Sci., 11:646, 1984.
4. Barbeau, A., Roy, M., and Paris, S.: Hair trace elements in Friedreich's disease. Can. J. Neurol. Sci., 11:620, 1984.
5. Barbeau, A., Sadibelouiz, M., Roy, M., Lemieux, B., Bouchard, J. P., and Geoffroy, G.: Origin of Friedreich's disease in Quebec. Can. J. Neurol. Sci., 11:506, 1984.
6. Bell, C. F., Kelly, J. M., and Jones, R. S.: Anaesthesia for Friedreich's ataxia. Case report and review of the literature. Anaesthesia, 41:296, 1986.
7. Berg, R. A., Kaplan, A. M., Jarrett, P. B., and Molthan, M. E.: Friedreich's ataxia with acute cardiomyopathy. Am. J. Dis. Child., 134:390, 1980.
8. Billimoria, M., Allard, P., Sibille, J., Sirois, J. P., Duhaime, M., and Geoffroy, G.: A simple device to obtain reliable foot radiographs of ambulatory and nonambulatory Friedreich's ataxia patients. Can. J. Neurol. Sci., 11:574, 1984.
9. Bird, T. M., and Strunin, L.: Hypotensive anesthesia for a patient with Friedreich's ataxia and cardiomyopathy. Anesthesiology, 60:377, 1984.
10. Bouthillier, D., Nestruck, A. C., Milne, R., Sing, C. F., Barbeau, A., and Davignon, J.: Distribution of apolipoprotein E phenotypes in Friedreich's ataxia. Can. J. Neurol. Sci., 11:626, 1984.
11. Boyer, S. H., Chisholm, A. W., and McKusick, V. A.: Cardiac aspects of Friedreich's ataxia. Circulation, 25:493, 1962.
12. Caruso, G., Santoro, L., Perretti, A., Serienga, L., Crisci, C., Rango, M., Barbieri, F., and Filla, A.: Friedreich's ataxia: Electrophysiological and histological findings. Acta Neurol. Scand., 67:26, 1983.
13. Child, J. S., Perloff, J. K., Bach, P. M., Wolfe, A. D., Perlman, S., and Kark, R. A.: Cardiac involvement in Friedreich's ataxia: A clinical study of 75 patients. J. Am. Coll. Cardiol., 7:1370, 1986.
14. Duchenne, G. B.: Physiologie des Mouvements. Paris, J. B. Ballière et Fils, 1867.
15. Fehrenbach, R. A., Wallesch, C. W., and Claus, D.: Neuropsychologic findings in Friedreich's ataxia. Arch. Neurol., 41:306, 1984.
16. Firenze, C., Trovarelli, G., Gallai, V., De Medio, G. E., and Porcellati, G.: Abnormalities of the erythrocyte membrane phospholipids in Friedreich's ataxia. Acta Neurol. Scand., 70:197, 1984.
17. Friedreich, N.: Uber degenerative Atrophie der spinalen Hinterstrange. Virchow Arch. Path. Anat., 26:391; 27:1, 1863.
18. Haidvogi, M., and Zweymuller, E.: So-called Friedreich's foot (author's transl.). Klin. Paediatr., 189:302, 1977.
19. Harayama, H., and Miyatake, T.: Polyneuropathy: Friedreich's ataxia. Nippon Rinsho, 40:1521, 1982.
20. Hart, R. P., Henry, G. K., Kwentus, J. A., and Leshner, R. T.: Information processing speed of children with Friedreich's ataxia. Dev. Med. Child Neurol., 28:310, 1986.
21. Hartman, J. M., and Booth, R. W.: Friedreich's ataxia. A neurocardiac disease. Am. Heart J., 60:716, 1960.
22. Heck, A. F.: A study of neural and extraneural findings in a large family with Friedreich's ataxia. J. Neurol. Sci., 1:226, 1961.
23. Hensinger, R. N., and MacEwen, G. D.: Spinal deformity associated with heritable neurological conditions: Spinal muscular atrophy, Friedreich's ataxia, familial dysautonomia and Charcot-Marie-Tooth disease. J. Bone Joint Surg., 58-A:13, 1976.
24. Hewer, R. L.: Study of fatal cases of Friedreich's ataxia. Br. Med. J., 3:649, 1968.
25. Huxtable, R. J., Johnson, P., and Lippincott, S. E.: Free amino acids and calcium, magnesium and zinc levels in Friedreich's ataxia. Can. J. Neurol. Sci., 11:616, 1984.
26. Labelle, H., Tohme, S., Suhaime, M., and Allard, P.: Natural history of scoliosis in Friedreich's ataxia. J. Bone Joint Surg., 68-A:564, 1986.
27. Lamarche, J. B., Lemieux, B., and Lieu, H. B.: The neuropathology of "typical" Friedreich's ataxia in Quebec. Can. J. Neurol. Sci., 11:592, 1984.
28. LaPresle, J.: Contribution a l'étude de la dystasie areflexique hereditaire. Etat actuel de quatre des sept cas princeps de Roussy et Mlle. Levy, trente ans après la premiere publication de ces auteurs. Sem. Hop. Paris, 32:2473, 1956.
29. Lemieux, B., Giguere, R., Barbeau, A., Melancon, S., and Shapcott, D.: Taurine in cerebrospinal fluid in Friedreich's ataxia. Can. J. Neurol. Sci., 5:125, 1978.
30. Lemieux, B., Giguere, R., and Shapcott, D.: Studies on the role of taurine in Friedreich's ataxia. Can. J. Neurol. Sci., 11:610, 1984.
31. Makin, M.: The surgical treatment of Friedreich's ataxia. J. Bone Joint Surg., 35-A:425, 1953.
32. Melancon, S. B., Cloutier, R., Potier, M., Dallaire, L., Vanasse, M., Geoffroy, G., and Barbeau, A.: Friedreich's ataxia: malic enzyme activity in cellular fractions of cultured skin fibroblasts. Can. J. Neurol. Sci., 11:637, 1984.
33. Millichap, J. G.: Friedreich's ataxia forme fruste and elevated creatine phosphokinase in a child with pseudohypoparathyroidism. Childs Brain, 6:170, 1980.
34. Nestruck, A. C., Huang, Y. S., Eid, K., Dufour, R., Boulet, L., Barbeau, A., and Davignon, J.: Plasma

cholesteryl sulfate in Friedreich's ataxia. Can. J. Neurol. Sci., 11:631, 1984.

35. Pelosi, L., Fels, A., Petrillo, A., Senatore, R., Russo, G., Lonegren, K., Calace, P., and Caruso, G.: Friedreich's ataxia: clinical involvement and evoked potentials. Acta Neurol. Scand., 70:360, 1984.

36. Pentland, B., and Fox, K. A.: The heart in Friedreich's ataxia. J. Neurol. Neurosurg. Psychiatry, 46:1138, 1983.

37. Podolsky, S., Pothier, A., Jr., and Krall, L. P.: Association of diabetes mellitus and Friedreich's ataxia. A study of two siblings. Arch. Intern. Med., 114:533, 1964.

38. Quebec Cooperative Study on Friedreich's Ataxia. Can. J. Neurol. Sci., 11:501, 1984.

39. Robinson, N.: An enzyme study of the myocardium in Friedreich's ataxia. Neurology, 16:1135, 1966.

40. Rodrigue, F., Belanger, F., van Gelder, N. M., and Barbeau, A.: Platelet taurine content in Friedreich's disease. Can. J. Neurol. Sci., 11:607, 1984.

41. Rodriguez-Budelli, M., and Kark, P.: Kinetic evidence for a structural abnormality of lipoamide dehydrogenase in two patients with Friedreich's ataxia. Neurology, 28:1283, 1978.

42. Rombold, C. R., and Riley, H. A.: The abortive type of Friedreich's disease. Arch. Neurol. Psychiatry, 16:301, 1926.

43. Romeo, G., Menozzi, P., Ferlini, A., Fadda, S., Di Donato, S., Uziel, G., Lucci, B., Capodaglio, L., Filla, A., and Campanella, G.: Incidence of Friedreich's ataxia in Italy estimated from consanguineous marriages. Am. J. Hum. Genet., 35:523, 1983.

44. Roth, M.: On a possible relationship between hereditary ataxia and peroneal muscular atrophy. With a critical review of the problem of "intermediate forms" in the degenerative disorders of the central nervous system. Brain, 71:416, 1948.

45. Roussy, G., and Levy, G.: Sept cas d'une maladie familiale particulaire; Troubles de la marche, pieds, bots et areflexie tendineuse generalisee, avec accessoirement, legrere maladresse des mains. Rev. Neurol. (Paris), 45:427, 1926.

46. Salisachs, P., Findley, L. J., Codina, M., La Torre, P., and Martinez-Lage, J. M.: A case of Charcot-Marie-Tooth disease mimicking Friedreich's ataxia: is there any association between Friedreich's ataxia and Charcot-Marie-Tooth disease? Can. J. Neurol. Sci., 9:99, 1982.

47. Saunders, J. T.: Etiology and treatment of clawfoot. Arch. Surg., 30:179, 1935.

48. Shapcott, D., Giguere, R., and Lemieux, B.: Zinc and taurine in Friedreich's ataxia. Can. J. Neurol. Sci., 11:623, 1984.

49. Sohi, G. S., Drake, C., and Flowers, N. C.: Friedreich's ataxia associated with hypertrophic cardiomyopathy and coronary vasospasm. Clin. Cardiol., 8:537, 1985.

50. Spillane, J. D.: Familial pes cavus and absent tendon jerks. Its relationship with Friedreich's disease and peroneal muscular atrophy. Brain, 63:275, 1940.

51. Steinsapir, K., and Lewis, W.: Dilated cardiomyopathy associated with Friedreich's ataxia. Arch. Pathol. Lab. Med., 109:454, 1985.

52. Sylvester, P. E.: Some unusual findings in a family with Friedreich's ataxia. Arch. Dis. Child., 33:217, 1958.

53. Symonds, C. P., and Shaw, M. E.: Familial claw-foot with absent tendon jerks. Brain, 49:387, 1926.

54. Therriault, L., Lamoureux, G., Cote, M., Plourde, G., and Lemieux, B.: The cardiomyopathy in Friedreich's ataxia: isotopic ventriculography and myocardial imaging with thallium-201. Can. J. Neurol. Sci., 11:588, 1984.

55. Thilenius, O. G., and Grossman, B. J.: Friedreich's ataxia with heart disease in children. Pediatrics, 27:246, 1961.

56. Yudell, A., Dyck, P. J., and Lambert, E. H.: A kinship with Roussy-Levy syndrome. Arch. Neurol., 13:432, 1965.

57. Zimmermann, M., Gabathuler, J., Adamec, R., and Pinget, L.: Unusual manifestations of heart involvement in Friedreich's ataxia. Am. Heart J., 111:184, 1986.

Affections of the Peripheral Nerves
Developmental and Degenerative Disorders

HEREDITARY MOTOR AND SENSORY NEUROPATHIES

Hereditary motor and sensory neuropathies (HMSN) are a heterogeneous group of familial distal muscular atrophy and weakness with relatively minor sensory deficit. These neuropathies are slowly progressive, but expectancy for life is normal. Females are more severely affected than males.

Classification

Based upon clinical, genetic, electrophysiologic, and neuropathologic criteria, Dyck and Lambert gave the following useful classification of hereditary peripheral neuropathies.[30, 31]

HMSN Type I. This is the form of Charcot-Marie-Tooth disease that is autosomal dominant in inheritance; has uniformly slow (half of normal) motor nerve conduction velocity (NCV); and exhibits hypertrophic changes—"onion bulb" formation—of the nerves on biopsy. HMSN Type I has, at present, at least two subgroups: HMSN *Type I-A* is not linked to the Duffy blood group focus on chromosome 1, in which the motor NCV is intermediately slow and moderate "onion bulb" changes are revealed on nerve biopsy. HMSN *Type I-B* is linked to Duffy blood group on chromosome 1, in which the motor NCV is very slow and the "onion bulb" changes on neural biopsy are very prominent. These two subgroups of HMSN are not allelic and represent mutations at separate genetic foci.[6] The Roussy-Lévy syndrome on neuropathologic and electrophysiologic grounds is included in the large group of HMSN Type I; it is not considered to be a separate entity.[5]

HMSN Type II is the neuronal form of Charcot-Marie-Tooth disease that is also inherited as an autosomal dominant trait, but the motor nerve conduction velocity is normal or slightly decreased, and on nerve biopsy hypertrophic changes are less pronounced.

HMSN Type III is Dejerine-Sottas disease—the familial hypertrophic interstitial neuritis of infancy and childhood. It is inherited as an autosomal recessive trait; the motor nerve conduction velocity is markedly slow, and nerve biopsy shows "onion bulb" formation with frequent segmental demyelinization.

HMSN Type IV is Refsum's disease. It is inherited as an autosomal recessive trait. Motor nerve conduction is slow, and nerve histology shows "onion bulb" formation. It is characterized by the serum elevation of phytanic acid.

HMSN Type V manifests as spastic paraplegia. Its inheritance is autosomal dominant. Electromyographic (EMG) and pathologic changes show the peripheral neuropathic nature of the disease.

HMSN Type VI is similar to Type I, but in addition it is characterized by optic atrophy.

HMSN Type VII comprises Type I patients who also have retinitis pigmentosa.

PERONEAL MUSCULAR ATROPHY (CHARCOT-MARIE-TOOTH DISEASE; HEREDITARY AND SENSORY NEUROPATHY TYPE I AND TYPE II)

Peroneal muscular atrophy of Charcot-Marie-Tooth may be defined as a hereditary and familial degenerative disorder of the peripheral nerves, the motor nerve roots, and frequently, the spinal cord. The process is slowly progressive and begins in the feet and legs and spreads to the hands and forearms after a lapse of several years. It is characterized by atrophy of certain muscle groups, particularly the peroneals and the intrinsic musculature of the hands and feet.

The condition was described in 1886, almost simultaneously, by Charcot and Marie of France and Tooth of England.[17, 18, 92] It was first considered to be a myopathy; however, Tooth and later Hoffmann emphasized its neuritic features.[49, 92] The radicular pathology was pointed out by England and Denny-Brown, who showed the pattern of sensory loss.[37] Herringham, in 1889, reported a study of four generations in one family in which only males were affected, stressing the hereditary aspects.[48]

Incidence

Its incidence is highly variable. In some geographic areas it is rare, with only one or two cases per year seen in large neurologic clinics, whereas in others it is one of the more common of the degenerative diseases of the peripheral nervous system. Boys are affected more frequently than girls. According to Jacobs and Carr, blacks appear to be exempt from Charcot-Marie-Tooth disease.[53]

Inheritance

HMSN Types I and II are inherited as an autosomal dominant trait. Sporadic cases do occur.

Pathology

The peripheral nerves and motor nerve roots show degenerative changes with loss of myelin and fragmentation of axis cylinders. In HMSN Type I, nerve biopsy (lateral sural) shows hypertrophic changes with "onion bulb" formation, which is histologic evidence of repetitive demyelinization and remyelinization. In Type II HMSN there are neuronal degenerative changes with minimal hypertrophy.

In the spinal cord, there may be secondary loss of anterior horn cells and degeneration of posterior roots and posterior columns. There is disagreement as to whether other spinal tracts are involved. Occasionally, degenerative changes occur in the lateral funiculi, which are not explainable on the basis of changes secondary to primary nerve root or peripheral nerve degeneration.

The muscle biopsy shows neuronal atrophy with changes in fiber-type groupings and blastic proliferation and infiltration of fat cells.

Clinical Picture

The age of onset of symptoms varies between Type I and Type II HMSN. In Type I it is between 5 and 15 years (usually the second decade of life), whereas in Type II it is usually deferred to the third decade of life. The type of Charcot-Marie-Tooth disease that the pediatric orthopedic surgeon encounters is motor sensory neuropathy Type I.

The presenting complaints may be muscle cramps in the legs and feet, abnormal shoe wear, difficulty in running on uneven ground, or discomfort under the metatarsal heads on prolonged standing or walking. Occasionally the patients complain of paresthesia in the legs.

The initial deformity is mild cavus of the foot with clawing of the toes. Gradually the cavus deformity of the foot and clawing of the toes increase in severity (Fig. 5–178).

The muscular atrophy is symmetrical and distal in distribution. The paralysis is flaccid, with fascicular twitchings often present in the wasting muscles. The peroneals and intrinsic muscles of the feet are affected first. As a result of muscular imbalance, pes cavovarus is the early deformity. Later, the atrophy spreads to the anterior compartment, involving the anterior tibial and the toe extensor muscles (Fig. 5–179). Equinus deformity of the forefoot and ankle gradually develops. The patient walks with a toe-heel gait. With steady progression of the disease, the gastrocnemius and other calf muscles are eventually atrophied. In Type II HMSN, early onset of paralysis of the triceps surae muscle causes calcaneus deformity of the ankle. The resultant foot deformity is calcaneocavovarus rather than cavovarus as in Type I.

The balance of the patient in stance and gait is unstable because of muscle weakness of the legs, foot deformity, and decreased proprioception. The patient may shift his feet or hold onto stationary objects in order to compensate for the decreased proprioception. Another mechanism is knee flexion, as this will activate the proprioceptive sensation of the knee joint itself and also lower the center of body gravity.

The upper limbs are involved at a later stage. In most cases, by the time there is atrophy of the calves, symmetrical atrophy of the intrinsic muscles of the hand and the forearm develops. The characteristic deformity of the hands is one of mild clawing, which becomes quite marked in severe cases. Opposition of the thumb may be lost. The patient develops progressive difficulty with fine motor activities. Upper limb involvement is less severe in Type II than in Type I. The pelvic and shoulder girdle musculatures and the muscles of the arms and thighs are usually not affected, and the face and trunk musculatures are practically always spared. Therefore, in the moderately advanced case, the legs, feet, forearms, and hands are wasted and very slender, whereas there is normal development of the thighs and upper arms. The contrast between the plump thighs and the slender legs with clawed toes gives the characteristic appearance of an inverted champagne bottle, which has been termed "ostrich legs." Weakness of the lower limb muscles is more pronounced in Type II HMSN than in Type I; therefore, the classic "stork leg" appearance is more commonly seen in Type II.

The deep tendon reflexes are decreased or absent. The ankle jerk is the first to be involved, followed by the radial periosteal reflex when the upper limbs are affected. The patellar, biceps, and triceps reflexes are usually preserved.

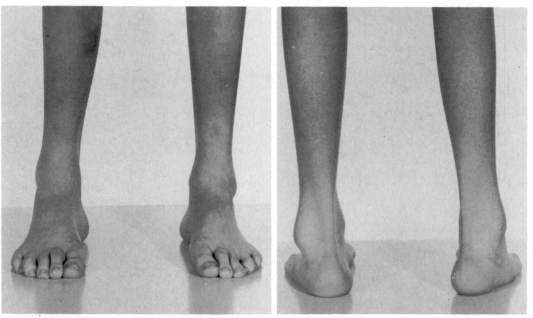

FIGURE 5–178. Charcot-Marie-Tooth disease.

Moderate varus and slight equinus deformity of both feet result from atrophy of peroneal, anterior tibial, and toe extensor muscles.

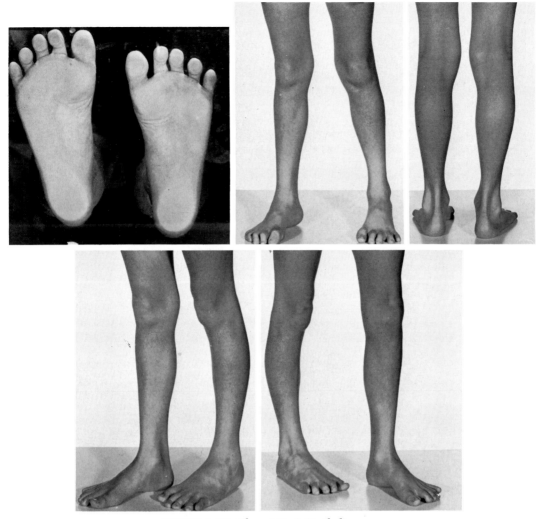

FIGURE 5–179. *Charcot-Marie-Tooth disease.*

There is moderate pes cavus deformity. Note the beginning of development of claw toes.

Sensory examination may reveal diminution in vibration and position senses, and in some cases, definite areas of hypoesthesia. Ataxia is not present. Sphincter tone is normal. Intelligence is not affected. The condition progresses slowly, with normal life expectancy. The patients are often ambulatory, and in many instances remain remarkably free of serious disability until well past the fourth decade of life.

Spinal deformity develops in 10 per cent of the cases of Charcot-Marie-Tooth disease. The scoliosis is usually mild to moderate and does not require surgical treatment.[24, 47]

Diagnosis

Peroneal muscular atrophy of Charcot-Marie-Tooth disease is suggested by the findings of (1) weakness and atrophy that begin in the peroneal group of muscles and extend slowly to other muscles of the anterior tibial compartment, intrinsic muscles of the hand, and muscles of the forearm, with the relative sparing of the muscles of the thigh and upper arm; (2) the slow course of the disease; and (3) the positive family history.

Motor nerve conduction velocity of peripheral nerve is slow (half of normal) in Type I, whereas it is either slightly reduced or normal in Type II.[34, 41]

Dyck, Lambert, and Mulder studied a total of 157 members of a family with peroneal muscular atrophy; 103 of these had neurologic examinations and studies of nerve conduction. Each of the 16 persons who showed definite evidence of Charcot-Marie-Tooth disease on clinical examination also had low conduction velocity of the peripheral motor nerves. In addition, seven persons who showed no certain clinical evidence of the disease had low conduction velocity. The investigators concluded that determination of conduction velocity was a valuable method for identifying carriers of the disease trait, at least in this family.[32]

The cerebrospinal fluid findings are normal, although occasionally the protein content may be slightly elevated. The electromyogram will disclose reduction of electrical reactions.

In the differential diagnosis, one should consider distal muscular dystrophy and various forms of HMSN—specifically Déjerine-Sottas hypertrophic interstitial neuritis and Refsum's disease, Roussy-Lévy syndrome, and Friedreich's ataxia.

Roussy-Lévy syndrome, characterized by familial bilateral pes cavus and absence of deep tendon reflexes, is very similar to peroneal muscular atrophy.[58, 74, 75, 97] Symonds and Shaw expressed the view that it is a forme fruste of Charcot-Marie-Tooth disease. Motor nerve conduction velocity is low in both conditions. Static tremor of the hands is the distinguishing feature of Roussy-Lévy syndrome. Cerebellar signs are absent.[90]

Friedreich's ataxia is characterized by the presence of cerebellar signs, speech disturbance, nystagmus, and positive Babinski response.

Treatment

In the early stages, treatment consists of passive stretching exercises and splinting the feet and legs at night in a neutral position to prevent the development of fixed deformities of pes varus, equinovarus, or cavus. Active exercises to maintain the strength of the weakened peroneals, toe extensors, and anterior tibial muscles are performed several times a day. Muscle testing at periodic intervals is essential to record the progress of the disease.

In the advanced case, properly chosen surgical procedures can correct and prevent deformities. Often, functional disability can be substantially diminished.[53, 56] The type of operation depends upon the muscle picture and the severity of foot deformity. When the peroneal muscles are of trace or zero strength, the anterior tibials are fair plus or good, and the posterior calf muscles are good or normal, the indicated procedure is anterior transfer of the posterior tibial tendon through the interosseous route to the base of the third metatarsal and the lateral transfer of the anterior tibial to the base of the second metatarsal. If the anterior tibial is weaker than fair in motor strength, the posterior tibial muscle only is transferred anteriorly through the interosseous route to the base of the third metatarsal.

Triple arthrodesis is performed to stabilize the hindfoot and to correct the cavovarus deformity. Plantar fasciotomy is performed if the fascia is contracted. It is best to correct equinus deformity by wedging casts rather than by lengthening the tendo Achillis.

References

1. Alajonanine, T. H., Castaigne, P., Cambier, J., and Escourolle, R.: Maladie de Charcot-Marie. Presse Med., 75:2745, 1967.
2. Allan, W.: Relation of hereditary pattern to clinical severity as illustrated by peroneal atrophy. Arch. Intern. Med., 63:1123, 1939.
3. Amick, L. D., and Lemmi, H.: Electromyographic studies in peroneal muscular atrophy (Charcot-Marie-Tooth disease). Arch. Neurol., 9:273, 1963.
4. Baker, R. S., and Upton, A. R.: Variation of phenotype in Charcot-Marie-Tooth disease. Neuropaeditrie, 10:290, 1979.
5. Barbieri, F., Filla, A., Ragno, M., Crisci, C., Santoro, L., Corona, M., and Campanella, G.: Evidence that Charcot-Marie-Tooth disease with tremor coincides with the Roussy-Lévy syndrome. Can. J. Neurol. Sci. (Suppl.), 4:534, 1984.
6. Bird, T., Ott, J., Giblett, E. R., Chance, P. F., Sumi, S. M., and Kraft, G. H.: Genetic linkage evidence for heterogeneity in Charcot-Marie-Tooth neuropathy (HMSN type I). Ann. Neurol., 14:679, 1983.
7. Blom, S., Hagbarth, K. F., and Lundberg, P. O.: Motor conduction velocities in amyotrophic lateral sclerosis, polyradiculoneuritis and Charcot-Marie-Tooth disease. Acta Neurol. Scand., 40:6, 1964.
8. Bourguignon, G.: Association of Friedreich's disease and atrophy of Charcot-Marie type. Rev. Neurol., 83:284, 1950.
9. Brihaye, M., Nenquin-Klaasen, E., and Berthdet, G.: Neurogenic muscular atrophy of Charcot-Marie-Tooth. Hoffman type combined with bilateral optic atrophy. Acta Neurol. Belg., 56:302, 1956.
10. Broda, A., and Refsum, S.: Progressive neural muscular atrophy. Acta Psychiatr. Neurol., 17:99, 1942.
11. Broda, A., Boyerson, S., and Frovig, A. G.: Progressive neuropathic atrophy (Charcot-Marie-Tooth). A.M.A. Arch. Neurol. Psychiatr., 70:1, 1953.
12. Brody, L. A., and Wilkins, R. H.: Charcot-Marie-Tooth disease. Arch. Neurol., 17:552, 1967.
13. Buchthal, F., and Pinelli, P.: Action potentials in muscular atrophy of neurogenic origin. Neurology, 3:591, 1953.
14. Bulgarelli, R., and Leva, R.: Are Friedreich, Charcot-Marie-Tooth and Dejerine-Sottas diseases distinct nosologic entities? Minerva Pediatr., 6:497, 1954.
15. Caccia, M. R.: Study of the dispersion of motor nerve conduction in Charcot-Marie-Tooth-Hoffmann disease and in the Steinert syndrome. Electromyogr. Clin. Neurophysiol., 12:91, 1972.
16. Carroll, W. M., Jones, S. J., and Halliday, A. M.: Visual evoked potential abnormalities in Charcot-Marie-Tooth disease and comparison with Friedreich's ataxia. J. Neurol. Sci., 61:123, 1983.
17. Charcot, J. M., and Marie, P.: Sur une forme particulaire d'atrophie musculaire progressive, souvent familiale, debutant par les pieds et les jambes et atteignant plus tard les mains. Rev. Med. (Paris), 6:97, 1886.

18. Charcot, J. M., and Marie, P.: Progressive muscular atrophy. Often familial, starting in the feet and legs and later reaching the hands. Arch. Neurol., *17*:553, 1967.

19. Christiaens, L., Poingt, O., and Farriaux, J. P.: Charcot-Marie disease in a four-year-old. Lille Med., *8*:513, 1963.

20. Christie, B. G.: Electrodiagnostic features of Charcot-Marie-Tooth disease. Proc. R. Soc. Med., *54*:321, 1961.

21. Cornell, J., Sellars, S., and Beighton, P.: Autosomal recessive inheritance of Charcot-Marie-Tooth disease associated with sensorineural deafness. Clin. Genet., 25:163, 1984.

22. Crank, H. H., and Reider, N.: Genetic features in the Charcot-Marie-Tooth type of muscular atrophy. Bull. Menninger Clin., *3*:88, 1939.

23. Currie, R. A.: Case of the Charcot-Marie-Tooth type of muscular atrophy with a note on the condition of the bones. Glasgow Med. J., *107*:28, 1927.

24. Daher, Y. H., Lonstein, J. E., Winter, R. B., and Bradford, D. S.: Spinal deformities in patients with Charcot-Marie-Tooth disease. A review of 12 patients. Clin. Orthop., *202*:219, 1986.

25. Dawson, C. W., and Roberts, J. B.: Charcot-Marie-Tooth disease. J.A.M.A., *188*:659, 1964.

26. Dejerine, et Armand-Delille: Un cas d'atrophie musculaire type Charcot-Marie, suivi d'autopsie. Rev. Neurol., *11*:1198, 1903.

27. Dyck, P. J.: Histologic measurements and fine structure of biopsied sural nerve: normal, and in peroneal muscular atrophy, hypertrophic neuropathy, and congenital sensory neuropathy. Mayo Clin. Proc., *41*:742, 1966.

28. Dyck, P. J., Kennel, A. J., Magal, I. V., and Draybill, E. N.: A virginal kinship with hereditary sensory neuropathy, peroneal muscular atrophy and pes cavus. Mayo Clin. Proc., *40*:685, 1965.

29. Dyck, P. J., and Lambert, E. H.: Numbers and diameters of nerve fibers and compound action potential of sural nerve: Controls and hereditary neuromuscular disorders. Trans. Am. Neurol. Assoc., *91*:214, 1966.

30. Dyck, P. J., and Lambert, E. H.: Lower motor and primary sensory neuron disease with peroneal muscular atrophy. I. Neurologic, genetic and electrophysiologic findings in hereditary polyneuropathies. Arch. Neurol., *18*:603, 1968.

31. Dyck, P. J., and Lambert, E. H.: Lower motor and primary sensory neurol disease with peroneal muscular atrophy. II. Neurologic, genetic and electrophysiologic findings in various neuronal degenerations. Arch. Neurol., *18*:619, 1968.

32. Dyck, P. J., Lambert, E. H., and Mulder, D. W.: Charcot-Marie-Tooth disease. Nerve conduction and clinical studies of a large kinship. Neurology, *13*:1, 1963.

33. Dyck, P. J., Winkelmann, R. K., and Bolton, C. F.: Quantitation of Meissner's corpuscles in hereditary neurologic disorders. Charcot-Marie-Tooth disease, Roussy-Lévy syndrome, Dejerine-Sottas disease, hereditary sensory neuropathy, spinocerebellar degeneration and hereditary spastic paraplegia. Neurology, *16*:10, 1966.

34. Earl, W. C., and Johnson, E. W.: Motor nerve conduction velocity in Charcot-Marie-Tooth disease. Arch. Phys. Med., *44*:247, 1963.

35. Editorial: Inherited neuropathies. Mayo Clin. Proc., *58*:476, 1983.

36. Eisenbud, A., and Grossman, M.: Peroneal form of progressive muscular atrophy. A clinical report of two families. Arch. Neurol. Psychiatr., *18*:766, 1927.

37. England, A. C., and Denny-Brown, D.: Severe sensory changes and trophic disorder, in peroneal muscular atrophy (Charcot-Marie-Tooth type). Arch. Neurol. Psychiatr., *67*:1, 1952.

38. Erwin, W. G.: A pedigree of sex-linked recessive peroneal atrophy. J. Hered., *35*:24, 1944.

39. Fenton, C. F., Schlefman, B. S., and McGlamry, E. D.: Surgical considerations in the presence of Charcot-Marie-Tooth disease. J. Am. Podiatr. Assoc., *74*:490, 1984.

40. Gherardi, R., Belghiti-Deprez, D., Hirbec, G., Bouche, P., Weil, B., and Lagrue, G.: Focal glomerulosclerosis associated with Charcot-Marie-Tooth disease. Nephron, *40*:357, 1985.

41. Gilliatt, R. W., and Thomas, P. K.: Extreme slowing of nerve conduction in peroneal muscular atrophy. Ann. Phys. Med., *4*:104, 1957.

42. Gould, N.: Surgery in advanced Charcot-Marie-Tooth disease. Foot Ankle, *4*:267, 1984.

43. Gutmann, L., Fakadej, A., and Riggs, J. E.: Evolution of nerve conduction abnormalities in children with dominant hypertrophic neuropathy of the Charcot-Marie-Tooth type. Muscle Nerve, *6*:515, 1983.

44. Gutrecht, J. A., and Dyck, P. J.: Segmental demyelinization in peroneal muscular atrophy: Nerve fibers teased from sural nerve biopsy specimens. Mayo Clin. Proc., *41*:775, 1966.

45. Haase, G. R., and Shy, G. M.: Pathological changes in muscle biopsies from patients with peroneal muscular atrophy. Brain, *83*:631, 1960.

46. Heimans, J. J., and Lindhout, D.: Charcot-Marie-Tooth disease. J. Med. Genet., *20*:77, 1983.

47. Hensinger, R. N., and MacEwen, G. D.: Spinal deformity associated with heritable neurologic conditions: Spinal muscular atrophy, Friedreich's ataxia, familial dysautonomia and Charcot-Marie-Tooth disease. J. Bone Joint Surg., *58-A*:13, 1976.

48. Herringham, W. P.: Muscular atrophy of the peroneal type affecting many members of a family. Brain, *11*:230, 1889.

49. Hoffmann, J.: Ueber progressive neurotische Muskelatrophie. Arch. Psychiatr. (Berlin), *20*:660, 1889.

50. Hoyt, W. F.: Charcot-Marie-Tooth disease with primary optic atrophy. A.M.A. Arch. Ophthalmol., *64*:925, 1960.

51. Hughes, J. T., and Browell, B.: Pathology of peroneal muscular atrophy (Charcot-Marie-Tooth disease). J. Neurol. Neurosurg. Psychiatry, *35*:648, 1972.

52. Humberstone, P. M.: Nerve conduction studies in Charcot-Marie-Tooth disease. Acta Neurol. Scand., *48*:176, 1972.

53. Jacobs, J. E., and Carr, C. R.: Progressive muscular atrophy of the peroneal type (Charcot-Marie-Tooth disease). Orthopedic management and end-result study. J. Bone Joint Surg., *32-A*:27, 1950.

54. Jammes, J. L.: The autonomic nervous system in peroneal muscular atrophy. Arch. Neurol., *27*:213, 1972.

55. Jones, S. J., Carroll, W. M., and Halliday, A. M.: Peripheral and central sensory nerve conduction in Charcot-Marie-Tooth disease and comparison with Friedreich's ataxia. J. Neurol. Sci., *61*:135, 1983.

56. Karlholm, S., and Nilsonne, U.: Operative treatment of the foot deformity in Charcot-Marie-Tooth disease. Acta Orthop. Scand., *39*:101, 1968.

57. Kimura, J.: An evaluation of the facial and trigeminal nerves in polyneuropathy: Electrodiagnostic study in Charcot-Marie-Tooth disease, Guillain-Barré syndrome and diabetic neuropathy. Neurology, *21*:745, 1971.

58. LaPresle, J.: Contribution à l'étude de la dystasie areflexique hereditaire. Etat actuel de quatre des sept cas princeps de Roussy et Mlle. Levy, trente ans après la premiere publication de ces auteurs. Sem. Hop. Paris, *32*:2473, 1956.

59. Levitt, R. L., Canale, S. T., Cooke, A. J., and Gartland, J. J.: The role of foot surgery in progressive neuromuscular disorders in children. J. Bone Joint Surg., *55-A*:1396, 1973.

60. Lidge, R. T., and Chandler, F. A.: Charcot-Marie-Tooth disease. J. Pediatr., 43:152, 1953.
61. Littler, W. A.: Heart block and peroneal muscular atrophy: A family study. Q. J. Med., 39:431, 1970.
62. Lloveras, J. J., Salles, J. P., Durand, D., Suc, J. M., and Rascol, A.: Focal glomerulosclerosis and Charcot-Marie-Tooth disease: not a chance association? Nephron, 43:231, 1986.
63. Lucas, G. J., and Forster, F. M.: Charcot-Marie-Tooth disease with associated myopathy: A report of a family. Neurology, 12:629, 1962.
64. MacKlin, M. T., and Bowman, J. T.: Inheritance of peroneal atrophy. J.A.M.A., 86:613, 1926.
65. Martini, A., Ravelli, A., and Burgio, G. R.: Focal segmental glomerulosclerosis and Charcot-Marie-Tooth disease. Int. J. Pediatr. Nephrol., 6:151, 1985.
66. Milhorat, A. T.: Progressive muscular atrophy of peroneal type associated with atrophy of the optic nerves. Arch. Neurol. Psychiatr., 50:279, 1943.
67. Myrianthopoulos, N. C., Lane, M. H., Silberberg, D. H., and Vincent, B. L.: Nerve conduction and other studies in families with Charcot-Marie-Tooth disease. Brain, 87:589, 1964.
68. Nielsen, V. K., and Pilgaard, S.: On the pathogenesis of Charcot-Marie-Tooth disease. A study of the sensory and motor conduction velocity in the median nerve. Acta Orthop. Scand., 43:4, 1972.
69. Panayiotopoulos, C. P.: F-wave conduction velocity in the deep peroneal nerve: Charcot-Marie-Tooth disease and dystrophia myotonica. Muscle Nerve, 1:37, 1978.
70. Popovian, M. D., Dubinskaia, E. E., and Ageeva, T. S.: Polymorphism of Charcot-Marie-Tooth neural amyotrophy in uniovular twins. Zh. Nevropatol. Psikhiatr., 77:1446, 1977.
71. Ross, A. T.: Combination of Friedreich's ataxia and Charcot-Marie-Tooth atrophy in each of two brothers. J. Nerv. Ment. Dis., 95:680, 1942.
72. Rossi, A., Paradiso, C., Cioni, R., Rizzuto, N., and Guazzi, G.: Charcot-Marie-Tooth disease: study of a large kinship with an intermediate form. J. Neurol., 232:91, 1985.
73. Rossi, A., Paradiso, C., DellAnna, P., and Mondelli, M.: Short latency somatosensory evoked potentials in Charcot-Marie-Tooth disease. A family with an intermediate form. Acta Neurol. Scand., 71:156, 1985.
74. Roussy, G., and Lévy, G.: Sept cas d'une maladie familiale particulière: Troubles de la march, pieds, bots, et aréflexie tendineuse generalisee avec accessoirement legere maladresse des mains. Rev. Neurol. (Paris), 45:427, 1926.
75. Roussy, G., and Lévy, G.: A propos de la dystasie areflexique hereditaire. Rev. Neurol. (Paris), 62:763, 1934.
76. Sabir, M., and Lyttle, D.: Pathogenesis of pes cavus in Charcot-Marie-Tooth disease. Clin. Orthop., 175:173, 1983.
77. Sabir, M., and Lyttle, D.: Pathogenesis of Charcot-Marie-Tooth disease. Gait analysis and electrophysiologic, genetic, histopathologic, and enzyme studies in a kinship. Clin. Orthop., 184:223, 1984.
78. Sachs, B.: The peroneal form or the leg-type of progressive muscular atrophy. Brain, 12:447, 1890.
79. Salisachs, P.: Wide spectrum of motor conduction velocity in Charcot-Marie-Tooth disease. An anatomicophysiological interpretation. J. Neurol. Sci., 23:25, 1974.
80. Salisachs, P.: Charcot-Marie-Tooth disease associated with "essential tremor." J. Neurol. Sci., 48:17, 1976.
81. Salisachs, P., Findley, L. J., Codia, M., La Torre, P., and Martinex-Lage, J. M.: A case of Charcot-Marie-Tooth disease mimicking Friedreich's ataxia: Is there any association between Friedreich's ataxia and Charcot-Marie-Tooth disease? Can. J. Neurol. Sci., 9:99, 1982.
82. Schneider, D. E., and Bels, M. M.: Charcot-Marie-Tooth disease with primary optic atrophy. Report of two cases occurring in brothers. J. Nerv. Ment. Dis., 85:541, 1937.
83. Schwartz, A. B.: Charcot-Marie-Tooth disease. A 45 year follow-up. Arch. Neurol., 9:623, 1963.
84. Schwartz, L. A.: Clinical histopathological and inheritance factors in peroneal muscular atrophy (Charcot-Marie-Tooth type). J. Mich. Med. Soc., 43:219, 1944.
85. Shannon, B. T., Williams, L. L., Fedrick, J. A., and Pandey, J. P.: Gm and Km allotypes in Charcot-Marie-Tooth disease. Immunogenetics, 12:175, 1985.
86. Siegel, I. M.: Charcot-Marie-Tooth disease. A diagnostic problem. J.A.M.A., 228:873, 1974.
87. Skre, H.: Genetic and clinical aspects of Charcot-Marie-Tooth's disease. Clin. Genet., 6:98, 1974.
88. Spillane, J. D.: Familial pes cavus and absent tendon jerks: Its relationship with Friedreich's disease and peroneal muscular atrophy. Brain, 63:275, 1940.
89. Stranak, V.: Charcot-Marie-Tooth-Hoffmann syndrome. Beitr. Orthop. Traumatol., 15:564, 1968.
90. Symonds, S. C. P., and Shaw, M. E.: Familial clawfoot with absent tendon-jerks. A "forme fruste" of the Charcot-Marie-Tooth disease. Brain, 49:387, 1926.
91. Thomas, P. K., Calne, D. B., and Stewart, G.: Hereditary motor and sensory polyneuropathy (peroneal muscular atrophy). Ann. Hum. Genet., 38:111, 1974.
92. Tooth, H. H.: The Peroneal Type of Progressive Muscular Atrophy. London, H. K. Lewis, 1886.
93. Van Bogaert, L., and Moreau, M.: Combinaison de l'amyotrophic de Charcot-Marie-Tooth et de la maladie de Friedreich, chez plusieurs membres d'une même famille. Encephale, 34:312, 1939–1941.
94. Vasilescu, C., Alexianu, M., and Dan, A.: Neuronal type of Charcot-Marie-Tooth disease with a syndrome of continuous motor unit activity. J. Neurol. Sci., 63:11, 1984.
95. Wagner, A.: Significance of sibship studies as demonstrated in a new family with neural muscular atrophy (Charcot-Marie-Tooth). Z. Arztl. Fortbild. (Jena), 66:621, 1972.
96. Weerdt, C. J., and Heerspink, W.: Family with Charcot-Marie-Tooth disease showing unusual biochemical-clinical and genetic features. Eur. Neurol., 12:253, 1974.
97. Yudell, A., Dyck, P. J., and Lambert, E. H.: A kinship with the Roussy-Lévy syndrome. Arch. Neurol., 13:432, 1965.

HYPERTROPHIC INTERSTITIAL NEURITIS (TYPE II HMSN)[1–29]

Déjerine and Sottas, in 1893, described a chronic familial polyneuropathy of childhood and adolescence.[10] This condition had been previously described by Gombault and Mallet, in 1889, as a pathologic variant of tabes dorsalis.[17] Déjerine-Sottas disease is inherited as an autosomal recessive trait.

The etiology of the condition is unknown. Disturbance of pyruvate metabolism was proposed by Joiner et al.; subsequent studies, however, have failed to show evidence of any thiamine deficiency.[16, 21, 22] Allergic or antigen-antibody immunologic factors may play a role in the pathogenesis.

Pathology

Peripheral nerves are enlarged as a result of the proliferation of perineural and endoneural connective tissue. The axis cylinders gradually decrease in size and eventually disappear. On cross section of nerve fibers the so-called onion bulb formation, a characteristic finding caused by proliferation of the Schwann cells, is seen. Muscles show atrophy of neural origin.

Clinical Features

Difficulty in locomotion is the usual presenting complaint. Walking is delayed. The child is unsteady, falls frequently, and has difficulty going up and down stairs. He is unable to run and to "keep up" with his playmates. His feet are weak and floppy. The abnormality of gait is similar to that of steppage gait. Subjective sensory disturbances, such as paresthesias and lightning type pains of the limbs, may occur. Pes cavus and muscle weakness in the lower limbs (which is distal in distribution) develop early, antedating the more florid findings by several years. Paralysis of the intrinsic muscles of the hand appears later. Flexion contracture of the fingers and wrist is usually present toward the end of the first decade. Scoliosis develops during the rapid growth of the spine in early adolescence.

The deep tendon reflexes are diminished or absent. Superficial skin reflexes such as abdominal and cremasteric reflexes are lost later. Sensory loss involves all modalities of sensation. Anesthesia to light touch and pinprick is of the "stocking-glove" type. Proprioceptive sensory disturbance is shown by loss of sensation of position and vibration and by the presence of a positive Romberg sign. Abnormalities of the pupil, such as Argyll Robertson phenomenon, result from involvement of the cranial nerves. Nystagmus and slurred speech occur in some cases. Incoordination and motor deficit result from the combination of muscle weakness and sensory deficit.

Enlargement of the peripheral nerves is a late manifestation; it develops first in the proximal segments of the nerves.

Diagnosis

The total protein level in the cerebrospinal fluid is elevated abnormally. On manometric tests there is no block to cerebrospinal fluid circulation. Total and differential cell counts are within normal range.

Serum aldolase and creatine phosphokinase levels are not increased. The serologic test for syphilis should be performed to rule out luetic infection of the central nervous system.

Radiograms and magnetic resonance imaging of the entire spine are obtained to rule out the possibility of an intraspinal tumor. Spinal nerve root enlargement may be demonstrated by computerized axial tomography or magnetic resonance imaging. Myelography should not be performed.

Pyruvate metabolism may be studied by determination of concentration of pyruvate in whole blood before and at intervals after the administration of glucose by mouth. Excessive accumulation of pyruvate in the blood, occurring as a response to a glucose load, is an indication that effective levels of thiamine are lacking in the body. In interstitial hypertrophic neuritis, there is no evidence of thiamine deficiency and the hydrochloric acid concentration of gastric contents is normal. Levels of blood glucose are determined to rule out diabetes. Lead or arsenic poisoning should also be ruled out.

Electromyography may disclose evidence of muscle atrophy of neural origin with reduced interference pattern, the presence of fibrillation potentials, and action potentials that are prolonged with normal or polyphasic potentials. Nerve conduction studies should be performed; evoked sensory and mixed nerve potentials will be absent or diminished in amplitude or will disclose a prolonged conduction time.

Muscle and nerve biopsies (usually of the lateral sural nerve) should be performed to confirm the diagnosis by histologic examination of the tissues.

Prognosis and Treatment

The course of the disease is one of slow progression with remissions and exacerbations. In mild cases, the disease may reach a plateau and life expectancy may be normal.

There is no specific treatment. Corticosteroids are reported to improve the condition and may be tried in severe cases or during acute exacerbations. Orthopedic management consists of passive stretching exercises and use of night splints to prevent the development of contractural deformity. In advanced cases, orthotic support to the lower limbs and spine may be indicated. Pes cavus may require surgical correction.

References

1. Andermann, F., Lloyd-Smith, S. L., Mavor, H., and Mathieson, G., Observations on hypertrophic neuropathy of Dejerine and Sottas. Neurology, *12*:712, 1962.

2. Anderson, R. M., Dennett, X., Hopkins, I. J., and Shield, L. K.: Hypertrophic interstitial polyneuropathy in infancy. Clinical and pathologic features in two cases. J. Pediatr., 82:619, 1973.

3. Austin, J. H.: Observations on the syndrome of hypertrophic neuritis (the hypertrophic interstitial radiculoneuropathies). Medicine, 35:187, 1956.

4. Bedford, P. D., and James, F. E.: A family with progressive hypertrophic polyneuritis of Dejerine and Sottas. J. Neurol. Neurosurg. Psychiatry, 19:46, 1956.

5. Byers, R. K., and Taft, L. T.: Chronic multiple peripheral neuropathy in childhood. Pediatrics, 20:517, 1957.

6. Cooper, E. L.: Progressive familial hypertrophic neuritis (Dejerine-Sottas). Br. Med. J., 1:793, 1936.

7. Craft, P. B., and Wadia, N. H.: Familial hypertrophic polyneuritis. Review of a previously reported family. Neurology, 7:356, 1957.

8. Creutzfeldt, H. G., Curtius, F., and Druger, K. H.: Zur Klinik histologie und genealogie der Dejerine-Sottasschen krankheit. Arch. Psychiatr. Nervenkr., 186:341, 1951.

9. DeBrwyn, R. S., and Stern, R. O.: A case of the progressive hypertrophic polyneuritis of Dejerine and Sottas, with pathological examination. Brain, 52:84, 1929.

10. Dejerine, J., and Sottas, J.: Sur la nevrite interstitielle, hypertrophique et progressive de l'enfance. C.R. Soc. Biol., 5:63, 1893.

11. Dyck, P. J.: Experimental hypertrophic neuropathy: pathogenesis of onion-bulb formations produced by related tourniquet applications. Arch. Neurol., 21:73, 1969.

12. Dyck, P. J., Ellefson, R. D., and Lais, A. C.: Histologic and lipid studies of sural nerves in inherited hypertrophic neuropathy. Preliminary report of lipid abnormality in nerve and liver in Dejerine-Sottas disease. Mayo Clin. Proc., 45:286, 1970.

13. Dyck, P. J., and Gomez, M. R.: Segmental demyelinization in Dejerine-Sottas disease: light phase contrast, and electron microscopic studies. Mayo Clin. Proc., 43:280, 1968.

14. Dyck, P. J., Lambert, E. H., and Sanders, K.: Severe hypomyelination and marked abnormality of conduction in Dejerine-Sottas hypertrophic neuropathy. Mayo Clin. Proc., 46:432, 1971.

15. Garcin, R., LaPresle, J., Fondeau, M., and de Recondo, J.: Etude en microscope electronique du nerf peripherique preleve par biopsie dans quatre cas de nevrite hypertrophique de Dejerine-Sottas. Rev. Neurol., 115:917, 1966.

16. Gilroy, J., Meyer, J. S., and Bauer, R. B.: Clinical, biochemical and neurophysiological studies of chronic interstitial hypertrophic polyneuropathy. Am. J. Med., 40:368, 1966.

17. Gombault, A., and Mallet: Un cas de tabes ayant debute dans l'enfance. Arch. Med. Exp., 1:385, 1889.

18. Green, L., Herzog, I., and Aberfeld, D.: Case of hypertrophic interstitial neuritis coexisting with dementia and cerebellar degeneration. J. Neuropathol. Exp., 24:682, 1965.

19. Hinck, V. C., and Sachdev, N. S.: Myelographic findings in hypertrophic interstitial neuritis. Am. J. Roentgenol. Radium Ther. Nucl. Med., 95:947, 1965.

20. Isaacs, H.: Familial chronic hypertrophic polyneuropathy with paralysis of the extremities in cold weather. S. Afr. Med. J., 34:758, 1960.

21. Joiner, C. L., McArdle, B., and Thompson, R. H. S.: Blood pyruvate estimations in the diagnosis and treatment of polyneuritis. Brain, 73:431, 1950.

22. Koeppen, A. H., Messmore, H., and Stehbens, W. B.: Interstitial hypertrophic neuropathy: Biomechanical study of the peripheral nervous system. Arch. Neurol., 24:340, 1971.

23. Krishna Rao, C. V. G., Fits, C. R., and Harwood-Nash, D. C.: Dejerine-Sottas syndrome in children (hypertrophic interstitial polyneuritis). A.J.R., 122:70, 1974.

24. Russell, W. R., and Garland, H. G.: Progressive hypertrophic polyneuritis, with case reports. Brain, 53:376, 1930.

25. Schaller, W. F.: Progressive interstitial hypertrophic neuritis of childhood of Dejerine and Sottas: Report of a case. Arch. Intern. Med., 10:399, 1912.

26. Thomas, P. K., and Llascellas, R. G.: Hypertrophic neuropathy. Q. J. Med., 36:223, 1967.

27. Weller, R. O.: An electron microscopic study of hypertrophic neuropathy of Dejerine and Sottas. J. Neurol. Neurosurg. Psychiatr., 30:111, 1967.

28. Weller, R. D., and Das Gupta, T. K.: Experimental hypertrophic neuropathy. An electron microscope study. J. Neurol. Neurosurg. Psychiatry, 31:34, 1968.

29. Zacks, S. I., Lipshutz, H., and Elliott, F.: Histochemical and electron microscopic observations on "onion bulb" formations in a case of hypertrophic neuritis of 25 years' duration with onset in childhood. Acta Neuropathol., 11:157, 1968.

REFSUM'S DISEASE (HEREDOPATHIA ATACTICA POLYNEURITIFORMIS)[1–48]

Heredopathia atactica polyneuritiformis is an extremely rare condition caused by a disorder of lipid metabolism. The basic defect seems to be in the enzyme that catalyzes the alpha-oxidative process by which phytanic acid is shortened by one carbon atom. Endogenous synthesis of phytanic acid is minimal, and the metabolic defect is one of degradation. In the serum and lipid deposits of the liver, kidney, and other organs is found an unusual fatty acid, 3,7,11,15-tetramethyl-hexadecanic acid. In patients with Refsum's disease, exogenous phytol is readily converted to phytanic acid. The inheritance is autosomal recessive.

Pathologic findings consist of interstitial hypertrophic polyneuritis and degenerative changes in the anterior horn cells and olivocerebellar tracts. Nerve biopsy will disclose "onion bulb" formation—increased endomesium with fat deposits.

In children, clinical symptoms are usually manifest between four and seven years of age. The cardinal features of the disease are chronic polyneuritis, retinitis pigmentosa, and signs of cerebellar involvement. The gait is unsteady, and the limbs show weakness and atrophy of the distal musculature. The deep tendon reflexes are absent. There is no spasticity. The Babinski sign is negative. Romberg's sign may be present, and vibration and position sense in the legs may be disturbed. Ichthyosis (especially on the limbs), night blindness, and retinal pigmentary changes are common. Some patients also complain of nerve deafness, anosmia, and nystagmus.

Laboratory Findings

The phytanic acid level of the serum is elevated. This finding is pathognomonic of Refsum's disease. Carriers can be detected by the phytol loading test. Motor nerve conduction velocity is slow. The protein level in the cerebrospinal fluid is markedly elevated.

Electrocardiographic changes, e.g., lengthening of systolic period, are present in most patients.

Diagnosis

In the differential diagnosis, one should consider Friedreich's ataxia, peroneal muscular atrophy, and Roussy-Lévy syndrome. Retinitis pigmentosa is the distinguishing clinical feature of Refsum's disease. The elevation of serum phytanic acid will establish the diagnosis.

Treatment

This consists of a diet that is free of chlorophyll and those foods that might contain phytol, phytanic acid, or their precursors. With such a diet, the level of phytanic acid in the blood can be reduced and clinical improvement effected. Pes cavus and other deformities of the limbs are managed according to the principles outlined in the section on Friedreich's ataxia.

Prognosis

It is guarded. The child may die because of cardiac disease or pulmonary infection.

References

1. Alexander, W. S.: Phytanic acid in Refsum's syndrome. J. Neurol. Neurosurg. Psychiatry, 29:412, 1966.
2. Ashenhurst, E. M., Millar, J. H. D., and Milliken, T. G.: Refsum's syndrome affecting a brother and two sisters. Br. Med. J., 2:415, 1958.
3. Baxter, J. H.: Absorption of chlorophyll phytol in normal man and in patients with Refsum's disease. J. Lipid Res., 9:636, 1968.
4. Blass, J. P., Avigan, J., and Steinberg, D.: Alpha-hydroxy fatty acids in hereditary ataxic polyneuritis (Refsum's disease). Biochem. Biophys. Acta, 187:36, 1969.
5. Campbell, A. M. G., and Williams, E. R.: Natural history of Refsum's syndrome in a Gloucestershire family. Br. Med. J., 3:777, 1967.
6. Dereux, J.: La maladie de Refsum. Rev. Neurol., 109:599, 1963.
7. Dubois-Dalcq, M., Menu, R., and Buyse, M.: Influence of fatty acid on fine structure of cultured neurons. An experimental approach to Refsum's disease. J. Neuropathol. Exp. Neurol., 31:645, 1972.
8. Dumas, J. L.: Refsum's disease. Presse Med., 77:2085, 1969.
9. Edstrom, R., Grontoff, D., and Sandring, H.: Refsum's disease—three siblings, one autopsy. Acta Psychiatr. Scand., 34:40, 1959.
10. Eldjarn, L., Try, K., Stokke, O., Munthe-Kaas, A. W., Refsum, S., Steinberg, D., Avigan, J., and Mize, C.: Dietary effects on serum phytanic acid levels and on clinical manifestations in heredopathia atactica polyneuritiformis. Lancet, 1:691, 1966.
11. Fardeau, M., Abelanet, B., Laudat, Ph., and Bonduelle, M.: Maladie de Refsum etude histologique, ultrastructurale et biochimique d'une biopsie de nerf peripherique. Rev. Neurol., 122:185, 1970.
12. Fardeau, M., and Engel, W. K.: Ultrastructural study of a peripheral nerve biopsy in Refsum's disease. J. Neuropathol. Exp. Neurol., 28:278, 1969.
13. Flament-Durand, J., Noel, P., Rutsaert, J., Toussant, D., Malmendier, C., and Lyon, G.: A case of Refsum's disease: Clinical, pathological, ultrastructural and biochemical study. Pathol. Eur., 6:172, 1971.
14. Fryer, D. G.: Refsum's disease. A clinical and pathological report. Neurology, 21:162, 1971.
15. Gamstorp, I.: Polyneuropathy in childhood. Acta Paediatr. Scand., 57:230, 1968.
16. Gibberd, F. B., Billimoria, J. D., Goldman, J. M., Clemens, M. E., Evans, R., Whitelaw, M. N., Retsas, S., and Sherratt, R. M.: Heredopathia atactica polyneuritiformis: Refsum's disease. Acta Neurol. Scand., 72:1, 1985.
17. Gilroy, J., and Meyer, J. S.: Hereditary neuropathies. In Medical Neurology. 2nd Ed. New York, Macmillan, 1975, pp. 661–664.
18. Goldman, J. M., Clemens, M. E., Gibberd, F. B., and Billimoria, J. D.: Screening of patients with retinitis pigmentosa for hereditary atactica polyneuritiformis (Refsum's disease). Br. Med. J., 290:1109, 1985.
19. Herndon, J. H., Steinberg, D., and Uhlendorf, B. W.: Refsum's disease: Defective oxidation of phytanic acid in tissue cultures derived from homozygotes and heterozygotes. N. Engl. J. Med., 281:1034, 1969.
20. Hungerbuhler, J. P., Meier, C., Rousselle, L., Quadri, P., and Bogousslavsky, J.: Refsum's disease: Management by diet and plasmapheresis. Eur. Neurol., 24:153, 1985.
21. Hutton, D., and Steinberg, D.: Localization of the enzymatic defect in phytanic acid storage disease (Refsum's disease). Neurology, 23:1333, 1973.
22. Kahke, W., and Wagner, H.: Conversion of H3-phytol to phytanic acid and its incorporation into plasma lipid fractions in heredopathia atactica polyneuritiformis. Metabolism, 15:687, 1966.
23. Laudat, P.: Phytol intolerance: Refsum's disease. Biochemie, 54:735, 1972.
24. Laurell, S., Nilsen, R., and Norden, A.: Incorporation of phytanic and linoleic acid into plasma lipids in Refsum's disease. Clin. Chim. Acta, 36:169, 1972.
25. Lenk, W.: Nutritional and metabolic aspects of heredopathia atactica polyneuritiformis (Refsum's syndrome). Nutr. Metabol., 16:366, 1974.
26. Lough, A. K.: The stereochemistry of phytanic acid in Refsum's syndrome. Lipids, 5:201, 1970.
27. Lovelock, J., and Griffith, H.: Case report 175: Refsum's syndrome. Skeletal Radiol., 7:214, 1981.
28. Lundberg, A., Lilja, L. G., Lundberg, P. O., and Try, K.: Heredopathia atactica polyneuritiformis (Refsum's disease). Experiences of dietary treatment and plasmapheresis. Eur. Neurol., 8:309, 1972.
29. Poll The, B. T., Ogier, H., Saudubray, J. M., Schutgens, R. B., Wanders, R. J., van den Bosch, H., and Schrakamp, G.: Impaired plasmalogen metabolism in infantile Refsum's disease (Letter). Eur. J. Pediatr., 144:513, 1986.
30. Poll The, B. T., Poulos, A., Sharp, P., Boue, J., Ogier, H., Odievre, M., and Saudubray, J. M.: Antenatal diagnosis of infantile Refsum's disease (Letter). Clin. Genet., 27:524, 1985.

31. Poulos, A., Sharp, P., and Whiting, M.: Infantile Refsum's disease (phytanic acid storage disease): A variant of Zellweger's syndrome? Clin. Genet., 26:579, 1984.
32. Quinlan, C. D., and Martin, E. A.: Refsum's syndrome: Report of three cases. J. Neurol. Neurosurg. Psychiatry, 33:817, 1970.
33. Rake, M., and Saunder, M.: Refsum's disease: A disorder of lipid metabolism. J. Neurol. Neurosurg. Psychiatry, 29:417, 1966.
34. Refsum, S.: Heredopathia atactica polyneuritiformis: A familial syndrome not hitherto described. Acta Psychiatr. Neurol. (Suppl.), 38, 1946.
35. Refsum, S.: Heredopathia atactica polyneuritiformis. J. Nerv. Ment. Dis., 116:1046, 1952.
36. Refsum, S.: Classification of some hereditary nervous diseases. The "heredo-ataxia." Nord. Med., 85:428, 1971.
37. Refsum, S., Salmonsen, L., and Skatvedt, M.: Heredopathia atactica polyneuritiformis in children. J. Pediatr., 35:335, 1949.
38. Richterich, R., Van Mechelen, P., and Rossi, E.: Refsum's disease (heredopathia atactica polyneuritiformis). An inborn error of lipid metabolism with storage of 3,7,11,15-tetramethyl hexadecanic acid. Am. J. Med., 39:230, 1965.
39. Rom, M. A.: Refsum's syndrome with normal phytate metabolism. Acta Neurol. Scand., 47:646, 1971.
40. Sahgal, V., and Olsen, W. O.: Heredopathia atactica polyneuritiformis (phytanic acid storage disease). A new case with special reference to dietary treatment. Arch. Intern. Med., 135:585, 1975.
41. Salisachs, P.: Ataxia and other data reviewed in Charcot-Marie-Tooth and Refsum's disease. J. Neurol. Neurosurg. Psychiatry, 45:1085, 1982.
42. Savettieri, G., Camarda, R., Galatioto, S., and Bonavita, V.: Refsum's disease. Clinical and morphological report on a case. Ital. J. Neurol. Sci., 3:241, 1982.
43. Steinberg, D.: Phytanic acid in patients with Refsum's syndrome and response to dietary treatment. Arch. Intern. Med., 125:75, 1970.
44. Steinberg, D., Herndon, J. H., Jr., Uhlendorf, B. W., Mize, G. E., Avigan, J., and Milne, C. W. A.: Refsum's disease. Nature of the enzyme defect. Science, 156:1740, 1967.
45. Steinberg, D., Herndon, J. H., Uhlendorf, J. A., Mize, C. E., and Fales, H. M.: The enzymatic defect in Refsum's disease. J. Clin. Invest., 46:1120, 1967.
46. Steinberg, D., Mize, C. E., Avigan, J., Fales, H. M., Eldjarn, L., Try, K., Stokke, O., and Refsum, S.: Studies on the metabolic error in Refsum's disease. J. Clin. Invest., 46:313, 1967.
47. Steinberg, D., Vroom, F. Q., Engel, W. K., Cammermeyer, J., Mize, C. E., and Avigan, J.: Refsum's disease—a recently characterized lipidosis involving the nervous system. Ann. Intern. Med., 66:365, 1967.
48. Wolf, L. M., Laudat, Ph., Chaumont, P., and Bonduelle, M.: Maladie de Refsum. Evolution clinique et bio-chimique sous regime sans phytol investigations bio-chimique complementaires. Rev. Neurol., 120:89, 1969.

ANALGIA—CONGENITAL OR HEREDITARY

In children, congenital or hereditary indifference to pain may be one of the following types: (1) congenital insensitivity to pain; (2) familial dysautonomia (Riley-Day syndrome); (3) congenital sensory neuropathy; (4) hereditary sensory radicular neuropathy; or (5) familial sensory neuropathy with anhidrosis.

Congenital Insensitivity to Pain[1-68]

This rare disorder is characterized by absence of normal subjective and objective responses to noxious stimuli in patients with intact central and peripheral nervous systems.

The condition was first reported by Dearborn, who described a "human pin cushion" performing vaudeville acts in which spectators thrust sterile needles into his limbs. The stage performance of this actor terminated with a special "crucifixion stunt" in which a lady in the audience fainted when spikes were driven through his palms. The neurologic examination of this person was entirely within normal limits except for the absence of pain sensation.

The etiology of the condition is unknown. There is no sex predilection.

CLINICAL AND PATHOLOGIC FEATURES

Although life without pain sounds ideal, in actuality the lack of protective reflexes handicaps the afflicted children in various ways.

As soon as the eruption of teeth takes place, the condition is first evidenced by biting of the tongue, lips, or fingers. Burns and multiple bruises are common occurrences. The infant often fails to cry when hurt. Dental sepsis causes early loss of teeth. Corneal opacity may result from trauma or foreign bodies in the eye. The intelligence of these patients is normal.

Skeletal manifestations vary, depending upon the nature of the injury and the age of the patient. Severe trauma causes ordinary fractures of the long bones, the skull, and the short tubular bones of the hands and feet. The bones are not unduly fragile (Fig. 5–180). However, delayed diagnosis and failure to treat these fractures result in gross deformities of the long bones and pseudarthrosis. Repeated injury to the same limb compounds fracture upon fracture. In infancy, epiphyseal separations occur; in early childhood the fractures take place at the metaphysis, and in later childhood, in the diaphysis. In adolescence and adult life, the incidence of acute fractures decreases, as with maturity and increasing awareness of analgia, the patient learns how to prevent injury. Aseptic necrosis of the talus and of the femoral head occurs frequently.

In the infant and the young child, widening of the epiphyseal plate develops from repeated minimal trauma, causing rachitic type changes

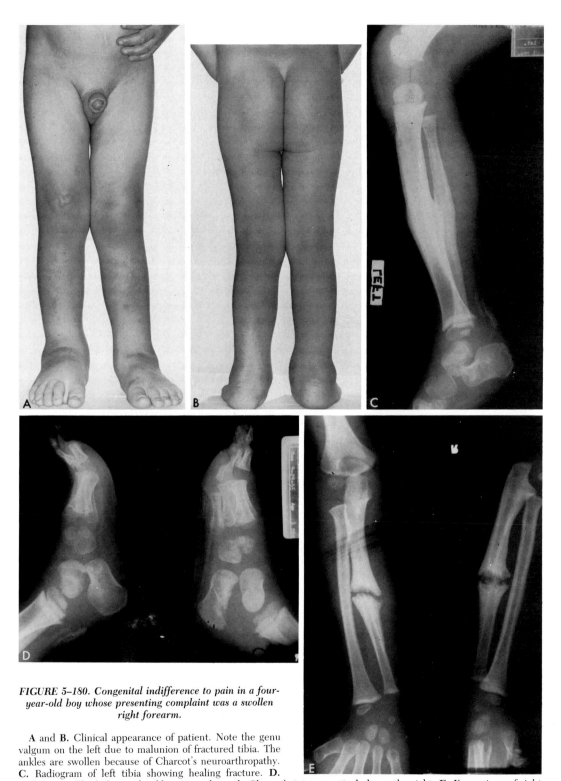

FIGURE 5-180. Congenital indifference to pain in a four-year-old boy whose presenting complaint was a swollen right forearm.

A and **B.** Clinical appearance of patient. Note the genu valgum on the left due to malunion of fractured tibia. The ankles are swollen because of Charcot's neuroarthropathy. **C.** Radiogram of left tibia showing healing fracture. **D.** Radiogram of both feet and ankles. Note the early Charcot's joints, particularly on the right. **E.** X-ray views of right forearm showing nonunion of fracture in the middle third of the ulna. After immobilization in an above-elbow cast for a period of three months there was no evidence of healing. Thus, an open reduction, intramedullary fixation with a Steinmann pin, and onlay bone grafting was performed.

Illustration continued on following page

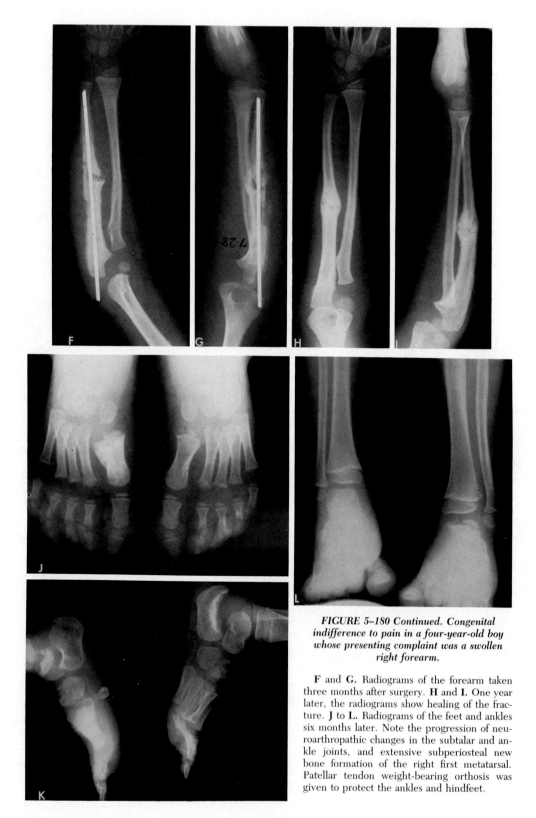

FIGURE 5–180 Continued. Congenital indifference to pain in a four-year-old boy whose presenting complaint was a swollen right forearm.

F and G. Radiograms of the forearm taken three months after surgery. H and I. One year later, the radiograms show healing of the fracture. J to L. Radiograms of the feet and ankles six months later. Note the progression of neuroarthropathic changes in the subtalar and ankle joints, and extensive subperiosteal new bone formation of the right first metatarsal. Patellar tendon weight-bearing orthosis was given to protect the ankles and hindfeet.

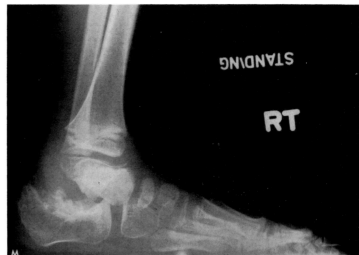

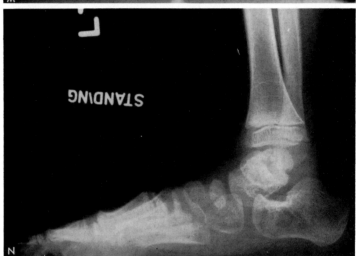

FIGURE 5-180 Continued. Congenital indifference to pain in a four-year-old boy whose presenting complaint was a swollen right forearm.

M and **N.** Lateral radiographs of the feet and ankles taken a year later show some improvement in the Charcot's joints.

in the radiogram. Direct injury and subperiosteal hemorrhage result in cortical thickening of long bones. Growth disturbances are produced by epiphyseal injury.

Joints respond to multiple injuries by effusion, hemarthrosis, synovial thickening, and ligamentous laxity. With continued chronic trauma, neuropathic arthropathy develops. Weight-bearing joints, especially the ankle, are common sites. The presence of Charcot's joints in a child should arouse suspicion of congenital indifference to pain.

Osteomyelitis of long bones is a common incidental finding in the radiogram, and is seen as an area of rarefaction in the metaphysis. The bone infection is usually discovered in its chronic stage, as it is indolent. Neglected foci of infection (such as infected teeth, burns, or bitten fingers) and local trauma are predisposing factors. Whenever a child is suspected of having congenital indifference to pain, a radiographic

skeletal survey should be obtained to rule out silent bone lesions and fractures. Electroencephalograms and psychologic and intelligence test scores are normal. There are no abnormalities of cutaneous nerve endings in the skin or periosteum, and the central, peripheral, and autonomic nervous systems are intact.

Familial Dysautonomia (Riley-Day Syndrome)[1-66]

This is very rare and is seen specifically in persons of Jewish ancestry. It is inherited as an autosomal recessive trait with varying expressivity. The disease manifests itself at birth with lack of lacrimation, excessive perspiration, and poor temperature control. The corneal reflex and the normal axon reflex responses to histamine are absent. There is a characteristic lack of fungiform papillae on the tongue. The afflicted children are emotionally unstable, and

Table 5–17. *Differential Diagnosis of Congenital Insensitivity to Pain**

Parameter	Congenital Indifference	Familial Dysautonomia	Congenital Sensory Neuropathy	Hereditary Sensory Radicular Neuropathy	Familial Sensory Neuropathy with Anhidrosis	Acquired Sensory Neuropathy (Toxic, Infectious)	Syringomyelia
Hereditary	None	Recessive	None, occasionally dominant	Dominant	Recessive	None	None
Age at onset	Birth	Birth	Birth	Early adolescence	Birth	Adult	Young adult
Physiologic pain reactions	Present	Absent	Absent	Absent	Absent	Absent	Absent
Touch perception	Normal	Normal	Lost	Lost	Normal	Normal	Normal
Temperature perception	Normal	Diminished	Lost	Lost	Diminished	Normal	Normal
Distribution of sensory loss	Universal	Incomplete	Islands of normal sensation	Legs and feet, occasionally hands	Islands of normal sensation	Legs and feet, occasionally hands	Arms and hands
Axon reflex	Normal	Absent	Absent	Absent	Absent	Absent	Normal

			Sensory absent Motor present	Sensory absent Motor normal	Sensory absent Motor normal	Motor and sensory abnormal	Normal or slightly reduced
Nerve conduction	Normal	Normal	Sensory absent	Sensory absent Motor normal	Sensory absent Motor normal	Motor and sensory abnormal	Normal or slightly reduced
Motor strength	Normal	Normal	Normal	Normal	Normal	Weak (atrophied)	Weak (atrophied)
Sensory nerve biopsy	Normal	Absence of fungiform papillae on tongue	No myelinated fibers	No myelinated fibers	Myelinated fibers present	Loss of myelinated fibers	Normal
Skin biopsy	Normal	Normal	No nerve endings No cholinesterase	—	Normal	Degeneration of nerve, normal cholinesterase	Normal
Brain and other	Normal	Normal *Autonomic N.S.* Lack of lacrimation Excessive perspiration Poor temperature control	Normal	Normal	Normal Absence of Lissauer's tract and small dorsal root axon	Normal	Normal
Intelligence	Normal	Dull to average	Dull to average	Normal	Defective	Normal	Normal

*Modified from Winkelmann, R. K., Lambert, E. H., and Hayles, A. B.: Congenital absence of pain. Report of a case and experimental studies. Arch. Dermatol., 85:334, 1962.

development of speech is abnormally delayed. The intelligence level is usually subnormal. Temperature perception is diminished, but touch perception is normal. There is lack of objective physiologic response to painful stimuli. The distribution of sensory loss is incomplete. These children may develop progressive structural scoliosis.

Congenital Sensory Neuropathy.[1-7] In this disorder the sensations of touch, temperature, and pain are lost.[1-7] Distribution of sensory loss is diffuse, but islands of normal sensation are usually present. Myelinated nerve fibers and dermal nerve networks are absent. The brain and spinal cord are intact. Motor nerve conduction is normal, but sensory nerve conduction is absent. Physiologic responses to pain stimuli cannot be elicited.

There is a lack of normal axon reflex response to histamine. Deep tendon reflexes are diminished or lost. Retinitis pigmentosa may be present. Occasionally the children are retarded mentally and are deaf.

Congenital sensory neuropathy is due to hypoplasia or aplasia of the dorsal root ganglion cells. It is nonprogressive. The condition is inherited as an autosomal recessive trait; sporadic cases do occur.

Hereditary Sensory Radicular Neuropathy.[1,2] In this autosomal dominant hereditary disorder, there is primary degenerative neuropathy of the dorsal root ganglia. All sensory modalities are affected with loss of axon reflex response. There is no disturbance of sweating. The Achilles tendon and patellar tendon reflexes are lost. The disorder manifests late in childhood, beginning distally in the lower limbs and gradually progressing proximally. Extension above the knee is rare. Occasionally, later in the course of the disease the upper limbs may be involved.

Familial Sensory Neuropathy with Anhidrosis.[1-5] In this autosomal recessive neuropathy there is decreased temperature sensation although sensation to touch is normal. Sweating is absent. The axon reflex to histamine is lost. Mentation is usually low.

DIAGNOSIS

When a patient is suspected of having loss of pain sensation, a systematic investigation of pain reaction should be made. Winkelmann et al. recommend the following: (1) a study of affective reaction or perception of the stimulus, (2) demonstration of the state of the peripheral receptors and pathways for pain appreciation, and (3) demonstration of integrated involuntary reflex responses to painful stimuli.[68]

Intelligence and psychometric tests are performed. A thorough neurologic examination, though difficult in a child, is essential. The neurologist possesses many devices to elicit pain; however, a sharp pin is as satisfactory as any sophisticated device, such as the square-wave electric pulse generator that gives shock at a definite milliamperage. Deep pain is tested by pressure on muscles or bones and by deep insertion of hypodermic needles. Various objectively recognizable physiologic responses to pain stimuli are studied: These include pupillary dilatation, blood pressure elevation, and a rise in the respiratory and pulse rates. The important determination is whether there is a lack of sensation when a painful stimulus is applied, or whether sensation is present but the patient is indifferent and does not recognize it as being a noxious one.

The integrity of peripheral nerves is assessed by nerve conduction studies. Sometimes a cutaneous nerve biopsy may be indicated. The presence of normal sudomotor and vasomotor reactions in the skin demonstrates an intact autonomic nervous system. Is the axon reflex response to histamine normal? A skin biopsy is performed to demonstrate whether the nerve end-organs are intact as well as the presence or absence of nonspecific cholinesterase activity in them. When cerebral organic disease is suspected, an electroencephalogram should be obtained. Magnetic resonance imaging of the central nervous system is performed to rule out organic disease.

The differential diagnosis between the major sensory syndromes with absence of pain perception is given in Table 5–17.

General analgesia is classified by Winkelmann et al. as follows:

I. Cerebral level
  A. Without lesions
    1. Congenital indifference to pain
    2. Oligophrenia
    3. Psychic states (hysteria, etc.)
  B. With lesions
    1. Asymbolia
    2. Postleukotomy state
II. Spinal cord level
  A. Syringomyelia
  B. Syringobulbia
III. Peripheral nerve
  A. Congenital sensory neuropathy
  B. Familial progressive neuropathy
  C. Acquired peripheral neuropathy (toxic or infectious)

Lesch-Nyhan syndrome must be distinguished from congenital indifference to pain. In

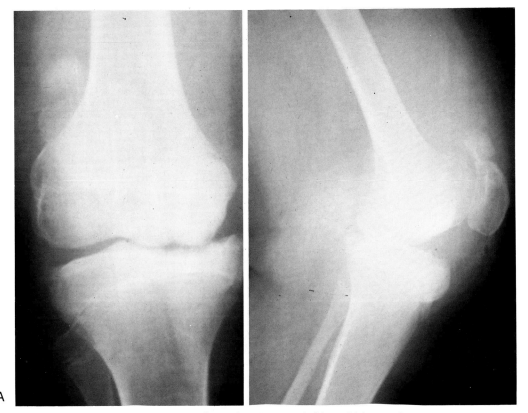

A   B

FIGURE 5–181. Charcot knee in congenital insensitivity to pain.

A and B. Anteroposterior and lateral views of the knee showing the subluxation and arthritic changes in the knee joint.

Lesch-Nyhan syndrome, activity of hypoxanthine guanine-phosphoribosyltransferase is absent; hyperuricemia results from disturbance of normal urate metabolism. The children with Lesch-Nyhan syndrome have an uncontrollable aggressive impulse; the patient is self-destructive, biting his fingers and lips; however, the destructive behavior can be directed toward others. There is no sensory disturbance. Other findings in Lesch-Nyhan syndrome are choreoathetosis with scissoring of the lower limbs, mental retardation, and hyperuricemia. In the diagnostic work-up of congenital indifference to pain, blood uric acid level should be determined.

TREATMENT

The patient and his parents should be educated to prevent injury. Early diagnosis and immediate treatment are important. Fractures ordinarily heal without difficulty. With delayed diagnosis and neglected treatment, pseudarthrosis may develop, necessitating a bone graft. Osteomyelitic lesions are treated in the usual manner.

Charcot joints are difficult to manage. The normal protective pain mechanism is absent; consequently, the joint is completely destroyed. The knee and hip joint may dislocate owing to secondary ligamentous hyperlaxity (Fig. 5–181). The unstable weight-bearing joints are protected by appropriate orthoses. Crutch protection is employed as indicated. Arthrodesis of joints may be attempted, but the results are poor; the joints fail to fuse, and an initially successful fusion breaks down with repeated trauma and develops pseudarthrosis.

References

CONGENITAL INSENSITIVITY TO PAIN

1. Abell, J. M., Jr., and Hayes, J. T.: Charcot knee due to congenital insensitivity to pain. J. Bone Joint Surg., 46-A:1287, 1964.
2. Appenzeller, O., and Kornfield, M.: Indifference to pain: A chronic peripheral neuropathy with mosaic Schwann cells. Arch. Neurol., 27:327, 1972.
3. Arbuse, D. I., Cantor, M. B., and Barenberg, P. A.: Congenital indifference to pain. J. Pediatr., 35:221, 1949.
4. Baxter, D. W., and Olszewski, J.: Congenital universal insensitivity to pain. Brain, 83:381, 1960.

5. Becak, W., Becak, M. L., and Andrade, J. D.: A genetical investigation of congenital analgesia: I. Cytogenic studies (Part I under Saldanaha, P.). Acta Genet. Statis. Med., 14:133, 1964.
6. Boyd, D. A., Jr., and Nie, L. W.: Congenital universal indifference to pain. Arch. Neurol. Psychiatr., 61:402, 1949.
7. Bourland, A., and Winkelman, R. K.: Study of cutaneous innervation in congenital anesthesia. Arch. Neurol., 14:233, 1966.
8. Chatrian, G. E., Farrell, D. G., Canfield, R. C., and Lettich, E.: Congenital insensitivity to noxious stimulation. Arch. Neurol., 32:141, 1975.
9. Comings, D. E., and Amromin, G. D.: Autosomal dominant insensitivity to pain with hyperplasia, myelinopathy and autosomal dominant indifference to pain. Neurology, 24:838, 1974.
10. Critchley, M.: Some aspects of pain. Br. Med. J., 4:891, 1934.
11. Critchley, M.: Congenital indifference to pain. Ann. Intern. Med., 45:737, 1956.
12. Dallosso, F. M.: Skeletal changes accompanying congenital indifference to pain in two Chinese children. Physiotherapy, 59:184, 1973.
13. Dearborn, G. V.: A case of congenital pure analgesia. J. Nerv. Ment. Dis., 75:612, 1932.
14. Dimon, J. H., Funk, F. J., Jr., and Wells, R. E.: Congenital indifference to pain with associated orthopedic abnormalities. South. Med. J., 58:524, 1965.
15. Drummond, R. P.: A twenty-one year review of a case of congenital indifference to pain. J. Bone Joint Surg., 57-B:241, 1975.
16. Dyck, P. J., and Stevens, J. C.: Charcot's joints associated with normal cutaneous sensations. Trans. Am. Neurol. Assoc., 101:240, 1976.
17. Ervin, F. R., and Sternbach, R. A.: Hereditary insensitivity to pain. Trans. Am. Neurol. Assoc., 85:70, 1960.
18. Fanconi, G., and Ferrazzini, F.: Kongenitale Analgie (Kongenitale generalisierte Schmerzzindifferenz). Helv. Paediatr. Acta, 12:79, 1957.
19. Farquhar, H. G., and Sutton, T.: Congenital indifference to pain. Lancet, 1:827, 1951.
20. Fath, M. A., Hassanein, M. R., and James, J. I.: Congenital absence of pain. A family study. J. Bone Joint Surg., 65-B:186, 1983.
21. Feindel, W.: Note on the nerve endings in a subject with arthropathy and congenital absence of pain. J. Bone Joint Surg., 35-B:402, 1953.
22. Fitzgerald, A. W., and Manning, C. W.: Neuropathic arthropathy secondary to atypical congenital indifference to pain. Proc. R. Soc. Med., 61:663, 1968.
23. Ford, F. R., and Wilkins, L.: Congenital universal insensitiveness to pain. Bull. Johns Hopkins Hosp., 62:448, 1938.
24. Fox, J. H., and Huott, A. D.: Congenital hemihypertrophy with indifference to pain. Arch. Neurol., 30:490, 1974.
25. Gillespie, J. B., and Perucca, L. G.: Congenital generalized indifference to pain. Am. J. Dis. Child., 100:124, 1960.
26. Gorlin, R. J., Sedano, H. O., and Boggs, W. S.: Congenital indifference to pain: The face in the diagnosis of dysmorphogenesis. Pediatr. Annu., 4:159, 1975.
27. Greider, T. D.: Orthopedic aspects of congenital insensitivity to pain. Clin. Orthop., 172:177, 1983.
28. Gristina, A. G., Thompson, W., Kester, N., Walsh, W., and Gristina, J.: Treatment of neuropathic conditions of the foot and ankle with a patellar-tendon-weight-bearing brace. Arch. Phys. Med. Rehabil., 54:562, 1973.
29. Haaxma, R., Korver, M. F., and Willemse, J.: Congenital indifference to pain associated with a defect in calcium metabolism. Acta Neurol. Scand., 47:194, 1971.
30. Ingwersen, O. S.: Congenital indifference to pain. J. Bone Joint Surg., 49-B:704, 1967.
31. Itoh, Y., Yagishita, S., Nakajima, S., Nakano, T., and Kawada, H.: Congenital insensitivity to pain with anhidrosis: morphological and morphometrical studies on the skin and peripheral nerves. Neuropediatrics, 17:103, 1986.
32. Jewesbury, E. C. O.: Insensitivity to pain. Brain, 74:336, 1951.
33. Johnson, J. T. H.: Neuropathic fractures and joint injuries. J. Bone Joint Surg., 49-A:1, 1967.
34. Kahn, S. A., and Peterkin, G. A. G.: Congenital indifference to pain. Trans. St. Johns Hosp. Dermatol. Soc., 56:122, 1970.
35. Kane, F. J., Downie, A. W., Marcotte, D. B., and Perez-Reyes, M.: A case of congenital indifference to pain. Dis. Nerv. Syst., 29:409, 1968.
36. Katz, I., Rabinowitz, J. G., and Dziadiw, R.: Early changes in Charcot's joints. A.J.R., 86:965, 1961.
37. Kidd, J. G.: The Charcot joint. South. Med. J., 67:597, 1974.
38. Kunkle, E. C.: Pain unfelt or pain unheeded: A distinction with a difference. Arch. Neurol., 5:579, 1961.
39. Kunkle, E. C., and Chapman, W. P.: Insensitivity to pain in man. Assoc. Res. Nerv. Ment. Dis. Proc., 23:100, 1943.
40. Lamy, J., Carcin, R., Jammet, M. L., Aussannaire, M., et al.: L'analgesia generalisée congenitale. Arch. Fr. Pediatr., 15:433, 1958.
41. Lau, T., Raw, I., Schmidt, B. J., and Piva, S.: Pain insensitivity, a metabolic disease. Lancet, 1:598, 1977.
42. Lesch, M., and Nylan, W. L.: A familial disorder of uric acid metabolism and central nervous system function. Am. J. Med., 36:561, 1964.
43. MacEwen, G. D., and Floyd, G. C.: Congenital insensitivity to pain and its orthopaedic implications. Clin. Orthop., 68:100, 1970.
44. McMurray, G. A.: Experimental study of a case of insensitivity to pain with neuropathic arthropathy. Arthritis Rheum., 9:820, 1966.
45. McMurray, G. A.: Theories of pain and congenital universal insensitivity to pain. Can. J. Psychol., 29:302, 1975.
46. Madonick, M. J.: Congenital insensitiveness to pain. J. Nerv. Ment. Dis., 120:87, 1954.
47. Magee, K. R.: Congenital indifference to pain. Arch. Neurol., 9:635, 1963.
48. Magee, K. R., Schneider, S. F., and Rosenzweig, N.: Congenital indifference to pain. J. Nerv. Ment. Dis., 132:249, 1961.
49. Mooney, V., and Mankin, H. J.: A case of congenital insensitivity to pain with neuropathic arthropathy. Arthritis Rheum., 9:820, 1966.
50. Murray, R. O.: Congenital indifference to pain with special reference to skeletal changes. Br. J. Radiol., 30:2, 1957.
51. Nellhaus, G.: Neurogenic arthropathies (Charcot's joints) in children. Clin. Pediatr., 14:647, 1975.
52. Ogden, T. E., Robert, F., and Carmichael, E. A.: Some sensory syndromes in children: Indifference to pain and sensory neuropathy. J. Neurol. Neurosurg. Psychiatry, 22:267, 1959.
53. Petrie, J. G.: A case of progressive joint disorders caused by insensitivity to pain. J. Bone Joint Surg., 35-B:399, 1953.
54. Pinsky, L., and DiGeorge, A. M.: Congenital familial sensory neuropathy with anhidrosis. J. Pediatr., 68:1, 1966.
55. Roberts, J. M., Taylor, J., and Burke, S.: Recurrent dislocation of the hip in congenital indifference to pain: Case report with arthrographic and operative findings. J. Bone Joint Surg., 62-A:829, 1980.

56. Roe, W.: Congenital indifference to pain. Proc. R. Soc. Med., *43*:250, 1956.
57. Rose, G. K.: Arthropathy of the ankle in congenital indifference to pain. J. Bone Joint Surg., *35-B*:408, 1953.
58. Sandell, L. J.: Congenital indifference to pain. J. Fac. Radiol. (London), *9*:50, 1958.
59. Siegelman, S. S., Heimann, W. G., and Manin, M. C.: Congenital indifference to pain. A.J.R., *97*:242, 1966.
60. Silverman, F. N., and Gilden, J. J.: Congenital insensitivity to pain: A neurologic syndrome with bizarre skeletal lesions. Radiology, *72*:176, 1959.
61. Swanson, A. G.: Congenital insensitivity to pain with anhidrosis. A unique syndrome in two male siblings. A.M.A. Arch. Neurol., *8*:299, 1963.
62. Swanson, A. G., Buchan, G. C., and Alvord, E. C., Jr.: Absence of Lissaer's tract and small dorsal root axons in familial congenital universal insensitivity to pain. Trans. Am. Neurol. Assoc., *88*:99, 1963.
63. Swanson, A. G., Buchan, G. C., and Alvord, E. C., Jr.: Anatomic changes in congenital insensitivity to pain. Arch. Neurol., *12*:12, 1965.
64. Thrush, D. C.: Autonomic dysfunction in four patients with congenital insensitivity to pain. Brain, *96*:591, 1973.
65. Thrush, D. C.: Congenital insensitivity to pain. Brain, *96*:369, 1973.
66. Van der Houwen, H.: A case of neuropathic arthritis caused by indifference to pain. J. Bone Joint Surg., *43-B*:314, 1961.
67. Westlake, E. K.: Congenital indifference to pain. Br. Med. J., *1*:144, 1952.
68. Winkelmann, R. K., Lambert, E. H., and Hayles, A. B.: Congenital absence of pain. Arch. Dermatol., *85*:325, 1962.

FAMILIAL DYSAUTONOMIA (RILEY-DAY SYNDROME)

1. Aguayo, A. J., Nair, C. P. V., and Bray, G. M.: Peripheral nerve abnormalities in the Riley-Day syndrome. Arch. Neurol., *24*:106, 1971.
2. Ariel, I., and Wells, T. R.: Structural abnormalities of the myenteric (Auerbach's) plexus in familial dysautonomia (Riley-Day syndrome) as demonstrated by flat-mount preparation of the esophagus and stomach. Pediatr. Pathol., *4*:89, 1985.
3. Axelrod, F. B., Branom, N., Becker, M., Nachtigal, R., and Dancis, J.: Treatment of familial dysautonomia with bethanechol (Urecholine). J. Pediatr., *81*:573, 1972.
4. Axelrod, F. B., and Dancis, J.: Intrauterine growth retardation in familial dysautonomia. Am. J. Dis. Child., *125*:379, 1973.
5. Axelrod, F. B., Nachtigal, R., and Dancis, J.: Familial dysautonomia: Diagnosis, pathogenesis and management. Adv. Pediatr., *21*:75, 1975.
6. Axelrod, F. B., and Pearson, J.: Congenital sensory neuropathies. Diagnostic distinction from familial dysautonomia. Am. J. Dis. Child., *138*:947, 1984.
7. Bartels, J., and Mazzia, V. D. B.: Familial dysautonomia. J.A.M.A., *212*:318, 1970.
8. Braun-Vallon, S., and Bessman, W.: La dysautonomia familiale (syndrome de Riley-Day). A propos de trois cas. Ann. Oculis (Paris), *193*:561, 1960.
9. Brown, J. C., and Johns, R. J.: Nerve conduction in familial dysautonomia (Riley-Day syndrome). J.A.M.A., *201*:200, 1967.
10. Brown, W. J., Beauchemin, J. A., and Linde, L. M.: A neuropathological study of familial dysautonomia (Riley-Day syndrome) in siblings. J. Neurol. Neurosurg. Psychiatry, *27*:131, 1964.
11. Brunt, P. W.: Unusual cause of Charcot joints in early adolescence (Riley-Day syndrome). Br. Med. J., *4*:277, 1967.
12. Brunt, P. W., and McKusick, V. A.: Familial dysautonomia: A report of genetic and clinical studies with review of the literature. Medicine, *49*:345, 1970.
13. Calvai, M., Giacanelli, M., Mongia, L., and Reynaud, G.: Dysautonomy, megasofago e ipotrofia musculare neurogena (sindrome de Riley-Day?) Presentazione di un caso. Minerva Pediatr., *21*:2466, 1969.
14. Cohen, P., and Solomon, N H.: Familial dysautonomia case report with autopsy. J. Pediatr., *46*:663, 1955.
15. Dancis, J., and Smith, A. A.: Familial dysautonomia. N. Engl. J. Med., *274*:207, 1966.
16. Dancis, J., and Smith, A. A.: Familial dysautonomia—What is in a name? J. Pediatr., *77*:174, 1970.
17. Fellner, M. J.: Manifestations of familial autonomic dysautonomia. Arch. Dermatol., *89*:190, 1964.
18. Fishbein, M.: Familial dysautonomia. Postgrad. Med., *38*:99, 1965.
19. Fogelson, M. H., Rorke, L. B., and Kaye, R.: Spinal cord changes in familial dysautonomia. Arch. Neurol., *17*:103, 1967.
20. Forster, W., and Tyndel, M.: The neuropsychiatric aspects of familial dysautonomia (the Riley-Day syndrome). J. Ment. Sci., *102*:345, 1956.
21. Freedman, A. M.: Psychiatric aspects of familial dysautonomia. Am. J. Orthopsychiatr., *27*:96, 1957.
22. Freedman, A. R.: Familial dysautonomia—Disease with a future. Clin. Pediatr., *5*:265, 1966.
23. Freedman, L. S., Ebstein, R. P., and Goldstein, M.: Serum dopamine-beta-hydroxylase in familial dysautonomia. J. Lab. Clin. Med., *85*:1008, 1975.
24. Ganz, S. B., Levine, D. B., Axelrod, F. B., and Kahanovitz, N.: Physical therapy management of familial dysautonomia. Phys. Ther., *63*:1121, 1983.
25. Geltzer, A. I., Gluck, L., Talner, N. S., and Polesky, H. F.: Familial dysautonomia. Studies in a newborn infant. N. Engl. J. Med., *271*:436, 1964.
26. Ginsberg, S. P.: Familial dysautonomia: The Riley-Day syndrome. Clin. Pediatr., *5*:308, 1966.
27. Gitlow, S. F., Bertani, I. M., and Wilk, E.: Excretion of catecholamine metabolites by children with familial dysautonomia. Pediatrics, *46*:513, 1970.
28. Goldstein-Nieviazhski, C., and Wallis, K.: Riley-Day syndrome (familial dysautonomia). Ann. Paediatr., *206*:188, 1966.
29. Goodall, J., Shinebourne, E., and Lake, B. D.: Early diagnosis of familial dysautonomia. Case report with special reference to primary pathophysiological finding. Arch. Dis. Child., *43*:455, 1968.
30. Grunebaum, M.: Radiological manifestations in familial dysautonomia. Am. J. Dis. Child., *128*:176, 1974.
31. Guzzetta, F., Tortorella, G., Cardia, E., and Ferriere, G.: Familial dysautonomia in a non-Jewish girl with histological evidence of progression in the sural nerve. Dev. Med. Child Neurol., *28*:62, 1986.
32. Hensinger, R. N., and MacEwen, G. D.: Spinal deformity associated with heritable neurolocal conditions: Spinal muscular atrophy, Friedreich's ataxia, familial dysautonomia, and Charcot-Marie-Tooth disease. J. Bone Joint Surg., *58-A*:13, 1976.
33. Hermier, M., Tanzy, M., Giley, J., Rosenberg, D., and Jeune, M.: La dysautonomie familiale. A propos d'un cas. Pediatre, *21*:943, 1966.
34. Howard, R. O.: Familial dysautonomia (Riley-Day syndrome). Am. J. Ophthalmol., *64*:392, 1961.
35. Hutchinson, J. H., and Hamilton, W.: Familial dysautonomia in two siblings. Lancet, *1*:1216, 1962.
36. Kaplan, M., Schiffman, R., and Shapira, Y.: Diagnosis of familial dysautonomia in the neonatal period. Acta Paediatr. Scand., *74*:131, 1985.
37. Keleman, G.: Familial dysautonomia (Riley-Day) aural histopathology. Pract. Otorhinolaryngol., *30*:194, 1968.

38. Kirkpatrick, R. H., and Riley, C. M.: Roentgenographic findings in familial dysautonomia. Radiology, 68:654, 1957.
39. Kritchman, M. M., Schwartz, H., and Papper, E. M.: Experience with general anesthesia in patients with familial dysautonomia. J.A.M.A., 170:529, 1959.
40. Kroops, I. G.: The production of tears in familial dysautonomia. J. Pediatr., 48:328, 1956.
41. Laxdal, D. E., Khera, S. A. K., and Haworth, D. H.: Familial dysautonomia (Riley-Day syndrome): Report of two siblings and review of literature. Can. Med. Assoc., 84:828, 1961.
42. Linde, L. M.: Dysautonomia (case report of a variant). J. Pediatr., 46:453, 1955.
43. Linde, L. M.: Diagnosis and management of dysautonomia. Pediatrics, 18:692, 1956.
44. McKendrick, T.: Familial dysautonomia. Arch. Dis. Child., 33:465, 1958.
45. McKusick, V. A., Norum, R. A., Farkas, H. J., Brunt, P. W., and Mahloudji, M.: The Riley-Day syndrome—Observations on genetics and survivorship. An interim report. Ir. J. Med. Sci., 3:372, 1967.
46. Mintzer, I. J., and Rubin, Z.: Dermatological manifestations of familial autonomic dysfunction (Riley-Day syndrome). Am. Arch. Derm. Syph., 67:561, 1953.
47. Pearson, J., Budzilovich, G., and Finegold, M. J.: Sensory motor and autonomic dysfunction: The nervous system in familial dysautonomia. Neurology, 21:486, 1971.
48. Rabinowitz, D., Landau, H., Rosler, A., Moses, S. W., Rotem, Y., and Freire, S.: Plasma renin activity and aldosterone in familial dysautonomia. Metabolism, 23:1, 1974.
49. Riley, C. M.: Familial dysautonomia. Adv. Pediatr., 9:157, 1957.
50. Riley, C. M., Day, R. L., Greeley, D. M., and Langford, W. S.: Central autonomic dysfunction with defective lacrimation. Pediatrics, 3:468, 1949.
51. Riley, C. M., Freedman, A. M., and Langford, W. S.: Further observations on familial dysautonomia. Pediatrics, 14:475, 1954.
52. Riley, C. M., and Moore, R. H.: Familial dysautonomia differentiated from related disorders. Pediatrics, 37:435, 1966.
53. Robin, G. C.: Scoliosis in familial dysautonomia. Bull. Hosp. Joint Dis. Orthop. Inst., 44:16, 1984.
54. Russell, A., and Avery, H. A.: Familial dysautonomia with other anomalies (Riley-Day syndrome). Three examples. Proc. R. Soc. Med., 56:291, 1963.
55. Siggers, D. C., Hacisca, T., and McKusick, V. A.: Vestibular dysfunction in familial dysautonomia. The Riley-Day syndrome. Arch. Dis. Child., 50:890, 1975.
56. Smith, A. A., and Dancis, J.: Response to intradermal histamine in familial dysautonomia. A diagnostic test. J. Pediatr., 63:889, 1963.
57. Smith, A. A., Farbman, A., and Dancis, J.: Absence of tastebud papillae in familial dysautonomia. Science, 147:1040, 1965.
58. Smith, A. A., Farbman, A., and Dancis, J.: Tongue in familial dysautonomia. A diagnostic sign. Am. J. Dis. Child., 110:152, 1965.
59. Smith, A. A., Hirsch, J. I., and Dancis, J.: Response to infused methacholine in familial dysautonomia. Pediatrics, 36:225, 1965.
60. Smithells, R. W.: Familial dysautonomia in the Riley-Day syndrome. Dev. Med. Child Neurol., 9:234, 1967.
61. Solitare, G. B., and Cohen, G. S.: Peripheral autonomic nervous system lesions in congenital or familial dysautonomia, Riley-Day syndrome. Neurology, 15:321, 1965.
62. St. Martin, D. A.: Familial autonomic dysfunction: Its occurrence in two siblings. Clin. Proc. Child. Hosp. Wash., D.C., 9:81, 1953.
63. Wolfe, S. M., and Henkin, R. I.: Absence of taste in the type II familial dysautonomia. Unresponsiveness to methacholine despite the presence of taste buds. J. Pediatr., 77:103, 1970.
64. Yatsu, F., and Zussman, W.: Familial dysautonomia (Riley-Day syndrome). Case report with postmortem findings of a patient at age 31. Arch. Neurol., 10:459, 1964.
65. Yoslov, W., Becker, M. H., Bartels, J., and Thompson, W. A. L.: Orthopaedic defects in familial dysautonomia. A review of sixty-five cases. J. Bone Joint Surg., 53-A:1541, 1971.
66. Ziegler, M. G., Lake, C. R., and Kopin, I. J.: Deficient sympathetic nervous response in familial dysautonomia. N. Engl. J. Med., 294:630, 1976.

CONGENITAL SENSORY NEUROPATHY

1. Axelrod, F. B., and Pearson, J.: Congenital sensory neuropathies. Diagnostic distinction from familial dysautonomia. Am. J. Dis. Child., 138:947, 1984.
2. Barry, J. E., Hopkins, I. J., and Neal, B. W.: Congenital sensory neuropathy. Arch. Dis. Child., 49:128, 1974.
3. Fedrizzi, E., D'Angelo, A., Negri, S., and Ermacora, E.: Peripheral sensory neuropathy in childhood. Dev. Med. Child Neurol., 14:501, 1972.
4. Haddow, J. E., Shapirao, S. R., and Gall, D. G.: Congenital sensory neuropathy in siblings. Pediatrics, 45:651, 1970.
5. Murray, T. J.: Congenital sensory neuropathy. Brain, 96:387, 1973.
6. Ogden, T. E., Robert, F., and Carmichael, E. A.: Some sensory syndromes in children. Indifference to pain and sensory neuropathy. J. Neurol. Neurosurg. Psychiatry., 22:267, 1959.
7. Taft, L. T.: Congenital sensory neuropathy. Dev. Med. Child Neurol., 13:109, 1971.

HEREDITARY SENSORY RADICULAR NEUROPATHY

1. Denny-Brown, D.: Hereditary sensory radicular neuropathy. J. Neurol. Neurosurg. Psychiatry, 14:237, 1951.
2. Turkington, R. W., and Stilfel, J. W.: Sensory radicular neuropathy. Arch. Neurol., 12:1924, 1965.

FAMILIAL SENSORY NEUROPATHY WITH ANHIDROSIS

1. Itoh, Y., Yagishita, S., Nakajima, S., Nakano, T., and Kawada, H.: Congenital insensitivity to pain with anhidrosis: morphological and morphometrical studies on the skin and peripheral nerves. Neuropediatrics, 17:103, 1986.
2. Lee, E. L., Oh, G. C., Lam, K. L., and Parameswann, N.: Congenital sensory neuropathy with anhidrosis. A case report. Pediatrics, 57:259, 1976.
3. Mazar, A., Herold, H. Z., and Vardy, P. A.: Congenital sensory neuropathy with anhidrosis: Orthopedic complications and management. Clin. Orthop., 118:184, 1976.
4. Pinsky, L., and DiGeorge, A. M.: Congenital familial sensory neuropathy with anhidrosis. J. Pediatr., 68:1, 1966.
5. Vasella, F., Emrich, H. M., Kraus-Ruppert, R., Aufdermaur, F., and Tonz, O.: Congenital sensory neuropathy with anhidrosis. Arch. Dis. Child., 43:124, 1968.

Infective Disorders

ACUTE POLYRADICULONEURITIS (GUILLAIN-BARRÉ SYNDROME)[1-116]

In this rare syndrome there is symmetrical motor and sensory paresis of the limbs, and in some cases, of the trunk. The paralysis, characteristically, ascends centripetally and may involve the cranial nerves. The etiology of the condition is unknown; most probably it is the result of a disturbance of the immune mechanism. A direct viral etiology has not been demonstrated. Landry, in 1859, described ten patients with ascending symmetrical weakness of the limbs, paresis of the respiratory muscles, and sensory disturbances; one of the patients was a 43-year-old man who died ten days after onset of the illness.[60] Guillain, Barré, and Strohl, in 1916, described two patients with motor weakness, hyperreflexia, and paresthesia; they found a dissociation between the level of spinal fluid protein and the cell count in the spinal fluid.[44] The syndrome is known by the eponyms *Guillain-Barré syndrome* and *Landry's paralysis*.

The pathophysiology is an acute demyelinization process. The posterior nerve roots and ganglia, the proximal portion of the peripheral nerves, and the anterior nerve roots are involved. Initially, pathologic changes consist of edema, followed by degeneration of axons and myelin, with some lymphocytic infiltration. In severe cases the peripheral nerves undergo wallerian degeneration. The anterior horn cells are involved only by retrograde extension of the demyelinizing process.

Clinical Features

There is great variation in the mode of onset, the severity of motor and sensory involvement, and the distribution of paresis. Ordinarily, the distal part of the limbs is involved initially, and the paresis ascends. Paralysis is usually symmetrical and is more marked distally than proximally. The deep tendon reflexes are absent or diminished. The motor weakness is accompanied by some degree of sensory disturbance, which may vary from minimal hypoesthesia to total loss of all modalities of sensation. In severe cases, sphincter disturbances and inability to urinate or defecate may be seen. Cranial nerves may be involved, usually the seventh or elev-

enth. On occasion, papilledema may be present. Autonomic disturbance is manifest as persistent tachycardia. Mentation is usually normal.

The course of the disease varies with the severity of the condition. In minimally involved patients, complete recovery may occur within one to two months, whereas in the severe forms it may take one to two years and varying grades of residual paralysis may persist. In the acute stage, paralysis of the limbs and trunk may be total, with the exception of some eye movement. In such cases, death may occur from cardiorespiratory collapse. Recurrent attacks may be encountered in an occasional patient.

Diagnosis

The cerebrospinal fluid shows an increase of proteins with a normal cellular picture. The concentration of cerebrospinal fluid protein reaches its maximal level in two to four weeks and starts to decline to normal values. Occasionally it may be abnormally high for several months.

Conduction in the motor and sensory fibers is slowed, as shown by nerve conduction studies, and evoked sensory potentials are absent or decreased in amplitude.

In the differential diagnosis, one should consider acute poliomyelitis, acute myelitis, acute porphyria, tick paralysis, and toxic neuropathy.

Treatment

Corticosteroids may be given during the acute paralytic phase; however, the results of such therapy are hard to assess.

Paralysis of the limbs is treated by supporting the parts in appropriate splints and passive and active assisted exercises to maintain the range of motion of the joints. When the antigravity weight-bearing muscles have regained fair motor strength, the patient is allowed to be ambulatory with the help of crutches. Orthotic devices are used as indicated. In severely involved patients in whom some degree of residual paralysis persists, orthopedic operations such as arthrodesis or tendon transfers are required for stabilization of joints and re-establishment of dynamic balance of muscles. In such instances, it is advisable to wait for two years to be sure that the paralysis is permanent.

Respiratory paralysis is a serious complication that occurs during the acute stage of the disease. It is treated by immediate tracheostomy and by the use of either tank type respirators or positive pressure systems.

References

1. Alvord, E. C., Jr.: Incubation period and severity of experimental allergic encephalomyelitis: analogy with swine-flu-vaccine-induced Guillain-Barré syndrome (Letter). Ann. Neurol., 19:100, 1986.
2. Andersson, T., and Siden, A.: A clinical study of the Guillain-Barré syndrome. Acta Neurol. Scand., 66:316, 1982.
3. Arbesman, C. E., Hyman, I., Dauzier, G., and Kantor, S. Z.: Immunologic studies of a Guillain-Barré syndrome following tetanus antitoxin. N.Y. J. Med., 58:2647, 1958.
4. Aylett, P.: Five cases of acute infective polyneuritis in children. Arch. Dis. Child., 29:531, 1954.
5. Baiocco, F., Bonora, G., Negri, A., Palma, A., and Rognoni, S.: Facila diplegia. Description of a post-varicella case classifiable as Guillain-Barré syndrome. Minerva Pediatr., 35:521, 1983.
6. Baoxun, Z., Yinchang, Y., Huifen, H., and Xiuqin, L.: Acute polyradiculitis (Guillain-Barré syndrome): an epidemiological study of 156 cases observed in Beijing. Ann. Neurol. (Suppl.), 9:146, 1981.
7. Bassoe, P.: Guillain-Barré syndrome and related conditions. Arch. Pathol., 26:289, 1938.
8. Beer, S. I., Avidan, G., and Viure, E.: Endotracheal intubation in Guillain-Barré syndrome. J.A.M.A., 244:2728, 1980.
9. Bendz, P.: Respiratory problems in acute Guillain-Barré syndrome. A.M.A. Arch. Neurol. Psychiatr., 73:22, 1955.
10. Bergamini, L., Durelli, L., Delsedime, M., and Cocito, D.: Therapeutic problems in the management of Guillain-Barré syndrome. Acta Neurol., 6:40, 1984.
11. Berlacher, F. J., and Abington, R. B.: ACTH and cortisone in Guillain-Barré syndrome. Review of the literature and report of a tested case following primary atypical pneumonia. Ann. Intern. Med., 48:1106, 1958.
12. Berman, A. T., and Tom, L.: The Guillain-Barré syndrome in children. Orthopedic management and patterns of recovery. Clin. Orthop., 116:673, 1976.
13. Bishop, N., Chakrabarti, A., Piercy, D., Harriman, D. G., and Pearce, J. M.: A case of sarcoma of the central nervous system presenting as a Guillain-Barré syndrome. J. Neurol. Neurosurg. Psychiatry, 46:352, 1983.
14. Blanco, K., and Cuomo, N.: From the other side of the bedrail: a personal experience with Guillain-Barré syndrome. J. Neurosurg. Nurs., 15:355, 1983.
15. Blood, A., Locke, W., and Carabasi, R.: Guillain-Barré syndrome tested with corticotropin. J.A.M.A., 152:139, 1953.
16. Boe, E., and Nyland, H.: Guillain-Barré syndrome after vaccination with human diploid cell rabies vaccine. Scand. J. Infect. Dis., 12:231, 1980.
17. Bradford, J. P., Bashford, E. F., and Wilson, J. A.: Acute infective polyneuritis. Q. J. Med., 12:88, 1918.
18. Brown, W. F., and Feasby, T. E.: Sensory evoked potentials in Guillain-Barré polyneuropathy. J. Neurol. Neurosurg. Psychiatry, 47:288, 1984.
19. Brumback, R. A.: Failure of oral versus parenteral corticosteroids in a case of acute inflammatory polyradiculoneuropathy (Guillain-Barré syndrome). Aust. N.Z. J. Med., 10:224, 1980.
20. Casamajor, L., and Lapert, G. R.: Guillain-Barré syndrome in children. Am. J. Dis. Child., 61:99, 1941.
21. Chung, H. O.: Infective polyneuritis (Guillain-Barré syndrome). Nurs. Times, 78:315, 1982.
22. Clement, M., and Ketelbant: Syndrome de Guillain et Barré et varicelle chez un enfant. J. Belge Neurol. Psychiatr., 38:240, 1938.
23. Cocito, D., Durelli, L., and Bergamini, L.: The treatment of Guillain-Barré syndrome. A comparison between steroid and plasmapheresis. Acta Neurol., 8:129, 1986.
24. Contreras Cortez, G., and Mora Gomaz, A.: Neonatal Landry-Guillain-Barré-Strohl syndrome. Bol. Med. Hosp. Infant Mex., 38:323, 1981.
25. Cook, S. D.: The Guillain-Barré syndrome. Relationship of circulating immunocytes. Its disease activity. Arch. Neurol., 22:470, 1970.
26. Corston, R. N., McGale, E. H., Stonier, C., Aber, G. M., and Hutchinson, E. C.: Abnormalities of cerebrospinal fluid amino acids in patients with the Guillain-Barré syndrome. J. Neurol. Neurosurg. Psychiatry, 44:86, 1981.
27. Crozier, R. E., and Ainley, A. B.: Guillain-Barré syndrome. N. Engl. J. Med., 252:83, 1955.
28. D'Ambrosia, G., De Angelis, G., and Vizioli, R.: Epidemiology of Guillain-Barré syndrome in Campania (south Italy). Preliminary results. Acta Neurol., 5:245, 1983.
29. Daniels, L., Williams, M., and Worthingham, C.: Muscle Testing. Techniques of Manual Examination. 2nd Ed. Philadelphia, W. B. Saunders, 1956.
30. Dureux, J. B., Gerard, A., Roche, G., Leheup, B., Canton, P., Schooneman, F., Jannot, C., and Streiff, F.: Treatment of Guillain-Barré syndrome by plasma exchange. 6 cases. Nouv. Presse Med., 9:3696, 1980.
31. Durocher, A., Servais, B., Caridroix, M., Chopin, C., and Wattel, F.: Autonomic dysfunction in the Guillain-Barré syndrome. Intensive Care Med., 6:3, 1980.
32. Durward, W. F., Burnett, A. K., Watkins, R., and Reid, J. M.: Plasma exchange in Guillain-Barré syndrome. Br. Med. J. (Clin. Res.), 283:794, 1981.
33. Dyck, P. J., and Kurtzke, J. F.: Plasmapheresis in Guillain-Barré syndrome (Editorial). Neurology, 35:1105, 1985.
34. Eberle, E., Brink, J., Azen, S., and White, D.: Early predictors of incomplete recovery in children with Guillain-Barré polyneuritis. J. Pediatr., 86:356, 1975.
35. Eden, A. N.: Guillain-Barré syndrome in a six-month-old infant. Am. J. Dis. Child., 102:224, 1961.
36. Eisen, A.: The Guillain-Barré syndrome. A clinical and electrodiagnostic study of 25 cases. Arch. Neurol., 30:438, 1974.
37. Fenichel, G. M.: Neurological complications of immunization. Ann. Neurol., 12:119, 1982.
38. Goldschmidt, B., Menonna, J., Fortunato, J., Dowling, P., and Cook, S.: Mycoplasma antibody in Guillain-Barré syndrome and other neurological disorders. Ann. Neurol., 7:108, 1980.
39. Gomirato, G., and Vignolo-Lutati, C.: Frequency and pathogenesis of Guillain-Barré-Strohl syndrome in children. Minerva Pediatr., 2:525, 1950.
40. Gordon, S. L., Morris, W. T., Stoner, M. A., and Greer, R. B.: Residual Guillain-Barré polyneuritis in children. J. Bone Joint Surg., 59-A:193, 1977.
41. Gracey, D. R., McMichan, J. C., Divertie, M. B., and Howard, F. M., Jr.: Respiratory failure in Guillain-Barré syndrome: a 6-year experience. Mayo Clin. Proc., 57:742, 1982.
42. Grattan, C. E., and Berman, P.: Chlamydial infection as a possible aetiological factor in the Guillain-Barré syndrome. Postgrad. Med. J., 58:776, 1982.

43. Guillain, G.: Radiculoneuritis with acellular hyperalbuminosis of the cerebrospinal fluid. Arch. Neurol. Psychiatr., *36*:975, 1936.

44. Guillain, G., Barré, J. A., and Strohl, A.: Sur un syndrome de radiculonevrite avec hyperalbuminose due liquide cephalorachidien sans reaction cellulaire. Bull. Soc. Med. Hop. Paris, *40*:1462, 1916.

45. Gupta, O. P., Kumar, N., and Agarwal, B. L.: Landry-Guillain-Barré syndrome. J. Indian Med. Assoc., *78*:43, 1982.

46. Haymaker, W., and Kernohan, J. W.: The Landry-Guillain-Barré syndrome, a clinicopathologic report of 50 fatal cases and a critique of the literature. Medicine, *28*:59, 1949.

47. Hecht, M. S.: Acute infective polyneuritis. J. Pediatr., *11*:743, 1937.

48. Heller, G. L., and DeJong, R. N.: Treatment of the Guillain-Barré syndrome. Arch. Neurol., *8*:179, 1963.

49. Hughes, R. A., Aslan, S., and Gray, I. A.: Lymphocyte subpopulations and suppressor cell activity in acute polyradiculoneuritis (Guillain-Barré syndrome). Clin. Exp. Immunol., *51*:448, 1983.

50. Hurwitz, E. S., Holman, R. C., Nelson, D. B., and Schonberger, L. B.: National surveillance for Guillain-Barré syndrome: January 1978–March 1979. Neurology, *33*:150, 1983.

51. Hurwitz, E. S., Schonberger, L. B., Nelson, D. B., and Holman, R. C.: Guillain-Barré syndrome and the 1978–1979 influenza vaccine. N. Engl. J. Med., *304*:1557, 1981.

52. Ince, L. P., and Leon, M. S.: Biofeedback treatment of upper extremity dysfunction in Guillain-Barré syndrome. Arch. Phys. Med. Rehabil., *67*:30, 1986.

53. Jones, I.: Facial diplegia in Guillain-Barré syndrome. Br. Med. J., *2*:84, 1954.

54. Kaplan, J. E., Katona, P., Hurwitz, E. S., and Schonberger, L. B.: Guillain-Barré syndrome in the United States, 1979–1980 and 1980–1981. Lack of an association with influenza vaccination. J.A.M.A., *248*:698, 1982.

55. Kaplan, J. E., Schonberger, L. B., Hurwitz, E. W., and Katona, P.: Guillain-Barré syndrome in the United States, 1978–1981: additional observations from the national surveillance system. Neurology, *33*:633, 1983.

56. Kaur, U., Chopra, J. S., Prabhakar, S., Radhakrishnan, K., and Rana, S.: Guillain-Barré syndrome. A clinical electrophysiological and biochemical study. Acta Neurol. Scand., *73*:394, 1986.

57. Keenlyside, R. A., Schonberger, L. B., Bregman, D. J., and Bolyai, J. Z.: Fatal Guillain-Barré syndrome after the national influenza immunization program. Neurology, *30*:929, 1980.

58. Kibel, M. A.: Guillain-Barré syndrome in childhood (Letter). S. Afr. Med. J., *63*:715, 1983.

59. Kurland, L. T., Wiederholt, W. C., Kirkpatrick, J. W., Potter, H. G., and Armstrong, P.: Swine influenza vaccine and Guillain-Barré syndrome. Epidemic or artifact? Arch. Neurol., *42*:1089, 1985.

60. Landry, O.: Note sur la paralysie ascendante aigue. Gaz. Hebd. Med., *6*:472, 1859.

61. Larsen, J. P., Kvale, G., and Nyland, H.: Epidemiology of the Guillain-Barré syndrome in the country of Hordaland, Western Norway. Acta Neurol. Scand., *7*:43, 1985.

62. Laufer, J., Passwell, J., Keren, G., Brandt, N., and Cohen, B. E.: Raised plasma renin activity in the hypertension of the Guillain-Barré syndrome. Br. Med. J. (Clin. Res.), *282*:1272, 1981.

63. Lejeune, B., Alix, D., LeFur, J. M., and Chastel, C.: Guillain-Barré syndrome and varicella (Letter). Arch. Fr. Pediatr., *38*:139, 1981.

64. LeLuyer, B., Devaux, A. M., Dailly, R., and Ensel, P.: Polyradiculoneuritis as a manifestation of childhood sarcoidosis. Arch. Fr. Pediatr., *40*:175, 1983.

65. Low, N. L., Schneider, J., and Carter, S.: Polyneuritis in children. Pediatrics, *22*:972, 1958.

66. McCarter, K. A.: Plasma exchange in Guillain-Barré syndrome. Nurs. Times, *78*:319, 1982.

67. McLeod, J. G.: Electrophysiological studies in the Guillain-Barré syndrome. Ann. Neurol. (Suppl.), *9*:20, 1981.

68. Marino, J. J., Motto, S., and Przypyszny, J. C.: Guillain-Barré syndrome in children. Illinois Med. J., *110*:73, 1956.

69. Markland, L. D., and Riley, H. D., Jr.: The Guillain-Barré syndrome in childhood. A comprehensive review, including observations on 19 additional cases. Clin. Pediatr., *6*:162, 1967.

70. Marshall, J.: The Landry-Guillain-Barré syndrome. Brain, *86*:55, 1963.

71. Massam, M., and Jones, R. S.: Ventilatory failure in the Guillain-Barré syndrome. Thorax, *35*:557, 1980.

72. Melnick, S. C.: Thirty-eight cases of the Guillain-Barré syndrome: An immunologic study. Br. Med. J., *1*:368, 1963.

73. Mendell, J. R., Kissel, J. T., Kennedy, M. S., Sahenk, Z., Grinvalsky, H. T., Pittman, G. L., Kyler, R. S., Roelofs, R. I., Witaker, J. N., and Bertorini, T. E.: Plasma exchange and prednisone in Guillain-Barré syndrome: a controlled randomized trial. Neurology, *35*:1551, 1985.

74. Merrill, R. E., and Fredrickson, D.: Landry-Guillain-Barré syndrome. J. Pediatr., *54*:816, 1959.

75. Merrill, R. E., and Fredrickson, D.: The distribution of paralysis in the Landry-Guillain-Barré syndrome. Am. Pract., *13*:450, 1962.

76. Mikati, M. A., and DeLong, G. R.: Childhood Guillain-Barré syndrome masquerading as a protracted pain syndrome (Letter). Arch. Neurol., *42*:839, 1985.

77. Miller, R. G.: Guillain-Barré syndrome. Current methods of diagnosis and treatment. Postgrad. Med., *77*:57, 1985.

78. Moore, P., and James, O.: Guillain-Barré syndrome: incidence, management and outcome of major complications. Crit. Care Med., *9*:549, 1981.

79. Moore, R. Y.: The Guillain-Barré syndrome. Develop. Med. Child Neurol., *9*:639, 1967.

80. Obiako, M. N.: The Landry-Guillain-Barré syndrome: the problem of establishing the right diagnosis. Practitioner, *224*:1293, 1980.

81. Osler, I. D., and Sidell, A. D.: The Guillain-Barré syndrome: The need for exact diagnostic criteria. N. Engl. J. Med., *262*:964, 1960.

82. Osterman, P. O., Fagius, J., Safwenberg, J., Danersund, A., Wallin, B. G., and Nordesjo, L. O.: Treatment of the Guillain-Barré syndrome by plasmapheresis. Arch. Neurol., *39*:148, 1982.

83. Parker, W., Wilt, J. C., Dawson, J. W., and Stackiu, W.: Landry-Guillain-Barré syndrome. The isolation of an ECHO virus type 6. Can. Med. Assoc. J., *82*:813, 1960.

84. Paulson, G. W.: The Landry-Guillain-Barré-Strohl syndrome in childhood. Dev. Med. Child Neurol., *12*:604, 1970.

85. Peterman, A. F., Daly, D. D., Dion, F. R., and Keith, H. M.: Infectious neuronitis (Guillain-Barré syndrome) in children. Neurology, *9*:533, 1959.

86. Plangues, J., and Mas, R.: Relapse 24 years after the first attack of a case of Guillain-Barré syndrome. Toulouse Med., *62*:445, 1961.

87. Posek, C. M., and Fowler, C. W.: The nosologic situation of the Landry-Guillain-Barré syndrome. Acta Neurol. Scand., *39*:187, 1963.

88. Poser, C. M.: Neurological complications of swine influenza vaccination. Acta Neurol. Scand., *66*:413, 1982.

89. Prydun, M.: Guillain-Barré syndrome: disease process. J. Neurosurg. Nurs., 15:27, 1983.
90. Radhakrishnan, K., Chopra, J. S., and Khattri, H. N.: Cardiovascular dysautonomia in Guillain-Barré syndrome. J. Assoc. Physicians India, 30:493, 1982.
91. Ravn, H.: The Landry-Guillain-Barré syndrome—a survey and a clinical report of 127 cases. Acta Neurol. Scand., 43:1, 1967.
92. Reichel, G., Perlwitz, R., and Wagner, A.: The prognostic significance of electromyographic and electroneurographic results in Landry-Guillain-Barré-Strohl polyradiculoneuritis. Psychiatr. Neurol. Med. Psychol., 33:281, 1981.
93. Reid, A. C., and Draper, I. T.: Pathogenesis of papilloedema and raised intracranial pressure in Guillain-Barré syndrome. Br. Med. J., 281:1393, 1980.
94. Reye, R. D. K.: Neuropathology of Landry-Guillain-Barré syndrome. Med. J. Aust., 2:386, 1954.
95. Ropper, A. H., and Chiappa, K. H.: Evoked potentials in Guillain-Barré syndrome. Neurology, 36:587, 1986.
96. Ropper, A. H., and Shahani, B. T.: Pain in Guillain-Barré syndrome. Arch. Neurol., 41:511, 1984.
97. Roquer, J., Herraiz, J., Maymo, J., Olive, A., and Carbonell, J.: Miller-Fisher syndrome (Guillain-Barré syndrome with ophthalmoplegia) during treatment with gold salts in a patient with rheumatoid arthritis (Letter). Arthritis Rheum., 28:838, 1985.
98. Schonberger, L. B., Hurwitz, E. S., Katona, P., Holman, R. C., and Bregman, D. J.: Guillain-Barré syndrome: its epidemiology and associations with influenza vaccination. Ann. Neurol. (Suppl.), 9:31, 1981.
99. Schuch, C. P., and Farmer, T. W.: Physical therapy in acute infectious polyneuritis. Phys. Ther. Rev., 35:238, 1955.
100. Siemes, H., Emerich, R., Merlin, M., and Reitter, B.: Acute polyradiculoneuritis (Guillain-Barré syndrome) in childhood. Klin. Padiatr., 195:38, 1983.
101. Singh, A., and Jolly, S. S.: Landry-Guillain-Barré syndrome. Report of 25 cases. Indian J. Med. Sci., 12:347, 1958.
102. Stillman, J. S., and Ganony, W. F.: Case of Guillain-Barré syndrome healed with ACTH and cortisone. N. Engl. J. Med., 246:293, 1952.
103. Takeuchi, H., Takahashi, M., Kang, J., Ueno, S., Yamada, A., Miki, H., and Tarui, S.: The Guillain-Barré syndrome: clinical and electroneuromyographic studies. J. Neurol., 231:6, 1984.
104. Tonnessen, T. I., Nyland, H., and Aarli, J. A.: Complement factors and acute phase reactants in the Guillain-Barré syndrome. Eur. Neurol., 21:124, 1982.
105. Toyka, K. V., Augspach, R., Paulus, W., Grabensee, B., and Hein, D.: Plasma exchange in polyradiculoneuropathy. Ann. Neurol., 8:205, 1980.
106. Vedeler, C. A., Nyland, H., Fagius, J., Osterman, P. O., Matre, R., Aarli, J. A., Jansen, R. W., Jacobsen, H., and Skre, H.: The clinical effect and the effect on serum IgG antibodies to peripheral nerve tissue of plasma exchange in patients with Guillain-Barré syndrome. J. Neurol., 228:59, 1982.
107. Von Hagen, K. O., and Baker, R. N.: Infectious neuronitis, present concepts of etiology and treatment. J.A.M.A., 151:1465, 1953.
108. Vranjesevic, D., Radojicic, B., Cvetkovic, D., and Dozic, S.: Recurrent polyradiculoneuritis in childhood. Clinical and biopsy findings. Srp. Arh. Celok. Lek., 110:901, 1982.
109. Vranjesevic, D., and Sinanovic, O.: Corticosteroids in polyradiculoneuritis therapy in childhood. Neurologija, 27:233, 1979.
110. Waksman, B. H., and Adams, R. D.: Experimental allergic neuritis produced in rabbits with nerve and adjuvants. Fed. Proc., 13:516, 1954.
111. Wexler, I.: Serial sensory and motor conduction measurement in Guillain-Barré syndrome. Electromyogr. Clin. Neurophysiol., 20:87, 1980.
112. Wiederholt, W. C., Mulder, D. W., and Lambert, E. H.: The Landry-Guillain-Barré-Strohl syndrome or polyradiculoneuropathy: Historical review, report on 97 patients and present concepts. Mayo Clin. Proc., 39:427, 1964.
113. Wisniewski, H., Terry, R. D., Whitaker, J. N., Cooh, S. D., and Dowling, P. C.: Landry-Guillain-Barré syndrome. Arch. Neurol., 21:269, 1969.
114. Wolfenden, W. H., and McGuinness, A. E.: The Guillain-Barré syndrome with special reference to respiratory paralysis and recurrence. Med. J. Aust., 45:163, 1958.
115. Zerbi, D., Celano, I., Forlani, G., Garelli, S., Mosconi, L., and Valbonesi, M.: Plasmapheresis in the treatment of four cases of Guillain-Barré syndrome (acute form). Ital. J. Neurol. Sci., 2:331, 1981.
116. Zhou, X. D.: Determination of nerve conduction speed in Guillain-Barré syndrome. Chung Hua Shen Ching Ching Shen Ko Tsa Chih, 12:65, 1979.

HERPES ZOSTER

Herpes zoster, commonly known as shingles, is an acute viral infection of one or more dorsal root ganglia or sensory ganglia of the cranial nerves. It is accompanied by a painful vesicular rash of the skin or mucous membrane that is distributed in the corresponding dermatome along the course of the peripheral sensory nerves arising in the affected ganglia. Herpes zoster and varicella appear to be caused by the same virus, varicella-zoster virus. Weller et al. have been able to propagate the etiologic agent in vitro in cultures of human tissues.[67, 68] The viral bodies from vesicles of varicella and zoster are identical in appearance, size, and serologic reactions. Infection with one disease may occur after contact with a patient suffering from the other. It seems that herpes zoster results from neurogenous spread of reactivated latent varicella virus in a partially immune individual, whereas varicella is caused by hematogenous spread of the virus in a nonimmune individual.[21]

Herpes zoster commonly occurs in individuals over 40 years of age; it is not, however, rare in children, in whom it is most frequently encountered in association with malignant neoplasms such as leukemia, lymphomas, or neuroblastoma. Other predisposing factors are poisoning with arsenic or other drugs, and trauma affecting the nerve roots, in which case herpes zoster develops in the involved dermatome.

Pathology

The lesions in the nervous system may be categorized as (1) inflammation of the spinal posterior root ganglia or the sensory ganglia of the cranial nerves (in the acute stage, there is marked lymphocytic reaction with a varying degree of cell necrosis, followed by secondary degeneration of the afferent fibers and eventual gliosis); (2) a "poliomyelitis-like" lesion involving both the anterior and the posterior horns and roots; (3) a relatively mild localized leptomeningitis; and (4) true peripheral mononeuritis.[25]

The involvement of the anterior horn cells of the spinal cord accounts for the motor manifestations of the disease. Broadbent, in 1866, is credited as being the first to describe paralysis of the upper limb due to herpes zoster.[13] Upper motor neuron involvement with hemiplegia was reported by Duncan in 1868, and a description of lower limb paralysis was published by Hardy in 1876.[27, 39]

The epithelial layer of the skin is markedly inflamed, and acidophilic intranuclear inclusion bodies are found in the epithelial cells of the vesicles.

Clinical Features

The manifestations of the disease are milder in children than in adults and the face is less frequently involved. There may be generalized malaise, low-grade fever, burning dysesthesia in the involved dermatome, or pain in the underlying muscles during the prodromal period, which may last three or four days. The regional lymph nodes may be enlarged. Neck stiffness and headache are occasional complaints.

The eruption develops suddenly, with characteristic distribution along the course of the sensory nerve. It is first papular, then vesicular, and eventually becomes crusted. The rash may form a complete girdle, or "cingulum," from which the name "shingles" is derived. The common site of the skin lesions is the trunk or face; they occur less frequently on the limbs, where they are more proximal than distal. Involvement is more often unilateral than bilateral.

Paralysis of the limbs occurs in about 5 per cent of cases. Gupta et al. have found limb paralysis in 15 of the 274 patients with zoster referred to the hospital—seven of the upper limbs, seven of the lower limbs, and one of both the upper and the lower limbs on the same side (lower motor neuron type).[37] Grant and Rowe reported 5 patients with paralysis of the limbs among 101 patients admitted to Massachusetts General Hospital (two of the upper, and three of the lower limbs).[33] Herpetic eruption frequently precedes the paralysis, the time interval between the two incidents being one to six days; however, it may take three and a half months for the paralysis to develop following the herpetic eruption. Occasionally the eruption and paralysis occur simultaneously.

The prognosis for full recovery is good in paralysis of the limbs in herpes zoster. Gupta et al. reported complete recovery in two thirds of the patients within a year. Permanent paralysis occurred in one sixth of the patients studied.[37] Permanent paralysis usually takes place in muscles that are mainly or wholly supplied from single segments of the spinal cord, such as the hemidiaphragm, the muscles of the anterior tibial compartment, and the intrinsic muscles of the hand.

The motor paralysis may suggest intraspinal tumor. The presence of herpetic rash should aid in the differential diagnosis.

Treatment

There is no specific remedy for herpes zoster. Relief of pain is afforded by analgesics. Local skin care is provided when the blisters become infected because of scratching. Therapy of paralysis of limbs follows the principles outlined for poliomyelitis.

References

1. Abercrombie, R. G.: Herpes zoster with muscular paralysis and disturbance of sensation. Br. Med. J., 1:778, 1941.
2. Adeniyi, A., Laditan, A. A., and Seriki, O.: Fatal herpes zoster in Burkitt's lymphoma following contact with chicken pox. J. Trop. Med. Hyg., 80:200, 1977.
3. Aimes, C. R.: The elementary bodies of zoster and their serological relationship to those of varicella. Br. J. Exp. Pathol., 15:314, 1934.
4. Asano, Y., Nakayama, H., Yazaki, T., Ito, S., and Isomura, S.: Protective efficacy of vaccination in children in four episodes of natural varicella and zoster in the ward. Pediatrics, 59:8, 1977.
5. Atkinson, K., Meyers, J. D., Storb, R., Prentice, R. L., and Thomas, E. D.: Varicella-zoster virus infection after marrow transplantation for aplastic anemia or leukemia. Transplantation, 29:47, 1980.
6. Baba, K., Yabuuchi, H., Takahashi, M., and Ogra, P. L.: Increased incidence of herpes zoster in normal children infected with varicella zoster virus during infancy: Community-based follow-up study. J. Pediatr., 108:372, 1986.
7. Bacon, G. E., Oliver, W. J., and Shapiro, D. A.: Factors contributing to the severity of herpes zoster in children. J. Pediatr., 67:768, 1965.
8. Bennet, R., Forsgren, M., and Herin, P.: Herpes zoster in a 2-week-old premature infant with possible congenital varicella encephalitis. Acta Pediatr. Scand., 74:979, 1985.
9. Benoit, Y., Laureys, G., Delbeke, M. J., and De-Clercq, E.: Oral BVDU treatment of varicella and zoster in children with cancer. Eur. J. Pediatr., 143:198, 1985.

10. Berlin, B. S., and Campbell, T.: Hospital acquired herpes zoster following exposure to chicken pox. J.A.M.A., *211*:1831, 1970.
11. Blank, H., Burgoon, C. F., Baldridge, G. D., McCarthy, P. L., and Urbach, F.: Cytologic smears in diagnosis of herpes simplex, herpes zoster and varicella. J.A.M.A., *146*:1410, 1951.
12. Brain, R. T.: The relationship between the viruses of zoster and varicella as demonstrated by the complement-fixation reaction. Br. J. Exp. Pathol., *14*:67, 1933.
13. Broadbent, W. H.: Case of herpetic eruption in the course of branches of the brachial plexus followed by partial paralysis in corresponding motor nerves. Br. Med. J., 2:460, 1866.
14. Brostoff, J.: Diaphragmatic paralysis after zoster. Br. Med. J., 2:1571, 1966.
15. Brunell, P. A., and Kotchmar, G. S., Jr.: Zoster in infancy: failure to maintain virus latency following intrauterine infection. J. Pediatr., 98:71, 1981.
16. Brunell, P. A., Miller, L. H., and Lovejoy, F.: Zoster in children. Am. J. Dis. Child., *115*:432, 1968.
17. Brunell, P. A., Ross, A., Miller, L. H., and Kuo, B.: Prevention of varicella by zoster immune globulin. N. Engl. J. Med., *280*:1191, 1969.
18. Brunell, P. A., Taylor-Wiedeman, J., Geiser, C. F., Frierson, L., and Lydick, E.: Risk of herpes zoster in children with leukemia: varicella vaccine compared with history of chickenpox. Pediatrics, 77:53, 1986.
19. Burgoon, C. F., Jr., Burgoon, J. S., and Baldridge, G. D.: The natural history of herpes zoster. J.A.M.A., *164*:265, 1957.
20. Carter, A. B., and Dunlop, J. B. W.: Paresis following herpes zoster. Br. Med. J., *1*:234, 1941.
21. Cheatham, W. J.: The relation of heretofore unreported lesions to pathogenesis of herpes zoster. Am. J. Pathol., 29:401, 1953.
22. Cheatham, W. J., Weller, T. H., Dolan, T. F., Jr., and Dower, J. C.: Varicella: report of two fatal cases with necropsy, virus isolation, and serologic studies. Am. J. Pathol., 32:1015, 1956.
23. Davis, C. M., Van Dersarl, J. V., and Coltman, C. A., Jr.: Failure of cytarabine in varicella-zoster infections. J.A.M.A., 224:122, 1973.
24. Dawber, R.: Idoxuridine in herpes zoster: further evaluation of intermittent topical therapy. Br. Med. J., 2:526, 1974.
25. Denny-Brown, D., Adams, R. D., and Fitzgerald, P. J.: Pathologic features of herpes zoster. Arch. Neurol. Psychiatr., *51*:216, 1944.
26. Devereaux, M. D., Hazelton, R. A.: Acute monarticular arthritis in association with herpes zoster. Arthritis Rheum., 26:236, 1983.
27. Duncan, J.: On herpes zoster. J. Cutan. Med., 2:241, 1868–9.
28. Fee, C. F., and Evarts, C. M.: Motor paralysis of the lower extremities in herpes zoster. Cleve. Clin. Q., 35:169, 1968.
29. Feldman, S., Hughes, W. T., and Kim, H. Y.: Herpes zoster in children with cancer. Am. J. Dis. Child., 126:178, 1973.
30. Frengley, J. D.: Herpes zoster: a challenge in management. Primary Care, 8:715, 1981.
31. Gershon, A. A.: Prevention and treatment of varicella-zoster virus infection. Pediatr. Infect. Dis., 3:34, 1984.
32. Gershon, A. A., Kalter, Z. G., and Steinberg, S.: Detection of antibody to varicella-zoster virus by immune adherence hemagglutination. Proc. Soc. Exp. Biol. Med., *151*:762, 1976.
33. Grant, B. D., and Rowe, C. R.: Motor paralysis of the extremities in herpes zoster. J. Bone Joint Surg., 43-A:85, 1961.
34. Greenberg, J.: Herpes zoster with motor involvement. J.A.M.A., *212*:322, 1970.
35. Grose, C.: Zoster in children with cancer: Radioimmune precipitation profiles of sera before and after illness. J. Infect. Dis., *147*:47, 1983.
36. Guess, H. A., Broughton, D. D., Melton, L. J., III, and Kurkland, L. T.: Epidemiology of herpes zoster in children and adolescents: A population-based study. Pediatrics, 76:512, 1985.
37. Gupta, S. K., Helal, B. H., and Kiely, P.: The prognosis in zoster paralysis. J. Bone Joint Surg., *51-B*:593, 1969.
38. Hanngren, K., Falksveden, L., Grandien, M., and Lidin Janson, G.: Zoster immunoglobulin in varicella prophylaxis. A study among high-risk patients. Scand. J. Infect. Dis., *15*:327, 1983.
39. Hardy, M.: Du zona. Gaz. Hop., *49*:827, 1876.
40. Hartley, W. J., and Mandal, B. K.: Herpes zoster in childhood. Practitioner, 226:766, 1982.
41. Hayne, S. T., and Mercer, J. B.: Herpes zoster: treatment with cimetidine. Can. Med. Assoc. J., 129:1284, 1983.
42. Helander, I., Arstila, P., and Terho, P.: Herpes zoster in a six-month-old infant. Acta Derm. Venereol., 63:180, 1983.
43. Hogan, E. L., and Krigman, M. R.: Herpes zoster myelitis. Arch. Neurol., 29:309, 1973.
44. Hutter, J. J., Jr., Minnich, L. L., and Ray, C. G.: Varicella-zoster antibody titers in children with leukemia and lymphoma. Relationship of titer to varicella-zoster infection. Am. J. Dis. Child., *138*:56, 1984.
45. Keiden, S. E., and Mainwaring, D.: Association of herpes zoster with leukemia and lymphoma in children. Clin. Pediatr., 4:13, 1965.
46. Kendall, D.: Motor complications of herpes zoster. Br. Med. J., 2:616, 1957.
47. Latif, R., and Shope, C.: Herpes zoster in normal and immunocompromised children. Am. J. Dis. Child., 137:801, 1983.
48. Lewkonia, I. A., and Jackson, A. A.: Infantile herpes zoster after intrauterine exposure to varicella. Br. Med. J., 3:149, 1973.
49. Lin, C. Y., Hsu, H. C., and Hung, H. Y.: Nephrotic syndrome associated with varicella infection. Pediatrics, 75:1127, 1985.
50. McClain, K., Warkentin, P., and Kay, N.: Spontaneous remission of Burkitt's lymphoma associated with herpes zoster infection. Am. J. Pediatr. Hematol. Oncol., 7:9, 1985.
51. Mietens, C.: Almost simultaneous occurrence of varicella and zoster in an otherwise healthy child. Pediatr. Infect. Dis., 5:482, 1986.
52. Mok, C. H.: Zoster-like disease in infants and young children. N. Engl. J. Med., 285:294, 1971.
53. Music, S. I., Fine, E. M., and Tago, Y.: Zoster-like disease in the newborn due to herpes simplex virus. N. Engl. J. Med., 284:24, 1971.
54. Nachman, A. R.: Neurological complications of herpes zoster. Pediatrics, 7:200, 1951.
55. Novelli, V. M., Marshall, W. C., Yeo, J., and McKendrick, G. D.: Acyclovir administered perorally in immunocompromised children with varicella-zoster infections. J. Infect. Dis., 149:478, 1984.
56. Ohsaki, M., Chiba, S., and Nakao, T.: Bell's palsy in infants associated with varicella-zoster virus infection. J. Pediatr., 84:103, 1974.
57. Paryani, S. G., and Arvin, A. M.: Intrauterine infection with varicella-zoster virus after maternal varicella. N. Engl. J. Med., *314*:1542, 1986.
58. Rodger, R. S., and Tindall, J. P.: Herpes zoster in children. Arch. Dermatol., *106*:204, 1972.
59. Skovby, F., and Sullivan, M. P.: Herpes zoster and varicella in children with Hodgkin's disease. Acta Pediatr. Scand., 71:269, 1982.
60. Sullinger, J. M., Imbach, P., Barandun, S., Gugler, E., Hirt, A., Luthy, A., Rossi, E., Tonz, O., and Wagner, H. P.: Varicella and herpes zoster in immu-

nosuppressed children: Preliminary results of treatment with intravenous immunoglobulin. Helv. Paediatr. Acta, 39:63, 1984.

61. Sutton, G.: Steroidstoss therapy in the treatment of herpes zoster. Br. J. Clin. Pract., 38:21, 1984.

62. Taterka, J. H., and O'Sullivan, M. E.: The motor complications of herpes zoster. J.A.M.A., 122:737, 1943.

63. Underwood, E. A.: The neurological complications of varicella: a clinical and epidemiological study. Br. J. Dis. Child., 32:83, 1977.

64. Verma, A. K., and Maheshwari, M. C.: Brachial monoparesis following herpes zoster. Acta Neurol., 7:32, 1985.

65. Waller, G.: Two cases of herpes with motor paralysis. Br. Med. J., 2:560, 1885.

66. Weintraub, I. I.: Treatment of herpes zoster with gamma globulin. J.A.M.A., 157:1611, 1955.

67. Weller, T. H., and Witton, H. M.: The etiologic agents of varicella and herpes zoster. Serologic studies with the viruses as propagated in vitro. J. Exp. Med., 108:869, 1958.

68. Weller, T. H., Witton, H. M., and Bell, E. J.: The etiologic aspects of varicella and herpes zoster. Isolation, propagation and cultural characteristics in vitro. J. Exp. Med., 108:843, 1958.

69. Weseley, M. S., and Barenfeld, P. A.: Motor involvement in herpes zoster. N.Y. J. Med., 65:913, 1965.

70. Williams, D. L., Gershon, A. A., Gelb, L. D., Spraker, M. K., Steinberg, S., and Ragab, A. H.: Herpes zoster following varicella vaccine in a child with acute lymphocytic leukemia. J. Pediatr., 106:259, 1985.

71. Winkelmann, R. K., and Perry, H. O.: Herpes zoster in children. J.A.M.A., 171:876, 1959.

72. Wright, E. T., and Winer, L. H.: Herpes zoster in malignancy. Arch. Dermatol., 84:242, 1961.

73. Wurzel, C. L., Kahan, J., Heitler, M., and Rubin, L. G.: Prognosis of herpes zoster in healthy children. Am. J. Dis. Child., 140:477, 1986.

74. Zaia, J. A., Levin, M. J., Preblud, S. R., Leszczynski, J., Wright, G. G., Ellis, R. J., Curtis, A. C., Valerio, M. A., and LeGore, J.: Evaluation of varicella-zoster immune globulin: protection of immunosuppressed children after household exposure to varicella. J. Infect. Dis., 147:737, 1983.

Traumatic Disorders

OBSTETRICAL BRACHIAL PLEXUS PALSY

Paralysis of the upper limb resulting from traction injury to the brachial plexus at birth was first mentioned by Smellie in 1764 in his textbook on midwifery.[115]

The incidence, severity, and extent of brachial plexus palsy have been minimized by better obstetrical care, i.e., earlier recognition of larger birth weight babies and induction of labor at an earlier gestational age, detection of intrauterine malposture by ultrasonography, and delivery of babies by cesarean section when they are at high risk of birth trauma. In spite of such preventative measures and improved obstetrical techniques, obstetrical brachial plexus paralysis has not been eliminated. It occurs in 0.4 to 2.5 per 1000 live births.[1, 45, 51, 60, 102, 123, 129, 135]

Etiology

The mechanism of trauma is forced stretching of one or more components of the brachial plexus by traction. The affected babies are large, their birth weight averaging two pounds heavier than normal.[1] Delivery is usually difficult. In breech delivery traction is applied on the brachial plexus at the stage when the head is extracted by strong lateral flexion of the trunk and neck, while in vertex presentation the brachial plexus is injured when the shoulders are delivered by forced lateral flexion of the head and neck (Fig. 5–182). Forceps used in delivery may directly contuse the brachial plexus.

In summary, the obstetrical risk factors for brachial plexus injury at birth are high birth weight, prolonged labor, breech position, and shoulder dystocia. During cesarean section, extraction of the fetus in breech position may injure the brachial plexus if traction forces are applied on the head and neck or on the shoulders.[48]

In experimental studies on the tensile strength of the brachial plexus, Wickstrom found the disruption of the lower plexus components occurred with approximately half the force required to disrupt the components of the upper plexus and that the soft-tissue structures surrounding the plexus contributed to the resistance to stretch of the tissues. Most of the disruptions occurred at the foramen or within the groove of the transverse process. Avulsion of the nerve roots from the spinal cord and cord disruption accounted for the upper motor neuron lesion findings often present in brachial plexus injuries.[137, 138]

Classification

Obstetrical brachial plexus palsy may be classified according to the severity of damage and according to the components of the plexus that are injured.

Injury to the nerves by increased traction on the plexus may vary from slight stretching (neurapraxia or axonotmesis) to complete rupture (neurotmesis). In *mild* lesions, failure of conduction results from simple stretching of the nerve fibers and associated perineural edema

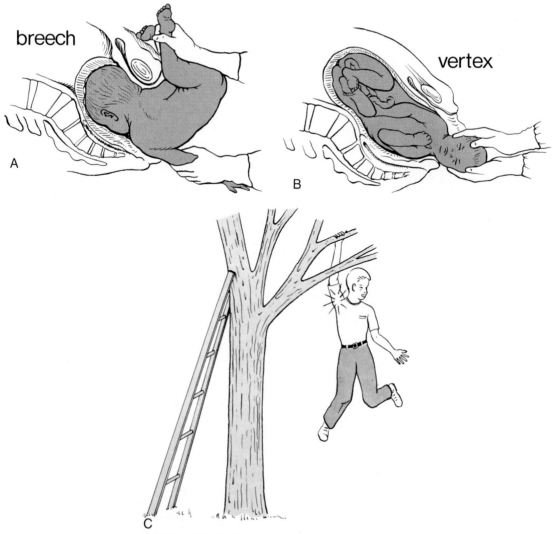

FIGURE 5–182. *Mechanism of injury to the brachial plexus.*

A. During delivery. In breech delivery traction is applied on the nerves by lateral flexion of the neck and trunk. **B.** In vertex presentation, traction on the nerves is applied when the shoulders are delivered by lateral flexion of the head and neck. **C.** In a fall from a tree.

and hemorrhage. In this type of injury, complete and early recovery usually takes place with absorption of the edema and hemorrhage. On occasion, however, cicatricial fibrosis occurs and recovery is slow and incomplete. In *moderate* lesions, some of the nerve fibers are stretched and others are torn, with associated intraneural and extraneural bleeding. Depending upon the severity of involvement, recovery of nerve conduction and function is slow and incomplete in this type. In *severe* lesions, there is almost complete rupture of the trunks of the plexus, or actual avulsion of the roots from the spinal cord. In this type, recovery is very poor.

According to the components of the plexus that are injured, obstetrical brachial plexus paralysis may be grouped into (1) the *upper arm paralysis of Erb-Duchenne*, in which the fifth and sixth cervical nerve roots or their derivatives are principally involved; (2) the *lower arm paralysis of Klumpke*, in which the eighth cervical and first thoracic roots are affected; and (3) *paralysis of the entire arm*, in which there is some involvement of all components of the plexus.[28, 31, 32, 61]

Clinical Features

Immediately following birth the injury is evident. The affected limb lies motionless at the side of the trunk with the elbow in extension

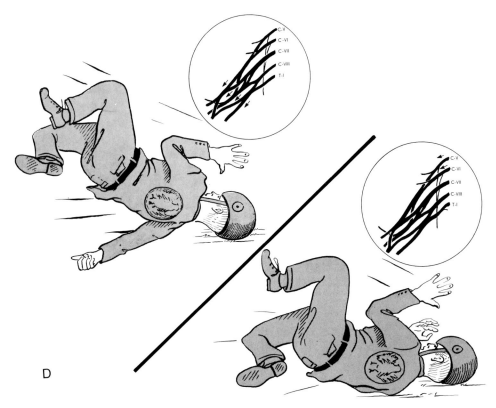

FIGURE 5–182 Continued. Mechanism of injury to the brachial plexus.

D. In a motorcycle accident.

(Fig. 5–183A). The Moro reflex is absent on the involved side (Fig. 5–184). In the lower arm and whole arm types of paralysis, there is loss of the grasp reflex. In the Klumpke type, the cervical sympathetic fibers in the first dorsal root may be involved, producing an ipsilateral Horner's syndrome characterized by enophthalmos, miosis, and ptosis. Phrenic nerve palsy with paralysis of the diaphragm may occur on rare occasions.

Avulsion of the nerve roots from the spinal cord may produce hematomyelia, which accounts for the presence of the transient spastic paralysis in the opposite upper limb and both lower limbs. There may be concomitant cerebral palsy due to injury of the central nervous system from dystocia and hypoxia at birth. In such cases, assessment by a pediatric neurologist is appropriate.

In some instances there may be supraclavicular swelling and ecchymosis and tenderness due to hemorrhage, or the nerve injury may be accompanied by a fractured clavicle (see Fig. 5–183B), traumatic separation of the upper humeral epiphysis, or a fracture of the humeral shaft. Passive movements of the affected limb may be painful owing to associated "neuritis."

Cephalohematoma or ecchymosis may be present owing to forceps injury.

The hips should be thoroughly examined to rule out hip dislocation; because of intrauterine malposition and breech delivery, these infants are at high risk for hip dysplasia. Re-examine the hips at six weeks and again at three months to rule out postnatal dislocation.

The distribution of motor paralysis depends upon the site of nerve injury. In the *upper arm or Erb-Duchenne type*, the deltoid muscle, the lateral rotator muscles of the shoulder (supraspinatus, infraspinatus, and teres minor), the biceps brachii, brachialis, supinator, and brachioradialis muscles are usually paralyzed. The fingers and wrist have normal active motion. There may be slight sensory deficit. The upper arm paralysis is the most frequent type.

In the *lower arm paralysis of Klumpke*, the wrist flexors, the long flexors of the fingers, and the intrinsic muscles of the hand are affected. The muscles controlling the shoulder and elbow are not involved. This is the rarest type. Sensation is ordinarily normal. When the *entire arm* is paralyzed, the upper limb is almost completely flaccid and there is often extensive sensory loss.

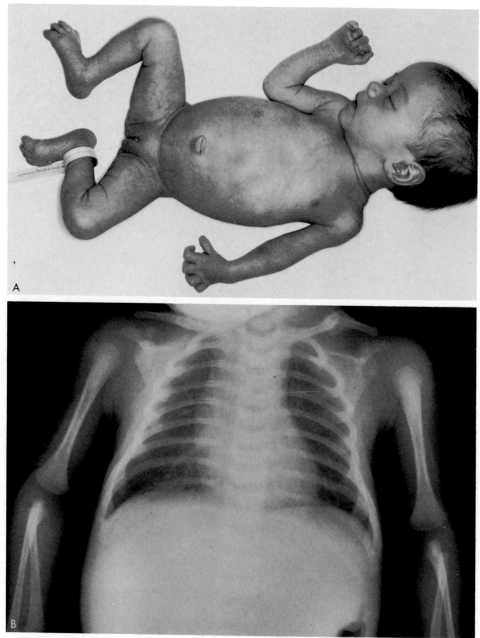

FIGURE 5–183. *Obstetrical brachial plexus paralysis on the left in a newborn infant.*

A. Clinical appearance of patient. The left upper limb lies at the side of the trunk with the elbow in extension. **B.** Radiogram shows healing fracture of left clavicle.

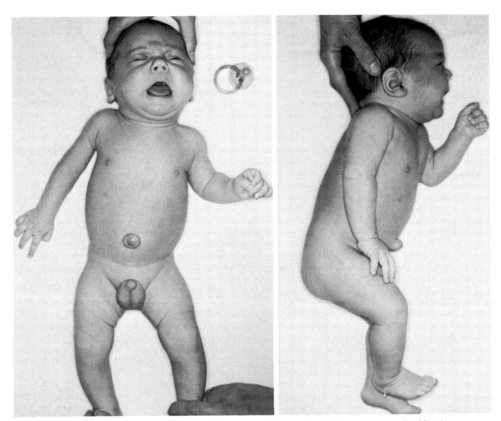

FIGURE 5–184. *Obstetrical brachial plexus paralysis on the right in a one-month-old infant.*

Note the lack of active motion in response to testing of asymmetrical tonic and Moro reflexes.

Prognosis and Natural History

The degree and rate of recovery vary with the type and severity of paralysis. It is difficult to estimate the end point of maximum spontaneous recovery, as it may vary from 1 to 18 months. In general, those patients with involvement of the entire plexus or lower plexus have a slower and more incomplete return than do those with only upper plexus involvement. Two other findings that herald a poor recovery are the presence of Horner's syndrome and paralysis of the parascapular muscles; both these findings indicate involvement of the roots before they form the trunks of the brachial plexus—a level of poor repair following nerve injury. Paralysis of the phrenic nerve is a poor prognostic sign.

With the advent of better obstetrical care and preventive measures the severity and extent of brachial plexus paralysis have markedly diminished. Reports in the literature prior to 1970 showed full recovery in 7 to 40 per cent of the cases.[1, 42, 137] Recent studies report full recovery in 80 to 95 per cent of the cases.[45, 48, 51, 123, 129]

The report of Greenwald et al. is of particular interest. They found 61 cases at Kaiser Foundation Hospital, San Francisco, in a ten-year period (1977–1987), an incidence of 2 per 1000 births. This study shows that the incidence has not declined; however, on follow-up they found full recovery in 95.7 per cent of the cases, indicating lessening of the severity of the paralysis. In 92 per cent of the cases, complete recovery occurred in three months; this was timely enough to ensure normal motor patterning and body imaging. Paralysis at birth did not preclude the development of the dominant use of the involved upper limb—73 per cent of the right-sided palsied patients were righthanded.[48]

Differential Diagnosis

In the neonatal period, in the differential diagnosis, one should consider fracture of the humerus, separation of the proximal humeral epiphysis, fracture of the clavicle, acute osteomyelitis of the humerus, and septic arthritis of the shoulder.

Clinically, in pseudoparalysis due to shoulder girdle fractures the Moro reflex is present, whereas in paralysis due to brachial plexus paralysis the Moro reflex is absent.

Radiograms of the upper limb, clavicle, and cervical spine should be routinely obtained in all suspected cases of obstetrical brachial plexus paralysis. A cervical myelogram is not indicated. When a patient is seen later in infancy, the possibility of a spinal cord tumor or cerebral palsy should be considered; however, when accurate delineation of brachial plexus and spinal cord pathology is desirable, nuclear magnetic resonance imaging is performed.

Residual Deformities

SHOULDER

Asynergy (or dyskinesia) of the muscles controlling the shoulder is a prominent feature. The normal scapulohumeral rhythm is disturbed. During attempted abduction, the scapula moves initially, and the greater part of the combined action at the shoulder is scapulocostal rather than scapulohumeral. When active shoulder abduction is attempted, hypertonicity of the flexor muscle groups is triggered and the shoulder and elbow joints simultaneously go into automatic flexion. The holding motor power of the deltoid muscle in abducted position is strong, but when the arm is in adducted position, the deltoid muscle is weak (usually fair minus) in motor strength. There are two possible etiologic factors in the pathogenesis of dyskinesia: the presence of retrograde upper motor neuron changes in the spinal cord as a result of avulsion of nerve roots from the cord, and the lack of development of functional cerebral motor patterns of coordination caused by paralysis occurring at birth.

Residual deformities of the shoulder can be classified, according to Zancolli, into various groups and subgroups depending upon the type of shoulder deformity, site of muscle contracture and pattern of flaccid paralysis, range of active and passive motion of the scapulohumeral joints, presence or absence of scapular elevation or Putti sign, and radiographic findings (Table 5–18).[143, 144]

In *Group I* (about 90 per cent of the cases), there is joint contracture, whereas in *Group II* there is pure flaccid paralysis without muscular contracture, joint deformity, or dislocation. Group I is subdivided into four subgroups: (A) medial rotation-adduction contracture without joint deformity or dislocation, i.e., the glenohumeral joint sphericity and congruity is preserved; (B) medial rotation-adduction contracture of the shoulder with joint deformity and posterior subluxation or dislocation; (C) lateral rotation-abduction contracture with anteroinfer-ior subluxation or dislocation; and (D) pure abduction contracture of the shoulder.

The most common deformity of the shoulder is medial rotation-adduction contracture of the shoulder. Clinically, the subgroup A (those without joint deformity or dislocation) and subgroup B (those with joint deformity and dislocation) can be distinguished by Putti's scapular elevation sign: With the elbow flexed 90 degrees the shoulder is adducted and laterally rotated; the upper medial corner of the scapula will be elevated when there is glenohumeral joint incongruity with posterior subluxation and contracture of the upper fibers of the subscapularis muscle (Figs. 5–185 and 5–186). In very severe medial rotation deformity of the shoulder, Putti's sign may be difficult to elicit.

Fixed medial rotation and adduction contracture of the shoulder is the most common deformity. Both active and passive abduction and lateral rotation of the shoulder are limited (Fig. 5–187). Biomechanically, the *prime movers* of the shoulder, i.e., those that supply power, are the deltoid and pectoralis major. The *steering muscles*, i.e., those that stabilize the humeral head against the glenoid, are the supraspinatus, infraspinatus, and subscapularis.[103]

Medial rotation-adduction deformity of the shoulder is caused by paralysis of the supraspinatus, infraspinatus, teres minor, and posterior and middle deltoid muscles and the unopposed action of strong subscapularis and pectoralis major muscles. Asynergy (dyskinesia) of the muscles controlling the shoulder is also a factor in the pathogenesis of shoulder deformity. The strong pectoralis major, subscapularis, teres major, and latissimus dorsi muscles develop myostatic contracture (Fig. 5–188 A and B). With the shoulder in the adducted and medially rotated position, dysplasia with broadening and flattening of the glenoid fossa of the scapula develops and the humeral head tends to be dislocated posteriorly. The coracoid process becomes elongated, hooks downward and laterally, and comes to rest in the position formerly occupied by the humeral head—and in fact, interferes with the return of the humeral head to its normal position. The acromion beaks downward as a result of the lack of shoulder abduction (Fig. 5–188 C). Retrotorsion of the upper humerus gradually develops (Fig. 5–189). These secondary bony abnormalities tend to obstruct lateral rotation and abduction of the shoulder. In obstetrical brachial plexus paralysis, the scapula tends to be smaller than normal, lies higher in position, and develops shortening of its neck.

Text continued on page 2021

Table 5–18. *Classification of Shoulder Sequelae in the Upper Arm Type of Birth Palsy*

Group	Subgroup	Scapular Elevation Sign	Muscle Contracture		Initial Obstetrical Lesion	Surgical Treatment
			Primary	Secondary		
Group 1: Joint contracture (90.2%)	1. Internal rotation-adduction contracture without joint deformity or dislocation (26.5%)*	Negative	Subscapularis	Pectoralis major Coracobrachialis		Anterior shoulder release plus external rotation transfer
	2. Internal rotation-adduction contracture with joint deformity and posterior subluxation or dislocation (67.4%)	Positive	Subscapularis	Short head of biceps Anterior deltoid	Upper brachial plexus and scapulohumeral joint	External rotation osteotomy
	3. External rotation-abduction contracture with anteroinferior subluxation or dislocation (4.8%)	Positive	Infraspinatus, teres minor	Posterior deltoid		Posterior shoulder release or internal rotation osteotomy
	4. Pure abduction contracture (1.2%)	Positive	Supraspinatus	—		Supraspinatus lengthening
Group 2: Pure flaccid paralysis (9.8%)	Shoulder abduction and rotation paralysis and elbow flexion paralysis	Negative	—	—	Upper brachial plexus	Shoulder arthrodesis and elbow flexoplasty

*Statistics in this classification are based on the evaluation of 92 patients with surgical reconstruction of the shoulder. (From Zancolli, E. A.: Classification and management of the shoulder in birth palsy. Orthop. Clin. North Am., *12:*433, 1981.)

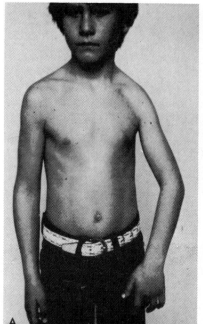
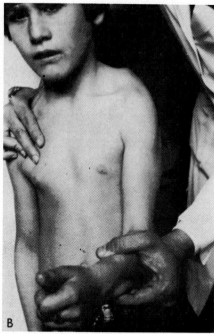
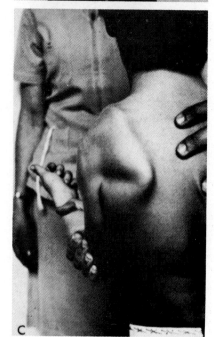

FIGURE 5–185. *Putti's sign.*

A. Severe medial rotation contracture in a ten-year-old boy with brachial plexus paralysis.

B. Passive abduction and lateral rotation shows a positive scapular sign.

C. Putti's maneuver will elicit winging of the scapula.

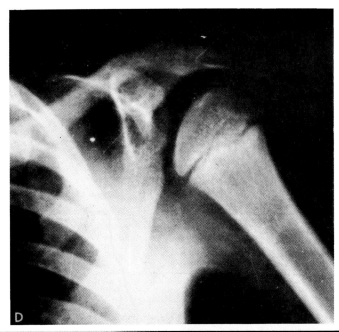

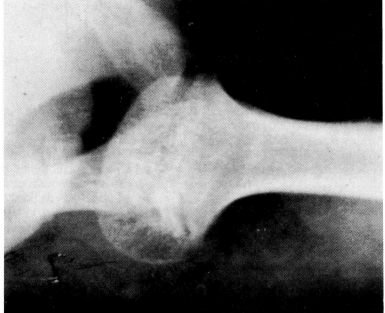

FIGURE 5–185 Continued.
Putti's sign.

D. In the AP view slight flattening of the humeral head is evident.

E. Axial view demonstrates severe enlargement and marked asymmetry of the humeral head.

(From Zancolli, E. A.: Classification and management of the shoulder in birth palsy. Orthop. Clin. North Am., *12*:433, 1981. Reprinted by permission.)

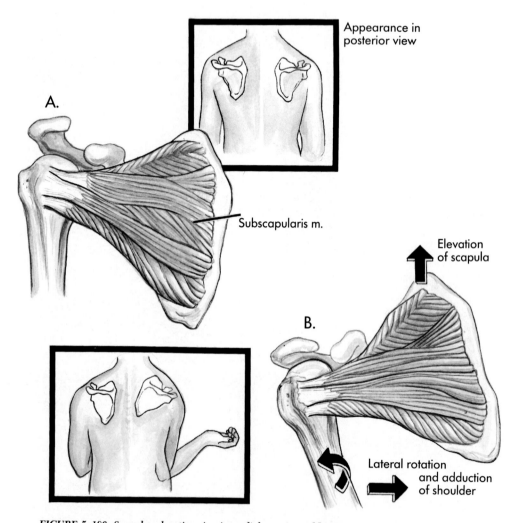

A.

Appearance in
posterior view

Subscapularis m.

Elevation
of scapula

B.

Lateral rotation
and adduction
of shoulder

FIGURE 5–186. *Scapular elevation sign in medial rotation–adduction contracture of the shoulder.*

A. Anterior view of scapular with arm and shoulder in neutral position and appearance of shoulders in the posterior view. **B.** On adduction and lateral rotation the medial upper corner of the scapula will be elevated. This is due to the glenohumeral joint incongruity with posterior subluxation and contracture of the upper fibers of the subscapularis muscle.

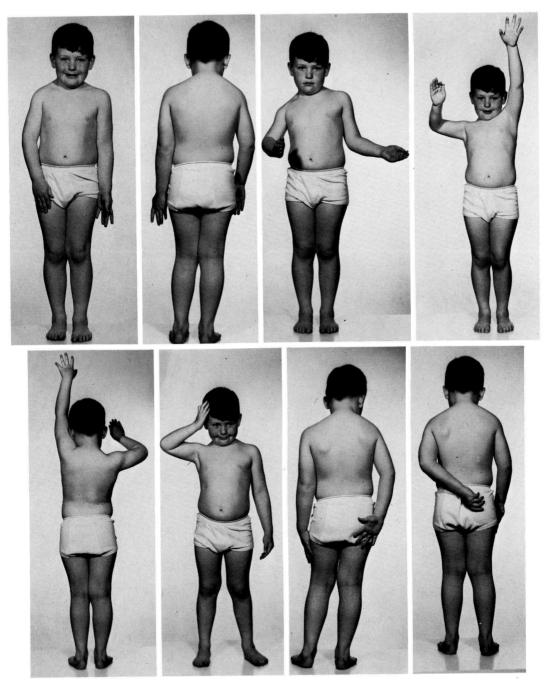

FIGURE 5–187. Obstetrical brachial plexus paralysis of the right upper limb in a six-year-old boy.

Note the limitation of active abduction and lateral rotation of the shoulder, and also the pronation contracture of the forearm.

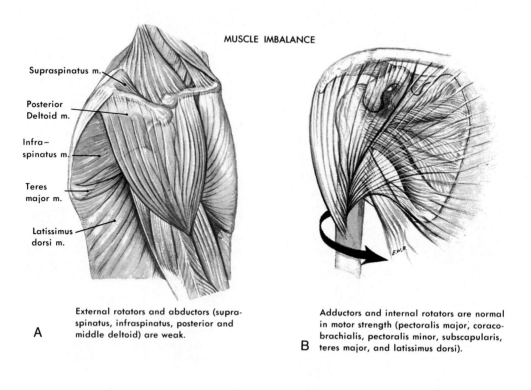

MUSCLE IMBALANCE

Supraspinatus m.

Posterior
Deltoid m.

Infra-
spinatus m.

Teres
major m.

Latissimus
dorsi m.

A   External rotators and abductors (supraspinatus, infraspinatus, posterior and
middle deltoid) are weak.

B   Adductors and internal rotators are normal
in motor strength (pectoralis major, coracobrachialis, pectoralis minor, subscapularis,
teres major, and latissimus dorsi).

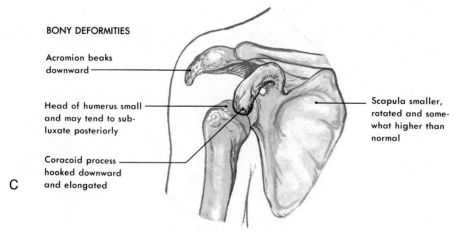

BONY DEFORMITIES

Acromion beaks
downward

Head of humerus small
and may tend to sub-
luxate posteriorly

Coracoid process
hooked downward
and elongated

Scapula smaller,
rotated and some-
what higher than
normal

C

*FIGURE 5–188. The muscle imbalance and residual bony deformities of the shoulder in obstetrical
brachial plexus paralysis.*

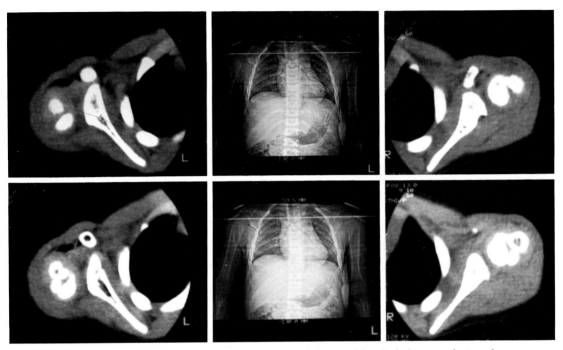

FIGURE 5–189. Retrotorsion of the proximal humerus in obstetrical brachial plexus paralysis as shown by computed tomography.

Functional use of the upper limb is greatly restricted as a result of limited abduction, lateral rotation, and extension of the shoulder. The asynergy of the muscles controlling the shoulder is an added factor in functional disability. The patient has difficulty in moving the hand to the mouth, to the top of the head, or to the back of the neck. Associated deformities of the forearm and paralysis of the hand compound the functional deficit. If the hand is normal, however, restoration of active lateral rotation and abduction of the shoulder serve to improve function of the limb immeasurably.

Abduction–Lateral Rotation Contracture of the Shoulder. This deformity may be associated with varying degrees of anteroinferior subluxation or dislocation of the glenohumeral joint. It may be caused by any, or a combination, of the following factors: (1) improper use of splints in the "Statue of Liberty" position in the early paralytic phase of the disease; (2) previous surgical procedures, namely, excessive release of medial rotators of the shoulder, anterior capsulotomy of the shoulder joint, lateral transfer of the latissimus dorsi and teres major, and an excessive degree of lateral rotation osteotomy of the proximal humerus; (3) fibrosis and contracture of the denervated abductors–lateral rotators of the shoulder—supraspinatus, infraspinatus, and teres minor: and (4) the constant

abduction of the shoulder required to compensate for the limited lateral rotation of the shoulder. The last two factors explain the occurrence of abduction–lateral rotation contracture of the shoulder without previous conservative and surgical treatment.

On clinical examination there is winging of the scapula when the arm is held at the side of the trunk. The Putti sign of scapular elevation is positive owing to contracture of the infraspinatus and teres minor; the maneuver to elicit the sign is different, however; i.e., the shoulder is passively rotated medially and adducted (Fig. 5–190). Passive range of abduction-adduction of the glenohumeral joint is very limited; it will be very stiff if dislocated. The humeral head may be palpated anteriorly and inferiorly. Functionally, the patient is disabled; he cannot bring the hand to the mouth or anterior aspect of the trunk.

Radiograms will depict the inferior and anterior subluxation of the glenohumeral joint. The humeral head is displaced inferiorly from the acromion process and overlaps the distal part of the glenoid fossa underneath the coracoid process. Anterior dislocation is well demonstrated by computerized axial tomography.

Pure Abduction Contracture of the Shoulder. This rare shoulder deformity is due to isolated contracture of the supraspinatus muscle. Clini-

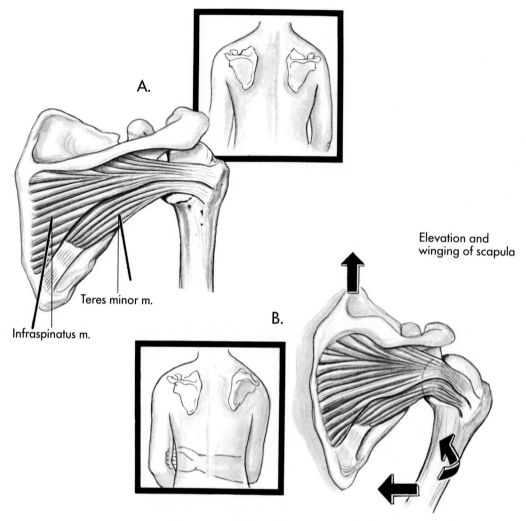

A.

Teres minor m.

Infraspinatus m.

B.

Elevation and
winging of scapula

FIGURE 5–190. Putti's scapular elevation sign in abduction–lateral rotation contracture of the shoulder in obstetrical brachial plexus paralysis.

A and **B.** The infraspinatous and teres minor muscles are contracted and the glenohumeral joint is subluxated anteriorly. On passive adduction and medial rotation of the shoulder the scapula is elevated. Note anteroinferior dislocation of the humeral head.

cally, on inspection there is winging of the superomedial angle of the scapula when the shoulder is passively adducted (positive Putti's sign) (Fig. 5–191).

Total Flaccid Paralysis of the Shoulder. In this group there is no contractural deformity of the muscles and joint capsule. The shoulder joint is flail. Often the elbow flexors are paralyzed.

ELBOW

Flexion contracture of the elbow joint frequently develops as a result of overaction of the flexors—the biceps and the brachialis. Another possible factor in its pathogenesis is constant use of the elbow in hyperflexed position because of limited abduction at the shoulder. Development of secondary bony changes, such as hypertrophy of the olecranon and coronoid process, further blocks extension of the elbow. In untreated cases in adolescence, the elbow joint may be in 45 to 90 degrees of flexion and can be very disturbing cosmetically.

Posterior dislocation of the radial head is a common deformity (Fig. 5–192). Aitken, in a survey of 107 cases of Erb's palsy, found 27 instances (25.5 per cent) of incipient or actual posterior dislocation of the radial head.[2] This is acquired, produced by muscle imbalance and improper rigid splinting over a long period of

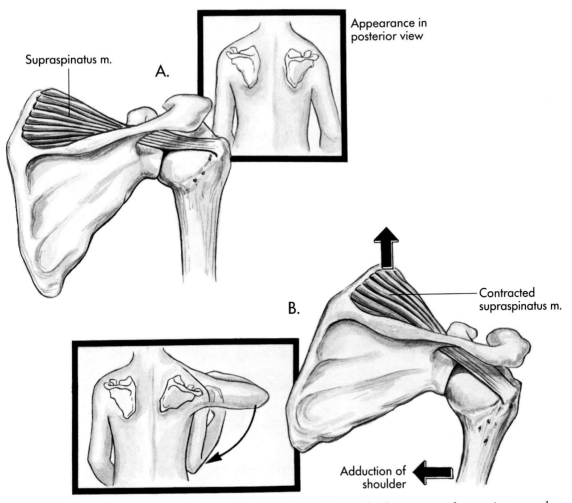

FIGURE 5–191. *Pure abduction contracture of glenohumeral joint due to isolated contracture of supraspinatus muscle.*

A and **B.** There is winging of the superomedial angle of the scapula on passive adduction of the shoulder.

time. Diagrammatic illustration of the progressive changes leading to posterior dislocation of the radial head is presented in Figure 5–193. Aitken proposes that when the paralyzed limb is rigidly immobilized over an unduly prolonged period in a Fairbank's splint, bowing of the ulna is produced as a result of forced flexion of the elbow against the pull of the strong triceps in the absence of a balancing biceps and brachialis pull (Fig. 5–194). Increased pressure is produced in the axis of the upper radius by forced supination against the pull of the spastic pronator teres muscle. This increased pressure of the proximal radial epiphysis against the capitellum causes abnormal bone growth and progressive osseous changes, namely, "clubbing," flattening, and anterior notching of the upper end of the radius, which begins to subluxate posteriorly and eventually becomes dislocated.

Contracture of the pronator teres and interosseous membrane is also a contributory force.

FOREARM AND HAND

The distribution and extent of paralysis determine the type of residual deformity at this level. Pronation deformity of the forearm is common. When the entire arm is paralyzed in the whole-arm type of obstetrical brachial plexus paralysis, supination contracture of the forearm may develop (Fig. 5–195). Paralysis of muscles of the hand is often present in the lower-arm type.

Treatment

Early Orthopedic Management. In the neonate and infant the objective of treatment is to prevent the development of contractural deformities during the period of spontaneous recovery.

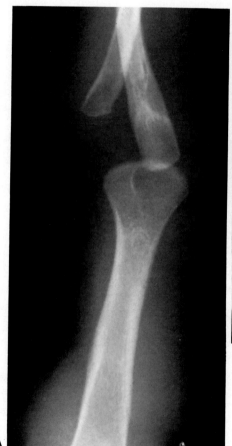

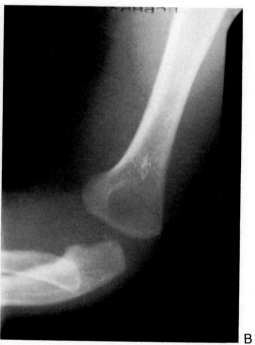

FIGURE 5-192. Posterior dislocation of the
radial head in obstetrical brachial plexus
paralysis.

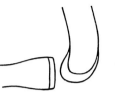
Seven weeks
"Clubbing" of metaphysis.

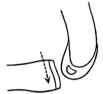
Two months
Flattening of radial metaphysis anteriorly. Commencing backward movement of upper radial shaft.

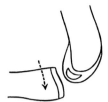
Seven months
Notching of previously flattened. area· Backward movement of shaft more obvious.

FIGURE 5–193. Diagrammatic illustration of the progressive changes leading to posterior dislocation of the radial head in obstetrical brachial plexus paralysis.

(From Aitken, J.: Deformity of the elbow joint as a sequel to Erb's obstetrical paralysis. J. Bone Joint Surg., *34-B*:361, 1952. Reprinted by permission.)

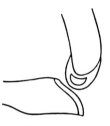
Two years
Notch spreading distally. Head subluxated.

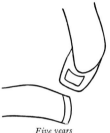
Five years
Head dislocated; capitulum begins to become flattened.

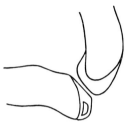
Eight years
Conical epiphysial centre appears. Head articulates by its anterior surface with the flattened capitulum.

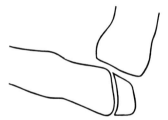
Fifteen years
Truncated-cone-shaped epiphysis about to fuse with shaft.

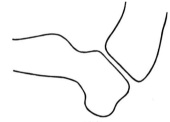
Adult
Final shape of dislocated head.

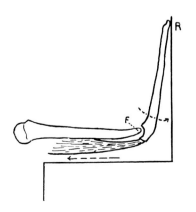

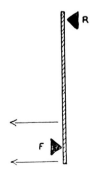

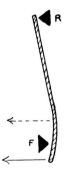

FIGURE 5–194. The bowing of the ulna in obstetrical brachial plexus paralysis.

The deformity results from imbalance between the spastic triceps and the paralyzed biceps and brachialis combined with firm corrective splinting. (From Aitken, J.: Deformity of the elbow joint as a sequel of Erb's obstetrical paralysis. J. Bone Joint Surg., *34-B*:361, 1952. Reprinted by permission.)

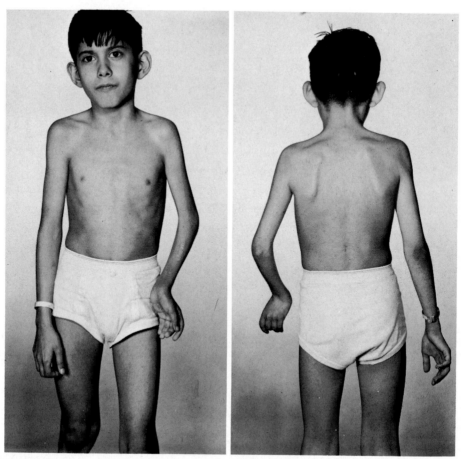

FIGURE 5–195. Supination contracture of the left forearm and flexion deformity of the elbow in the whole arm type of obstetrical brachial plexus paralysis.

In the past it was customary in the nursery to pin the arm in abduction and lateral rotation with the help of a diaper; at present the use of such immobilization of the shoulder in the neonate is discouraged, as inadvertent lifting of the infant from the bed may dislocate the shoulder. The potential risk outweighs the possible advantages. Also, at present, this author does not recommend the use of a shoulder splint. In the past a light splint was made that held the shoulder in about 70 degrees of abduction, 10 degrees of forward flexion, and 90 degrees of lateral rotation, with the elbow in 60 degrees of flexion, the forearm in midpronation, and the wrist in neutral position. The improper and rigid immobilization of the shoulder in such a splint is dangerous. Too much forward flexion at the shoulder will cause posterior dislocation of the humeral head. Forced full supination of the forearm against the pull of the taut pronator teres may cause bowing of the ulna and posterior dislocation of the radial head. The improper

use of a shoulder splint may cause abduction contracture of the shoulder. Because of these inherent dangers this author has abandoned the use of the shoulder orthosis (the so-called Statue of Liberty splint).

Physical therapy is performed three to four times a day. Parents are instructed to perform it at home with the periodic supervision of the therapist, who checks once or twice a month. Passive exercises are performed *gently* by the parents, putting all joints of the upper limb through their full range of motion. By the use of stimulation techniques, guided active exercises are performed to develop normal cerebral motor patterns.

When the infant is four to six weeks old, with paralysis of the elbow flexors and supinators of the forearm, the resting posture of the elbow is in extension, and of the forearm full pronation. In such an instance the part-time use of an elbow-wrist orthosis, holding the elbow in 60 degrees of flexion and the forearm in neutral rotation to 45 degrees supination, is recommended. The limb should be out of the splint several hours in the morning and the afternoon; when the splint is off, passive and active exercises are performed by the parents. It is vital that the orthopedic surgeon carefully examine the elbow to rule out dislocation of the radial head. The orthosis is used for gradually decreasing periods as recovery takes place. Within three months, its use is discontinued during the day; it is usually needed for night use for an additional two to four months, depending upon the rate of recovery. Improper and rigid use of orthosis is condemned.

Passive and active exercises should be performed during the period of growth. If paralysis and residual deformity persist after three years of age, surgical correction may be indicated.

Early Neurosurgical Repair of Brachial Plexus by Microsurgical Techniques. Historically Kennedy and Clark and Taylor et al. were pioneers in early surgical intervention for obstetrical traction injuries of the brachial plexus.[19, 58, 59, 130] With resection of the neuroma and primary suture of the nerves under tension, Sharpe reported 30 to 60 per cent "success."[114] On critical analysis, however, the results prior to the advent of microsurgical and modern neurosurgical technique were poor; therefore, the procedure was abandoned.

In 1960, microsurgical repair of peripheral nerves was developed.[117, 118] Millesi recommended early microsurgical repair when there is failure of rapid recovery.[78–81] Lesions distal to the intervertebral foramen may be amenable to surgical repair. The level and type of nerve injury are determined by electromyography, by myelography, and recently, by magnetic resonance imaging.

Gilbert, utilizing microsurgical technique, has improved the results of repair of brachial plexus in obstetrical paralysis. He recommends observation for 12 weeks; if there is no return of function, the level and type of nerve injury is determined. If the nerves are not avulsed at the spinal cord, they are repaired with appropriate intercostal nerve graft. The results reported by Gilbert are 50 per cent return of satisfactory function.[40]

Teot recommends exploration and repair if there is no return of function in two months.[131]

This author does not recommend microsurgical repair prior to three months of age, because adequate time is not given for demonstration of healing potential by spontaneous recovery. Also, this author does not recommend microsurgical intervention in cases of partial paralysis of the brachial plexus—because in such cases the results of early microsurgical repair functionally are not better than those achieved by reconstructive surgery later on in childhood. It is the policy of this author to explain to the family the feasibility of microsurgical repair of the nerves by early microsurgical intervention and discuss with them its indications, results, and drawbacks. The parents are given the opportunity to obtain expert neurosurgical consultation.

Management of Residual Deformities

Zancolli et al. classified residual deformities of the upper limb in obstetrical brachial plexus paralysis into three types: first, *upper arm type* (34.2 per cent), with predominant involvement of the shoulder and occasionally also of the elbow and forearm; second, *predominant lower arm type* (65.1 per cent), in which the hand is always involved, with varying degrees of paralysis of the forearm, elbow, and shoulder; third, *flaccid paralysis whole-arm type* (0.7 per cent), in which all the muscles of the upper limb are paralyzed with minimal or no muscular contractures or joint deformity.[143] The trapezius is the only muscle that moves the upper limb. In the upper-arm and predominant lower-arm types, there is always muscle contracture or joint deformity.[144, 145]

SHOULDER

Medial Rotation-Adduction Contracture of the Shoulder Without Joint Deformity or Dislocation. In this subgroup the adductors and medial rotators of the shoulder (subscapularis, pectoralis major–minor, latissimus dorsi, and teres major) are normal in motor strength, whereas the lateral rotators and abductors of the shoulder are weak. The active range of shoulder abduction is limited to 60 to 90 degrees. The primary muscles with contracture are the subscapularis and pectoralis major; the coracobrachialis and short head of the biceps are also shortened. The glenohumeral joint is congruous and concentrically reduced. The coracoid process and acromion are normal or minimally deformed.

Various operations have been described in the literature for correction of medial rotation-adduction deformity of the shoulder. Fairbank sectioned the upper portion of the pectoralis major, the subscapularis, and the anterior capsule of the shoulder.[33] Sever modified the Fairbank procedure; he performed a complete division of the pectoralis major and subscapularis but did not open the joint capsule (as the latter caused anterior dislocation of the shoulder).[112, 113] L'Episcopo described transfer of the teres major to a lateral position, making it a lateral rotator of the shoulder.[65, 66] Zachary added the latissimus dorsi to the transfer, a modification subsequently adopted by L'Episcopo.[140] To assist in lateral rotation of the shoulder, Moore suggested posterior transfer of the origin of the anterior deltoid.[83] Green and Tachdjian adopted a technique in which the pectoralis major and subscapularis are lengthened and balanced by the active lateral rotation of the transferred latissimus dorsi and teres major.[47]

Zancolli further modified the L'Episcopo procedure; he recommended transfer of only the latissimus dorsi; this tendon, which is about 10 cm. long, is completely dissected and divided in a long Z, forming proximal and distal tendinous segments. The distal tendon strip is passed around the humerus under the deltoid muscle, exiting posteriorly through the quadrilateral space. The distal tendon strip is firmly sutured to the proximal tendon strip with the shoulder in 90 degrees of abduction and maximal lateral rotation. The teres major is left intact to function as a medial rotator of the shoulder. Zancolli also sectioned the pectoralis major near its humeral attachment, the subscapularis, coracobrachialis, and short head of the biceps. He recommended transfer of the pectoralis major to the distal tendon of subscapularis, thereby relatively lengthening the pectoralis major and preserving its action as a medial rotator of the shoulder.[143]

Ingram recommended lengthening of the subscapularis through a posterior lateral parascapular approach, by (1) stripping it from the ventral surface of the scapula and sectioning the teres major; (2) rerouting and transferring to the tendon of supraspinatus at its insertion; and (3) sectioning, rerouting, and transferring the teres minor to the tendon of infraspinatus at its insertion.[54]

Transfer of the teres major and latissimus dorsi to the rotator cuff was suggested by Roper and later described by Hoffer et al.[52, 99] Carlioz described recession of the origin of subscapularis muscle to correct medial rotation deformity of the shoulder with simultaneous transfer of the latissimus dorsi and teres major muscles to the rotator cuff.[16]

Rotation osteotomy of the humerus to place the distal segment in lateral rotation has been advocated.[137, 138] Green recommended excision of the coracoid process if it is long and hooked, and resection of the lateral portion of the acromion process, if indicated.[47]

The *objectives* of the preceding operative procedures are (1) to release fixed myostatic contracture of the medial rotators and adductors of the shoulder that limit lateral rotation and abduction and hinder effective action of the weakened muscles; and (2) to increase the power of active lateral rotation of the shoulder, provide stability to the rotator cuff, and increase glenohumeral abduction by enabling the deltoid to be more effective. Functional goals are to enable the patient to bring his hand to the mouth and other parts of the head and neck and to improve appearance of the upper limb. The posture of the trunk is improved, as medial rotation contracture of the shoulder accentuates lumbar hyperlordosis.

Author's Recommendation for Correction of Medial Rotation-Adduction Deformity of the Shoulder. The Sever procedure (sectioning of subscapularis and pectoralis major) compromises the appearance of the individual, creating a large defect due to the retraction of the muscle and its subsequent scarring. When the pectoralis major and subscapularis are detached and the remaining medial rotators (latissimus dorsi and teres major) are transferred, there is marked weakness of medial rotation of the shoulder. This can be functionally quite disabling; there should be proper dynamic balance between medial rotators and lateral rotators of the shoulder. The pectoralis major should be elongated and not sectioned; this author recommends the Z-lengthening technique as described by Green (see Plate 76), as it increases the range of shoulder abduction as well as lateral rotation.

The Zancolli technique of transferring detached pectoralis major to the distal-lateral stump of sectioned subscapularis does not increase range of shoulder abduction. The subscapularis muscle should be lengthened and not sectioned; this author has utilized the technique of Green, an oblique cut splitting the tendon into anterior and posterior halves (see Plate 76). It should be noted that the most contracted fibers of the subscapularis are the upper ones. The anterior capsule of the shoulder joint should not be divided, as this will result in anterior dislocation of the humeral head. Recession of the subscapularis at its origin from the ventral surface of the scapula (see Plate 77) is technically more difficult, but the scar is cosmetically much more pleasing. This author utilizes it when the pectoralis major is not contracted and shoulder abduction is not limited. When simultaneous lengthening of the pectoralis major is indicated, the subscapularis is lengthened anteriorly.

The classic deltopectoral groove incision should not be employed; it produces an ugly, hypertrophic scar. Use the axillary approach, extending from the coracoid process to the posterior border of the axilla, which is formed by the latissimus dorsi and teres major tendons.

Author's Recommendations for Increase of Motor Power of Lateral Rotators of the Shoulder. This involves transfer of the teres major and latissimus dorsi to the rotator cuff. The operative technique is described and illustrated in Plate 78.

In the 11 cases reported by Hoffer et al., the average gain in abduction was 64 degrees, and in lateral rotation 45 degrees (Fig. 5–196). All transfers functioned at fair (Grade 3) or better motor strength two or more years postoperatively.[52] In the personal experience of this author the results have been equally good.

Requisites for surgery are the following: (1) concentrically reduced shoulder—there should be no subluxation or dislocation. (2) Normal passive range of shoulder motion. If there is medial rotation-adduction contracture of the shoulder, it should be corrected by passive stretching exercises and/or serial application of stretching shoulder spica casts. If full passive abduction and lateral rotation of the shoulder cannot be obtained, the first step of the operative procedure is the release of the tendinous insertions of the pectoralis major through a short anterior axillary incision. Hoffer does not

Text continued on page 2046

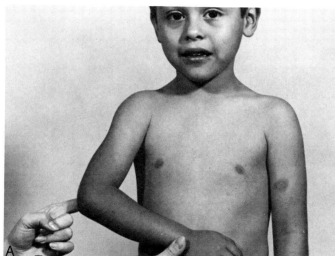

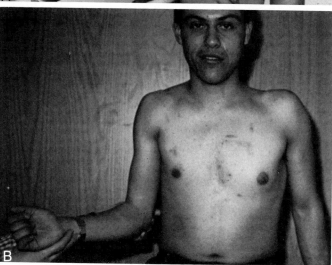

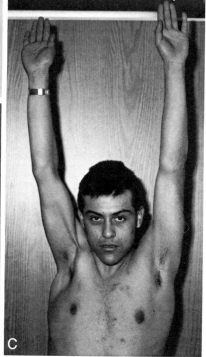

FIGURE 5–196. *Results of transfer of the latissimus dorsi and teres major muscles to the rotator cuff in obstetrical brachial plexus paralysis.*

A. Preoperative photograph of patient showing attempted abduction and lateral rotation. **B** and **C.** Postoperative photographs. Note the range of abduction and lateral rotation. (Courtesy of Dr. M. Hoffer.)

Modified Sever-L'Episcopo Procedure (After Green)

OPERATIVE TECHNIQUE

A sandbag is placed under the upper part of the chest for proper exposure. The entire upper limb, the front and back of the shoulder, and the lateral half of the chest are prepared and draped sterile. An adequate amount of whole blood should be available for transfusion.

A. An anterior incision is made, beginning over the coracoid process and extending distally along the deltopectoral groove for 12 cm. When exposure of the acromion is indicated, the incision extends superiorly and laterally.

B. The cephalic vein is identified. It may be ligated or retracted out of the way with a few fibers of deltoid muscle. By blunt dissection, the interval between the pectoral and deltoid muscles is developed and the coracobrachialis, the short head of the biceps, the coracoid process, the insertion of the tendinous portion of the subscapularis, and the insertion of the pectoralis major are exposed by adequate retraction.

C. The short head of the biceps and coracobrachialis are detached from their origin from the coracoid process and reflected downward. In the distal part of the wound, the insertion of the pectoralis major is exposed at its humeral attachment. Both its anterior and posterior surfaces are well-defined and separated from the adjacent tissues.

Plate 76. Modified Sever-L'Episcopo Procedure (After Green)

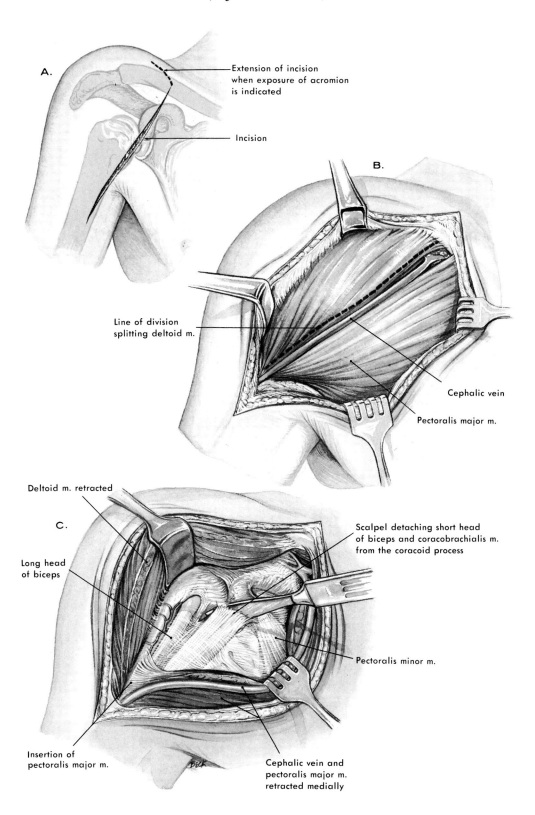

A.

Extension of incision when exposure of acromion is indicated

Incision

B.

Line of division splitting deltoid m.

Cephalic vein

Pectoralis major m.

Deltoid m. retracted

C.

Scalpel detaching short head of biceps and coracobrachialis m. from the coracoid process

Long head of biceps

Pectoralis minor m.

Insertion of pectoralis major m.

Cephalic vein and pectoralis major m. retracted medially

2031

Modified Sever-L'Episcopo Procedure (After Green)
(Continued)

D to F. With a periosteal elevator, the muscle fibers of the pectoralis major are reflected medially in order to expose as much as possible the tendinous portion of its insertion. Z-lengthening is obtained by dividing the distal half of the tendinous insertion of the pectoralis major immediately on the humeral shaft. The upper half of the tendinous portion of the pectoralis major is divided as far medially as good aponeurotic tendinous material exists, usually 4 to 5 cm. from its insertion. Later, the distal tendon stump is to be attached to the proximal tendon left inserted on the humerus, thus providing further length to the pectoralis major. The reattachment of the tendon more proximally permits a greater degree of shoulder abduction, but still allows rotary function. At this time whip sutures are applied to the tendon still attached to the shaft and to the portion of the tendon attached to the muscle.

Plate 76. *Modified Sever-L'Episcopo Procedure (After Green)*

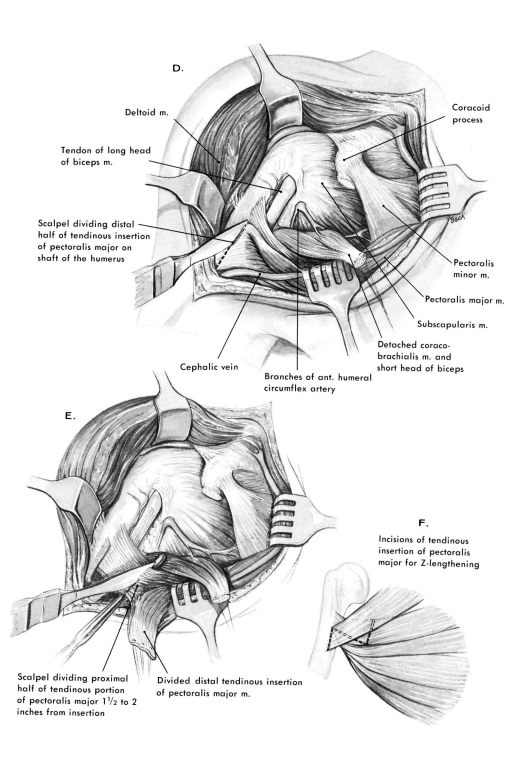

D.

Deltoid m.

Tendon of long head of biceps m.

Scalpel dividing distal half of tendinous insertion of pectoralis major on shaft of the humerus

Coracoid process

Pectoralis minor m.

Pectoralis major m.

Subscapularis m.

Detached coraco-brachialis m. and short head of biceps

Cephalic vein

Branches of ant. humeral circumflex artery

E.

F.

Incisions of tendinous insertion of pectoralis major for Z-lengthening

Scalpel dividing proximal half of tendinous portion of pectoralis major 1½ to 2 inches from insertion

Divided distal tendinous insertion of pectoralis major m.

Modified Sever-L'Episcopo Procedure (After Green)
(Continued)

G. Next, the subscapularis muscle is exposed over the head of the humerus. Starting medially with a blunt instrument, the subscapularis muscle is separated and elevated from the capsule. The shoulder capsule should not be opened; if, inadvertently, it is incised, it should be repaired.

H. With a knife, the subscapularis tendon is lengthened on the flat by an oblique cut starting medially, splitting the tendon into anterior and posterior halves, becoming more superficial laterally, and completing the division at the insertion of the subscapularis into the humerus. Again, meticulous care should be taken not to open the capsule. Ordinarily, once the subscapularis is divided, the shoulder joint will abduct and externally rotate freely. The coracoid process is excised to its base if it is elongated, hooked downward and laterally, and limits external rotation. The acromion process is partially resected if it is beaked downward, obstructing shoulder abduction.

I. Next, the insertions of the latissimus dorsi and teres major are identified and exposed by separating them from adjacent tissues both anteriorly and posteriorly. The attachment of the latissimus dorsi is superior and anterior to that of the teres major. Both tendons are divided immediately on bone, and into each tendon 0 silk is sutured by a whip stitch.

Plate 76. Modified Sever-L'Episcopo Procedure (After Green)

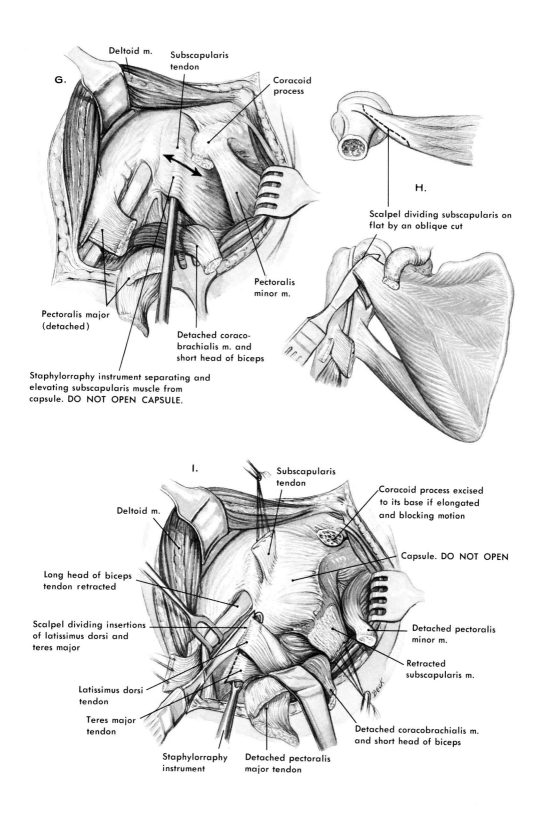

G.

Deltoid m.

Subscapularis tendon

Coracoid process

Pectoralis minor m.

Pectoralis major (detached)

Detached coraco-brachialis m. and short head of biceps

Staphylorraphy instrument separating and elevating subscapularis muscle from capsule. DO NOT OPEN CAPSULE.

H.

Scalpel dividing subscapularis on flat by an oblique cut

I.

Subscapularis tendon

Coracoid process excised to its base if elongated and blocking motion

Deltoid m.

Capsule. DO NOT OPEN

Long head of biceps tendon retracted

Scalpel dividing insertions of latissimus dorsi and teres major

Detached pectoralis minor m.

Retracted subscapularis m.

Latissimus dorsi tendon

Teres major tendon

Detached coracobrachialis m. and short head of biceps

Staphylorraphy instrument

Detached pectoralis major tendon

Modified Sever-L'Episcopo Procedure (After Green)
(Continued)

J. Then, with the patient turned over on his side and his arm adducted across the chest, a 7 to 8 cm. long incision is made over the deltoid-triceps interval.

K. The deltoid muscle is retracted anteriorly and the long head of the triceps, posteriorly. One should be careful not to damage the radial and axillary nerves. The lateral surface of the proximal diaphysis of the humerus is subperiosteally exposed. A 5 cm. long longitudinal cleft is made, using drills, osteotome, and curet.

L to N. Four drill holes are made from the depth of the cleft coming out on the medial surface of the humeral shaft at the site of the former insertion of the teres major and latissimus dorsi muscles. The tendons of the latissimus dorsi and teres major are identified in the anterior wound and are delivered into the posterior incision so that their line of pull is straight from their origins to the proposed site of attachment on the lateral humerus. The latissimus dorsi and teres major tendons are drawn into the slot in the humerus and tied securely in position with 0 silk sutures in the front.

Plate 76. Modified Sever-L'Episcopo Procedure
(After Green)

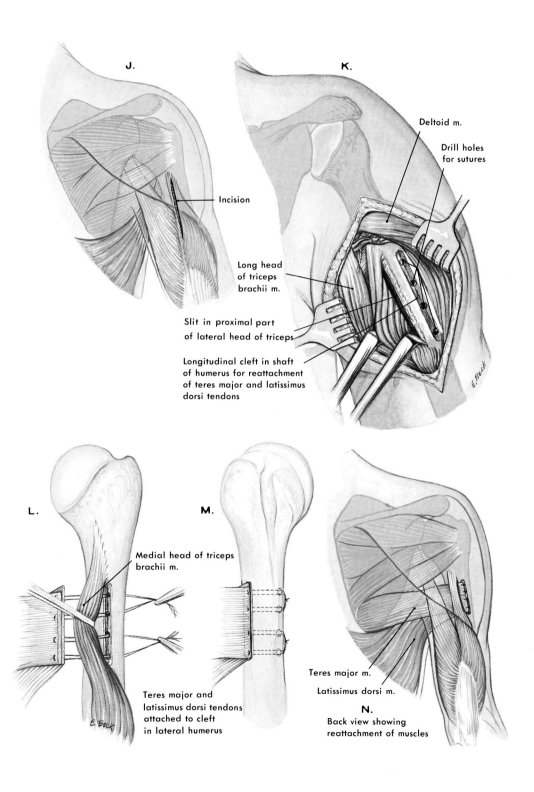

J.

K.

Incision

Deltoid m.

Drill holes
for sutures

Long head
of triceps
brachii m.

Slit in proximal part
of lateral head of triceps

Longitudinal cleft in shaft
of humerus for reattachment
of teres major and latissimus
dorsi tendons

L.

M.

Medial head of triceps
brachii m.

Teres major and
latissimus dorsi tendons
attached to cleft
in lateral humerus

Teres major m.

Latissimus dorsi m.

N.
Back view showing
reattachment of muscles

Modified Sever-L'Episcopo Procedure (After Green)
(Continued)

O to Q. The subscapularis tendon, which is lengthened "on the flat," is sutured at its divided ends so as to provide maximal lengthening. The pectoralis major is reconstituted in a similar way. The coracobrachialis and short head of the biceps are reattached to the coracoid process at its base. If the coracobrachialis and short head of the biceps are short, they are lengthened at their musculotendinous junction. The lengthened muscles should be of sufficient length to permit complete external rotation in abduction without undue tension. The wound is closed in the usual manner and the upper limb is immobilized in a previously prepared bivalved shoulder spica cast that holds the shoulder in 90 degrees of abduction, 90 degrees of external rotation, and 20 degrees of forward flexion. The elbow is in 80 to 90 degrees of flexion. The forearm and hand are placed in a functional neutral position.

An alternate method is to utilize a single anterior incision. The teres major and latissimus dorsi tendons, after detachment at their insertion, are passed posteriorly about the humerus from the anterior incision and reattached to the humerus immediately lateral to the course of the long head of the biceps lateral to the bicipital groove. Another variation in technique is employed when the teres major is markedly contracted; in such an instance, the teres major tendon may be attached to the latissimus dorsi tendon in a recessed position, which, in turn, is attached to the humerus. This allows greater scapulohumeral motion.

POSTOPERATIVE CARE

Almost three weeks after surgery, exercises are begun to develop abduction and external rotation of the shoulder, as well as shoulder adduction and internal rotation. Particular emphasis is given to developing function and strength of the transferred muscles. When the arm adducts satisfactorily, a sling is used during the day and the bivalved shoulder spica cast at night. The night support is continued for three to six more months. Exercises are performed for many months or years to preserve functional range of motion of the shoulder and to maintain muscle control.

Plate 76. Modified Sever-L'Episcopo Procedure
(After Green)

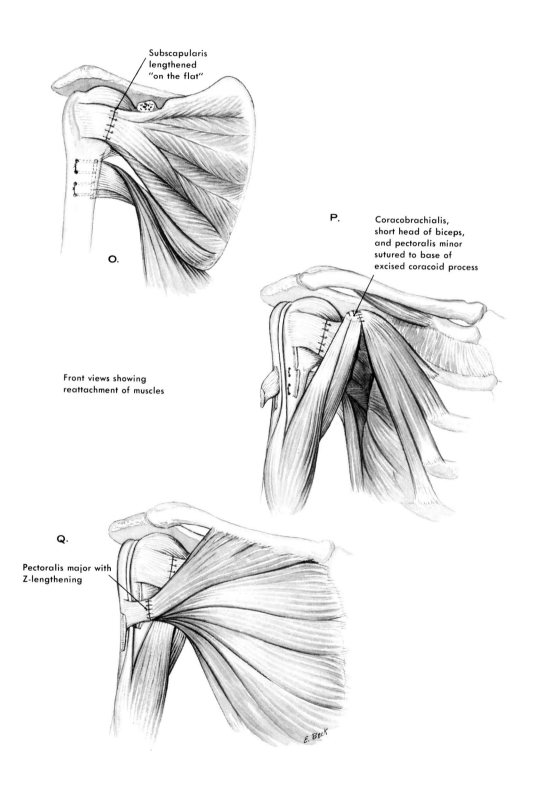

Subscapularis lengthened "on the flat"

O.

P.

Coracobrachialis, short head of biceps, and pectoralis minor sutured to base of excised coracoid process

Front views showing reattachment of muscles

Q.

Pectoralis major with Z-lengthening

E. Beck

Recession of Subscapularis Muscle at Its Origin

OPERATIVE TECHNIQUE

A. The patient is placed in supine position. The shoulder is flexed and adducted across the chest, with an assistant holding the arm in that position from the opposite side of the table. A posterior incision is made parallel to the axillary border of the scapula, extending from its inferior angle to the posterosuperior corner of the shoulder joint. (The surgical approach should allow simultaneous lateral transfer of the latissimus dorsi muscle, if necessary.)

B. The subcutaneous tissue and deep fascia are divided in line with the skin incision. The wound edges are retracted. The latissimus dorsi covers the lateral edge of the scapula, with its fibers originating from the inferior angle of the scapula. The latissimus dorsi is undermined by blunt dissection and retracted inferiorly.

C. The scapula is stabilized and pulled distally by placing Mersilene traction suture through its inferior angle, with the help of periosteal elevators. The subscapularis muscle is elevated from its origin, beginning inferiorly and going upward. All dissection should be extraperiosteal. There is no danger of injury to neurovascular structures, as they are kept out of the way.

D. The upper part of the subscapularis muscle near the posterior capsule of the shoulder joint is freed.

E. On external rotation of the shoulder the subscapularis muscle will recess and advance, releasing the medial rotation contracture of the shoulder. Tubes for closed suction are placed, and the wound is closed in the usual fashion.

POSTOPERATIVE CARE

It is not necessary to immobilize the shoulder in abduction–lateral rotation. As soon as the patient is comfortable, guided active and passive exercises are performed to increase and maintain the range of shoulder motion. It is best to make a splint holding the shoulder in 30 to 40 degrees of lateral rotation with the arm in 20 degrees of abduction. The child wears it part of the day and at night for three to four weeks. Then the day-wearing is discontinued, and it is worn only at night for another six to eight weeks.

Carlioz, in 1976, reported the results of subscapularis recession at its origin in 31 patients with a maximum follow-up of five years. In two cases the results were poor; in one case there was incongruity of the shoulder joint and deformity of the humeral head and glenoid. Radiograms of the shoulder, in the anteroposterior and lateral projections, should be throughly studied to rule out articular deformations. When indicated, arthrography of the shoulder joint is performed.

When the humeral head is flattened medially, advancement of the subscapularis muscle by recession at its origin is contraindicated; derotation osteotomy of the proximal humerus is performed in such cases.

The second case was a failure because of poor postoperative care. In the remaining 29 cases the range of lateral rotation of the shoulder was maintained or improved.

Plate 77. Recession of Subscapularis Muscle at Its Origin

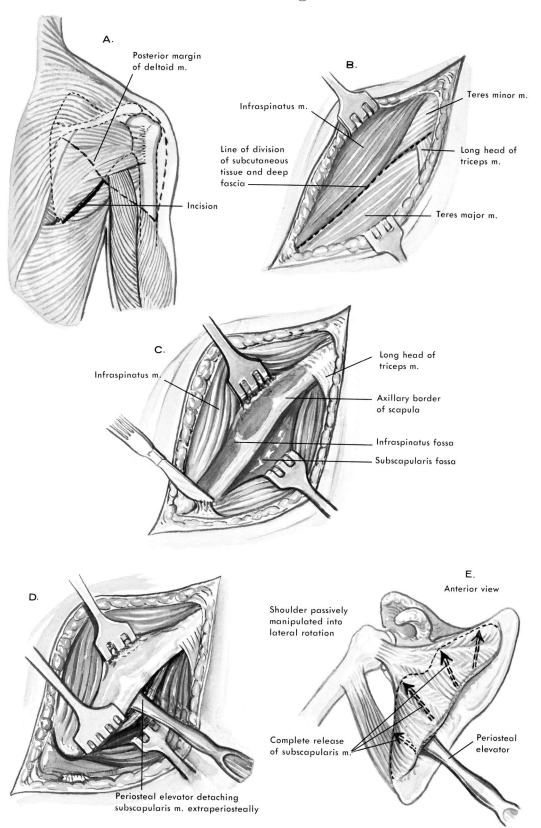

A.

Posterior margin of deltoid m.

B.

Infraspinatus m.

Teres minor m.

Line of division of subcutaneous tissue and deep fascia

Long head of triceps m.

Incision

Teres major m.

C.

Infraspinatus m.

Long head of triceps m.

Axillary border of scapula

Infraspinatus fossa

Subscapularis fossa

D.

E.
Anterior view

Shoulder passively manipulated into lateral rotation

Complete release of subscapularis m.

Periosteal elevator

Periosteal elevator detaching subscapularis m. extraperiosteally

2041

Latissimus Dorsi and Teres Major Transfer to the Rotator Cuff

OPERATIVE TECHNIQUE

In order to save anesthesia time in the operating room it is desirable to manufacture a bivalved shoulder spica cast with the shoulder and upper limb in appropriate position for postoperative immobilization. This is relatively simple in the cooperative patient.

The patient is positioned in side-lying lateral posture, and the paralyzed upper limb, shoulder, and neck are prepared and draped. The upper limb should be draped free, and the sterile area of preparation should extend to the midline anteriorly and posteriorly. If there is persistent adduction–medial rotation deformity of the shoulder, the pectoralis major is sectioned at its insertion through a short anterior axillary incision. This author prefers to lengthen and not section the pectoralis major (see Plate 76) because the cosmetic appearance is much more pleasing and it saves power of medial rotation of the shoulder.

A. The arm is adducted across the chest, and a 7 to 8 cm. long incision is made over the deltoid-triceps interval. The incision should be proximal enough to expose the rotator cuff. Retract the deltoid muscle anteriorly and the long head of the triceps posteriorly. Avoid injury to the radial and axillary nerves and posterior circumflex humeral vessels.

B. Next, the tendinous insertions of the latissimus dorsi and teres major are identified, sectioned at their insertions, and passed posterior to the long head of the triceps.

Plate 78. Latissimus Dorsi and Teres Major Transfer to the Rotator Cuff

A.

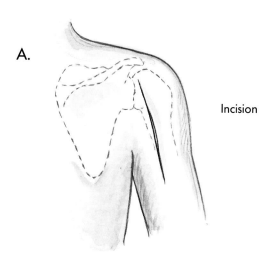

Incision

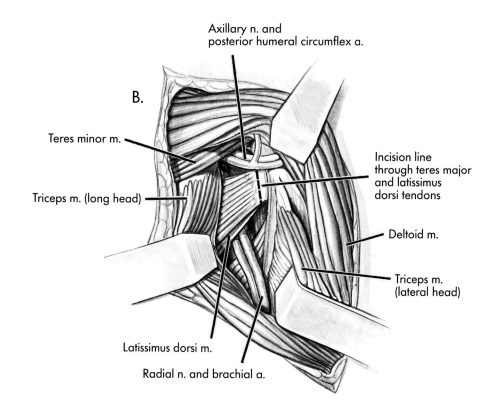

Axillary n. and
posterior humeral circumflex a.

B.

Teres minor m.

Triceps m. (long head)

Incision line
through teres major
and latissimus
dorsi tendons

Deltoid m.

Triceps m.
(lateral head)

Latissimus dorsi m.

Radial n. and brachial a.

Latissimus Dorsi and Teres Major Transfer to the Rotator Cuff (Continued)

C to E. The interval between the posterior border of the deltoid and rotator cuff is then developed by blunt dissection. The shoulder is maximally abducted and laterally rotated, and the tendons of latissimus dorsi and teres major are passed through two incisions in the rotator cuff and sutured to itself. The transferred latissimus dorsi and teres major function as lateral rotators instead of medial rotators of the shoulder. The wounds are closed in the routine fashion. The preoperatively manufactured bivalved shoulder spica cast is applied for immobilization.

POSTOPERATIVE CARE

The spica cast is bivalved four weeks postoperatively and the tendon transfer trained as a lateral rotator. Shoulder abduction and medial rotation exercises are performed to mobilize the elbow, forearm, and wrist. In between exercise periods the shoulder is maintained in abduction–lateral rotation until the transferred muscles are fair or better in motor strength. Thereafter, new shoulder splints are made, gradually adducting the shoulder. The shoulder splint is worn at night for a period of six months.

Plate 78. Latissimus Dorsi and Teres Major Transfer to the Rotator Cuff

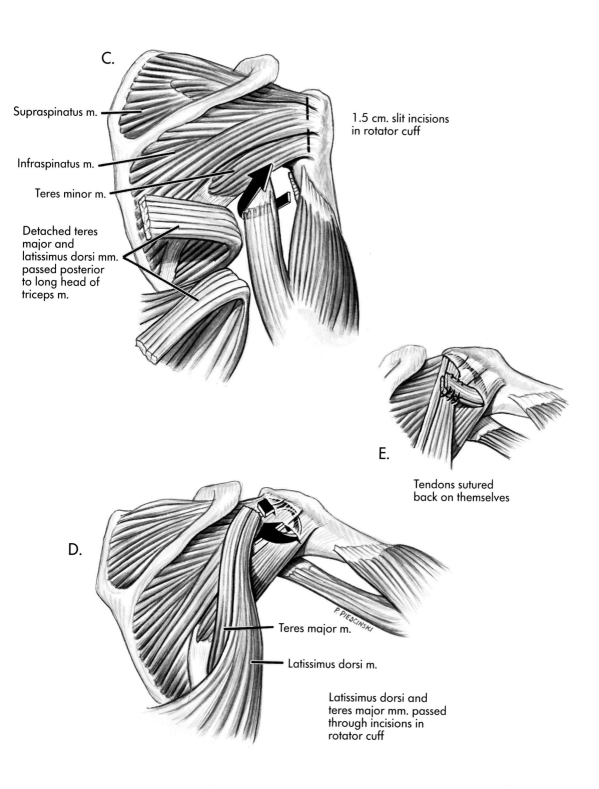

C.

Supraspinatus m.

Infraspinatus m.

Teres minor m.

Detached teres major and latissimus dorsi mm. passed posterior to long head of triceps m.

1.5 cm. slit incisions in rotator cuff

E.

Tendons sutured back on themselves

D.

P. PIESCINSKI

Teres major m.

Latissimus dorsi m.

Latissimus dorsi and teres major mm. passed through incisions in rotator cuff

2045

recommend release of the subscapularis muscle. (3) Normal or good motor strength of latissimus dorsi and teres major muscles. (4) The deltoid muscle should be at least fair in motor strength. When the deltoid muscle is poor or less in motor strength, the procedure is contraindicated. (5) The motor function and sensation of the hand and pronation-supination of the forearm should be normal. Impaired sensation and motor function in the hand is a contraindication to the operation.

When scapulohumeral motion is markedly limited and teres major is very taut, the teres major tendon is detached at its insertion and attached to the latissimus dorsi tendon in a recessed position, which in turn is attached to the rotator cuff. This variation of technique allows greater scapulohumeral motion.

Zancolli's technique of Z-lengthening of the latissimus dorsi tendon and suturing of the transferred tendon to tendon is technically simple and easy to perform; an additional advantage is that it increases range of glenohumeral abduction.

Often it is best to transfer only the latissimus dorsi; leaving the teres major intact maintains some strength of medial rotation of the shoulder.

Lateral Rotation Osteotomy of the Humerus

Indications. Lateral rotation osteotomy of the humerus is performed (1) when medial rotation-adduction deformity of the shoulder is fixed and teres major–latissimus dorsi are paralyzed and not strong enough for transfer to function as lateral rotators of the shoulder; (2) when there is marked retrotorsion of the humerus (as demonstrated by CT scan); and (3) when there is structural deformity of the glenohumeral joint with instability and posterior subluxation or dislocation; clinically the Putti sign is positive in these cases.

Lateral rotation osteotomy of the humerus does not change the incongruency of the glenohumeral joint and does not locate a subluxated or dislocated shoulder joint. It greatly improves the posture and function of the arm by increasing the range of lateral rotation and abduction of the shoulder. Rotation osteotomy is ordinarily carried out when the child is three to four years of age.

Operative technique of proximal humeral osteotomy is described and illustrated in Plate 79.

When there is severe flexion deformity of the elbow, the osteotomy is performed through the distal humeral diaphysis, tilting the distal segment into hyperextension as it is rotated laterally.

Abduction–Lateral Rotation Contracture of the Shoulder. When the glenohumeral joint is congruous or minimally subluxated, the contracted lateral rotator muscles of the shoulder are lengthened through a posterior approach. This author recommends the Zancolli technique.[143] Make a posterior skin incision from the spine of the scapula to the posterior border of the axilla, in line with the glenohumeral joint. The subcutaneous tissue and fascia are divided in line with the skin incision. The wound edges are dissected, elevated, and retracted, exposing the teres minor and infraspinatus (Fig. 5–197). The teres minor tendon is sectioned at its insertion and infraspinatus tendon is divided 2.5 to 4.0 cm. proximal to its insertion. The posterior capsule of the shoulder is not opened. On medial rotation, the anteriorly displaced humeral head can be easily reduced. With the shoulder located, the teres minor tendon is sutured to the distal tendon of the infraspinatus. The recessed proximal segment of infraspinatus is sutured to the teres minor. The wound is closed, and a shoulder Velpeau cast is applied with the arm in medial rotation for a period of four weeks. When the glenohumeral joint is reducible and not deformed, the results are good.

When the glenohumeral joint is incongruous and deformed, a medial rotation osteotomy of the proximal humerus is performed. The results are satisfactory (Fig. 5–198).

Pure Abduction Contracture of the Shoulder. This is treated by Z-lengthening of the contracted supraspinatus muscle.

In severe flaccid paralysis of the whole-arm type, if there is adequate sensation of the hand, elbow flexion is obtained by Bunnell's sternocleidomastoid transfer or Clark's pectoralis major transfer. Shoulder fusion is performed if there is muscular control of the scapula, and an automatic hinge hand is given. If sensory loss of the upper limb is extensive, functional improvement is best obtained by performing a below- or above-elbow amputation and fitting the patient with a prosthetic limb.

When the shoulder is luxated posteriorly, a posterior capsuloplasty is performed and the long head of the triceps is transferred to the posterior acromion and the spine of the scapula.

DEFORMITIES OF THE ELBOW

Flexion Deformity of the Elbow. It is managed by passive stretching exercises and active exercises to strengthen the triceps brachii. Persistent physical therapy by the parents will usually check progression of the deformity be-

Text continued on page 2053

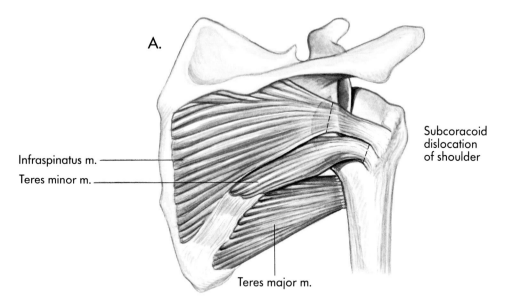

A.

Infraspinatus m.

Teres minor m.

Subcoracoid
dislocation
of shoulder

Teres major m.

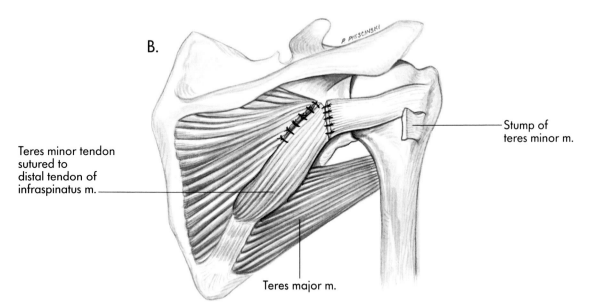

B.

P. PIESCINSKI

Teres minor tendon
sutured to
distal tendon of
infraspinatus m.

Stump of
teres minor m.

Teres major m.

FIGURE 5–197. Lengthening of the lateral rotators of the shoulder.

A. Lines of division of infraspinatus and teres minor muscles near their insertion. **B.** The teres minor tendon is sutured to the distal tendon of the infraspinatus muscle and the proximal part of the infraspinatus is sutured to the teres minor.

Lateral Rotation Osteotomy of the Humerus

OPERATIVE TECHNIQUE

A. The skin incision begins at the coracoid process, extends to the middle of the axilla, and then curves distally on the medial aspect of the arm, terminating at its upper third. Surgical exposure of the proximal humerus by this axillary approach results in minimal visibility of the operative scar.

B. The lateral skin margin is retracted laterally; with the shoulder in medial rotation, the upper humeral shaft is exposed. Avoid injury to the cephalic vein and anterior humeral circumflex vessels. The proximal humeral physis should not be disturbed.

C. The level of osteotomy is distal to the insertion of the pectoralis major and proximal to that of the deltoid. The pectoralis major tendon is lengthened as described in Plate 76.

Plate 79. Lateral Rotation Osteotomy
of the Humerus

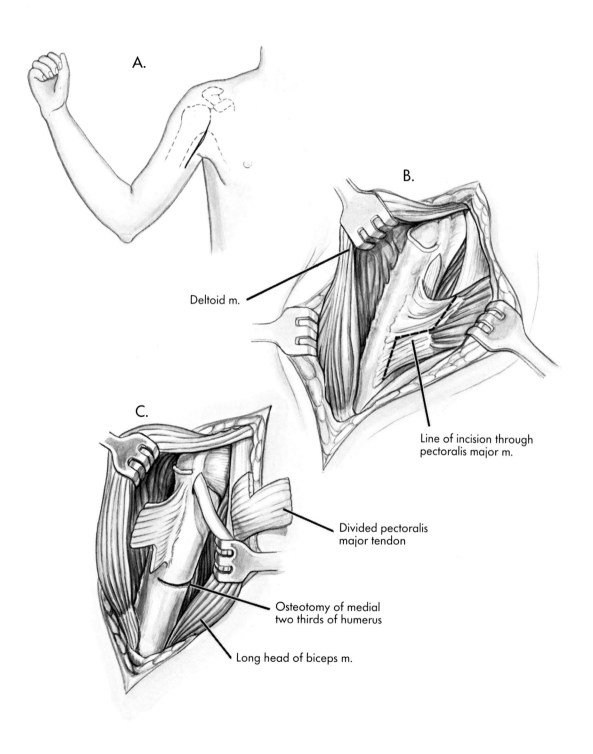

A.

B.

Deltoid m.

Line of incision through
pectoralis major m.

C.

Divided pectoralis
major tendon

Osteotomy of medial
two thirds of humerus

Long head of biceps m.

Lateral Rotation Osteotomy of the Humerus (Continued)

D to **F**. This increases range of shoulder abduction and also facilitates exposure of the humeral shaft. This author recommends internal fixation with a four- or five-hole plate. First, perform an incomplete osteotomy of the humeral diaphysis three fourths of the way through the anteromedial aspect. Second, fix the upper humeral segment to the plate by two screws (**D**). Then complete the osteotomy with an electric saw, rotate the arm laterally to the desired degree, and temporarily fix with a bone-holding forceps (**E**). Next, test passive range of shoulder rotation. The ideal position of the shoulder is complete lateral rotation of the shoulder in 90 degrees of abduction. Then, with the shoulder in adduction, the hand should touch the anterior abdomen without elevating the scapula. Avoid the pitfall of overcorrection, as it will produce lateral rotation-abduction contracture of the shoulder. Finally, once the desired degree of lateral rotation is obtained, complete internal fixation of the osteotomy by insertion of the distal two or three screws (**F**). The wound is closed as usual. The shoulder is immobilized in a shoulder spica cast. In order to save operating room time the shoulder spica cast may be manufactured preoperatively, bivalved, and fitted at completion of surgery.

POSTOPERATIVE CARE

Six weeks following surgery the cast is removed, and range-of-motion exercises of the shoulder and elbow are performed.

The results of lateral rotation osteotomy of the humerus are very satisfactory; the improved rotational posture of the shoulder increases range of shoulder abduction.

Plate 79. Lateral Rotation Osteotomy of the Humerus

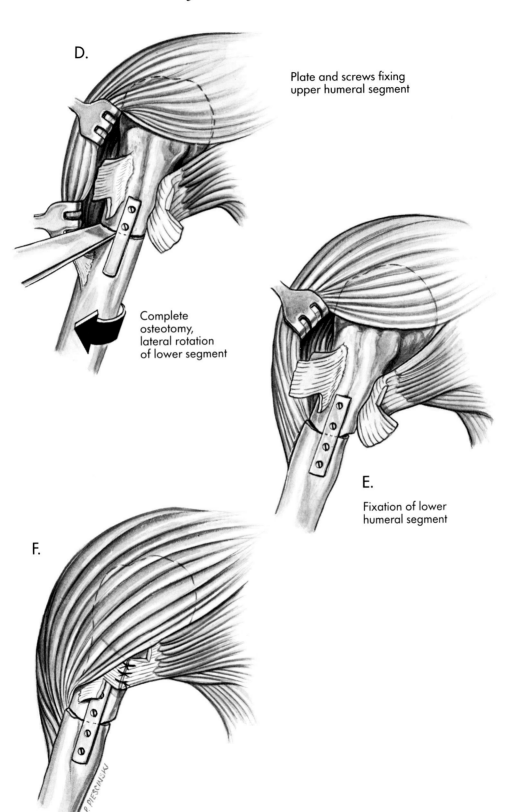

D.

Plate and screws fixing
upper humeral segment

Complete
osteotomy,
lateral rotation
of lower segment

E.

Fixation of lower
humeral segment

F.

P. PIESCINSKI

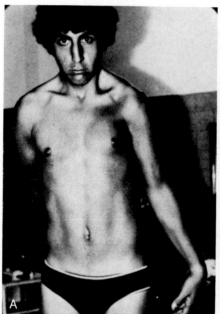
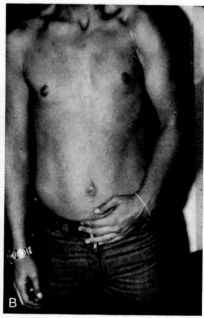
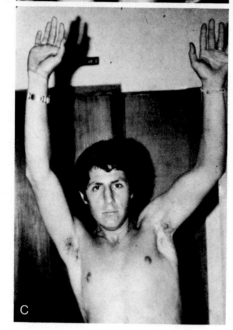

FIGURE 5–198. Abduction–lateral rotation deformity of the shoulder in obstetrical brachial plexus paralysis in an 18-year-old boy.

A. Preoperative appearance of 18-year-old with marked abduction–lateral rotation contracture. Scapular elevation was severe, and he was unable to touch the anterior aspect of his body with his hand. **B.** Postoperative appearance after medial rotation osteotomy of the humerus. Note that the patient regained medial rotation of the upper limb. **C.** View showing that elevation of the shoulder is maintained. (From Zancolli, E. A.: Classification and management of the shoulder in birth palsy. Orthop. Clin. North Am., *12*:433, 1981. Reprinted by permission.)

yond 20 to 25 degrees, which is both cosmetically and functionally acceptable.

In the more severe deformities, a plastic elbow extension orthosis that serves to hold the elbow in maximal extension is worn at night. The wearing of a cast or extension orthosis ordinarily has its problems, as it keeps sliding and coming off the arm. This can be prevented by anchoring the cast to shoulder straps and putting the wrist in extension. On occasion, a turnbuckle cast is applied, stretching the elbow into extension; the degree of correction obtained is then maintained in a bivalved cast.

When flexion deformity of the elbow exceeds 40 to 50 degrees and does not respond to the foregoing conservative measures, surgical correction is indicated. Correction of shoulder deformities should precede elbow surgery, as mentioned previously. Hyperflexion of the elbow is often a mechanism to compensate for limited shoulder abduction. The hypertrophied portion of the olecranon process blocking extension is resected. The brachialis muscle is fractionally lengthened by transverse division of its tendinous portion at two levels. It is best to avoid damage to the muscle fibers of the brachialis and the periosteum in order to prevent myositis ossificans. The biceps tendon is lengthened, if indicated; power of elbow flexion, however, should be preserved, as the functional deficit will be greater if the patient loses functional range and strength of elbow flexion. On occasion, the pronator teres and common flexor muscle mass are lengthened at their tendinous origin from the medial epicondyle of the humerus.

Posterior Dislocation of the Radial Head. This presents a difficult problem. When detected early, it can be reduced by shortening the radius at its mid-diaphysis (Fig. 5–199) (see Chapter 2, under Congenital Dislocation). If the patient is older with structural deformation of the radial head and capitellum of the humerus, it is best to await completion of growth, at which time the radial head is resected, if so indicated.

FOREARM DEFORMATION

Pronation Contracture of the Forearm. This deformity will gradually develop when the pronators of the forearm are normal or good in motor strength and the supinators of the forearm are paralyzed. Initially this is treated by passive stretching exercises, manipulating the forearm into full supination, thereby elongating the contracted forearm pronators. An above-elbow plastic splint is worn at night and part of the day, maintaining the forearm in maximal supination and the elbow in 45 degrees of flexion. An attempt is made to correct rigid pronation deformities that do not respond to passive exercises and splinting by stretching cast. When full supination cannot be obtained, the pronator teres is lengthened by division of its tendinous fibers. This is usually combined with a flexor carpi ulnaris transfer to give power of active supination. If the wrist dorsiflexors are normal in motor strength, a Steindler procedure is performed; i.e., the flexor carpi ulnaris tendon is attached to the distal radius (in growing children it is anchored to the tendon of the brachioradialis at its insertion to the radial styloid). If there is weakness of wrist dorsiflexion, the Green modification is utilized; i.e., the flexor carpi ulnaris tendon is attached to the extensor carpi radialis brevis. On occasion, bony deformity of the ulna and radius is present to such a degree that there is a bony block to rotation of the forearm; in such an instance, osteotomy of the radius is performed at the site of pronator teres insertion and the forearm immobilized in neutral rotation. Ordinarily, simultaneous osteotomy of the ulna is not required. The pronator teres is lengthened in order to prevent recurrence of the deformity. The operative technique recommended by this author is multiple drilling of the radius and osteoclasis without disturbing the periosteal sleeve. Internal fixation is usually not required, thereby making the entire procedure relatively simple.

When pronation deformity is uncorrected, posterior dislocation of the radial head may develop. In its early stages the radial head is reducible by supinating the forearm; later the deformity becomes fixed and the dislocation irreducible by manipulation; in such an instance, treatment consists of open reduction and shortening-derotation of the radius at its mid-diaphysis.

Supination Contracture of the Forearm

This is encountered in the whole-arm type of paralysis. It is caused by dynamic muscle imbalance—strong supinators (primarily biceps brachii) versus paralyzed pronators. In the beginning, the contractural deformity involves only the interosseous membrane and shortening of the biceps brachii and supinator brevis and longus muscles. With growth, the radius becomes curved and tends to spiral around the ulna as a result of the progressive contracture of the interosseous membrane and the unopposed action of the biceps brachii. This alteration in the bony configuration of the radius

Soft-Tissue Release to Correct Supination Deformity of the Forearm

OPERATIVE TECHNIQUE

A. A longitudinal dorsal incision is made midway between the radius and ulna; it begins at the radial head and terminates at the distal one fourth of the forearm. When release of the dorsal distal radioulnar ligament is indicated, the incision is extended to the wrist. The subcutaneous tissue and fascia are divided in line with the skin incision.

B. The interosseous nerve is protected by retracting radially the dorsal muscles of the forearm. The interosseous membrane and oblique descending band are exposed.

C. The contracted interosseous membrane and the oblique descending band are sectioned near their ulnar attachment.

D. Check passive range of pronation of the forearm; if it is not full, by gentle dissection expose the interosseous nerve and release the supinator brevis muscle near its ulnar insertion.

E. Range of passive pronation of the forearm is tested again; if hyperpronation of the forearm is not achieved, the dorsal ligaments of the distal radioulnar joint are sectioned. If necessary, also divide the pronator quadratus.

POSTOPERATIVE CARE

An above-elbow cast is applied with the elbow in 60 degrees of flexion, the forearm in full pronation, and the wrist-hand in functional position. The cast is removed in three to four weeks, and range-of-motion exercises are commenced.

Plate 80. Soft-Tissue Release to Correct Supination Deformity of the Forearm

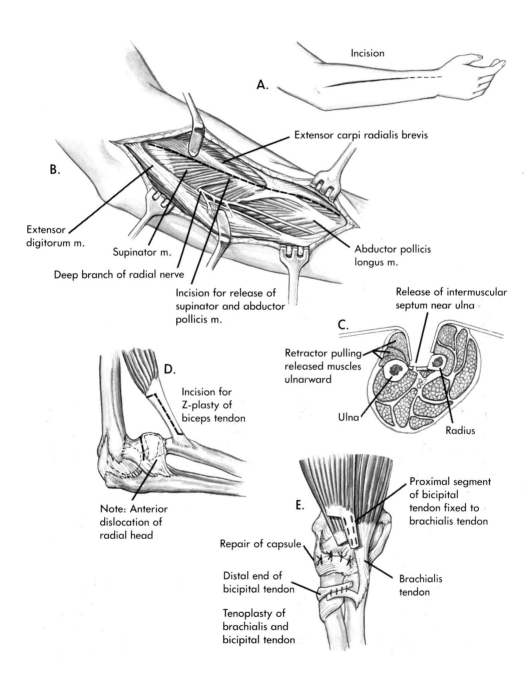

A.

Incision

B.

Extensor carpi radialis brevis

Extensor digitorum m.

Supinator m.

Deep branch of radial nerve

Incision for release of supinator and abductor pollicis m.

Abductor pollicis longus m.

C.

Release of intermuscular septum near ulna

Retractor pulling released muscles ulnarward

Ulna

Radius

D.

Incision for Z-plasty of biceps tendon

Note: Anterior dislocation of radial head

E.

Proximal segment of bicipital tendon fixed to brachialis tendon

Repair of capsule

Distal end of bicipital tendon

Tenoplasty of brachialis and bicipital tendon

Brachialis tendon

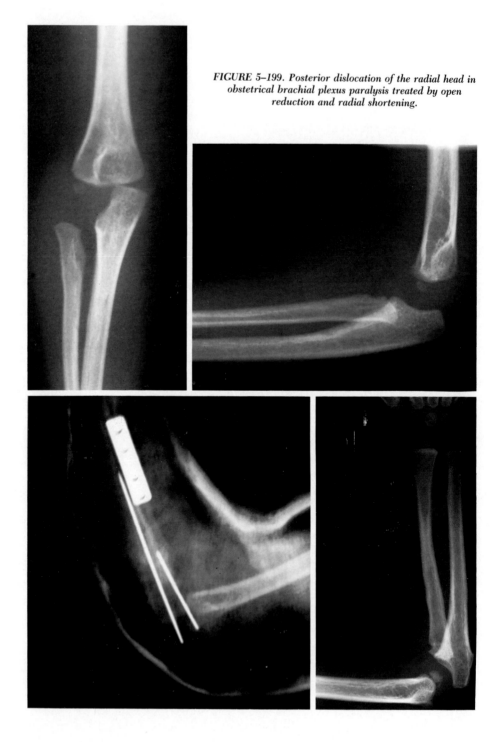

FIGURE 5–199. Posterior dislocation of the radial head in obstetrical brachial plexus paralysis treated by open reduction and radial shortening.

further increases and fixes the supination deformity of the forearm. The contracted biceps may cause anterior dislocation of the radial head. The dorsal ligaments of the distal radioulnar articulation become shortened, and the distal end of the ulna may displace anteriorly. Initially, the anterior dislocation of the radial head and dorsal dislocation of the distal ulna are reducible, as shown by a palpable jump or clunk on pronation-supination of the forearm. Eventually, with increasing contractural deformity the dislocation becomes irreducible.

Functionally, loss of active pronation of the forearm causes serious disability. It impairs and limits use of the hand in functions that require active pronation of the forearm—namely, writing, dressing, and eating. Coordinated elbow flexion and forearm pronation are lost as active flexion of the elbow by the biceps simultaneously supinates the forearm.

Treatment

In the infant and young child, passive stretching exercises are performed to retain full range of passive pronation of the forearm. Above-elbow plastic splints are worn at night and part of the day to maintain the forearm in pronation. With growth, when the supination contracture becomes fixed, a series of stretching casts is applied to correct the deformity.

When the child is four to six years old, muscle tendon transfers are performed for dynamic balance of muscles controlling rotation of the forearm.

Rerouting of Biceps Brachii Tendon. This procedure was originally mentioned by Schottstaedt, Larsen, and Bost, and later described by Grilli.[49, 105] Zancolli reported the results of 16 biceps tendon rerouting in 14 patients.

Indication for the procedure is paralytic supination contracture of the forearm with the biceps brachii normal or good in motor function and the pronators of the forearm paralyzed. *Requisites* for the operation are, *first,* full range of passive pronation and supination of the forearm. When there is fixed supination deformity, an attempt is made to correct it by a stretching cast; if it fails, surgical release of the interosseous membrane and the supinator is performed. The *second* requisite is normal anatomic relationship of the proximal and distal radioulnar joint. When there is anterior dislocation of the radial head or dorsal dislocation of the distal ulna, it should be reduced at the time of interosseous membrane release. *Third,* there should be no bowing of the anatomic configuration of the radius. If the deformed radius is blocking pronation of the forearm, it should be corrected

by osteotomy and, if indicated, by shortening at its mid-diaphysis. *Fourth,* the child should be old enough to be cooperative and motivated; the tendon transfer requires meticulous postoperative training.

Operative Technique. Preoperatively, carefully assess all the pathogenic factors: first, *contractures and shortening* of the (1) interosseous membrane, (2) biceps, (3) supinator brevis, and (4) dorsal ligament of the distal radioulnar joint; and second, *structural deformity of bones and joints,* namely (1) anterior subluxation or dislocation of the radial head, and (2) dorsal displacement of the distal ulna.

The first phase of surgery is soft-tissue release to correct supination contracture of the forearm, and anatomic reduction of the anteriorly dislocated radial head and dorsally subluxated distal radioulnar joint (Plate 80). When the forearm is postured in supination but passively can be pronated fully with no dislocation of the radial head or distal ulna, the first stage of soft-tissue release is not necessary. The second phase is biceps tendon rerouting—it is described and illustrated in Plate 81.

Surgical procedures for correction of paralytic deformities of the hand depend upon the distribution and extent of paralysis.

For opposition of the thumb the procedures recommended are either the Riordan technique (Plate 82) or the Brand modification (Plate 83). If the flexor sublimis of the ring finger is not strong, then abductor digiti quinti may be utilized to restore thumb opposition (Plate 84). When the thumb adductors are paralyzed, this author recommends the Boyes technique, in which a free tendon graft is utilized that is transferred to brachioradialis tendon (Plate 85).

When the thumb abductors are paralyzed, the extensor pollicis brevis is transferred to the extensor carpi ulnaris tendon (Plate 86).

Paralysis of the index finger abductors is restored by the Phalen technique (Plate 87). For complete paralysis of the thenar muscles, this author recommends intermetacarpal bone block (Plate 88).

References

1. Adler, J. B., and Patterson, R. L.: Erb's palsy. Long-term results of treatment in eighty-eight cases. J. Bone Joint Surg., 49-A:1052, 1967.
2. Aitken, J.: Deformity of the elbow joint as a sequel to Erb's obstetrical paralysis. J. Bone Joint Surg., 34-B:352, 1952.
3. Annovazzi, F.: Sur l'étiologie de la paralysis obstetricale du plexus brachial. Arch. Orthop., 38:41, 1922.
4. Babbitt, D. P., and Cassidy, R. H.: Obstetrical paralysis and dislocation of the shoulder in infancy. J. Bone Joint Surg., 50-A:144, 1967.

Text continued on page 2080

Rerouting of Biceps Brachii Tendon to Convert Its Motion from Supinator to Pronator of the Forearm (Zancolli Procedure) (Continued)

OPERATIVE TECHNIQUE

A. An S-shaped incision is made on the volar surface of the elbow. Begin 3 to 5 cm. above the elbow joint and extend to the antecubital crease, then laterally to the radial head and distally into the forearm for a distance of 5 cm. The subcutaneous tissue and deep fascia are divided in line with the skin incision.

B. Expose the biceps tendon and trace it distally to its insertion to the bicipital tuberosity of the radius. Identify and trace brachial vessels and median nerve.

Plate 81. Rerouting of Biceps Brachii Tendon to Convert Its Motion from Supinator to Pronator of the Forearm (Zancolli Procedure)

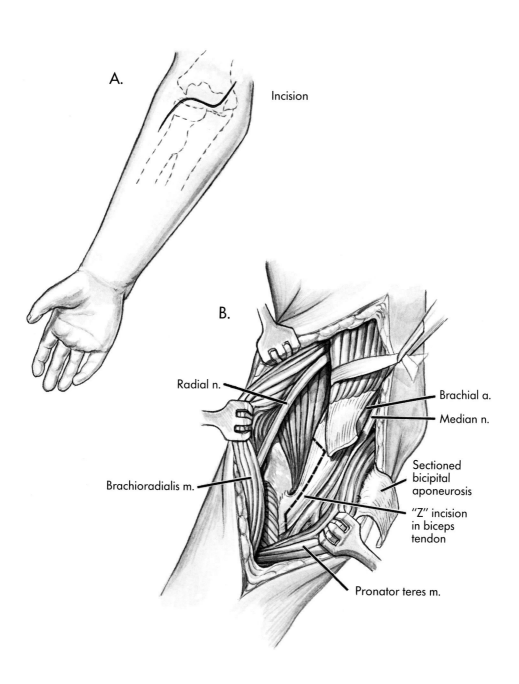

A.

Incision

B.

Radial n.

Brachial a.

Median n.

Brachioradialis m.

Sectioned bicipital aponeurosis

"Z" incision in biceps tendon

Pronator teres m.

Rerouting of Biceps Brachii Tendon to Convert Its Motion from Supinator to Pronator of the Forearm (Zancolli Procedure) (Continued)

C. Perform a long Z-plasty of the biceps tendon.

D. Reroute the distal segment of the biceps tendon around the neck of the radius, passing it mediolaterally.

E. Then resuture the divided biceps tendon segments side to side at that length which will maintain full pronation of the forearm and extension of the elbow.

Avoid excessive tension on the tendon in young children and when the forearm is hyperflexible into pronation. The wounds are closed in the routine fashion. An above-elbow cast is applied with the elbow in 30 degrees of flexion and the forearm in full pronation.

POSTOPERATIVE CARE

Four weeks after surgery the cast is removed, and active assisted exercises are performed three to four times a day to develop pronation and supination of the forearm and elbow flexion-extension. Gentle passive exercises are carried out to maintain full pronation and supination of the forearm and complete flexion and extension of the elbow. At night a plastic splint is worn, maintaining the forearm in full pronation and the elbow in 30 degrees of flexion.

Plate 81. Rerouting of Biceps Brachii Tendon to Convert Its Motion from Supinator to Pronator of the Forearm (Zancolli Procedure)

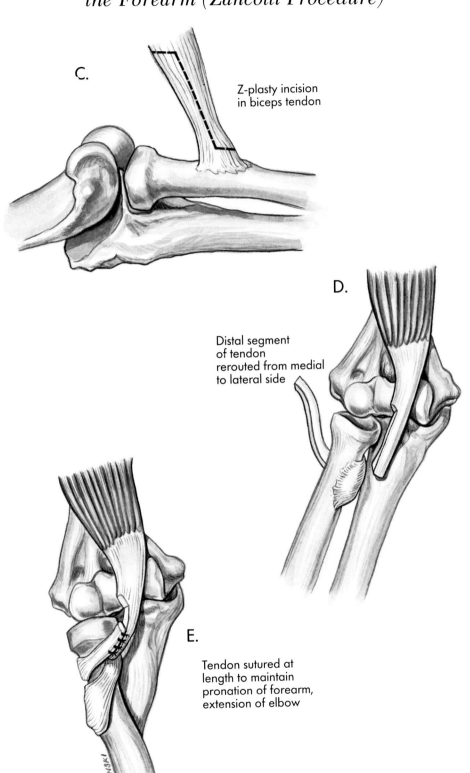

C.

Z-plasty incision
in biceps tendon

D.

Distal segment
of tendon
rerouted from medial
to lateral side

E.

Tendon sutured at
length to maintain
pronation of forearm,
extension of elbow

R. PIESCINSKI

Restoration of Thumb Opposition by the Riordan Technique (Continued)

OPERATIVE TECHNIQUE

A. A midlateral incision is made on the ulnar aspect of the ring finger centered over the proximal interphalangeal joint. The skin incision begins immediately dorsal to the flexor skin crease and extends distally and proximally for a distance of 3 cm. The volar and dorsal skin flaps are developed, taking great care not to injure the neurovascular bundle.

B and **C.** The sublimis tendon of the ring finger is isolated, and its two slips are sectioned at the level of the joint.

D. Next, an L-shaped skin incision is made over the flexor carpi ulnaris tendon. Subcutaneous tissue is divided in line with the skin incision and the flexor carpi ulnaris tendon is identified. Do not injure the ulnar nerve and vessels.

E. The flexor carpi ulnaris tendon is split into two longitudinal halves from its insertion to the pisiform bone and extending proximally for a distance of 3 to 4 cm. Then the radial part of the split tendon is divided proximally and sutured to the remaining half at its distal insertion, creating a loop. The loop should be large enough for the sublimis tendon to glide through easily.

Plate 82. Restoration of Thumb Opposition by the Riordan Technique

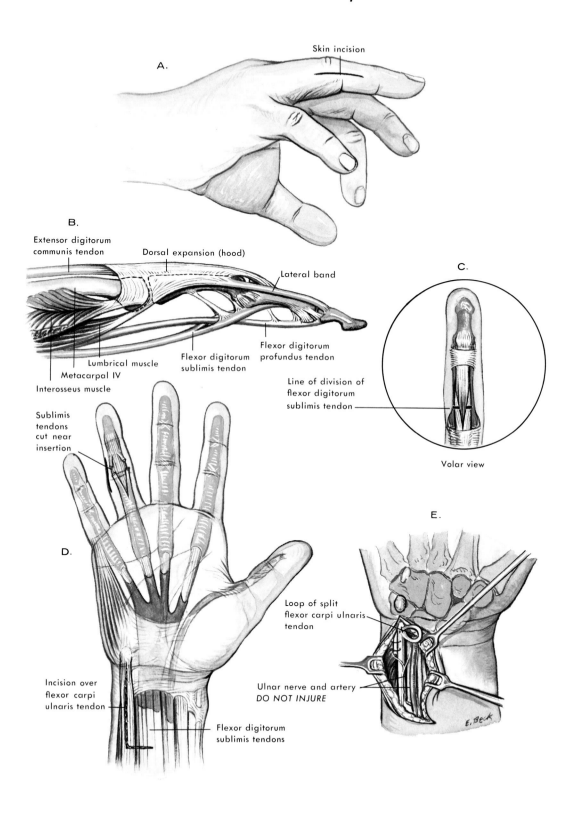

A.

Skin incision

B.

Extensor digitorum communis tendon

Dorsal expansion (hood)

Lateral band

Flexor digitorum profundus tendon

Flexor digitorum sublimis tendon

Lumbrical muscle

Metacarpal IV

Interosseus muscle

C.

Line of division of flexor digitorum sublimis tendon

Volar view

Sublimis tendons cut near insertion

D.

Incision over flexor carpi ulnaris tendon

Flexor digitorum sublimis tendons

E.

Loop of split flexor carpi ulnaris tendon

Ulnar nerve and artery
DO NOT INJURE

E. Beck

Restoration of Thumb Opposition by the Riordan Technique *(Continued)*

F. Make a C-shaped incision on the dorsolateral aspect of the thumb. The incision begins on the dorsum of the thumb 1 cm. proximal to the interphalangeal joint and then it extends proximally and volarward around the radial aspect of the thumb; at the metacarpal phalangeal joint the incision curves distally in line with the creases of the thenar eminence. Do not injure the sensory nerve branches from the superficial branch of the radial nerve.

G. Identify the tendons of extensor pollicis longus, extensor pollicis brevis, and abductor pollicis brevis.

H. At the wrist, the flexor sublimis tendon to the ring finger is identified through the forearm incision and the tendon is pulled and delivered into the wound in the wrist.

I. Next, pass the sublimis tendon through the loop fashioned from the flexor carpi ulnaris and, with a tendon passer, pass the tendon subcutaneously across the thenar eminence in line with the fibers of the abductor pollicis brevis. A small tunnel is fashioned by making two parallel incisions in the abductor pollicis brevis tendon. Next, split the distal part of the sublimis tendon for approximately 3 cm.

Plate 82. Restoration of Thumb Opposition by the Riordan Technique

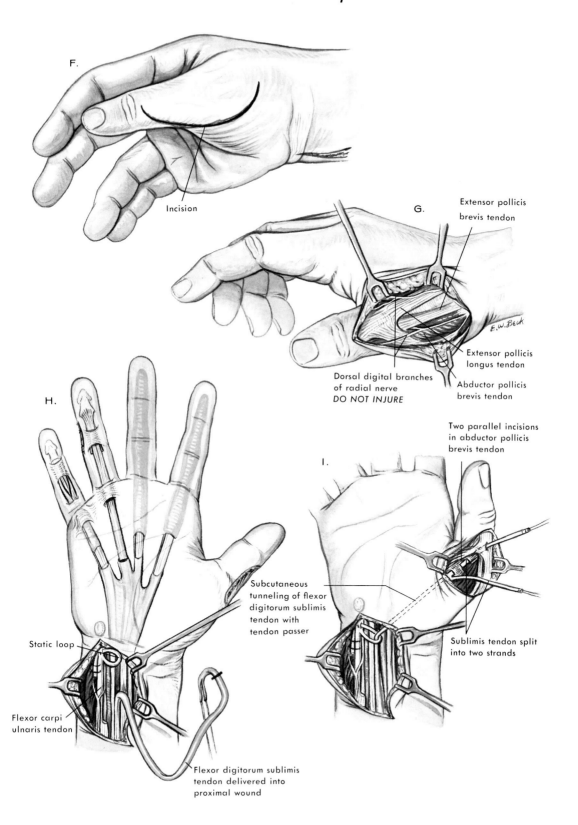

F.

Incision

G.

Extensor pollicis brevis tendon

E.W.Beck

Extensor pollicis longus tendon

Dorsal digital branches of radial nerve
DO NOT INJURE

Abductor pollicis brevis tendon

H.

Two parallel incisions in abductor pollicis brevis tendon

I.

Subcutaneous tunneling of flexor digitorum sublimis tendon with tendon passer

Sublimis tendon split into two strands

Static loop

Flexor carpi ulnaris tendon

Flexor digitorum sublimis tendon delivered into proximal wound

Restoration of Thumb Opposition by the Riordan Technique (Continued)

J. Separate the extensor aponeurosis from the periosteum of the proximal phalanx of the thumb; make a small incision through the aponeurosis and pass one half of the split sublimis tendon through it.

K to N. The proper tension for the transferred sublimis tendon is determined next. The two slips of the tendon are held together with a hemostat. With the wrist passively flexed, releasing the thumb should completely relax the transfer (**K**). Dorsiflexion of the wrist to 45 degrees should apply enough traction on the transfer to bring the thumb into complete opposition and the interphalangeal joint into complete extension. The tension of the tendon is readjusted if insufficient. When appropriate tension has been determined, the two slips of the sublimis tendon are sutured together. The transferred tendon should pass in the middle of the metacarpal head. If necessary, apply a single nonabsorbable suture fixing the tendon to the abductor pollicis brevis and the joint capsule.

The wounds are closed in the usual fashion, and an above- or below-elbow cast is applied holding the wrist in 30 degrees of flexion and the fingers in functional position. The thumb should be in full opposition with the interphalangeal joint in complete extension.

POSTOPERATIVE CARE

The cast is removed in three to four weeks, and physical therapy is performed to train the transferred tendon. A removable opponens splint is used during the night and part of the day for an additional two to three months.

Plate 82. Restoration of Thumb Opposition by the Riordan Technique

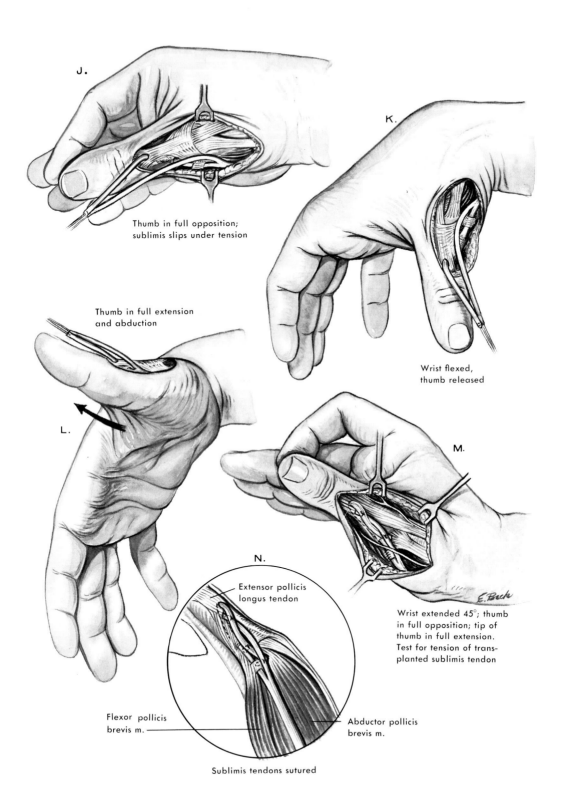

J.

Thumb in full opposition; sublimis slips under tension

K.

Wrist flexed, thumb released

Thumb in full extension and abduction

L.

M.

Wrist extended 45°; thumb in full opposition; tip of thumb in full extension. Test for tension of transplanted sublimis tendon

N.

Extensor pollicis longus tendon

Flexor pollicis brevis m.

Abductor pollicis brevis m.

Sublimis tendons sutured

E. Beck

Restoration of Thumb Opposition by the Brand Technique

OPERATIVE TECHNIQUE

The sublimis tendon of the ring finger is divided, and the incision over the thenar eminence of the thumb is similar to that described in the Riordan technique (see Plate 82).

A. A small incision is made on the volar surface of the forearm about 6 cm. proximal to the wrist, and the sublimis tendon from the ring finger is transferred into the forearm wound. Next, a 2 cm. longitudinal incision is made immediately distal and lateral to the pisiform bone. The subcutaneous tissue is divided in line with the skin incision, and the dissection is deepened until loose fatlike tissue is exposed. Do not injure a branch of the ulnar nerve that is in this fibrofatty tissue. Through the incision near the pisiform bone insert a tendon passer that exits in the forearm wound.

B. Sublimis tendon to the ring finger is pulled into the palmar wound with the help of the tendon passer.

C and **D.** The sublimis tendon is passed subcutaneously to the metacarpophalangeal joint of the thumb. The fibrous septa in the fat of the palm act as a pulley. The distal end of the sublimis tendon is split into two halves. The proximal slip of the sublimis tendon is sutured to the ulnar side of the metacarpophalangeal joint and the distal slip is sutured to the tendons of abductor pollicis brevis and extensor pollicis longus; this step prevents shifting in the position of the tendon as it crosses the metacarpophalangeal joint.

The tourniquet is released, and after complete hemostasis the wounds are closed in the usual fashion; a below-elbow cast is applied holding the thumb in opposition with the interphalangeal joint completely extended and the wrist in 30 degrees of flexion.

POSTOPERATIVE CARE

The cast is removed in three weeks, and physical therapy is performed to train the transferred tendon. A removable opponens splint is used during the night and part of the day for an additional two months.

Plate 83. Restoration of Thumb Opposition by the Brand Technique

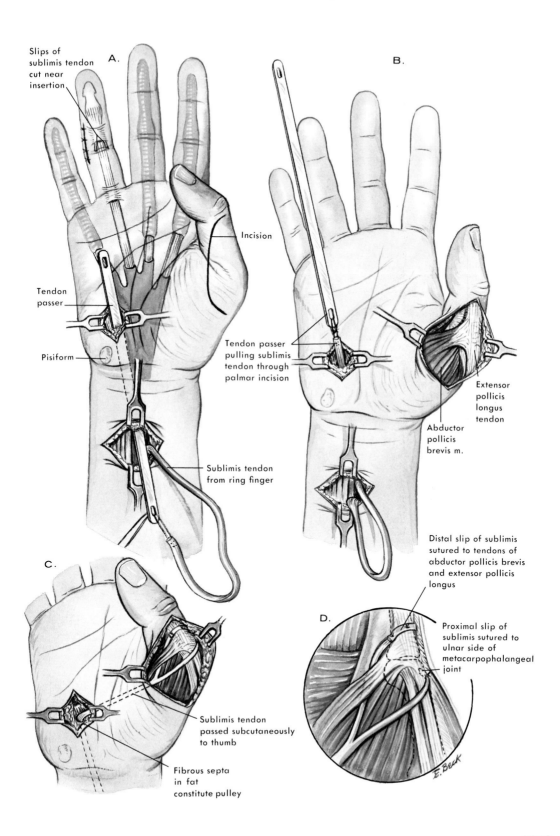

A.

Slips of sublimis tendon cut near insertion

Incision

Tendon passer

Pisiform

Tendon passer pulling sublimis tendon through palmar incision

Sublimis tendon from ring finger

B.

Extensor pollicis longus tendon

Abductor pollicis brevis m.

C.

Sublimis tendon passed subcutaneously to thumb

Fibrous septa in fat constitute pulley

D.

Distal slip of sublimis sutured to tendons of abductor pollicis brevis and extensor pollicis longus

Proximal slip of sublimis sutured to ulnar side of metacarpophalangeal joint

E. Beck

Transfer of Abductor Digiti Quinti Manus Muscle to Restore Opposition (Littler's Technique)

OPERATIVE TECHNIQUE

A. A curvilinear incision is made in the palm along the radial border of the abductor digiti quinti muscle belly. The incision begins from the radial side of the pisiform and terminates on the ulnar border of the middle phalanx of the little finger. Subcutaneous tissue is divided in line with the skin incision.

B. The abductor digiti quinti is exposed distally until its two tendon slips of insertion are identified and divided. One of the tendinous insertions inserts to bone and the other to the extensor apparatus of the little finger.

C. The abductor digiti quinti muscle is lifted from its fascial compartment and elevated proximally until its neurovascular pedicle is identified and isolated. Avoid tension on muscle and neurovascular pedicle while freeing.

D. Proximally, the abductor digiti quinti is released from the pisiform bone, but its origin from flexor carpi ulnaris tendon is left intact. Do not injure the ulnar nerve and artery.

E. Abductor digiti quinti muscle is folded over about 170 degrees like the page of a book, and passed subcutaneously to its new position on the thumb. Avoid tension and angulation of the neurovascular bundle.

F. Next, the tendons of the abductor digiti quinti muscle are sutured to abductor pollicis brevis tendon at its insertion. The tourniquet is released, and after complete hemostasis the wound is closed in the usual manner. A below-elbow cast is applied supporting the wrist in neutral position and the thumb in relaxed palmar abduction.

POSTOPERATIVE CARE

The cast is removed in three weeks, and active exercises are performed to oppose the thumb. An opponens splint is worn at night and part of the day for several months.

Plate 84. Transfer of Abductor Digiti Quinti Manus Muscle to Restore Opposition (Littler's Technique)

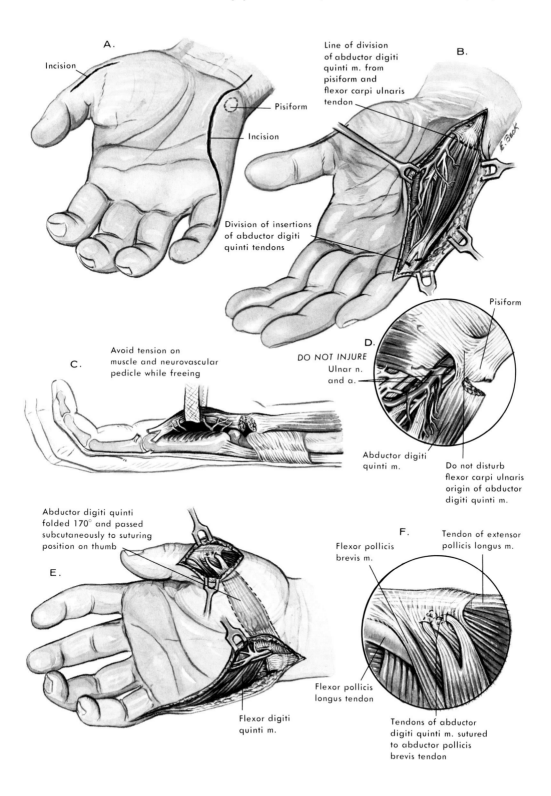

A.

Incision

Pisiform

Incision

Line of division
of abductor digiti
quinti m. from
pisiform and
flexor carpi ulnaris
tendon

B.

E. Beck

Division of insertions
of abductor digiti
quinti tendons

C.

Avoid tension on
muscle and neurovascular
pedicle while freeing

D.

Pisiform

DO NOT INJURE
Ulnar n.
and a.

Abductor digiti
quinti m.

Do not disturb
flexor carpi ulnaris
origin of abductor
digiti quinti m.

Abductor digiti quinti
folded 170° and passed
subcutaneously to suturing
position on thumb

E.

F.

Flexor pollicis
brevis m.

Tendon of extensor
pollicis longus m.

Flexor pollicis
longus tendon

Flexor digiti
quinti m.

Tendons of abductor
digiti quinti m. sutured
to abductor pollicis
brevis tendon

Boyes Technique

OPERATIVE TECHNIQUE

A. A longitudinal incision is made beginning at the radial styloid process and extending proximally for a distance of 7 to 10 cm. The subcutaneous tissue is divided in line with the skin incision; the wound flaps are undermined, mobilized, and retracted. The flat tendon of the brachioradialis is identified at its insertion and sectioned. The tendon is dissected, and its muscle is freed and mobilized proximally as far as its nerve supply permits. Next, on the dorsum of the hand, two incisions are made: a 3 cm. longitudinal incision between the third and fourth metacarpals, and a curvilinear 2.5 cm. incision between the first and second metacarpals. An alternative surgical approach to expose the adductor tubercle of the thumb is by a 2.5 cm. incision in the palm in line with the skin crease of the metacarpophalangeal joint of the thumb.

B. Then a free tendon graft is taken either from the palmaris longus in the forearm or from the plantaris in the leg. First, the tendon graft is sutured to the adductor tubercle of the thumb and the insertion of adductor pollicis; next with an Ober tendon passer the tendon graft is passed along the adductor muscle belly in the palm to exit through the third interosseous space on the dorsum of the hand in the incision between the third and fourth metacarpals.

C. Next, a tendon passer is inserted deep to the extensor digitorum communis tendons, and the free tendon graft is delivered from the incision on the dorsum of the hand to the radial incision on the forearm.

D. The proximal end of the tendon graft is sutured to the brachioradialis tendon.

The tourniquet is released and after complete hemostasis is obtained, the wounds are closed in routine fashion. A below-elbow cast is applied holding the wrist in 45 degrees of dorsiflexion and the thumb in adduction.

POSTOPERATIVE CARE

The cast is removed in four to six weeks following surgery. Active exercises are performed to develop thumb adduction.

Plate 85. Boyes Technique

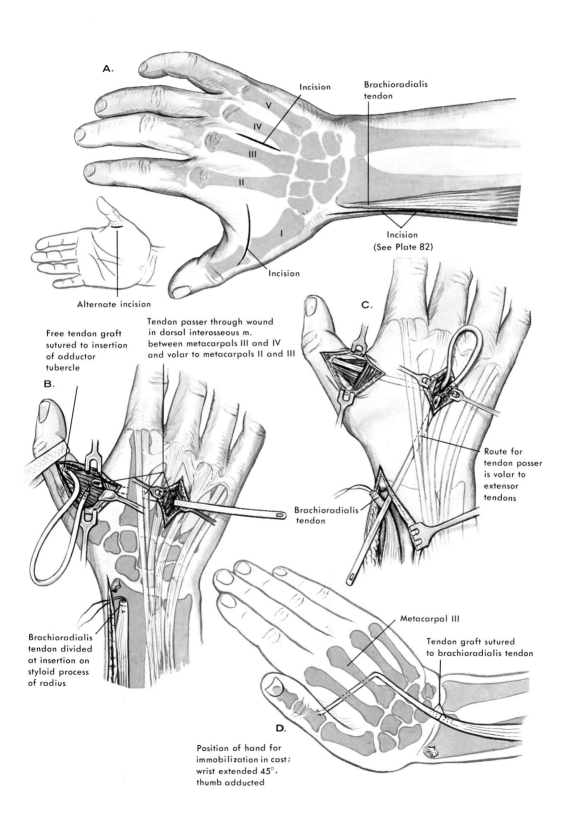

A.

Incision

Brachioradialis tendon

V

IV

III

II

I

Incision
(See Plate 82)

Incision

Alternate incision

B.

Free tendon graft sutured to insertion of adductor tubercle

Tendon passer through wound in dorsal interosseous m. between metacarpals III and IV and volar to metacarpals II and III

C.

Route for tendon passer is volar to extensor tendons

Brachioradialis tendon

Brachioradialis tendon divided at insertion on styloid process of radius

Metacarpal III

Tendon graft sutured to brachioradialis tendon

D.

Position of hand for immobilization in cast; wrist extended 45°, thumb adducted

Restoration of Thumb Abduction by Transfer of Extensor Pollicis Brevis Tendon to Extensor Carpi Ulnaris Tendon

OPERATIVE TECHNIQUE

A. Make a 3 cm. transverse incision on the dorsoradial aspect of the distal forearm immediately proximal to the extensor retinaculum of the wrist over the musculotendinous junction of extensor pollicis tendon. The subcutaneous tissue is divided in line with the skin incision. The fasciae are divided by longitudinal incision and the tendon of extensor pollicis brevis is identified and divided at its musculotendinous junction.

Next, a 3 cm. long incision is made on the dorsolateral aspect of the metacarpophalangeal joint of the thumb. The subcutaneous tissue is divided in line with the skin incision. The tendon of extensor pollicis brevis is identified at its insertion and pulled into the thumb wound from the wrist wound.

B. A curvilinear incision is made on the ulnar aspect of the wrist. It begins at the base of the fourth metacarpal and extends ulnarward and palmarward immediately distal to the ulnar styloid and then extends proximally for a distance of 3 cm. along the volar surface of the wrist. The extensor carpi ulnaris tendon is identified and divided at its insertion and freed proximally.

C. The extensor pollicis brevis tendon is passed subcutaneously toward the palmar surface of the hand and sutured to extensor carpi ulnaris tendon with the thumb in maximal abduction.

The tourniquet is released, and after complete hemostasis the wound is closed in the usual fashion. A below-elbow cast is applied holding the wrist in neutral position and the thumb in maximal abduction.

POSTOPERATIVE CARE

The cast is removed four weeks following surgery. Active exercises are performed for active thumb abduction. A plastic splint is worn at night and part of the day holding the thumb in maximal abduction.

Plate 86. Restoration of Thumb Abduction by Transfer of Extensor Pollicis Brevis Tendon to Extensor Carpi Ulnaris Tendon

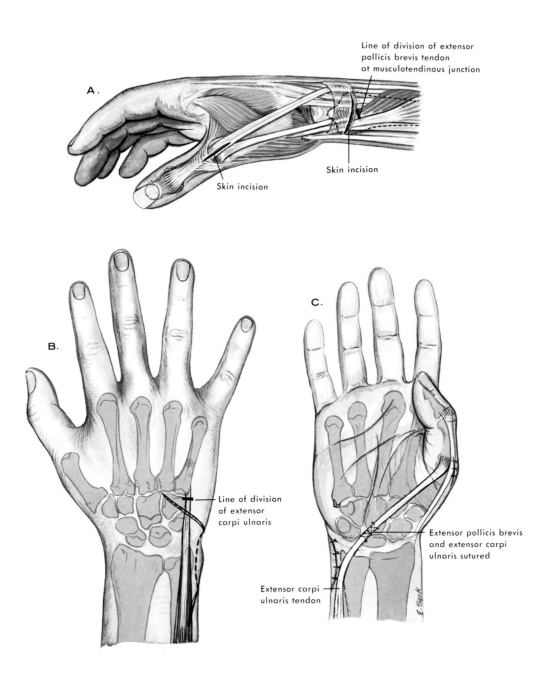

A.

Line of division of extensor pollicis brevis tendon at musculotendinous junction

Skin incision

Skin incision

B.

C.

Line of division of extensor carpi ulnaris

Extensor pollicis brevis and extensor carpi ulnaris sutured

Extensor carpi ulnaris tendon

E. Beck

Restoration of Abduction of Index Finger
(Phalen Technique)

OPERATIVE TECHNIQUE

A. Make a curved incision on the midlateral aspect of the index finger extending from the proximal phalanx to the radial aspect of the metacarpophalangeal joint; then extend it dorsally to the middle third of the index metacarpal.

B. The dorsal expansion over the metacarpophalangeal joint is incised. The extensor indicis proprius muscle is identified and sectioned at its insertion and pulled proximally. Do not injure dorsal digital branches of the radial artery and nerve.

C. Next, the tendon of extensor indicis proprius is passed distally to the radial and palmar aspects of the index finger and sutured to the tendon of the first dorsal interosseous muscle. The incision in the dorsal expansion is closed.

The tourniquet is released, and after complete hemostasis the wound is closed in the usual fashion. A below-elbow cast is applied holding the wrist in neutral position and the index finger in 10 degrees of abduction.

POSTOPERATIVE CARE

The cast is removed three to four weeks following surgery, and active exercises are performed to provide abduction of the index finger.

Plate 87. Restoration of Abduction of Index Finger
(Phalen Technique)

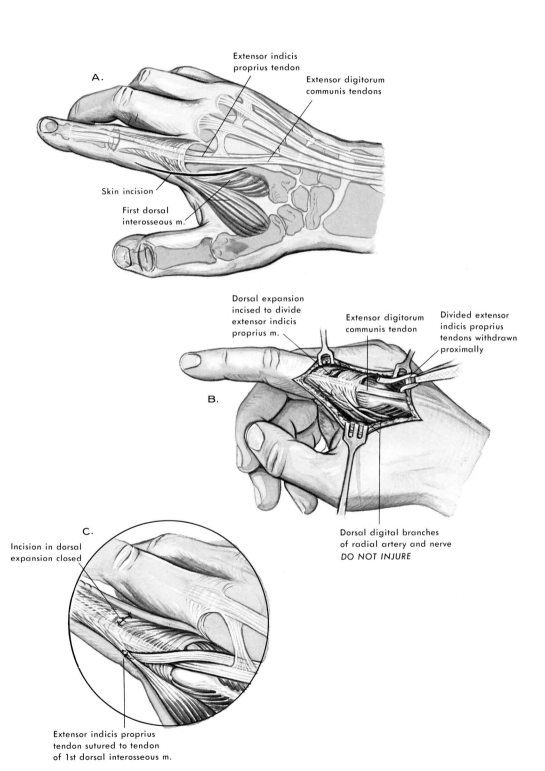

A.

Extensor indicis proprius tendon

Extensor digitorum communis tendons

Skin incision

First dorsal interosseous m.

Dorsal expansion incised to divide extensor indicis proprius m.

Extensor digitorum communis tendon

Divided extensor indicis proprius tendons withdrawn proximally

B.

Dorsal digital branches of radial artery and nerve
DO NOT INJURE

C.

Incision in dorsal expansion closed

Extensor indicis proprius tendon sutured to tendon of 1st dorsal interosseous m.

Intermetacarpal Bone Block for Thenar Paralysis

OPERATIVE TECHNIQUE

A. A curvilinear incision is made between the index and thumb metacarpals at the juncture of their distal third and proximal two thirds. The subcutaneous tissue is divided in line with the skin incision. The first dorsal interosseous muscle is elevated from the index and thumb metacarpals. The radial artery between the bases of the first and second metacarpals should not be injured.

B. The thumb metacarpal is rotated into full opposition, and the interspace between the thumb and index metacarpals is measured for length of iliac bone graft.

C. The interosseous muscle is split on the volar surface of the index and thumb metacarpals; a slot is made with a hand drill and gouges. The physes of the index and thumb metacarpals should not be injured.

D. The iliac bone graft is taken and shaped so that its ends are tapered to fit into the previously prepared slots.

E. The thumb metacarpal is fully abducted and rotated into neutral opposition, and the bone graft is inserted into the previously prepared slots. Chips of cancellous bone are placed at each end. A threaded Steinmann pin is used for internal fixation, transfixing the iliac graft to the metacarpals.

The tourniquet is released, and after complete hemostasis the wound is closed in the usual fashion; a below-elbow cast is applied holding the thumb in maximal abduction and opposition.

POSTOPERATIVE CARE

The cast is changed in one month and radiograms are made. If there is adequate healing, the pin is removed; if not, the pin is left for another month. Usually the graft will heal within two to three months. When there are problems with bone healing, the Steinmann pin is left in as an internal fixator until bony union takes place.

Plate 88. Intermetacarpal Bone Block for Thenar Paralysis

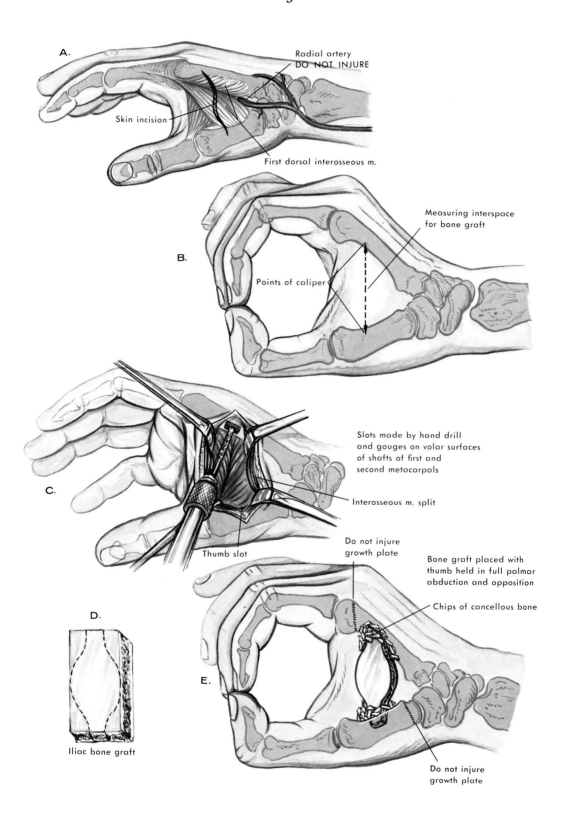

A.

Radial artery
DO NOT INJURE

Skin incision

First dorsal interosseous m.

B.

Measuring interspace
for bone graft

Points of caliper

C.

Slots made by hand drill
and gouges on volar surfaces
of shafts of first and
second metacarpals

Interosseous m. split

Thumb slot

D.

Iliac bone graft

E.

Do not injure
growth plate

Bone graft placed with
thumb held in full palmar
abduction and opposition

Chips of cancellous bone

Do not injure
growth plate

5. Bale, J. F., Jr., Thompson, J. A., Petajan, J. H., and Ziter, F. A.: Childhood brachial plexus neuropathy. J. Pediatr., 95:741, 1979.

6. Bateman, J. E.: The Shoulder and Neck. 2nd. Ed. (With special assistance of Fournasier, V. L.) Philadelphia, W. B. Saunders, 1978.

7. Bennet, G. C., and Harrold, A. J.: Prognosis and early management of birth injuries to the brachial plexus. Br. Med. J., 1:1520, 1976.

8. Blount, W. P.: Osteoclasis for supination deformities in children. J. Bone Joint Surg., 22:300, 1940.

9. Bonney, G.: The value of axon responses in determining the site of lesion in traction injuries of the brachial plexus. Brain, 2:588, 1954.

10. Bonney, G.: Prognosis in traction lesions of the brachial plexus. J. Bone Joint Surg., 41-B:4, 1959.

11. Bozhko, O. L.: Obstetrical paralysis of the arm in infants. Med. Sestra., 38:40, 1979.

12. Bozhko, O. L.: Paralysis of the arm in newborn infants. Feldsher Akush., 44:25, 1979.

13. Brown, K. L.: Review of obstetrical palsies. Nonoperative treatment. Clin. Plast. Surg., 11:181, 1984.

14. Bullard, W. N.: Obstetric paralysis. Am. J. Med. Sci., 134:93, 1907.

15. Burman, M.: Paralytic supination contracture of the forearm. J. Bone Joint Surg., 38-A:303, 1956.

16. Carlioz, H., and Brahimi, L.: La place de la desinsertion interne du sous-scapulaire dans le traitement de la paralysie obstetricale du membre superieur chez l'enfant. Ann. Chir. Infant., 12:159, 1971.

17. Castaing, J., and Delplace, J.: Paralysie obstetricale du plexus brachiale. S.O.F.C.O.T., XLVI Reunion Annuelle. Rev. Chir. Orthop., 59(Suppl.):133, 1972.

18. Chung, S. M. K., and Nissenbaum, M. M.: Obstetrical paralysis. Orthop. Clin. North Am., 6:393, 1975.

19. Clark, I. P., Taylor, A. S., and Prout, T. P.: A study of brachial birth palsy. Am. J. Med. Sci., 130:670, 1905.

20. Danos, E.: Obstetrical palsy. J. Bone Joint Surg., 47-B:805, 1965.

21. Dautry, P., Apoil, A., Moinet, F., and Koechlin, P.: Paralysie radiculaire superieure du plexus brachial. Traitement par transpositions musculaires associees. Resultat de sept cas. Rev. Chir. Orthop., 63:399, 1977.

22. DeGuidi, G., Garelli, R., and Nicosia, U.: Le paralisi ostetriche dell'arto superiore: contributo clinico statistico. Minerva Pediatr., 19:119, 1967.

23. Dolnitski, O. V., Iatsenko, V. P., and Dolnitski, I. O.: Birth injuries to the brachial plexus in infants (clinical and morphological parallels). Klin. Khir., 6:46, 1981.

24. Dolnitski, O. V., and Karchemski, V. I.: Functional disorders of the upper extremity as a consequence of total birth paralysis of the brachial plexus in children. Klin. Khir., 6:50, 1978.

25. Dolnitski, O. V., and Klimmenko, M. D.: L'Episcopo's operation in the Duchenne-Erb type of brachial plexus birth paralysis in children. Ortop. Travmatol. Protez., 7:42, 1978.

26. Dubousset, J.: Paralysie obstetricale du plexus brachiale. S.O.F.C.O.T., XLVI Reunion Annuelle. Rev. Chir. Orthop., 59(Suppl):159, 1972.

27. Dubousset, J. F.: Paralysie obstetricale du plexus brachiale. Paris, Journées de l'hôpital Cochin, Nov. 1979.

28. Duchenne, G. B. A.: De l'Electrisation Localisée et de Son Application à la Pathologic et à la Therapeutique. 3rd Ed. Paris, Bailliere, 1872, p. 357.

29. Eng, G. D.: Brachial plexus palsy in newborn infants. Pediatrics, 48:18, 1971.

30. Eng, G. D., Koch, B., and Smokvina, M. D.: Brachial plexus palsy in neonates and children. Arch. Phys. Med. Rehabil., 59:458, 1978.

31. Erb, W. H.: Ueber eine Eigenthumliche Localisation von Lahmungen im Plexus Brachialis. Verhandl. Naturhist. Med. Heidelberg, N. F., 2:130, 1874.

32. Erb, W.: On a characteristic site of injury in the brachial plexus (Reprinted). Arch. Neurol., 21:433, 1969.

33. Fairbank, H. A. T.: Birth palsy: Subluxation of shoulder joints in infants and young children. Lancet, 1:1217, 1913.

34. Faysse, R.: Paralysie obstetricale du plexus brachial. Traitement, II: Therapeutique, (d) l'osteotomie du derotation de l'humerus dans les sequelles. Rev. Chir. Orthop., 58(Suppl):187, 1972.

35. Fishchenko, P. I., Ovsiankin, N. A., and Malenkov, N. N.: Myolavsanplasty of the trapezius muscle in children with the sequelae of the Erb type of birth injury to the brachial plexus. Ortop. Travmatol. Protez., 7:38, 1978.

36. Frankel, M. E., Goldner, J. L., and Stelling, F. H.: Partial shoulder girdle paralysis. Surgical treatment. South. Med. J., 62:1502, 1969.

37. Frot, B.: La myelographie cervicale opaque dans les paralysies traumatiques du plexus brachial. Rev. Chir. Orthop., 63:67, 1977.

38. Frot, B., Filipe, G., Olivier, H., Alnot, J. Y., and Duparc, J.: Interet de la myelographie cervicale à contraste positif brachial chez l'adulte. Ann. Radiol., 16:715, 1973.

39. Gerard, Y.: Les paralysies obstetricales du membre superieur. Thèse Médecine, Paris, 1955.

40. Gilbert, A., Khouri, N., and Carlioz, H.: Exploration chirurgicale du plexus brachial dans la paralysie obstetricale. Constatations anatomiques chez 21 maladies opères. Rev. Chir. Orthop., 66:33, 1980.

41. Gilmour, J.: Notes on the surgical treatment of brachial birth palsy. Lancet, 2:696, 1925.

42. Gjorup, L.: Obstetrical lesions of the brachial plexus. Acta Neurol. Scand. (Suppl. 18), 42:1, 1966.

43. Glez Cuesta, F. J., Prats, F. L., Glez Lopez, F. J., and Sitja, J. B.: The role of bone operations as palliative surgical treatment for the sequelae of obstetrical brachial paralysis in the shoulder. Acta Orthop. Belg., 48:757, 1982.

44. Goddard, N. J., and Fixsen, J. A.: Rotation osteotomy of the humerus for birth injuries of the brachial plexus. J. Bone Joint Surg., 66-B:257, 1984.

45. Gordon, M., Rich, H., Deutschberger, J., and Green, M.: The immediate and long-term outcome of obstetrical birth trauma. Am. J. Obstet. Gynecol., 117:51, 1973.

46. Granberry, W. M., and Lipscomb, P. R.: Tendon transfers to the hand in brachial palsy. Am. J. Surg., 108:840, 1964.

47. Green, W. T., and Tachdjian, M. O.: Correction of residual deformities of the shoulder in obstetrical palsy. J. Bone Joint Surg., 45-A:1544, 1963.

48. Greenwald, A. G., Schute, P. C., and Shiveley, J. L.: Brachial plexus birth palsy: A 10-year report on the incidence and prognosis. J. Pediatr. Orthop., 4:689, 1984.

49. Grilli, F. P.: Il trapianto del bicipite brachiale in funzione pronatoria. Arch. Putti, 12:359, 1959.

50. Hambly, E.: Should a brachial plexus injury be explored? Lancet, 22:360, 1945.

51. Hardy, A. E.: Birth injuries of the brachial plexus: Incidence and prognosis. J. Bone Joint Surg., 63-B:98, 1981.

52. Hoffer, M. M., Wickenden, R., and Roper, B.: Brachial plexus birth palsies. Results of tendon transfers to the rotator cuff. J. Bone Joint Surg., 60-A:691, 1978.

53. Hsu, J. D., Perry, J., and Barber, L.: The use of orthoses in patients with brachial plexus lesions (Abstract). Arch. Phys. Med. Rehabil., 53:583, 1972.

54. Ingram, A. J. (ed.): Campbell's Operative Orthopedics. St. Louis, C. V. Mosby, 1971, p. 1722.
55. Jolly, A.: Traitement chirurgical direct des lesions par elongation du plexus brachial de l'adulte. Paris, Thèse, 1980.
56. Jones, B. N., Manske, P. R., Schoenecker, P. L., et al.: Latissimus dorsi transfer to restore elbow extension in obstetrical palsy. J. Pediatr. Orthop., 5:287, 1985.
57. Jones, S. J.: Investigation of brachial plexus traction lesions by peripheral and spinal somatosensory evoked potentials. J. Neurol. Neurosurg. Psychiatry, 42:107, 1979.
58. Kennedy, R.: Suture of the brachial plexus in birth paralysis of the upper extremity. Br. Med. J., 1:298, 1903.
59. Kennedy, R.: Further notes on the treatment of birth paralysis of the upper extremity by suture of the fifth and sixth cervical nerves. Br. Med. J., 2:1065, 1904.
60. Khatree, M. H., Gamsu, H. R., Rudd, P., and Studd, J. W.: Features predictive of brachial plexus injury during labour. S. Afr. Med. J., 61:232, 1982.
61. Klumpke, A.: Contribution à l'étude des paralysies radiculaires du plexus brachial. Paralysies radiculaires totales. Paralysies radiculaires inferieures. De la participation des filets sympathiques oculo-pupillaires dans ces paralysies. Rev. Med. (Paris), 5:591, 1885.
62. Kowalski, M., and Weiss, M.: Osteotomia derotacyjna kosci ramiennej w rehabilitacji porodowego porazenia splotu ramiennego u dzieci. (With English abstract.) Chir. Narzadow Ruchu Ortop. Pol., 40:445, 1975.
63. Kwast, O.: F wave study in children with birth brachial plexus paralysis. Electromyogr. Clin. Neurophysiol., 24:457, 1984.
64. Landi, A., Copeland, S. A., Wynn Parry, C. B., and Jones, S. J.: The role of somatosensory evoked potentials and nerve conduction studies in the surgical management of brachial plexus injuries. J. Bone Joint Surg., 62-B:492, 1980.
65. L'Episcopo, J. B.: Tendon transplantation in obstetrical paralysis. Am. J. Surg., 25:122, 1934.
66. L'Episcopo, J. B.: Restoration of muscle balance in the treatment of obstetrical paralysis. N.Y. J. Med., 39:357, 1939.
67. Liebolt, F. L., and Furry, J. G.: Obstetrical paralysis with dislocation of the shoulder. J. Bone Joint Surg., 35-A:227, 1953.
68. Lovett, R.: The surgical aspect of the paralysis of newborn children. Boston Med. Surg. J., 127:8, 1892.
69. Malenkov, N. N., Moroz, I. N., Syracheva, I. S., and Lakovleva, M. I.: Functional rehabilitation of the upper extremity in children with sequelae of birth injuries to the brachial plexus using the method of adaptive bioregulation. Zh. Nevropatol. Psikhiatr., 77:516, 1977.
70. Mallet, J.: Symposium sur la paralysie obstetricale du plexus brachial. Rev. Chir. Orthop., 58:117, 1972.
71. Manfrini, M., and Valdiserri, L.: Proximal radio-ulnar arthrosis in the treatment of supination deformity resulting from obstetrical paralysis. Ital. J. Orthop. Traumatol., 11:309, 1985.
72. Marakas, A.: Brachial plexus surgery. Orthop. Clin. North Am., 12:303, 1981.
73. Mastandrea, G.: Il traplanto del muscolo tricipite brachiale sul bicipite negli esiti della paralisi obstetrica. Ortop. Traumatol., 23:953, 1953.
74. Menzel, K., Genssler, W., Gottschlak, E., Linke, M., and Topke, B.: Paralysis of phrenic nerve due to birth injury. Acta Pediatr. Acad. Sci. Hung., 18:69, 1977.
75. Merger, R., and Judet, J.: Paralysie obstetricale du plexus brachial. Prevention et traitement. Nouv. Presse Med., 2:1935, 1973.
76. Metaizeau, J. P., Gayet, C., and Plenat, F.: Brachial plexus birth injuries. An experimental study (author's transl.). Chir. Pediatr., 20:159, 1979.
77. Meyer, R. D.: Treatment of adult and obstetrical plexus injuries. Orthopedics, 9:899, 1986.
78. Millesi, H.: Resultats tardifs de la greffe nerveuse interfasciculaires. Chirurgie reparatrice des lesions du plexus brachial. Rev. Med. Suisse Romande, 1973, p. 935.
79. Millesi, H.: Indications et resultats des interventions directes dans la paralysie traumatique du plexus brachial chez l'adulte. Rev. Chir. Orthop., 63:82, 1977.
80. Millesi, H.: Surgical management of brachial plexus injuries. J. Hand Surg., 2:367, 1977.
81. Millesi, H., Meissl, G., and Berger, A.: The interfascicular nerve grafting of the median and ulnar nerves. J. Bone Joint Surg., 54-A:727, 1972.
82. Moldaver, J.: Tinel's sign. Its characteristics and significance. J. Bone Joint Surg., 60-A:412, 1978.
83. Moore, B. H.: A new operation for brachial birth palsy—Erb's paralysis. Surg. Gynecol. Obstet., 61:832, 1935.
84. Moore, B. H.: Brachial birth palsy. Am. J. Surg., 43:338, 1939.
85. Morison, J. E.: Peripheral brachial paralysis in infants and children. Arch. Dis. Child., 13:310, 1938.
86. Mugica, E. E.: Traumatologia y Ortopedia de las Lesiones Obstetricas en el Nino. Madrid, Editorial Marban, 1976.
87. Narakas, A.: Indications et resultats du traitement chirurgical direct dans les lesions par elongation du plexus brachial de l'adulte. Rev. Chir. Orthop., 63:88, 1977.
88. Narakas, A.: Surgical treatment of traction injuries of the brachial plexus. Clin. Orthop., 133:71, 1978.
89. Narakas, A.: Editorial: Why is my peripheral nerve surgery so poor? Int. J. Microsurg., 1:150, 1979.
90. Narakas, A.: Brachial plexus surgery. Orthop. Clin. North Am., 12:303, 1981.
91. Neuenschwander, S., Brauner, M., Gilbert, A., and Faure, C.: Cervical myelography with metrizamide in brachial birth palsies. Ann. Radiol. (Paris), 23:93, 1980.
92. Palacios Suarez, E. M., Martinez Bracamontes, G., Sandoyal Moron, O. J., Orozco Sanches, J., Jimenez Rojas, D., and Aguilar Lopez de Nava, L. L.: Diaphragmatic and Erb-Duchenne's paralysis: an infrequent obstetric trauma. Bol. Med. Hosp. Infant. Mex., 37:63, 1980.
93. Parry, C. B.: The Roscoe Clarke Memorial Lecture, 1979. The management of traction lesions of the brachial plexus and peripheral nerve injuries in the upper limb: A study in teamwork. Injury, 11:265, 1980.
94. Perricone, G.: Lesioni Ostetriche dei Neonati. Bologna, Capelli Editore, 1963.
95. Perry, J., Hsu, J., Barber, L., and Hoffer, M. M.: Orthoses in patients with brachial plexus injuries. Arch. Phys. Med. Rehabil., 55:134, 1974.
96. Putti, V.: Due sindromi paralitiche del'arto superiore. Note di fisiopatologia della rotazione antibrachiale. Chir. Organi Mov., 26:215, 1940.
97. Robles, J.: Brachial plexus avulsion: A review of diagnostic procedures and report of six cases. J. Neurosurg., 28:434, 1968.
98. Rogers, M. H.: An operation for the correction of the deformity due to "obstetrical paralysis." Boston Med. Surg. J., 174:163, 1916.
99. Roper, B.: A new operation to improve weakness of the abductors and external rotators of the shoulder. *In* Orthopedic Seminars. Downey, Calif., Rancho Los Amigos Hospital, 4:347, 1971.
100. Rorabeck, C. H.: The management of flail upper

extremity in brachial plexus injuries. J. Trauma, 20:491, 1980.

101. Rorabeck, C. H., and Harris, W. R.: Factors affecting the prognosis of brachial plexus injuries. J. Bone Joint Surg., 63-B:404, 1981.

102. Rossi, L. N., Vassella, F., and Mumenthaler, M.: Obstetrical lesions of the brachial plexus: Natural history in 34 personal cases. Eur. Neurol., 21:1, 1982.

103. Saha, A. K.: Surgery of the paralyzed and flail shoulder. Acta Orthop. Scand., (Suppl.):97, 1907.

104. Scaglietti, O.: The obstetrical shoulder trauma. Surg. Gynecol. Obstet., 66:868, 1938.

105. Schottstaedt, E. R., Larsen, L. J., and Bost, F. C.: The surgical reconstruction of the upper extremity paralyzed by poliomyelitis. J. Bone Joint Surg., 40-A:633, 1958.

106. Seddon, H. J.: Brachial plexus injuries. J. Bone Joint Surg., 31-B:3, 1949.

107. Seddon, H. J.: Surgical Disorders of the Peripheral Nerves. London, Churchill Livingstone, 1972.

108. Sedel, L.: The results of surgical repair of brachial plexus injuries. J. Bone Joint Surg., 64-B:54, 1982.

109. Serratrice, G.: Le syndrome de Claude Bernard Horner. Revue Prat., 11:2109, 1961.

110. Sever, J. W.: Obstetric paralysis. Its etiology, pathology, clinical aspects, and treatment, with a report of 470 cases. Am. J. Dis. Child., 12:541, 1916.

111. Sever, J. W.: The results of a new operation for obstetrical paralysis. Am. J. Orthop. Surg., 16:248, 1918.

112. Sever, J. W.: Obstetrical paralysis. J.A.M.A., 85:1862, 1925.

113. Sever, J. W.: Obstetrical paralysis. Surg. Gynecol. Obstet., 44:547, 1927.

114. Sharpe, W.: The operative treatment of brachial plexus paralysis. J.A.M.A., 66:876, 1916.

115. Smellie, W.: Collection of Preternatural Cases and Observations in Midwifery. Compleating the Design of Illustrating His First Volume on That Subject. Vol. III. London, Wilson and Durham, 1764, p. 504.

116. Smith, F. M.: The concealed incision for surgical approach of the upper humerus. Surg. Gynecol. Obstet., 108:756, 1959.

117. Smith, J. W.: Microsurgery of peripheral nerves. Plast. Reconstr. Surg., 33:317, 1964.

118. Smith, J. W.: Factors influencing nerve repair. Arch. Surg., 93:335, 1966.

119. Solonen, K. A., Teleranta, T., and Ryoppy, S.: Early reconstruction of birth injuries of the brachial plexus. Pediatr. Orthop., 1:367, 1981.

120. Solonen, K. A., Teleranta, T., and Vilkki, S.: Reconstruction of the median and ulnar nerves in the forearm. In Lie, T. S. (ed.): Microsurgery. Amsterdam, Excerpta Medica International Congress Series 465, 1979, pp. 81–84.

121. Solonen, K. A., et al.: Surgery of the brachial plexus. Acta Orthop. Scand., 55:436, 1984.

122. Soni, A. L., Mir, N. A., Kishan, J., Faquih, A. M., and Elzouki, A. Y.: Brachial plexus injuries in babies born in hospital: An appraisal of risk factors in a developing country. Ann. Trop. Paediatr., 5:69, 1985.

123. Specht, E.: Brachial plexus palsy in the newborn: Incidence and prognosis. Clin. Orthop., 110:32, 1975.

124. Stefanova-Uzunova, M., Stamatova, L., and Gatev, V.: Dynamic properties of partially denervated muscle in children with brachial plexus birth palsy. J. Neurol. Neurosurg. Psychiatry, 44:497, 1981.

125. Stojcevic-Polovina, M.: Risk factors in infants with paresis of the brachial plexus. Acta Med. Iugosi, 40:3, 1986.

126. Sugioka, H.: Evoked potentials in the investigation of traumatic lesions of the peripheral nerve and the brachial plexus. Clin. Orthop., 184:85, 1984.

127. Sunderland, S.: Repair of the brachial plexus directed to restoring elbow flexion. Bull. Hosp. Jt. Dis. Orthop. Inst., 44:485, 1984.

128. Tada, K., Tsuyuguchi, Y., and Kawai, H.: Birth palsy: Natural recovery course and combined root avulsion. J. Pediatr. Orthop., 4:279, 1984.

129. Tan, K. L.: Brachial palsy. J. Obstet. Gynaecol. Br. Commonw., 80:60, 1973.

130. Taylor, A. S.: Results from the surgical treatment of brachial birth palsy. J.A.M.A., 48:96, 1907.

131. Teot, L.: Etude anatomon clinique des lesions neonatales du plexus brachial. These: Presentee à Faculté de Médicine, Universite du Montpellier, France.

132. Thomas, T. T.: The relation of posterior subluxation of the shoulder joint to obstetrical palsy of the upper extremity. Ann. Surg., 59:197, 1914.

133. Tsai, T. M., et al.: Restoration of elbow flexion by pectoralis major and pectoralis minor transfer. J. Hand Surg., 8:186, 1983.

134. Vannini, F.: Il quadro radiografico del trauma ostetrico dell'artro superiore. Atti della XXIII Riunione dei Radiologi Emiliani. Radiol. Med., 1933.

135. Vassalos, E., Prevedourakis, C., and Paraschopoulou, P.: Brachial plexus paralysis in the newborn. Am. J. Obstet. Gynecol., 101:554, 1968.

136. Wickstrom, J.: Birth injuries of the brachial plexus. J. Bone Joint Surg., 42-A:1448, 1960.

137. Wickstrom, J.: Birth injuries of the brachial plexus. Treatment of defects in the shoulder. Clin. Orthop., 23:187, 1962.

138. Wickstrom, J., Haslam, E. T., and Hutchinson, R. H.: The surgical management of residual deformities of the shoulder following birth injuries of the brachial plexus. J. Bone Joint Surg., 37-A:27, 1955.

139. Wolman, B.: Erb's palsy. Arch. Dis. Child., 23:129, 1948.

140. Zachary, R. B.: Transplantation of teres major and latissimus dorsi for loss of external rotation at the shoulder. Lancet, 2:757, 1947.

141. Zachary, R. B.: Results of nerve suture. In Seddon, H. J. (ed.): Peripheral Nerve Injuries. London, Her Majesty's Stationery Office, 1954, pp. 354–388.

142. Zancolli, E. A.: Paralytic supination contracture of the forearm. J. Bone Joint Surg., 49-A:1275, 1967.

143. Zancolli, E. A.: Classification and management of the shoulder in birth palsy. Orthop. Clin. North Am., 12:433, 1981.

144. Zancolli, E. A., Aponte, F., and Zancolli, E. R.: Paralisis obstetrica. Clasificacion de las secuelas. Bol. y Trab. de la Sociedad Arg. de Ortopedia y Traumatologia, Ano XLIV, No. 3, 1979.

145. Zancolli, E. A., Aponte, F., and Zancolli, E. R.: Paralisis obstetrica de tipo braquial superior. Clasificacion de sus secuelas y su correcion quirurgica. Bol. y Trab. de la Sociedad Arg. de Ortopedia y Traumatologia. Aano XLIV, No. 5, 1979.

146. Zaoussis, A. L.: Osteotomy of the proximal end of the radius for paralytic supination deformity in children. J. Bone Joint Surg., 45-B:523, 1963.

SCIATIC NERVE PALSY[1–43]

Etiology

The common cause of sciatic nerve injury in infants and children is intramuscular injection of antibiotics or other medications into the gluteal region. The noxious agent is placed directly in or immediately adjacent to the nerve trunk as it emerges from the sciatic notch and is crossed by the piriformis muscle. The unfortunate victim may be an emaciated and sick child with marked gluteal atrophy, or he may be a robust uncooperative infant who is crying and kicking at the time of inoculation. Such a mishap can also occur when the site of injection is inadequately exposed in an anesthetized patient covered by surgical drapes or when the physician or nurse is simply careless or ignorant.

Parenteral administration of therapeutic agents through the umbilical vessels in a newborn may cause thrombosis of the inferior gluteal arteries and damage to both sciatic nerves. The skin over the buttocks may slough in such an instance. The sciatic nerve may stretch and become paralyzed during closed or open reduction of congenital dislocation of the hip or during femoral lengthening. Posterior traumatic dislocation of the hip is very rare in children; however, when it does occur, it can cause sciatic nerve palsy. Avulsion fracture of the lesser trochanter can injure the sciatic nerve. The sciatic nerve may also be injured during Salter Chiari's innominate osteotomy, during closed intramedullary nailing of the femur, or during delivery as a result of traction. Heterotopic ossification may cause entrapment and paresis of the sciatic nerve.

Pathologic Anatomy

Of the two components of the sciatic nerve, the common peroneal nerve is the most frequently injured, as its superficial and more lateral location at the level of the piriformis muscle makes it more susceptible to the iatrogenic insult of the needle. It is rare that the posterior tibial component of the sciatic nerve is solely involved; if this does occur, the prognosis for its recovery is good. Mechanical trauma of the needle, intraneural hemorrhage, and the toxic effects of the high local concentration of the chemical agents are all factors to consider in the pathogenesis of injection palsy. Pathologically, an acute inflammation of the intraneural and perineural tissues develops first, followed by destruction of the axons and disappearance of the myelin sheaths and eventual fibrosis of the nerve.

On exploration, one may find a 2 to 3 cm. long segment of the nerve trunk shrunk to a fibrous band. Characteristic features of injection palsy are the marked local hypervascularity and adhesion of the nerve to neighboring areolar and muscular tissues.

Clinical Picture

Loss of motor function and sensory function in the sciatic nerve distribution is present immediately following injection. This is usually accompanied by intense local and referred pain that can be controlled only by strong analgesics. After several days, the hypersensitivity radiating along the course of the involved nerves gradually subsides. On deep palpation of the gluteal region there may be local tenderness. If the paresis involves the common peroneal nerve, the patient will be unable to dorsiflex and evert the foot actively, and the lateral aspect of the leg and foot will be anesthetic; if the entire sciatic nerve is paralyzed, however, the foot and ankle will be flail, with anesthesia of the sole of the foot, the lateral aspect of the leg, and the dorsum of the foot. The ankle jerk will be absent. The neurologic deficit is maximal immediately following the injury. The paresis may either diminish or remain static, but it will not increase. Destruction of nerve tissue is not progressive.

Imaging Findings

Routine radiography will disclose possible causes such as fracture of the lesser trochanter, posterior hip dislocation, or myositis ossificans. Computed axial tomography and nuclear magnetic resonance imaging will show the inflamed sciatic nerve.

Treatment

A thorough assessment of neurologic deficit is made initially and repeated at monthly intervals. Prognosis for satisfactory recovery is good if paralysis is incomplete at the beginning and if some improvement of motor function is shown on the monthly examinations. Prognosis is poor, however, if there is total paralysis at the onset and periodic examination does not disclose any return of neurologic function.

If, within three months following injury, there is no improvement, the sciatic nerve should be surgically explored. During this period of observation, it is important to perform passive and active stretching exercises, to maintain the ankle and foot in neutral position in a bivalved cast at night, and to support the ankle in a below-knee orthosis during the day. Every effort should be made to prevent the development of contractural deformity. If there is progressive improvement of function, observation for 12 months is recommended, at the end of which time the residual motor and sensory picture is assessed. If adequate function is not restored, exploration of the sciatic nerve is again indicated.

The patient is placed in prone position, and the entire lower limb and gluteal region are prepared and draped sterile in order to permit evaluation of function by electrical stimulation during surgery. Beginning over the posterior superior iliac spine, the incision extends toward the greater trochanter and then distally over the posterior aspect of the thigh to terminate 5 cm. above the popliteal crease. The subcutaneous tissue and deep fascia are divided in line with the skin incision. The gluteus maximus and gluteus medius muscles are detached from their insertions and reflected medially to expose the sciatic nerve. This surgical approach permits exposure of the entire sciatic nerve from the sciatic notch to the popliteal space. The status of the nerve is determined by gross inspection and by direct electrical stimulation. If the pathologic change is simple perineural scarring, a meticulous neurolysis is carried out. In the presence of total destruction of the nerve, however, the damaged segment is resected and end-to-end anastomosis is performed utilizing microsurgical technique. Relative length of the sciatic nerve is obtained by mobilizing it subcutaneously and by placing the hip in hyperextension and the knee in flexion. Following closure of the wound, the patient is placed in a bivalved hip spica cast, which is made preoperatively with the hip in hyperextension, the knee in 90 degrees of flexion, and the ankle in neutral position. Immobilization in the cast is continued for a period of six to eight weeks, at which time gentle range-of-motion exercises of the hip and knee are instituted. Care of the muscles in the recovery period follows the principles outlined for poliomyelitis.

Measures to prevent sciatic nerve injury in infants and children include the following: (1) Give intramuscular injections in the anterior and lateral portions of the midthigh (quadriceps femoris muscle). (2) If multiple intramuscular injections are to be administered, rotate them from the right to the left side. (3) Inject into the upper and outer quadrant of the buttocks if the gluteal muscle is to be used. (4) Expose the site of injection adequately, and have an assistant securely immobilize the child in prone position. (5) Always have both hands free, "picking up" the muscle with one hand and introducing the needle with the other. (6) Do not use a long intramuscular needle, and always control the depth of needle penetration. (7)

Make it a routine habit to double-check the point of the needle both before and following injection. (8) If repeated parenteral medications are to be given to a sick child, use the intravenous route through an indwelling catheter.

References

1. Bates, C., and Page, A. P. M.: A new neonatal syndrome. Br. Med. J., 2:756, 1949.
2. Bay, E.: Injection injury to the sciatic nerve. Dtsch. Med. Wochenschr., 86:505, 1961.
3. Benson, M. K., and Jameson Evans, D. C.: The pelvic osteotomy of Chiari: an anatomical study of the hazards and misleading radiographic appearances. J. Bone Joint Surg., 58-B:164, 1976.
4. Bigos, S. J., and Coleman, S. S.: Foot deformities secondary to gluteal injection in infancy. J. Pediatr. Orthop., 4:560, 1984.
5. Brown, B. A.: Sciatic injection neuropathy. Calif. Med., 116:13, 1972.
6. Clark, K., Williams, P. E., Willis, W., and McGavran, J.: Injection injury of the sciatic nerve. Clin. Neurosurg., 17:111, 1970.
7. Coumbes, M. A., Clark, W. K., Gregory, C. F., and James, J. A.: Sciatic nerve injuries in infants. Recognition and prevention of impairment resulting from intragluteal injections. J.A.M.A., 173:1336, 1960.
8. Curtiss, P. H., Jr., and Tucker, H. J.: Sciatic palsy in premature infants—a report and follow-up study of 10 cases. J.A.M.A., 174:586, 1960.
9. DiMargo, A.: On paralysis of the sciatic nerve caused by intragluteal injection of drugs. Clin. Pediatr., 43:230, 1961.
10. Dingeman, R. D., and Mutz, S. B.: Hemorrhagic neuropathy of the sciatic, femoral and obturator nerves: case report and review of the literature. Clin. Orthop., 127:133, 1977.
11. Fahrenfest, H.: Birth Injuries of the Child. 2nd Ed. New York, D. Appleton & Co., 1931.
12. Fahrni, W. H.: Neonatal sciatic palsy. J. Bone Joint Surg., 32-B:42, 1950.
13. Fleming, R. E., Michelsen, C. B., and Stinchfield, F. E.: Sciatic paralysis. A complication of bleeding following hip surgery. J. Bone Joint Surg., 61-A:37, 1979.
14. Frykman, G. K.: Peripheral nerve injuries in children. Orthop. Clin. North Am., 7:701, 1976.
15. Giles, F. H., and French, J. H.: Post injection sciatic nerve palsies in infants and children. J. Pediatr., 58:195, 1961.
16. Harper, M. C.: Closed intramedullary nailing of femoral shaft fractures (Letter). J. Bone Joint Surg., 64-A:474, 1982.
17. Hirasawa, Y., Oda, R., and Nakatani, K.: Sciatic nerve paralysis in posterior dislocation of the hip. A case report. Clin. Orthop., 126:172, 1977.
18. Hudson, F. P., McCandless, A., and O'Malley, A. G.: Sciatic paralysis in newborn infants. Br. Med. J., 1:223, 1950.
19. Johnson, E. W., Jr.: Sciatic nerve palsy following delivery. Postgrad. Med., 30:495, 1961.
20. Johnson, E. W., and Raptou, A. D.: A study of intragluteal injections. Arch. Phys. Med. Rehabil., 46:167, 1965.
21. Jones, B. V., and Ward, M. W.: Myositis ossificans in the biceps femoris muscles causing sciatic nerve palsy. A case report. J. Bone Joint Surg., 62-B:506, 1980.
22. Kleiman, S. G., Stevens, J., Kolb, L., and Pankovich, A.: Late sciatic-nerve palsy following posterior fracture-dislocation of the hip. A case report. J. Bone Joint Surg., 53-A:781, 1971.
23. Lachman, E.: Applied anatomy of intragluteal injections. Am. Surg., 29:236, 1963.

24. Lanzieri, C. F., and Hilal, S. K.: Computed tomography of the sacral plexus and sciatic nerve in the greater sciatic foramen. A.J.R., *143*:165, 1984.
25. Meyer, M.: Paralysie obstetricale des membres inferieurs. Rev. Orthop. (Paris), *18*:767, 1931.
26. Miller, A., Stedman, G. H., Beisaw, N. E., and Gross, P. T.: Sciatica caused by an avulsion fracture of the ischial tuberosity. A case report. J. Bone Joint Surg., *69-A*:143, 1987.
27. Mills, W. G.: A new neonatal syndrome. Br. Med. J., *2*:464, 1949.
28. Owen, C. A., Woody, P. R., Mubarak, S. J., and Hargens, A. R.: Gluteal compartment syndrome: a report of three cases and management utilizing the Wick catheter. Clin. Orthop., *132*:57, 1978.
29. Purohit, D. M., Levkoff, A. H., and deVito, P. C.: Gluteal necrosis with foot-drop. Complications associated with umbilical artery catheterization. Am. J. Dis. Child., *132*:897, 1978.
30. Richlin, D. M., Carron, H., and Rowlingson, J. C.: Reflex sympathetic dystrophy: successful treatment by transcutaneous nerve stimulation. J. Pediatr., *93*:84, 1978.
31. San Augustin, M., Nitowsky, H. M., and Borden, J. N.: Neonatal sciatic palsy after umbilical vessel injection. J. Pediatr., *60*:408, 1962.
32. Scheinberg, L., and Allensworth, M.: Sciatic neuropathy in infants related to antibiotic injections. Pediatrics, *19*:261, 1957.
33. Schindera, F.: Skin necrosis and sciatic nerve paralysis following injections of tris buffer into the umbilical artery of a newborn infant. Monatschr. Kinderheilkd., *118*:137, 1970.
34. Shaw, N. E.: Neonatal sciatic palsy from injection into the umbilical cord. J. Bone Joint Surg., *42-B*:736, 1960.
35. Sogaard, I.: Sciatic nerve entrapment. Case report. J. Neurosurg., *58*:275, 1983.
36. Solheim, L. F., Siewers, P., and Paus, B.: The piriformis muscle syndrome. Sciatic nerve entrapment treated with section of the piriformis muscle. Acta Orthop. Scand., *52*:73, 1981.
37. Sriram, K., and Sakthivel, A.: Sciatic nerve palsy in the newborn. Ann. Acad. Med. Singapore, *10*:472, 1981.
38. Thakker, D. H., and Porter, R. W.: Heterotopic ossification enveloping the sciatic nerve following posterior fracture-dislocation of the hip: a case report. Injury, *13*:207, 1981.
39. Triano, J. J., and Luttges, M. W.: Nerve irritation: a possible model of sciatic neuritis. Spine, *7*:129, 1982.
40. Turner, G. G.: The site of intramuscular injections. Lancet, *2*:819, 1920.
41. Tuvo, F., and Bouquet, F.: Clinical and instrumental contribution to the knowledge of painful iatrogenic paralyzing sciatica (PIPS) in the adult and pediatric age. Minerva Med., *62*:784, 1971.
42. von Hochstetter, A.: Problems and technique of intragluteal injections, part 2. Influence of injection technique on the development of the syringe injuries. Schweiz. Med. Wochenschr., *86*:69, 1956.
43. Weisseman, G. J.: Tendon transfers for peripheral nerve injuries of the lower extremity. Orthop. Clin. North Am., *12*:459, 1981.

MISCELLANEOUS AFFECTIONS OF PERIPHERAL NERVES[1-14]

Neuropathy Associated with Diabetes Mellitus

In severely diabetic children, neuropathy may develop as early as ten years of age. It may be manifest in several forms.[4, 10, 12] In *Type I*, the lower limbs are primarily involved, with loss of deep tendon reflexes and a variable degree of anesthesia. Motor weakness and disability are minimal. In *Type II*, the autonomic system is predominantly affected. The presenting symptoms are incontinence of urine, diarrhea, orthostatic hypotension, and anhidrosis. *Type III* is characterized by sudden onset of asymmetrical cranial nerve palsy (commonly of the third and seventh) and complete or partial paralysis of one or several of the lumbar nerve roots. Nerve conduction studies will disclose a diminution of the conduction rate in both motor and sensory fibers or absence of evoked potentials. There is no specific therapy. Vitamin B_{12} injections are often given. Adequate control of diabetes mellitus is imperative.

Acute Intermittent Porphyria[7]

This disorder of porphyrin metabolism usually has its onset in adult life, but it may occur in children. The symptoms are acute. Colicky abdominal pain, constipation, mental confusion varying from neurosis to psychosis, and polyneuropathy characterize the condition. Sensory loss and paresthesia are uncommon. Involvement is predominantly motor, with paralysis of the proximal muscle groups and cranial nerves. The clinical picture may simulate polyradiculoneuritis. The urine contains excessive amounts of uroporphyrins and coproporphyrins, Types I and III. The freshly voided urine is normal in color but turns reddish brown on standing. The proteins may be increased in cerebrospinal fluid. Death may occur from respiratory paralysis.

Toxic Neuropathy

Toxic neuropathy may result from the administration of various drugs such as isoniazid and nitrofurantoin, or from accidental poisoning with toxins such as arsenic, insecticides, lead, and mercury. Neuropathy may also follow prophylactic inoculations.[1-3, 6, 8, 11] In the differential diagnosis, the preceding conditions should be considered.

References

1. Campbell, A. M. C.: Neurological complications associated with insecticide and fungicides. Br. Med. J., *2*:415, 1952.
2. Cassady, J. R., Tonnesen, G. L., Wolfe, L. C., and Sallan, S. E.: Augmentation of vincristine neurotoxicity by irradiation of peripheral nerves. Cancer Treat. Rep., *64*:963, 1980.

3. Collings, H.: Polyneuropathy associated with nitrofuran therapy. Arch. Neurol., 3:656, 1960.
4. Dreyfus, P. M., Hakim, S., and Adams, R. D.: Diabetic ophthalmoplegia. Arch. Neurol. Psychiatr., 77:337, 1957.
5. Fischer, C. M., and Adams, R. D.: Diphtheritic polyneuritis, a pathological study. J. Neuropathol. Exp. Neurol., 15:243, 1956.
6. Gallassi, R., Monagna, P., Pazzaglia, P., Cirignotta, F., and Lugaresi, E.: Peripheral neuropathy due to gasoline sniffing—A case report. Eur. Neurol., 19:419, 1980.
7. Goldberg, A.: Acute intermittent porphyria. Q. J. Med., 28:183, 1959.
8. Heyman, A., Pfeiffer, J. B., Willet, R. W., and Taylor, H. M.: Peripheral neuropathy caused by arsenical intoxication. N. Engl. J. Med., 254:401, 1956.
9. Jacobs, R. L., and Karmody, A. M.: Office care of the insensitive foot. Foot Ankle, 2:230, 1982.
10. Lawrence, D. G., and Locke, S.: Neuropathy in children with diabetes mellitus. Br. Med. J., 1:784, 1963.
11. Miller, H. G., and Stanton, J. B.: Neurological sequelae of prophylactic inoculation. Q. J. Med., 23:1, 1954.
12. Rundles, R. W.: Diabetic neuropathy. Medicine, 24:111, 1945.
13. Wells, J., and Templeton, J.: Femoral neuropathy associated with anticoagulant therapy. Clin. Orthop., 124:155, 1977.
14. Wilgis, E. F.: Techniques for diagnosis of peripheral nerve loss. Clin. Orthop., 163:8, 1982.

ARTHROGRYPOSIS MULTIPLEX CONGENITA (MULTIPLE CONGENITAL CONTRACTURE)

Arthrogryposis multiplex congenita (AMC) is a syndrome complex characterized by contracture (limitation of motion) of several joints in different parts of the body due to varying degrees of fibrosis of the affected muscles and thickening and shortening of periarticular capsular and ligamentous tissues of the affected joints; the basic pathologic process is nonprogressive.

The term arthrogryposis (derived from two Greek words—curved or hooked joint) is a descriptive sign and not a diagnosis.[71] In the literature, a variety of conditions with contractural deformity of joints have been referred to as arthrogryposis. It is vital to recognize the heterogeneity of the condition and distinguish the various forms of congenital multiple contractures of joints; each entity has different genetic background and natural history, requiring special modalities of treatment.

Historical Perspective

Otto, in 1841, was first to describe a full-term infant with multiple congenital contractures; he believed the pathologic process was due to congenital myodystrophy.[157] In 1897,

Schanz referred to the condition as multiple congenital contracture.[184] The descriptive term multiple congenital articular rigidity was used by Nové-Josserand and Rendu in 1906, and Rocher in 1913.[154, 176] The term arthrogryposis was first used by Rosencranz; Stern later used the term arthrogryposis multiplex congenita.[177, 203] These authors believed that the joint deformity was the cause of the contracture. However, it became evident that the fibrosis and fibrofatty change in muscles were the primary cause of deformity—the joints contracted because of lack of motion and normal development. Therefore, Sheldon, in 1932, proposed the term *amyoplasia congenita*, with the suggestion that the primary lesion is hypoplasia or aplasia of certain muscle groups.[194] However, the term amyoplasia is not correct because multiple congenital contractures do not result from primary aplasia of muscles; initially the muscles are formed normally, but later they are replaced by fibrofatty or fibrous tissue.[71, 72] Middleton preferred the term myodystrophia foetalis deformans to denote the condition.[147, 148]

In the orthopedic literature, arthrogryposis multiplex congenita is commonly used to describe the condition. Swinyard and Bleck prefer the use of the term multiple congenital contractures, which was first used by Schanz.[184, 204]

Prevalence. The classic arthrogryposis (amyodysplasia congenita) is quite rare; it is estimated to be present in 0.03 per cent of neonates.[205]

Etiology

The basic pathomechanism of multiple congenital joint contracture appears to be lack of fetal movement—*fetal akinesia*. A heterogeneous group of factors may cause decrease or cessation of movements of a fetus in the uterus. Drachman and Coulombre temporarily immobilized the chick embryo by infusion of the chorioallantoic vessels with d-tubocurarine at a constant rate for two days; this resulted in ankylosis of the various joints, clawing of the toes, and immobility of the necks and wings.[45] Fuller immobilized fetal joints and caused progressive prenatal deformity.[60] Jago has described arthrogryposis in an infant of a mother who was treated for clinical tetanus with muscle relaxants for the first 10 to 12 weeks of pregnancy.[102]

Moessinger paralyzed rat fetuses by daily intrauterine injection of curare from the eighteenth day of gestation until term (twenty-first day). The following deformities were noted at birth—multiple joint contractures, pulmonary hypoplasia, micrognathia, fetal growth retardation, short umbilical cord, and polyhydramnios. He termed these sets of anomalies the "fetal akinesia sequence." Lack of movement in utero leads to a set of anomalies of various organ systems, of which contracture of joints is only one feature.[151] Clinically, in the human these sets of deformities already have been described, such as in the Pena-Shokeir syndrome.[162, 163]

Experimentally in chick embryos, prenatal contraction of joints can be caused by the Newcastle disease virus and by Coxsackie virus.[175] Akabane virus has been implicated as a cause of multiple congenital joint contracture in cattle.[204]

Classification

Hall critically analyzed 350 cases of congenital multiple nonprogressive joint contractures and subdivided them into three broad categories.[71–73] The first group had involvement primarily of the limbs with no other abnormalities (about 50 per cent of the cases); the second group had involvement of the limbs with congenital joint contracture, but in addition had anomalies in some other areas such as the viscera or craniofacies; the third group had congenital contractures of the limbs and severe central nervous system dysfunction (Table 5–19).

CONGENITAL JOINT CONTRACTURES PRIMARILY INVOLVING THE LIMBS

This first category can be subdivided into two specific entities: (1) amyoplasia, and (2) distal arthrogryposis.

Amyoplasia is the classic arthrogryposis multiplex congenita well recognized by the orthopedic surgeon. It is probably not a hereditary condition; there is no recurrence risk in the family. There are no affected children born to affected parents. The clinical appearance and position of the limbs are typically symmetrical; the condition is present at birth (Figs. 5–200 and 5–201). Flexion or extension contractures or any combination of contractural deformity may occur in the limbs. All four limbs are affected in 46 per cent of the patients, only the lower limbs in 43 per cent, and only the upper limbs in 11 per cent. The frequency of joint involvement increases from proximal to distal. No synovial joint is exempt from contracture. Any group, or all, of the craniospinal motor units may be affected.[204]

Hall has designated the condition as amyodysplasia because of the apparent absence or hypoplasia of the muscles; however, embryologically the muscles are actually formed normally but during the fetal period are replaced by fibrous and fatty tissue.[71–73] Diminished muscle substance gives the appearance of wasting. There is decreased active and passive motion of the joints, which are fixed in either extension or flexion. The rigidity of joints is unique, in that there are always a few degrees of free passive and painless motion between the extremes of motion. The normal skin creases are usually absent, and the skin is tense and glossy. Dimpling may be present at the joints, usually at the elbows, patellae, and wrists. In the infant, port-wine facial stains, frequently on the forehead between the eyebrows, are common; in the infant they fade in time. When the joints are fixed in flexion, there may be definite webbing of the skin and subcutaneous tissues. On deep palpation of the limbs, subcutaneous tissues and muscle are found to be diminished in substance. The atrophy of the limbs, combined with the cylindrical shape of the knees and elbows, gives the patient a "wooden doll" appearance. There is no sensory deficit, but the deep tendon reflexes may be diminished or absent.

In the lower limbs the feet are often in equinovarus, and the knees in flexion or extension contracture (Fig. 5–202). When the hips are not dislocated, they are usually in the posture of flexion–lateral rotation and abduction, or the hips may be in flexion-adduction contracture with unilateral or bilateral dislocation. Femoropelvic obliquity may result because of the hip contractural deformity. A long C thoracolumbar scoliosis develops in childhood or adolescence in about one fifth of the patients.

In the upper limbs, the shoulders are medially rotated, the elbows in extension or flexion contracture, the radial heads possibly dislocated, the forearms pronated, the wrists often in flexion contracture and occasionally in extension contracture, the thumbs clenched in the palm, and the fingers in flexion at the proximal interphalangeal joints. The intelligence is usually normal. The prognosis is good. With proper management, most patients live independently and hold useful jobs. It is surprising how they develop dexterity and adapt to their multiple deformities (Fig. 5–203).

Distal Arthrogryposis

This is the second entity in the large category of patients with multiple congenital joint contracture primarily involving the limbs. In this

Text continued on page 2097

Table 5–19. Areas of Involvement

Primarily Limbs	Limbs Plus Other Body Areas	Limbs Plus CNS
Absence of dermal ridges	Camptomelic dysplasia	Adducted thumbs
Absence of DIP creases	Conradi-Hünermann (chondrodysplasia punctata)	Cerebro-oculo-facio-skeletal (COFS)
Amniotic bands (Streeter)		Cloudy corneae, diaphragmatic defects, distal limb deformities
Amyoplasia	Contractural arachnodactyly	
Antecubital webbing	Craniocarpotarsal dystrophy (whistling face, Freeman-Sheldon)	Craniofacial/brain anomalies/IUGR
Camptodactyly		Cryptorchidism, chest deformity, contractures
Clasped thumbs, congenital	Diastrophic dysplasia	
Coalition	Focal femoral dysplasia	Faciocardiomelic
Contractures, continuous muscle discharge and titubation	Hand muscle wasting and sensorineural deafness	Fetal alcohol syndrome
		FG syndrome
Distal arthrogryposis	Holt-Oram	Marden-Walker
Humeroradial synostosis (HRS)	Kniest syndrome	Meningomyelocele
Impaired pronation, supination of forearm (familial)	Kuskokwim syndrome	Mietens
	Larsen dysplasia	Miller-Dieker (lissencephaly)
Liebenberg syndrome	Leprechaunism	Multiple pterygium, lethal
Nievergelt-Pearlman	Megalocornea with multiple skeletal anomalies	Myotonic dystrophy-severe congenital (SCMD)
Poland anomaly		
Radioulnar synostosis	Metaphyseal dysostosis (Jansen)	Neu laxova
Symphalangism/brachydactyly	Metatropic dysplasia	Neuromuscular disease of larynx
Tel Hashomer camptodactyly	Moebius	Nezelof syndrome
Trismus pseudocamptodactyly	Multiple pterygium syndrome	Pena-Shokeir (ankylosis, facial anomalies and pulmonary hypoplasia)
	Nail patella (hereditary onycho-osteodysplasia)	Popliteal pterygium with facial clefts
	Nemaline myopathy	Potter syndrome
	Neurofibromatosis	Pseudotrisomy 18
	Oculodentodigital syndrome	Zellweger syndrome (cerebrohepatorenal)
	Ophthalmomandibulomelic dysplasia	
	Oral cranial digital syndrome	46,XXY/48,XXXY
	Osteogenesis imperfecta, congenital lethal "crumpled bone type" (type II)	49,XXXXX and 49,XXXXY
		4p trisomy
		trisomy 8/trisomy 8 mosaicism
	Otopalatodigital	trisomy 9
	Pfeiffer	trisomy 9q
	Popliteal pterygium	10q trisomy
	Prader-Willi habitus, osteoporosis, hand contractures	trisomy 10p
		11q trisomy
	Pseudothalidomide syndrome (Roberts syndrome)	trisomy 13
		partial trisomy 14 (proximal)
	Puertic syndrome	15 trisomy (proximal)
	Sacral agenesis	trisomy 18
	Schwartz-Jampel	
	SED congenita	
	Sturge-Weber	
	Tuberous sclerosis	
	VATER association	
	Weaver syndrome	
	Winchester syndrome	
	X-trapezoidocephaly, midfacial hypoplasia, cartilage abnormalities	

From Hall, J. G.: Genetic aspects of arthrogryposis. Clin. Orthop., *194*:44, 1985. Reprinted with permission.

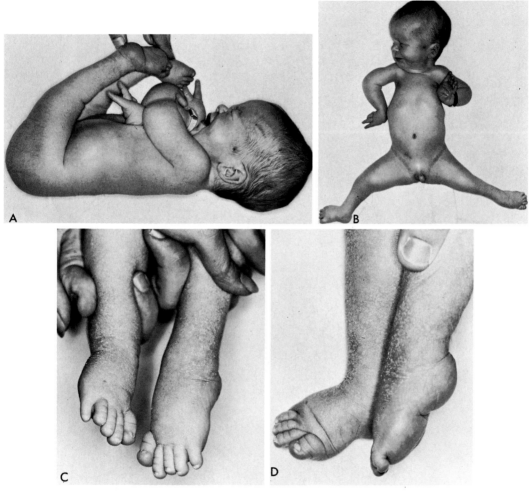

FIGURE 5-200. Arthrogryposis multiplex congenita.

A and **B.** Clinical appearance at birth, showing typical deformities. **C** and **D.** Close view of the feet, showing equinovalgus deformity.

Illustration continued on following page

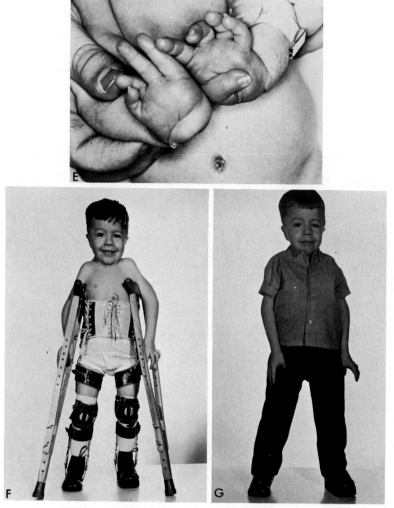

FIGURE 5–200 Continued. Arthrogryposis multiplex congenita.

E. Palmar view of the hands of the same patient. Note the adducted thumbs. **F** and **G.** The patient, three years later, is able to walk with the help of braces. He had bilateral heel cord lengthening and flexion release of both hips.

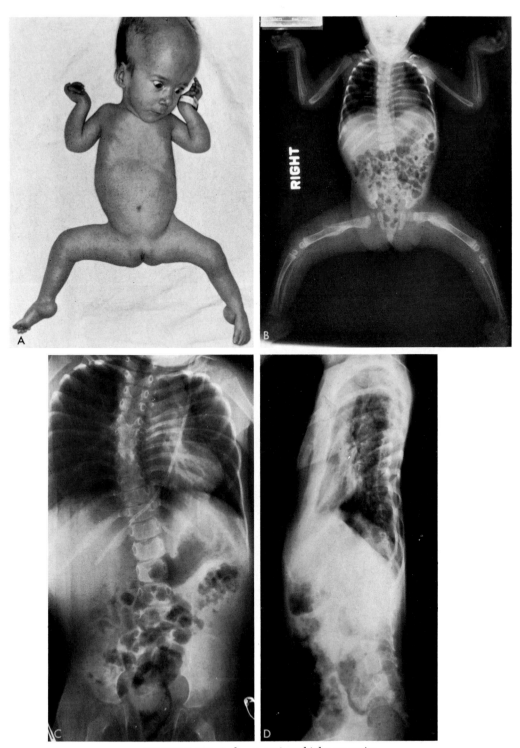

FIGURE 5–201. Arthrogryposis multiplex congenita.

A. The infant at three weeks of age. Note the severe hydrocephalus and the pectus excavatum. The deformities of the limbs are characteristic. **B.** Anteroposterior radiogram of entire body. The healed fractures of both femoral shafts and right humerus are evident. **C** and **D.** Radiograms of spine of same patient at age two years, showing the structural right dorsal scoliosis and the dorsal lordosis with decrease in the anteroposterior diameter of the chest.

Illustration continued on following page

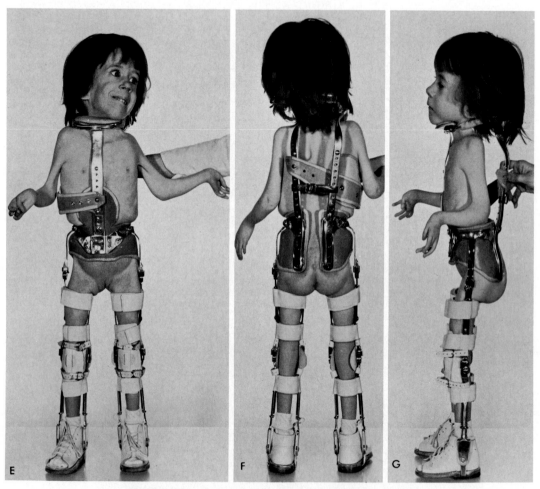

FIGURE 5–201 Continued. *Arthrogryposis multiplex congenita.*

E to G. A Milwaukee brace and bilateral long leg braces were fitted to the patient. She is able to walk with crutches. Despite the hydrocephalus, her intelligence is normal.

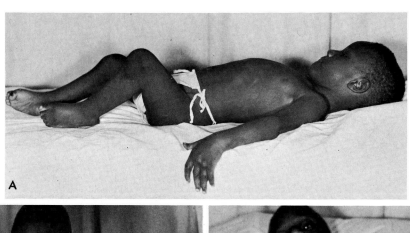

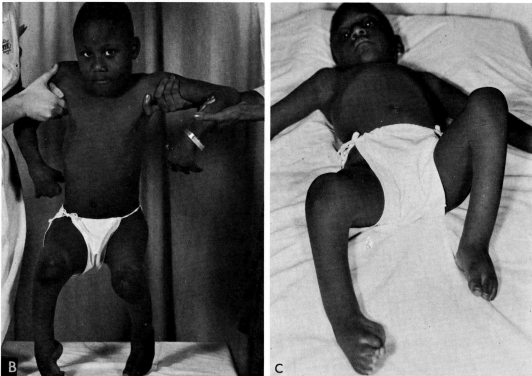

FIGURE 5–202. Arthrogryposis multiplex congenita with severe flexion contracture of the knees.

A to **C.** Lateral, standing, and anteroposterior recumbent views of patient. Because of the severity of the equinovarus deformity of the feet and flexion contracture of the knees, he is unable to bear weight on his lower limbs. Below the knee, the musculature is poor in motor strength. Bilateral knee disarticulation was performed.

Illustration continued on following page

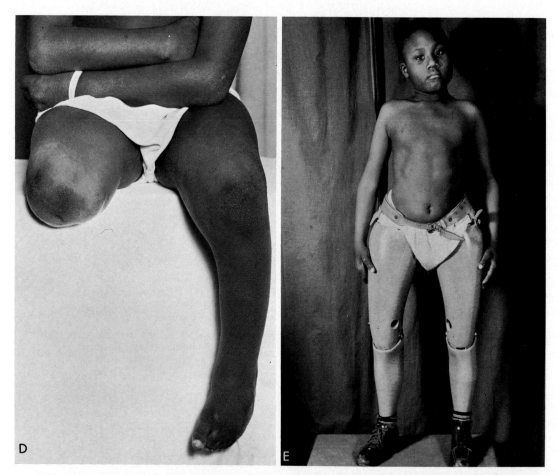

FIGURE 5–202 Continued. Arthrogryposis multiplex congenita with severe flexion contracture of the knees.

D. The patient following knee disarticulation on the right. **E.** The patient standing with bilateral prostheses. He is able to walk.

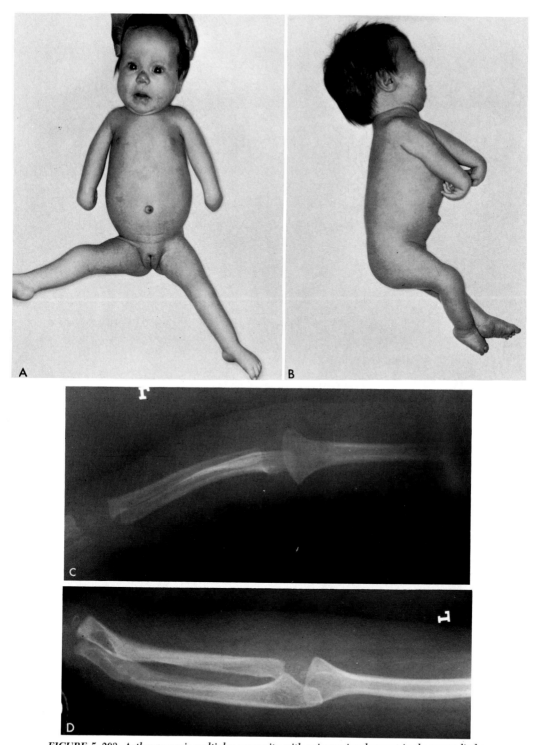

FIGURE 5–203. Arthrogryposis multiplex congenita with primary involvement in the upper limbs.

A and **B.** The patient at three months of age. Note the severe flexion deformity of the wrists and fingers, and extension contracture of the elbows. Treatment consisted of stretching casts, and at age two years a dorsiflexion close-up osteotomy of the distal radius and ulna was performed. **C** and **D.** Lateral radiograms of the wrists and forearms before and after osteotomy.

Illustration continued on following page

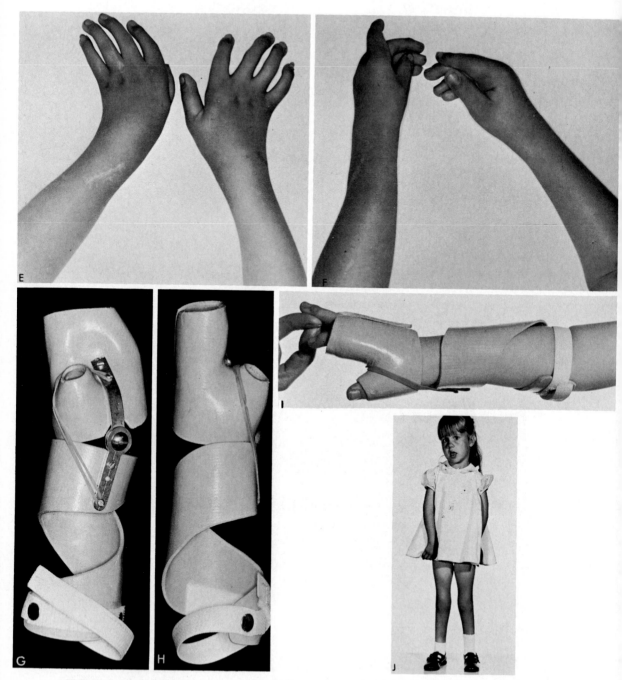

FIGURE 5–203 Continued. *Arthrogryposis multiplex congenita with primary involvement in the upper limbs.*

E and F. Postoperative photographs. G to I. The type of splint used to maintain correction in various views and on the patient. J. Clinical appearance of patient at four years of age.

condition it is the hands and feet that are involved, hence the term distal arthrogryposis. The clinical picture is very typical. In the hand the thumb is flexed and adducted across the palm; the fingers are clenched in the palm and tend to overlap each other. In the newborn the deformity of the hands resembles that of trisomy 18. The feet are in either equinovarus or calcaneovalgus with varying degrees of flexion contracture of the toes. Distal arthrogryposis is inherited as an autosomal dominant trait.[77]

MULTIPLE CONGENITAL JOINT CONTRACTURES WITH INVOLVEMENT IN OTHER BODY AREAS

This broad category involves a wide diversity of conditions in which joint contractures are associated with anomalies in other areas of the body. Most of these conditions are specific entities and syndromes—such as contractural arachnodactyly, cranio-carpo-tarsal dysplasia (Freeman-Sheldon syndrome), diastrophic dysplasia, and pterygium syndromes (see Table 5–19). These conditions are described in Chapters 2 and 3.

MULTIPLE CONGENITAL JOINT CONTRACTURES WITH CENTRAL NERVOUS SYSTEM DYSFUNCTION

This large group comprises entities with chromosomal abnormalities. These are detected by peripheral blood karyotypes and a second tissue (such as fibroblast) study. Most of the affected infants fail to thrive, and about 50 per cent die within the first few years of life.

Pathology

Histologic changes are nonspecific because arthrogryposis multiplex congenita is not a distinct pathologic entity but rather a symptom complex of multiple nonprogressive congenital joint contracture. It is associated with neurogenic and myopathic disorders in which motor weakness in varying stages of the development of the fetus immobilizes the joints, resulting in contracture. The pathologic findings of the neuropathic form are distinguished from those of the myopathic form by Adams et al.[3] The neurogenic form is much more common than the myopathic. In a pathologic study of 74 children with features of arthrogryposis, Banker found in 93 per cent that the deformities were of neurogenic origin, 7 per cent being myopathic.[8] The neuropathic form is often associated with other congenital anomalies such as dysgenesis of the anterior horn cells and with apparent involvement of the brain in some cases, whereas in the myopathic form there are few associated defects. Creatine kinase is often normal in both the neuropathic and the myopathic forms of the disease.

In determination of the pathologic type of arthrogryposis, chromosomal studies should be carried out and a muscle biopsy should be performed with complete muscle study (routine histology, electron microscopy, and histochemistry) to distinguish the dysgenesis of anterior horn cell form from primary myopathy.

In the neuropathic form, the most important finding is the disappearance, degeneration, or decrease in the size of the anterior horn cells of the central nervous system. The diameter of the spinal cord is usually decreased, particularly in the lumbar and cervical regions. The number of anterior nerve roots is less than normal, whereas that of the posterior nerve roots is usually average. There are no abnormal findings in the nerve cells, the posterior and the lateral horns, Clarke's columns, or the dorsal root ganglion cells. Cerebral lesions include underdevelopment, incomplete fissurations, large lateral ventricles, and reduction of the number of Betz cells in the motor cortex.[44, 53, 58, 106] The muscles in the limbs show varying changes, depending upon the severity of involvement. They may be normal in size, color, and texture; or they may be decreased in size or even not be found at all, having been replaced by fat and connective tissue. On microscopic examination, there is a diminution in the number of muscle fibers and a decrease in the transverse diameter of the individual fibers. Transverse and longitudinal striations are retained in most of the small fibers. There is variation in the size and diameter of the affected muscle fibers. Fat cells may be present in some and not in others. In the early stages the articular hyaline cartilage is normal, but later on in older children, destruction of the joint surfaces and secondary degenerative changes take place. Thickening and fibrosis of the capsule of the affected joints is common.

In the *myopathic form* of arthrogryposis, as contrasted to the neuropathic type, there are no changes in the brain and no primary changes in the anterior horn cells.[3, 57, 106] Motor roots and intramuscular nerves are normal. The affected muscles are of a firm, fibrous consistency and are pale in appearance. On microscopic examination, there is fibrous and fatty degeneration of the involved muscles. There is great variation of individual muscle fibers, with haphazard distribution of large and small fibers. The endomyseal connective tissue is increased.

The joint changes are similar to those of the neuropathic form.

In the neuropathic and myopathic forms, Banker demonstrated 17 specific disorders depending on the site of the pathologic lesion—whether in the anterior horn cells, nerve roots, peripheral nerves, end-plates, or muscle. In the *neurogenic form* Banker found the following subtypes:

1. Muscle fiber predominance or disproportion (26 per cent).
2. Dysgenesis of the motor nuclei of spinal cord and brain stem (7 per cent).
3. Dysgenesis of the central nervous system (23 per cent).
4. Dysgenesis of the central nervous system—trisomy 18 (10 per cent).
5. Dysgenesis of the central nervous system—the partial deletion of the long arm of chromosome 18 (1 per cent).
6. Dysgenesis of the brain stem (Pierre Robin syndrome) and the spinal cord (1 per cent).
7. Dysgenesis of the motor muscles of the brain stem (Möbius syndrome) and the spinal cord (1 per cent).
8. Dysgenesis of the spinal cord and the prune-belly syndrome (3 per cent).
9. Encephalocele, arhinencephaly (Meckel-Gruber syndrome), and dysgenesis of anterior horn cells (3 per cent).
10. Anencephaly and dysgenesis of the anterior horn cells (9 per cent).
11. Myelomeningocele and dysgenesis of the central nervous system (Chiari-Arnold syndrome) (7 per cent).
12. Agenesis of lumbosacral cord and vertebrae (1 per cent).
13. Dysgenesis of the central nervous system and the hepatorenal syndrome (Zellweger syndrome) (3 per cent).
14. Spinal muscular dystrophy (Werdnig-Hoffmann disease) (3 per cent).

In the myopathic form of arthrogryposis multiplex congenita, Banker reported three subtypes:

15. Central core disease.
16. Nemeline myopathy.
17. Congenital muscular dystrophy.

The reader is referred to Banker's original article for a description of the pathologic findings in these 17 subtypes of arthrogryposis multiplex congenita.[8]

Treatment

Management of arthrogryposis multiplex congenita is complex and difficult but rewarding.

Often these children are above average in intelligence. Despite the severity of their deformities, they are able to walk. It is surprising how they develop a functional degree of dexterity for performance of activities of daily living such as self-feeding, dressing, and toilet needs. The efficacy of performance is hampered by abnormal patterns of substitution and use of bimanual activities; however, most of these children in adult life become independent and gainfully employed. Initially, the parents of the affected patients should be reassured of the fair to good prognosis. The goals of treatment are ambulation, independent or assisted, and maximum functional use of the upper limbs. The degree of involvement varies. The care of each child should be individualized.

The following are the basic principles of management of arthrogryposis multiplex congenita. *First*, the obstruction to joint motion is almost entirely extra-articular by the contracted capsule, ligaments, and fibrosed muscles. Once these extra-articular obstacles are released the affected joints will move through a useful, if not normal, range of motion. The contracted soft tissues are so rigid that they do not yield to manipulative stretching and casts. In fact, such forceful measures may be harmful, as they cause compression necrosis of the delicate hyaline articular cartilage, intra-articular fibrous adhesions, and ankylosis. *Early surgical release of contracted soft tissues* is the *conservative* method of correction of deformity. The capsule, ligaments, and shortened muscles should all be sectioned to provide maximum arc of joint motion. *Second*, physiotherapy alone rarely achieves significant improvement; however, it is crucial to perform daily physical therapy for a prolonged period to maintain the correction obtained by surgical release. *Third*, it is crucial to splint the limb in the improved position at night. Orthoses may be used during the day for ambulation. *Fourth*, the deformities in arthrogryposis multiplex congenita have a propensity for recurrence. Therefore, whenever possible, muscle-tendon transfers should be performed to replace the absent or the pale, small fibrosed muscles that are functionally ineffective. It should be realized, however, that muscle-tendon transfers in arthrogryposis do not work as well as in poliomyelitis. Expectations should be realistic.

Osteotomy of the long bones to correct angular or rotational deformity does not stop recurrence of deformity unless contracted soft tissues are sectioned or excised and muscle imbalance is corrected by muscle-tendon transfer coupled with prolonged physiotherapy and splinting. In the arthrogrypotic child the contracted joint capsule and rigid periarticular soft tissues do not stretch as the limbs grow. Prior to surgery, it is best to explain to the parents that because of the recalcitrant nature of the disease the deformities will recur and require further surgical correction. These children require persistent vigilant care until completion of skeletal growth.

With these principles in mind the management of deformities will be discussed next. In the lower limbs the deformities of the hips, knees, and ankles-feet should be assessed together as one functional unit, because deformity at one level will affect function and posture at another level.

FOOT-ANKLE

Talipes equinovarus is the most common deformity, and congenital convex pes valgus is the second most common; other infrequent deformities of the foot-ankle in arthrogryposis multiplex congenita are calcaneovalgus, cavovarus, metatarsus adductus, and pure ankle equinus. Management of these foot deformities is described in Chapter 7. The arthrogrypotic deformities are difficult to treat because of the thickened and contracted capsule and ligaments and fibrosis and shortening of the muscles. Calcaneovalgus or simple metatarsus adductus may be corrected by serial manipulative stretching cast and retention in splints. Talipes equinovarus and congenital convex pes valgus require open surgical treatment at an early age by an experienced pediatric orthopedic surgeon. Initially (birth to three months of age) casts are applied to stretch the skin, but caution should be exercised in order not to produce secondary iatrogenic deformities. There is a high incidence of recurrence of deformity; therefore, tendons of nonfunctioning muscles are resected and not simply divided. Perform capsulectomy and not capsulotomy! Identification of individual joints is difficult; when in doubt, use radiographic control in the operating room. Injury to the physes should be avoided. It is vital to perform complete peritalar release. The importance of adequate lateral release cannot be overemphasized. The talus should be repositioned in the ankle mortise, and in the true lateral radiogram made intraoperatively the talocalcaneal angle should be restored to normal. Do not accept inadequate correction of equinus—either in the ankle or in the forefoot! Plantar release should always be performed. In rigid talipes equinovarus the lateral column of the foot is shortened by resection of anterior

end of calcaneus (Lichtblau procedure), or calcaneocuboid joint resection with fusion (Evan's operation), or cuboid decancellation (Verebelyi-Ogston procedure), or closing wedge osteotomy of the calcaneus. Following concentric reduction of medial-plantar displacement of the talocalcaneonavicular and calcaneocuboid joints in talipes equinovarus, maintain anatomic reduction by threaded pins across both the talonavicular and the calcaneocuboid joints. Correct rotation at the subtalar joint; if the talocalcaneal interosseous ligament has to be sectioned, transfix the subtalar joint with one or two threaded Steinmann pins. The objective of surgery in the arthrogrypotic talipes equinovarus is to provide an asymptomatic plantigrade foot for locomotion. Often there are varying degrees of stiffness of the talocalcaneonavicular and midtarsal joints and limitation of ankle motion. The nature of arthrogryposis is such that full mobility of tarsal and ankle joints cannot be provided. Triple arthrodesis in the skeletally mature deformed foot will give a satisfactory plantigrade foot.

Talectomy is a salvage procedure. It should not be employed as a primary measure in the treatment of the rigid arthrogrypotic clubfoot. Excise the entire talus! If cartilaginous parts of the talus are left behind, the deformity will recur. Displace the calcaneus posteriorly; this may require excision of the navicular and partial resection of the cuboid. Fix internally the calcaneus to the tibia by one or two Steinmann pins, which are removed four weeks postoperatively; cast immobilization should be carried out for a minimum of two, and preferably three, months, however.

In the treatment of *congenital convex pes valgus*, often the medial column of the foot has to be shortened by excision of the navicular. Avoid avascular necrosis of the talus.

Cavovarus deformity of the foot requires extensive plantar-medial release for correction. Often, bony procedures such as dorsal wedge osteotomy of the midtarsus and/or the first metatarsal are performed in the adolescent. The severe rigid cavovarus feet are corrected by triple arthrodesis. The operative techniques of the foregoing surgical procedures are described in detail in Chapter 7.

KNEE

A variety of deformities may be present at the knee, occurring in isolation or in conjunction. *Flexion deformity* may be mild, moderate, or severe. A fixed knee flexion deformity of less than 20 degrees is classified as mild; this does not interfere with functional ambulation.[89] Ordinarily this can be adequately treated by stretching cast, night splinting, and physical therapy in the form of passive stretching of knee flexors and active exercises to strengthen quadriceps femoris. *Moderate knee flexion deformity* (20 to 60 degrees) may be slightly improved by cast and manipulative stretching; however, often these measures are ineffective and may result in posterior dislocation of the knee. Early surgical release of the rigid contracted soft tissues is the treatment of choice. The hamstrings (both medial and lateral) are lengthened (if functional) or sectioned (if fibrosed and nonfunctional), and posterior capsulotomy of the knee joint is performed. Simple hamstring release without posterior capsulotomy has a very high recurrence rate. The minimum posterior soft-tissue release should be posterior capsulotomy of the knee with hamstring tenotomy. In some cases, when surgical release of posterior structures fails to fully correct flexion deformity, the anterior aspect of the knee joint should be explored. There may be a mass of undifferentiated fibrofatty tissue filling the joint and blocking full extension.

Contracture of collateral and cruciate ligaments may prevent complete extension of the knee; should they be sectioned? The problem is the resultant anteroposterior and mediolateral instability of the knee, which will require orthotic support for ambulation. This author recommends elongation rather than complete division of the ligaments in the young child, and extension osteotomy of the distal femur (at the metaphyseal-diaphyseal juncture) with anteriorly based closing wedge in the adolescent near skeletal maturity. Bony deformity with square or posteriorly tilted femoral condyles may be present in long-standing knee flexion deformity; in such cases the knee cannot be fully extended with soft-tissue release, no matter how extensive anteriorly or posteriorly.

In untreated, long-standing *severe flexion deformity* (over 60 degrees), neurovascular structures behind the knee will develop contracture; after soft-tissue release the tautest structures will be sciatic nerve and popliteal vessels. This problem can be solved only by shortening of the femur by excision of a trapezoid segment (based anteriorly) from the distal metaphyseal-diaphyseal region in order to relatively lengthen contracted soft tissues. Anterior epiphysiodesis of the distal femoral and proximal tibial physis is another method of correction of knee flexion deformity. However, results in moderate or severe deformity have not been satisfactory,

and its use is not recommended. In very severe flexion deformity in the older child, knee disarticulation may be performed; with appropriate prosthetic fitting, the patient will be able to walk (Fig. 5–203).

Extension deformity (genu recurvatum and anterior dislocation of the knee) is often bilateral. Management of these deformities is discussed in detail in the section on congenital deformities. They should be treated as early as possible, as soft-tissue contractural deformities are least rigid immediately after birth. Mild recurvatum and extension deformity may respond to gentle manipulative stretching and serial splinting; however, if they fail to correct within a few weeks, quadricepsplasty should be performed, preferably before the age of six months. Moderate genu recurvatum and anterior dislocation of the knee almost always requires quadricepsplasty and open reduction of the dislocated knee. Recurrence is minimized by splinting the knee in flexion at night over prolonged periods.

Pure *genu valgum* in arthrogryposis multiplex congenita is rare; it is almost always associated with flexion or hyperextension deformity of the knee and/or dislocation of the patellofemoral joint. Treatment consists of correction of associated deformities, realignment of quadriceps mechanism, and reduction of the patellofemoral joint.

Instability of the knee in the anteroposterior or mediolateral plane may occur, especially after reduction of anterior dislocation of the knee. Medial instability of the knee will require external orthotic support; in the experience of this author, ligamentous reconstruction has not been satisfactory.

HIP

Deformities of the hip may be subdivided into two broad categories: (1) those without dislocation, and (2) those with dislocation.

Dislocation of the hip may be unilateral or bilateral; also, the dislocated hip may be mobile or stiff. Management of hip dislocation is presented in Chapter 2. Only general principles of treatment of the arthrogrypotic hip will be discussed. First, if both hips are dislocated and stiff, they should not be treated because open reduction will result in two nondislocated or nonconcentrically reduced subluxated *stiff* hips, which functionally are no better than the original stiff dislocated hips. Asymmetrical contractural deformities of the hip may develop postoperatively; this will cause troublesome fixed pelvic obliquity and scoliosis. If *one hip* is dislocated and stiff, this author recommends mobilization of the stiff hip by soft-tissue release followed by open reduction with femoral shortening. This method of management affords a reasonable chance of provision of a reduced hip with functional mobility. In other words, this author recommends one attempt of reduction of the unilateral dislocated stiff arthrogrypotic hip; it is combined with femoral shortening and preceded by extensive soft-tissue release (both hips and knees). Always mobilize the extension contracture of the knee prior to open reduction of the hip. Timing of open reduction is important; it is best to wait until the infant is four to six months of age.

If one or both hips are dislocated but mobile, they should be treated. Again, be sure that the knees are mobile. In unilateral dislocation it is relatively simple to achieve a good result; in bilateral dislocation, one hip is usually more difficult to reduce than the other. The problem is asymmetry and pelvic obliquity. Treat the difficult hip first. In the postoperative period, congruity of the hip may be enhanced by the use of a Scottish-Rite hip abduction orthosis during the day and night. In some patients, because of noncompliance or because of socioeconomic conditions, a broomstick plastic or plaster cast may be used six weeks after surgery; it is followed by the part-time use of abduction hip orthosis for an additional three to six months. Frequently, secondary procedures will be required to improve results.

Deformities of the Hips Without Dislocation. These contractural deformities are (1) abduction, lateral rotation-flexion; (2) simple abduction; (3) flexion; and (4) extension. *Flexion abduction–lateral rotation contractures* of the hips are the most common deformity; if involvement is unilateral, the resultant infrapelvic obliquity causes scoliosis and subluxation of the contralateral hip. In bilateral cases the gait is awkward, orthotic fitting difficult, and lumbar lordosis excessive. Treatment consists of surgical release of the contracted iliotibial band and lengthening or sectioning of the tensor fasciae femoris and iliopsoas. *Simple abduction contracture* is infrequent; it is treated by surgical release of the fibrosed gluteus mediusminimus and gluteal fascia. *Pure flexion deformity* of the hip is usually minimal or moderate and can be easily controlled by splinting at night and prone posture during sleep. Severe flexion deformity will require surgical release of the hip flexors. Extension osteotomy of the proximal femur in the subtrochanteric region is rarely indicated; it should be performed toward the end of skeletal growth in order to prevent recurrence of deformity. *Extension contracture of the hip* is very rare but it does occur, preventing sitting in the severely involved child. Treatment consists of surgical release of gluteus maximus and posterior fascial and ligamentous structures.

ELBOW

The elbow joint may be fixed in extension or stiff in varying degrees of flexion. The *elbow with flexion deformity* usually has a functionally useful arc of motion. The biceps brachii and brachialis muscles are functioning with antigravity motor strength, whereas the triceps brachii is weak. The anterior aspect of the joint capsule and ligaments is thickened and contracted. In the young patient there are no changes in the bony configuration of the articulation of the elbow joint.

Treatment. Treatment is conservative, consisting of intensive physical therapy—repeated passive stretching of the elbow into extension. In the rigid deformity, stretching cast may be employed. An extension elbow orthosis is utilized at night to maintain the correction. Surgical measures usually are not employed; occasionally, however, musculotendinous lengthening of the biceps brachii brachialis with anterior capsulotomy of the elbow joint is indicated. Maintenance of correction is the problem; in the presence of muscle imbalance there is a high rate of recurrence of flexion deformity of the elbow.

Extension Contracture of the Elbow Joint. This deformity is usually associated with pronation contracture of the forearm, flexion deformity of the wrist, and a varying degree of involvement of the thumb and fingers (Fig. 5–204). The triceps brachii is strong in its motor power, whereas biceps brachii and brachialis are weak or absent. The natural history of the rigid extended elbow is such that improvement in range of flexion is minimal with growth. Forceful manipulation and stretching casts may cause cartilage necrosis and intra-articular adhesions and stiffness. Extra-articular soft tissues block elbow flexion; the soft tissues (i.e., the fibrosed musculotendinous structures and thick capsule) are hard, and the hard tissues (hyaline articular cartilage) are soft. Gentleness is extremely important. Continuous passive elbow motion, in the experience of this author, has not been effective to mobilize the elbow joint when there are only a few degrees of passive motion to begin with. Surgery is the most conservative method of management.

Functional disability of the extended rigid

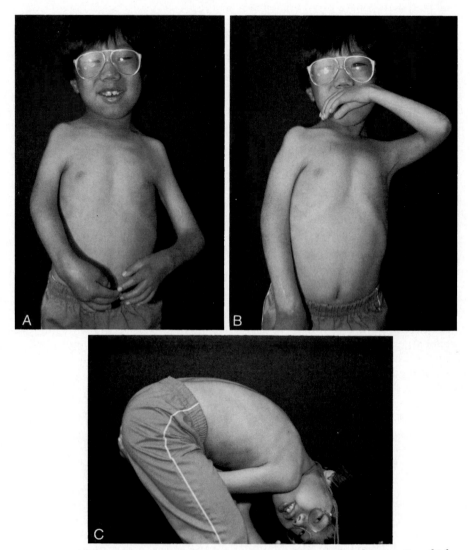

FIGURE 5–204. Extension deformity of the right elbow in a seven-year-old boy with arthrogryposis multiplex congenita.

A. Clinical appearance. **B.** Left elbow was treated by anterior transfer of the triceps brachii muscle. He can bring his left hand to his mouth. **C.** The right elbow is in extension. He uses his right hand for his toilet needs.

elbow is severe; the patient is unable to feed himself. It is crucial, however, to postpone surgical mobilization of the elbows until independent walking without crutches is achieved. In the wheelchair-bound patient, the ability to transfer to the wheelchair and in and out of bed should be assessed. Loss of triceps brachii function may cause inability to walk with crutches or transfer. The two prime objectives of restoration of upper limb function are independent self-feeding and independent toilet care; in order to achieve these goals it is best to provide active flexion in one elbow with the contralateral elbow capable of extension. Muscle-tendon transfers to restore elbow flexion should not be performed on both elbows unless the patient is capable of extending both elbows against gravity.

Proper timing of surgery is essential. In general, muscle-tendon transfers to restore elbow flexion are best deferred until five or six years of age—in the postoperative training period it is essential for the child to be motivated and cooperative. Simple soft-tissue lengthening and release for mobilization of the elbow into flexion can be performed in the younger age group.

A vital requisite for muscle-tendon transfer is functional (preferably normal) range of joint motion. The first step of treatment of extension contracture of the elbow is mobilization of the elbow joint by lengthening of the triceps tendon and posterior capsulotomy. This is relatively simple and, if performed early, can achieve full motion. The problem, however, is to maintain the correction. In the absence of active elbow flexion the extension deformity tends to recur. Passive range-of-motion exercises and splinting of the elbow are crucial in the postoperative period. With persistent splinting over the years, varying degrees of flexion deformity of the elbow may develop; however, this is usually of mild degree, and functional range of elbow motion can be maintained. Continuous passive elbow motion can be used to maintain mobility.

Following mobilization of the elbow, muscle-tendon transfers are performed to provide active elbow flexion. Anterior transfer of the triceps brachii may be carried out at the same time as the posterior elbow release. The drawback of triceps transfers is the loss of active extension against gravity. As stated earlier, triceps brachii transfer should not be performed when the support of crutches is required for walking, or when active elbow extension power is required for wheelchair or bed transfer. In bilateral extension contractures of the elbow, posterior release of the capsule and triceps

lengthening is carried out on one side (toilet arm), and anterior transfer of the triceps on the other (the feeding limb); this combination, according to Williams, achieves the optimum functional result.[223, 225] In addition to toilet care and self-feeding, the hands can be brought together for bimanual activity.

The operative technique of anterior transfer of triceps brachii is illustrated and described in Plate 89. The long-term results of this procedure reported in the literature are not that good. Initially, Williams reported improvement in 19 cases, but reassessment of his cases at completion of growth showed that instead of improving with age, nearly all lost function owing to progressive flexion deformity and loss of the arc of motion. The average range of elbow motion was only 20 degrees. One of the serious problems of flexion deformity of the elbows was the loss of ability to reach the perineum. In some patients, Williams had to perform extension osteotomy of the humerus in order to change the arc of motion to one in extension range.[223, 225] Carroll and Hill reported improvement of upper limb function in five of eight patients.[23] This author has performed ten anterior transfers of triceps in arthrogryposis. The long-term results have been better than those reported by Williams—with an average arc of motion of 70 degrees and flexion deformity of 20 degrees. It is crucial to provide meticulous care until skeletal maturity by part-time splinting of the elbow and an intensive physical therapy program. When range of elbow motion is being lost, a continuous passive-motion machine is utilized to increase the arc of motion. The author has performed only unilateral transfer (the feeding arm), and that only when the child is old enough to cooperate; it is diligent, persistent postoperative care that has achieved the good results.

Steindler's flexorplasty of the elbow, in which forearm flexor muscles are transferred from the origin in the medial epicondyle to a proximal and lateral position in the lower humeral shaft, is not recommended by this author in arthrogryposis, primarily because it aggravates the flexion deformity of the wrist and digits; it also has the drawback of inadequate strength of flexion and progressive flexion deformity of the elbow with skeletal growth.

Pectoralis major transfer is the most effective in restoring elbow flexion.[16, 25] It is recommended that the entire pectoralis major be transferred. The operative technique is described and illustrated in Plate 90. Other muscles available to provide elbow flexion are the

Text continued on page 2112

Anterior Transfer of Triceps Brachii (Carroll's Modification of Bunnell's Technique)

OPERATIVE TECHNIQUE

A. The patient is placed in lateral position. A midline incision is made on the posterior aspect of the arm, beginning in its middle half and extending distally to a point lateral to the olecranon process; then the incision is carried over the subcutaneous surface of the shaft of the ulna for a distance of 5 cm. The subcutaneous tissue is divided, and the wound flaps are mobilized.

B. The ulnar nerve is identified and mobilized medially to protect it from injury. The intermuscular septum is exposed laterally.

C. The triceps tendon is detached from its insertion with a long tail of periosteum.

Plate 89. Anterior Transfer of Triceps Brachii (Carroll's Modification of Bunnell's Technique)

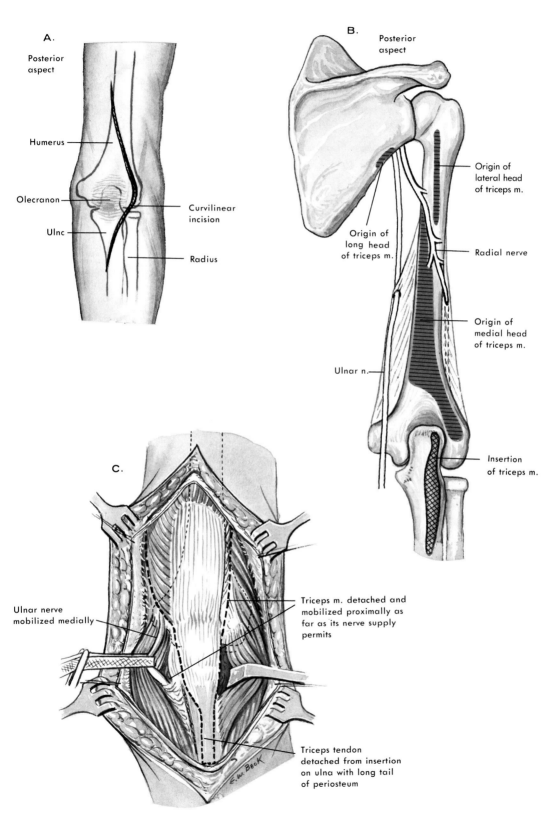

A.

Posterior aspect

Humerus

Olecranon

Ulna

Curvilinear incision

Radius

B.

Posterior aspect

Origin of lateral head of triceps m.

Origin of long head of triceps m.

Radial nerve

Origin of medial head of triceps m.

Ulnar n.

Insertion of triceps m.

C.

Ulnar nerve mobilized medially

Triceps m. detached and mobilized proximally as far as its nerve supply permits

Triceps tendon detached from insertion on ulna with long tail of periosteum

Anterior Transfer of Triceps Brachii (Carroll's Modification of Bunnell's Technique) (Continued)

D. Then the triceps muscle is freed and mobilized proximally as far as its nerve supply permits. The motor branches of the radial nerve to the triceps enter the muscle in the interval between the lateral and medial heads as the radial nerve enters the musculospiral groove. The distal portion of the detached triceps is then sutured to itself to form a tube.

E and **F.** Through a curvilinear incision in the antecubital fossa, the interval between the brachioradialis and the pronator teres is developed.

G. With an Ober tendon passer, the triceps tendon is passed into the anterior wound subcutaneously, superficial to the radial nerve.

H. With the elbow in 90 degrees of flexion and the forearm in full supination, the triceps tendon is either sutured to the biceps tendon or anchored to the radial tuberosity by a suture passed through a drill hole.

The wound is closed in routine fashion. An above-elbow cast is applied with the elbow in 90 degrees of flexion and full supination.

POSTOPERATIVE CARE

Four weeks after surgery the cast is removed and active exercises are performed to develop elbow flexion. Gravity provides extension to the elbow.

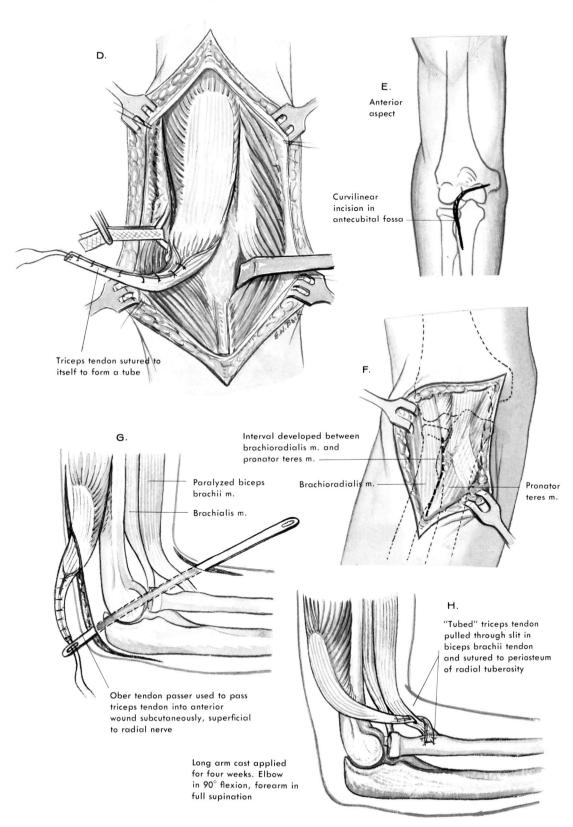

D.

Triceps tendon sutured to itself to form a tube

E.

Anterior aspect

Curvilinear incision in antecubital fossa

F.

Interval developed between brachioradialis m. and pronator teres m.

Brachioradialis m.

Pronator teres m.

G.

Paralyzed biceps brachii m.

Brachialis m.

Ober tendon passer used to pass triceps tendon into anterior wound subcutaneously, superficial to radial nerve

Long arm cast applied for four weeks. Elbow in 90° flexion, forearm in full supination

H.

"Tubed" triceps tendon pulled through slit in biceps brachii tendon and sutured to periosteum of radial tuberosity

Pectoralis Major Transfer for Paralysis of Elbow Flexors

OPERATIVE TECHNIQUE

A. The patient is positioned supine with the upper limb supported on a hand table with the shoulder in 45 degrees of abduction and 30 degrees of external rotation. Two incisions are made, the first one following the deltopectoral groove extending from the clavicle down to the junction of the upper and middle thirds of the arm. The second incision is centered over the anteromedial aspect of the elbow.

B. Through the first incision the subcutaneous tissue and deep fascia are divided, and the cephalic vein is ligated if necessary.

C. The pectoralis major tendon is identified and divided at its insertion, as close to the bone as possible. By blunt dissection, the muscle is mobilized from the chest wall toward the clavicle. The deltoid muscle is then retracted laterally and the tendon of the long head of the biceps exposed running upward toward the shoulder joint. It is severed at the upper end of the bicipital groove and pulled distally into the wound.

Plate 90. Pectoralis Major Transfer for Paralysis of Elbow Flexors

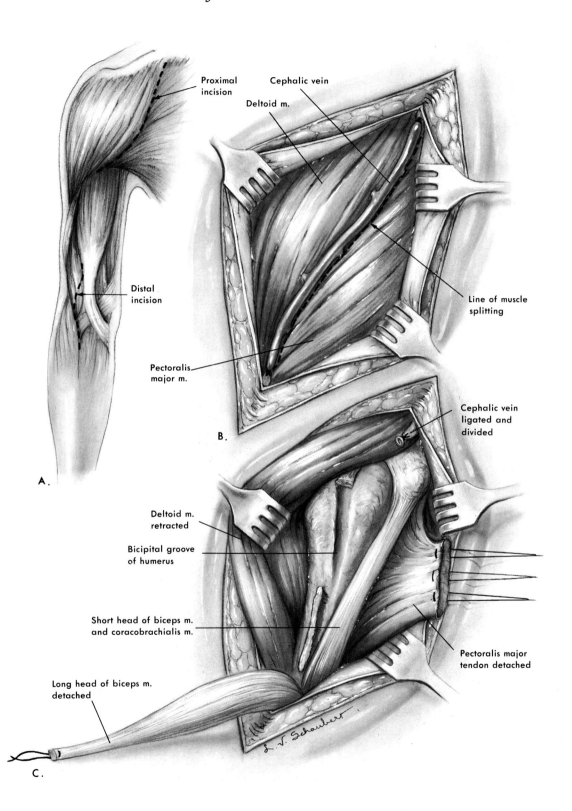

Proximal incision

Cephalic vein

Deltoid m.

Distal incision

Line of muscle splitting

Pectoralis major m.

B.

A.

Cephalic vein ligated and divided

Deltoid m. retracted

Bicipital groove of humerus

Short head of biceps m. and coracobrachialis m.

Pectoralis major tendon detached

Long head of biceps m. detached

L. V. Schaubert

C.

Pectoralis Major Transfer for Paralysis of Elbow Flexors
(Continued)

D. By blunt and sharp dissection, the muscle belly of the long head of the biceps is mobilized to the lowest third of the arm by freeing it from the short head. The vessels and nerves entering the muscle belly are divided and ligated as necessary. The tendon and muscle of the long head are delivered into the distal second incision and freed down to the tuberosity of the radius. Often, freeing the muscle from adhesions to the overlying fascia requires sharp dissection. After complete mobilization of the long head of the biceps by traction on its proximal end, one should be able to flex the elbow.

E. The long head of the biceps is pulled into the upper wound. Two slits are made in the tendon of the mobilized pectoralis major through which the tendon of the long head is passed, looped on itself, and brought down again into the distal wound. With the elbow acutely flexed, the proximal end of the tendon is sutured to its own tendon of insertion through a slit in the distal tendon. Silk sutures are also inserted at the level of the tendon of the pectoralis major. The incisions are then closed in the routine manner. A plaster of Paris reinforced Velpeau bandage is applied with the elbow acutely flexed.

POSTOPERATIVE CARE

Plaster of Paris immobilization is continued for three weeks. At the end of this time active flexion and extension exercises of the elbow are started, first with gravity eliminated and then against gravity. A sling is used to protect the transferred tendon from stretching. Care should be taken to extend the elbow gradually so that active flexion above the right-angle position is maintained. Extension of the elbow is regained slowly.

Plate 90. Pectoralis Major Transfer for Paralysis of Elbow Flexors

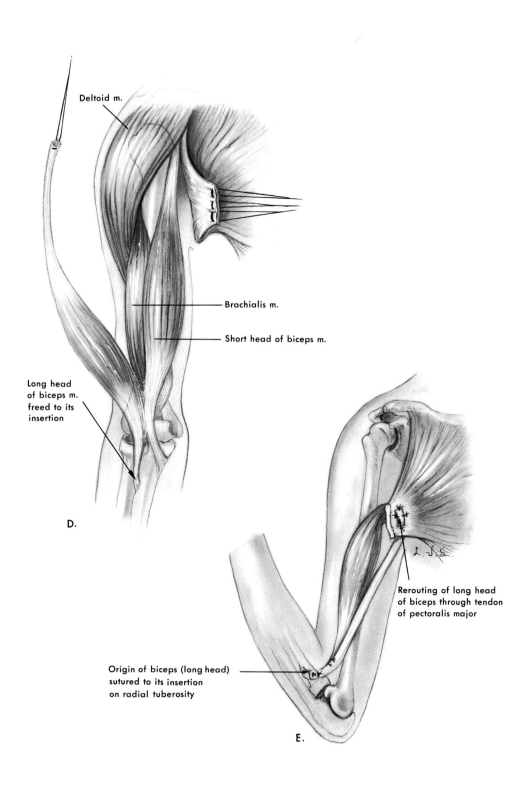

Deltoid m.

Brachialis m.

Short head of biceps m.

Long head of biceps m. freed to its insertion

D.

Rerouting of long head of biceps through tendon of pectoralis major

Origin of biceps (long head) sutured to its insertion on radial tuberosity

E.

latissimus dorsi and sternocleidomastoid muscles (see section on poliomyelitis). This author has not utilized these motors to provide elbow flexion in arthrogryposis.

WRIST

The common deformity of the wrist is severe flexion (sometimes up to 90 degrees) and varying degrees of ulnar deviation. Often the wrist deformity is associated with a varying extent of thumb and finger involvement. Correction of the wrist deformity will improve the function of the entire upper limb. Treatment should begin as soon as possible, preferably during the first few days of life. Passive stretching exercises are followed by serial splinting with the wrist in progressive dorsiflexion. The finger and thumb deformities are corrected simultaneously—the function of the digits is closely related to the position of the wrist, and the care of the fingers and thumb is coordinated with that of the wrist. When the wrist deformity is very rigid, one may have to employ serial casts. Ordinarily the wrist deformity will correct by exercise and splint or serial casts; however, in the absence of functioning active wrist dorsiflexors, it will tend to recur very rapidly despite attempts at splinting. Muscle imbalance should be corrected early—a functioning flexor carpi ulnaris is transferred to the extensor carpi radialis longus and brevis; often the wrist extensors are absent or hypoplastic, and one has to attach the flexor carpi ulnaris tendon to the base of the second or third metacarpal, or on the carpus as far distally as possible. The tendon transfer may be reinforced with Mersilene or free fascial graft tenodesis, attaching to the radius proximally and the second and third metacarpal bones distally. This provides stability to the wrist in functional position, and at the same time some mobility of the wrist joint is allowed, which functionally is advantageous.

Williams recommends stabilization of the wrist in the skeletally immature patient (six years of age and older) by an intramedullary rod that traverses from the third metacarpal and the radius. He leaves the rod in situ until skeletal maturity, at which time he performs wrist fusion. The optimum position of wrist fusion is individualized; it is determined by preoperative splinting. Often it is in five degrees of palmar flexion. The technique of wrist fusion recommended by Williams is simple excision of a wedge from the radiocarpal articulation and immobilization of the wrist-forearm in a cast for six weeks.[225]

This author does not recommend wrist fusion, because a certain degree of mobility of the wrist stabilized in functional neutral position or 5 to 10 degrees of palmar flexion is functionally desirable. The arc of motion is restricted by tendon transfers, tenodesis, or fasciodesis. Some degree of wrist flexion is maintained to enable self-care for feeding and toileting. It is always essential to provide elbow mobility with correction of wrist deformity.

The rigid flexion deformity of the wrist can be corrected in several ways. This author prefers dorsal wedge osteotomy of the distal radius and ulna (as advocated by Meyn and Ruby, and Weeks).[146, 217] The procedure corrects the flexion deformity and relatively lengthens the contracted volar soft-tissue structures; however, it does not improve the range of wrist motion. Positioning of the wrist in better anatomic position improves hand function. Other methods are volar soft-tissue release and proximal row carpectomy. This author finds dorsal wedge osteotomy of the radius-ulna much simpler; the procedure is combined with tendon transfers and dorsal tenodesis. Soft-tissue release or dorsal wedge osteotomy of the radius alone often will end in failure with recurrence of deformity.

Pronation Contracture of the Forearm. This is corrected by section of pronator teres tendon at its insertion to the radius; this is simple and effective. An alternative method is to reverse the action of pronator teres from pronation to supination when the pronator teres is good in motor strength. This is achieved by a step-cut of the pronator teres tendon near its insertion. The distal segment of the tendon that is left attached to the radius is rerouted around the radial border of the radius and through the interosseous membrane and resutured to the proximal segment of the pronator tendon. This author has had no personal experience with this procedure.

THUMB

The objective of surgery of the thumb is to increase span, provide opposition between the pulps of the thumb and index–long fingers, and enable the patient to grasp with the fingers by having the thumb out of the palm.

In arthrogryposis with upper limb involvement, the thumb is usually adducted with contracture of the soft tissues in the first web interspace and adductor pollicis; the thumb is also flexed at the metacarpophalangeal joint with varying degrees of flexion of the interphalangeal and carpometacarpal joints because of contracture of flexor pollicis longus. The extensor pollicis longus and brevis and abductor pollicis may be hypoplastic or absent. The volar skin of the first web space is contracted. This clutched thumb deformity blocks grasp and hinders opposition between the thumb and fingers.

In infancy, treatment consists of passive stretching exercises and splinting and stretching casts to elongate the shortened soft tissue and get the clutched thumb out of the palm. One should be cautious not to subluxate the metacarpophalangeal joint and cause instability. Often, surgical intervention is indicated. It consists of deepening of the first web space by double Z-plasty. In severe deformities, dorsal rotation flap and skin graft may be required. Often, one has to release the adductor pollicis at its origin in the palm and fractionally lengthen the flexor pollicis longus at its musculotendinous juncture in the distal forearm. When the metacarpophalangeal part of the thumb is unstable, it is stabilized by fusion.

FINGERS

Flexion deformity of the proximal interphalangeal joints of the digits is the most common problem; this is usually minimal or moderate, requiring no surgical treatment. Passive stretching exercises are performed, and a splint is worn at night in an attempt to checkrein progression of flexion deformity. In moderate flexion deformity that cannot be controlled by nonsurgical means, volar soft-tissue release is indicated; often one has to release adhesions of flexor sublimis and section accessory collateral ligaments to correct the joint contracture. Internal fixation with Kirschner wires for a period of three weeks maintains the correction obtained at surgery. Ordinarily, the arc of motion of the proximal interphalangeal joint is not improved. When range of extension of the finger joints improves with palmar flexion of the wrist, the flexion deformity of digits is due to contracture of flexor digitorum profundus and sublimis—in such an instance the long finger flexors are fractionally lengthened at their musculotendinous juncture in the distal forearm.

Ulnar Drift of the Fingers. This should be corrected at the same time as correction of thumb-in-palm deformity, in order to allow the corrected thumb to pinch against the index and long fingers. Treatment consists of release of ulnar lateral bands and tendon transfer of the ulnar intrinsic muscles to the radial side in the young child and radial angulation osteotomy of the distal metacarpal shaft. In the growing child between 8 and 11 years of age, asymmetrical

growth arrest (partial epiphysiodesis of the radial half) of the metacarpals and proximal phalanges will correct ulnar drift at skeletal maturity.

SPINE

The incidence of scoliosis in arthrogryposis reported in the literature varies from 2.5 to 34 per cent; the 20 per cent incidence reported by Herron et al. is probably representative of the average figure.[86, 183]

The age of onset of scoliosis varies; it may be noted at birth, in childhood, or in adolescence. In the severe arthrogrypotic, scoliosis is more prevalent and is detected during the first four years of life.

The predominant curve pattern in arthrogryposis is a long-C thoracolumbar structural curve extending to the sacrum; this is typical of neuromuscular scoliosis. Often the scoliosis is associated with hyperlordosis and pelvic obliquity (due to unilateral contractural deformity or dislocation of the hip).

Associated congenital anomalies of the spine may be present or absent. In the series of Drummond and MacKenzie, of 14 cases of scoliosis in arthrogryposis, 7 had congenital scoliosis, 3 nonprogressive, and 4 progressive. Herron et al. reported 18 arthrogrypotic patients with scoliosis, and none of them had congenital anomalies of the spine.[49, 86] Sarwark et al. reported a 35 per cent incidence of scoliosis in amyelodysplasia congenita (23 of 65 patients). In 5 of the patients (7.7 per cent) the scoliosis was infantile, and in 18 patients (27.8 per cent) it was juvenile or adolescent. Congenital anomalies of the vertebrae were not noted in any of these patients.[183]

The natural history of the neuromuscular long thoracolumbar scoliosis in arthrogryposis is steady progression, the curves being rigid and fixed at an early age.

Treatment. Scoliosis, when noted in infancy in arthrogryposis, is often due to intrauterine malposture (related to oligohydramnios, transverse lie, or breech position). In the infant, treatment consists of passive stretching exercises and, in the moderately severe case, corrective custom-made spinal orthosis. Often the spinal deformity will respond to such therapy.

In the juvenile and adolescent period, in curves up to 20 to 40 degrees an attempt can be made to control by orthosis. Often nonsurgical measures are unsuccessful. Herron et al. reported results of orthotic or corrective cast treatment in five patients—all of them failed to respond, and the curves progressed and eventually required spinal fusion.[86] Sarwark et al. reported two cases of juvenile scoliosis in arthrogryposis treated by orthosis. In one of these, there was no progression of the 20 degree curve at age 17 years, whereas the other patient had progressed from 25 to 58 degrees at age 19 years.[183] This author recommends a trial of orthosis for one to two years for a curve less than 35 degrees; if the curve progresses while being treated by orthosis, it should be corrected and fused surgically.

For curves greater than 35 to 40 degrees, spinal fusion and internal fixation with instrumentation is indicated. The curve should extend distally to include the sacrum if the sacrum is included in the lumbar portion of the curve.

References

1. Aaro, S., Gottfries, B., Krapelieu, T., and Troell, S.: Teratologic congenital dislocation of the hip. Acta Orthop. Scand., 54:178, 1983.
2. Abraham, R. D., and Vanace, P. W.: Mobility for a multidisabled child. Arch. Phys. Med. Rehabil., 56:365, 1975.
3. Adams, R. D., Denny-Brown, D., and Pearson, C. M.: Diseases of Muscle. New York, Paul B. Hoeber, 1953, pp. 229–235.
4. Arstila, P.: Quantitative studies on absorption, dilution and haemagglutination of vesicular stomatitis virus. Arch. Virol., 51:51, 1976.
5. Arthrogryposis multiplex congenita (Editorial). Br. Med. J. (Clin. Res.), 283:2, 1981.
6. Badgley, C. E.: Correlation of clinical and anatomical facts leading to a conception of the etiology of congenital hip dysplasias. J. Bone Joint Surg., 25:503, 1943.
7. Badgley, C. E.: Primary and secondary congenital deformities. A.A.O.S. Instr. Course Lect. 10:147, 1953.
8. Banker, B. Q.: Neuropathologic aspects of arthrogryposis mutiplex congenita. Clin. Orthop., 194:30, 1985.
9. Banker, B. Q., Victor, M., and Adams, R. D.: Arthrogryposis multiplex due to congenital muscular dystrophy. Brain, 80:319, 1957.
10. Bayne, L. G.: Hand assessment and management of arthrogryposis multiplex congenita. Clin. Orthop., 194:68, 1985.
11. Beckerman, R. C., and Buchino, J.: Arthropgryposis multiplex congenita as part of an inherited symptom complex: two case reports and a review of the literature. Pediatrics, 61:417, 1978.
12. Bennett, J. B., Hansen, P. E., Granberry, W. M., and Cain, T. E.: Surgical management of arthrogryposis in the upper extremity. J. Pediatr. Orthop., 5:281, 1985.
13. Bharucha, E. P., Pandya, S. S., and Dastur, D. K.: Arthrogryposis multiplex congenita. Part I. Clinical and electromyographic aspects. J. Neurol. Neurosurg. Psychiatry, 35:425, 1972.
14. Blery, M., Pannier, S., and Barre, J. L.: Etude radiologique de l'arthrogrypose. A propos de 20 cas. J. Radiol. Electrol., 58:597, 1977.
15. Brandt, S.: A case of arthrogryposis multiplex congenita anatomically appearing as foetal spinal muscular atrophy. Acta Paediatr., 34:365, 1947.
16. Brooks, D. M., and Seddon, H. J.: Pectoral transplantation for paralysis of the flexor of the elbow. A new technique. J. Bone Joint Surg., 41-B:36, 1959.
17. Brown, L. M., Robson, M. J., and Sharrard, W. J.: The pathophysiology of arthrogryposis multiplex congenita neurologica. J. Bone Joint Surg., 62-B:291, 1980.
18. Bunnell, S.: Restoring flexion to the paralyzed elbow. J. Bone Joint Surg., 33-A:566, 1951.
19. Bunnell, S.: Surgery of the Hand. Philadelphia, J. B. Lippincott, 1970.
20. Call, W. H., and Strickland, J. W.: Functional hand reconstruction in the whistling-face syndrome. J. Hand Surg., 6:148, 1981.
21. Carlson, W. O., Speck, G. J., Urcari, U., and Wenger, D. R.: Arthrogryposis multiplex congenita—a long-term follow-up study. Clin. Orthop., 194:115, 1985.
22. Carroll, R. E.: Restoration of flexion power in the flail elbow by transplantation of the triceps tendon. Surg. Gynecol. Obstet., 95:685, 1952.
23. Carroll, R. E., and Hill, N. A.: Triceps transfer to restore elbow flexion. J. Bone Joint Surg., 52-A:239, 1970.
24. Carter, C. O., and Fairbank, T. J.: The Genetics of Locomotor Disorders. London, Oxford University Press, 1974, p.124.
25. Clark, J. M. P.: Reconstruction of biceps brachii by pectoral muscles transplantation. Br. J. Surg., 34:180, 1946.
26. Clarren, S. K., and Hall, J. G.: Neuropathologic findings in spinal cords of 10 infants with arthrogryposis. J. Neurol. Sci., 58:89, 1983.
27. Cohen, S. R., and Isaacs, H.: Otolaryngological manifestations of arthrogryposis multiplex congenita. Ann. Otol. Rhinol. Laryngol., 85:484, 1976.
28. Cognee: Contribution à l'étude des syndromes arthrogryposiques. A propos de 9 observations. Grenoble, These, 1978.
29. Cook, C. C.: Amyoplasia congenita associated with mongolism. Arch. Dis. Child., 11:261, 1936.
30. Cote, G. B., Adamopoulos, D., and Pantelakis, S.: Arthrogryposis and ectodermal dysplasia. Hum. Hered., 32:71, 1982.
31. Cotton, J. B., and Robert, J. M.: Etio-pathogenie de l'arthrogrypose multiple congenitale. Conseil genetique. Ann. Med. Phys., 19:17, 1976.
32. Crowe, M. W.: Congenital arthrogryposis in offspring of sows fed tobacco (Nicotiana tabacum). Am. J. Vet. Res., 35:1071, 1974.
33. Damrongsak, D., Srichomkwan, A., and Techakvmpuch, S.: Arthrogryposis multiplex congenita: roentgenographic features of 3 cases. J. Med. Assoc. Thai., 56:302, 1973.
34. Dangles, C. J., and Bilos, Z. J.: Surgical correction of thumb deformity in arthrogryposis multiplex congenita. Hand, 13:55, 1981.
35. Dastur, D. K., Razzak, Z. A., and Bharucha, E. P.: Arthrogryposis multiplex congenita. Part 2. Muscle pathology and pathogenesis. J. Neurol. Neurosurg. Psychiatry, 35:435, 1972.
36. Davidson, J., and Beighton, P.: Whence the arthrogrypotics? J. Bone Joint Surg., 58-B:492, 1976.
37. Della-Porta, A. J.: Congenital bovine epizootic arthrogryposis and hydranencephaly in Australia. Aust. Vet. J., 52:496, 1976.
38. Delplace, J.: Faut-il une luxation de hanche sur arthrogrypose? Ann. Orthrop. Quest, 8:51, 1976.
39. Derkaloustian, V. M., Affifi, A. K., and Mire, J.: The myopathic variety of arthrogryposis multiplex congenita; a disorder with massive inheritance. Pediatrics, 81:76, 1972.
40. Diamond, L. S., and Alegado, R.: Perinatal fractures in arthrogryposis multiplex congenita. J. Pediatr. Orthop., 1:189, 1981.
41. Dimmick, J. E., Berry, K., MacLeod, P. M., and Hardwick, D. F.: Syndrome of ankylosis, facial anom-

alies, and pulmonary hypoplasia: A pathologic analysis of one infant. Birth Defects, *13*:133, 1977.

42. Drachman, D. B.: Atrophy of skeletal muscle in chick embryos treated with botulism toxin. Science, *145*:719, 1964.

43. Drachman, D. B.: The syndrome of arthrogryposis multiplex congenita. Birth Defects (Original Article Series, Vol. VII), 2:90, 1971.

44. Drachman, D. B., and Banker, B. Q.: Arthrogryposis multiplex congenita. A case due to disease of the anterior horn cells. Arch. Neurology, 5:77, 1961.

45. Drachman, D. B., and Coulombre, A.: Experimental club foot and arthrogryposis multiplex congenita. Lancet, 2:523, 1962.

46. Drachman, D. B., and Sokoloff, L.: The role of movement in embryonic joint development. Dev. Biol., *14*:401, 1966.

47. Drachman, D. B., Weiner, L. P., Price, D. L., and Chase, J.: Experimental arthrogryposis multiplex congenita caused by viral myopathy. Arch. Neurol., *33*:362, 1976.

48. Drummond, D. S., and Cruess, R. L.: The management of the foot and ankle in arthrogryposis multiplex congenita. J. Bone Joint Surg., *60-B*:96, 1978.

49. Drummond, D. S., and MacKenzie, D. A.: Scoliosis in arthrogryposis multiplex congenita. Proceedings of the Scoliosis Research Society. J. Bone Joint Surg., *56-A*:1763, 1974.

50. Drummond, D. S., Siller, T. N., and Cruess, R. L.: Management of arthrogryposis multiplex congenita. A.A.O.S. Instructional Course Lectures. St. Louis, C. V. Mosby, 1974, p. 79.

51. Dubowitz, V., and Brooke, M. H.: Muscle Biopsy: A Modern Approach. Philadelphia, W. B. Saunders, 1973.

52. Edwards, M. J.: Experimental production of arthrogryposis multiplex congenita in guinea pig by maternal hyperthermia. J. Pathol., *104*:221, 1971.

53. Ek, J. I.: Cerebral lesions in arthrogryposis multiplex congenita. Acta Paediatr., *47*:302, 1958.

54. Evans, E. L.: Astragalectomy. In The Robert Jones Birthday Volume: A Collection of Surgical Essays. London, Oxford Medical Publications, 1928, pp. 375–394.

55. Ferguson, A. B., Jr.: Orthopaedic Surgery in Infancy and Childhood. Baltimore, Williams & Wilkins, 1975, pp. 704–706.

56. Fisher, R. L., Johnstone, W. T., Fisher, W. H., and Goldkamp, O. G.: Arthrogryposis multiplex congenita: a clinical investigation. J. Pediatr., *76*:255, 1970.

57. Fitti, R. M., and D'Auria, T. M.: Arthrogryposis multiplex congenita. J. Pediatr., *48*:797, 1956.

58. Fowler, M.: A case of arthrogryposis multiplex congenita with lesions in the nervous system. Arch. Dis. Child., *34*:505, 1959.

59. Friedlander, H. L., Westin, G. W., and Wood, W. L., Jr.: Arthrogryposis multiplex congenita. J. Bone Joint Surg., *50-A*:89, 1968.

60. Fuller, D. J.: Immobilisation of foetal joints: a cause of progressive prenatal deformity. J. Bone Joint Surg., *57-B*:115, 1975.

61. Geny Chanson, L., Hoeffel, J. C., Merle, M., and Barthelet, P.: Radiological appearances of congenital malformations of the hand. J. Radiol., *61*:353, 1980.

62. Gibson, D. A., and Urs, N. D. K.: Arthrogryposis multiplex congenita. J. Bone Joint Surg., *52-B*:483, 1970.

63. Gilmour, J. R.: Amyoplasia congenita. J. Pathol. Bacteriol., *58*:675, 1946.

64. Giroud, A.: Syndromes arthro-myodysplasiques et leurs causes chez l'homme et l'animal. Acad. Natl. Med., *156*:814, 1972.

65. Green, A. D. L., Fixsen, J. A., and Lloyd-Roberts, G. C.: Talectomy for arthrogryposis multiplex congenita. J. Bone Joint Surg., *66-B*:697, 1984.

66. Grossiord, A., Held, J. P., Lacert, P., Panniers, S., Beaupère-Duval, G., and Quinet, I.: L'arthrogrypose: aspects cliniques (à propos de 15 cas). Ann. Med. Phys., *19*:1, 1976.

67. Gruttola, G. L., and Ferrara, M.: Considerazioni etiopatogenetiche, cliniche e studio cromosomico in un caso di arthrogripose multipla congenita. Pediatria (Napoli), *83*:773, 1975.

68. Guillamat, M., and Bedouelle, J.: Le membre inferieur de l'arthrogrypose. Ann. Med. Phys., *19*:51, 1976.

69. Hageman, G., and Willemse, J.: Arthrogryposis multiplex congenita. Review with comment. Neuropediatrics, *14*:6, 1983.

70. Hahn, G.: Arthrogryposis. Pediatric review and habilitation aspects. Clin. Orthop., *194*:104, 1985.

71. Hall, J. G.: An approach to congenital contracture. Pediatr. Annu., *10*:15, 1981.

72. Hall, J. G.: An approach to research on congenital contractures. In Strategies in Genetic Counseling: Clinical Investigative Studies. Birth Defects (Original Article Series, Vol. 20), 6:8, 1984. (White Plains, N.Y., March of Dimes Birth Defects Foundation.)

73. Hall, J. G.: Genetic aspects of arthrogryposis. Clin. Orthop., *194*:44, 1985.

74. Hall, S. D., McGillivray, B. C., Herrmann, J., Partington, M. W., Schinzel, A., Shapiro, J., and Weaver, D. D.: Part II. Amyoplasia: Twinning in amyoplasia—A specific type of arthrogryposis with an apparent excess of discordantly affected identical twins. Am. J. Genet., *15*:591, 1983.

75. Hall, J. G., and Reed, S. D.: Teratogens associated with congenital contractures in humans and in animals. Teratology, *25*:173, 1982.

76. Hall, J. G., Reed, S. D., and Driscoll, E. P.: Part I. Amyoplasia: A common sporadic condition with congenital contractures. Am. J. Med. Genet., *15*:571, 1983.

77. Hall, J. G., Reed, S. D., and Greene, G.: The distal arthrogryposes: delineation of new entities—review and nosologic discussion. Am. J. Med. Genet., *11*:185, 1982.

78. Hall, J. G., Reed, S. D., Rosenbaum, K. N., Chen, H., and Wilson, K. M.: Limb pterygium syndromes: a review and report of eleven patients. Am. J. Med. Genet., *12*:377, 1982.

79. Hall, J. G., Truog, W. E., and Plowman, D. L.: A new arthrogryposis syndrome with facial and limb anomalies. Am. J. Dis. Child., *129*:120, 1975.

80. Hamada, T.: Serum creatine phosphokinase levels in calves with arthrogryposis-hydranencephaly syndrome. Vet. Rec., *95*:441, 1974.

81. Handelsman, J. E.: Lumbosacral agenesis. In Delchef, E. J., de Marneffe, R., and Vander Elst, E. (eds.): Orthopaedic Surgery and Traumatology, International Congress Series No. 291. Amsterdam, Excerpta Medica, 1973, pp. 421–422.

82. Handelsman, J. E.: Lumbo-sacral agenesis. J. Bone Joint Surg., *53-B*:564, 1971.

83. Hansen, O. M.: Surgical anatomy and treatment of patients with arthrogryposis. J. Bone Joint Surg., *43-B*:855, 1961.

84. Hanset, R., Leroy, P., and Michaux: Le syndrome arthrogrypose et palatoschisis dans un troupeau de croises charolais. Ann. Med. Vet., *122*:591, 1978.

85. Hartley, W. J., and Wanner, R. A.: Serological evidence for the association of Akabane virus with epizootic bovine congenital arthrogryposis and hydranencephaly syndromes in New South Wales. Aust. Vet. J., 5:103, 1975.

86. Herron, L. D., Westin, G. W., and Dawson, E. G.: Scoliosis in arthrogryposis multiplex congenita. J. Bone Joint Surg., *60-A*:293, 1978.

87. Hildanus, F.: Observationum et curationum medico-chirurgarum centurae sex 1641. Cited in Bick, E. M.:

Source Book of Orthopaedics. 2nd Ed. Baltimore, Williams & Wilkins, 1948, p. 52.

88. Hillman, J. W., and Johnson, J. T. H.: Arthrogryposis multiplex congenita in twins. J. Bone Joint Surg., *34-A*:211, 1952.

89. Hoffer, M. M., Swank, S., Eastman, R., Clark, D., and Teige, R.: Ambulation in severe arthrogryposis. J. Pediatr. Orthop., *3*:293, 1983.

90. Holmdahl, H. C.: Astragalectomy as a stabilising operation for foot paralysis following poliomyelitis: results of a followup investigation of 153 cases. Acta Orthop. Scand., *25*:207, 1956.

91. Hoosmand, H., Martinez, A. J., and Roseblum, W. I.: Arthrogryposis multiplex congenita, simultaneous involvement of peripheral nerve and skeletal muscle. Arch. Neurol., *24*:561, 1971.

92. Houston, C. S., Reed, M. H., and Desautels, J. E.: Separating Larsen syndrome from the "arthrogryposis basket." J. Can. Assoc. Radiol., *32*:206, 1981.

93. Hsu, L. C., Jaffray, D., and Leong, J. C. Y.: Talectomy for clubfoot in arthrogryposis. J. Bone Joint Surg., *66-B*:694, 1984.

94. Hughes, S.: Orthopaedics. 2. Telling them apart. Nurs. Mirror, *151*:20, 1980.

95. Huurman, W. H., and Jacobson, S. T.: The hip in arthrogryposis multiplex congenita. Clin. Orthop., *194*:81, 1985.

96. Imamura, M., Yamanaka, N., Nakamura, F., and Oyanagi, K.: Arthrogryposis multiplex congenita: an autopsy case of a fatal form. Hum. Pathol., *12*:699, 1981.

97. Inaba, Y., Kurogi, H., and Omori, T.: Akabane disease: Epizootic abortion, premature birth, stillbirth and congenital arthrogryposis hydranencephaly in cattle, sheep and goats, caused by Akabane virus. Aust. Vet. J., *51*:584, 1975.

98. Ionasescu, V., Zellweger, H., Filer, L. J., and Conway, T. W.: Increased collagen synthesis in arthrogryposis multiplex congenita. Arch. Neurol., *23*:128, 1970.

99. Isaacs, H., and Barlow, M. B.: Central core disease associated with elevated creatine phosphokinase levels. Two members of a family known to be susceptible to malignant hyperpyrexia. S. Afr. Med. J., *48*:640, 1974.

100. Isaacs, H., Heffrom, J. J. A., and Badenhorst, M.: Central core disease. A correlated genetic, histochemical, ultramicroscopic, and biochemical study. J. Neurol. Neurosurg. Psychiatry, *38*:1177, 1975.

101. Jacobsen, H., Herbert, E. A., and Poppel, M. H.: Arthrogryposis multiplex congenita. Radiology, *65*:8, 1955.

102. Jago, R. H.: Arthrogryposis following treatment of maternal tetanus with muscle relaxants: case report. Arch. Dis. Child., *45*:277, 1970.

103. James, T.: Multiple congenital articular rigidities. Edinb. Med. J., *58*:565, 1951.

104. Jones, L. E., Schutt, A. M., and Sawtell, R. R.: Arthrogryposis multiplex congenita: a review of 40 cases seen at the Mayo Clinic between 1966 and 1976. Rev. Med. Child. Neurol., *20*:239, 1978.

105. Kalyanaraman, K., and Kalyanaraman, U. P.: Myopathic arthrogryposis with seizures and abnormal electroencephalogram. J. Pediatr., *100*:247, 1982.

106. Kanof, A., Aronson, S. M., and Volk, B. W.: Arthrogryposis. A clinical and pathological study of three cases. Pediatrics, *17*:532, 1956.

107. Katzeff, M.: Arthrogryposis multiplex congenita. Arch. Surg., *46*:673, 1943.

108. Katz, J. F.: Teratological hip dislocation. Isr. J. Med. Sci., *16*:238, 1980.

109. Keeler, R. F.: Congenital defects in calves from maternal ingestion of Nicotiana glauca of high anabasine content. Clin. Toxicol., *15*:417, 1979.

110. Khera, K. S., LaHam, Q. M., Ellis, C. F. G., and Zawidska, Z. Z.: Foot deformity in ducks from injection of EPN during embryogenesis. Toxicol. Appl. Pharmacol., *8*:540, 1966.

111. Kite, J. H.: Arthrogryposis multiplex congenita. Review of 54 cases. South. Med. J., *48*:1141, 1955.

112. Konno, S., Moriwaki, M., and Nakagawa, M.: Congenital abnormality of calves with arthrogryposis and hydranencephaly in Japan in 1972–1973. Natl. Inst. Anim. Health Q., *15*:52, 1975.

113. Krieger, I.: Arthrogryposis multiplex congenita and the Turner phenotype. Am. J. Dis. Child., *12*:141, 1972.

114. Krugliak, L., Gadoth, N., and Behar, A. J.: Neuropathic form of arthrogryposis multiplex congenita. Report of 3 cases with complete necropsy including the first reported case of agenesis of muscle spindles. J. Neurol. Sci., *37*:179, 1978.

115. Kullman, L., and Szijj, E.: Electromyographische und histologische veranderungen bei Arthrogryposis. Arch. Orth. Unfallchir., *76*:235, 1973.

116. Lajos, K.: Possibilities of treatment of arthrogryposis. Magy. Traum. Orthop., *18*:189, 1975.

117. Lauvergne, J. J.: Etat present des connaissances sur le syndrome d'arthrogrypose et de palatoschisis dans le betail charolais en France. Ann. Genet. Sel. Anim., *7*:321, 1975.

118. Lauvergne, J. J., and Faucon, A.: Le syndrome d'arthrogrypose et de palatoschisis en race bovine charolaise. Ann. Genet. Sel. Anim., *8*:51, 1976.

119. Lebard, J. P., Queneau, P., and Dubousset, J. F.: Membres superieurs de l'arthrogrypose. Ann. Med. Phys., *19*:33, 1976.

120. Lebenthal, E., Bembassat, M., Reisner, S. H., and Seelemfreund, M.: Arthrogryposis multiplex congenita, myopathic type. Isr. J. Med. Sci., *9*:463, 1973.

121. Lebenthal, E., Shockhet, S. B., Adan, A., Seelenfreund, M., Fried, A., Najenson, T., Sandbank, U., and Mathothy: Arthrogryposis multiplex congenita. 23 cases in an Arab family. Kindred Pediatr., *46*:891, 1970.

122. Lecoeur, P.: Anatomie chirurgicale. Ann. Med. Phys., *1*:29, 1976.

123. Lefort, G., Lauvergne, J. J., and Fabregues, P.: Frequence et penetrance du gene responsable du syndrome d'arthrogrypose et de palatoschisis dans le betail charolais en France. Ann. Genet. Sel. Anim., *9*:283, 1977.

124. Leikkonen, O.: Astragalectomy as ankle stabilizing operation in infantile paralysis sequelae: with special reference to astragalectomies and total arthrodeses performed in Finland. Acta Chir. Scand., *100*:668, 1950.

125. Leipold, H. W.: Arthrogryposis and palatoschisis in neonatal Charolais calves. Vet. Med. Small Anim. Clin., *68*:1140, 1973.

126. Leipold, H. W., Cates, W. F., Radostits, O. M., and Howell, W. E.: Arthrogryposis and associated defects in newborn calves. Am. J. Vet. Res., *31*:1367, 1970.

127. Leipold, H. W., Oehme, F. W., and Cook, J. E.: Congenital arthrogryposis associated with ingestion of Jimson weed by pregnant sows. J.A.V.M.A., *162*:1059, 1973.

128. Leskiewicz, W., and Milewska, B.: Arthrogryposis multiplex congenita. Pediatr. Pol., *48*:1505, 1973.

129. Lewin, P.: Arthrogryposis multiplex congenita. J. Bone Joint Surg., *7*:630, 1925.

130. Lipton, F. L., and Morgenstern, S. A.: Arthrogryposis multiplex congenita in identical twins. Am. J. Dis. Child., *89*:233, 1955.

131. Lloyd-Roberts, G. C., and Lettin, A. W. F.: Arthrogryposis multiplex congenita. J. Bone Joint Surg., *52-B*:494, 1970.

132. Lukes, J., Marten, J., and Kopecky, J.: Arthrogryposis

multiplex congenita se soucasnym vyskytem atrezie ilea. Cesk. Pediatr., 29:542, 1974.

133. McCormack, M. K., Coppola-McCormack, P. J., and Lee, M. L.: Autosomal-dominant inheritance of distal arthrogryposis. Am. J. Med. Genet., 6:163, 1980.

134. MacKenzie, D. H.: Arthrogryposis multiplex congenita. Proc. Soc. Med., 52:1106, 1959.

135. Magnus, F.: Ein Fall von multiplex congenitalen contracturen mit Muskeldefecten. Z. Orthop. Chir., 11:424, 1903.

136. Markusfeld, O.: An outbreak of arthrogryposis and hydranencephaly syndrome affecting calves in Israel: a retrospective epidemiological study. Adv. Exp. Med. Biol., 27:527, 1972.

137. Martin, C. L., Vital, C. L., Babin, J. P., Vallat, J. M., and Heheunstre, J. P.: Etude clinique et ultra-structurale d'un cas d'arthrogrypose. Arch. Fr. Pediatr., 28:445, 1971.

138. Masse, P.: Indications operatoires dans l'arthrogry-pose. Ann. Med. Phys., 19:60, 1976.

139. Mead, N. G., Lithgow, W. C., and Sweeney, H. J.: Arthrogryposis multiplex congenita. J. Bone Joint Surg., 40-A:1285, 1958.

140. Mease, A. D., Yeatman, G. W., and Pettett, G.: A syndrome of ankylosis, facial anomalies and pulmonary hypoplasia secondary to foetal neuromuscular dysfunction. Birth Defects, 12:193, 1976.

141. Medrea, O., Gorun, N., and Nailescu, N.: Artrogri-poza multipla congenitala. Rev. Chir., 24:339, 1975.

142. Meerbach, W.: Changes in the skeletal muscles in arthrogryposis multiplex congenita. Zentralbi Allg. Pathol., 115:163, 1972.

143. Mendell, J. R., Engel, W. K., and Derrer, E. C.: Ischemic myopathy reproducing the histological pattern of Duchenne dystrophy. Neurology, 21:451, 1971.

144. Menelaus, M. B.: Talectomy for equinovarus deformity in arthrogryposis and spina bifida. J. Bone Joint Surg., 53-B:468, 1971.

145. Merlini, L., Gualtieri, I., and Gualtieri, G.: Arthro-griposi multipla congenita. Rilievi clinici ed elettro-miografici. Chir. Organi Mov., 62:347, 1975.

146. Meyn, M., and Ruby, L.: Arthrogryposis of the upper extremity. Orthop. Clin. North Am., 7:501, 1976.

147. Middleton, D. S.: Occurrence of incomplete development of the striated muscle fibre as a cause of certain congenital deformities of the extremities. Edinb. Med. J., 39:389, 1932.

148. Middleton, D. S.: Studies on prenatal lesions of striated muscle as a cause of congenital deformity. Edinb. Med. J., 41:401, 1934.

149. Miskin, M., Rothberg, R., Rudd, N. L., Benzie, R. J., and Shime, J.: Arthrogryposis multiplex congenita—prenatal assessment with diagnosis ultrasound and fetoscopy. Brief Clin. Lab. Obs., 95:463, 1979.

150. Miura, Y.: Neutralizing antibody against Akabane virus in procolostral sera from calves with congenital arthrogyposis-hydranencephaly syndrome. Arch. Gesamte Virus-forscn, 46:377, 1974.

151. Moessinger, A. C.: Fetal akinesia deformation sequence: An animal model. Pediatrics, 72:857, 1983.

152. Moriguchi, R., Izawa, H., and Soekawa, M.: A pathological study on calves with arthrogryposis and hydranencephaly. Zbl. Vet. Med., 23:190, 1976.

153. Nezelof, C., Dupart, J. F., and Eliachar, E.: A lethal familial syndrome associating arthrogryposis multiplex congenita, renal dysfunction, and a cholestatic and pigmentary liver disease. J. Pediatr., 94:258, 1979.

154. Nové-Josserand, G., and Rendu, A.: Résultats eloigné et valeur de la methode de Finck dans le traitement prococe de pieds bots congenitaux. Lyon Chir., 8:121, 1918.

155. Oh, W. H.: Arthrogryposis multiplex congenita of the lower extremity; report of two siblings. Orthop. Clin. North Am., 7:511, 1976.

156. Osterberger, M., and Bourret, J.: Le reeducation de l'arthrogrypose (a propos de 4 cas). Ann. Med. Phys., 19:24, 1976.

157. Otto, A. W.: Monstrum humanum extremitatibus incurvatus. Monstrorum Sexcentorum descriptio Anatomica in Vratislaviae Museum. Anatomico-Patholo-gieum Breslau. 1841, p. 322. English translation in Clin. Orthop., 194:4, 1985.

158. Padovani, J. P., Rigault, P., Pouliquen, J. C., Guyon-varch, G., and Durand, Y.: L'astragalectomie chez l'enfant, resultats, technique, indications d'apres notre experience de 33 cas. Rev. Chir. Orthop., 62:475, 1976.

159. Paez, J. H., Tuulonen, A., Yaro, R., Arad, I., Zeli-kovitch, A., and Ben Ezra, D.: Ocular findings in arthrogryposis multiplex congenita. J. Pediatr. Ophthalmol. Strabismus, 19:75, 1982.

160. Palmer, P. M., MacEwen, G. D., Bowen, J. R., and Mathews, P. A.: Passive motion therapy for infants with arthrogryposis. Clin. Orthop., 194:54, 1985.

161. Pedreira, F. A., Long, R. E.: Arthrogryposis multiplex congenita, in one of identical twins. Am. J. Dis. Child., 121:64, 1971.

162. Pena, S. D. J., and Shokeir, M. H. K.: Syndrome of camptodactyly, multiple ankyloses, facial anomalies, and pulmonary hypoplasia: A lethal condition. J. Pediatr., 85:373, 1974.

163. Pena, S. D. J., and Shokeir, M. H. K.: Autosomal recessive cerebro-oculo-facio-skeletal (COFS) syndrome. Clin. Genet., 5:285, 1974.

164. Pilotti, G., Avanzini, P., Castelli, G., et al.: Aspwetti ultrastrutturali del muscolo nell artrogriposi multipla congenita. Minerva Pediatr., 27:1400, 1975.

165. Popihn, H.: Contribution to the surgical treatment of congenital multiple arthrogryposis of the lower extremity. Beitr. Orthop. Traumatol., 27:580, 1980.

166. Pouliquen, J. C., Duval-Beaupere, G., Louvogoy, J., Barois, A., Lebard, J. P., and Rigault, P.: Deviations rachidiennes dans l'arthrogrypose. Am. Med. Phys., 19:42, 1976.

167. Pous, J. G.: Arthrogryposis in childhood. Arthrogryposis multiplex congenita. Chir. Pediatr., 22:289, 1981.

168. Poznanski, A. K., and Larowe, P. C.: Radiographic manifestations of the arthrogryposis syndrome. Radiology, 95:353, 1970.

169. Price, D. L.: The influence of the periphery on spinal motor neurons. Ann. N.Y. Acad. Sci., 228:355, 1976.

170. Price, D. S.: A case of amyoplasia congenita, with pathological report. Arch. Dis. Child., 8:343, 1933.

171. Redard, P.: Contribution a l'étude des contractures congenitales. Gaz. Med. Paris, 8:217, 1913.

172. Reed, S. D., Hall, J. G., Riccardi, V. M., Aylsworth, A., and Timmons, D.: Chromosomal abnormalities associated with congenital contractures (arthrogry-posis). Clin. Genet., 27:353, 1985.

173. Ritsila, V.: Experimental foot deformities. Acta Orthop. Scand., 36:351, 1965.

174. Roberts, J. A. F.: The inheritance of a lethal muscle contracture in sheep. J. Genet., 21:57, 1929.

175. Robertson, G. G., Williamson, A. P., and Blattner, R. J.: A study of abnormalities in early chick embryos inoculated with New Castle disease virus. J. Exp. Zool., 129:5, 1955.

176. Rocher, H. L.: Les raideurs articulaires congenitales multiples. J. Med. Bordeaux, 84:722, 1913.

177. Rosencranz, E.: Ueber kongenitale Kontraturen der oberen Extremitaten. Z. Orthop. Chir., 14:52, 1905.

178. Rosenmann, A., and Arad, I.: Arthrogryposis multiplex congenita: neurogenic type with autosomal recessive inheritance. J. Med. Genet., 11:91, 1974.

179. Rosenkranz, V.: Malformations and anomalies of the foot. Wien Med. Wochenschr., 131:39, 1981.

180. Rossi, E.: Le syndrome arthromyodysplasique congenital. Helv. Paediatr. Acta, 2:82, 1947.

181. Ryckewaert, P. H., Corette, L., Vanhove, J., and Bombart, E.: Syndrome de Marfan et arthrogrypose chez un nouveau-né. Arch. Fr. Pediatr., 32:492, 1975.
182. Sage, F. P.: Congenital anomalies. In Edmondson, A. S., and Crenshaw, A. H. (eds.): Campbell's Operative Orthopedics. 6th Ed. St. Louis, C. V. Mosby, 1980, pp. 1922–1926.
183. Sarwark, J. F., MacEwen, G. D., and Scott, C. I.: Scoliosis in amyoplasia congenita (classic arthrogryposis). Paper No. 51, presented at Scoliosis Research Society, 20th Annual Meeting. Coronado, Calif., September 1985.
184. Schanz, A.: Ein Fall von Multiplen Kongenitalen Kontracturen. Z. Orthop. Chir., 5:9, 1898.
185. Scher, M. A., Handelsman, J. E., and Isaacs, H.: The effect on muscle of immobilisation under tension and relaxation. J. Bone Joint Surg., 59-B:257, 1977.
186. Schmidt, M. A., and Bowers, A.: Avenues—A national support group for arthrogryposis multiplex congenita newsletter: 5430 East Harbor Heights Drive, Port Orchard, Washington 98366.
187. Schnabel, R.: Intrauterine coxsackie B infection in arthrogryposis multiplex congenita syndrome. Verh. Dtsch. Ges. Pathol., 65:311, 1981.
188. Schultz, K., and Weisenbach, J.: Arthrogryposis multiplex congenita. Orv. Hetil., 113:315, 1972.
189. Sedel, L., and Masse, P.: Orthopedie de l'arthrogrypose. Rev. Chir. Orthop., 56:537, 1970.
190. Segawa, M., Mizuno, Y., Itoh, K., and Uono, M.: Neuropathic and myopathic arthrogryposis multiplex congenita. In Kakulas, B. A. (ed.): Clinical Studies in Myology. Amsterdam, Excerpta Medica, 1971, pp. 717–721.
191. Serratrice, G., Gastault, J. L., Pellissier, J. F., and Cros, D.: Etude de deux cas d'arthrogrypose. Rev. Rhum., 44:5, 1977.
192. Shapiro, F., and Brenan, M. J.: Orthopaedic management of childhood neuromuscular disease. Part II: Peripheral neuropathies, Friedreich's ataxia, and arthrogryposis multiplex congenita. J. Bone Joint Surg., 64:949, 1982.
193. Shariff, F. K., Horoupian, D., and Greenlaw, R. K.: Arthrogryposis multiplex congenita. Clin. Orthop., 94:263, 1973.
194. Sheldon, W.: Amyoplasia congenita. (Multiple congenital articular rigidity: Arthrogryposis multiplex congenita.) Arch. Dis. Child., 7:117, 1932.
195. Shepard, M. K.: Arthrogryposis multiplex congenita in sibs. Birth Defects, 7:127, 1971.
196. Siebold, R. M., Winter, R. B., and Moe, J. H.: The treatment of scoliosis in arthrogryposis multiplex congenita. Clin. Orthop., 103:191, 1974.
197. Smith, E. M., Bender, L. F., and Stover, C. N.: Lower motor neuron deficit in arthrogryposis. Arch. Neurol., 8:97, 1963.
198. Smith, R. J.: Hand deformities with arthrogryposis multiplex congenita. J. Bone Joint Surg., 55-A:883, 1973.
199. Soriano, J.: Multiple congenital arthrogryposis as a cause of learning and communicating problems. Bol. Med. Hosp. Infant. Mex., 33:179, 1976.
200. St. Clair, H. S., and Zimbler, S.: A plan of management and treatment results in the arthrogrypotic hip. Clin. Orthop., 194:74, 1985.
201. Steindler, A.: A muscle plasty for the relief of the flail elbow in infantile paralysis. Interstate Med. J., 5:235, 1918.
202. Steindler, A.: Arthrogryposis. J. Int. Coll. Surg., 12:21, 1949.
203. Stern, W. G.: Arthrogryposis multiplex congenita. J.A.M.A., 81:1507, 1923.
204. Swinyard, C. A., and Bleck, E. E.: The etiology of arthrogryposis (multiple congenital contractures). Clin. Orthop., 194:15, 1985.

205. Swinyard, C. A., and Mayer, V.: Multiplex congenital contractures. Public health considerations of arthrogryposis multiplex congenita. J.A.M.A., 183:23, 1963.
206. Szabo, L., and Perjes, K.: Uber die Differenzierung der Arthrogryposis multiplex congenita und des Larsen-Syndroms. Z. Orthop., 112:1275, 1974.
207. Thompson, G. H., and Bilenko, R. M.: Comprehensive management arthrogryposis multiplex congenita. Clin. Orthop., 194:6, 1985.
208. Tompkins, S. F., Miller, R. J., and O'Donoghue, D. H.: An evaluation of astragalectomy. South. Med. J., 49:1128, 1956.
209. Trellu, M.: Arthrogrypose chez des jumelles. Ann. Med. Phys., 19:11, 1976.
210. Turkel, S. B., Iseri, A. L., and Fujimoto, A. O.: Malformation complex. Spondylohypoplasia, arthrogryposis, and popliteal pterygium. Am. J. Dis. Child., 134:42, 1980.
211. Twomey, M. R.: Arthrogryposis multiplex congenita. Nurs. Times, 72:1117, 1976.
212. Vallat, J. M.: Les hypotonies congenitales d'origine myogene ou myopathies congenitales. Bordeaux, These Med., 1972.
213. Vallat, J. M., and Vital, C.: Etude anatomique et ultrastructurale d'un cas d'arthrogrypose. Acta Pathol. Neuro-Musc., L'Expansion, Paris, 1971.
214. Verger, P., Vital, Cl., Guillard, J. M., Vallat, J. M., and Leblanc: Etude ultra-structurale de certaines amyotrophies neurogenes precoces. Pediatrics, 25:377, 1970.
215. Verhagen, A. D.: Gastroschisis and congenital contractures: Coincidence or syndrome? J. Pediatr. Surg., 16:605, 1981.
216. Warkany, J.: Congenital Malformations. Chicago, Year Book Medical Publishers, 1971, p. 1011.
217. Weeks, P. M.: Surgical correction of upper extremity deformities in arthrogrypotics. Plast. Reconstr. Surg., 36:459, 1965.
218. Whitman, R.: The operative treatment of paralytic talipes of the calcaneus type. Trans. Am. Orthop. Assoc., 14:178, 1901.
219. Whitman, R.: The operative treatment of paralytic talipes of the calcaneus type. Am. J. Med. Sci., 122:593, 1901.
220. Whitman, R.: Further observations on the treatment of paralytic talipes calcaneus by astragalectomy and backward displacement of the foot. Ann. Surg., 47:264, 1908.
221. Whitman, R.: Further observations on the operative treatment of paralytic talipes of the calcaneus type. Am. J. Orthop. Surg., 8:137, 1910.
222. Whittem, J. H.: Congenital abnormalities in calves: Arthrogryposis and hydranencephaly. J. Pathol. Bacteriol., 73:375, 1957.
223. Williams, P. F.: The elbow in arthrogryposis. J. Bone Joint Surg., 55-B:834, 1973.
224. Williams, P. F.: The management of arthrogryposis multiplex. Orthop. Clin. North Am., 9:67, 1978.
225. Williams, P. F.: Management of upper limb problems in arthrogryposis. Clin. Orthop., 194:60, 1985.
226. Wolf, A., Roverud, E., Poser, C.: Amyoplasia congenita. Neuropathol. Exp. Neurol., 14:112, 1955.
227. Wyatt, S., Beach, R. C., Stuart, C., and Hallett, R. J.: Cluster of cases of arthrogryposis (Letter). Lancet, 1:713, 1983.
229. Wyckoff, E., and Mitani, M.: The spoon plate: a self feeding device. Am. J. Occup. Ther., 36:333, 1982.
230. Wynne-Davies, R.: Heritable disorders in orthopedics. Orthop. Clin. North Am., 9:39, 1978.
231. Wynne-Davies, R., and Lloyd-Roberts, G. C.: Search for prenatal factor in 66 sporadic cases of arthrogryposis multiplex congenita. Arch. Dis. Child., 51:618, 1976.

232. Wynne-Davies, R., Williams, P. F., and O'Connor, J. C.: The 1960's epidemic of arthrogryposis multiplex congenita: a survey from the United Kingdom, Australia and the United States of America. J. Bone Joint Surg., *63-B*:76, 1981.

233. Yonenobu, K., Tada, K., and Swanson, A. B.: Arthrogryposis of the hand. J. Pediatr. Orthop., *4*:599, 1984.

234. Yuill, G. M., and Lynch, P. G.: Congenital non-progressive peripheral neuropathy with arthrogryposis multiplex. J. Neurol. Neurosurg. Psychiatry, *37*:316, 1974.

235. Zimbler, S., and Craig, C. L.: The arthrogrypotic foot plan of management and results of treatment. Foot Ankle, *3*:211, 1983.

Affections of Muscles
Congenital Anomalies of Muscles

CONGENITAL ABSENCE OF MUSCLES

Developmental abnormalities in the fetus may lead to hypoplasia or aplasia of various skeletal muscles. Any of the voluntary muscles may be congenitally absent in whole or in part, but certain muscles are deficient more frequently than others. The pectoralis, particularly the sternocostal part of the pectoralis major, is most commonly involved.[7, 25] Next in order of frequency are the trapezius, quadratus femoris, serratus magnus, omohyoideus, semimembranosus, brachioradialis, abdominis, deltoid, latissimus dorsi, sternocleidomastoid, rhomboid, supraspinatus and infraspinatus, biceps brachii, thenar or hypothenar of the hand, and quadriceps femoris.[4, 18]

Usually the abnormality is discovered at birth or soon afterward. It tends to be unilateral and may involve a single muscle or a related group of muscles. The resulting functional disability remains static.

Congenital absence of a muscle may be combined with congenital abnormalities of the organs. Some of the best known examples of these are agenesis of the pectoral muscles in conjunction with syndactyly or microdactyly, and malformation of the genitourinary and alimentary tracts associated with congenital absence of the abdominal musculature (prune belly).[3, 6, 7, 17, 30, 31, 33]

References

1. Armendares, S.: Absence of pectoralis major muscle in two sisters associated with leukemia in one of them. J. Pediatr., *85*:436, 1974.
2. Bailey, J. A.: Gross anatomy of a congenitally deformed upper limb. Bull. Hosp. Joint Dis., *29*:48, 1968.
3. Beals, R. K., and Crawford, S.: Congenital absence of the pectoral muscles. A review of twenty-five patients. Clin. Orthop., *119*:166, 1976.
4. Bing, R.: Ueber angeborene Muskeldefecte. Virchows Arch. Pathol. Anat., *170*:175, 1902.
5. Boaz, D., Mace, J. W., and Gotlin, R. W.: Poland's syndrome and leukemia. Lancet, *1*:349, 1971.
6. Brown, J. B., and McDowell, I.: Syndactylism with absence of the pectoralis major. Surgery, *7*:599, 1940.
7. Christopher, F.: Congenital absence of the pectoral muscles. J. Bone Joint Surg., *10*:350, 1928.
8. Clarkson, P.: Poland's syndactyly. Guys Hosp. Rep., *111*:335, 1962.
9. David, T. J.: Nature and etiology of the Poland anomaly. N. Engl. J. Med., *287*:487, 1972.
10. Dellon, A. L., and Rayan, G.: Congenital absence of the thenar muscles. Report of two cases. J. Bone Joint Surg., *63-A*:1014, 1981.
11. Gordon, H.: A case of Poland's syndrome: congenital unilateral brachysyndactyly with partial absence of the pectoralis major muscle. S. Afr. Med. J., *14*:285, 1970.
12. Gorlin, J. R., and Sedano, H.: Mobius syndrome. Mod. Med., *40*:110, 1972.
13. Hoefnagel, D., Rozycki, A., Wurster-Hill, D., Stern, P., and Gregory, D.: Leukemia and Poland's syndrome. Lancet, *2*:1038, 1972.
14. Horan, F. T., and Bonafede, R. P.: Bilateral absence of the trapezius and sternal head of the pectoralis major muscles. A case report. J. Bone Joint Surg., *59-A*:133, 1977.
15. Ireland, D. C., Takayama, N., and Flatt, A. E.: Poland's syndrome. J. Bone Joint Surg., *58-A*:52, 1976.
16. Joller, R., and Scheier, H.: Complete thoracic segment insensibility accompanying prune belly syndrome with scoliosis. Spine, *11*:496, 1986.
17. Krabbe, K.: Les lesions embryonnaires à la lumière des defectuosites mammaire et pectorale de la syndactylie et de la microdactylie. Acta Psychiatr. Neurol., *24*:539, 1949.
18. LeDouble, A. F.: Traite des Variations de Systeme Musculaire de l'Homme et Leur Signification au Point de Vue de l'Anthropologie Zoologique. Paris, Schleicher Frères, 1897.
19. Lewis, K. B., Bruce, R. A., Baum, D., and Motulsky, A. G.: The upper limb-cardiovascular syndrome. J.A.M.A., *193*:1080, 1965.
20. McCarroll, H. R., Jr., and Manske, P. R.: Congenital absence of the thenar muscles (Letter). J. Bone Joint Surg., *64-A*:153, 1982.
21. Mace, J. W., Kaplan, J. M., Schanberger, J. E., and Gotlin, R. W.: Poland's syndrome report of seven cases and review of the literature. Clin. Pediatr., *11*:98, 1972.
22. Menelaus, M. B.: Radial club hand with absence of the biceps muscle treated by centralixation of the ulna and triceps transfer. Report of two cases. J. Bone Joint Surg., *58-B*:488, 1976.
23. Miller, R. A., and Miller, D. R.: Congenital absence of the pectoralis major muscle with acute lymphoblastic leukemia and genitourinary anomalies. J. Pediatr., *87*:146, 1975.
24. Miura, T.: Congenital absence of the flexor pollicis longus—a case report. Hand, *9*:272, 1977.
25. Morley, E. B.: Congenital defect of pectoral muscle. Lancet, *1*:1101, 1923.
26. Neviaser, R. J.: Congenital hypoplasia of the thumb with absence of the extrinsic extensors, abductor pollicis longus and thenar muscles. J. Hand Surg., *4*:301, 1979.

27. Peterson, B. P., Pardo, J. M., and Bond, E. C.: Poland syndrome: a new presentation (Letter). J. Pediatr., 90:843, 1977.
28. Poland, A.: Deficiency of the pectoral muscles. Guys Hosp. Rep., 6:191, 1841.
29. Rayan, G. M.: Congenital hypoplastic thumb with absent thenar muscles: anomalous digital neurovascular bundle. J. Hand Surg., 9-A:665, 1984.
30. Resnick, E.: Congenital unilateral absence of the pectoral muscles of often associated with syndactylism. J. Bone Joint Surg., 24:925, 1942.
31. Silverman, F. N., and Huang, N.: Congenital absence of the abdominal muscles associated with malformations of the genitourinary and alimentary tracts: Report of cases and review of literature. Am. J. Dis. Child., 80:91, 1950.
32. Temtamy, S., and McKusick, V. A.: Synopsis of hand malformations with particular emphasis on genetic factors. Birth Defects, 5:125, 1969.
33. Tuch, B. A., and Smith, T. K.: Prune-belly syndrome: a report of twelve cases and review of the literature. J. Bone Joint Surg., 60-A:109, 1978.
34. Uchida, M., Kojima, T., and Sakurai, N.: Congenital absence of flexor pollicis longus without hypoplasia of thenar muscles. Plast. Reconstr. Surg., 75:413, 1985.
35. Walters, T. R., Reddy, B. N., Ballon, A., and Vitale, L. F.: Poland's syndrome associated with leukemia. Pediatrics, 82:889, 1973.
36. Wolfson, R. B.: Syndactyly. A review of 122 cases. Proc. Western Orthop. Assoc. J. Bone Joint Surg., 53-A:395, 1971.

ACCESSORY MUSCLES

Supernumerary muscles are rare. In the limbs, they often simulate soft-tissue tumors, and because of the possibility of malignancy, surgical exploration is carried out. Dunn reported two cases of soleus accessorius muscles, both of which appeared bilaterally as a mass anteromedial to the Achilles tendon (Fig. 5–205).[8] An anomalous accessory hamstring muscle may be manifest as a popliteal swelling (Fig. 5–206). This usually originates from the linea aspera of the femur and passes medially to insert into the dorsal part of the capsule of the knee joint.[8, 14]

In the hand, Lipscomb described a duplication of the hypothenar muscle that was explored on the assumption that it was a tumor.[19] Anomalies of the extensor indicis muscle have been described.[6] When it is a short muscle and arises from the distal end of the radius, proximal carpal bones, or related ligaments, it is called extensor digitorum brevis manus. This usually is mistaken for a ganglion or other soft-tissue tumor.

An accessory palmaris muscle may present clinically as a mass that produces symptoms by compression of the subjacent nerves and tendons.[25] This anomalous muscle usually arises from the palmaris longus tendon and inserts into the ulnar border of the hand. The mass will enlarge on flexion and ulnar deviation of the wrist, and will decrease in size or disappear on wrist extension.

References

1. Apple, J. S., Martinez, S., Khoury, M. B., and Nunley, J. A.: Case report 376: Accessory (anomalous) soleus muscle. Skeletal Radiol., 15:398, 1986.
2. Bardeen, C. R.: Development and variation of nerves and musculature of the inferior extremity and neighboring regions of the trunk in man. J. Anat., 6:259, 1907.
3. Beasley, A. W.: The accessory soleus. Aust. N.Z. J. Surg., 49:86, 1969.
4. Bejjani, F. J., and Jahss, M. H.: Le Double's study of muscle variations of the human body. Part II: Muscle variations of the foot. Foot Ankle, 6:157, 1986.
5. Bonnell, J., and Cruess, R.: Anomalous insertion of the soleus muscle as a cause of fixed equinus deformity (Case report). J. Bone Joint Surg., 51-A:999, 1969.
6. Cauldwell, E. W., Anson, B. J., and Wright, R. R.: The extensor indicis proprius muscle. A study of 263 consecutive specimens. Q. Bull. Northwestern Univ. Med. School, 17:267, 1943.
7. Dokter, G., and Linclau, L. A.: The accessory soleus muscle: symptomatic soft tissue tumour or accidental finding. Neth. J. Surg., 33:146, 1981.
8. Dunn, A. W.: Anomalous muscles simulating soft tissue tumors in the lower extremities. Report of three cases. J. Bone Joint Surg., 47-A:1397, 1965.
9. Dunn, A. W., and Evarts, C. M.: The extensor digitorum brevis manus muscle: A case report. Clin. Orthop., 28:210, 1963.
10. Ger, R., and Sedlin, E.: The accessory soleus muscle. Clin. Orthop., 116:200, 1976.
11. Gordon, S. L., and Matheson, D. W.: The accessory soleus. Clin. Orthop., 97:129, 1973.
12. Graham, C. E.: Accessory soleus muscle. Med. J. Aust., 2:574, 1980.
13. Graham, C. E.: The accessory soleus muscle (Letter). Clin. Orthop., 205:311, 1986.
14. Gray, D. J.: Some anomalous hamstring muscles. Anat. Rec., 91:33, 1945.
15. Humphrey, G. M.: Observations in Myology. London, Macmillan & Co., 1872.
16. Jones, B. W.: An anomalous extensor indicis muscle. J. Bone Joint Surg., 41-B:763, 1959.
17. King, T. S., and O'Rahilly, R.: Muscle palmaris accessorius and duplication of muscle palmaris longus. Acta Anat. (Basel), 10:327, 1950.
18. LeDouble, A. F.: Traite de Variations du Systeme Musculaire de l'Homme et deleur Signification au Point de Vue de l'Anthropologie Zoologique. Paris, Schleicher Freres, 1897.
19. Lipscomb, P. R.: Duplication of hypothenar muscles simulating soft tissue of the hand. Report of a case. J. Bone Joint Surg., 42-A:1058, 1960.
20. Nichols, G. W., and Kalenak, A.: The accessory soleus muscle. Clin. Orthop., 190:279, 1984.
21. Nidecker, A. C., von Hochstetter, A., and Fredenhagen, H.: Accessory muscles of the lower calf. Radiology, 151:47, 1984.
22. Percy, E. C., and Telep, G. N.: Anomalous muscle in the leg: soleus accessorium. Am. J. Sports Med., 12:447, 1984.
23. Romanus, B., Lindahl, S., and Stener, B.: Accessory soleus muscle. A clinical and radiographic presentation of eleven cases. J. Bone Joint Surg., 68-A:731, 1986.
24. Thomas, C. G., Jr.: Clinical manifestation of an accessory palmaris muscle. J. Bone Joint Surg., 40-A:929, 1958.
25. Tountas, C. P., and Halikman, L. A.: An anomalous flexor digitorum sublimis muscle. A case report. Clin. Orthop., 121:230, 1976.

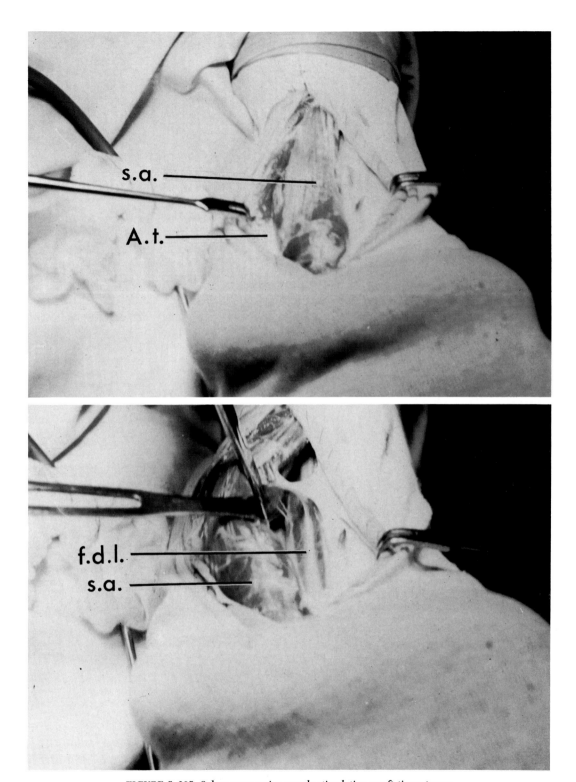

FIGURE 5–205. Soleus accessorius muscle stimulating a soft-tissue tumor.

Gross appearance at surgery. s.a., Soleus accessorius muscle; A.t., Achilles tendon; f.d.l., flexor digitorum longus muscle and tendon. (From Dunn, A. W.: Anomalous muscles simulating soft tissue tumors in the lower extremities. J. Bone Joint Surg., *47-A*:1398, 1965. Reprinted by permission.)

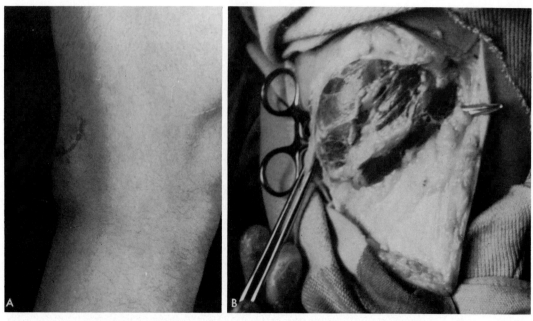

FIGURE 5–206. Anomalous hamstring muscle presenting as a popliteal mass.

A. Clinical appearance. **B.** Findings at operation. Note that muscle crosses the popliteal fossa from the lateral to the medial side. The thumb forceps is pulling the semitendinosus tendon medially. (From Dunn, A. W.: Anomalous muscles simulating soft tissue tumors in the lower extremities. J. Bone Joint Surg., 47-A:1399, 1965. Reprinted by permission.)

IDIOPATHIC FIBROSIS OF MUSCLES

Progressive Fibrosis of Quadriceps Muscle

In this rare affliction of early childhood there is insidious development of extension contracture of the knee due to progressive fibrosis of one or more components of the quadriceps muscle. The condition is preponderant in girls. The exact cause is unknown. Hnevkovsky, who first described the entity in 1961, believed the fibrosis to be the result of muscular dysplasia of congenital origin.[33] Because of the resemblance of its histologic picture to that of contracture of the sternocleidomastoid muscle in congenital muscular torticollis, a similar pathogenesis for the two conditions has been suggested by others.[14, 20, 22] A number of authors have proposed the cause to be multiple injections of antibiotics into the thigh muscles in early infancy.[26, 44, 76]

The distal portion of the quadriceps muscle is principally involved, the vastus intermedius being affected most frequently. There is fibrosis within and between the muscle fibers. The subcutaneous adipose tissue may be decreased over the affected area. A dimple in the skin produced by the rigid fibrous septa that extend between the skin and deep fascia may be pres-

ent and will deepen on forced flexion of the knee. Painless and progressive limitation of knee flexion is the principal clinical finding (Figs. 5–207 and 5–208). The patella will be high-riding.

The contracture does not respond to passive stretching exercises or to other conservative measures. Treatment is by surgical division and lengthening of the fibrotic portion of the quadriceps muscle. Postoperatively the knee is immobilized in 90 degrees of flexion for three weeks. Active and passive exercises are then performed to obtain full range of knee motion.

This author has seen one case of idiopathic fibrosis of the proximal part of the rectus femoris muscle. The resultant deformity was flexion contracture of the hip and limited flexion of the knee.

Deltoid Muscle

A similar condition occurring in the deltoid muscle has been described by several authors.[4, 9, 23, 43, 75] Abduction contracture of the shoulder is produced when the intermediate part of the deltoid muscle is fibrosed, whereas fibrosis of the anterior part of the deltoid muscle will result in flexion contracture of the shoulder. Treatment is by surgical division of the fibrous band.

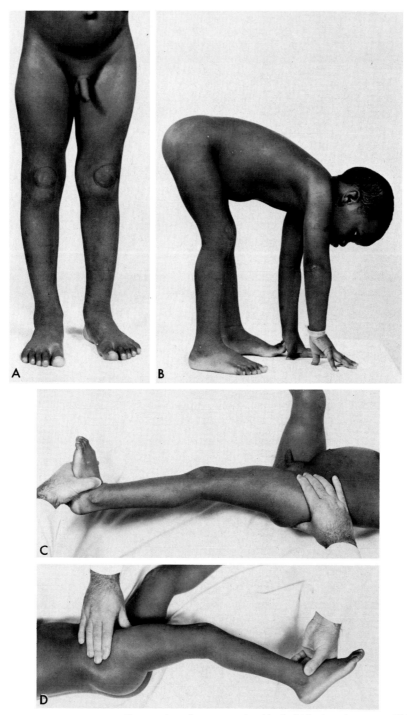

FIGURE 5–207. *Progressive fibrosis of quadriceps muscle of both thighs in a three-year-old boy.*

In early infancy this child had multiple injections of antibiotics in both thighs for treatment of pneumonia. **A.** Standing view showing the high-riding patellae. **B.** He cannot flex his knees to squat. **C** and **D.** These demonstrate the maximum range of passive flexion of both knees. At surgery, fibrosis of the vastus intermedius and vastus lateralis muscles was found.

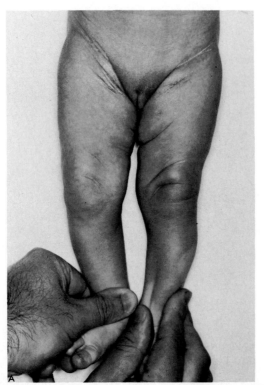

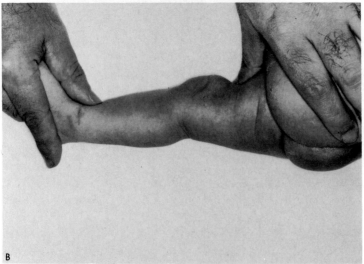

FIGURE 5–208. Progressive fibrosis of left quadriceps muscle in a five-month-old child who was the product of a premature birth.

A. Note the scars of bilateral femoral vein cutdowns for infusion. She also received multiple antibiotic injections in her thighs. **B.** The maximum range of passive flexion of the left knee. Passive exercises and corrective casts failed to improve range of left knee motion. At surgery, the vastus lateralis, vastus intermedius, and rectus femoris were found to be fibrosed.

References

1. Alvarez, E. V., Munters, M., Lavne, L. S., Manes, H., and Waxman, J.: Quadriceps myofibrosis. A complication of intramuscular injections. J. Bone Joint Surg., 62-A:58, 1980.
2. Aparo, C. J. P.: Ginocchio rigido fell'infanzia retrazione del quadricipite du iniezioni. Chir. Organi Mov., 59:506, 1971.
3. Babhulkar, S. S.: Triceps contracture caused by injections. A report of 11 cases. J. Bone Joint Surg., 67-B:94, 1985.
4. Bhattacharyya, D.: Abduction contracture of the shoulder from contracture of the intermediate part of the deltoid. J. Bone Joint Surg., 48-B:127, 1966.
5. Blum, J. L.: Contracture of the vastus intermedius in children. A review of the literature and presentation of two cases. South. Med. J., 65:1501, 1972.
6. Bose, K., and Chong, K. C.: The clinical manifestations and pathomechanics of contracture of the extensor mechanism of the knee. J. Bone Joint Surg., 58-B:478, 1976.
7. Calandriello, B., and Beltrami, P.: Ginocchio rigido del bambino da retrazione del quadricipite. Chir. Organi Mov., 56:427, 1968.
8. Canadell, J., Beguiristain, J. L., Gili, J., Reparaz, B., Itiurri, G., and Ayala, H.: Fibrose du quadriceps. Acta Orthop. Belg., 41:299, 1975.
9. Cellarius, T. L.: Die Abduktionskonkraktur im Schultergelenk. Chirurg, 19:221, 1948.
10. Chiu, S. S., Furuya, K., Arai, T., Nakagawa, M., and Iida, M.: Congenital contracture of the quadriceps muscle: four case reports in identical twins. J. Bone Joint Surg., 56-A:1054, 1974.
11. Chiu, S. S., Mano, J., Yukawa, Y. N., Kamakura, T. K., and Hyama, T.: Contracture of the quadriceps muscle caused by injection. Acta Orthop. Belg., 41:306, 1975.
12. Coleman, S. S., and Simpson, S.: Gait disturbances due to idiopathic contracture of thigh musculature. In Proceedings. J. Bone Joint Surg., 49-A:1481, 1967.
13. Cozen, L. N.: Pentazocine injections as a causative factor in dislocation of the shoulder. J. Bone Joint Surg., 59-A:979, 1977.
14. Csink, L., and Imrie, J.: Isolated contracture of rectus femoris muscle. J. Bone Joint Surg., 45-B:145, 1963.
15. Daoud, H., O'Farrell, T., and Cruess, R. L.: Quadricepsplasty. The Judet technique and results of six cases. J. Bone Joint Surg., 64-B:194, 1982.
16. Dufek, M.: Contribution à la discussion sur l'etiologie de la fibrose du muscle crural chez l'enfant. Acta Chir. Ortop. Traumatol. Cech., 29:149, 1962.
17. Duran, S. H., Sanchez-Barba, A., Lopez-Duran Stern, L., Mendez Martin, J., Linan, C., and Ferrandez, L.: Fibrosis of the gluteal muscles. Report of three cases. J. Bone Joint Surg., 56-A:1510, 1974.
18. Engel, W. K.: Focal myopathic changes produced by electromyographic and hypodermic needles: "needle myopathy." Arch. Neurol., 16:509, 1967.
19. Euliano, J. J.: Fibrosis of the quadriceps mechanism in children. Clin. Orthop., 70:181, 1970.
20. Fairbank, T. J., and Barett, A. M.: Vastus intermedius contracture in early childhood. Case report of identical twins. J. Bone Joint Surg., 43-B:326, 1961.
21. Fernandez de Valderrama, J. A., et al.: Fibrosis of the gluteus maximus: a cause of limited flexion and adduction of the hip in children. Clin. Orthop., 156:67, 1981.
22. Gammie, W. F. P., Taylor, J. H., and Ursch, H.: Contracture of the vastus intermedius in children. A report of two cases. J. Bone Joint Surg., 45-B:370, 1963.
23. Goodfellow, J. W., and Nade, S.: Flexion contracture of the shoulder from fibrosis of the anterior part of the deltoid muscle. J. Bone Joint Surg., 51-B:356, 1969.
24. Gray, J. E.: Local histological changes following long-term intramuscular injections. Arch. Pathol. Lab. Med., 84:522, 1967.
25. Gunn, D. R.: Contracture of the quadriceps muscle. J. Bone Joint Surg., 46-B:492, 1964.
26. Hagen, R.: Contracture of the quadriceps muscle in children. Acta Orthop. Scand., 39:565, 1968.
27. Hang, Y. S., et al.: Abduction contracture of the shoulder. A report of two patients. Acta Orthop. Scand., 49:154, 1978.
28. Harrold, A. J.: Rigid valgus foot from fibrous contracture of the peronei. J. Bone Joint Surg., 47-B:743, 1965.
29. Hashimoto, M.: A case of congenital deltoid contracture. Orthop. Surg. (Tokyo), 19:1259, 1968.
30. Hayashi, T., and Sugiura, Y.: Three cases of the deltoid contracture. Tohoku Arch. Orthop. Surg. Traumatol. (Sendai), 15:383, 1970.
31. Hessel, G., Martens, M., Thibaut, H., Fabry, G., and Mullier, J. C.: Progressive contracture of the quadriceps in children. Acta Orthop. Belg., 41:274, 1975.
32. Hill, N. A., Liebler, W. A., Wilson, H. J., and Rosenthal, E.: Abduction contracture of both glenohumeral joints and extension contracture of one knee secondary to partial muscle fibrosis. J. Bone Joint Surg., 49-A:961, 1967.
33. Hnevkovsky, O.: Progressive fibrosis of the vastus intermedius muscle in children. A cause of limited knee flexion and elevation of the patella. J. Bone Joint Surg., 43-B:318, 1961.
34. Hollaert, P., Adijns, P., Destoop, N., De Witte, E., and Claessens, H.: Review of the literature on quadriceps fibrosis and study of 11 cases. Acta Orthop. Belg., 41:255, 1975.
35. Howard, R. C.: Iatrogenic quadriceps and gluteal fibrosis. In Proceedings. J. Bone Joint Surg., 53-B:354, 1971.
36. Jackson, A. M., and Hutton, P. A. N.: Injection-induced contractures of the quadriceps in childhood. A comparison of proximal release and distal quadricepsplasty. J. Bone Joint Surg., 67-B:97, 1985.
37. Jerotic, R., Nikolic, G., Rajic, D., and Stojanovic, L.: Rehabilitation of post-injection contractures of the quadriceps tissues in children. Srp. Arh. Celok. Lek., 103:59, 1975.
38. Kaneko, M., and Maeda, H.: A case of the deltoid contracture. J. Jpn. Orthop. Assoc., 42:912, 1968.
39. Karlen, A.: Congenital fibrosis of the vastus intermedius muscle. J. Bone Joint Surg., 46-B:488, 1964.
40. Katz, M. M., and Mubarak, S. J.: Hereditary tendo Achilles contractures. J. Pediatr. Orthop., 4:711, 1984.
41. Konkel, K. F., and Lucas, G. L.: Abduction contracture of the shoulders. A case report. Clin. Orthop., 104:224, 1974.
42. Lehart, G., and Killmann, L.: Isolated contracture of the rectus femoris muscle. Clin. Orthop., 99:125, 1974.
43. Lerch, H.: Die Abduktions Kontraktur im Schultergelenk. Chirurg, 20:675, 1949.
44. Lloyd-Roberts, G. C., and Thomas, T. G.: The etiology of quadriceps contracture in children. J. Bone Joint Surg., 46-B:498, 1964.
45. Ludescher, E.: Infantile quadratus femoris kontraktur nach intramusculaten injektionen. Padiatr. Padol., 7:288, 1972.
46. Makhani, J. S.: Quadriceps fibrosis: a complication of intra-muscular injections in the thigh. Indian J. Pediatr., 38:54, 1971.
47. Makhani, J. S.: Osteoarticular lesions in quadriceps fibrosis. Indian J. Radiol., 25:179, 1971.
48. Malek, R.: Retractions quadricipitales et injections intra-musculaires chez l'enfant. Ann. Chir. Infant., 7:85, 1966.
49. Malek, R., and Arama, S.: Retractions quadricipitales chez l'enfant. Acta Orthop. Belg., 41:267, 1975.

50. Manske, P. R.: Deltoid muscle abduction contracture. Clin. Orthop., *128*:165, 1977.
51. Masse, P.: Fibrose du quadriceps ou des fessiers chez l'enfant. Signes radiologiques des fibroses du quadriceps. Acta Orthop. Belg., *41*:316, 1975.
52. Masse, P., Poujol, J., and Bigan, R.: A propos de trois cas d'enradissement en extension du genou par fibrose progressive du quadriceps chez l'enfant. Arch. Fr. Pediatr., *22*:697, 1965.
53. Minami, M., Ishii, S., Usui, M., and Terashima, Y.: The deltoid contracture. Clin. Orthop. Surg. (Tokyo), *11*:493, 1976.
54. Minami, M., Yamazaki, J., Minami, A., and Ishii, S.: A postoperative long-term study of the deltoid contracture in children. J. Pediatr. Orthop., *4*:609, 1984.
55. Mukherjee, P. K., and Das, K.: Injection fibrosis in the quadriceps femoris muscle in children. J. Bone Joint Surg., *62-A*:453, 1980.
56. Murakami, H., Kumagai, S., Mizushima, T., Ando, K., and Katada, S.: Fourteen cases of the deltoid contracture. *In* Proceedings of the 24th East Japanese Clinical Orthopedic Meeting, Niigata, 1975.
57. Nakaya, M., Kumon, Y., and Fujiwara, M.: Two cases of the congenital deltoid contracture. Orthop. Surg. (Tokyo), *22*:814, 1971.
58. Nielsen, A. H. O., and Nielsen, J. L.: Contracture of the quadriceps muscle in children. A complication of intramuscular injections. Ugeskr. Laeger, *136*:2690, 1974.
59. Norman, M. G., Temple, A. R., and Murphy, J. V.: Infantile quadriceps-femoris contracture resulting from intramuscular injections. N. Engl. J. Med., *282*:964, 1970.
60. Ogawa, S., Abe, Y., and Fujita, S.: Two cases of the deltoid contracture. J. Jpn. Orthop. Assoc., *43*:178, 1969.
61. Oh, I., Smith, J. A., Spencer, G. E., Jr., Frankel, V. H., and Mack, R. P.: Fibrous contracture of muscles following intramuscular injections in adults. Clin. Orthop., *127*:214, 1977.
62. Oh, S. J., Rollins, J. L., and Lewis, I.: Pentazocine-induced fibrous myopathy. J.A.M.A., *231*:271, 1975.
63. Oyoshi, K., and Minami, M.: Two cases of the deltoid contracture. Hokkaido J. Orthop. Trauma Surg. (Sapporo), *13*:165, 1968.
64. Paralkar, A. N.: Genu recurvatum in quadriceps contracture following intramuscular injection in thigh. Indian J. Surg., *39*:295, 1977.
65. Pavillon, P., and Chabrol, J.: Paralysies du quadriceps. Traitement chirurgical. Resultats et indications therapeutiques. Rev. Chir. Orthop., *59*:263, 1973.
66. Peiro, A., Ildefonso, F. C., and Gomar, F.: Gluteal fibrosis. J. Bone Joint Surg., *57-A*:987, 1975.
67. Pipino, F., et al.: Gluteal fibrosis. Ital. J. Orthop. Traumatol., *3*:75, 1977.
68. Pouliquen, J. C., Figault, P., and Judet, J.: Retraction du quadriceps apres injections medicamenteuses chez l'enfant. Ann. Pediatr., *19*:613, 1972.
69. Roberson, J. R., and Dimon, J. H.: Myofibrosis and joint contractures caused by injections of pentazocine. A case report. J. Bone Joint Surg., *65-A*:1007, 1983.
70. Roland, R., and Warren, D.: Abduction deformity of the shoulder secondary to fibrosis of the central portion of the deltoid muscle. Read at the Annual Meeting of the A.A.O.S., Washington, D.C., 1972.
71. Sacristan, M., Sanchez-Barba, A., Stern, L. L-D., and Martin, J. M.: Fibrosis of gluteal muscles. Report of three cases. J. Bone Joint Surg., *56-A*:1510, 1974.
72. Sanmugasundaran, T. K.: Fibrosis of the quadriceps. J. Bone Joint Surg., *49-B*:801, 1967.
73. Sanmugasundaran, T. K.: Post-injection fibrosis of skeletal muscle: a clinical problem. A personal series of 169 cases. Int. Orthop., *4*:31, 1980.
74. Sarkar, P. K., and Das Gupta, S.: Management of stiff knee in children. J. Indian Med. Assoc., *69*:195, 1977.
75. Sato, M., Honda, S., and Inoue, H.: Three cases of abduction contracture of the shoulder caused by fibrosis of the deltoid muscle. Orthop. Surg. (Tokyo), *16*:1052, 1965.
76. Saunders, F. P., Hoefnagel, D., and Staples, O. S.: Progressive fibrosis of the quadriceps muscle. J. Bone Joint Surg., *47-A*:380, 1965.
77. See, G., Briard, J., and Czernichoq, P.: Fibrose du quadriceps consecutive a des injections intra-musculaires pratiquees chez le prematute et le nourrisson. Ann. Pediatr., *15*:104, 1968.
78. Seibold, J. R.: Digital sclerosis in children with insulin-dependent diabetes mellitus. Arthritis Rheum., *25*:1357, 1982.
79. Sengupta, S.: Pathogenesis of infantile quadriceps fibrosis and its correction by proximal release. J. Pediatr. Orthop., *5*:187, 1985.
80. Shahane, M. N.: Quadriceps contracture. J. Bone Joint Surg., *49-B*:800, 1967.
81. Shen, Y. S.: Gluteus maximus contracture. Clin. Orthop., *162*:185, 1982.
82. Stark, W. A.: Quadriceps contracture in children. Am. J. Dis. Child., *120*:349, 1970.
83. Steiner, J. C., Winkelman, A. C., and De Jesus, P. V., Jr.: Pentazocine-induced fibrous myopathy. Arch. Neurol., *28*:408, 1973.
84. Takagi, K., and Tsuyama, N.: The quadriceps contracture. Ijin. Yakujin (Tokyo), *24*:25, 1975.
85. Theodorou, S. D.: Fibrosis and contracture of the quadriceps muscle in children. Acta Orthop. Belg., *41*:285, 1975.
86. Thompson, T. C.: Quadriceps plasty to improve knee function. J. Bone Joint Surg., *26*:366, 1944.
87. Todd, J. V.: Intramuscular injections. Br. Med. J., *2*:1362, 1961.
88. Tokarowski, A., and Skawinska, E.: Progressive scarring of quadriceps muscle in children. Chir. Narzadow Ruchu Ortop. Pol., *33*:385, 1968.
89. Verma, B. P., and Chandra, U.: Bilateral ankylosis of elbows in extension due to contracture of the triceps: a case report. Int. Surg., *52*:337, 1969.
90. Viladot, A., et al.: Gluteal fibrosis. Ital. J. Orthop. Traumatol., *2*:239, 1976.
91. Williams, P. H.: Quadriceps contracture. J. Bone Joint Surg., *50-B*:278, 1968.
92. Wolbrink, A. J., Hsu, Z., and Bianco, A. J.: Abduction contracture of the shoulders and hips secondary to fibrous bands. J. Bone Joint Surg., *55-A*:844, 1973.
93. Wrighton, J. J.: Quadriceps contracture in infancy and childhood. Acta Orthop. Belg., *41*:259, 1975.
94. Yamaguchi, M., Izumida, S., Murakami, H., and Kumagai, S.: Three cases of the deltoid contracture after intermuscular injections. Orthop. Surg. (Tokyo), *21*:1105, 1970.
95. Ziegert, D.: Progressive kindliche Kniestrecksteife nach intramuskularen Injektionen. Beitr. Orthop. Traumatol., *20*:119, 1973.

PROGRESSIVE MUSCULAR DYSTROPHY

Definition

Progressive muscular dystrophy is a genetically determined primary degenerative noninflammatory disease of skeletal muscle. It is generally classified as a *myopathy*, a broad term that encompasses diseases caused by pathologic, biochemical, or electrical changes in the muscle fibers or in the interstitial tissues of the voluntary musculature, and in which there is no abnormality of the innervation of the affected muscles; the central nervous system and peripheral nerves are normal.

Historical Aspects

Probably the first true observation of muscular dystrophy as such was made by Meryon, in 1852, who described in detail a family in which four boys had developed progressive atrophy and weakness of muscles in childhood. He lucidly narrated the progressive course of muscle weakness: "In May, 1847 when nearly nine years of age, he walked from Brutton Street to Westminster Bridge, but in November, 1848, he could neither walk not stand, and in 1850 his arms were fast losing power." In two of these patients, pathologic examination at autopsy disclosed the spinal cord and nerves to be normal, but the muscles showed a form of "granular degeneration." Meryon unfortunately still confused the condition with progressive neural muscular atrophy.[108]

In 1868, Duchenne published his definitive treatise on *"le paralysie musculaire pseudo-hypertrophique ou paralysie myosclerosique"* (pseudohypertrophic or myelosclerotic muscular paralysis). He clearly delineated the entity as a muscle disease of childhood or adolescence, more common in boys than girls and characterized by the following features: (1) progressive weakness of muscles that begins initially in the lower limbs and then gradually spreads to the trunk and upper limbs; (2) enlargement (pseudohypertrophy) of the weakened muscles; and (3) hyperplasia of interstitial connective tissue and increase in fat cells in the affected muscles, but preservation of striation. In later postmortem studies he demonstrated that the pathologic findings were present only in the interstitial tissues of muscles and that there were no changes in the nervous system.[33]

Gowers, in 1879, in an excellent treatise on pseudohypertrophic dystrophy in young boys, described his sign of "climbing up the legs" and wrote: "It is a disease of early life and of early growth. Manifesting itself commonly at the transition from infancy to childhood, it develops with the child's development, grows with his growth—so that every increase in stature means an increase in weakness, and each year takes him a step further on the road to a helpless infirmity, and in most cases to an early and

inevitable death." Gowers also recognized that muscular hypertrophy and atrophy could occur in variable proportions in the same family.[47]

Both Leyden and Mobius, in 1876 and 1879, respectively, described a familial form of dystrophy of the pelvic girdle musculature.[96, 115] Landouzy and Dejerine, in 1834, gave a classic description of the facioscapulohumeral form[88]; Erb later published a report on the juvenile or scapulohumeral form of the disorder.[41]

Gowers, in 1902, described another form of the disease in which the distal muscles of the limbs were primarily affected.[48]

Batten, in 1909, suggested that the simple atrophic variety of muscular dystrophy could simulate amyotonia congenita.[10] Hutchinson and Fuchs reported involvement of the external ocular muscles.[44, 65]

During this period, another disorder of skeletal muscles, myotonia, was recognized. Myotonia is characterized by a delay in muscular relaxation. Thomsen, in 1876, described individuals in whom all the skeletal muscles were affected from birth; this condition is now known as *myotonia congenita* or *Thomsen's disease*.[200] Eulenberg, in 1886, described a condition in which myotonia occurred from exposure to cold and there were associated attacks of disabling muscle weakness.[42] Another more common condition known as dystrophia myotonica was reported later, in which there is progressive atrophy and weakness of the distal muscles of the limbs and of the facial muscles associated with myotonia, which is less severe and localized to only a few muscles.[10, 59, 189]

Classification

The classification of progressive muscular dystrophy that is most adequate from the clinical and genetic standpoints is the one given by Walton:[218]

I. The pure muscular dystrophies
   A. X-linked recessive
      1. Duchenne muscular dystrophy—severe
      2. Becker muscular dystrophy—benign
      3. Emery-Dreifus dystrophy—benign with early contracture
   B. Autosomal recessive
      1. Scapulohumeral—"limb girdle," "quadriceps myopathy"
      2. Early onset in childhood—"Duchenne-like"
      3. Congenital muscular dystrophies
   C. Autosomal dominant
      1. Facioscapulohumeral

2. Scapuloperoneal
3. Late-onset proximal
4. Distal (adult onset)
5. Distal (infantile onset)
6. Ocular
7. Oculopharyngeal

II. Dystrophies with myotonia
   A. Myotonia congenita
   B. Dystrophia myotonica
   C. Paramyotonia congenita[218]

Etiology

The cause of muscular dystrophy is unknown. It is a hereditary disease. Genetic aspects of the various specific forms are mentioned in the section on clinical features.

Several abnormalities in the chemistry of dystrophic muscle have directed research efforts toward a search for a fundamental biochemical defect or defects in muscular dystrophy. To date, a specific relationship between the biochemical aberrations and the dystrophic process has not been established. By analogy with other hereditary diseases, the basic defect in muscular dystrophy is probably complete or partial failure to synthesize a particular enzyme, the activity of which is essential for the maintenance of normal cell structure. The site of the primary defect is yet undetermined. Abnormalities of the erythrocyte membrane have been shown.[6, 179]

Pathology

Histopathologic examination does not reliably distinguish between the various types of muscular dystrophy. Essential changes in the muscles are the same in all types. The subdivision of dystrophic diseases is based upon the type of inheritance, the pattern of muscle involvement, the age of onset, and the pace of the natural course of the disease.

Gross appearance depends on the relative amounts of fat and fibrous tissue that replace the muscle fibers. In pseudohypertrophic muscular dystrophy, the enlarged calf muscles look like a fatty tumor at autopsy. Other affected muscles show varying degrees of atrophy and change in color from yellowish to pinkish gray.

The most important histologic feature of muscle dystrophy is the loss of muscle fibers, which appears to result from atrophy and the eventual fragmentation of fibers.

The following histologic changes are found in varying degrees (Fig. 5–209):

Great variation in the size of individual muscle fibers. The largest fibers may reach a size of 230 μ and the smallest fibers may be as narrow as 10 μ. These large and small muscle fibers, along with the normal-sized ones, are scattered in haphazard arrangements throughout the muscle in all stages of the disease. The enlargement of fibers may be due simply to simple hypertrophy, or it may represent the primary change of dystrophy.[2, 41]

Retraction of the muscle fibers from the endomysial sheaths.

Forking or branching of fibers.[228] A common feature in all dystrophies is actual splitting of muscle fibers into daughter fibers, each with distinct sarcolemma within the same endomysial tube. This could represent a regenerative response.

Necrosis of single fibers or groups of fibers with signs of phagocytosis. Recent degeneration of muscle fibers is represented by clusters of histiocytes. There is diminution in the complement of muscle fibers.

Increase in size of sarcolemmal nuclei with prominent nucleation. There is central nucleation in some muscle fibers. Long chains of central nuclei are more characteristic of myotonic dystrophy.

Increase in endomysial connective tissue. This fibrosis could be secondary to loss of muscle fibers.

Hyperplasia of adipose tissue in the form of fat cells. Fat cell infiltration may be due to reduced volume and number of muscle fibers. In the severely involved muscle one will see a few scattered atrophic muscle fibers in a vast field of fatty and connective tissue. Thus, in the terminal stage of muscular dystrophy, there is disappearance of muscle fibers; muscle is reduced to fat and connective tissue, with a few stray surviving fibers. This is the basis for paralysis.

There are no significant changes in the motor and sensory peripheral nerve fibers or in the central nervous system.

In the cardiovascular system, fibrosis of the myocardium is the most striking finding, varying from finely diffused sclerosis to large areas of scarring. There is no evidence of a specific inflammatory reaction.

The prominent histologic findings in the various types of muscular dystrophy are reflected by the pace of the disease and the age of onset. For example, in the Duchenne pseudohypertrophic type, the rapid progression of the disease is evidenced by the prominent necrosis, phagocytosis, abortive regeneration, and forking of fibers. Enlargement of fibers is also a

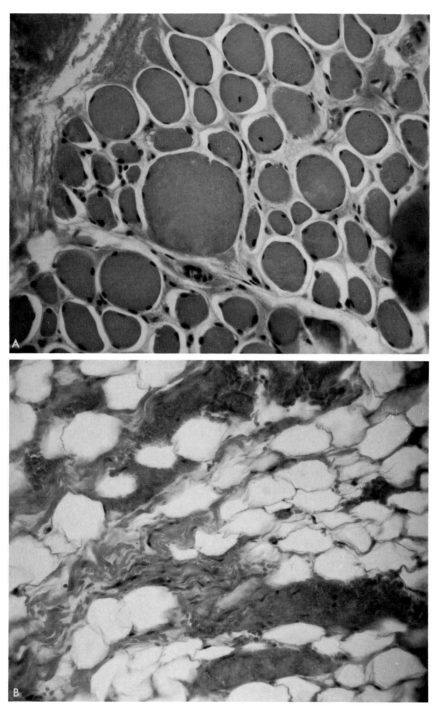

FIGURE 5–209. Histologic changes in progressive muscular dystrophy.

A. Transverse section taken from vastus lateralis muscle of seven-year-old boy. Early stage (× 400, hematoxylin and eosin stain). Note the great variation in the size of individual muscle fibers and retraction of the muscle fibers from the endomysial sheaths. **B.** Longitudinal section from enlarged gastrocnemius muscle. Note the accumulation of adipose tissue and the reduction in number of muscle fibers (× 250, hematoxylin and eosin stain).

prominent feature of the pseudohypertrophic type, whereas in the slowly advancing general adolescent and adult types (Landouzy-Dejerine facioscapulohumeral, limb girdle, and distal), there is little necrosis—the usual findings are variation in fiber size, central nucleation, and fibrosis and fat cell infiltration, and enlargement of fibers is less frequent than that seen in the Duchenne type. In the late adult and restricted muscular dystrophies (such as the ocular form) necrosis is rare; the dominant findings are variation in size of muscle fibers, fibrosis, and increase in fat cells. In myotonic dystrophy, the distinctive features are the rows of central nuclei and annulets (Ringbinden) and peripheral masses of clear sarcoplasm devoid of myofibrils.

Electron microscopic examination shows nonspecific changes of degeneration of muscle fibers. Histochemistry reveals a predominance of Type I fibers and relative loss of clear-cut differentiation into the fiber types with standard ATPase reaction at pH 9.4.

Biochemical Considerations

CHANGES IN BODY FLUID

Creatine and Creatinine. Historically, the first biochemical defect observed in muscular dystrophy was a decrease in urinary creatinine excretion reported by Rosenthal in 1870.[154] Levine and Kristeller, in 1909, noted an increase in urinary excretion of creatine in addition to a diminished creatinine output.[93]

Creatine, an amino acid, is synthesized from glycine, arginine, and methionine, largely in tissues other than muscle; the liver, kidney, and pancreas are probably the most important sites. Skeletal muscle contains the largest amount of creatine (more than any other organ or tissue). Most of the creatine formed is delivered to the muscle. In the muscle cell, creatine is phosphorylated by the action of creatine kinase, with the help of adenosine triphosphate, to form creatine phosphate, which represents an important reserve of energy for muscular contraction.

Creatinine, an anhydride of creatine, is a degradation product of it. Creatinine content of muscle is low (about 5 mg. per 100 gm.), since it is readily diffused from the muscle fiber into serum and is then completely disposed of by the kidneys. The normal serum values for creatinine range from 0.8 to 1.4 per cent and are increased only in kidney failure. The daily excretion of creatinine in the urine is considerable and constant (1 to 2 gm. per day).

The normal serum values for creatine are 0.2 to 0.6 mg. per 100 ml. in the adult male, and 0.4 to 0.9 mg. per 100 ml. in the adult female. The renal threshold for creatine is about 0.5 mg. per 100 ml.; hence, the urine of normal adults contains little or no creatine (the average 24-hour urine excretion of creatine is 60 to 150 mg. in the adult male, and 120 to 300 mg. in the adult female).

In muscular dystrophy there is a disturbance in creatine and creatinine excretion, namely (1) a decrease in creatinine content of the urine, (2) an increase in urinary creatine, and (3) often a mild hypercreatinemia. In the past, it was speculated that muscular dystrophy was caused by a disturbance of creatine metabolism; however, these claims have now been abandoned, and it is generally accepted that decreased urinary output of creatinine and hypercreatinuria is a nonspecific manifestation of muscle atrophy. If the amount of muscular bulk is diminished because of atrophy, creatine will be removed less rapidly from the blood, the blood level will be higher, and excretion by the kidneys will be increased.

Van Pilsum and Wolin reported the following mean figures for creatine excretion (in milligrams per kilogram of body weight per day) in various conditions.[206]

Normal adults	0
Pseudohypertrophic muscular dystrophy	18
Adult muscular dystrophy	18
Poliomyelitis	14
Amyotonia congenita	9
Paraplegia	5
Quadriplegia	5
Polymyositis	9
Disuse atrophy	4
Charcot-Marie-Tooth peroneal atrophy	4
Amyotrophic lateral sclerosis	4
Dermatomyositis	14
Myotonia dystrophica	3
Myasthenia gravis	0
Progressive muscular dystrophy	8

These figures demonstrate that an increase in creatine excretion is found in almost all types of muscle disease.

Creatine tolerance is decreased in muscular dystrophy.[27] This finding is nonspecific and indicates a reduction in functional muscle mass. If a test dose (1 to 3 gm.) is given orally to a normal subject, most of the creatine will be taken up by skeletal muscle and little or no creatinuria will result. In muscular dystrophy or in muscle diseases in which the muscle mass is decreased, the creatine tolerance is disturbed because the remaining musculature is not capable of absorbing all the creatine and some spills out into the urine.

SERUM ENZYMES

Creatine Kinase. A very pronounced increase in creatine kinase activity in the serum of patients with muscular dystrophy was reported by Ebashi, Toyokura, Momoi, and Sugita in 1959.[34] It is known that creatine kinase reversibly transfers a phosphate group from creatine phosphate to adenosine diphosphate, forming creatine and adenosine triphosphate. The average serum level of creatine kinase in normal persons is about 2 units, i.e., μM of creatine formed per hour per milliliter of serum. In children with the early Duchenne type of muscular dystrophy, values up to several hundred units have been found. In fact, the increase may occur long before any overt clinical signs of the disease are apparent. To a varying degree, elevation of the serum creatine kinase level is found in the great majority of mothers who transmit the Duchenne type of dystrophy; this demonstrates that clinically normal carriers of the abnormal gene may show biochemical abnormalities characteristic of the disease to a minor degree. Normal values of creatine kinase do not rule out the possibility that the mother is a carrier, for only two thirds of probable of known carriers have an abnormally high level of creatine kinase.[135] Creatine kinase is a more specific indicator than aldolase, as it does not appear to increase in liver disease.

Another practical advantage of measuring creatine kinase is that erythrocytes contain very little of this enzyme and serum assays are not disturbed by hemolysis of the sample. Its disadvantages are the requirement that the blood specimens reach the laboratory for freezing more quickly and also the possibility of greater pitfalls due to certain technical difficulties. However, these are outweighed by its advantages of specificity and sensitivity. The reliable techniques of determining the serum levels of creatine kinase are those of Hughes and Rosalki.[64, 152]

A micromethod of determining serum creatine phosphokinase (CPK) was developed by Zellweger and Antonik.[237] A drop of blood is dried on filter paper; the test is based upon the amount of light released by the ATP of the reaction process of bn luci ferin-lucirase. The value of this micromethod of testing is for general screening of newborns for muscle dystrophy.

Aldolase. High levels of serum aldolase are found in muscular dystrophy. The enzyme aldolase is found in most tissues and catalyzes one of the steps in the breakdown of glucose—the splitting of fructose 1:6-diphosphate. The normal serum values are less than 10 (expressed in the most commonly used Bruns units). In the Duchenne type of muscular dystrophy, values of over 100 are frequently found. In adult types of muscular dystrophy and in myotonic dystrophy, the elevation in serum aldolase is much less and is often absent.

The increase of serum aldolase and creatine kinase is most marked in the early stages of the disease. Their serum values decline as the disease progresses, and in fact, in the end stages of the disease, they may be just above the normal range.[22] One can often correlate the level of the enzymes with the duration of the disease.

A rise in serum aldolase is often seen in polymyositis and dermatomyositis, but in neural atrophies, elevated levels have been encountered only very rarely. The real value of the test is in the diagnosis of primary myopathy.

Other enzymes may appear in increased amounts in the blood in muscular dystrophy. Of these, lactate dehydrogenase and the two aminotransferases—aspartate aminotransferase and alanine aminotransferase-GOT and -GPT—have been studied most extensively.[137] The source of increased amounts of the aforementioned serum enzymes is largely or wholly the muscle tissue itself; they leak out of the fibers as the latter are disturbed and damaged by the disease.

There are other reported changes in body fluids in muscular dystrophy. Increased aminoaciduria is often present and seems to result from protein breakdown associated with muscle wasting. Another significant change is an increase in serum-2-globulin, for further discussion of which the reader is referred to Oppenheimer and Milhorat.[128]

CHANGES IN MUSCLE

Research in this area is proceeding at an increasing pace. A decrease, relative to noncollagen nitrogen, in the amount of the main contractile protein, myosin, in dystrophic muscle was found by Vignos and Lefkowitz.[209] In dystrophic muscle the myoglobin content is diminished, and there are qualitative alterations in myoglobin.[225] An elevated sodium and decreased potassium content has been found in dystrophic muscles.[60]

Studies of the activity of various enzymes in

dystrophic muscles have been carried out. Dreyfus et al. found a decrease in the rate of glycolysis in specimens of the transversus abdominis muscle from patients with muscular dystrophy on comparing them with corresponding normal muscles obtained during appendectomy, using noncollagen protein as a reference base. The extent of the decrease paralleled the severity of the disease.[30, 31] Other workers, using histochemical techniques, have shown increased activity of dephosphorylating enzymes in dystrophic muscle.[45] Elevated levels of cathepsins (intracellular proteolytic enzymes) in muscle biopsies from boys with the Duchenne type of dystrophy are reported by Pennington.[137]

Specific Forms of Muscular Dystrophy

The principal types of muscular dystrophy differ with respect to heredity, age of onset, groups of muscles involved by the disease process, and the rate of progression of muscular weakness.

DUCHENNE TYPE MUSCULAR DYSTROPHY—SEVERE

This is the most common type of the disorder. The prevalence in the general population is about 3 per 100,000. The incidence is not exactly known—it is probably 13 to 33 per 100,000 live male births.

Heredity. The severe form of Duchenne muscular dystrophy is inherited as an X-linked recessive trait; therefore, it is confined to boys. The rare severe muscular dystrophy encountered occasionally in girls represents the severe form of limb girdle muscular dystrophy, which is inherited as an autosomal recessive trait. There are exceptionally rare cases of severe Duchenne muscular dystrophy associated with Turner's syndrome. There is a high mutation rate—about 43 per million genes per generation.[215] In about three fifths of the cases there is a positive family history. The statistical data are changing with the advent of screening methods for detection of muscular dystrophy in the neonatal period.[237]

Clinical Features. The *onset* is insidious. The initial symptoms of the disease are usually apparent within the first three years of life and are manifest as slowness in learning to walk at the usual age. On specific inquiry there is delay in development of motor milestones—holding the head up, sitting unsupported, crawling, standing, and independent ambulation. The presenting complaint is abnormal gait, such as walking on toes or a waddling gait on a wide base. The child is prone to falling frequently and has difficulty in climbing stairs and rising from the floor. He has difficulty standing on one leg, hopping, and jumping, and running is clumsy with a marked Trendelenburg lurch.

In a few cases the disease may commence between the third and sixth years, and rarely, in early or late adolescence. Symptoms due to weakness of the shoulder musculature appear in the later stages.

Involvement of muscles is symmetrical, initially of the pelvic girdle, followed after three to five years by affection of the muscles of the shoulder girdle. A predominant feature of the condition is pseudohypertrophy, which is caused by accumulation of fat.

On examination, the child stands with a protuberant abdomen and excessive lumbar lordosis. The shoulders are carried behind the pelvis. The calf muscles are enlarged. The shoulders have a sloping appearance because of the weakness of the shoulder girdle musculature.

The gait is waddling, with a gluteus maximus, gluteus medius, and quadriceps limp. If the anterior tibial and peroneal muscles are weak and there is contracture of the triceps surae, the child will have a toe-heel or toe-toe gait. When caught off balance, he will tend to fall because his knees give way. He may walk and stand by placing his feet wide apart to increase his base of support, and often will utilize trick movements to maintain equilibrium.

The difficulty in climbing stairs or in rising from the floor is due to bilateral weakness of the gluteus maximus and the quadriceps muscles. The affected child "climbs up on his legs" when rising from the floor, i.e., he first puts his hands on his knees (to keep them extended) and then pushes his trunk upward by working the hands up the thighs, a finding referred to as *Gowers' sign* (Fig. 5–210).[147, 48]

The muscle weakness is proximal in distribution; it is usually first evident in the gluteus maximus, later on the hip abductors and adductors, iliopsoas, anterior abdominal, and quadriceps muscles are progressively involved, and eventually the anterior crural group is involved. The muscles of the neck and upper limbs involved in the early stages include the lower and middle parts of the trapezius, the rhomboids, the latissimus dorsi, and the inward rotators. The shoulder girdle weakness is shown by Meryon's sign—upon lifting the patient under his armpits, he slides through the examiner's

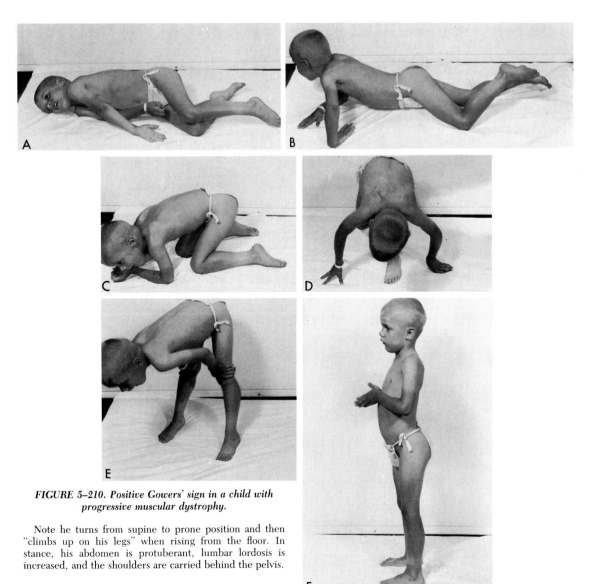

FIGURE 5–210. Positive Gowers' sign in a child with progressive muscular dystrophy.

Note he turns from supine to prone position and then "climbs up on his legs" when rising from the floor. In stance, his abdomen is protuberant, lumbar lordosis is increased, and the shoulders are carried behind the pelvis.

hands.[108] Later, the biceps and brachioradialis are affected. The neck muscles are involved comparatively late in the course of the disease, and the gastrocnemius-soleus, tibialis posterior, and toe flexors may remain comparatively strong for several years. The intercostal muscles are eventually affected. With progression of the disease, muscle weakness spreads to the periphery of the limbs with ultimate loss of the entire motor strength of the hip, knee, shoulder, elbow, and ankle joints. The hamstring muscles in the lower limbs and the muscles of the hand, face, jaw, pharynx, larynx, and eyes are relatively spared to the end. Diaphragmatic movement is usually normal. Complete manual muscle tests should be performed on all patients

with muscular dystrophy and should be repeated at regular intervals to determine the course of muscle weakness.

The affected muscles may be increased or decreased in size. Pseudohypertrophy caused by accumulation of fat attracts attention first and is present in about 80 per cent of cases. It is frequently seen in calf muscles, but sometimes also in the quadriceps and deltoid muscles. The pseudohypertrophied muscles have a typical firm rubbery texture and are not as strong as healthy muscles of the same size. Macroglossia is commonly present.

Muscular atrophy eventually sets in during the course of the disease. It usually begins near the insertion of the muscles and then spreads proximally. Excessive deposition of subcutaneous fat may hide the muscle atrophy and tends to preserve the contour of the limbs. In the terminal stages of the disease, all the muscles of the limbs, pelvic and shoulder girdles, and trunk become atrophic, giving the appearance of severe inanition.

The deep tendon reflexes are normal or hypoactive early in the disease, but later disappear as the muscles involved become too weak to respond to the stimuli. Superficial reflexes are usually present. With loss of muscle tone, venous insufficiency develops, causing mottling and cyanosis of the limbs.

Early in the disease the joints have full range of motion, and the limbs are loose and flaccid. Weakness of one group of muscles, but not of their antagonists, results in permanent shortening of the stronger muscles and subsequently the development of contractures. These are commonly seen in the triceps surae muscle, with equinus deformity of the ankles and feet. Later in the course of the disease, when the affected children are confined to a wheelchair or bed, contractures develop because of remaining in one position for prolonged periods; these are commonly seen in the hamstrings, the hip flexors, and the iliotibial band.

Scoliosis and kyphoscoliosis are common in the late stages of muscular dystrophy, especially in the wheelchair-bound patient. Changes in the skeleton develop as a result of disuse and the maintenance of abnormal postures of the trunk and limbs. The bones undergo demineralization, with narrowing of the shafts and rarefaction of the ends of long bones. The appearance of the centers of ossification is delayed. Fractures as a result of minimal trauma are not unusual.

Myocardial degeneration with fatty infiltration and fibrosis eventually develops. Cardiomegaly and persistent tachycardia are frequently present in the late stages. The electrocardiogram will disclose prolongation of the PR interval, slurring of the QRS complex, bundle branch block, elevation or depression of the ST segment, and other changes, indicating conduction defects or myocardial failure.

Intellectual impairment is common in patients with the Duchenne type of muscular dystrophy, the mean intelligence quotient being approximately 15 to 20 per cent lower than that of normal peers. The personality pattern of these children is characterized by dependency, withdrawal, passivity, and lack of ambition and spontaneity.

Clinical Course. This is defined by three landmarks: (1) age at onset of symptoms; (2) age at loss of ambulation; and (3) age at death. In Duchenne muscular dystrophy the course is one of steady, rapid, and relentless progression. Periods of bed rest, necessitated by febrile illness or surgical procedures, will result in rapid deterioration. The child is usually confined to a wheelchair by the age of 10 to 15 years, which leads to the development of severe flexion contractures of the hips, knees, and elbows. Scoliosis results from weakness of the trunk and abdominal muscles. Eventually the patient is unable to sit and is confined to bed with little or no residual active movement in his limbs, except some weak grasp with his hands and flexion of his toes and feet. The muscles of the face and those involved in respiration and swallowing are relatively spared. Survival beyond the age of 20 years is a rarity. Most patients die from sudden cardiac failure, pulmonary infection, or inanition. A few in whom the onset of disease was comparatively late may survive until the fourth or fifth decade.

Laboratory Findings

Serum Enzymes. In the early stages of severe Duchenne muscular dystrophy there is marked elevation (as high as 50 times normal value) of serum creatine phosphokinase (CPK). This probably is due to leakage of the enzyme from the muscle cell. The level of serum CPK does not reflect the severity of the dystrophy. With progression of the disease there is gradual decline of the serum CPK values; this is due to loss of muscle tissue. The serum levels of aldolase and aminotransferase (transaminase) are also raised; however, these enzymes are not as sensitive as CPK.

Electromyographic Findings. The EMG changes are nonspecific; they consist of a pattern of low amplitude, short duration, and polyphoric motor unit potentials. The same changes occur in various forms of myopathy. The diagnostic value of EMG is in distinguishing myopathy from neuropathy.

Muscle Biopsy. The histologic findings depend upon the stage of the dystrophic process, the pattern changing with progression of the disease. Early the muscle appears to be "normal," but on close scrutiny, variation in fiber size and focal area of degenerating or regenerating fibers will be seen. Later on, the variation in fiber size becomes more marked with moderate proliferation of endomysial connective tissue and adipose tissue; also, there will be round dark-staining fibers. With progression of the dystrophy the muscle fibers are gradually lost and replaced by connective tissue and fat. Toward the end, the muscle is replaced by fat with scattered isolated clusters of residual weak fiber.

Ultrastructural studies will disclose the degenerated muscle fibers with nonspecific changes. Histochemistry will show loss of differentiation into fiber types and predominance of Type I fibers.

BECKER'S BENIGN MUSCULAR DYSTROPHY

The benign form of muscular dystrophy, first described by Becker, has X-linked recessive inheritance.[12, 13] The genes for Becker's and Duchenne's muscular dystrophy, however, are distinct and not alleles.

Clinically, it is characterized by late onset of symptoms, usually after seven years of age. The presenting complaint is toe-walking or a waddling gait. The distribution of muscle weakness in the Becker type is similar to that of Duchenne. Calf pseudohypertrophy is present in both. In the Becker type, the course of the disease is more benign (ambulation being maintained until early adulthood). These patients are usually disabled by middle age. Cardiac involvement is less common, with half the patients having a normal EKG. Mental retardation is rare. Creatine phosphokinase (CPK) levels are elevated; in general, they are lower than in the Duchenne type. There are subtle histopathologic differences between the Becker and Duchenne types, but these are not reliable in distinguishing between the two forms of X-linked recessive muscular dystrophy. The diagnosis should be based upon clinical criteria.

EMERY-DREIFUSS X-LINKED RECESSIVE MUSCULAR DYSTROPHY

This rare type is characterized by variable disability, development of early contractures, and a benign course. Some of the patients, however, eventually die of cardiomyopathy.[38]

LIMB GIRDLE MUSCULAR DYSTROPHY

This type of autosomal recessive muscular dystrophy was delineated by Walton and Nattrass in 1954.[219] It is characterized by involvement of the proximal muscles of the limbs. In the pelvic-femoral type the muscle weakness predominantly involves the pelvic girdle musculature, whereas in the scapulohumeral type the shoulder girdle muscles are primarily affected. It occurs in both sexes. Inheritance pattern is autosomal recessive; however, sporadic cases do occur.

Age of Onset. There is marked variability. In general, the onset is during the second or third decade of life, and a course of slow progression ensues, severe disability occurring 20 years after onset of the symptoms. Life expectancy may be shortened. In severe cases the onset is early with rapid progression, resembling the Duchenne type. This accounts for the occasional presence of "Duchenne" type muscular dystrophy in the female. Sometimes limb girdle muscular dystrophy commences later, after 40 years of age, with rapid, relentless progression of muscle weakness and confinement to bed within three years.

The pelvic girdle type was originally described by Leyden in 1876.[96] Initially the muscles involved are the gluteus maximus, iliopsoas, and quadriceps; later on the muscle weakness spreads to a lesser degree to the shoulder girdle region.

The initial symptoms develop slowly. Depending on where the disease begins, the early symptoms consist of hunched shoulders and difficulty in lifting the arms above the head or difficulty in climbing stairs and rising from the floor or low chairs. Usually, if the shoulder girdle is affected initially, the pelvic girdle musculature will not be involved for quite some time. However, if the dystrophy begins in the muscles of the pelvic girdle, the shoulder girdle muscles will be affected soon.

Pseudohypertrophy of the calf and anterior thigh muscles occurs in less than a third of these patients. Enlargement of the muscles of the upper limbs, particularly the deltoid muscles, is rare. The pattern of muscle weakness is proximal, but not unique, as it is also seen in Duchenne dystrophy. In the upper limb, the muscles most commonly affected early include the lower and middle parts of the trapezius, rhomboids, latissimus dorsi, and medial rotators of the shoulder. In the lower limb, the gluteus maximus, iliopsoas, hip adductors, and quadriceps are usually involved early in the course of the disease. The disease spreads distally, affecting the anterior tibial and peroneal muscles. The calf muscles are usually spared until later in the course. On occasion, there is comparatively early involvement of the muscles of the forearm and hand. Contractures and skeletal changes develop late and are similar to, but less severe than, those of the Duchenne type. The knee jerk and biceps and radial periosteal reflexes are often diminished or absent, but the Achilles tendon and triceps reflexes remain normal until late in the disease.

The intellectual level is normal in this type of muscular dystrophy. Cardiac involvement is very rare.

Limb girdle muscular dystrophy can be easily misdiagnosed as the late-onset (Kugelberg-Welander) form of spinal muscular atrophy. Congenital myopathies and metabolic myopathies should also be excluded. Because of problems of delineation and confusion in diagnosis, thorough laboratory investigation should be carried out. The electromyogram will disclose myopathic patterns of abnormalities, i.e., low amplitude with polyphasic potentials. The creatine phosphokinase is usually elevated. The histologic picture on muscle biopsy will confirm the diagnosis of muscular dystrophy.

CONGENITAL MUSCULAR DYSTROPHY

This type of muscular dystrophy is present at birth or noted soon afterward. Inheritance is autosomal recessive. Presenting complaints are hypotonia and motor weakness of the limbs, trunk, and facial muscles. Sucking and swallowing may be difficult. The deep tendon reflexes are depressed or absent. The pharyngeal muscles are not affected. Contractural deformities such as talipes equinovarus are often present at birth; in some cases they develop later. The deformities tend to increase with growth and are aggravated by immobility.[238]

In contradistinction to other muscular dystrophies of childhood, this condition is relatively static. It may progress slightly or may improve with time. Ordinarily, the affected children are able to walk independently at about two years of age.

The electromyographic studies show myopathic changes. The creatine phosphokinase is elevated. Muscle biopsy reveals dystrophic changes that are strikingly similar to those of muscular dystrophy.

FACIOSCAPULOHUMERAL MUSCULAR DYSTROPHY OF LANDOUZY AND DÉJERINE

This benign form of muscular dystrophy predominantly affects the muscles of the shoulder girdle and the face. Males and females are affected with equal frequency. Inheritance is autosomal dominant with almost complete penetrance by the fourth decade of life. The prevalence is about 1 in 20,000.[129]

Partially affected or abortive cases are common in this type of muscular dystrophy.[60, 64, 79] In the mild form, the patient may even be unaware that he is suffering from the disease; in the abortive forms, the disease may remain limited to one or two muscles or muscle groups.

The condition begins at any age from early childhood until adult life, but usually the onset is in the second decade. Initially the face and shoulder girdle muscles are affected, but later on the disease spreads to the pelvic girdle.

The characteristic appearance of the face is due to weakness of the facial muscles (Fig. 5–211). Wrinkles are often absent from the forehead and around the eyes. The patient cannot close the eyes properly, whistle, or pout the lips. There may be a transverse smile. As muscle weakness progresses, speech becomes indistinct.

The pattern of muscle involvement in the early stages of facioscapulohumeral dystrophy is unique. The upper part of the pectoralis major in the neck and shoulder area and the anterior tibial in the lower limb are affected early, while the trunk extensors, iliopsoas, gluteus medius, tensor fasciae latae, and quadriceps are spared. This pattern is somewhat similar to that of the limb girdle type.

Pseudohypertrophy is rare, but on occasion it is seen in the calf musculature and the deltoids.

Contractural and bony deformities are mild and occur late. The intelligence level is normal, and cardiac involvement is rare.

The disease progresses insidiously with prolonged periods of apparent arrest. Occasionally, however, there is unusually rapid progression. Most patients survive and remain ambulatory to a normal age.

In the differential diagnosis of facioscapulohumeral muscular dystrophy, one should consider myasthenia and other types of myopathy—such as myotubular, nemaline, mitochondrial, and central core disease.[206]

Histologic findings on muscle biopsy are not striking. The most constant finding is the presence of isolated small atrophic fibers intermixed with hypertrophic muscle fibers.

SCAPULOPERONEAL DYSTROPHY

This is a variant of facioscapulohumeral dystrophy characterized by involvement of the peroneal and tibialis anterior muscles. The presenting complaint is a toe-heel or toe-toe gait. There is associated weakness of the shoulder girdle and facial muscles. Muscle biopsy is performed to confirm the diagnosis.

DISTAL MUSCULAR DYSTROPHY

First described by Gowers in 1902, this is distinguished from the limb girdle type by initial involvement of the distal limb muscles rather than the proximal ones.[48] Welander's extensive experience, in Sweden, of 250 cases

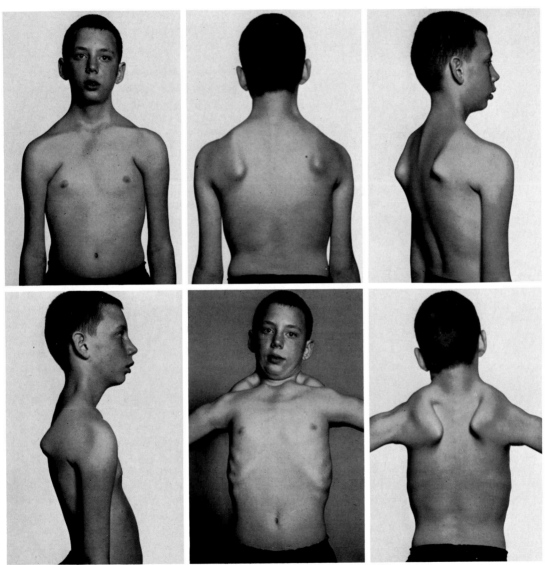

FIGURE 5–211. *An adolescent boy with facioscapulohumeral muscular dystrophy of Landouzy and Déjerine.*

Appearance of the face and weakness of scapulohumeral muscles are characteristic.

of distal muscular dystrophy is unique, as the disorder is considered to be very rare.[224] It is inherited as an autosomal dominant trait and affects both sexes. The age of onset varies from 20 to 77 years, with a mean of 47 years. The small muscles in the hands and feet are affected. In the hand the presenting complaint is clumsiness and loss of fine motor coordination. In the lower limbs, drop-foot gait results from weakness of the anterior tibial muscle. Later the weakness slowly spreads proximally. The course of the disease is comparatively benign. Distal muscular dystrophy should be differentiated from dystrophia myotonica. Also, one should rule out spinocerebellar degenerative tract and anterior horn cell disorders.

OCULAR DYSTROPHY OR PROGRESSIVE DYSTROPHIA OPHTHALMOPLEGIA

This is a rare and very slowly progressive dystrophy involving primarily, and usually limited to, the external ocular muscles and levators of the eyelids. This disease may develop at any age from infancy to over 50 years but usually occurs in adolescence. It begins with ptosis and diplopia or strabismus. It slowly progresses to complete bilateral ophthalmoplegia in most cases. The facial muscles become involved. Dysphagia occurs in about 50 per cent of the cases. Eventually the dystrophy progresses to involve the muscles of the shoulder girdle.

OCULOPHARYNGEAL DYSTROPHY

This is a rare disorder that is inherited as an autosomal dominant trait. Its onset is in the third decade of life. In addition to weakness of the extraocular muscles, the pharyngeal muscles are involved with resultant dysarthria and dysphagia. The dystrophy progresses to involve the muscles of the shoulder and pelvic girdle.[55]

DYSTROPHIA MYOTONICA (MYOTONIC DYSTROPHY)

This is a steadily progressive familial disease in which a myopathy involving the face, jaw,

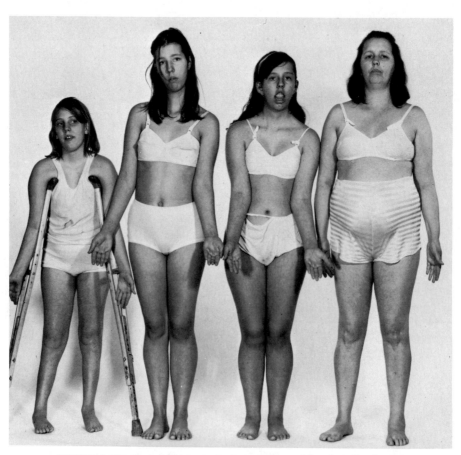

FIGURE 5–212. Dystrophia myotonica in a mother and her three daughters.

The condition is transmitted as a mendelian dominant character.

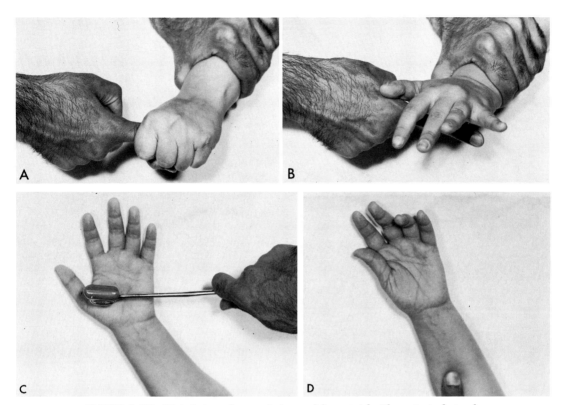

FIGURE 5–213. *Clinical signs of myotonia in an adolescent girl with myotonic dystrophy.*

A and B. Relaxation of the hand grip is slow. C and D. After a sharp blow on the belly of the thenar muscles in the thenar eminence a dimple is formed and the thumb is adducted.

eye, neck, and distal limb muscles is associated with myotonia. The onset is usually in late adolescence or early adult life. The condition is transmitted as an autosomal dominant trait (Fig. 5–212). In the second generation, the dystrophia myotonica is much more severe and begins at an earlier age, commonly in childhood.

Myotonia, the striking feature of the disease, is characterized by failure of the voluntary muscles to relax immediately, and persistence of contraction following voluntary movement or mechanical or electrical stimulation. Myotonia is evidenced clinically by apparent slowness in relaxation of the hand grip and is best demonstrated as a persistent dimpling after a sharp blow on a muscle belly, such as the thenar eminence, tongue, or deltoid (Fig. 5–213).

There is great variation in the clinical picture. The muscles affected by myotonia are those of the hands, the face and tongue, and occasionally the limbs. Upon tight closure of the eyes, there is a delay in relaxation. The degree of myotonia is lessened with repetition of motion. Tripping, falling, and difficulty in walking are other manifestations of the disease.

The pattern of muscle weakness in the limbs, in contrast to most myopathies, is distal, rather than proximal, in distribution. The long flexors and extensors of the fingers, small muscles of the hand, tibialis anterior, and peroneal muscles are involved early. Soon the disease affects the calf muscles, and later it spreads proximally to involve the quadriceps and hamstrings. The deep tendon reflexes are diminished or absent. Contractural deformities are mild and occur late (Fig. 5–214).

The face is expressionless (Fig. 5–215). Ptosis is invariable. The patient has difficulty in closing the eyes, in pursing the lips, and in whistling. The voice is monotonous and nasal owing to involvement of the laryngeal muscles. Dysarthria is common.

The characteristic facial appearance, called "myopathic facies," is haggard, being produced by atrophy of the masseters, narrowing of the lower half of the face and mandible, bilateral ptosis, and general weakness of the facial musculature. The sternocleidomastoids are frequently wasted, resulting in increased cervical lordosis ("swan neck").

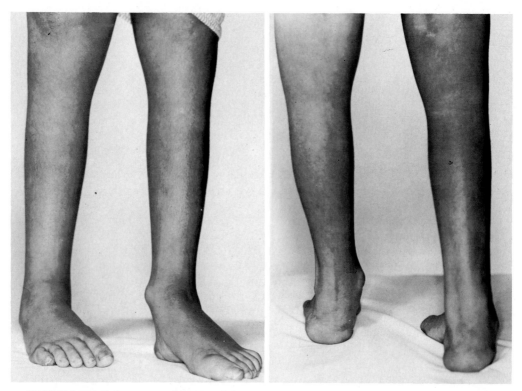

FIGURE 5–214. *Calcaneovarus deformity of the right foot in a 12-year-old girl with myotonic dystrophy.*

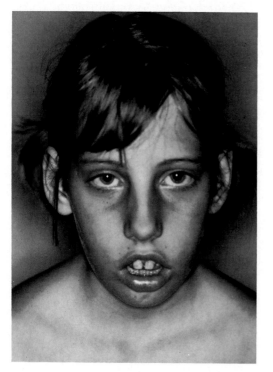

FIGURE 5–215. *Expressionless face in dystrophia myotonica.*

The patient has difficulty in pursing the lips, closing the eyes, and whistling.

Most patients with dystrophia myotonica develop cataracts, frontal baldness (in the male), and gonadal atrophy. Mental retardation is not uncommon.

The course of the disease is one of steady progression; within 20 years of the onset of symptoms, most patients are severely disabled and unable to walk. The majority die before the normal age.

MYOTONIA CONGENITA AND PARAMYOTONIA CONGENITA

There is some controversy about whether dystrophia myotonica and myotonia congenita are separate diseases or clinical variants of the same disease.[199] Intermediate cases do occur, but they are generally regarded as different clinical syndromes. Myotonia congenita (Thomsen's disease) and paramyotonia congenita (Eulenburg's disease) are not associated with dystrophy and are discussed later.[200]

The differential diagnosis of the principal types of muscular dystrophy is presented in Table 5–20.

Diagnosis

The established case of muscular dystrophy with its characteristic pattern of muscular weakness rarely represents a diagnostic problem. It is in the early stages of disease, when the complaints are clumsiness of gait and difficulty in climbing stairs, that diagnosis is more difficult. Often the patient has consulted a number of physicians and has been treated for unrelated conditions, such as retarded development, before the correct diagnosis is made. A careful analysis of the physical, genetic, biochemical, electromyographic, and histologic findings is essential to make the diagnosis of muscular dystrophy.

When a child is presented with muscle weakness, it should first be determined whether this is caused by a primary myopathic or by a neuropathic disease. Electromyography is of great value in distinguishing the two. The distinguishing clinical and laboratory features of disorders of the anterior horn cells, peripheral nerves, and muscles is presented in Table 5–1.

A manual muscle test is performed to localize the specific pattern of muscle involvement. Distal weakness is the first indication of neurogenic disease, in contrast to proximal involvement, which is characteristic of the various types of muscular dystrophy; however, one must be cautious about too rigid categorization of diseases solely on the basis of distal or proximal involvement. Distal myopathy and dystrophia myotonica should be distinguished from peroneal muscular atrophy. The loss of vibratory sense at the ankles in Charcot-Marie-Tooth disease and the associated cataracts, frontal baldness, and sternocleidomastoid weakness in dystrophia myotonica are valuable distinguishing findings.

Other diagnostic signs of neuropathic disease are the presence of fasciculation (rarely, if ever, seen in muscular dystrophy), and changes in deep tendon reflexes (which are usually preserved until late in the course of muscular dystrophy).

The differential diagnosis between muscular dystrophy and polymyositis is sometimes a difficult one. The diagnostic criteria that are of value in differentiating the two diseases are listed in Table 5–21.

Determination of serum levels of creatine phosphokinase is an important diagnostic screening tool. It is elevated in most muscular dystrophies but is not diagnostic.

Histologic examination of muscle obtained by open biopsy is important in establishing the diagnosis of muscular dystrophy. A muscle biopsy clamp will maintain the length of the muscle as it is being fixed (Fig. 5–216). In addition to routine histology, ultrastructure of the muscle tissue and histochemistry should be performed.

Treatment

There is no specific medical treatment for muscular dystrophy; many agents have been tried without benefit.

The severity of muscle weakness, the pattern of muscle involvement, and the type of deformity and functional impairment vary according to the specific form of muscular dystrophy and from patient to patient.

Though severe Duchenne progressive muscular dystrophy almost always results in complete loss of ambulation, there is reason to believe that its loss is premature in many cases. It is imperative that independent ambulation be maintained as long as possible. Progressive muscle weakness eventually leads to the inevitable wheelchair and bed confinement; there is no specific remedy for it. However, there are a variety of contributory factors that can be controlled to delay this loss of independence as much as possible.

In view of these facts, patients with muscular dystrophy are assessed as to their total motor performance on the basis of the degree of

Table 5–20. *Differential Diagnosis of the Principal Types of Muscular Dystrophy*

Clinical Features	Duchenne Type Muscular Dystrophy	Limb Girdle Muscular Dystrophy	Facioscapulo-humeral Muscular Dystrophy	Distal Muscular Dystrophy	Progressive Dystrophia Ophthalmoplegia	Congenital or Infantile Muscular Dystrophy
Incidence	Commonest	Less common, but not infrequent	Not common	Rare	Rare	Rare
Age at onset	Usually prior to 3 yr., some between 3 and 6 yr.	Variable (usually by second decade, occasionally later)	Variable (usually in second decade)	20–77 yr. (mean 47 yr.)	At any age (infancy to over 50 yr.)	At or soon after birth
Sex preponderance	Male	Either sex	Male and female equally affected	Either sex	Either sex	Not yet determined
Inheritance	Sex-linked recessive, autosomal less than 10 per cent	Autosomal recessive, on rare occasions autosomal dominant	Autosomal dominant usually, autosomal recessive very rarely	Autosomal dominant	Simple dominant or simple recessive	Unknown
Pattern of muscle involvement	Proximal (pelvic and shoulder girdle muscles affected early, spreads to periphery of limbs late in course)	Proximal (shoulder and pelvic girdle, spreads to periphery late)	Face and shoulder girdle; later spreads to pelvic girdle	Distal (hand first, anterior tibial, and calf in leg)	Usually limited to extend ocular muscles	Generalized
Muscle spared until late	Gastrocnemius, toe flexors posterior tibial, hamstrings, hand muscles, upper trapezius, biceps, triceps, face, jaw pharyngeal, laryngeal, and ocular	In upper extremity brachioradialis and hand, calf muscles	Back extensors, iliopsoas, hip abductors, quadriceps	Proximal until late	See above	—

Pseudohypertrophy	80 per cent of cases (calf muscles)	Less than 33 per cent of cases	Rare	Not seen	Not seen	Not seen
Myotonia	Absent	Absent	Absent	Absent	Absent	Absent
Contractural deformities	Common	Develop late in course, less severe than Duchenne	Mild, occur late	Mild, late	—	Severe
Scoliosis and kyphoscoliosis	Common in late stage	Mild, in late stage	Mild, occur late	—	—	?
Heart involvement	Hypertrophy and tachycardia common; in late stages widespread degeneration, fibrosis, and fatty infiltration	Very rare	Very rare	Very rare	Not seen	Not observed
Endocrine changes	Not seen	Not seen	Not seen	Not seen	Not seen	?
Intellectual level	Commonly decreased	Normal	Normal	Normal	Normal	?
Course	Steady rapid progression	Slow progression, considerable variation in pace of disease	Progresses insidiously	Comparatively benign	Slow progression	Steady progression

Table 5–21. *Differential Diagnosis of Progressive Muscular Dystrophy and Polymyositis*

Features	Duchenne Type Progressive Muscular Dystrophy	Polymyositis
Sex preponderance	Males	Females
Inheritance	Sex-linked recessive Autosomal recessive less than 10 per cent	None
Pattern of muscle involvement	Proximal, much more selective	Proximal, sometimes distal
Facial muscle weakness	May be present in some forms	Almost never
Weakness of neck and back extensors	Rare except very late	Common
Dysphagia	Very rare except terminally	Frequent
Muscular atrophy	Severe	Mild (with tenderness)
Pseudohypertrophy	Common	Rare
Deep tendon reflexes	Preserved until late	Preserved longer
Skin changes	Not observed	Present
Electromyography	Short low-amplitude potentials	Short low-amplitude potentials Fibrillations
Serum enzymes (creatine kinase and aldolase)	Elevated	Elevated
Muscle biopsy	Variable fiber size degeneration	Degeneration and inflammatory cells
Specific treatment	None	Steroids (definite clinical response if given early in high dosage)
Course	Steady progression	More rapid progression
Prognosis	Usually death within 20 years	Spontaneous remission in 80%

functional capacity that they still possess. Vignos has given a functional classification graded on a scale of 1 through 10, with the higher classifications representing progressively more severe involvement:[207]

1. Obvious defect in posture and walking stance, but walks and climbs stairs without assistance.
2. Walks, but climbs steps only with aid of railing.
3. Walks, but climbs eight standard steps with aid of railing in over 25 seconds.
4. Walks, but cannot climb steps.
5. Walks unassisted, but cannot climb steps or get out of chair.
6. Walks only with assistance of braces.
7. In wheelchair. Sits erect, can roll chair and perform bed or chair activities of daily living.
8. In wheelchair. Sits erect, unable to perform bed and chair activities without assistance.
9. In wheelchair. Sits erect only with support. Able to do only minimal activities of daily living.
10. In bed. Can do no activities of daily living without assistance.

Of the multiple factors involved in the loss of ambulation, *muscle power* is the most important. The antigravity muscles essential for independent walking are the gluteus maximus, quadriceps, and triceps surae. When these muscles become poor in motor strength, some external support, such as knee-ankle-foot orthoses (KAFO) or hip-knee-ankle-foot orthoses (HKAFO), is usually necessary to maintain independent ambulation.

Contractural deformity is another important factor affecting walking. In muscular dystrophy, contractures result from a dynamic imbalance of the agonist-antagonist muscles and from maintenance of limbs in faulty postures for prolonged periods. The most common contractural deformity is an equinus deformity of the foot and ankle, caused by permanent shortening of the triceps surae muscle. As the motor strength of the posterior tibial muscle persists until later in the course of the disease, the foot often tends to assume a varus posture. The equinovarus deformity of the feet interferes with locomotion, as it is difficult to balance oneself on one's toes and lateral border of the foot.

Flexion contracture of the knee, another se-

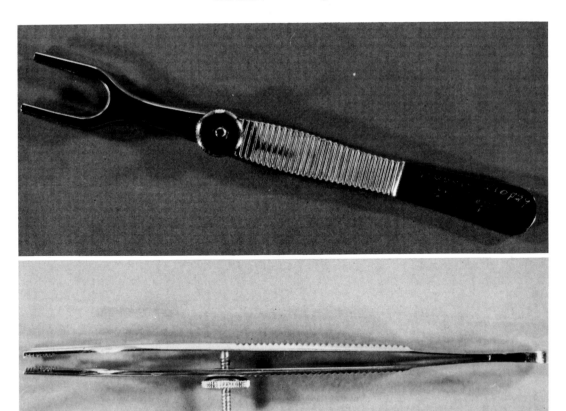

FIGURE 5–216. *Muscle biopsy clamp used to maintain the length of the muscle as it is being fixed.*

rious deformity, causes instability and impedes mechanical efficiency of the quadriceps muscle, thus weakening it further. It is usually minimal when the child is still walking; however, when he is confined to a wheelchair, it becomes progressively severe.

Hip flexion contracture results in anterior shifting of the center of gravity of body weight, making standing balance precarious, particularly in the presence of poor gluteus maximus muscles.

The development of contractures can be prevented or minimized through passive stretching exercises and the use of lightweight orthotic devices.

Inactivity is detrimental, as it will cause disuse atrophy of the muscles. Patients with muscular dystrophy should be encouraged to walk and use their limbs as much as possible. When the dystrophic child suffers a fracture or has a febrile illness, he should not remain in bed any longer than is absolutely necessary. A fractured tibia should be treated in a walking cast. Prolonged bed rest will result in marked loss of motor strength, eventually leading to permanent wheelchair or bed confinement.

Obesity—A sizable weight gain greatly increases the difficulties in ambulation. Because of the inactivity and decreased energy needs, the caloric intake should be limited and carefully controlled by an appropriate dietary regimen. This is a difficult problem, however, due to a combination of psychic overeating and pampering.

Many *emotional factors* influence the regression of locomotion. Most children with muscular dystrophy are withdrawn and exhibit extreme passivity and dependency. A fear of falling produces increased anxiety. A restrained optimism and positive encouragement will boost the morale of these children and motivate walking. Parents and teachers frequently are responsible for too rapid a transition from ambulation to wheelchair status. This premature confinement is a definite deterrent to the child's psychological and intellectual development.

Text continued on page 2150

Scapulocostal Stabilization for Scapular Winging (Ketenjian) (Continued)

OPERATIVE TECHNIQUE

In winging of the scapula in facioscapulohumeral muscular dystrophy, the scapula is malrotated, with its longitudinal axis deviated medially and its inferomedial angle displaced toward the spinous process of the vertebrae.

First determine the position in which the scapula is to be fixed to the thoracic wall. This is done prior to surgery, with the patient standing and the surgeon behind the patient.

A. Between your thumb and fingers, hold the superomedial border of the scapula steady with one hand; with the thumb of your opposite hand, hook the inferior angle of the scapula with the palm and fingers grasping the thoracic cage laterally. The patient's arm hangs loosely at his side.

B. Laterally displace the inferior angle of the scapula until the medial border of the scapula is parallel with the longitudinal axis of the spinous processes of the vertebrae. With the scapula fixed on the thoracic cage, the patient actively abducts the shoulder, and the degree of glenohumeral active abduction is measured. (In this illustration active shoulder abduction is 80 degrees.)

C. Next, laterally displace the inferior angle of the scapula, thus laterally rotating the scapula in the coronal (scapular) plane. (In this illustration the medial border of the scapula is tilted laterally 40 degrees in relation to the vertebral spines.) The patient is asked to actively abduct the shoulder, and the total range of thoracoglenohumeral abduction is measured and correlated with the scapuloaxial angle, i.e., the angle formed by the medial border of the scapula with the longitudinal line connecting the spinous processes of the vertebrae.

At surgery the scapula is fixed to the thoracic cage at the scapuloaxial angle obtained at the maximum desired position of shoulder abduction. The operation is performed with the patient in prone position. The neck, entire thorax, and involved upper limb are prepared and carefully draped to allow free manipulation of the shoulder.

D. With the scapula in position to be fixed to the thoracic cage a longitudinal incision is made at its medial border. The subcutaneous tissue and superficial fascia are divided in line with the skin incision.

Plate 91. Scapulocostal Stabilization for Scapular Winging (Ketenjian)

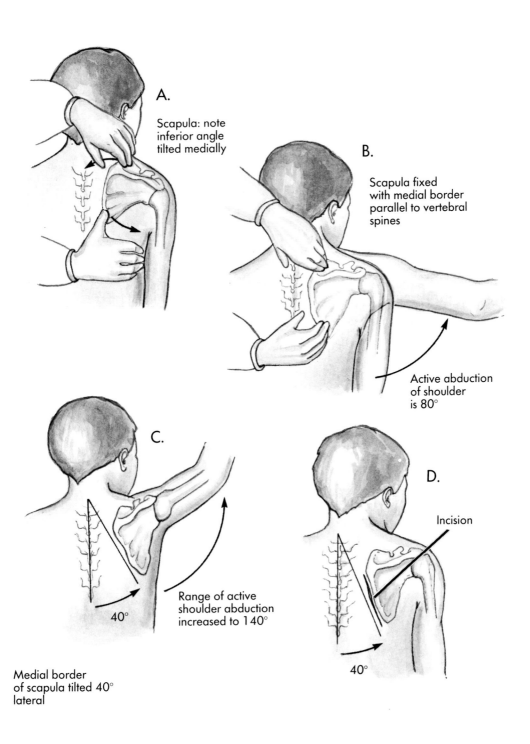

A.

Scapula: note inferior angle tilted medially

B.

Scapula fixed with medial border parallel to vertebral spines

Active abduction of shoulder is 80°

C.

Range of active shoulder abduction increased to 140°

40°

Medial border of scapula tilted 40° lateral

D.

Incision

40°

Scapulocostal Stabilization for Scapular Winging
(Ketenjian) (Continued)

E. The trapezius, levator scapulae, and rhomboids are sectioned from the medial border of the scapula; these muscles will be atrophic and replaced by fibrous or fibrofatty tissue. With a periosteal elevator the supraspinatus, infraspinatus, and subscapularis are elevated for a distance of 2.5 cm. from the medial border of the scapula.

F. Next, make four drill holes 1.3 cm. from the medial border of the scapula at the levels of the adjacent ribs when the scapula is placed in the desired position for stabilization. The scapula is tilted approximately to 20 degrees of lateral rotation.

G. Expose the ribs underlying the drill holes in the scapula subperiosteally. Caution! Do not injure the intercostal vessels and nerves at the inferior margin of the ribs. Then pass Mersilene or fascia lata strips around the ribs.

H. Pass the strips through the drill holes and tie them snugly, with the scapula maintained at 20 degrees of lateral rotation. Then test the stability of fixation of the scapula to the rib cage. The wound is closed in the usual fashion.

POSTOPERATIVE CARE

The upper limb is supported in a sling. Several days postoperatively active assisted and gentle passive range of motion exercises are performed several times a day. Codman pendulum exercises are begun seven days post surgery. The sling support is discontinued four to five weeks after operation.

Plate 91. Scapulocostal Stabilization for Scapular Winging (Ketenjian)

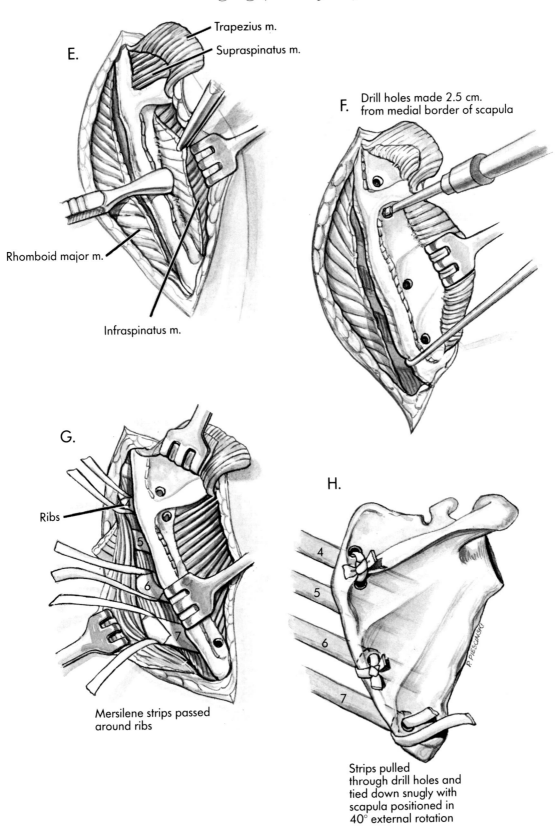

E.
Trapezius m.
Supraspinatus m.
Rhomboid major m.
Infraspinatus m.

F. Drill holes made 2.5 cm. from medial border of scapula

G.
Ribs
5
6
7
Mersilene strips passed around ribs

H.
4
5
6
7
Strips pulled through drill holes and tied down snugly with scapula positioned in 40° external rotation

P. PIESCINSKI

ORTHOTIC SUPPORT

Orthotic devices should be used judiciously, as they are cumbersome and heavy and interfere with trick movements to maintain balance. They should be used toward the end of independent ambulation, i.e., when the child reaches the stage at which he walks less and less and uses furniture and walls for support in getting from place to place. Above-knee orthoses should be used before the child is confined to the wheelchair and prior to development of flexion contractures of the hips and knees. One should not expect a child who has been nonambulatory for more than a month to begin walking after contractural deformities are corrected and he is braced. Orthoses, when used at the appropriate stage in the disease, improve the functional capacity of the dystrophic child and extend the period of ambulation. When the patient is not able to walk even with the help of orthoses, he can stand with assistance, thus preventing the development of flexion deformities of the knees and hips as well as improving his general stamina. Below-knee orthoses do not contribute to functional improvement; their only value lies in preventing contractural deformities of the foot and ankle by supporting them in a functional position.

A *wheelchair* is required for mobility in the later stages of the disease, when the patient becomes incapable of independent ambulation. It should be of the folding type, with brakes, extensible leg rests, and a seat belt (to obviate falls). Hyperextension of the neck may be prevented with an extended back and head rest. With progressive weakness of the shoulders and arm muscles, a lapboard or an overhead device can be added to the wheelchair to assist in bringing the hands to the mouth, as hand function usually persists until very late in the course of the disease. In the wheelchair, appropriate support to the spine should be provided to checkrein the development of scoliosis and lordosis.

Adequate support should be provided to the trunk, as paralytic scoliosis usually develops late in the disease, with the spine collapsing under the strain of body weight. A well-molded plastic body jacket is ordinarily adequate to support and balance the trunk. When spinal deformity is already present, special spinal orthotics are applied, the type depending on the nature of the deformity.

SURGICAL MEASURES

Soft-tissue surgery for release of contractural deformities followed by immediate support in orthoses and ambulation has proved to be of definite value. It is indicated when the contractural deformity interferes with walking and when standing without support becomes precarious. Following surgical correction of deformities of the lower limb in muscular dystrophy, above-knee (KAFO or HKAFO) orthoses will be required for unsupported standing and independent or assisted walking. Preoperatively this should be made clear to the patient and his parents; arrangements should be made so that the child can be fitted with the orthosis on the day of operation and start ambulating immediately. Knee flexion contracture will make proper fitting of the orthosis difficult; in such an instance, when the knee flexion deformity is corrected, above-knee casts made of light plastic tape and with walking heels are applied. The patient is placed upright on a tilt table on the day of surgery. The casts are removed as soon as the orthoses are manufactured, and the child starts walking.

Equinus and Equinovarus Deformity. If the ankle foot deformity is simple equinus and is not severe, percutaneous heel cord lengthening with a sharp Ryerson tenotome is performed. If the deformity is severe and fixed, an open tenotomy is carried out. Often, equinus of the ankle is associated with varus deformity of the hindfoot and forefoot because the posterior tibial muscle function persists until late in the course of the disease. In such an instance, in combination with the heel cord release, two options are available: first, anterior transfer of the posterior tibial through the interosseous route to the dorsum of the foot, as recommended by Spencer.[186] The advantage of this procedure is that it provides active dorsiflexion of the foot; however, such a tendon transfer is not in phase, and the patient needs orthotic support following surgery. In the personal experience of the author, the anteriorly transferred posterior tibial functions only as a tenodesis, not providing active forces for ankle dorsiflexion. For this reason, this procedure is not recommended except in special circumstances when the child does not have severe involvement. The second option is simple release of the posterior tibial tendon combined with heel cord sectioning. The procedure is very simple and fast. If the long toe flexors are contracted, they can be divided at the same time.

Cavus deformity (forefoot equinus) is encountered particularly in Becker type muscular dystrophy. It is corrected by plantar release. The severe rigid cavus deformity requires dorsal wedge resection.

Knee-Hip Flexion Contracture. These are minimal when the patient still is a walker and is splinted at night with the knee in extension and in prone position; when the patient is confined to a wheelchair, however, hip-knee flexion deformity becomes severe. At this stage in the course of the disease, there is no reason to perform surgical release unless the patient complains of low back pain due to the excessive lumbar lordosis.

Scapulocostal Stabilization. In facioscapulohumeral muscular dystrophy, limited shoulder abduction and scapular winging can be corrected by fixation of the scapula to the thoracic cage. The operative technique of scapulocostal fasciodesis as described by Ketenjian is described and illustrated in Plate 91. This surgical procedure is effective in increasing range of shoulder abduction and strength. It also prevents scapular winging.

Screening and Genetic Counseling

Early diagnosis of muscular dystrophy is vital if one is to prevent further affected siblings by means of genetic counseling.[43] Zellweger's micromethod for creatine phosphokinase (CPK) determination has made routine screening of newborn infants relatively simple.[237] Preclinical cases can be detected. Unfortunately, it has not found general appeal. Antenatal diagnosis of muscular dystrophy has been attempted by testing for CPK and carbonic anhydrase III of fetal blood obtained by direct fetoscopy.[56, 57, 190] It appears to be promising, especially when normal values of CPK of fetal blood are standardized in the future.

In X-linked severe Duchenne muscular dystrophy the female carrier is clinically asymptomatic. Serum creatine phosphokinase (CPK) levels are determined to detect female carriers; raised values of CPK are found in about 70 per cent of the carriers.[34] In suspected carrier cases, electromyography and needle muscle biopsy (which is relatively atraumatic) are performed for confirmation. A carrier status is not ruled out by a normal CPK.

In genetic counseling of X-linked Duchenne muscular dystrophy a female carrier has a 50 per cent risk of any son being affected and a 50 per cent risk of any daughter being a carrier. If a female carrier becomes pregnant, it is feasible to sex the fetus at 14 weeks' gestation and, if it is a boy, to perform selective abortion. Prenatal diagnosis is not reliable at present.

Becker's muscular dystrophy is inherited as an X-linked recessive trait; therefore, the principles of genetic counseling are similar to those for Duchenne muscular dystrophy.

Limb girdle dystrophy, being transmitted as an autosomal recessive trait, carries a 25 per cent risk of any further child being affected if both parents are heterozygous. The affected patient, however, will not transmit to his or her children when he or she marries a carrier of the same gene. It is best not to marry a blood relative.

Facioscapulohumeral dystrophy is transmitted as an autosomal dominant trait; therefore, the risk of any child being affected is 50 per cent. Careful examination of the relative is important because about a third are asymptomatic.[129]

For a recent review of the genetics of muscular dystrophies the reader is referred to the excellent article by Harper.[54]

References

1. Aberion, G., Alba, A., Lee, M. H., and Solomon, M.: Pulmonary care of Duchenne type muscular dystrophy. N.Y. State J. Med., 73:1206, 1973.
2. Adams, R. D., Denny-Brown, D., and Pearson, C. M.: Diseases of Muscle: A Study of Pathology. 2nd Ed. New York, Hoeber, 1962.
3. Alderson, M. K., and Ziter, F. A.: Distal muscular dystrophy (Letter). Muscle Nerve, 8:723, 1985.
4. Alexander, M. A., Johnson, E. W., Petty, J., and Stauch, D.: Mechanical ventilation of patients with late stage Duchenne muscular dystrophy: Management in the home. Arch. Phys. Med. Rehabil., 60:289, 1979.
5. Allen, J. E., and Rodgin, D. W.: Mental retardation in association with progressive muscular dystrophy. Am. J. Dis. Child., 100:208, 1960.
6. Appenzeller, O., and Orgin, G.: Pathogenesis of muscular dystrophies. Arch. Neurol., 32:2, 1975.
7. Archibald, K. C., and Vignos, P. J., Jr.: A study of contractures in muscular dystrophy. Arch. Phys. Med., 40:150, 1959.
8. Arthur, H., de-Niese, M., Jeffrey, P. L., and Austin, L.: Plasma lipoprotein in Duchenne muscular dystrophy. Biochem. Int., 6:307, 1983.
9. Aston, J. P., Kingston, H. M., Ramasamy, I., Walters, E. G., and Stansbie, D.: Plasma pyruvate kinase and creatine kinase activity in Becker muscular dystrophy. J. Neurol. Sci., 65:307, 1984.
10. Batten, F. E.: The myopathies or muscular dystrophies: Critical review. Q. J. Med., 3:313, 1909.
11. Batten, F. E., and Gibb, H. P.: Myotonia atrophica. Brain, 32:187, 1909.
12. Becker, P. E.: Two new families of benign sex-linked recessive muscular dystrophy. Rev. Can. Biol., 21:551, 1962.
13. Becker, P. E., and Kiener, F.: Eine neve x-chromasomale Muskeldystrophie. Arch. Psychiatr. Nerven., 193:427, 1955.
14. Bohannon, R. W., and Jones, P. L.: Results of manual resistance exercise on a manifesting carrier of Duchenne muscular dystrophy. A case report. Phys. Ther., 66:973, 1986.
15. Bowker, J. H., and Halpin, P. J.: Factors determining success in reambulation of the child with progressive muscular dystrophy. Orthop. Clin. North Am., 9:431, 1978.

16. Bowyer, S. L., Blane, C. E., Sullivan, D. B., and Cassidy, J. T.: Childhood dermatomyositis: Factors predicting functional outcome and development of dystrophic calcification. J. Pediatr., *103*:882, 1983.

17. Bradley, W. G., Jones, M. Z., Mussini, J. M., and Fawcett, P. R.: Becker type muscular dystrophy. Muscle Nerve, *1*:111, 1978.

18. Brownell, A. K., Paasuke, R. T., Elash, A., Fowlow, S. B., Seagram, C. G., Diewold, R. J., and Friesen, C.: Malignant hyperthermia in Duchenne muscular dystrophy. Anesthesiology, *58*:180, 1983.

19. Burke, S. S., Grove, N. M., Houser, C. R., and Johnson, D. M.: Respiratory aspects of pseudohypertrophic muscular dystrophy. Am. J. Dis. Child., *121*:230, 1971.

20. Call, G., and Ziter, F. A.: Failure to thrive in Duchenne muscular dystrophy. J. Pediatr., *106*:939, 1985.

21. Carter, H. W.: A modified clamp for striated muscle biopsies. Am. J. Clin. Pathol., *51*:516, 1969.

22. Chung, C. S., Morton, N. E., and Peters, H. A.: Serum enzymes and genetic carriers in muscular dystrophy. Am. J. Hum. Genet., *12*:52, 1960.

23. Classics in Neurology: Congenital facioscapulohumeral muscular dystrophy described by Duchenne in 1862. Neurology, *34*:647, 1984.

24. Cohen, L., Morgan, J., Babbs, R., Jr., Karrison, T. G., and Giacomoni, M.: Fast walking velocity in health and Duchenne muscular dystrophy: A statistical analysis. Arch. Phys. Med. Rehabil., *65*:573, 1984.

25. Currie, S.: Inflammatory myopathies. Practitioner, *226*:1039, 1982.

26. Daher, Y. H., Lonstein, J. E., Winter, R. B., and Bradford, D. S.: Spinal deformities in patients with muscular dystrophy other than Duchenne. A review of 11 patients having surgical treatment. Spine, *10*:614, 1985.

27. Danowski, T. S., Wirth, P. M., Leinberger, M. H., Randall, A., and Peters, J. H.: Muscular dystrophy. III. Serum and blood solutes and other laboratory indices. Am. J. Dis. Child., *91*:346, 1956.

28. Delaporte, C., Dehaupas, M., and Fardeau, M.: Comparison between the growth pattern of cell cultures from normal and Duchenne dystrophy muscle. J. Neurol. Sci., *64*:149, 1984.

29. Dorando, C., and Newman, M. K.: Bracing for severe scoliosis of muscular dystrophy patients. Phys. Ther. Rev., 37:230, 1957.

30. Dreyfus, J. C., Schapira, G., and Schapira, F.: Biochemical study of muscle in progressive muscular dystrophy. J. Clin. Invest., 33:794, 1954.

31. Dreyfus, J. C., Schapira, G., and Schapira, F.: Serum enzymes in the pathophysiology of muscle. Ann. N.Y. Acad. Sci., 75:235, 1958.

31a. Dubowitz, V.: Muscle Disorders in Childhood. Philadelphia, W. B. Saunders, 1978.

32. Dubowitz, V., and Brooke, M. H.: Muscle Biopsy: A Modern Approach. Philadelphia, W. B. Saunders, 1973.

33. Duchenne, G. B.: Recherches sur le paralysie musculaire pseudo-hypertrophique ou paralysie myosclerosique. Arch. Gen. Med., *11*:5, 179, 305, 421, 552, 1868.

34. Ebashi, S., Toyokura, Y., Momoi, H., and Sugita, H.: High creatin phosphokinase activity of sera of progressive muscular dystrophy patients. J. Biochem. (Tokyo), *46*:103, 1959.

35. Edwards, R. H., Round, J. M., Jackson, M. J., Griffiths, R. D., and Lilburn, M. F.: Weight reduction in boys with muscular dystrophy. Dev. Med. Child Neurol., *26*:384, 1984.

36. Edwards, R. J., Watts, D. C., Watts, R. L., and Rodeck, C. H.: Creatine kinase estimation in pure fetal blood samples for the prenatal diagnosis of Duchenne muscular dystrophy. Prenat. Diagn., *4*:267, 1984.

37. Egger, J., Kendall, B. E., Erdohazi, M., Lake, B. D., Wilson, J., and Brett, E. M.: Involvement of the central nervous system in congenital muscular dystrophies. Dev. Med. Child Neurol., *25*:32, 1983.

38. Emery, A. E. H., and Dreifuss, F. E.: Unusual type of benign x-linked muscular dystrophy. J. Neurol. Neurosurg. Psychiatry, *29*:138, 1966.

39. Emery, A. E. H., and Skinner, R.: Clinical studies in benign (Becker-type) x-linked muscular dystrophy. Clin. Genet., *10*:189, 1976.

40. Erb, W. H.: Uber die "juvenile form" der progressiven muskelatrophie ihre beziehungen zur sogennanten pseudohypertrophie der muskeln. Dtsch. Arch. Klin. Med., *34*:467, 1884.

41. Erb, W. H.: Dystrophia Muscularis Progressive. Klinische und Pathologischanatomische Studien. Dtsch. Nervenheilk, *1*:13, 1891.

42. Eulenberg, A.: Uber eine familiare, durch 6 Generationen verfolgbare Form kongenitaler Paramyotonie. Zbl. Neurol., *5*:265, 1886.

43. Firth, M. A., and Wilkinson, E. J.: Screening the newborn for Duchenne muscular dystrophy: Parents' views. Br. Med. J., *286*:6382, 1983.

44. Fuchs, E.: Ueberisolieren dopelseitige Ptosia. Arch. Ophthalmol., *36*:234, 1890.

45. Golarz, M. N., Bourne, G. H., and Richardson, H. D.: Histochemical studies on human muscular dystrophy. J. Histochem. Cytochem., *9*:132, 1961.

46. Goodfellow, P. N.: Duchenne muscular dystrophy. Collaboration and progress (News). Nature, *322*:12, 1986.

47. Gowers, W. R.: Pseudohypertrophic Muscular Paralysis. London, Churchill Livingstone, 1879.

48. Gowers, W. R.: A lecture on myopathy of a distal form. Br. Med. J., 2:89, 1902.

49. Gregoric, M., Pecak, F., Tronteli, J. V., and Dimitrijevic, M. R.: Postural control in scoliosis. A statokinesimetric study in patients with scoliosis due to neuromuscular disorders and in patients with idiopathic scoliosis. Acta Orthop. Scand., *52*:59, 1981.

50. Griggs, R. C., Mendell, J. R., Brooke, M. H., Fenichel, G. M., Miller, J. P., Province, M., Moxley, R. T., III, Huntzinger, D., Vaughn, A., and Cohen, M.: Clinical investigation in Duchenne dystrophy: V. Use of creatine kinase and pyruvate kinase in carrier detection. Muscle Nerve, *8*:60, 1985.

51. Grimm, T.: Genetic counseling in Becker type X-linked muscular dystrophy. I. Theoretical considerations. Am. J. Med. Genet., *18*:713, 1984.

52. Grimm, T.: Genetic counseling in Becker type X-linked muscular dystrophy. II. Practical considerations. Am. J. Med. Genet., *18*:719, 1984.

53. Gucker, T., III: The orthopedic management of progressive muscular dystrophy. J. Am. Phys. Ther. Assoc., *44*:243, 1964.

54. Harper, P. S.: The genetics of muscular dystrophies. Prog. Med. Genet., *6*:53, 1985.

55. Hayes, R., London, W., Seidman, J., and Embree, L.: Oculopharyngeal muscular dystrophy. N. Engl. J. Med., *268*:163, 1963.

56. Health, R., Carter, N. D., Jeffrey, S., Edwards, R. J., Watts, D. C., Watts, R. L., and Rodeck, C.: Fetal plasma carbonic anhydrase III in prenatal diagnosis of Duchenne muscular dystrophy. Am. J. Med. Genet., *20*:115, 1985.

57. Health, R., Carter, N. D., Jeffrey, S., Edwards, R. J., Watts, D. C., and Watts, R. L.: Evaluation of carrier detection of Duchenne muscular dystrophy using carbonic anhydrase III and creatine kinase. Am. J. Med. Genet., *21*:291, 1985.

58. Heckmatt, J. Z., Dubowitz, V., Hyde, S. A., Florence, J., Gabain, A. C., and Thompson, N.: Prolongation of walking in Duchenne muscular dystrophy with lightweight orthoses: A review of 57 cases. Dev. Med. Child Neurol., 27:149, 1985.

59. Hoffman, J.: Ein Fall von Thomsen'scher Krankheit, complicert durch Neuritis multiplex. Dtsch. Nervenheilk., 9:272, 1897.

60. Horvath, B., Berg, L., Cummings, D. J., and Shy, G. M.: Muscular dystrophy cation concentrations in residual muscle. J. Appl. Physiol., 8:22, 1955.

61. Houten, R., and De Visser, M.: Histopathological findings in Becker-type muscular dystrophy. Arch. Neurol., 41:729, 1984.

62. Hsu, J. D.: The natural history of spine curvature progression in the nonambulatory Duchenne muscular dystrophy patient. Spine, 8:771, 1983.

63. Hudgson, P., Pearce, G. W., and Walton, J. N.: Preclinical muscular dystrophy: Histopathological changes observed on muscle biopsy. Brain, 90:565, 1967.

64. Hughes, B. P.: A method for the estimation of serum creatine kinase and its use in comparing creatine kinase and aldolase activity in normal and pathological sera. Clin. Chim. Acta, 7:597, 1962.

65. Hutchinson, J.: An ophthalmoplegia externa or symmetrical immobility (partial) of the eye with ptosis. Trans. Med. Chir. Soc. Edinb., 62:307, 1879.

66. Inkley, S. R., Oldenburg, F. C., and Vignos, P. J., Jr.: Pulmonary function in Duchenne muscular dystrophy related to stage of disease. Am. J. Med., 56:197, 1974.

67. Jones, D. A., Round, J. M., Edwards, R. H., Grindwood, S. R., and Tofts, P. S.: Size and composition of the calf and quadriceps muscles in Duchenne muscular dystrophy. A tomographic and histochemical study. J. Neurol. Sci., 60:307, 1983.

68. Jones, G. E., and Witkowski, J. A.: Analysis of skin fibroblast aggregation in Duchenne muscular dystrophy. J. Cell Sci., 48:291, 1981.

69. Jones, G. L.: Plasma anti-proteases in Duchenne muscular dystrophy. Biochem. Med., 27:1, 1982.

70. Karagan, N. J., Richman, L. C., and Sorenson, J. P.: Analysis of verbal disability in Duchenne muscular dystrophy. J. Nerv. Ment. Dis., 168:419, 1980.

71. Kavtaradze, N. P., Mindadze, B. A., and Natriashvili, G. D.: Clinico-genealogic analysis of the malignancy of Duchenne's progressive muscular dystrophy. Zh. Nevropatol. Psikhiatr., 82:26, 1982.

72. Kelfer, H. M., Singer, W. D., and Reynolds, R. N.: Malignant hyperthermia in a child with Duchenne muscular dystrophy. Pediatrics, 71:118, 1983.

73. Kelly, C. R., Redford, J. B., Zilber, S., and Madden, P. A.: Standing balance in healthy boys and in children with Duchenne muscular dystrophy. Arch. Phy. Med. Rehabil., 62:324, 1981.

74. Ketenjian, A. Y.: Muscular dystrophy: Diagnosis and treatment. Orthop. Clin. North Am., 9:25, 1978.

75. Ketenjian, A. Y.: Scapulocostal stabilization for scapula winging in facioscapulohumeral muscular dystrophy. J. Bone Joint Surg., 60-A:476, 1978.

76. Kiessling, W. R., and Beckman, R.: Duchenne muscular dystrophy: Does serum myoglobin correlation with serum creatine kinase? (Letter). Muscle Nerve, 4:257, 1981.

77. Kingston, H. M.: Clinical and genetic studies of Becker muscular dystrophy. M.D. Thesis, University of Manchester, 1983.

78. Kingston, H. M., Sarfarazi, M., Newcombe, R. G., Willis, N., and Harper, P. S.: Carrier detection in Becker muscular dystrophy using creatine kinase estimation and DNA analysis. Clin. Genet., 27:383, 1985.

79. Kinoshita, M., Iwasaki, Y., Wada, F., and Segawa, M.: A case of congenital polymyositis—A possible pathogenesis of "Fukuyama type congenital muscular dystrophy." Rinsho Shinkeigaku, 20:911, 1980.

80. Kobayashi, Y., Suzuki, H., Iinuma, K., Tada, K., and Yamanoto, T. Y.: Endothelial alterations of skeletal muscle capillaries in childhood myopathies. Tohoku J. Exp. Med., 140:381, 1983.

81. Konagaya, M., Takayanagi, T., Kamiya, T., and Takamatsu, S.: Genetic linkage study of Duchenne muscular dystrophy and hemophilia A. Neurology, 32:1046, 1982.

82. Korf, B. R., Bresnan, M. J., Shapiro, F., Sotrel, A., and Abroms, I. F.: Facioscapulohumeral dystrophy presenting in infancy with facial diplegia and sensorineural deafness. Ann. Neurol., 17:513, 1985.

83. Kornfeld, M. S., and Siegel, I. M.: Parental group therapy in the management of two fatal childhood diseases: A comparison. Health Soc. Work, 5:28, 1980.

84. Kousseff, B.: Linkage between chronic granulomatous disease and Duchenne's muscular dystrophy? (Letter). Am. J. Dis. Child., 135:1149, 1981.

85. Kulakowski, S., Renoirte, P., and de Bruyn, C. H.: Dynamometric and biochemical observations in Duchenne patients receiving allopurinol. Neuropediatrics, 12:92, 1981.

86. Kunze, D., Rustow, B., and Olthoff, D.: Studies of selected enzymes of phospholipid metabolism in the dystrophic human muscle. Clin. Chim. Acta, 108:211, 1980.

87. Kurz, L. T., Mubarak, S. J., Schultz, P., Park, S. M., and Leach, J.: Correlation of scoliosis and pulmonary function in Duchenne muscular dystrophy. J. Pediatr. Orthop., 3:347, 1983.

88. Landouzy, L., and Dejerine, J.: De la myopathie atrophique progressive (myopathie hereditaire), debutant, dans l'enfance, par la face, sans alteration du systeme nerveux. C. R. Acad. Sci. (Paris), 98:53, 1884.

89. Laurent, M., Daveloose, D., Leterrier, F., Fischer, S., and Schapira, G.: A spin label study of the erythrocyte membranes on Duchenne muscular dystrophy. Clin. Chim. Acta, 105:183, 1980.

90. Legge, M., and Potter, H. C.: Elevated second trimester amniotic fluid myoglobin from a fetus with Duchenne muscular dystrophy. Aust. N.Z. J. Obstet. Gynaecol., 25:107, 1985.

91. Leibowitz, D., and Dubowitz, V.: Intellect and behavior in Duchenne muscular dystrophy. Dev. Med. Child Neurol., 23:577, 1981.

92. Leth, A., Wulff, K., Corfitsen, M., and Elmgreen, J.: Progressive muscular dystrophy in Denmark. Natural history, prevalence and incidence. Acta Paediatr. Scand., 74:881, 1985.

93. Levine, P. A., and Kristeller, L.: Factors regulating the creatinine output in man. Am. J. Physiol., 24:45, 1909.

94. Lewandowski, K. B.: Strabismus as a possible sign of subclinical muscular dystrophy predisposing to rhabdomyolysis and myoglobinuria: A study of an affected family. Can. Anaesth. Soc. J., 29:372, 1982.

95. Lewis, J. A., and Bertorini, T. E.: Duchenne muscular dystrophy and Tourette syndrome (letter). Neurology, 32:329, 1982.

96. Leyden, E.: Klinik der Ruckenmarks-Krankheiten. Berlin, Hirschwald, 2:531, 1876.

97. Liechti-Gallati, S., Moser, H., Siegrist, H. P., Wiesmann, U., and Herschkowitz, N. N.: Abnormal growth kinetics and 5'-nucleotidase activities in cultured skin fibroblasts from patients with Duchenne muscular dystrophy. Pediatr. Res., 15:1411, 1981.

98. Lopez-Estrada, E., and Lopez, E.: Evoked muscle action potentials in patients with muscular dystrophy. Arch. Phys. Med. Rehabil., 65:717, 1984.

99. Luz Aviles, C., Gutierrez, C., Novoa, F., Gil, E., and Stuardo, A.: Steroid treatment of Duchenne's muscular dystrophy. Rev. Chil. Pediatr., 53:187, 1982.

100. Magotra, M. L., Likhare, R. S., and Sircar, P. K.: Congenital muscular dystrophy. A case report. Indian J. Pediatr., 17:983, 1980.

101. Malarbi, R., and Marenduzzo, A.: Orodental aspects in patients with progressive muscular dystrophy. Arch. Stomatol., 20:535, 1979.

102. Mandon, C., and Colin, D.: The adolescents with myopathies become young adults at Brasset. Rev. Infirm., 32:19, 1982.

103. Manning, G. W., and Cropp, G. J.: The electrocardiogram in progressive muscular dystrophy. Br. Heart J., 20:416, 1958.

104. Marescaux, C., Rumbach, L., Ramdane, S., Galmiche, J., and Warter, J. M.: Combination of a myopathy and involvement of the central and peripheral nervous system. Rev. Otoneuroophthalmol., 54:61, 1982.

105. Matkovics, B., Laszlo, A., and Szabo, L.: A comparative study of superoxide dismutase, catalase and lipid peroxidation in red blood cells from muscular dystrophy patients and normal controls. Clin. Chim. Acta, 118:289, 1982.

106. Matsuishi, T., Yano, E., Terasawa, K., Nonaka, I., Ishihara, O., Yamaguchi, Y., and Okudera, T.: Basilar artery occlusion in a case of Duchenne muscular dystrophy. Brain Dev., 4:379, 1982.

107. Mattioli, L., and Melhorn, M.: Duchenne's muscular dystrophy: The diagnosis and management of cardiac involvement. J. Kans. Med. Soc., 83:115, 1982.

108. Meryon, E.: On granular or fatty degeneration of the voluntary muscles. Trans. Med. Chir. Soc. Edinb., 35:72, 1852.

109. Mgone, C. S., and Kimati, V. P.: Duchenne muscular dystrophy. A case report. Cent. Afr. J. Med., 27:174, 1981.

110. Miike, T., Tamari, H., Ohtani, Y., Nakamura, H., Matsuda, I., and Miyoshino, S.: A fluorescent microscopic study of biopsied muscles from infantile neuromuscular disorders. Acta Neuropathol., 59:48, 1983.

111. Millefiorini, M., and Cortesani, F.: Functional and clinical selectivity in myodystrophic deficits. Rev. Neurol., 52:198, 1982.

112. Miller, G., and O'Connor, J.: Spinal bracing and respiratory function in Duchenne muscular dystrophy (Letter). Clin. Pediatr., 24:94, 1985.

113. Milne, B., and Rosales, J. K.: Anaesthetic considerations in patients with muscular dystrophy undergoing spinal fusion and Harrington rod insertion. Can. Anaesth. Soc. J., 29:250, 1982.

114. Miyazaki, S., Fukuda, S., Shibata, R., Kurokawa, T., Goya, N., Kobayashi, T., and Fukuda, T.: A case of autoimmune hemolytic anemia associated with Duchenne's muscular dystrophy. Nippon Ketsueki Gakkai Zasshi, 43:685, 1980.

115. Möbius, P. J.: Ueber die hereditaren Nervenkrankheiten. Samml. Vortr., 171:1505, 1879.

116. Mollica, F., LiVolti, S., Rapisarda, A., Longo, G., Pavone, L., and Vanella, A.: Increased erythrocytic spermine in Duchenne muscular dystrophy. Pediatr. Res., 14:1196, 1980.

117. Mollman, J. E., Cardenas, J. C., and Pleasure, D. E.: Alteration of calcium transport in Duchenne erythrocytes. Neurology, 30:1236, 1980.

118. Moosa, A.: Duchenne's muscular dystrophy in six siblings. The case for early diagnosis and neonatal screening. S. Afr. Med. J., 62:765, 1982.

119. Mortier, W.: Duchenne's muscular dystrophy—possible therapy. Monatsschr. Kinderheilkd., 128:673, 1980.

120. Moser, H.: Duchenne muscular dystrophy: Pathogenetic aspects and genetic prevention. Hum. Genet., 66:17, 1984.

121. Nesvadba, Z., Hoskova, L., Zdansky, P., and Groh, J.: Functional and biochemical responses of children with progressive muscular dystrophy on standard physical exertion. Sb. Ved. Pr. Lek. Fak. Univ. Karlovy, 24:215, 1981.

122. Nicholson, G. A., and Sugars, J.: Decreased A23187-induced chemiluminescence in Duchenne muscular dystrophy granulocytes. J. Neurol., 56:11, 1982.

123. Nonaka, I., Une, Y., Ishihara, T., Miyoshino, S., Nakashima, T., and Sugita, H.: A clinical and histological study of Ullrich's disease (congenital atonic-sclerotic muscular dystrophy). Neuropediatrics, 12:197, 1981.

124. O'Brien, T., Harper, P. S., Davies, K. E., Murray, J. M., Sarfarazi, M., and Williamson, R.: Absence of genetic heterogeneity in Duchenne muscular dystrophy shown by a linkage study using two cloned DNA sequences. J. Med. Genet., 20:249, 1983.

125. Oguchi, K., and Tsukagoshi, H.: An electron-microscopic study of the T-system in progressive muscular dystrophy (Duchenne) using lanthanum. J. Neurol. Sci., 44:161, 1980.

126. Olney, K. K., and Miller, R. G.: Inflammatory infiltration in Fukuyama type congenital muscular dystrophy (Letter). Muscle Nerve, 6:75, 1983.

127. Olson, B. J., and Fenichel, G. M.: Progressive muscle disease in a young woman with a family history of Duchenne's muscular dystrophy. Arch. Neurol., 39:378, 1982.

128. Oppenheimer, H., and Milhorat, A. T.: Serum proteins, lipoproteins and glycoproteins in muscular dystrophy and related diseases. Ann. N.Y. Acad. Sci., 94:308, 1961.

129. Padberg, G.: Facioscapulohumeral disease. Thesis, University of Leiden, 1982.

130. Padberg, G., Eriksson, A. W., Volkers, W. S., Bernini, L., Van Loghem, E., Meera-Khan, P., Nijenhuis, L. E., Pronk, J. C., and Schreuder, G. M.: Linkage studies in autosomal dominant facioscapulohumeral muscular dystrophy. J. Neurol. Sci., 65:261, 1984.

131. Pandya, S., Florence, J. M., King, W. M., Robison, J. D., Oxman, M., and Province, M. A.: Reliability of goniometric measurements in patients with Duchenne muscular dystrophy. Phys. Ther., 65:1339, 1985.

132. Passos, M. R., Gonzales, C. H., and Zatz, M.: Creatine-kinase and pyruvate-kinase activities in normal children: Implications in Duchenne muscular dystrophy carrier detection. Am. J. Med. Genet., 22:255, 1985.

133. Passos, M. R., and Zatz, M.: Creatine-kinase (CK) and pyruvate-kinase (PK) activities in cord blood of normal newborn infants: Application to Duchenne muscular dystrophy screening programs. Am. J. Med. Genet., 16:367, 1983.

134. Patten, B. M., and Zeller, R. S.: Clinical trials of vasoactive and antiserotonin drugs in Duchenne muscular dystrophy. Ann. Clin. Res., 15:164, 1983.

135. Pearce, J. M. S., Pennington, R. J. T., and Walton, J. N.: Serum enzyme studies in muscle disease. III. Serum creatine kinase activity in relatives of patients of the Duchenne type muscular dystrophy. J. Neurol. Neurosurg. Psychiatry, 27:181, 1964.

136. Pearce, P. H., Johnsen, R. D., Wysocki, S. J., and Kaklas, B. A.: Muscle lipids in Duchenne muscular dystrophy. Aust. J. Exp. Biol. Med. Sci., 59:77, 1981.

137. Pennington, R. J.: Some enzyme studies in muscular dystrophy. Proc. Assoc. Clin. Biochem., 2:17, 1962.

138. Perloff, J. K.: Cardiac rhythm and conduction in

Duchenne's muscular dystrophy: A prospective study of 20 patients. J. Am. Coll. Cardiol., 3:1263, 1984.

139. Pineda, M., Fabregues, I., Campistol, J., Fernandez Alvarez, E., and Alvarez, M.: Therapeutic trial with allopurinol in progressive muscular dystrophy. Ann. Esp. Pediatr., 16:42, 1982.

140. Prick, M. J., Gabreels, F. J., Trijbels, J. M., Janssen, A. J., Le Coultre, R., van Dam, K., Jasper, H. H., Ebels, E. J., and Op de Coul, A. A.: Progressive poliodystrophy (Alpers' disease) with a defect in cytochrome aa3 in muscle: A report of two unrelated patients. Clin. Neurol. Neurosurg., 85:57, 1983.

141. Rabbi Bortolini, E., and Zatz, M.: Investigation on genetic heterogeneity in Duchenne muscular dystrophy. Am. J. Med. Genet., 24:111, 1986.

142. Radhakrishnan, K., Sridharan, R., and Ashok, P. P.: Duchenne muscular dystrophy in monozygotic twins. Indian J. Pediatr., 51:251, 1984.

143. Rayport, M.: A disposable isometric muscle biopsy clamp. J.A.M.A., 210:1451, 1969.

144. Reich, D. R., and Neff, J.: Oral-surgical management of an odontogenic keratocyst in a patient with Duchenne muscular dystrophy. Pediatr. Dent., 3:343, 1981.

145. Rennie, M. J.: Muscle wasting in the muscular dystrophies Dev. Med. Child Neurol., 27:524, 1985.

146. Rideau, Y., Gatin, G., Bach, J., and Gines, G.: Prolongation of life in Duchenne muscular dystrophy. Acta Neurol. (Napoli), 5:118, 1983.

147. Rideau, Y., Glorion, B., Delaubier, A.: The treatment of scoliosis in Duchenne muscular dystrophy. Muscle Nerve, 7:281, 1984.

148. Rideau, Y., Glorion, B., and Duport, G.: Prolongation of ambulation in the muscular dystrophies. Acta Neurol. (Napoli), 5:390, 1983.

149. Riku, S., Konagaya, M., Ibi, T., and Sobue, I.: Unusual sibling cases of Fukuyama type congenital muscular dystrophy. Rinsho Shinkeigaku, 22:216, 1982.

150. Riku, S., Kumagai, T., and Sobue, I.: Familial occurrence of Fukuyama type congenital muscular dystrophy and limb-girdle syndrome. Rinsho Shinkeigaku, 23:711, 1983.

151. Rodriquez, J., and Ferriere, G.: Progressive muscular dystrophies in children. Rev. Chil. Pediatr., 53:379, 1982.

152. Rosalki, S. B.: An improved procedure for serum creatine phosphokinase determination. J. Lab. Clin. Med., 69:696, 1967.

153. Rosenberg, H., and Heiman-Patterson, T.: Duchenne's muscular dystrophy and malignant hyperthermia: Another warning (Letter). Anesthesiology, 59:362, 1983.

154. Rosenthal, M.: Handbuch der Diagnostik und Therapie der Newrvenkrankheiten. Erlangen, F. Enke, 1870.

155. Roses, A. D., Hartwig, G. B., Mabry, M., Nagano, Y., and Miller, S. E.: Red blood cell and fibroblast membranes in Duchenne and myotonic muscular dystrophy. Muscle Nerve, 3:36, 1980.

156. Roses, A. D., Roses, M. J., Miller, S. E., Hull, K. L., and Appel, S. H.: Carrier detection in Duchenne muscular dystrophy. N. Engl. J. Med., 294:193, 1976.

157. Rott, H. D., Breimesser, F. H., and Rodl, W.: Imaging technics in muscular dystrophies. J. Genet. Hum., 33:397, 1985.

158. Rott, H. D., and Mulz, D.: Duchenne's muscular dystrophy: Carrier detection by muscle ultrasound. J. Genet. Hum., 31:63, 1983.

159. Sakai, D. N., Hsu, J. D., Bonnett, C. A., and Brown, J. C.: Stabilization of the collapsing spine in Duchenne muscular dystrophy. Clin. Orthop., 128:256, 1977.

160. Sandyk, R.: Congenital fibre type disproportion. A case report. S. Afr. Med. J., 60:833, 1981.

161. Sanyal, S. K., and Johnson, W. W.: Cardiomyopathy in children with Duchenne's progressive muscular dystrophy. Indian Heart J. Teach. Ser., 6:258, 1980.

162. Sanyal, S. K., Johnson, W. W., Dische, M. R., Pitner, S. E., and Beard, C.: Dystrophic degeneration of papillary muscle and ventricular myocardium. A basis for mitral valve prolapse in Duchenne muscular dystrophy. Circulation, 62:430, 1980.

163. Sanyal, S. K., Leung, R. K., Tierney, R. C., Gilmartin, R., and Pitner, S.: Mitral valve prolapse syndrome in children with Duchenne's progressive muscular dystrophy. Pediatrics, 63:116, 1979.

164. Sanyal, S. K., Tierney, R. C., Rao, P. S., Pitner, S. E., George, S. L., and Givins, D. R.: Systolic time interval characteristics in children with Duchenne's progressive muscular dystrophy: A serial section study. Neurology, 34:60, 1984.

165. Sayli, B. S., Yaltkaya, K., and Cin, S.: Facioscapulohumeral muscular dystrophy concentrated in the village Cullar, Nevsehir, Turkey. Hum. Genet., 67:201, 1984.

166. Scheuerbrandt, G., Lundin, A., Lovgren, T., and Mortier, W.: Screening for Duchenne muscular dystrophy: An improved screening test for creatine kinase and its application in an infant screening program. Muscle Nerve, 9:11, 1986.

167. Schmalbruch, H.: Regenerated muscle fibers in Duchenne muscular dystrophy: A serial section study. Neurology, 34:60, 1984.

168. Schmidt, A., and Hassler, A.: Lipid storage myopathy—a contribution to the problem of the differential diagnosis of muscle dystrophy (Duchenne). Zentralbl. Allg. Pathol., 127:229, 1983.

169. Schober, R.: An unusual cytoplasmic organelle of the perineurium in a case of Duchenne muscular dystrophy. Acta Neuropathol. (Berlin), 61:311, 1983.

170. Scholte, H. R., and Busch, H. F.: Early changes of muscle mitochondria in Duchenne dystrophy. Partition and activity of mitochondrial enzymes in fractionated muscle of unaffected boys and adult patients. J. Neurol. Sci., 45:217, 1980.

171. Secchi, M. B., Wu, S. C., Obbiassi, M., Oltrona, L., and Folli, G.: Evaluation of systolic intervals in Duchenne cardiomyopathy. Arch. Mal Coeur, 75:1291, 1982.

172. Seeger, B. R., Caudrey, D. J., and Little, J. D.: Progression of equinus deformity in Duchenne muscular dystrophy. Arch. Phys. Med. Rehabil., 66:286, 1985.

173. Seeger, B. R., and Sutherland, A. D.: Modular seating for paralytic scoliosis: Design and initial experience. Prosthet. Orthot. Int., 5:121, 1981.

174. Seeger, B. R., Sutherland, A. D., and Clark, M. S.: Orthotic management of scoliosis in Duchenne muscular dystrophy. Arch. Phys. Med. Rehabil., 65:83, 1984.

175. Seiler, J., and Bope, E. T.: The muscular dystrophies. Am. Fam. Physician, 34:123, 1986.

176. Sekiya, E., Yoshida, K., Eguchi, T., Sato, K., and Takahashi, I.: Community care practiced at the Shinagawa Ward: An example of the care of the child with muscular dystrophy. Hokenfu. Zasshi., 39:90, 1983.

177. Serratrice, G., and Pellissier, J. F.: A forgotten muscular dystrophy: Ullrich's disease. Rev. Neurol. (Paris), 139:523, 1983.

178. Serratrice, G., Pellissier, J. F., and Pouget, J.: Distal myopathies: Critical study and report on one case. Ann. Med. Interne (Paris), 133:192, 1982.

179. Siegel, I. M.: Scoliosis in muscular dystrophy. Clin. Orthop., 93:235, 1973.

180. Siegel, I. M.: Spinal stabilization in Duchenne muscular dystrophy: rationale and method. Muscle Nerve, 5:417, 1982.

181. Smith, C. L., and Bush, G. H.: Anaesthesia and

progressive muscular dystrophy. Br. J. Anaesth., 57:1113, 1985.

182. Smyth, D. P.: Quantitative electromyography in babies and young children with primary muscle disease and neurogenic lesions. J. Neurol. Sci., 56:199, 1982.

183. Socol, M. L., Sabbagha, R. E., Elias, S., Tamura, R. K., Simpson, J. L., Dooley, S. L., and Depp, R.: Prenatal diagnosis of congenital muscular dystrophy producing arthrogryposis (Letter). N. Engl. J. Med., 313:1230, 1985.

184. Sollee, N. D., Latham, E. E., Kindlon, D. J., and Bresnan, M. J.: Neuropsychological impairment in Duchenne muscular dystrophy. J. Clin. Exp. Neuropsychol., 7:486, 1985.

185. Somer, H.: Enzyme release from isolated erythrocytes and lymphocytes in Duchenne muscular dystrophy. J. Neurol. Sci., 48:445, 1980.

186. Spencer, G. E., Jr.: Orthopaedic care of progressive muscular dystrophy. J. Bone Joint Surg., 49-A:1201, 1967.

187. Spencer, G. E., Jr., and Vignos, P. J., Jr.: Bracing for ambulation in childhood progressive muscular dystrophy. J. Bone Joint Surg., 44-A:234, 1962.

188. Staheli, L. T.: A clamp for isometric muscle biopsies. Surgery, 59:1154, 1966.

189. Steinert, H.: Myopathologische Beitrage: I. Ueber das klinische und anatomische Bild des Muskelschwunds der Myotoniker. Dtsch. Nervenheilk., 37:58, 1909.

190. Stengel-Rutkowski, L., Scheuerbrandt, G., Beckmann, R., and Pongratz, D.: Prenatal diagnosis of Duchenne's muscular dystrophy. (Letter). Lancet, 1:1359, 1977.

191. Stern, L. M., Caudrey, D. J., Clark, M. S., Perrett, L. V., and Boldt, D. W.: Carrier detection in Duchenne muscular dystrophy using computed tomography. Clin. Genet., 27:392, 1985.

192. Stern, L. M., Caudrey, D. J., Perrett, L. V., and Boldt, D. W.: Progression of muscular dystrophy assessed by computed tomography. Dev. Med. Child Neurol., 26:569, 1984.

193. Sussman, M. D.: Treatment of scoliosis in Duchenne muscular dystrophy. Dev. Med. Child Neurol., 27:522, 1985.

194. Swank, S. M., Brown, J. C., and Perry, R. E.: Spinal fusion in Duchenne's muscular dystrophy. Spine, 7:484, 1982.

195. Swinyard, C. A., Deaver, G. G., and Greenspan, L.: Gradients of functional ability of importance in rehabilitation of patients with progressive muscular and neuromuscular diseases. Arch. Phys. Med., 38:574, 1957.

196. Szentistvanyi, F., Janka, Z., and Heiner, L.: Calcium-dependent potassium transport in progressive muscular dystrophy. Eur. Neurol., 19:39, 1980.

197. Tamari, H., Ohtani, Y., Higashi, A., Miyoshino, S., and Matsuda, I.: Xanthine oxidase inhibitor in Duchenne muscular dystrophy. Brain Dev., 4:137, 1982.

198. Taylor, D. A., Carroll, J. E., Smith, M. E., Johnson, M. O., Johnston, G. P., and Brooke, M. H.: Facioscapulohumeral dystrophy associated with hearing loss and Coats syndrome. Ann. Neurol., 12:395, 1982.

199. Thomasen, E.: Myotonia: Thomsen's Disease (Myotonia congenita), Paramyotonia and Dystrophia Myotonica: A Clinical and Heredobiologic Investigation. Aarhus, Denmark, Universitetsforlaget, 1948.

200. Thomsen, J.: Tonische Krampfe in willkurlich beweglichen muskeln in Folge von Ererbter psychischer Disposition (Ataxia muscularis?). Arch. Psychiatr. Nervenkr., 6:706, 1876.

201. Thornell, L. E., Edstrom, L., Eriksson, A., Henriksson, K. G., and Angqvist, K. A.: The distribution of intermediate filament protein (skeletin) in normal and diseased human skeletal muscle—an immunohisto-

chemical and electron-microscopic study. J. Neurol. Sci., 47:153, 1980.

202. Turner, J. W. A.: The relationship between amytonia congenita and congenital myopathy. Brain, 63:163, 1940.

203. Turner, J. W. A.: On amyotonia congenita. Brain, 72:25, 1949.

204. Tyler, K. L., and McHenry, L. C., Jr.: Classics in neurology. Fragments of neurologic history: Pseudohypertrophic muscular dystrophy and Gowers' sign. Neurology, 33:88, 1983.

205. Valikova, T. A.: Clinical results of thymectomy in myopathy patients depending on the degree of muscular weakness. Vrach. Delo, 5:89, 1981.

206. van Wijngaarden, G. K., and Bethlem, J.: The facioscapulohumeral syndrome. In Kakulas, B. A.: The Second International Congress on Muscle Diseases. Perth, Australia, 1971. Abstracts. Amsterdam, Excerpta Medica, I.C.S. No. 237, 1971, p. 54.

207. Vignos, P. J., Jr.: Diagnosis of progressive muscular dystrophy. J. Bone Joint Surg., 49-A:1212, 1967.

208. Vignos, P. J., Jr., and Archibald, K. C.: Maintenance of ambulation in childhood muscular dystrophy. J. Chron. Dis., 12:273, 1960.

209. Vignos, P. J., Jr., and Lefkowitz, M.: A biochemical study of certain skeletal muscle constituents in human progressive muscular dystrophy. J. Clin. Invest., 38:873, 1959.

210. Vignos, P. J., Jr., Spencer, G. E., Jr., and Archibald, K. C.: Management of progressive muscular dystrophy in childhood. J.A.M.A., 184:89, 1963.

211. Vignos, P. J., Jr., and Wagner, M. B.: More about muscular dystrophy (Letter). Phys. Ther., 60:810, 1980.

212. Vignos, P. J., Jr., Wagner, M. B., Kaplan, J. S., and Spencer, G. E., Jr.: Predicting the success of reambulation in patients with Duchenne muscular dystrophy. J. Bone Joint Surg., 65-A:719, 1983.

213. Vignos, P. J., Jr., and Watkins, M. P.: The effect of exercise in muscular dystrophy. J.A.M.A., 197:843, 1966.

214. Wakayama, Y., Bonilla, E., and Schotland, D. L.: Muscle plasma membrane abnormalities in infants with Duchenne muscular dystrophy. Neurology, 33:1368, 1983.

215. Walton, J. N.: On the inheritance of muscular dystrophy. Ann. Hum. Genet., 20:1, 1955.

216. Walton, J. N.: The inheritance of muscular dystrophy. Further observations. Ann. Hum. Genet., 21:40, 1956.

217. Walton, J. N.: Clinical aspects of human muscular dystrophy. In Bourne, G. H., and Golarz, N., (eds.): Muscular Dystrophy in Man and Animals. New York, S. Karger, 1962.

218. Walton, J. N., and Gardner-Medwin, D.: Progressive muscular and myotonic disorders. In Disorders of Voluntary Muscle. 4th Ed. Edinburgh, Churchill Livingstone, 1981, pp. 481–524.

219. Walton, J. N., and Nattrass, F. J.: On the classification, natural history and treatment of the myopathies. Brain, 77:169, 1954.

220. Waters, R. L., Perry, J., McDaniels, J. M., and House, K.: The relative strength of the hamstrings during hip extension. J. Bone Joint Surg., 56-A:1592, 1974.

221. Watkins, S. C., and Cullen, M. J.: Muscle fiber size and shape in Duchenne muscular dystrophy. Neuropathol. Appl. Neurobiol., 8:11, 1982.

222. Watters, G. V., and Williams, T. W.: Early-onset myotonic dystrophy. Clinical and laboratory findings in five families and a review of the literature. Arch. Neurol., 17:137, 1967.

223. Weimann, R. L., Gibson, D. A., Moseley, C. F., and Jones, D. C.: Surgical stabilization of the spine in Duchenne muscular dystrophy. Spine, 8:776, 1983.

224. Welander, L.: Myopathia distalis tarda hereditaria. Acta Med. Scand. (Suppl.), 265:1, 1951.
225. Whorton, C. M., Hudgins, P. C., and Connors, J. J.: Abnormal spectrophotometric absorption spectrums of myoglobin in two forms of progressive muscular dystrophy. N. Engl. J. Med., 265:1242, 1961.
226. Wilkins, K. E., and Gibson, D. A.: The patterns of spinal deformity in Duchenne muscular dystrophy. J. Bone Joint Surg., 58-A:24, 1976.
227. Williams, E. A., Read, L., Ellis, A., Morris, P., and Galasko, C. S. B.: The management of equinus deformity in Duchenne muscular dystrophy. J. Bone Joint Surg., 66-B:546, 1984.
228. Wohlfart, G.: Aktuelle Probleme der Muskelpathologie. Dtsch. Nervenheilk., 173:426, 1955.
229. Worden, D. K., and Vignos, P. J., Jr.: Intellectual function in childhood progressive muscular dystrophy. Pediatrics, 29:968, 1962.
230. Yasin, R., Walsh, F. S., Landon, D. N., and Thompson, E. J.: New approaches to the study of human dystrophic muscle cells in culture. J. Neurol., 58:315, 1983.
231. Yokochi, K., Tanaka, T., and Nonaka, I.: Congenital muscular dystrophy with severe infantile scoliosis. Brain Dev., 7:492, 1985.
232. Young, A., Johnson, D., O'Gorman, E., Macmillan, T., and Chase, A. P.: A new spinal brace for use in Duchenne muscular dystrophy. Dev. Med. Child Neurol., 26:808, 1984.
233. Zalmann, F., Perloff, J. K., Durant, N. N., and Campion, D. S.: Acute respiratory failure following intravenous Verapamil in Duchenne's muscular dystrophy. Am. Heart J., 105:510, 1983.
234. Zatuchni, J., Aegerter, E. E., Molthan, L., and Shuman, C. R.: The heart in progressive muscular dystrophy. Circulation, 3:846, 1951.
235. Zatz, M., and Betti, R. T.: Benign Duchenne muscular dystrophy in a patient with growth hormone deficiency: A five year follow-up. Am. J. Med. Genet., 24:567, 1986.
236. Zatz, M., Betti, R. T., and Frota-Pessoa, O.: Treatment of Duchenne muscular dystrophy with growth hormone inhibitors. Am. J. Med. Genet., 24:549, 1986.
237. Zellweger, H., and Antonik, A.: Newborn screening for Duchenne muscular dystrophy. Pediatrics, 5:30, 1975.
238. Zellweger, H., Afifi, A., McCormick, W. F., and Mergner, W.: Severe congenital muscular dystrophy. Am. J. Dis. Child., 114:591, 1967.
239. Ziter, F. A., Allsop, K. G., and Tyler, F. H.: Assessment of muscle strength in Duchenne muscular dystrophy. Neurology, 27:981, 1977.

MYOTONIA CONGENITA (THOMSEN'S DISEASE)

Myotonia congenita is a congenital affliction characterized by myotonia of the entire voluntary musculature—a state of delayed relaxation of the muscle following voluntary contraction or mechanical or electrical stimulation; i.e., active contraction of the muscle continues. In the electromyograph there is an afterdischarge. The condition is extremely rare. It was first described by Julius Thomsen, who himself suffered from the disease and could trace it through five generations of his family. About one fourth of the reported cases are inherited by autosomal dominant transmission.[1] A recessive pattern of inheritance has been reported.[25] Males and females are affected equally.

Etiology and Pathology

The cause of Thomsen's disease is unknown. The basic defect resides in the sarcoplasm of the muscle itself. The myotonic response may be the result of blockage of potassium transfer across the cell membrane, or it may be produced by defective formation or utilization of energy-rich phosphates.

The only significant pathologic finding is hypertrophy of the muscle fibers. There is no evidence of degenerative or dystrophic changes. The central nervous system is found to be normal at autopsy.[6, 12] Myotonia occurs independently of the nerve supply to the muscles or its motor end-plate.

Clinical Features

Myotonia, the cardinal feature of Thomsen's disease, may be noted in infancy or early childhood. Often a history of delay in motor development is given by the parents. The presenting complaints are difficulty and stiffness in initiating any active movements following rest, difficulty in walking or running after prolonged sitting, frequent falling, and clumsiness. Myotonia is usually more marked in the lower limbs. It is also worse with the initial motion; after repetitive movements, the myotonia decreases and successive movements are executed with greater ease. Repetitive movement of one group of muscles, however, does not prevent myotonia from taking place in a separate group of adjacent muscles. Thus, limbering of the legs by walking does not prevent myotonia when attempting to ascend a flight of stairs.

The characteristic physical finding is myotonia, which can be observed when the surface of any muscle is sharply percussed with a reflex hammer or pencil. The stimulated area of the muscle will contract and will remain contracted for several seconds before relaxing (see Fig. 5–213 C and D). Another way to demonstrate myotonia is to ask a patient to open a tightly clenched fist rapidly (see Fig. 5–213 A and B). Muscle weakness and endocrine abnormalities are not found in myotonia congenita. Neurologic examination is normal. As the child grows older, diffuse hypertrophy of the muscles develops, giving the patient a so-called Herculean appearance.

Laboratory Findings

The electromyogram will disclose a rapid volley of action potentials. The sound of rhythmic myotonic discharges emanating from the electromyographic loudspeaker exhibits a crescendo and decrescendo quality that has been likened to that of a diving airplane. These electromyographic findings are similar in all myotonic disorders.[11]

The levels of serum enzymes, creatine phosphokinase and aldolase, are normal. In myotonia congenita, however, creatine clearance is increased, reflecting the increased metabolism and greater production of creatinine by hypertrophic muscles. Creatine is not excreted in urine.

Differential Diagnosis and Treatment

Myotonia congenita should be distinguished from myotonic dystrophy and paramyotonia congenita of Eulenburg (Table 5–22).

Quinine sulfate (300 mg. orally two or three times a day) or procaine amide will ameliorate the myotonia. Prednisone is equally effective in

Table 5–22. Differential Diagnosis of Myotonia in Children

	Myotonia Congenita (Thomsen's Disease)	Paramyotonia Congenita (Paramyotonia of Eulenberg)	Myotonic Dystrophy
Age at onset	Childhood or infancy	Infancy or early childhood	Childhood to adulthood
Inheritance	Autosomal dominant (¼ of cases) Recessive gene often (Becker)	Autosomal dominant	Autosomal dominant
Sex incidence	Males and females equally affected	Males and females equally affected	Males and females equally affected
Precipitating factors	Voluntary movement after prolonged sitting or inactivity	Exposure to cold	Voluntary movement
Clinical findings			
Muscle group involved	Generalized	Proximal muscles of limbs, eyelids, and tongue	Muscles in face, tongue, and distal limbs, particularly upper
	Difficulty in walking or running after prolonged sitting Clumsiness	Intermittent attacks of weakness may last from few minutes to 24 hr. Myotonia precedes weakness	
Response to activity	Improves myotonia	Aggravates myotonia	Aggravates myotonia and fatigue-affected muscles
Muscle hypertrophy	Present ("Herculean appearance")	Absent	Muscle atrophic
Endocrine, cardiac, other abnormalities	None	None	Testicular atrophy, EKG changes Frontal baldness, mental retardation
Laboratory findings			
Serum potassium level	Normal	High normal or elevated	Normal
Creatine phosphokinase, aldolase levels	Normal	Normal	Elevated
Creatine clearance	Increased	Normal	Decreased
EMG	Rapid volley of action potentials on insertion of electrode in myotonic muscle	Rapid volley of action potentials on insertion of electrode in myotonic muscle	Rapid volley of action potentials of varying amplitude on insertion of electrode in myotonic muscle
Histologic findings	Hypertrophy of muscle fibers No dystrophic changes	Similar to myotonic dystrophy	Dystrophic changes (see text)
Treatment	Quinine hydrochloride and procaine amide effective	Not available Calcium gluconate may abort an attack	No specific treatment
Prognosis	Disability minimal Condition remains static	Improves with age Nonprogressive	Progressive, moderate disability over a period of many years.

relieving myotonia; however, it should be used with caution because of its side effects.

Disability is minimal, and often patients learn to live satisfactorily with the disease by "warming up" to limber the muscles before activity. Drug therapy should be reserved for use only in severe cases.

References

1. Adams, R.D., Denny-Brown, D., and Pearson, C.M.: Diseases of Muscle. A Study in Pathology. 2nd Ed. New York, Harper and Bros., 1962, p. 650.
2. Becker, P.E.: *In* Proceedings, Third International Congress Human Genetics. Baltimore, Johns Hopkins Press, 1967.
3. Birt, A.: A study of Thomsen's disease (congenital myotonia) by a sufferer from it. Montreal Med., 37:771, 1908.
4. Bourne, G.H.: The Structure and Function of Muscle. Vol. III. Pharmacology and Disease. New York, Academic Press, 1960.
5. Celesia, G.G., Andermann, F., Wiglesworth, F.W., and Robb, J.P.: Monomelic myopathy—congenital hypertrophic myotonic myopathy limited to one extremity. Arch. Neurol., 17:69, 1967.
6. Déjerine, J., and Sotas, J.: Sur un cas de maladie de Thomsen, suivi d'autopsie. Rev. Med., 15:241, 1895.
7. Denny-Brown, D., and Nevin, S.: The phenomenon of myotonia. Brain, 64:1, 1941.
8. Ellis, F.R.: Inherited muscle disease. Br. J. Anaesth., 52:153, 1980.
9. Erb: Ueber die Thomsen'sche Krankheit. Wien Klin. Wochenschr., 2:931, 1889.
10. Flora, G.C.: Differential diagnosis of myotonia. Postgrad. Med., 41:148, 1967.
11. Floyd, W.F., Kent, P., and Page, F.: An electromyographic study of myotonia. Electroencephalogr. Clin. Neurophysiol., 7:621, 1955.
12. Foix, C., and Nicoleson, I.: Note sur les alterations du systeme nerveux dans un cas de maladie de Thomsen. C.R. Soc. Biol. (Paris), 89:1095, 1923.
13. Gerschwind, N., and Simpson, J.A.: Procaine amide in the treatment of myotonia. Brain, 78:81, 1955.
14. Haass, A., Ricker, K., Rudel, R., Lehmann-Horn, F., Bohlen, R., Dengler, R., and Mertens, H.G.: Clinical study of paramyotonia congenita with and without myotonia in a warm environment. Muscle Nerve, 4:388, 1981.
15. Harper, P.S.: Myotonic disorders. Practitioner, 226:1065, 1982.
16. Hausmanowa-Petrusewicz, I.: Diagnostic value of the electromyography in myopathies. Neurol. Neurochir. Pol., 5–6:370, 1982.
17. Howeler, C.J., Busch, H.F., Bernini, L.F., van Loghem, E., Khan, P.M., and Nijenhuis, L.E.: Dystrophia myotonia and myotonia congenita concurring in one family. A clinical and genetic study. Brain, 103:497, 1980.
18. Isaacs, H.: The treatment of myotonia congenita. S. Afr. Med. J., 33:984, 1959.
19. Jiddane, M., Gastaut, J.L., Pellissier, J.F., Pouget, J., Serratrice, G., and Salamon, G.: CT of primary muscle diseases. A.J.N.R., 4:773, 1983.
20. Johnsen, T., and Frilis, M.L.: Paramyotonia congenita (von Eulenburg) in Denmark. Acta Neurol. Scand., 61:78, 1980.
21. Johnson, J.: Thomsen and myotonia congenita. Med. Hist., 12:190, 1968.
22. Johnson, R., Somer, H., Karli, P., and Saris, N.E.: Erythrocyte flexibility, ATPase activities and CA efflux in patients with Duchenne muscular dystrophy, myo-
23. Kuhn, E.: Liegt den Erbkranheiten Myotonia congenita und Dystrophia myotonica eine biochemisch fassbare Storung zugrunde? Aerztl. Forsch., 15:6, 1961.
24. Kuzuhara, S.: Myotonia and related diseases. Nippon Rinsho, 40:1547, 1982.
25. Liebenam, L.: Zwillingspathologische Beobachtung bei Myotonia congenita (Thomsen'sche Krankheit). Z. Mensch. Vererb. Konstitutionslehre, 24:13, 1939.
26. Maas, O., and Paterson, A.S.: The identity of myotonia congenita (Thomsen's disease), dystrophia myotonica (myotonia atrophica) and paramyotonia. Brain, 62:198, 1939.
27. Nissen, K.: Beitrage zur Kenntnis der Thomsenschen Krankheit (Myotonia congenita) mit Besonderer Berucksichtigung des hereditaren Momentes und seinen Beziehungen zu den Mendelschen Vererbungsregeln. Z. Klin. Med., 97:58, 1923.
28. Sanders, J.: Eine Familie mit Myotonia congenita. (Thomsen'sche Krankheit). Genetica, 17:253, 1935.
29. Streib, E.W., and Sun, S.F.: EMG detection of heterozygote carriers of recessive generalized myotonia (Letter). Muscle Nerve, 5:179, 1982.
30. Swash, M., and Schwartz, M.S.: Normal muscle spindle morphology in myotonia congenita: the spindle abnormality in myotonic dystrophy is not due to myotonia alone. Clin. Neuropathol., 2:75, 1983.
31. Thomasen, E.: Myotonia. Universitatis hafniensis. Copenhagen, Munksgaard, 1948.
32. Thomsen, J.: Tonische Kranfe in willkurlich beweglichen Muskein in Folge von erebier psychischer Disposition. Arch. Psychiat. Nervenkr., 6:706, 1876.
33. Van Der Meulen, J.P., Gilbert, G.J., and Kane, C.A.: Familial hyperkalemic paralysis with myotonia. N. Engl. J. Med., 264:1, 1961.
34. Wagner, A., and Zett, L.: Results of electromyographical and mechanographical investigations in myotonia congenita (author's transl.). EEG EMG, 13:14, 1982.
35. Winters, J.L., and McLaughlin, L.A.: Myotonia congenita. J. Bone Joint Surg., 52-A:1345, 1970.
36. Wohlfart, G.: Dystrophia myotonica and myotonia congenita. Histopathologic studies with special reference to changes in the muscle. J. Neuropathol. Exp. Neurol., 10:109, 1951.
37. Wroblewski, T., and Wesolek, D.: Case of Thomsen's myotonia with an atypical course. Pediatr. Pol., 55:1161, 1980.
38. Zellweger, H., Pavone, L., Biondi, A., Cimino, V., Gullotta, F., Hart, M., Ionasescu, V., Mollica, F., and Schieken, R.: Autosomal recessive generalized myotonia. Muscle Nerve, 3:176, 1980.

MYOSITIS

Myositis is a general term used to describe several inflammatory conditions of muscles, such as suppuration myositis, traumatic myositis, parasitic infestation of muscles (trichinosis), and polymyositis. Often, what may be interpreted as myositis is due to a spasm or sensitivity in the muscles arising from lesions in other tissues in related structures such as adjacent joints or from the nervous system.

POLYMYOSITIS AND DERMATOMYOSITIS

Polymyositis is a nonhereditary myopathy characterized by nonsuppurative inflammation of voluntary muscles associated with degenerative changes and motor weakness. It was first described by Wagner in 1863.[133] When it occurs in conjunction with nonsuppurative inflammation of the skin and erythematous skin rash, the term *dermatomyositis* is used to describe the condition. Unverricht (1887) is credited as being the first to delineate the subgroup of dermatomyositis.[130] Polymyositis and dermatomyositis are variants of the same disorder. Banker and Victor, in 1966, described a childhood form of dermatomyositis with vascular complications.[9]

Age-Sex

About one sixth of the cases of polymyositis occur in children, and the condition is twice as common in females as in males.

Classification

Pearson has subdivided polymyositis into six types: polymyositis in adults (Type I); typical dermatomyositis in adults (Type II); typical dermatomyositis (occasionally polymyositis) with malignancy (Type III); childhood dermatomyositis (Type IV); acute myolysis (Type V); and polymyositis in Sjögren's syndrome (Type IV).[106-109]

The World Federation of Neurology Research Group on Neuromuscular Disorders gave the following classification of polymyositis and dermatomyositis:[143]

Group I. Simple or uncomplicated polymyositis
Group II. Dermatomyositis and myositis associated with connective tissue disorders
    A. Adult dermatomyositis
    B. Childhood dermatomyositis
    C. Polymyositis associated with
        a. Rheumatoid arthritis
        b. Sjögren syndrome
        c. Progressive systemic sclerosis
        d. Systemic lupus erythematosus
Group III. Polymyositis and dermatomyositis associated with malignancy

It should be noted that dermatomyositis is the more common form observed in children. Childhood dermatomyositis with vasculitis involving the gastrointestinal tract is a distinct entity with characteristic clinical and pathologic features.[8, 9] Acute myolysis is frequently a disease of childhood, although it may occur in adults.

Etiology

The exact cause of polymyositis and dermatomyositis is unknown. It most probably is an autoimmune disorder. The hypersensitivity may be due to an "altered" muscle protein or to a tumor antigen. Some cases of polymyositis may be the result of an as yet unrecognized infectious, toxic, or metabolic cause.

In some cases one can identify precipitating factors, such as connective tissue disorders, neoplasms, viral exanthemas, drugs, and agammaglobulinemia.

Neoplasms. In adults there is a significant association between malignant tumors and polymyositis or dermatomyositis. The overall incidence of the disease found in the combined form is reported to be 20 per cent; simultaneous occurrence of these two pathologic conditions is not found in children. An adult male over 40 years of age with dermatomyositis, according to Arundell et al., has a 50 per cent chance of developing a neoplasm, and according to De Vere and Bradley, a 66 per cent chance.[7, 48] It should be noted, however, that such an association does not denote a causal relationship.

Connective Tissue Disease. Polymyositis and dermatomyositis occur in systemic lupus erythematosus, rheumatoid arthritis, Sjögren's syndrome, progressive systemic sclerosis, and periarteritis nodosa. In childhood dermatomyositis, vasculitis in muscles is commonly found, and there are associated joint manifestations in the form of arthralgia and overt arthritis.

Dermatomyositis may be associated with hereditary X-linked or primary acquired agammaglobulinemia. The immunocompromised child is susceptible to viral infections such as echovirus.

Polymyositis and dermatomyositis may be precipitated by viral exanthema, toxoplasmosis, and a febrile illness such as a viral upper respiratory infection or gastroenteritis. Other precipitating factors are drugs such as sulfonamides and penicillin.

Pathology

The involved skeletal muscles may be pale red, grayish red, or yellowish, and on palpation their consistency is either soft and friable or rubbery and firm, depending on the duration of the disease. The principal histologic abnormalities are widespread degeneration of muscle fibers with some regenerative activity, perivascular collections of chronic inflammatory cells, and phagocytosis of necrotic muscle fibers. In the later stages of the disease, interstitial fibrosis takes place. Vasculitis with hyperplasia of the intima of the arteries and veins may be present.[1, 136]

In order to observe typical histologic changes, it is essential to choose the site for muscle biopsy carefully; the muscle should be neither markedly weakened and atrophic nor of normal strength.

In dermatomyositis, the epidermis is thinned, and there is edema and vasculitis in the dermis.

Clinical Features

Polymyositis is a kaleidoscopic disease with great diversity in its symptoms and variable modes of onset and rate of progression, with exacerbation and remissions. It is difficult to portray a unified clinical picture of the disease.

The symptoms may become manifest following exposure to sunlight, an exanthem, febrile illness, or injury and following ingestion of drugs such as the sulfonamides or penicillin. Often a precipitating cause cannot be found, and most likely the preceding "inciting factors" are coincidental, occurring during the subclinical stage of the disease. In dermatomyositis, however, photosensitivity is common, with sunlight initiating or aggravating the eruption on the face, upper limbs, and trunk.

Dermatomyositis in children may have a sudden onset and acute course, or an insidious beginning and chronic course.

Muscle weakness of varying severity is present in all cases. In its absence, the diagnosis of polymyositis should not be made. In the subacute and chronic forms of the disease, muscular weakness develops insidiously, similar to that seen in progressive muscular dystrophy. The muscles of the pelvic and shoulder girdles are affected first. Initial symptoms consist of difficulty in arising from the floor or in climbing up steps without holding the hand rails. Soon the patient is unable to comb his hair and cannot abduct the shoulders to 90 degrees. As the disease progresses and the sternocleidomastoid muscle becomes affected, he is unable to flex his neck and lift his head against gravity while supine. Involvement of the muscles of the pharynx and deglutition causes dysphagia and difficulty in eating. The patient may develop dysphagia with a nasal voice. In severe cases, weakness may extend to involve all the muscles of the body. The patient becomes confined to a wheelchair or bed. Progressive involvement of the respiratory muscles may lead to death; however, a fatal outcome is very rare.

The affected muscles become tender, brawny, and indurated. Pain is more prominent about the shoulders, upper back, arms, and thighs.

The *skin lesions* of dermatomyositis are quite characteristic. The rash consists of a dusky, violaceous, or faint erythema over the bridge of the nose and the malar areas in a butterfly distribution. A dark lilac discoloration of the upper eyelids can be seen, which is called heliotrope eyelids; this is believed to be pathognomonic for dermatomyositis. The periorbital rash may spread to the neck and upper chest. The skin on the extensor surfaces of the elbows, knees, and metacarpophalangeal joints and on the medial malleoli often becomes erythematous, atrophic, and scaly. There may be linear hyperemic streaks on the dorsa of the hands and fingers. There may be hyperemia at the base of the fingernails; the skin of the fingertips may be shiny, red, and atrophic. In the acute stage of the disease, the skin and subcutaneous tissue frequently develop nonpitting edema. Later, the skin over the involved parts becomes tight and glossy. During the chronic stage, the skin becomes atrophic and adherent to underlying structures. Calcium deposits eventually develop in the subcutaneous tissues, muscles, and fasciae (Fig. 5–217).

Mild transient nonspecific *synovitis* of the knees, wrists, and metacarpophalangeal and interphalangeal joints occurs in about 40 per cent of patients. Occasionally, articular manifestations are present prior to the appearance of muscle weakness. *Raynaud's phenomenon* may be present, with the fingers becoming cyanotic or blanched following emotional stress or exposure to cold temperature. *Visceral manifestations* of polymyositis are rare. Dysphagia results from weakness of the pharyngeal muscles and hypotonicity of the esophagus. Occasionally, there may be associated pneumonitis, myocarditis, pericarditis, and nephritis. In Table 5–23 a summary of signs and symptoms of polymyositis-dermatomyositis is given.

Laboratory Findings

In acute polymyositis the serum levels of the various enzymes that normally reside in voluntary muscle are elevated. Of particular value are creatine phosphokinase, aldolase, and glutamic and pyruvic transaminases. The biochemical changes are not pathognomonic for polymyositis, but serial determinations of these enzyme levels are of definite diagnostic and

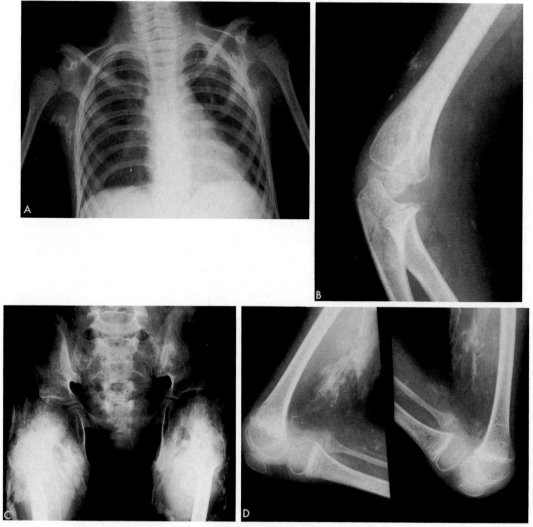

FIGURE 5–217. Dermatomyositis in a child.

A and **B.** Radiograms of shoulders and elbow showing calcification of subcutaneous tissues. **C** and **D.** Radiograms of hips and knees. Note the progression of calcification involving the muscles of the proximal thigh and pelvic girdle.

prognostic help. When the acute inflammation of the muscle responds to corticosteroid therapy, the elevated levels of serum enzymes decline toward normal, and within four to six weeks the muscles gradually recover motor strength. In muscular dystrophy, serum creatine phosphokinase and aldolase values are increased, but they do not decrease following any form of treatment. In neural atrophy, these serum enzymes remain normal. In the late stages of polymyositis, when the muscle fibers have degenerated and are replaced by fibrous tissue, the serum enzyme levels are normal or slightly elevated.

Nonspecific changes reflecting the underlying myopathic process are elevation of x and y globulins of serum proteins and abnormal levels of creatine and creatinine in the serum and urine. The sedimentation rate is elevated. Rheumatoid factor is sometimes present, but lupus erythematosus (LE) cells are usually not found.

The electromyogram will disclose the following abnormalities: (1) spontaneous fibrillation and positive or sawtooth potentials at complete rest or after mild mechanical irritation; (2) complex polyphasic or short-duration potentials of low amplitude, which occur on voluntary contraction; and (3) salvos of repetitive potentials of high frequency occurring after mechanical stimulation or use of the electrode.[105-109] According to Pearson, these changes in the electromyogram are quite characteristic but not absolutely specific for polymyositis.[108]

Table 5–23. Signs and Symptoms of Polymyositis-Dermatomyositis

Signs and Symptoms	Incidence (Approximate Percentage)
Muscular	
Muscle weakness	100
Proximal muscles	
Shoulder girdle	75–100
Pelvic	75–100
Distal muscles	30
Sternocleidomastoid	65
Posterior pharyngeal	50
Facial muscles	Rare
Respiratory muscles	Rare
Muscle pain-tenderness	50–75
Atrophy	50
Contracture	25
Skin	30
Other	
Arthralgia-arthritis	50
Raynaud's phenomenon	25
Gastrointestinal	Rare
Pulmonary	Rare
Cardiac	Rare
Peripheral nerves	Rare

Diagnosis

The following are the criteria for diagnosis of polymyositis and dermatomyositis: (1) symmetrical progressive weakness of limb-girdle and sternocleidomastoid muscles; (2) histologic evidence on muscle biopsy of Type I and Type II fibronecrosis, phagocytosis, regeneration, and atrophy in a perifascicular distribution with perivascular inflammatory exudate; (3) elevated serum phosphokinase; (4) electromyographic findings of small polyphasic motor units, fibrillation, and repetitive discharges; and (5) skin rash of dermatomyositis as seen on the face, neck, and extensor surface of the limbs.[24, 25] In order to make a definitive diagnosis of polymyositis the first four criteria must be present, whereas for a definitive diagnosis of dermatomyositis the rash plus three other criteria must be present. The positive response to steroid therapy should not be used as a criterion for diagnosis. In dermatomyositis, skin biopsy specimens taken from clinically involved areas will disclose a noninflammatory edema type of poikiloderma and deposits of mucin; these histologic findings in the affected skin are distinctive of dermatomyositis. In polymyositis a muscle biopsy is vital for definitive diagnosis, whereas in dermatomyositis only skin biopsy is indicated, as the above-mentioned histologic findings in the presence of muscle weakness, characteristic rash, elevated serum creatine phosphokinase, and EMG findings are diagnostic.

In summary, the principal laboratory tests to perform for diagnostic work-up of polymyositis and dermatomyositis are, first, determination of serum creatine phosphokinase (CPK); second, electromyography; and third, muscle and/or skin biopsy. Ancillary laboratory investigations include erythrocyte sedimentation rate (ESR); blood count; tests for connective tissue disease, such as rheumatoid (Rh) factor, lupus erythematosus (LE) cell, positive direct Coombs test, and antibodies to cell constituents; and serum urinary levels of myoglobulins.

In the differential diagnosis one should consider (1) muscular dystrophy, (2) benign chronic spinal muscular atrophy, (3) hereditary metabolic myopathies such as McArdle's disease, (4) myasthenia gravis, (5) rhabdomyolysis, and (6) inflammatory myopathies such as viral myositis, parasitic myositis, granulomatous and giant-cell myopathy, and sarcoid myopathy.

Treatment

In the acute stage of polymyositis and dermatomyositis, when the muscles are painful, tender, and edematous, the patient is placed on bed rest and moist heat is applied over the sore muscles to alleviate the discomfort. Corticosteroids (prednisone is preferred) are usually given, though their effect on the course of the myopathy is debatable.[137] They ameliorate the acute inflammatory reaction and diminish pain. Serum enzyme levels are determined at regular intervals; their return to normal is a favorable prognostic sign, indicating a good chance of recovery of motor strength. The dosage of corticosteroids is slowly reduced until an effective maintenance dose is reached. In children, dermatomyositis runs a self-limited course and the value of corticosteroid therapy seems to be primarily for symptomatic relief.[107]

Immunosuppressant drugs, such as methotrexate, may be given occasionally, especially if there have been problems with steroid therapy. Thymectomy has been performed occasionally in the treatment of polymyositis and dermatomyositis.

Active and passive exercises are performed gently to preserve normal range of joint motion. If contractural deformities develop, the affected limbs are supported in functional position in well-padded splints.

In the later stages of the disease, when contracture and calcification of the deep fascia, intermuscular septa, and subcutaneous tissue have taken place, the thickened calcified tissues are excised. This author has found the procedure to be very satisfactory; it will increase the circulation and function of the muscles and improve nutrition of the skin.

References

1. Adams, R.D., Denny-Brown, D., and Pearson, C.M.: Diseases of Muscle. 2nd Ed. New York, Harper & Row, 1962.
2. Alexander, S., and Foreman, L.: Dermatomyositis and carcinoma. A case report and immunological investigations. Br. J. Dermatol., 80:86, 1968.
3. Ames, E.L., and Posch, J.L.: Calcinosis of the flexor and extensor tendons in dermatomyositis. Case report. J. Hand Surg., 9:876, 1984.
4. Anderson, B.A., Young, P.V., Kean, W.F., Ludwin, S.K., Galbraith, P.R., and Anastassiades, T.P.: Polymyositis in chronic graft vs host disease. A case report. Arch. Neurol., 39:188, 1982.
5. Anderson, L., and Ziter, F.A.: Plasmapheresis via central catheter in dermatomyositis: A new method for selected pediatric patients. J. Pediatr., 98:240, 1981.
6. Ansel, B.M.: Management of polymyositis and dermatomyositis. Clin. Rheum. Dis., 10:205, 1984.
7. Arundell, F.D., Wilkinson, R.D., and Haserick, J.R.: Dermatomyositis and malignant neoplasms in adults. Arch. Derm. Syph., 82:772, 1960.
8. Banker, B.Q.: Dermatomyositis of childhood. Ultrastructural alterations of muscle and intramuscular blood vessels. J. Neuropathol. Exp. Neurol., 34:46, 1975.
9. Banker, B.Q., and Victor, M.: Dermatomyositis (systemic angiopathy) of childhood. Medicine, 45:261, 1966.
10. Bardelas, J.A., Winkelstein, J.A., Seto, D.S.Y., Tsai, T., and Rogol, A.D.: Fatal Echo 24 infection in a patient with hypogammaglobinaemia: Relationship to dermatomyositis-like syndrome. J. Pediatr., 90:396, 1977.
11. Barnes, A.B., and Link, D.A.: Childhood dermatomyositis and pregnancy. Am. J. Obstet. Gynecol., 146:335, 1983.
12. Barnes, B.E.: Dermatomyositis and malignancy. A review of the literature. Ann. Intern. Med., 84:68, 1976.
13. Bates, D.S., Stevens, J.C., and Hudgson, P.: "Polymyositis" with involvement of facial and distal musculature. J. Neurol. Sci., 19:105, 1973.
14. Bazhenova, L.K., Zhvanilia, M.A., and Kopeva, T.N.: Characteristics of the pathological changes in the heart in dermatomyositis in children. Vopr. Okhr. Materin. Det., 25:23, 1980.
15. Behan, W.M.H., and Behan, P.O.: Complement abnormalities in polymyositis. J. Neurol. Sci., 34:241, 1977.
16. Behan, W.M.H., Behan, P.O., and Dick, H.: HLA-B8 in polymyositis. N. Engl. J. Med., 298:1260, 1978.
17. Behan, W.M.H., McQueen, A., and Behan, P.O.: Immunogenetic findings in polymyositis. In preparation.
18. Benbassat, J., Gefel, D., Larholt, K., Sukenik, S., Morgenstern, V., and Zlotnick, A.: Prognostic factors in polymyositis/dermatomyositis. A computer-assisted analysis of ninety-two cases. Arthritis Rheum., 28:249, 1985.
19. Ben-Bassat, M., and Machtey, I.: Picorna virus–like structures in acute dermatomyositis. Am. J. Clin. Pathol., 58:245, 1972.
20. Ben-Youssef, L., and Schmidt, T.L.: Battered child

21. syndrome simulating myositis. J. Pediatr. Orthop., 3:392, 1983.
21. Bitnum, S., Daeschner, C.W., Travis, L.B., Dodge, W.F., and Hopps, H.C.: Dermatomyositis. J. Pediatr., 64:101, 1964.
22. Blane, C.E., White, S.J., Braunstein, E.M., Bowyer, S.L., and Sullivan, D.B.: Patterns of calcification in childhood dermatomyositis. A.J.R., 142:397, 1984.
23. van Bogaert, L., Radermecker, M.A., Lowenthal, A., and Ketelaer, C.J.: VII. Le polymyosite chronique (essais avec la cortisone). Acta Neurol. Belg., 11:869, 1955.
24. Bohan, A., and Peter, J.B.: Polymyositis and dermatomyositis. N. Engl. J. Med., 292:344, 1975.
25. Bohan, A., Peter, J.B., Bowman, R.L., and Person, C.M.: A computer-assisted analysis of 153 patients with polymyositis and dermatomyositis. Medicine, 56:255, 1977.
26. Bowyer, S.L., Blane, C.E., Sullivan, D.B., and Cassidy, J.T.: Childhood dermatomyositis: Factors predicting functional outcome and development of dystrophic calcification. J. Pediatr., 108:882, 1983.
27. Boylan, R.C., and Sokoloff, L.: Vascular lesions in dermatomyositis. Arthritis Rheum., 3:379, 1960.
28. Braunstein, E.M., and White, S.J.: Pneumatosis intestinalis in dermatomyositis. Br. J. Radiol., 53:1011, 1980.
29. Brewer, E.J., Jr., Giannini, E.H., Rossen, R.D., Patten, B., and Barkley, E.: Plasma exchange therapy of a childhood onset dermatomyositis patient. Arthritis Rheum., 23:509, 1980.
30. Brooke, M.H., and Kaplan, H.: Muscle pathology in rheumatoid arthritis, polymyalgia rheumatica and polymyositis. A histochemical study. Arch. Pathol., 94:101, 1972.
31. Brown, M., Swift, T.R., and Spies, S.M.: Radioisotope scanning in inflammatory muscle disease. Neurology, 26:517, 1976.
32. Camp, A.V., Lane, D.J., and Mowat, A.G.: Dermatomyositis with parenchymal lung involvement. Br. Med. J., 1:155, 1972.
33. Carlisle, J.W., and Good, R.A.: Dermatomyositis in childhood: Report of studies on seven cases and a review of the literature. Lancet, 79:266, 1959.
34. Carpenter, S., Karpati, G., Rothman, S., and Watters, G.: The childhood type of dermatomyositis. Neurology, 26:952, 1976.
35. Carton Sanchez, J.A., Diaz Fernandez, J.L., and Llorente de Jesus, R.: Pure red cell aplasia associated with polymyositis. Rev. Clin. Esp., 159:221, 1980.
36. Caspary, E.A., Gubbay, S.S., and Stern, G.M.: Circulating antibodies in polymyositis and other muscle-wasting disorders. Lancet, 2:941, 1964.
37. Chadda, V.S., Solanki, R., Chadda, S., Jain, N.C., and Misra, S.N.: Dermatomyositis. J. Indian Med. Assoc., 79:142, 1982.
38. Chou, S.M.: Myxovirus-like structures and accompanying nuclear changes in chronic polymyositis. Arch. Pathol., 86:649, 1968.
39. Chou, S.M., and Gutmann, L.: Picorna virus–like crystals in subacute polymyositis. Neurology, 20:205, 1970.
40. Chou, S.M., and Miike, T.: Ultrastructural abnormalities and perifascicular atrophy in childhood dermatomyositis with special reference to transverse tubular system–sarcoplasmic reticulum junctions. Arch. Pathol. Lab. Med., 105:76, 1981.
41. Christianson, H.B., O'Leary, P.A., and Power, M.H.: Urinary excretion of creatine and creatinine in dermatomyositis. J. Invest. Dermatol., 27:431, 1956.
42. Cook, C.D., Rosen, F.S., and Banker, B.Q.: Dermatomyositis and focal scleroderma. Pediatr. Clin. North Am., 10:976, 1963.
43. Currie, S.: Destruction of muscle cultures by lympho-

cytes from cases of polymyositis. Acta Neuropathol. (Berlin), *15*:11, 1970.

44. Currie, S.: Experimental myositis. The in-vivo and in-vitro activity of lymph-node cells. J. Pathol., *105*:169, 1971.

45. Datz, F.L., Lewis, S.E., Conrad, M.R., Maravilla, A., and Parkey, R.W.: Pyomyositis diagnosed by radionuclide imaging and ultrasonography. South. Med. J., *73*:649, 1980.

46. Dau, P.C., and Bennington, J.L.: Plasmapheresis in childhood dermatomyositis. J. Pediatr., *98*:237, 1981.

47. Denisiewicz-Rostropowicz, K., and Romicka, H.: Systemic lupus erythematosus and dermatomyositis in children. Rev. Rhum. Mal. Osteoartic., *47*:93, 1980.

48. De Vere, R., and Bradley, W.G.: Polymyositis: its presentation, morbidity and mortality. Brain, *98*:637, 1975.

49. Diessner, G.R., Howard, F.M., Winkelmann, R.K., Lambert, E.H., and Mulder, D.W.: Laboratory tests in polymyositis. Arch. Intern. Med., *117*:757, 1966.

50. Donoghue, F.D., Winkelmann, R.K., and Moersch, J.H.: Esophageal defects in dermatomyositis. Ann. Otol., *69*:1139, 1960.

51. Dowling, G.B.: Scleroderma and dermatomyositis. Br. J. Dermatol., *67*:275, 1955.

52. Dubowitz, V.: Prognostic factors in dermatomyositis (Letter). J. Pediatr., *105*:336, 1984.

53. Dupre, A., Viraben, R., Bonafe, J.L., Touron, P., and Lamon, P.: Zebra-like dermatomyositis (Letter). Arch. Dermatol., *117*:63, 1981.

54. Eaton, L.M.: The perspective of neurology in regard to polymyositis. Study of 41 cases. Neurology, *4*:245, 1954.

55. Esiri, M., MacLennan, I.C.M., and Hazelman, B.L.: Lymphocyte sensitivity to skeletal muscle in patients with polymyositis and other disorders. Clin. Exp. Immunol., *14*:25, 1973.

56. Everett, M.M., and Curtis, A.C.: Dermatomyositis: A review of 19 cases in adolescents and children. Arch. Intern. Med., *100*:70, 1957.

57. Frazier, A.R., and Miller, R.D.: Interstitial pneumonitis in association with polymyositis and dermatomyositis. Chest, *65*:403, 1974.

58. Friedman, J.M., Pachman, L.M., Maryjowski, M.L., Radvany, R.M., Crowe, W.E., Hanson, V., Levinson, J.E., and Spencer, C.H.: Immunogenetic studies of juvenile dermatomyositis: HLA-DR antigen frequencies. Arthritis Rheum., *26*:214, 1983.

59. Fries, J.F., Sharp, G.C., McDevitt, H.O., and Holman, H.R.: Cyclophosphamide therapy in systemic lupus erythematosus and polymyositis. Arthritis Rheum., *16*:154, 1973.

60. Fudman, E.J., and Schnitzer, T.J.: Dermatomyositis without creatine kinase elevation. A poor prognostic sign. Am. J. Med., *80*:329, 1986.

61. Gamstorp, I.: Non-dystrophic, myogenic myopathies with onset in infancy or childhood. A review of some characteristic syndromes. Acta Paediatr. Scand., *71*:881, 1982.

62. Garcin, R., LaPresle, J., Gruner, J., and Scherrer, J.: Les polymyosites. Rev. Neurol. (Paris), *92*:465, 1955.

63. Gelderman, A.H., Levine, R.A., and Arndt, K.A.: Dermatomyositis complicated by generalized amyloidosis. N. Engl. J. Med., *267*:858, 1962.

64. Gonzales-Angulo, A., Fraga, A., Mintz, G., and Zavala, B.J.: Submicroscopic alterations in capillaries of skeletal muscles in polymyositis. Am. J. Med., *45*:873, 1968.

65. Gotoff, S.P., Smith, R.D., and Sugar, O.: Dermatomyositis with cerebral vasculitis in a patient with agammaglobinaemia. Am. J. Dis. Child., *123*:53, 1972.

66. de Groot, A.C.: Childhood dermatomyositis (Proceedings). Br. J. Dermatol., *102*:478, 1980.

67. Guillet, G.Y., Guillet, J.A., Blanquet, P., and Maleville, J.: A new noninvasive evaluation of muscular lesions in dermatomyositis: Thallium 201 muscle scans. J. Am. Acad. Dermatol., *5*:670, 1981.

68. Guillet, J., Blanquet, P., Guillet, G., Mollard, S., Massicot, P., and Maleville, J.: The use of technetium (Tc-99m) medronate scintigraphy as a prognostic guide in childhood dermatomyositis (Letter). Arch. Dermatol., *117*:451, 1981.

69. Haas, R.H., Dyck, R.F., Dubowitz, V., and Pepys, M.B.: C-reactive protein in childhood dermatomyositis. Ann. Rheum. Dis., *41*:483, 1982.

70. Hanauer, L.B.: "Chronic" dermatomyositis: Response to corticosteroids. J. Med. Soc. N.J., *77*:121, 1980.

71. Harati, Y., Niakan, E., and Bergman, E.W.: Childhood dermatomyositis in monozygotic twins. Neurology, *36*:721, 1986.

72. Hochberg, M.C., Lopez-Acuna, D., and Gittelsohn, A.M.: Mortality from polymyositis and dermatomyositis in the United States, 1968–1978. Arthritis Rheum., *26*:1465, 1983.

73. Isaeva, L.A., and Zhvaniia, M.A.: Working classification of dermatomyositis in children. Vopr. Revm., *1*:55, 1980.

74. Johns, R.A., Finhoit, D.A., and Stirt, J.A.: Anaesthetic management of a child with dermatomyositis. Can. Anaesth. Soc. J., *33*:71, 1986.

75. Kagen, L.J.: Dermatomyositis and polymyositis: Clinical aspects. Clin. Exp. Rheumatol., *2*:271, 1984.

76. Kalmanti, M., and Athanasiou, A.: Neuroblastoma occurring in a child with dermatomyositis. Am. J. Pediatr. Hematol. Oncol., *7*:387, 1985.

77. Kesseler, A., and Greninger, G.: Dermatomyositis with predominantly atypical skin manifestations. Ann. Pediatr. (Paris), *27*:227, 1980.

78. Kinoshita, M., Iwasaki, Y., Wada, F., and Segawa, M.: A case of congenital polymyositis—A possible pathogenesis of "Fukuyama type congenital muscular dystrophy" (author's transl.). Rinsho Shinkeigaku, *20*:191, 1980.

79. Lambert, E.H., Sayre, G.P., and Eaton, L.M.: Electrical activity of muscles in polymyositis. Trans. Am. Neurol. Assoc., *79*:64, 1954.

80. Le Guillou, M., Richard, F., L'Henaff, F., Ferriere, J.M., Durand, J., Lacert, P., and Kuss, R.: Bilateral ureteral necrosis in a child with dermatomyositis. Eur. Urol., *6*:190, 1980.

81. Lucci, B., Govoni, E., Bragaglia, M.M., Martinelli, G., and Benatti, C.: Case of universal calcinosis in dermatomyositis in childhood. Riv. Neurobiol., *27*:783, 1981.

82. Magid, D., Fishman, E.K., and Siegelman, S.S.: Dermatomyositis with calcinosis cutis. Case report 317. Skeletal Radiol., *14*:126, 1985.

83. Malleson, P.: Juvenile dermatomyositis: A review. J. R. Soc. Med., *75*:33, 1982.

84. Manchul, L.A., Jin, A., Pritchard, K.L., Tenebaum, J., Boyd, N.F., Lee, P., Germanson, T., and Gordon, D.A.: The frequency of malignant neoplasm in patients with polymyositis-dermatomyositis. A controlled study. Arch. Intern. Med., *145*:1835, 1985.

85. Martini, A., and Raelli, A.: Unusual case of childhood dermatomyositis (Letter). Ann. Rheum. Dis., *44*:356, 1985.

86. Mastaglia, F.L., and Currie, S.: Immunological and ultrastructural observations on the role of lymphoid cells in the pathogenesis of polymyositis. Acta Neuropathol. (Berlin), *18*:1, 1971.

87. Mastaglia, F.L., and Kakulas, B.A.: A histological and histochemical study of skeletal muscle regeneration in polymyositis. J. Neurol. Sci., *10*:471, 1970.

88. Mastaglia, F.L., and Walton, J.N.: Coxsackie virus–like particles in skeletal muscle in polymyositis. J. Neurol. Sci., *11*:593, 1970.

89. Mastaglia, F.L., and Walton, J.N.: A ultrastructural study of skeletal muscle in polymyositis. J. Neurol. Sci., *12*:473, 1971.

90. Mechler, F.: Changing electromyographic findings during chronic course of polymyositis. J. Neurol. Sci., *23*:237, 1974.

91. Medsger, T.A., Dawson, W.N., and Masi, A.T.: The epidemiology of polymyositis. Am. J. Med., *48*:715, 1970.

92. Metzger, A.L., Bohan, A., Goldberg, L.S., Bluestone, R., and Pearson, C.M.: Polymyositis and dermatomyositis: combined methotrexate and corticosteroid therapy. Ann. Intern. Med., *81*:182, 1974.

93. Miike, T., Ohtani, Y., Hattori, S., Ono, T., Kageshita, T., and Matsuda, I.: Childhood-type myositis and linear scleroderma. Neurology, *33*:928, 1983.

94. Miller, G., Heckmatt, J.Z., and Dubowitz, V.: Drug treatment of juvenile dermatomyositis. Arch. Dis. Child., *58*:445, 1983.

95. Miller, M., and Carton, F.X.: Vasculitis in children's dermatomyositis (author's transl.). Ann. Dermatol Venereol., *107*:841, 1980.

96. Moran-Vazquez, J.O., Santana-Lomeli, O., Viruete-Alcaraz, M., Garcia-Perez, J., and Jasso-Urzua, H.: Infantile dermatomyositis: A propos of 2 cases. Bol. Med. Hosp. Infant. Mex., *39*:617, 1982.

97. Newman, A.J., and Lee, C.: Hypothyroidism simulating dermatomyositis. J. Pediatr., *97*:772, 1980.

98. Niakan, E., Pitner, S.E., Whitaker, J.N., and Bertorini, T.E.: Immunosuppressive agents in corticosteroid-refractory childhood dermatomyositis. Neurology, *30*:286, 1980.

99. O'Leary, P.A., and Waisman, M.: Dermatomyositis: A study of forty cases. Arch. Dermatol. Syph., *41*:1001, 1940.

100. O'Neill, M., and Basheer, S.M.: Childhood dermatomyositis case report. Ir. Med. J., *76*:243, 1983.

101. Pachman, L.M., and Cooke, N.: Juvenile dermatomyositis: A clinical and immunologic study. J. Pediatr., *96*:226, 1980.

102. Pachman, L.M., Jonasson, O., Cannon, R.A., and Friedman, J.M.: HLS-B8 in juvenile dermatomyositis. Lancet, *2*:567, 1977.

103. Pachman, L.M., and Maryjowski, M.C.: Juvenile dermatomyositis and polymyositis. Clin. Rheum. Dis., *10*:95, 1984.

104. Patrone, N.A.: Steroid therapy of dermatomyositis (Letter). J. Pediatr., *105*:176, 1984.

105. Pearson, C.M.: Rheumatic manifestations of polymyositis and dermatomyositis. Arthritis Rheum., *2*:127, 1959.

106. Pearson, C.M.: Polymyositis: Clinical forms, diagnosis and therapy. Postgrad. Med., *31*:450, 1962.

107. Pearson, C.M.: Patterns of polymyositis and their response to treatment. Ann. Intern. Med., *59*:827, 1963.

108. Pearson, C.M.: Polymyositis and related disorders. *In* Walton, J.N. (ed.): Disorders of Voluntary Muscle. Boston, Little, Brown, 1964, p. 305.

109. Pearson, C.M., and Bohan, A.: The spectrum of polymyositis and dermatomyositis. Med. Clin. North Am., *61*:439, 1977.

110. Pirofsky, B., and Bardana, E.J.: Immunosuppressive therapy in rheumatic disease. Med. Clin. North Am., *61*:419, 1977.

111. Reichlin, M., and Mattioli, M.: Description of a serological reaction characteristic of polymyositis. Clin. Immunol. Immunopathol., *5*:12, 1976.

112. Renault, F., and Raimbault, J.: Muscle latency in polymyositis in children. Electrodiagn. Ther., *17*:87, 1980.

113. Renault, F., Raimbault, J., Roy, C., Harpey, J.P., and Laget, P.: Electromyography in children with polymyositis (author's transl). Sem. Hop. Paris, *58*:220, 1982.

114. Resnick, J.S., Mammel, M., Mundale, M.O., and Kottke, F.J.: Muscular strength as an index of response to therapy in childhood dermatomyositis. Arch. Phys. Med. Rehabil., *62*:12, 1981.

115. Roberts, H.M., and Brunsting, L.A.: Dermatomyositis in childhood: Summary of 40 cases. Postgrad. Med., *16*:396, 1954.

116. Rose, A.L., and Walton, J.N.: Polymyositis: A survey of 89 cases with particular reference to treatment and prognosis. Brain, *89*:747, 1966.

117. Rothstein, T.L., Carlson, C.B., and Sumi, S.M.: Polymyositis with facioscapulohumeral distribution. Arch. Neurol., *25*:313, 1971.

118. Ruff, R.L., and Secrist, D.: Viral studies in benign acute childhood myositis. Arch. Neurol., *39*:261, 1982.

119. Sammartino, A., Lucariello, A., Esposito, L., Coluccino, V., and Loffredo, A.: A rare presentation of bilateral membranous conjunctivitis in dermatomyositis in young age. J. Pediatr. Ophthalmol. Strabismus, *18*:47, 1981.

120. Sammartino, A., Lucariello, A., Esposito, L., Vetrano, A., and Loffredo, A.: A rare presentation of bilateral membranous conjunctivitis in dermatomyositis. Ophthalmologica, *184*:97, 1982.

121. Sarrat, P.: Periungual capillaroscopy in children with scleroderma and dermatomyositis. J. Med. Vasc., *8*:175, 1983.

122. Selander, P.: Dermatomyositis in early childhood. Acta Med. Scand. (Suppl.), *246*:187, 1950.

123. Sheard, C.: Dermatomyositis. Arch. Intern. Med., *88*:640, 1951.

124. Shearin, J.C., and Pickrell, K.: Surgical treatment of subcutaneous calcifications of polymyositis or dermatomyositis. Ann. Plast. Surg., *5*:381, 1980.

125. Skuterud, E., Sydness, O.A., and Haavik, T.K.: Calcinosis in dermatomyositis treated with probenecid. Scand. J. Rheumatol., *10*:92, 1981.

126. Smyth, D.P.: Quantitative electromyography in babies and young children with primary muscle disease and neurogenic lesions. J. Neurol. Sci., *56*:199, 1982.

127. Solomon, S.D., and Maurer, K.H.: Association of dermatomyositis and dysgerminoma in a 16-year-old patient (Letter). Arthritis Rheum., *26*:572, 1983.

128. Spencer, C.H., Hanson, V., Singsen, B.H., Bernstein, B.H., Kornreich, H.K., and King, K.K.: Course of treated juvenile dermatomyositis. J. Pediatr., *105*:399, 1984.

129. Thompson, C.E.: Polymyositis in children. Clin. Pediatr., *7*:24, 1968.

130. Unverricht, H.: Polymyositis acuta progressiva. Z. Klin. Med., *12*:533, 1887.

131. Vaughan, S.M., and Whittle, E.: Caring for the child with dermatomyositis. Issues Compr. Pediatr. Nurs., *7*:255, 1984.

132. Vignos, P.J., and Goldwyn, J.: Evaluation of laboratory tests in diagnosis and management of polymyositis. Am. J. Med. Sci., *263*:291, 1972.

133. Wagner, E.: Fall einer seltnen Muskelkrankheit. Arch. Heilk., *4*:288, 1863.

134. Wagner, E.: Ein Fall von akuter Polymyositis. Dtsch. Arch. Klin. Med., *40*:241, 1887.

135. Wallace, D.J., Metzger, A.L., and White, K.K.: Combination immunosuppressive treatment of steroid-resistant dermatomyositis/polymyositis. Arthritis Rheum., *28*:590, 1985.

136. Walton, J.N., and Adams, R.D.: Polymyositis. Baltimore, Williams & Wilkins, 1958.

137. Wedgwood, R.J.P., Cook, C.D., and Cohen, J.: Dermatomyositis: Report of 26 cases with a discussion of endocrine therapy in 13. Pediatrics, *12*:447, 1953.

138. Williams, R.C.: Dermatomyositis and malignancy: A review of the literature. Ann. Intern. Med., *50*:1174, 1959.

139. Wilshire, M.L., Holdaway, I.M., and North, J.D.:

Hypercalcemia during resolution of calcinosis in juvenile dermatomyositis. Br. Med. J., *288*:1345, 1984.

140. Winkelmann, R.K.: Dermatomyositis in childhood. Clin. Rheum. Dis., 8:353, 1982.

141. Winkelmann, R.K., Mulder, D.W., Lambert, E.H., Howard, F.M., and Diessner, G.R.: Course of dermatomyositis-polymyositis. Comparison of untreated and cortisone treated patients. Proc. Mayo Clin., *43*:545, 1968.

142. Wolfe, J.F., Adelstein, E., and Sharp, G.C.: Antinuclear antibody with distinct specificity for polymyositis. J. Clin. Invest., *59*:176, 1977.

143. World Federation of Neurology Research Group on Neuromuscular Disorders. Classification of polymyositis and dermatomyositis. J. Neurol. Sci., *6*:165, 1968.

144. Young, J.W., and Haney, P.J.: Case report 314. Diagnosis: juvenile dermatomyositis with changes of the hallux typical of fibrodysplasia (myositis) ossificans progressiva. Skeletal Radiol., *13*:318, 1985.

145. Yousefzadeh, D.K., Schumann, E.M., Mulligan, G.M., Bosworth, D.E., Young, C.S., and Pringle, K.C.: The role of imaging modalities in diagnosis and management of pyomyositis. Skeletal Radiol., *8*:285, 1982.

SUPPURATIVE MYOSITIS[1-30]

Pyomyositis is rare because normal muscle is resistant to bacterial infection. Ordinarily, it is encountered in patients with severe septicemia, in whom bacterial emboli result in multiple acute abscesses in muscles. Immunosuppressed patients are particularly susceptible to suppurative myositis. It may also arise by direct extension from an adjacent infectious process.

In children, pyomyositis occurs usually in early childhood (two- to five-year age group). The quadriceps and other large muscles are the common sites of involvement.

Etiology

Staphylococcus aureus is the most common pathogenic organism. Occasionally, pyomyositis is due to beta-hemolytic and nonhemolytic streptococci. Streptococcal pyomyositis is usually very acute and fulminating in its course, whereas staphylococcal pyomyositis develops gradually over a period of days or weeks.

Traumatically devitalized muscles are prone to infection with *Clostridium welchii*, which results in gas gangrene. In tuberculosis, cold abscesses may directly extend into adjacent muscles.

Clinical Features

There are three stages in the course of pyomyositis: (1) The *early, invasive stage* is characterized by acute local pain that is aggravated by motion. On palpation the involved muscle is swollen and indurated. There is no fluctuation and no pus on aspiration. Erythema is not common in the early stages. (2) The *suppurative stage* develops in one to three weeks. There is increased pain, edema, and systemic symptoms in the form of high fever and leukocytosis. On palpation there is local fluctuation. On aspiration, pus is obtained. (3) The third and final phase is the *toxic or systemic stage;* if untreated it may result in a fatal outcome.

Diagnosis

Most infections that are suspected of being myositis are in reality osteomyelitis, particularly in the infant; the pus perforates the cortex at the metaphysis and breaks through the periosteum to lie in the soft tissues. Acute osteomyelitis must always be the first consideration in the differential diagnosis when suppurative myositis is suspected. In the diagnostic work-up a bone scan with technetium-99m and, if indicated, gallium-67 is performed.

Pyomyositis should be considered in the differential diagnosis in a febrile child with muscle pain and tenderness or swelling. Suppurative myositis may be mistaken for hematoma, tumor, cellulitis, septic arthritis, or fasciitis. A CT scan should be performed, as it will confirm the diagnosis of pyomyositis and delineate the anatomic site, which may require surgical drainage.

Treatment

This follows the same principles of treatment as for soft-tissue infections. Appropriate antibiotics are given. Local heat is applied, and the part is immobilized with splints. As the process localizes, if it does not regress and fluctuation is present, simple incision and drainage are indicated.

Tetanus must be considered as a possible complication in all traumatic wounds, particularly in those that are grossly contaminated and in which debridement and cleaning are delayed. Appropriate measures against tetanus must be adopted as indicated.

VIRAL MYOSITIS

Muscle ache and tenderness are common in viral infections such as influenza, poliomyelitis, and pleurodynia or Bornholm disease. Coxsackie B virus is the etiologic agent of *pleurodynia,* which is a benign and self-limited entity characterized by fever, headache, and acute chest pain. Treatment is symptomatic. In children with diffuse muscle weakness and tenderness, Coxsackie B virus titer may be raised. The causal relationship of viral myopathy to polymyositis is not clear.

PARASITIC MYOSITIS

In the tropics, skeletal muscle may be affected by a number of parasitic infections. *Trichinosis* caused by *Trichinella spiralis* is the most common. Other forms of parasitic infestations of muscles are *cysticercosis* (due to *Taenia solium*), *toxoplasmosis*, and *sarcosporidiosis*. In the modern age of jet travel, parasitic myositis should be considered in the differential diagnosis of muscle pain and weakness in children.

References

1. Altrocchi, P.H.: Spontaneous bacterial myositis. J.A.M.A., 217:819, 1971.
2. Anand, S.V., and Evans, K.T.: Pyomyositis. Br. J. Surg., 51:917, 1964.
3. Ashken, M.H., and Cotten, R.E.: Tropical skeletal muscle abscesses: Pyomyositis tropicans. Br. J. Surg., 50:846, 1963.
4. Barrett, A.M., and Gresham, G.A.: Acute streptococcal myositis. Lancet, 1:347, 1958.
5. Bosworth, D.E., Young, C.S., and Pringle, K.C.: The role of imaging modalities in diagnosis and management of pyomyositis. Skeletal Radiol., 8:285, 1982.
6. Chacha, P.B.: Muscle abscesses in children. Clin. Orthop., 70:174, 1970.
7. Chaitow, J., Martin, H.C., Knight, P., and Buchanan, N.: Pyomyositis tropicans: A diagnostic dilemma. Med. J. Aust., 2:512, 1980.
8. Chiedozi, L.C.: Pyomyositis. Review of 205 cases in 112 patients. Am. J. Surg., 137:255, 1979.
9. Echeverria, P., and Vaughn, M.C.: Tropical pyomyositis. A diagnostic problem in temperate climates. Am. J. Dis. Child., 129:856, 1975.
10. Goldberg, J.S., London, W.L., and Nagel, D.M.: Tropical pyomyositis. A case report and review. Pediatrics, 63:298, 1979.
11. Grose, C.: Staphylococcal pyomyositis in South Texas. J. Pediatr., 93:457, 1978.
12. Gross, S., and First, J.: Thorn-induced non-specific granulomatous left biceps myositis with left subareolar lymphadenopathy. Arch. Orthop. Trauma Surg., 103:142, 1984.
13. Hirano, T., Srinivasan, G., Janakiraman, N., Pleviak, D., and Mukhopadhyay, D.: Gallium 67 citrate scintigraphy in pyomyositis. J. Pediatr., 97:596, 1980.
14. Kallen, P., Nies, K.M., Louie, J.S., Keller, M., Worthen, N., and Bayer, A.S.: Tropical pyomyositis. Arthritis Rheum., 25:107, 1982.
15. Lamki, L., and Willis, R.B.: Radionuclide findings of pyomyositis. Clin. Nucl. Med., 7:465, 1982.
16. Levin, M.J., Gardner, P., and Waldvogel, F.A.: Tropical pyomyositis. An unusual infection due to Staphylococcus aureus. N. Engl. J. Med., 284:196, 1971.
17. Ludwig, I., and Tomsak, R.L.: Acute recurrent orbital myositis. J. Clin. Neurol. Ophthalmol., 3:41, 1983.
18. MacLaurin, J.P.: Spontaneous streptococcal myositis associated with disseminated intravascular coagulopathy. J. Am. Osteopath. Assoc., 76:675, 1977.
19. McLoughlin, M.J.: CT and percutaneous fine-needle aspiration biopsy in tropical pyomyositis. A.J.R., 134:167, 1980.
20. Mattingly, P.C., and Mowat, A.G.: Streptococcal pyomyositis following a sore throat. Rheumatol. Rehabil., 20:151, 1981.
21. Moore, D.L., Delage, G., Labelle, H., et al.: Peracute streptococcal pyomyositis: report of two cases and review of the literature. J. Pediatr. Orthop., 6:232, 1986.
22. O'Brien, D.D.: Pyomyositis in London. Br. Med. J., 1:78, 1974.
23. Ramirez, H., Jr., Brown, J.D., and Evans, J.W., Jr.: Case report 225. Myonecrosis of left leg (simulating gas) due to gram-negative organisms. Skeletal Radiol., 9:223, 1983.
24. Schlech, W.F., Moulton, P., and Kaiser, A.B.: Pyomyositis: tropical disease in a temperate climate. Am. J. Med., 71:900, 1981.
25. Shepherd, J.J.: Tropical myositis: is it an entity and what is its cause? Lancet, 2:1240, 1983.
26. Sirinavin, S., and McCracken, G.H.: Primary suppurative myositis in children. Am. J. Dis. Child., 133:263, 1979.
27. Smith, I.M., and Vickers, A.B.: Natural history of treated and untreated staphylococcal septicemia. Lancet, 1:1818, 1960.
28. Svane, S.: Peracute spontaneous streptococcal myositis. Acta Chir. Scand., 137:155, 1971.
29. Tucker, R.E., Winter, W.G., Del Valle, C., et al.: Pyomyositis mimicking malignant tumor. Three case reports. J. Bone Joint Surg., 60-A:701, 1978.
30. Yousefzaden, D.K., Schumann, E.M., Mulligan, G.M., et al.: The role of imaging modalities in diagnosis and management of pyomyositis. Skeletal Radiol., 8:285, 1982.

TRAUMATIC MYOSITIS, "MUSCLE CRAMPS"

Fibrillary tears of muscles and contusions of muscles are often sustained by healthy, active youngsters, but usually they are of little significance. A "charley horse" represents a hemorrhage into the muscle belly arising from a tear of fibers or from contusion. The clinical findings are swelling, sensitivity to palpation, and pain on use of the muscle. Fluctuation is present if the hematoma is large. Treatment is by rest and immobilization. Elevation of the part and application of ice packs for the first few hours after the injury will reduce the inflammation. As the symptoms subside, function should be resumed gradually. If the hematoma is large, it may require aspiration. Usually, little treatment is necessary except for protection until the symptoms subside.

A muscle working at a mechanical disadvantage because of faulty body mechanics, whether in the back, foot, or elsewhere, is subject to abnormal fatigue. If the handicap to function is sufficient, the muscle atrophies rather than hypertrophies, with the result that the strain may be progressive.

Persistent abnormal muscle function in a growing child tends to produce permanent structural abnormality. Such alterations are promoted not only by mechanical factors but also by factors of general health that contribute to muscular fatigue.

Muscle cramps and "growing pains" seem to be a manifestation of chronic muscle strain and fatigue. The most common site of muscle cramps is in the calves and in the intrinsic muscles of the feet. These are usually associated with pronated feet and foot strain with "tight heel cords" in which there is myostatic contracture of the triceps surae muscle. Tight posterior structures, including contracted hamstrings, are often present. Muscle cramps are probably initiated by overexertion of muscle with tissue anoxia; it has been asserted that they are associated with "the accumulation of nitrogenous wastes." The exact relation of vasospasms to the phenomenon has not been clarified.

Treatment is aimed at correcting the mechanical abnormality and adapting the structures to better functional position. For example, in instances in which foot strain is the factor, the child should be given support for his feet, and the contracted triceps surae muscles should be stretched.

TRAUMATIC MYOSITIS OSSIFICANS (MYOSITIS OSSIFICANS CIRCUMSCRIPTA)[1-55]

Traumatic myositis ossificans is characterized by heterotopic calcification and ossification in muscle tissue; it may or may not be associated with periosteum. Injury is an important factor in its pathogenesis. Most likely the process represents metaplasia of fibroblasts at the site of injury. There seems to be an individual diathesis for the abnormal ossification in soft tissue.

The condition may be subdivided into (1) the traumatic myositis ossificans that follows a severe single injury such as that seen following dislocation and fractures at the elbow (this is the most common form seen in children); and (2) the myositis ossificans that follows repeated minor injuries and occupational strain of certain muscles. This type usually occurs in adolescents and young adults. Common examples are heterotopic bone formation in the soleus muscle in ballerinas (toe dancer's bone), in the brachialis anticus in fencers, and in the thigh adductors in equestrians.

Pathology

Ackerman has reviewed the pathologic findings, emphasizing the presence of four histologic zones: (1) a central, undifferentiated zone, which is highly cellular, with mitotic figures and with extreme variation in the size and shape of the cells (cytologic differentiation of this zone from sarcoma is extremely difficult); (2) an adjacent zone in which there are well-oriented zones of cellular osteoid separated by loose cellular stroma; (3) a more peripheral zone showing new bone formation with osteoblasts and fibrous tissue undergoing trabecular organization; and (4) an outermost zone of well-delimited and oriented bone encapsulated by fibrous tissue. The benign nature of the lesion is established by the presence of the zone phenomenon, i.e., the innermost undifferentiated area merging into oriented osteoid formation and finally into well-formed bone in the periphery. As the bone matures, the area involved becomes smaller.

Clinical Features

Physical findings consist of tenderness over the area, palpable swelling, and pain on motion. Often in children a history of acute trauma is obtained, with symptoms and signs of the injury that gradually regress over a period of 7 to 14 days, only to recur with increasing severity in the third week. Persistence of local discomfort and marked limitation of joint motion noted at three weeks following posterior dislocation of the elbow suggest the possibility of myositis ossificans.

Imaging Findings

Bone scan with technetium-99m will disclose increased local uptake. In its initial stage, routine radiograms may be normal; soon, however, discrete calcification of delicate texture will be observed in the mass. Computerized tomography is of great value in delineating the nature of the lesion. After a variable interval, the acuteness of the symptoms subsides, the ossified mass tends to regress, and the calcification becomes smaller and of greater density (Fig. 5–218). The process is self-limiting, with the period of acute activity lasting from a few weeks to several months.

In the neurogenic form, the process is likely to be much more extensive, and often no history of trauma is obtained. In the absence of normal innervation of the part, trauma may occur without its being appreciated.

Differential Diagnosis

Myositis ossificans must be distinguished from calcifying hematoma, interstitial calcinosis, and osteogenic sarcoma. Calcification in myositis ossificans is diaphyseal in location, lying parallel to the surface of the bone and often

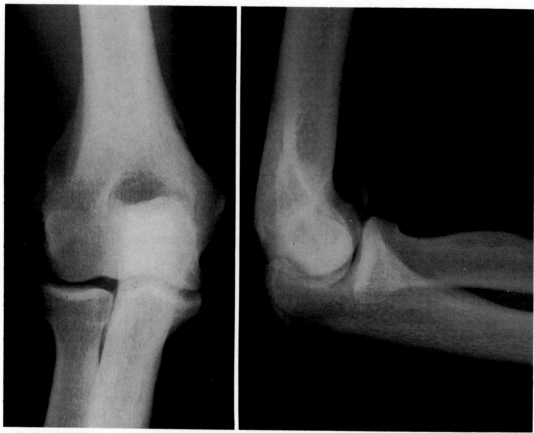

FIGURE 5–218. Traumatic myositis ossificans following posterior dislocation of the elbow joint.

Note the new bone formation in the brachialis muscle and in the capsule.

separated from it by a distinct area in which the cortex and periosteum have a normal appearance; osteogenic sarcoma, on the other hand, is likely to show some evidence of involvement of the cortex and periosteum, and it is metaphyseal in location. Computerized tomography will delineate the nature of the pathology. In doubtful cases, serial radiograms taken at short intervals should demonstrate the difference between the two processes. Occasionally, the differentiation is difficult, and even the histologic examination may be misinterpreted.

Treatment

Rest of the affected part during the period while the process is active is the basic principle of treatment. All physiotherapeutic measures should be avoided. Nonsteroidal anti-inflammatory drugs, such as Tolectin and Naprosyn, can provide sufficient relief. Immobilization to a greater or lesser degree is desirable, with gradual resumption of motion and activity as the acute phase subsides. Myositis ossificans about the elbow is greatly aggravated by stren

uous attempts to develop motion; prophylactically, all physiotherapeutic measures to increase motion of the elbow should be minimal, consisting only of gentle active assisted exercises. Radiation should not be given to children and adolescents.

Once the process has matured, it may be excised if the location or the size of the residual mass interferes with function; otherwise, it is left alone. Excision is not performed until a year or so after the acute stage at a time when, as judged from the radiograms, the bone is fully mature.

References

1. Ackerman, L.V.: Extra-osseous localized non-neoplastic bone and cartilage formation (so-called myositis ossificans). Clinical and pathological confusion with malignant neoplasms. J. Bone Joint Surg., *40-A:*279, 1958.
2. Amendola, M.A., Glazer, G.M., Agha, F.P., Francis, I.R., Weatherbee, L., and Martel, W.: Myositis ossificans circumscripta: computerized tomographic diagnosis. Radiology, *149:*775, 1983.
3. Angervall, L., Stener, I., and Ahren, C.: Pseudomalignant osseous tumour of soft tissue: a clinical, radiological and pathological study of five cases. J. Bone Joint Surg., *51-B:*654, 1969.

4. Bassett, C.A.L., and Ruedi, T.P.: Transformation of fibrous tissue to bone in vivo. Nature, 209:988, 1966.

5. Binnie, J.F.: On myositis ossificans traumatica. Ann. Surg., 38:423, 1903.

6. Bulstrode, C., Helal, B., and Revell, R.: Pseudo-malignant osseous tumour of soft tissue. J. Hand Surg., 9-B:345, 1984.

7. Campanacci, M., Gardini, G.F., Guinti, A., et al: Pseudo-tumoral ossification of the muscles and/or periosteum. (A study of 57 cases.) Ital. J. Orthop. Traumatol., 6:385, 1980.

8. Carlson, W.O., and Klassen, R.A.: Myositis ossificans of the upper extremity: A long-term follow-up. J. Pediatr. Orthop., 4:693, 1984.

9. Coley, W.B.: Myositis ossificans traumatica. A report of three cases illustrating the difficulties of diagnosis from sarcoma. Ann. Surg., 57:305, 1912.

10. Constance, T.J.: Localized myositis ossificans. J. Pathol. Bacteriol., 68:381, 1954.

11. De Smet, L., and Vercauteren, M.: Fast-growing pseudomalignant osseous tumour (myositis ossificans) of the finger. A case report. J. Hand Surg., 9-B:93, 1984.

12. Dickerson, R.C.: Myositis ossificans in early childhood. Report of an unusual case. Clin. Orthop., 79:42, 1971.

13. Drane, W.E.: Myositis ossificans and the three-phase bone scan. A.J.R., 142:179, 1984.

14. Ellis, M., and Frank, H.G.: Myositis ossificans traumatica: with special reference to the quadriceps femoris muscle. J. Trauma, 6:724, 1966.

15. Fay, O.J.: Traumatic parosteal bone and callus formation. The so-called traumatic ossifying myositis. Surg. Gynecol. Obstet., 19:174, 1914.

16. Fout, L.R., and McLeod, T.L.: Heterotopic ossification in the brachium secondary to unusual trauma. Milit. Med., 142:622, 1977.

17. Geschickter, C.F., and Maseritz, I.H.: Myositis ossificans. J. Bone Joint Surg., 20:661, 1938.

18. Goldman, A.B.: Myositis ossificans circumscripta: a benign lesion with a malignant differential diagnosis. A.J.R., 126:32, 1976.

19. Hait, G., Boswick, J.A., Jr., and Stone, N.H.: Heterotopic bone formation secondary to trauma (myositis ossificans traumatica): an unusual case and a review of current concepts. J. Trauma, 10:405, 1970.

20. Heiken, J.P., Lee, J.K.T., Smathers, R.L., Totty, W.G., and Murphy, W.A.: CT of benign soft-tissue masses of the extremities. A.J.R., 142:575, 1984.

21. Hierton, C.: Regional blood flow in experimental myositis ossificans. A microsphere study in conscious rabbits. Acta Orthop. Scand., 54:58, 1983.

22. Hirsch, E.F., and Morgan, R.H.: Causal significance to traumatic ossification of the fibrocartilage in tendon insertions. Arch. Surg., 39:824, 1939.

23. Howard, C.: Traumatic ossifying myositis. U.S. Naval Med. Bull., 46:724, 1946.

24. Huss, C.D., and Puhl, J.J.: Myositis ossificans of the upper arm. Am. J. Sports Med., 8:419, 1980.

25. Ivey, M.: Myositis ossificans of the thigh following manipulation of the knee. A case report. Clin. Orthop., 198:102, 1985.

26. Jackson, D.W., and Feagin, J.A.: Quadriceps contusion in young athletes: Relation of severity of injury to treatment and prognosis. J. Bone Joint Surg., 55-A:95, 1973.

27. Jajic, I., and Rulnjevic, J.: Myositis ossificans localista as a complication of tetanus. Acta Orthop. Scand., 50:547, 1979.

28. Johnson, L.C.: Histogenesis of myositis ossificans (Abstract). Am. J. Pathol., 24:681, 1948.

29. Johnson, P.H.: Traumatic myositis ossificans. J. Arkansas Med. Soc., 74:249, 1977.

30. Jones, B.V., and Ward, M.W.: Myositis ossificans in the biceps femoris muscles causing sciatic nerve palsy. A case report. J. Bone Joint Surg., 62-B:506, 1980.

31. Kramer, F.L., Kurtz, A.B., Rubin, C., et al.: Ultrasound appearance of myositis ossificans. Skeletal Radiol., 4:19, 1979.

32. Lewis, D.: Myositis ossificans. J.A.M.A., 80:1281, 1923.

33. Liefeld, P.A., Ferguson, A.B., Jr., and Fu, F.H.: Focal myositis: a benign lesion that mimics malignant disease. A case report. J. Bone Joint Surg., 64-A:1371, 1982.

34. Makins, G.H.: Traumatic myositis ossificans. Proc. R. Soc. Med., 4:Part 3 (Surg. Sec.):133, 1911.

35. Merkow, S.J., St. Clair, H.S., and Goldberg, M.J.: Myositis ossificans masquerading as sepsis. J. Pediatr. Orthop., 5:601, 1985.

36. Michelson, J.E., Granroth, G., and Andersson, L.C.: Myositis ossificans following forcible manipulation of the leg. A rabbit model for the study of heterotopic bone formation. J. Bone Joint Surg., 62-A:811, 1980.

37. Mitra, A., Sen, A.K., and Deb, H.K.: Myositis ossificans traumatica: a complication of tetanus. Report of a case and review of the literature. J. Bone Joint Surg., 58-A:885, 1976.

38. Molley, J.C., and McGuirk, R.A.: Treatment of traumatic myositis ossificans circumscripta: use of aspiration and steroids. J. Trauma, 16:851, 1976.

39. Nielsen, B.F.: Myositis ossificans articulating with the pelvis. A case report. Acta Orthop. Scand., 56:86, 1985.

40. Norman, A., and Dorfman, H.D.: Juxtacortical circumscribed myositis ossificans: evolution and radiographic features. Radiology, 96:301, 1970.

41. Ogilvie-Harris, D.J., and Fornasier, V.L.: Pseudomalignant myositis ossificans: heterotopic new-bone formation without a history of trauma. J. Bone Joint Surg., 62-A:1274, 1980.

42. Pack, G.T., and Braund, R.R.: The development of sarcoma in myositis ossificans. Report of three cases. J.A.M.A., 119:776, 1942.

43. Paterson, D.C.: Myositis ossificans circumscripta: report of four cases without history of injury. J. Bone Joint Surg., 52-A:296, 1970.

44. Pazzaglia, U.E., Beluffi, G., Colombo, A., Marchi, A., Coci, A., and Ceciliani, L.: Myositis ossificans in the newborn. J. Bone Joint Surg., 68-A:456, 1986.

45. Pinter, J., Lenart, G., and Rischak, G.: Histologic, physical and chemical investigation of myositis ossificans traumatica. Acta Orthop. Scand., 51:899, 1980.

46. Pohle, E.A., and Tomlinson, C.: Roentgen therapy in traumatic myositis ossificans. Am. J. Med. Sci., 215:372, 1948.

47. Roberts, P.H.: Heteropic ossification complicating paralysis of intracranial origin. J. Bone Joint Surg., 50-B:70, 1968.

48. Sazbon, L., Najenson, T., Tartakovsky, M., Becker, E., and Grosswasser, Z.: Widespread periarticular new-bone formation in long-term comatose patients. J. Bone Joint Surg., 63-B:120, 1981.

49. Schecter, W.P., Wong, D., Kilgore, E.S., et al.: Peripartum pseudomalignant myositis ossificans of the finger. J. Hand Surg., 7:43, 1982.

50. Thakkar, D.H., and Porter, R.W.: Heterotopic ossification enveloping the sciatic nerve following posterior fracture-dislocation of the hip: a case report. Injury, 13:207, 1981.

51. Thompson, H.C., III, and Garcia, A.: Myositis ossificans: aftermath of elbow injuries. Clin. Orthop., 50:129, 1967.

52. Thorndike, A.: Myositis ossificans traumatica. J. Bone Joint Surg., 22:315, 1940.

53. Vas, W., Cockshott, W.P., Martin, R.F., Pai, M.K., and Walker, I.: Myositis ossificans in hemophilia. Skeletal Radiol., 7:27, 1981.

54. Wilkes, L.L.: Myositis ossificans traumatica in a young child: a case report. Clin. Orthop., 118:151, 1976.

55. Zeanah, W.R., and Hudson, T.M.: Myositis ossificans: radiologic evaluation of two cases with diagnostic computed tomograms. Clin. Orthop., 168:187, 1982.

Metabolic Diseases of Muscle

PERIODIC PARALYSIS

Transient and recurring weakness or paralysis of skeletal muscles may occur in familial or sporadic forms. The plasma level of potassium may be low (hypokalemia), elevated (hyperkalemia), or normal (normokalemia).

Familial or Hypokalemic Periodic Paralysis

This rare disorder is usually inherited as an autosomal dominant trait, with complete penetrance in the male and variable penetrance in the female. Sporadic cases or autosomal recessive or sex-linked recessive forms may occur on occasion.

The exact etiology of the disease is unknown. During an attack, the plasma potassium falls as a result of shift of potassium from the extracellular to the intracellular compartments.[59] There is no loss of potassium from the body.[1, 17] During paralysis the potassium moves into the muscle cells, and during spontaneous recovery it is re-released into the plasma. The basis of pathogenesis appears to be an enzyme defect that causes an excessive accumulation of indiffusible intermediates of carbohydrate metabolism, with the resultant passage of potassium and water into the cells.[33] This theory is supported by the finding of hyperdilatation of the endoplasmic reticulum on microscopy. During paralysis, neuromuscular transmission is blocked and there is failure of spread of electrical action potential along muscle fibers. This was originally ascribed to hyperpolarization or to an increase in potential of the muscle fiber membrane; however, direct measurements of the resting membrane potential in patients with familial periodic paralysis during attacks of paralysis revealed this to be normal.[9, 25, 49] Why the membrane potential does not rise with sharp reduction in the extracellular potassium concentration has not been explained.

The onset of periodic attacks of paralysis is usually in early adolescence; the episodes tend to decrease in number and severity with advancing years and may completely disappear after 40 years of age.

The paralytic episodes are usually induced by prolonged inactivity following vigorous exercise or after a meal consisting largely of carbohydrates. Anxiety, emotional stress, and exposure to extreme cold may be other predisposing factors. The patient awakes in the night to find himself paralyzed. The proximal muscles of the lower limbs are affected first, followed by those of the upper limbs. Paralysis of the muscles of the neck, trunk, and face occurs next. The respiratory and ocular muscles are rarely involved. The sphincters are not affected. The mentation is normal. Attacks are usually self-limiting, lasting several hours. Severe paralysis in a child, however, may last two or three days, and very occasionally, a patient may die because of total paralysis.

Urinary output is decreased and thirst increased during paralysis; abnormal sweating and diuresis follow recovery. These symptoms most probably result from the concomitant shift of water and potassium into and out of the cells. The muscles of the paralyzed limbs appear enlarged during an attack and fail to respond to direct mechanical or electrical stimulation. The deep tendon reflexes are absent. The heart may be enlarged, and bradycardia and cardiac arrhythmia occasionally occur. In later life, permanent muscle weakness and atrophy may develop in the severe case.

The electrocardiogram during a paralytic episode will show findings characteristic of hypokalemia—prominent U waves, flattening of the T waves, and prolongation of the PR, QRS, and QT intervals with depression of the RST segment. The plasma potassium level falls during an attack, usually to about 2 to 2.5 mEq per liter.

TREATMENT

Potassium will abort or control a hypokalemic paralytic attack. It is usually administered orally in water in doses of 0.2 gm. per kg. of body weight, up to a maximum dose of 10 gm. If, within one to two hours, there has been no improvement, half of the preceding dose may be repeated. When attacks are frequent, preventive measures should be taken in the form of a prophylactic dose of potassium at night, restriction of sodium intake, and avoidance of excessive exercise and heavy intake of carbohydrates. Spironolactone in doses of 100 to 200 mg. each day orally may be effective in controlling the attacks. If cardiac arrhythmia develops, the attacks are controlled by infusion of 50 mg. of potassium. Digitalis should not be given.

Hyperkalemic Periodic Paralysis

Gamstorp gave the name *adynamia episodica hereditaria* to a rare disease characterized by periodic attacks of paralysis of the limbs and trunk in which the serum potassium concentration is increased during an attack.[18] Tyler et al. previously had investigated a family in which the serum potassium did not fall during attacks and in which paralysis failed to respond to potassium.[53]

The condition is inherited as an autosomal dominant trait. Its exact etiology is unknown. Paralysis is due to an abnormally low resting muscle membrane potential.[9] Potassium leaks from the muscle during attacks, with resultant lowering of the concentration of potassium in the muscle, and an increase in that of the sodium chloride.[33] The serum potassium level is increased to as much as 7.0 mEq per liter during an attack, with concomitant increase in urinary output of potassium. In normal individuals, muscle weakness does not develop until the serum potassium is elevated to 8.0 mEq per liter, indicating an undue susceptibility in the affected patients.

The attacks usually start in infancy and early childhood. They are induced by rest after heavy exercise. The muscles involved first are the gluteals, lower erector spinae, quadriceps, and triceps surae. Gradually, the paralysis spreads to the musculature of the upper limb. The neck muscles may be affected in severe attacks. The muscles supplied by the cranial nerves are occasionally involved; transient blurring of vision and diplopia have been noted. Bulbar and respiratory paralysis rarely occurs.

The paralytic attacks occur during the day and are frequent and short, lasting from 20 to 60 minutes. Exercise accelerates recovery; rest following exercise induces paralysis. During the attacks, especially in mild cases, myotonia may be elicited by direct percussion of a muscle. When the attack is severe, the muscles fail to respond to direct stimulation and the deep tendon reflexes are diminished or absent. The presence of myotonia in some families links the condition with paramyotonia congenita.

During an attack, the serum potassium level is elevated, and electromyography shows action potential change indicating loss of both individual fibers and the whole motor units. Hyperirritability of the myotonic type may be present in some fibers.

The mild or moderate attacks usually do not require treatment, for they are very short. If they are too frequent, their incidence can be reduced or they can be prevented by administering diuretics that promote excretion of potassium and sodium. Dichlorphenamide in 50 to 100 mg. daily dosage is usually very effective in preventing attacks. The severe and prolonged episodes are treated by intravenous administration of calcium gluconate (1 to 2 gm.). The attacks usually abate and disappear with increasing age.

Normokalemic Periodic Paralysis

In this very rare type of periodic paralysis, the attacks are severe and may last for days or even weeks, occurring mainly at night. The serum concentration of potassium is normal, even during the most severe attack. Potassium is retained rather than lost. Attacks are neither provoked nor made worse by administration of potassium; they may be improved by large doses of sodium chloride and prevented by daily administration of a combination of 250 mg. of acetazolamide and 0.1 mg. of 9α-fluorohydrocortisone.

References

1. Allot, E.W., and McArdle, B.: Further observations on familial periodic paralysis. Clin. Sci., 3:229, 1938.
2. Armstrong, F.S.: Hyperkalemic familial periodic paralysis (adynamia episodica hereditaria). Ann. Intern. Med., 57:455, 1962.
3. Bergman, R.A., Afifi, A.K., Dunkle, L.M., and Johns, R.J.: Muscle pathology in hypokalemic periodic paralysis with hyperthyroidism. I. High resolution light microscopic study of a case. Johns Hopkins Med. J., 126:88, 1970.
4. Bergman, R.A., Afifi, A.K., Dunkle, L.M., and Johns, R.J.: Muscle pathology in hypokalemic periodic paralysis with hyperthyroidism. II. A light and electron microscopic study. Johns Hopkins Med. J., 126:100, 1970.
5. Biczyskowa, W., Fidzianska, A., and Jedrzejowska, H.: Light and electron microscopic study of the muscles in hypokalemic periodic paralysis. Acta Neuropathol. (Berlin), 12:329, 1969.
6. Bradley, W.G.: Adynamia episodica hereditaria. Clinical, pathological and electrophysiological studies in an affected family. Brain, 92:345, 1969.
7. Bradley, W.G.: Ultrastructural changes in adynamia episodica hereditaria and normokalemic familial periodic paralysis. Brain, 92:379, 1969.
8. Buruma, O.J., Bots, G.T., and Went, L.N.: Familial hypokalemic periodic paralysis. 50-year follow-up of a large family. Arch. Neurol., 42:28, 1985.
9. Creutzfeldt, O.D., Abbott, B.C., Fowler, W.M., and Pearson, C.M.: Muscle membrane potentials in episodic adynamia. Electroencephalogr. Clin. Neurophysiol., 15:508, 1963.
10. Dunkle, L.M., Diggs, Ch.H., Bergman, R.A., and Johns, R.J.: A light and electron microscopic study of a second case of hypokalemic periodic paralysis with hyperthyroidism. Johns Hopkins Med. J., 126:225, 1970.
11. Egan, T.J., and Klein, R.: Hyperkalemic familial periodic paralysis. Pediatrics, 24:761, 1959.
12. Engel, A.G.: Evolution and content of vacuoles in primary hypokalemic periodic paralysis. Mayo Clin. Proc., 45:774, 1970.
13. Engel, A.G., Potter, C.S., and Rosevear, J.W.: Nucleotides and adenosine monophosphate deaminase activity of muscle in primary hypokalemic periodic paralysis. Nature (London), 202:670, 1964.

14. Fernandez Sein, A., and Vazquez, M.: Hypokalemic periodic paralysis: a rarely considered diagnosis in the pediatric patient. Bol. Assoc. Med., 77:66, 1985.
15. Fozard, J.R.: Anaesthesia and familial periodic paralysis (Letter). Anaesthesia, 38:293, 1983.
16. Fudema, J.J., Oester, Y.T., Talso, P.J., and Glynn, M.F.: Electromyography and electrodiagnosis in familial periodic paralysis. Bull. Am. Assoc. Electromyogr. Electrodiagn., 9:7, 1962.
17. Gammon, G.D., Austin, J.A., Blithe, M.D., and Reid, G.G.: The relation of potassium to periodic paralysis. Am. J. Med. Sci., 197:326, 1939.
18. Gamstorp, I.: Adynamia episodica hereditaria. Acta Paediatr. (Suppl. 108), 45:1, 1956.
19. Gamstorp, I.: A study of transient muscular weakness. Acta Neurol. Scand., 38:3, 1962.
20. Gobbi, G., Armani, M., Pierobon-Bormioli, S., Giovanardi-Rossi, P., and Angelini, C.: A childhood case of hypokalemic periodic paralysis. Acta Neurol. (Napoli), 6:147, 1984.
21. Gordon, A.M., Green, J.R., and Langunoff, D.: Studies on a patient with hypokalemic familial periodic paralysis. Am. J. Med., 48:185, 1970.
22. Graeff, J. de, and Lameijer, L.D.: Periodic paralysis. Am. J. Med., 39:70, 1965.
23. Griggs, R.C., Engel, W.K., and Resnick, J.S.: Acetazolamide treatment of hypokalemic periodic paralysis. Prevention of attacks and improvement of persistent weakness. Ann. Intern. Med., 73:39, 1970.
24. Griggs, R.C., Resnick, J., and Engel, W.K.: Intravenous treatment of hypokalemic periodic paralysis. Arch. Neurol., 40:539, 1983.
25. Grob, D., Lijestrand, A., and Johns, R.J.: Potassium movement in patients with familial periodic paralysis. Am. J. Med., 23:356, 1957.
26. Hofmann, W.W., and Smith, R.A.: Hypokalemic periodic paralysis studied in vitro. Brain, 93:445, 1970.
27. Ionescu, V., Radu, H., and Nicolescu, P.: Ultrastructural changes in hypokalemic periodic paralysis. Rev. Roum. Neurol., 8:419, 1971.
28. Iverson, T.O.: Familial episodic adynamia. Acta Med. Scand., 171:737, 1962.
29. Johnson, V., and Winternitz, W.W.: Hypokalemic periodic paralysis. South. Med. J., 77:1207, 1984.
30. Klein, R., Egan, T., and Usher, P.: Changes in sodium, potassium, and water in hyperkalemic familial periodic paralysis. Metabolism, 9:1005, 1960.
31. Knochel, J.P.: Hypokalemia. Adv. Intern. Med., 30:317, 1984.
32. McArdle, B.: Le role du potassium dans la paralysie periodique familiale. Sem. Hop. Paris, 30:3724, 1954.
33. McArdle, B.: Familial periodic paralysis. Br. Med. Bull., 12:226, 1956.
34. McArdle, B.: Adynamia episodica hereditaria and its treatment. Brain, 85:121, 1962.
35. McArdle, B.: Metabolic myopathies: The glycogenoses affecting muscle and hypo- and hyperkalemic periodic paralysis. Am. J. Med., 35:661, 1963.
36. McArdle, B.: Metabolic and endocrine myopathies. In Walton, J.N. (ed.): Disorders of Voluntary Muscle. J. and A. Churchill, 1964, pp. 607–638.
37. MacDonald, R.D., Rewcastle, N.B., and Humphrey, J.G.: The myopathy of hyperkalemic periodic paralysis. An electron microscopic study. Arch. Neurol., 19:274, 1968.
38. MacDonald, R.D., Rewcastle, N.B., and Humphrey, J.G.: Myopathy of hypokalemic periodic paralysis. Arch. Neurol., 20:566, 1969.
39. Martin, J.J., Ceuterick, C., Mercelis, R., and Amrom, D.: Familial periodic paralysis with hypokalemia. Study of a muscle biopsy in the myopathic stage of the disorder. Acta Neurol. Belg., 84:233, 1984.
40. Melnick, B., Chang, J.L., Larson, C.E., and Bedger, R.C.: Hypokalemic familial periodic paralysis. Anesthesiology, 58:263, 1983.

41. Pearson, C.M.: The periodic paralysis: Differential features and pathological observations in permanent myopathic weakness. Brain, 87:341, 1964.
42. Poskanzer, D.C., and Kerr, D.N.S.: Periodic paralysis with response to spironolactone. Lancet, 2:511, 1961.
43. Poskanzer, D.C., and Kerr, D.N.S.: A third type of periodic paralysis with normokalemia and favorable response to sodium chloride. Am. J. Med., 31:328, 1961.
44. Resnick, J.S., and Engel, W.K.: Myotonic lid lag in hypokalemic periodic paralysis. J. Neurol. Neurosurg. Psychiatry, 30:47, 1967.
45. Resnick, J.S., Engel, W.K., Griggs, R.C., and Stam, A.C.: Acetazolamide prophylaxis in hypokalemic periodic paralysis. N. Engl. J. Med., 278:582, 1968.
46. Ricker, K., Bohlen, R., and Rohkamm, R.: Different effectiveness of tocainide and hydrochlorothiazide in paramyotonia congenita with hyperkalemic episodic paralysis. Neurology, 33:1615, 1983.
47. Rollman, J.E., and Dickson, C.M.: Anesthetic management of a patient with hypokalemic familial periodic paralysis for coronary artery bypass surgery. Anesthesiology, 63:526, 1985.
48. Saunders, M., Ashworth, B., Emery, A.E.H., and Benedikz, J.E.G.: Familial myotonic periodic paralysis with muscle wasting. Brain, 91:295, 1968.
49. Shy, G.M., Wanko, T., Rowley, P.T., and Engel, A.G.: Studies in familial periodic paralysis. Exp. Neurol., 3:53, 1961.
50. Streeten, D.H.P., Dalakos, T.G., and Fellerman, H.: Studies on hyperkalemic periodic paralysis. Evidence of changes in plasma Na and Cl and induction of paralysis by adrenal glucocorticoids. J. Clin. Invest., 50:142, 1971.
51. Subramony, S.H., and Wee, A.S.: Exercise and rest in hyperkalemic periodic paralysis. Neurology, 36:173, 1986.
52. Troni, W., Doriguzzi, C., and Mongini, T.: Interictal conduction slowing in muscle fibers in hypokalemic periodic paralysis. Neurology, 33:1522, 1983.
53. Tyler, I.H., Stephens, F.E., Gunn, F.D., and Perkoff, G.T.: Studies on disorders of muscle. VII. Clinical manifestations and inheritance of a type of periodic paralysis without hypopotassemia. J. Clin. Invest., 30:492, 1951.
54. Van der Muelen, J.P., Gilbert, G.J., and Kane, C.A.: Familial hyperkalemic paralysis with myotonia. N. Engl. J. Med., 264:1, 1961.
55. Van't Hoff, W.: Familial myotonic periodic paralyses. Q. J. Med., 31:385, 1962.
56. Vastola, E.F., and Bertrand, C.A.: Intracellular water and potassium in periodic paralysis. Neurology, 6:523, 1956.
57. Weller, R.O., and McArdle, B.: Calcification within muscle fibres in the periodic paralyses. Brain, 94:263, 1971.
58. Wiggers, P., and Nrregaard Hansen, K.: Myoglobin, creatine kinase and creatine kinase subunit-beta in serum from patients with relatives with hypokalaemic familial periodic paralysis. Acta Neurol. Scand., 71:69, 1985.
59. Zierler, K.L., and Andres, R.: Movement of potassium into skeletal muscle during spontaneous attack in family periodic paralysis. J. Clin. Invest., 36:730, 1957.

McARDLE'S SYNDROME (MYOPHOSPHORYLASE DEFICIENCY)

This rare disorder of muscle glycogen metabolism is characterized by muscular pain, stiffness, and weakness following exercise. The symptoms are relieved by rest. It was first described by McArdle in 1951.[16] The condition is transmitted by an autosomal recessive gene and is caused by absence in muscles of myophosphorylase—an enzyme that splits off the terminal glucose molecule from the arborizations of glycogen.

Any muscle in the body may be affected. The muscles that are exercised most develop the most severe symptoms; for example, in walking, the calf and thigh muscles are involved; and in chewing, the masseter muscles. The affected muscles are abnormally stiff and remain in a contracted state for varying periods (the more strenuous the exercise, the longer the duration of affection). Muscular ischemia induces symptoms more rapidly.

A characteristic laboratory finding is failure of the level of blood lactate and pyruvate to rise following exercise. Muscle glycogen is increased. Diagnosis is confirmed by biochemical study, which shows absence of myophosphorylase activity. On occasion, the condition may be associated with myoglobinuria, in which case the prognosis must be more guarded. The disease, when not associated with myopathy, does not appear to be progressive.

Treatment consists of limitation of physical activity. Oral administration of glucose, or preferably fructose, prior to strenuous activity will increase the tolerance to exercise.

References

1. Bank, W.J., DiMauro, S., and Rowland, L.P.: Renal failure in McArdle's disease (lack of muscle phosphorylase). N. Engl. J. Med., 287:1102, 1972.
2. Brody, I.A.: Muscle contracture induced by exercise. A syndrome attributed to decreased relaxing factor. N. Engl. J. Med., 281:187, 1969.
3. Brownell, B., Hughes, J.T., Goldby, F.S., and Woods, H.F.: McArdle's myopathy. A report of a case with observations on the muscle ultrastructure. J. Neurol. Sci., 9:515, 1969.
4. Dawson, D.M., Spong, L.F., and Harrington, J.F.: McArdle's disease. Lack of muscle phosphorylase. Ann. Intern. Med., 69:229, 1968.
5. Diamond, J.: Phosphorylase, calcium and cyclic AMP in smooth-muscle contraction. Am. J. Physiol., 225:930, 1973.
6. Dyken, M.L., Smith, D.M., and Peake, R.L.: An electromyographic diagnostic screening test in McArdle's disease and a case report. Neurology, 17:45, 1967.
7. Engel, W.K., Eyerman, E.L., and Williams, H.E.: Late-onset type of skeletal-muscle phosphorylase deficiency: New familial variety with completely and partially affected subjects. N. Engl. J. Med., 268:135, 1963.
8. Fattah, S.M., Rubulis, A., and Faldon, W.W.: McArdle's disease: metabolic studies in a patient and review of the syndrome. Am. J. Med., 48:693, 1970.
9. Gruener, R., McArdle, B., Ryman, B.E., and Weller, R.O.: Contracture of phosphorylase deficient muscle. J. Neurol. Neurosurg. Psychiatry, 31:268, 1968.
10. Grunfeld, J.P., Ganeval, D., Chanard, J., Fardeau, M., and Dreyfus, J.C.: Acute renal failure in McArdle's disease. Report of two cases. N. Engl. J. Med., 286:1237, 1972.
11. Haller, R.G., and Lewis, S.F.: Abnormal ventilation during exercise in McArdle's syndrome: modulation by substrate availability. Neurology, 36:716, 1986.
12. Harris, R.A., and Dowben, R.M.: McArdle's disease in an elderly woman. South. Med. J., 78:191, 1985.
13. Hockaday, T.D., and Downey, J.A.: McArdle's syndrome. Lancet, 1:1185, 1962.
14. Hockaday, T.D.R., Downey, J.A., and Nottram, R.F.: A case of McArdle's syndrome with a positive family history. J. Neurol. Neurosurg. Psychiatry, 27:186, 1964.
15. Layzer, R.B.: McArdle's disease in the 1980's (Editorial). N. Engl. J. Med., 312:370, 1985.
16. McArdle, B.: Myopathy due to a defect in muscle strengcogen breakdown. Clin. Sci., 10:13, 1951.
17. Mellick, R.S., Mahler, R.E., and Hughes, B.P.: McArdle's syndrome: Phosphorylase-deficient myopathy. Lancet, 1:1045, 1962.
18. Mommaerts, W.F.H.M., Illingsworth, B., Pearson, C.M., Guillory, R.J., and Saraydarian, K.: A functional disorder of muscle associated with the absence of phosphorylase. Proc. Natl. Acad. Sci. U.S.A., 46:791, 1959.
19. Opie, L.H., Evans, J.R., and Renold, A.E.: Fructose in McArdle's syndrome. Lancet, 2:358, 1962.
20. Pearson, C.H., Rimer, D.G., and Mommaerts, N.M.: Defect in muscle phosphorylase. A newly defined human disease. Clin. Res., 7:298, 1959.
21. Pearson, C.M., Rimer, D.G., and Mommaerts, W.F.H.M.: A metabolic myopathy due to absence of muscle phosphorylase. Am. J. Med., 30:502, 1961.
22. Pernow, B.B., Havel, R.J., and Jennings, D.B.: The second wind phenomenon in McArdle's syndrome. Acta Med. Scand., 472:294, 1967.
23. Porte, D., Jr., Crawford, D.W., Jennings, D.M., Aber, O., and McIlroy, M.B.: Cardiovascular and metabolic responses to exercise in a patient with McArdle's syndrome. N. Engl. J. Med., 275:406, 1966.
24. Rowland, L.P., Araki, S., and Carmel, P.: Contracture in McArdle's disease: stability of adenosine triphosphate during contracture in phosphorylase-deficient human muscle. Arch. Neurol., 13:541, 1964.
25. Rowland, L.P., Fahn, S., and Schotland, D.L.: McArdle's disease: hereditary myopathy due to absence of muscle phosphorylase. Arch. Neurol., 9:325, 1963.
26. Salter, R.H., Adamson, D.G., and Pearce, G.W.: McArdle's syndrome (myophosphorylase deficiency). A study of a family. Q. J. Med., 36:565, 1967.
27. Schmid, R., and Hammaker, L.: Hereditary absence of muscle phosphorylase (McArdle's syndrome). N. Engl. J. Med., 264:223, 1961.
28. Schotland, D.L., Spiro, D., Rowland, L.P., and Carmel, P.: Ultrastructure of phosphorylase-deficient human muscle (McArdle's disease). J. Neuropathol. Exp. Neurol., 24:629, 1965.
29. Slonim, A.E., and Goans, P.J.: Myopathy in McArdle's syndrome. Improvement with a high-protein diet. N. Engl. J. Med., 312:355, 1985.
30. Thompson, P.D., and Flynn, M.M.: Myopathy in McArdle's syndrome (Letter). N. Engl. J. Med., 312:1518, 1985.
31. Tobin, R.B., and Coleman, W.A.: A family study of phosphorylase-deficiency in muscle. Ann. Intern. Med., 62:313, 1965.

IDIOPATHIC PAROXYSMAL MYOGLOBINURIA

This rare condition was first described by Meyer-Betz in 1911.[18] It is characterized by recurrent transient acute attacks of severe pain and cramping in the muscles associated with weakness or paralysis, and followed within a few hours by myoglobinuria. The muscles of the lower limbs are more frequently affected. With rest, the attack subsides within a few days. In severe cases, oliguria and anuria may be present owing to renal damage from myoglobin.

In myoglobinuria, the urine is reddish brown and does not contain erythrocytes; the urine becomes burgundy in color on exposure to light. The presence of myoglobin in the urine is confirmed by spectrophotometric examination.

Paroxysmal myoglobinuria is differentiated into two types. In the first, the attacks occur primarily in childhood, often following an acute infectious disease, and are frequently accompanied by fever, leukocytosis, and renal insufficiency. Familial incidence is low. In the other type, symptoms usually begin between the second and third decades. The attacks are induced by exercise. There is a high familial incidence, and recurrent severe attacks may result in permanent muscle atrophy.

Treatment is symptomatic, consisting of rest and alkalization of urine. Kidney function should be carefully observed, as uremia and death may occur in the childhood form.

References

1. Bailie, M.D.: Primary paroxysmal myoglobinuria. N. Engl. J. Med., 271:186, 1964.
2. Berenbaum, M.C., Birch, C.A., and Moreland, J.D.: Paroxysmal myoglobinuria. Lancet, 1:892, 1955.
3. Borman, J.B., Davidson, J.T., and Blondsheim, S.H.: Idiopathic rhabdomyolysis (myoglobinuria) as an acute respiratory problem. Br. Med. J., 2:726, 1963.
4. Borolan, T.V., and Attwoods, G.R.: Myoglobinuria. J. Pediatr., 67:69, 1965.
5. Buchanan, D., and Steiner, P.R.: Myogloginuria with paralysis (Meyer-Betz disease). A.M.A. Arch. Neurol. Psychiatr., 66:107, 1951.
6. Comings, D.E., and Rosenfeld, H.: Idiopathic paroxysmal myoglobinuria. Ann. Intern. Med., 55:647, 1967.
7. Farmer, T.A., Hammack, W.J., and Frommeyer, W.B., Jr.: Idiopathic recurrent rhabdomyolysis associated with myoglobinuria. N. Engl. J. Med., 264:60, 1961.
8. Favara, B.E., Wagner, G.F., Kevy, S., and Porter, E.: Familial paroxysmal rhabdomyolysis in children. Am. J. Med., 42:196, 1967.
9. Gillett, R.L.: Primary myoglobinuria. N. Engl. J. Med., 260:1156, 1959.
10. Kaufman, R.P., and Barry, P.E.: Rhabdomyolysis with myoglobinuria. N. Engl. J. Med., 260:430, 1959.
11. Kohler, H.J.: Die Myoglobinurien. Ergeb. Inn. Med. Kinderheilkd., 11:1, 1959.
12. Korein, J., Coddon, D.R., and Mowrey, F.H.: The clinical syndrome of paroxysmal paralytic myoglobinuria. Neurology, 9:767, 1959.
13. Kossman, R.J., Camp, W.A., and Engel, R.L., Jr.: Idiopathic recurrent rhabdymyolysis: myoglobinuria. Am. J. Med., 34:554, 1963.
14. de Langen, C.D.: Myoglobin and myoglobinuria. Acta Med. Scand., 124:213, 1946.
15. Lee, T., and Goodley, E.L.: Myoglobinuria and renal failure with myopathy. Penn. Med., 74:56, 1971.
16. Louw, A., and Nielson, H.E.: Paroxysmal paralytic hemoglobinuria. Acta Med. Scand., 117:424, 1944.
17. Marks, A.D., and Haase, G.: Medical grand rounds: myoglobinuria. Am. J. Med. Sci., 261:351, 1971.
18. Meyer-Betz, F.: Beobachtungen an einem eigenartigen mit Muskellahmungen verbundenem Fall von Hamoglobinurie. Dtsch. Arch. Klin. Med., 101:85, 1911.
19. Pearson, C.M., Beck, W.S., and Blahd, W.H.: Idiopathic paroxysmal myoglobinuria. Detailed study of a case including radioisotope and serum enzyme evaluation. A.M.A. Arch. Intern. Med., 99:376, 1957.
20. Savage, D.C.L.: Forbes, M., and Pearce, G.W.: Idiopathic rhabdomyolysis. Arch. Dis. Child., 46:594, 1971.
21. Schaar, F.E., LaBree, J.W., and Gleason, D.F.: Paroxysmal myoglobinuria with fatal renal tubular injury. Cent. Soc. Clin. Res. Proc., 22:71, 1949.
22. Tavill, A.S., Evanson, J.M., Baker, S.B., and Hewitt, V.: Idiopathic paroxysmal myoglobinuria with acute renal failure and hypercalcemia. N. Engl. J. Med., 271:283, 1964.
23. Wheby, M.S., and Miller, H.S., Jr.: Idiopathic paroxysmal myoglobinuria. Am. J. Med., 29:599, 1960.
24. Whisnant, C.L., Jr., Owings, R.H., Cantell, G.G., and Cooper, G.R.: Primary idiopathic myoglobinuria. Ann. Intern. Med., 51:141, 1959.
25. Wissler, H.: Paroxysmale myoglobinurie. Helv. Paediatr. Acta, 3:334, 1948.

STIFF-MAN SYNDROME [1-35]

This extremely rare entity of unknown etiology occurs primarily in the adult but does occur in children. It is characterized by stiffness and rigidity of skeletal muscles induced by a sudden stimulus or a voluntary movement. A neurologic and metabolic abnormality has not been found. Quinine and procaine are not effective in relieving the muscle spasms.

References

1. Asher, R.: A woman with the stiff-man syndrome. Br. Med. J., 1:265, 1958.
2. Black, J.T., Garcia-Mullin, R., Good, E., and Brown, S.: Muscle rigidity in a newborn due to continuous peripheral nerve activity. Arch. Neurol., 27:413, 1972.
3. Bowler, D.: The stiff-man syndrome in a boy. Arch. Dis. Child., 35:289, 1960.
4. Buckner, W.J.: Stiff man syndrome. Progressive fluctuating muscular rigidity and spasm. Calif. Med., 87:336, 1957.
5. Cobb, J.J.: Stiff man syndrome: Is the lesion at spinal cord or brain-stem level? Proc. R. Soc. Med., 67:1065, 1974.
6. Cohen, L.: Stiff man syndrome: two patients treated with diazepam. J.A.M.A., 195:222, 1966.
7. Drake, M.E., Jr.: Stiff-man syndrome and dementia. Am. J. Med., 74:1085, 1983.
8. Editorial: Stiff-man syndromes. Br. Med. J., 2:1478, 1956.
9. Editorial: New stiff-muscle syndrome. Annotation. Br. Med. J., 1:168, 1962.
10. George, T.M., Burke, J.M., Sobotka, P.A., Greenberg, H.S., and Vinik, A.I.: Resolution of stiff-man syndrome with cortisol replacement in a patient with deficiencies

of ACTH, growth hormone and prolactin. N. Engl. J. Med., *310*:1511, 1984.

11. Goodall, M.C., and Szent-Gyorgy, A.G.: Relaxation factor in muscle. Nature, *172*:84, 1953.

12. Gordon, E., Jamisko, D.M., and Kaufman, L.: A critical survey of stiff-man syndrome. Am. J. Med., *42*:582, 1967.

13. Howard, F.M.: A new and effective drug in the treatment of stiff-man syndrome. Proc. Staff Meet. Mayo Clin., *38*:203, 1963.

14. Huhnstock, V.K., Brock, R., and Kuhn, E.: On stiff-man syndrome. Report of a case and review of the literature. Dtsch. Med. Wochenschr., *87*:1388, 1962.

15. Isaacs, H.: A syndrome of continuous muscle fiber activity. J. Neurol. Neurosurg. Psychiatry, *24*:319, 1961.

16. Klein, R., Haddow, J.E., and DeLuca, C.: Familial congenital disorder resembling stiff-man syndrome. Am. J. Dis. Child., *124*:730, 1972.

17. Kugelmass, W.: Stiff-man syndrome in a child. N.Y. State J. Med., *61*:2483, 1961.

18. Meinck, H.M., Ricker, K., and Conrad, B.: The stiff-man syndrome: new pathophysiological aspects from abnormal exteroceptive reflexes and the response to clomipramine, clonidine, and tizanidine. J. Neurol. Neurosurg. Psychiatry, *47*:280, 1984.

19. Moersch, F.P., and Woltman, H.W.: Progressive fluctuating muscular rigidity ("stiff-man syndrome"). Proc. Staff Meet. Mayo Clin., *31*:421, 1956.

20. Nakumura, N., Fujiya, S., Yahara, O., Fujioka, Y., and Kawakami, Y.: Stiff-man syndrome with spinal cord lesion. Clin. Neuropathol., *5*:40, 1986.

21. O'Connor, D.C.J.: Stiff man syndrome. Br. Med. J., *1*:645, 1958.

22. Olafson, R.A., Mulder, D.W., and Howard, F.M.: Stiff man syndrome: a review of the literature, report of three additional cases and discussion of pathophysiology and therapy. Proc. Staff Meet. Mayo Clin., *39*:131, 1964.

23. Price, T.M.L., and Allott, E.M.: The stiff-man syndrome. Br. Med. J., *2*:682, 1958.

24. Seitz, D.: An unusual muscle affection characterized by progressive contractures. Dtsch. Z. Nernenk., *178*:492, 1958.

25. Shukla, K.L., and Sikand, P.: Stiff man syndrome. J. Indian Med. Assoc., *37*:610, 1961.

26. Sigwald, J., Rondot, P., Raverdy, P., and Singer, B.: Le syndrome de l'homme raide (stiff man syndrome): particulaires cliniques, electrologiques, et therapeutiques. Sem. Hop. (Paris), *44*:1705, 1968.

27. Sikes, Z.S.: Stiff-man syndrome. (Analysis and case report with spinal cord autopsy.) Dis. Nerv. Syst., *20*:254, 1959.

28. Trethowan, W.H., Allsop, J.L., and Turner, B.: The "stiff-man" syndrome. Arch. Neurol., *3*:448, 1960.

29. Valli, G., Barbieri, S., Cappa, S., Pellegrini, G., and Scarlato, G.: Syndromes of abnormal muscular activity: overlap between continuous muscle fiber activity and the stiff man syndrome. J. Neurol. Neurosurg. Psychiatry, *46*:241, 1983.

30. Wallis, W.E., Van Poznak, A., and Plum, F.: Generalized muscular stiffness, fasciculations, and myokymia of peripheral nerve origin. Arch. Neurol., *22*:430, 1970.

31. Warneke, L.: Stiff-man syndrome. Can. Psychiatr. Assoc. J., *19*:399, 1974.

32. Whalen, R.E., Combs, J.J., and Deiss, W.J., Jr.: "Stiff-man" syndrome. Am. J. Med., *27*:678, 1959.

33. Whiteley, A.M., Swash, M., and Urich, H.: Progressive encephalomyelitis with rigidity. Its relation to subacute myoclonic spinal neuronitis and to the stiff man syndrome. Brain, *99*:27, 1976.

34. Yarom, R., Chaco, J., and Steigbuegel, D.: Ultrastructure of muscle in "stiff-man" syndrome. Virchows Arch., *362*:207, 1974.

35. Young, W.: The stiff man syndrome. Br. J. Clin. Pract., *20*:507, 1966.

MYASTHENIA GRAVIS

Myasthenia gravis is a chronic autoimmune disorder in which there is sustained production of an antibody to the nicotinic acetylcholine receptor at the neuromuscular junction, affecting the transmission of impulses at the myoneural junction. It is characterized by excessive fatigability and apparent paralysis of voluntary muscles following repetitive activity or prolonged tension, with a marked tendency to recovery of motor power after a period of inactivity or diminution of muscular tension.[95] The first case was described by Willis in 1672.[101] The characteristics of the disease were fully described by Erb (1879) and Goldflam (1893); hence the eponym Erb-Goldflam disease.[27, 32] Jolly applied the term myasthenia gravis.[40] A historical review of myasthenia gravis from 1672 to 1900 is given by Viets.[94] Walker noted the similarity of a myasthenic patient to a curarized normal individual, and knowing the antagonism of physostigmine for curare, demonstrated the remarkable therapeutic effect of neostigmine (a synthetic analogue of physostigmine) on a myasthenic patient.[98, 99] Viets and Schwab devised a definitive neostigmine test.[96]

The incidence of myasthenia gravis is variously reported as from 1 in 50,000 to 1 in 10,000 of the population. The disease may become manifest at any age. About 10 per cent of the patients have symptoms in infancy and childhood.[54, 67] There is a preponderance of the disease in the female, the female to male ratio being 4.5:1 in the first decade but reversing in later life.

The exact cause of the disorder is unknown. Myasthenia gravis is considered to be an autoimmune disorder in which an antibody is produced against an end-plate protein antigen, which is alleged to interfere with normal neuromuscular transmission. The thymus gland is thought to be the site of this antibody production. The muscles appear normal to the naked eye; however, lymphocytic infiltrations of muscles (termed lymphorrhages) are found in some muscles on histologic examination. Recently, "dystrophic" and "dysplastic" type changes have been observed in the motor end-plates.[85]

Abnormalities of the thymus gland, such as benign tumors, hyperplasia, and persistence of the gland, are frequently found in patients with myasthenia gravis, but the relation of these changes to the disease is uncertain.

Clinical Features

Myasthenia gravis in children has been subdivided into three groups by Millichap and Dodge.[54] Depending upon the age at onset and features of the disease, they are (1) neonatal transient, (2) neonatal persistent (congenital), and (3) juvenile myasthenia gravis.

NEONATAL TRANSIENT MYASTHENIA GRAVIS

In this type, all infants are born to mothers with myasthenia gravis. Symptoms begin soon after birth. They consist of generalized muscular weakness with little spontaneous movement, weak Moro response, weak suck, facial weakness, ptosis, respiratory weakness, and dysphagia. These symptoms are transient, lasting less than four weeks. It seems that the antibody passed through the placenta to the fetus is slowly excreted or destroyed by the neonate. Death may occur if the infant is untreated. Therapy with neostigmine will result in recovery.

NEONATAL PERSISTENT (CONGENITAL) MYASTHENIA GRAVIS

In this form the mothers do not suffer from myasthenia gravis. The clinical features consist of ptosis, weak cry, and generalized weakness. In later life, external ophthalmoplegia develops. Involvement of the bulbar musculature and respiratory difficulty are uncommon, and in general, the symptoms are of mild degree. The disease runs a protracted course and is somewhat resistant to drug therapy, but neostigmine will relieve symptoms in most cases.

JUVENILE MYASTHENIA GRAVIS

Symptoms usually begin after ten years of age. A family history of myasthenia gravis is usually not obtained. Ptosis is the most common presenting sign and is usually bilaterally symmetrical; however, it may be unilateral or bilaterally asymmetrical. Weakness in the upper and lower limbs occurs commonly. The child is unable to walk for long distances without rest. He has difficulty in climbing stairs and falls frequently because his knees collapse. There may be bilateral gluteus maximus and gluteus medius limp. The Trendelenburg test may be positive.

Weakness of the facial muscles gives a sad expression to the face, often out of line with the true emotional state. Weakness in mastication results from easy fatigability of the jaw muscles. Weakness of the tongue muscles causes dysarthria. The patient will pronounce several sentences clearly and then, complaining that his tongue feels thick, talk as though he had a mouthful of food. Difficulty in deglutition arises from weakness of the voluntary muscles of the upper pharynx. Respiratory difficulty is not uncommon. Involvement of the bulbar muscles and respiratory failure may occur in myasthenia gravis and cause sudden death.

Fatigability of the voluntary muscles is always less in the morning, but as the day progresses, the weakness becomes more marked. Neurologic examination will disclose normal sensation and deep tendon reflexes. Pathologic reflexes are absent.

The natural history of the disease is extremely variable. There may be periods of remission that last for several months or even years. Ordinarily, the disease becomes most severe in 83 per cent of the patients within three years after onset. The patients are at risk for progression during the first and second years after the onset of the disease.

Diagnosis

The cardinal feature of myasthenia gravis is a history of muscular weakness that is precipitated by activity. A positive edrophonium chloride (Tensilon) test will confirm the diagnosis. Edrophonium chloride is an analogue of neostigmine (Prostigmin). Of the two agents, Tensilon is preferred because of its shorter duration of action and rapid excretion. The intravenous test dose is 1 mg. (in children up to 75 lb.) and 2 mg. in children above 75 lb.; when administered intramuscularly, the test dose is 2 mg. (in children up to 75 lb.) and 5 mg. for children above this weight. In normal individuals, edrophonium chloride has no effect on muscle strength but has marked cholinergic side effects, such as excessive perspiration and salivation, lacrimation, and fasciculations. In the myasthenic patient, however, within the first minute after injection there is marked improvement in motor strength of weak muscles, and cholinergic side reactions are minimal. Five minutes following administration of the drug the beneficial effects disappear.

Faradic stimulation will produce brisk, strong muscle contractions initially, but on repeated stimulation the contractions diminish and eventually disappear (the so-called myasthenic reaction of Jolly).[40]

This easy fatigability of voluntary muscles also can be demonstrated in the electromyogram, in which the action potentials from the repeatedly stimulated muscles show a gradual diminution in amplitude as the stimulation is continued.

In the differential diagnosis, various conditions should be considered, such as brain tumor, poliomyelitis, encephalitis, tuberculous meningitis, chronic barbiturate or bromide intoxication, muscular dystrophy, polyneuropathy, tumors of the larynx or esophagus, and psychoneurosis, particularly globus hystericus and the so-called nervous fatigue syndrome. Myasthenia gravis is distinguished from these disorders by the positive Tensilon test and progressive weakness of voluntary muscles following activity or faradic stimulation.

Treatment

Immunosuppressive therapy, especially with cyclosporine, is very effective.[10, 93] Patients who do not respond to drug therapy may require thymectomy. Neostigmine (Prostigmin bromide), pyridostigmine bromide (Mestinon), and ambenonium chloride (Mytelase) usually provide partial or complete relief of the symptoms. The dosage of these drugs is variable, depending upon the age of the patient, the severity of the disease, and the response to medication.

When the muscles of respiration are involved, the assistance of a mechanized respirator may be required. Tracheostomy is indicated when there is marked pooling of secretions due to weakness of the pharyngeal muscles.

Prognosis

The outlook for children and adolescents with myasthenia gravis is generally favorable, although myasthenia crises may occur in about one of six patients, necessitating the use of a mechanical respirator. Occasionally the outcome may be fatal.[54]

References

1. Ahuja, G.K., Verman, A., Ghosh, P., and Nagaraj, M.N.: Stapedius reflexometry. A diagnostic test of myasthenia gravis. J. Neurol. Sci., 46:311, 1980.
2. Albers, J.W., Faulkner, J.A., Dorovini-Zis, K., Barald, K.F., Must, R.E., and Ball, R.D.: Abnormal neuromuscular transmission in an infantile myasthenic syndrome. Ann. Neurol., 16:28, 1984.
3. Allen, N., Kissel, P., Pietrasiuk, D., and Perlow, M.J.: Myasthenia gravis in monozygotic twins. Clinical follow-up nine years after thymectomy. Arch. Neurol., 41:994, 1984.
4. Alt, W., and Hochman, H.I.: Thyrotoxicosis and myasthenia gravis. Case reports and discussion of immunologic similarities. Clin. Pediatr., 21:749, 1982.
5. Ashok, P.P., Ahuja, G.K., Manchanda, S.C., and Jalal, S.: Cardiac involvement in myasthenia gravis. Acta Neurol. Scand., 68:113, 1983.
6. Baptist, E.C., Landes, R.V., and Sturman, J.K., Jr.: Familial infantile myasthenia gravis: a preventable cause of sudden death. South. Med. J., 78:201, 1985.
7. Barlow, C.F.: Neonatal myasthenia gravis. Am. J. Dis. Child., 135:309, 1981.
8. Biesecker, G., and Koffler, D.: Immunology of myasthenia gravis. Hum. Pathol., 14:419, 1983.
9. Binet, J.P., Pouliquen, E., Razafinombana, A., Le-Brigand, H., and Lasfargues, G.: Thymectomy for myasthenia in young children. Apropos of 2 cases. Bull. Acad. Natl. Med. (Paris), 164:665, 1980.
10. Bjerre, I., and Hallberg, A.: Myasthenia gravis. Immunological studies in a young child treated with thymectomy and immunosuppressive drugs. Neuropediatrics, 14:106, 1983.
11. Bowman, J.R.: Myasthenia gravis in young children. Pediatrics, 1:472, 1948.
12. Brown, L.R., Muhm, J.R., Sheedy, P.F., Unni, K.K., Bernatz, P.E., and Hermann, R.C., Jr.: The value of computed tomography in myasthenia gravis. A.J.R., 140:31, 1983.
13. Burke, W.J.: Myasthenia gravis: a clinical review. Clin. Exp. Neurol., 17:1, 1981.
14. Campbell, J.R., Bisio, J.M., Harrison, M.W., and Campbell, T.J.: Surgical treatment of myasthenia gravis in childhood. J. Pediatr. Surg., 18:857, 1983.
15. Cavanagh, N.P.: The role of thymectomy in childhood myasthenia. Dev. Med. Child Neurol., 22:668, 1980.
16. Chan Lui, W.Y., and Hawkins, B.R.: Infantile myasthenia. Neuropediatrics, 16:24, 1985.
17. Chutorian, A.M.: Corticosteroids and corticotrophin in the treatment of neurologic disorders, with emphasis on neurologic disorders of childhood. Clin. Neuropharmacol., 5:239, 1982.
18. Cohen, M.S., and Younger, D.: Aspects of the natural history of myasthenia gravis: crisis and death. Ann. N.Y. Acad. Sci., 377:670, 1981.
19. Cobeel, L., Lacquet, A., Casteels-Van Daele, M., Melchoir, S., and Igodt-Ameye, L.: Myasthenia gravis, clinical findings before and after thymectomy. Acta Paediatr. Belg., 31:95, 1978.
20. Cox, A., Lisak, R.P., Skolnik, P., and Zweiman, B.: Effect of thymectomy on blood T-cell subsets in myasthenia gravis. Ann. Neurol., 19:297, 1986.
21. Cruz Martinez, A., Ferrer, M.T., Perez Conde, M.C., Diez Tejedor, E., Barreiros, P., and Ribacoba, R.: Diagnostic yield of single fiber electromyography and other electrophysiological techniques in myasthenia gravis. II. Jitter and motor unit fiber density studies. Clinical remission and thymectomy evaluation. Electromyogr. Clin. Neurophysiol., 22:395, 1982.
22. Donat, J.F., Donat, J.R., and Lennon, V.A.: Exchange transfusion in neonatal myasthenia gravis. Neurology, 31:911, 1981.
23. Donnelly, R.J., Laquaglia, M.P., Fabri, B., Hayward, M., and Florence, A.M.: Cervical thymectomy in the treatment of myasthenia gravis. Ann. R. Coll. Surg., 66:305, 1984.
24. Eaton, L.M.: Diagnostic tests for myasthenia with Prostigmin and quinine. Proc. Staff Meet. Mayo Clin., 18:230, 1943.
25. Emery, E.J., and Szymanski, H.V.: Psychological symptoms preceding diagnosed myasthenia gravis. Psychosomatics, 22:993, 1981.
26. Engel, A.G., Lambert, E.H., and Gomez, M.R.: End-plate acetylcholinesterase deficiency associated with small nerve terminals and reduced acetylcholine release. A new syndrome. Int. J. Neurol., 14:73, 1980.
27. Erb, W.: Zur Casuistik der bulbaren Lahmungen. Ueber einen neuen, wanrscheinlich bulbaren Symptomen-complex. Arch. Psychiatr., 9:336, 1879.
28. Fenichel, G.M.: Clinical syndromes of myasthenia in infancy and childhood. A review. Arch. Neurol., 35:97, 1978.

29. Furman, W.L., Buckley, P.J., Green, A.A., Stokes, D.C., and Chien, L.T.: Thymoma and myasthenia gravis in a 4-year-old child. Case report and review of the literature. Cancer, 56:2703, 1985.

30. Gieron, M.A., and Korthals, J.K.: Familial infantile myasthenia gravis. Report of three cases with follow-up until adult life. Arch. Neurol., 42:143, 1985.

31. Gilhus, N.E., Aarli, J.A., and Matre, R.: Myasthenia gravis: the specificities of skeletal muscle and thymus antibodies. Acta Neurol. Scand., 68:328, 1983.

32. Goldflam, S.: Ueber einen scheinbar heilbaren bulbarparalytischen Symptomencomplex mit Betheiligung der Extremitaten. Dtsch. Z. Nervenheilkd., 4:312, 1893.

33. Grob, D.: Course and management of myasthenia gravis. J.A.M.A., 153:529, 1953.

34. Guthrie, L.G.: Myasthenia gravis in the seventeenth century. Lancet, 1:330, 1903.

35. Harvey, A.M., and Johns, R.J.: Myasthenia gravis and the thymus. Am. J. Med., 32:1, 1962.

36. Hawkins, B.R., Chan Lui, W.Y., Choi, E.K., and Ho, A.Y.: Strong association of HLA BW46 with juvenile onset myasthenia gravis in Hong Kong Chinese. J. Neurol. Neurosurg. Psychiatry, 47:555, 1984.

37. Hofstad, H., Ohm, O.J., Mrk, S.J., and Aarli, J.A.: Heart disease in myasthenia gravis. Acta Neurol. Scand., 70:176, 1984.

38. Janssen, R.S., Kaye, A.D., Lisak, R.P., Schatz, N.J., Arger, P.A., and Savino, P.J.: Radiologic evaluation of the mediastinum in myasthenia gravis. Neurology, 33:534, 1983.

39. Jauregui, W.O., DiGressia, C., Herrera, M.E., and Muchnik, S.: Plasmapheresis in myasthenia gravis. Medicina (Buenos Aires), 41:511, 1981.

40. Jolly, F.: Ueber Myasthenia gravis pseudoparalytica. Berlin Klin. Wochenrschr., 32:1, 1895.

41. Keesey, J., Bein, M., Mink, J., Sample, F., Sarti, D., Mulder, D., Herrmann, C., Jr., and Peter, J.B.: Detection of thymoma in myasthenia gravis. Neurology, 30:233, 1980.

42. Keesey, J., Buffkin, D., Kebo, D., Ho, W., and Herrmann, C., Jr.: Plasma exchange alone as therapy for myasthenia gravis. Ann. N.Y. Acad. Sci., 377:729, 1981.

43. Kibrick, S.: Myasthenia gravis in the newborn. Pediatrics, 14:365, 1954.

44. Kissling, W.R., Finke, R., Kotulla, P., and Schleusener, H.: Circulating TSH-binding inhibiting immunoglobulins in myasthenia gravis. Acta Endocrinol. (Copenhagen), 101:41, 1982.

45. Korn, I.L., and Abramsky, O.: Myasthenia gravis following viral infection. Eur. Neurol., 20:435, 1981.

46. Kornstein, M.J., Brooks, J.J., Anderson, A.O., Levinson, A.I., Lisak, R.P., and Zweiman, B.: The immunohistology of the thymus in myasthenia gravis. Am. J. Pathol., 117:184, 1984.

47. Kunze, K.: Thymectomy in the treatment of myasthenia. Thorac. Cardiovasc. Surg., 28:380, 1980.

48. Lefvert, A.K., and Osterman, P.O.: Newborn infants to myasthenic mothers: a clinical study and an investigation of acetylcholine recepter antibodies in 17 children. Neurology, 33:133, 1983.

49. Lin, J.T., and Singer, P.A.: Myasthenia gravis. Its pathophysiology, diagnosis, and treatment. J. Kans. Med. Soc., 84:53, 1983.

50. MacRae, D.D.: Myasthenia gravis in early childhood. Pediatrics, 13:511, 1954.

51. Maret, G., and Gamondes, J.P.: Thymectomy for myasthenia gravis without thymoma. Long term results. Ann. Chir., 34:173, 1980.

51a. Mendell, J.R., Warmolts, J.R., and Bass, J.C.: Caution urged in childhood thymectomy for myasthenia gravis (Letter). Neurology, 27:1182, 1977.

52. Mennuni, G., Morante, M., Scoppetta, C., and Bergonzi, P.: First REM latency in patients with myasthenia gravis: an observation, an hypothesis. Acta Neurol. (Napoli), 5:253, 1983.

53. Mier, A.K., and Havard, C.W.: Diaphragmatic myasthenia in mother and child. Postgrad. Med. J., 61:725, 1985.

54. Millichap, J.G., and Dodge, P.R.: Diagnosis and treatment of myasthenia gravis in infancy, childhood, and adolescence. Neurology, 10:1007, 1960.

55. Mintz, S., Petersen, S.R., MacFarland, D., Petajan, J., and Richards, R.C.: The current role of thymectomy for myasthenia gravis. Am. J. Surg., 140:734, 1980.

56. Moore, A.V., Korobkin, M., Olanow, W., Heaston, D.K., Ram, P.C., Dunnick, N.R., and Silverman, P.M.: Age-related changes in the thymus gland: CT-pathologic correlation. A.J.R., 141:241, 1983.

57. Morel, E., Bach, J.F., Briard, M.L., and Aubry, J.P.: Neonatal myasthenia gravis. Anti-acetylcholine receptor antibodies in the amniotic fluid. Neuroimmunology, 6:313, 1984.

58. Murphy, J., and Murphy, S.F.: Myasthenia gravis in identical twins. Neurology, 36:78, 1986.

59. Musiol, A., Szczechowski, L., Arkuszewski, Z., and Dawidowicz-Sobczak, K.: Case of myasthenia gravis preceded by viral encephalitis in a 13-year-old girl. Neurol. Neurochir. Pol., 15:345, 1981.

60. Nakao, Y., Matsumoto, H., Miyazaki, T., Nishitani, H., Ota, K., Fujita, T., and Tsuji, K.: Gm allotypes in myasthenia gravis. Lancet, 1:677, 1980.

61. Nazarian, J., and O'Leary, D.: Corneal sensitivity in myasthenia gravis. Br. J. Ophthalmol., 69:519, 1985.

62. Niakan, E., Harati, Y., and Rolak, L.A.: Arch. Neurol., 43:155, 1986.

63. Nicholson, G.A., McLeod, J.G., and Griffiths, L.R.: Comparison of diagnostic tests in myasthenia gravis. Clin. Exp. Neurol., 19:45, 1983.

64. Noroian, E.L.: Myasthenia gravis: a nursing perspective. J. Neurosci. Nurs., 18:74, 1986.

65. Olanow, C.W., Lane, R.J., Hull, K.L., Jr., and Roses, A.D.: Neonatal myasthenia gravis in the infant of an asymptomatic thymectomized mother. Can. J. Neurol. Sci., 9:85, 1982.

66. Oosterhuis, H.J., Ritsma, R.J., and Horst, J.W.: Failure of stapedius reflexometry in the diagnosis of myasthenia gravis (Letter). Ann. Neurol., 18:519, 1985.

67. Osserman, K.E.: Myasthenia Gravis. New York, Grune & Stratton, 1958.

68. Palencia, R., Hermoso, F., Blanco, A., and Sanchez Villares, E.: Congenital and hereditary myasthenia. Eur. J. Pediatr., 138:349, 1982.

69. Pascuzzi, R.M., Sermas, A., Phillips, L.H., II, and Johns, T.R.: Familial autoimmune myasthenia gravis and thymoma: occurrence in two brothers. Neurology, 36:423, 1986.

70. Pasternak, J.F., Hageman, J., Adams, M.A., Philip, A.G., and Gardner, T.H.: Exchange transfusion in neonatal myasthenia. J. Pediatr., 99:644, 1981.

71. Penn, A.S., Jaretzki, A., III, Wolff, M., Chang, H.W., and Tennyson, V.: Thymic abnormalities: antigen or antibody? Response to thymectomy in myasthenia gravis. Ann. N.Y. Acad. Sci., 377:786, 1981.

72. Pritchard, E.A.B.: "Prostigmin" in the treatment of myasthenia gravis. Lancet, 1:432, 1935.

73. Rauch, H.C., Montgomery, I.N., and Kaplan, J.: Natural killer cell activity in multiple sclerosis and myasthenia gravis. Immunol. Invest., 14:427, 1985.

74. Richman, D.P.: Treatment of myasthenia gravis (Editorial). J. Neurol., 232:202, 1985.

75. Robertson, W.C., Chun, R.W., and Kornguth, S.E.: Familial infantile myasthenia. Arch. Neurol., 37:117, 1980.

76. Robinson, C.L.: The role of surgery of the thymus for myasthenia gravis. Ann. R. Coll. Surg. Engl., 65:145, 1983.
77. Rodriguez, M., Gomez, M.R., Howard, F.M., Jr., and Taylor, W.F.: Myasthenia gravis in children: long-term follow-up. Ann. Neurol., 13:504, 1983.
78. Rowland, L.P.: Fatalities in myasthenia gravis. J. Am. Neurol. Assoc., 78:158, 1953.
79. Rowland, L.P.: Prostigmin responsiveness in the diagnosis of myasthenia gravis. Neurology, 5:612, 1955.
80. Rowland, L.P., and Eskenzai, A.M.: Myasthenia gravis with features resembling muscular dystrophy. Neurology, 6:667, 1956.
81. Rubin, J.W., Ellison, R.G., Moore, H.V., and Pai, G.P.: Factors affecting response to thymectomy for myasthenia gravis. J. Thorac. Cardiovasc. Surg., 82:720, 1981.
82. Scoppetta, C., Casali, C., and Piantelli, M.: Congenita myasthenia gravis (Letter). Muscle Nerve, 5:493, 1982.
83. Secher, N.H., and Petersen, S.: Fatigue of voluntary contractions in normal and myasthenic human subjects. Acta Physiol. Scand., 122:243, 1984.
84. Seybold, M.E.: The office Tensilon test for ocular myasthenia gravis. Arch. Neurol., 43:842, 1986.
85. Simpson, J.A.: Myasthenia gravis and myasthenic syndromes. *In* Walton, J.A. (ed.): Disorders of Voluntary Muscle. New York, Churchill Livingstone, 1981.
86. Seybold, M.E., and Lindstrom, J.M.: Myasthenia gravis in infancy. Neurology, 31:476, 1981.
87. Snead, O.C., III, Benton, J.W., Dwyer, D., Morley, B.J., Kemp, G.E., Bradley, R.J., and Oh, S.J.: Juvenile myasthenia gravis. Neurology, 30:732, 1980.
88. Spence, P.A., Morin, J.E., and Katz, M.: Role of plasmapheresis in preparing myasthenic patients for thymectomy: initial results. Can. J. Surg., 27:303, 1984.
89. Stortebecker, T.P.: Signs of myositis in myasthenia gravis and in myopathy clinically resembling progressive muscular dystrophy. Acta Med. Scand., 151:451, 1955.
90. Strickroot, F.L., Schaeffer, R.L., and Bergs, H.L.: Myasthenia gravis occurring in an infant born of a myasthenic mother. J.A.M.A., 120:1207, 1942.
91. Teng, P., and Osserman, K.E.: Studies in myasthenia gravis: Neonatal and juvenile types. A report of 21 and a review of 188 cases. J. Mt. Sinai Hosp., 23:711, 1956.
92. Tindall, R.S.: Diagnosis and treatment of myasthenia gravis. Compr. Ther., 7:33, 1981.
93. Tindall, R.S., Rollins, J.A., Phillips, T., Green, R.G., Wells, L., and Blendiuk, G.: Preliminary results of a double-blind, randomized, placebo-controlled trial of cyclosporine in myasthenia gravis. N. Engl. J. Med., 316:719, 1987.
94. Viets, H.R.: A historical review of myasthenia gravis from 1672 to 1900. J.A.M.A., 153:1273, 1953.
95. Viets, H.R., and Brown, M.R.: Medical progress: Diseases of muscles. N. Engl. J. Med., 245:647, 1951.
96. Viets, H.R., and Schwab, R.S.: Prostigmin in the diagnosis of myasthenia gravis. N. Engl. J. Med., 213:1280, 1935.
97. Vincent, A., and Newsom Davis, J.: Acetylcholine receptor antibody as a diagnostic test for myasthenia gravis: results in 153 validated cases and 2967 diagnostic assays. J. Neurol. Neurosurg. Psychiatry, 48:1246, 1985.
98. Walker, M.B.: Treatment of myasthenia gravis with prostigmin. Lancet, 1:1200, 1934.
99. Walker, M.B.: Case showing effect of prostigmin on myasthenia gravis. Proc. R. Soc. Med., 28:759, 1935.
100. Westerberg, M.R., and MaGee, K.R.: Treatment review: Myasthenia gravis. Neurology, 5:728, 1955.
101. Willis, T.: De anima brutorum. Oxford: Theatro Sheldoniano, 1672, pp. 404–406.
102. Wilkes, S.: On cerebritis, hysteria, and bulbar paralysis as illustrative of arrest of function of the cerebrospinal centers. Guys Hosp. Rep., 22:7, 1877.
103. Wyllie, W.G., Bodian, M., and Burrows, N.F.E.: Myasthenia gravis in children. Arch. Dis. Child., 26:457, 1951.
104. Youssef, S.: Thymectomy for myasthenia gravis in children. J. Pediatr. Surg., 18:537, 1983.

Affections of Bursae

Bursae are thin-walled sacs lined by synovial membrane that are usually located about joints and serve to decrease friction. Some of them communicate with the articular cavity. The synovial membranes of bursae are subject to the same pathologic processes that affect the synovial membranes of joints. Adventitious bursae develop secondarily from friction, as occurs in a bunion over the first metatarsal head.

BURSITIS[1–28]

Bursitis may be traumatic, suppurative, tuberculous, gouty, or rheumatoid. Various tumorous processes, such as villonodular synovitis, osteochondromatosis, or synovioma, may involve the bursae. Nonspecific bursitis secondary to calcified tendinitis does not occur in children.

Traumatic Bursitis

Injury usually affects bursae that are superficial in location, such as those over the olecranon or over the patella. The onset of symptoms is sudden following a direct injury such as a fall on the knee. There is distention of the bursa with hemorrhage, local pain, tenderness, and restriction of motion in the adjacent joint. If the bursa is deep in relation to tendons, pain on motion is the principal symptom, with protective muscle spasm restricting the motion. If the bursa is subcutaneous, tenderness to pressure is the salient finding.

Traumatic bursitis may be associated with ligamentous injury of neighboring joints. Radiograms should be taken to rule out fracture of adjacent bones. Treatment consists of aspiration of the fluid, compression bandage, and rest to the part in a splint or sling. If the condition is very acute, hot packs may be applied intermittently to enhance absorption. Local injection of hydrocortisone is usually not indicated. In "adventitious" bursitis the underlying cause must be determined and, if possible, corrected, for instance, by improving the fit of the shoe or orthosis that is causing undue irritation, by using protective pads, or by excising the subadjacent bony protuberance.

Chronic bursitis may follow an acute process but frequently develops insidiously. It occurs in children very occasionally; in the adult, however, chronic bursitis is a common disease, occurring in several specific and familiar locations, such as subdeltoid bursitis, olecranon bursitis, prepatellar bursitis (housemaid's knee), ischial bursitis (weaver's or tailor's bottom), iliopectineal bursitis, and pes anserinus bursitis. It is beyond the scope of this textbook to discuss calcareous tendinitis.

Infectious or Suppurative Bursitis

This is common in the superficial bursae, such as the prepatellar and olecranon bursae. It commonly occurs in children. Pyogenic organisms are implanted within the bursal sac as a result of direct inoculation from a penetrating wound or by hematogenous metastatic spread. Local pain and tenderness on direct pressure and marked swelling of the affected bursa are the outstanding findings. There may be systemic signs of infection. The condition should be distinguished from pyogenic arthritis of a subjacent joint.

The exudate from the swollen bursa is aspirated and the pathogenic organism and sensitivity to antibiotics are determined by culture studies. (During aspiration of the bursa, care should be taken not to contaminate the subjacent joint.) Systemic antibiotics are administered. Antibiotics may be injected locally. The affected part of the limb is splinted, and hot packs are applied. Often, incision and drainage are necessary. If the process becomes chronic, excision of the bursa may be indicated.

References

1. Abeles, M.: Anserine bursitis (Letter). Arthritis Rheum., 29:812, 1986.
2. Alario, A.J., Su, E.Y., and Ho, G., Jr.: Septic prepatellar bursitis in a child. R.I. Med. J., 65:279, 1982.
3. Broderick, A., Perlman, S., and Dietz, F.: Pseudomonas bursitis: inoculation from a catfish. Pediatr. Infect. Dis., 4:693, 1985.
4. Canoso, J.J.: Idiopathic or traumatic olecranon bursitis. Clinical features and bursal fluid analysis. Arthritis Rheum., 20:1213, 1977.
5. Canoso, J.J., and Scheckman, P.R.: Septic subcutaneous bursitis: Report of sixteen cases. J. Rheumatol., 6:96, 1979.
6. Child, D.L., Sturrock, R.G., and Lawrie, J.H.: Massive prepatellar bursitis. J. R. Coll. Surg. Edinb., 26:101, 1981.
7. Ege-Rasmussen, K.J., and Fan, N.: Trochanteric bursitis. Treatment by corticosteroid injection. Scand. J. Rheumatol., 14:417, 1985.
8. Esposito, L.: Calcifying traumatic bursitis. Arch. Putti Chir. Organi Mov., 28:97, 1977.
9. Fisher, R.H.: Conservative treatment of distended patellar and olecranon bursae. Clin. Orthop., 123:98, 1977.
10. Heneghan, M.A., and Wallace, T.: Heel pain due to retrocalcaneal bursitis—radiographic diagnosis (with a historical footnote on Sever's disease). Pediatr. Radiol., 15:119, 1985.
11. Ho, G., Jr., and Su, E.Y.: Antibiotic therapy of septic bursitis. Its implications in the treatment of septic arthritis. Arthritis Rheum., 24:905, 1981.
12. Ho, G., Jr., and Tice, A.D.: Comparison of nonseptic and septic bursitis. Arch. Intern. Med., 139:1269, 1979.
13. Ho, G., Jr., Tice, A.D., and Kaplan, S.R.: Septic bursitis in the prepatellar and olecranon bursae: an analysis of 25 cases. Ann. Intern. Med., 89:21, 1978.
14. Holder, S.F., et al.: Tuberculous arthritis of the elbow presenting as chronic bursitis of the olecranon. A case report. J. Bone Joint Surg., 67-A:1127, 1985.
15. Larsen, R.L., and Osternig, L.R.: Traumatic bursitis and artificial turf. J. Sports Med., 2:183, 1974.
16. Marchildon, A., Slonim, R.R., Brown, H.E., and Howell, D.S.: Primary septic bursitis. Fla. Med. Assoc. J., 50:139, 1963.
17. Meyers, S., Lonon, W., and Shannon, K.: Suppurative bursitis in early childhood. Pediatr. Infect. Dis., 3:156, 1984.
18. Nardella, F.A.: Blood patch treatment for prepatellar bursitis (housemaid's knee) (Letter). N. Engl. J. Med., 306:1553, 1982.
19. Paisley, J.W.: Septic bursitis in childhood. J. Pediatr. Orthop., 2:57, 1982.
20. Pavlov, H., Heneghan, M.A., Hersh, A., Goldman, A.B., and Vigorita, V.: The Haglund syndrome: initial and differential diagnosis. Radiology, 144:83, 1982.
21. Pravda, V.A.: Antescapular bursitis in children. Vestn. Khir., 125:97, 1980.
22. Quayle, J.B.: A useful procedure in the treatment of chronic olecranon bursitis. Injury, 9:299, 1978.
23. Quayle, J.B., et al.: An operation for chronic prepatellar bursitis. J. Bone Joint Surg., 58-B:504, 1976.
24. Sartorius, D.J., Danzig, L., Gilula, L., Greenway, G., and Resnick, D.: Synovial cysts of the hip joint and iliopsoas bursitis: a spectrum of imaging abnormalities. Skeletal Radiol., 14:85, 1985.
25. Thompson, G.R., Manshady, B.M., and Weiss, J.J.: Septic bursitis. J.A.M.A., 240:2280, 1978.
26. Tollerud, D.J., Albano, L., and Bia, F.J.: Anaerobic septic bursitis (Letter). Ann. Intern. Med., 91:494, 1979.
27. Viggiano, D.A., et al.: Septic arthritis presenting as olecranon bursitis in patients with rheumatoid arthritis. A report of three cases. J. Bone Joint Surg., 62-A:1011, 1980.
28. Winter, F.E., and Runyon, E.H.: Prepatellar bursitis caused by Mycobacterium marinum. J. Bone Joint Surg., 47:375, 1965.

Appendix

Anterior Transfer of Peroneus Longus Tendon to Base
of Second Metatarsal

OPERATIVE TECHNIQUE

The patient is placed in semilateral position with a sandbag under the hip on the affected side.

A. A 3 to 4 cm. long incision is made over the lateral aspect of the foot, extending from the base of the fifth metatarsal to a point 1 cm. distal to the tip of the lateral malleolus. Subcutaneous tissue is divided, and the tendons of the peroneus longus and brevis are exposed. Then a second incision is made over the fibular aspect of the leg; it begins 3 cm. above the lateral malleolus and extends proximally for a distance of 7 cm. Subcutaneous tissue and deep fascia are incised, and the peroneal tendons are exposed by dividing their sheath. The peroneus longus tendon lies superficial to that of the peroneus brevis. The muscle is inspected to ensure that it is of normal gross appearance.

B. Next, the peroneus brevis muscle is detached from the base of the fifth metatarsal and a whip suture is inserted into its distal end.

C and **D.** The peroneus longus tendon is divided as far distally as possible. The peroneus brevis is sutured to the distal stump of the peroneus longus to preserve the longitudinal arch and depression of the first metatarsal.

Plate A. Anterior Transfer of Peroneus Longus Tendon to Base of Second Metatarsal

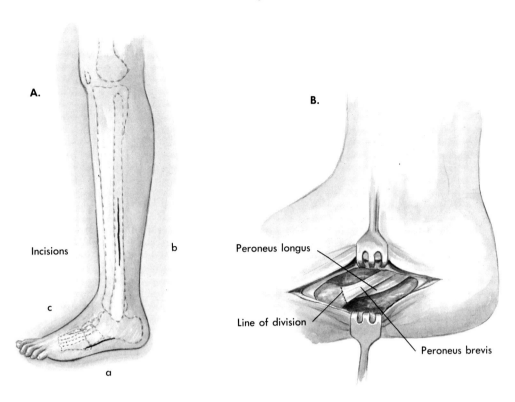

A.

Incisions

b

c

a

B.

Peroneus longus

Line of division

Peroneus brevis

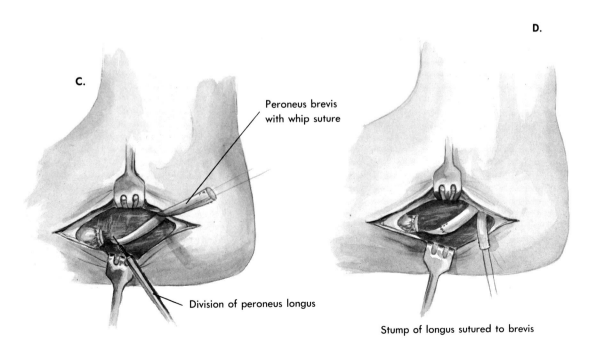

D.

C.

Peroneus brevis
with whip suture

Division of peroneus longus

Stump of longus sutured to brevis

2182C

Anterior Transfer of Peroneus Longus Tendon to Base of Second Metatarsal *(Continued)*

E and **F.** The peroneus longus tendon is mobilized, and with the two-hand technique, it is gently pulled into the proximal wound in the leg. The origin of the peroneus brevis from the fibula should not be disrupted. An adequate opening is made in the intermuscular septum, taking care not to injure neurovascular structures.

G and **H.** A 2 to 3 cm. long longitudinal incision is made over the dorsum of the foot, centering over the base of the second metatarsal bone. The deep fascia is divided, and the extensor tendons are retracted to expose the proximal one fourth of the second metatarsal bone. The periosteum is divided longitudinally and the cortex of the recipient bone is exposed.

With an Ober tendon passer, the peroneus longus tendon along with its sheath is passed into the anterior tibial compartment, deep to the cruciate crural and tarsal ligaments, and delivered into the incision on the dorsum of the foot. The author does not recommend a subcutaneous route. It should be ensured that there is a direct line of pull of the peroneus longus tendon from its origin to its insertion.

I and **J.** A drill hole is made in the base of the second metatarsal. A star-head hand drill is used to enlarge the hole to receive the tendon adequately. The peroneus longus tendon is passed through the recipient hole and sutured on itself under correct tension. If the peroneus longus tendon is not of adequate length, two small holes are made 1.5 cm. distal to the large hole at each side of the metatarsal shaft. The silk sutures at the end of the tendon are passed from the large central hole to the lateral distal small holes and the tendon is securely sutured to the bone. The ankle joint should be in neutral position or 5 degrees of dorsiflexion. The pneumatic tourniquet is released and hemostasis is obtained. The wounds are closed in routine manner. A long leg cast is applied with the ankle in 5 degrees of dorsiflexion and the knee in 45 degrees of flexion. Postoperative care follows the guidelines outlined in the section on principles of tendon transfer.

Plate A. Anterior Transfer of Peroneus Longus Tendon to Base of Second Metatarsal

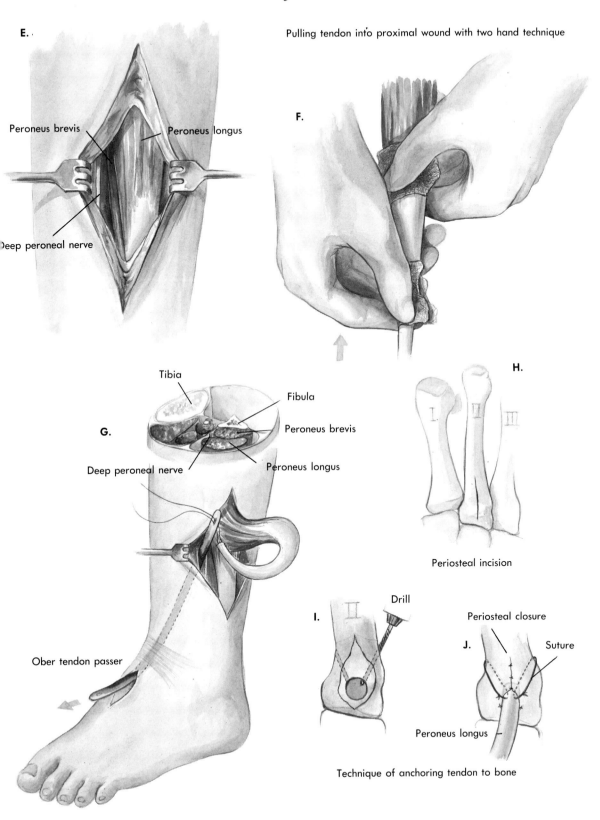

E.

Peroneus brevis

Peroneus longus

Deep peroneal nerve

Pulling tendon into proximal wound with two hand technique

F.

Tibia

G.

Fibula

Peroneus brevis

Deep peroneal nerve

Peroneus longus

Ober tendon passer

H.

Periosteal incision

Drill

I.

J. Periosteal closure

Suture

Peroneus longus

Technique of anchoring tendon to bone

2182E

Anterior Transfer of Posterior Tibial Tendon Through Interosseous Membrane

OPERATIVE TECHNIQUE

A. A 4 cm. long incision is made over the medial aspect of the foot, beginning posterior and immediately distal to the tip of the medial malleolus and extending to the base of the first cuneiform bone. A second longitudinal incision is made 1.5 cm. posterior to the subcutaneous medial border of the tibia, beginning at the center of the middle third of the leg and ending 3 cm. from the tip of the medial malleolus.

B. The posterior tibial tendon is identified at its insertion and its sheath is divided. The tendon is freed and sectioned at its attachment to the bone, preserving maximal length. The peritenon of the distal 3 cm. of the tendon is excised, and a 00 silk whip suture is inserted in its distal end.

C. The posterior tibial muscle is identified in the leg incision and its sheath opened and freed. Traction on the stump in the foot incision will aid in its identification. Moist sponges and the two-hand technique are used to deliver the posterior tibial tendon into the proximal wound. The muscle belly is freed well up the tibia. One should be careful to preserve the nerve and blood supply to the posterior tibial muscle.

D. Next, a longitudinal skin incision is made anteriorly, one fingerbreadth lateral to the crest of the tibia, starting at the proximal margin of the cruciate ligament of the ankle and extending 7 cm. proximally. Then a 4 cm. long longitudinal incision is made over the dorsum of the foot, centering over the base of the second metatarsal.

Plate B. Anterior Transfer of Posterior Tibial Tendon Through Interosseous Membrane

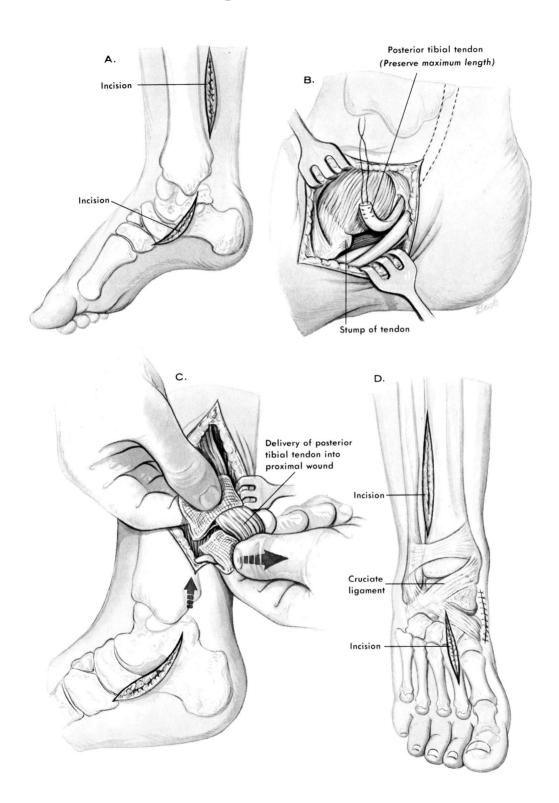

A.

Incision

Incision

B.

Posterior tibial tendon
(Preserve maximum length)

Stump of tendon

C.

Delivery of posterior
tibial tendon into
proximal wound

D.

Incision

Cruciate
ligament

Incision

Anterior Transfer of Posterior Tibial Tendon Through Interosseous Membrane (Continued)

E. The anterior tibial muscle is exposed and elevated from the anterolateral surface of the tibia together with the anterior tibial artery and extensor hallucis longus muscle. It is retracted laterally, exposing the interosseous membrane. Next, a large rectangular window is cut in the interosseous membrane. One should avoid stripping the periosteum from the tibia or fibula.

F and **G.** Then, with an Ober tendon passer, the posterior tibial tendon is passed through the window in the interosseous membrane from the posterior into the anterior tibial compartment. One should be careful not to twist the tendon or to damage its nerve or blood supply. Next, with the aid of an Ober tendon passer, the posterior tibial tendon is passed beneath the cruciate ligament and the extensors and delivered into the wound on the dorsum of the foot. It is anchored to the base of the second metatarsal bone according to the method described in anterior transfer of peroneal tendons (see Plate A). The wounds are closed in layers in the usual manner. A long leg cast is applied, holding the foot in neutral position at the ankle joint and the knee in 45 degrees of flexion.

The principles of postoperative care are the same as for any tendon transfer.

Plate B. Anterior Transfer of Posterior Tibial Tendon Through Interosseous Membrane

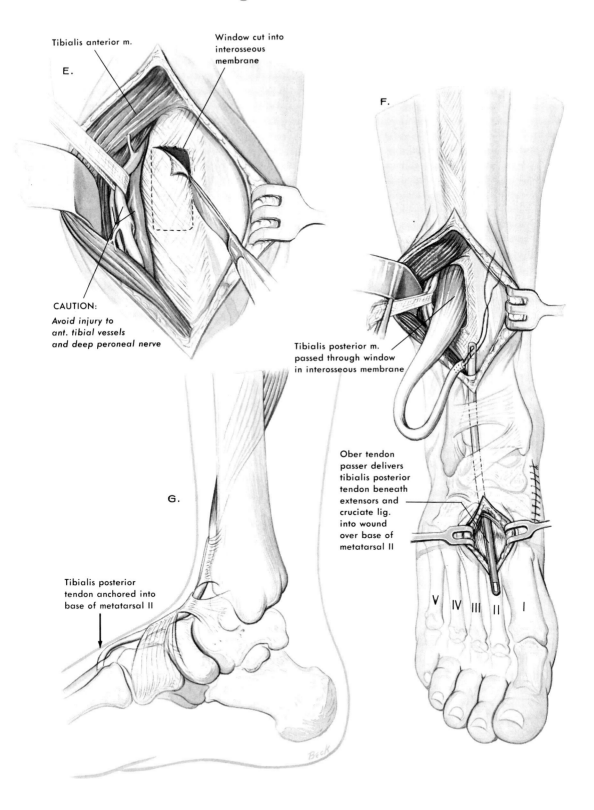

E.

Tibialis anterior m.

Window cut into interosseous membrane

CAUTION:
Avoid injury to ant. tibial vessels and deep peroneal nerve

F.

Tibialis posterior m. passed through window in interosseous membrane

G.

Tibialis posterior tendon anchored into base of metatarsal II

Ober tendon passer delivers tibialis posterior tendon beneath extensors and cruciate lig. into wound over base of metatarsal II

V IV III II I

Beck

Triple Arthrodesis

OPERATIVE TECHNIQUE

A pneumatic tourniquet is placed on the proximal thigh, and the patient is positioned semilaterally with a large sandbag under the hip on the affected side.

A. A curvilinear incision is made, centering over the sinus tarsi. It starts one finger-breadth distal and posterior to the tip of the lateral malleolus and extends anteriorly and distally to the base of the second metatarsal bone.

B. Skin flaps should not be developed. The incision is carried to the floor of the sinus tarsi. By sharp dissection, with scalpel and periosteal elevator, the periosteum of the calcaneus, the adipose tissue contents of the sinus tarsi, and the tendinous origin of the exterior digitorum brevis are elevated in one mass from the calcaneus and lateral aspect of the neck of the talus and retracted distally. It is essential to provide a viable soft-tissue pedicle to obliterate the dead space remaining at the end of the operation.

Next, an incision is made superiorly over the periosteum of the talus, and the head and neck of the talus are carefully exposed. The upper flap of the skin, subcutaneous tissue, and periosteum should be kept as thick as possible to avoid necrosis. Traction sutures are placed on the periosteum. At no time are the skin edges to be retracted. It is not necessary to divide the peroneal tendons or their sheaths. By subperiosteal dissection, the peroneal tendons are retracted posteriorly for exposure of the subtalar joint.

C and D. The capsules of the calcaneocuboid, talonavicular, and subtalar joints are incised. These joints are opened and their cartilaginous surfaces clearly visualized by turning the foot into varus position. A laminar spreader placed in the sinus tarsi will aid in exposure of the posterior subtalar joint. Before excision of articular cartilaginous surfaces, one should review the deformity of the foot and decide on the wedges of bone to be removed to correct the deformity. Circulation of the talus and the complications of avascular necrosis of the talus and arthritis of the ankle following triple arthrodesis should always be kept in mind. The height of the foot is another consideration. A low lateral malleolus will cause difficulty with wearing shoes. At times, it is best to add a bone graft rather than resect wedges of bone. With a sharp osteotome, the cartilaginous surfaces of the calcaneocuboid joint are excised. Next, the articular cartilage surface of the talonavicular joint is exposed, the plane of osteotomy being perpendicular to the long axis of the neck of the talus and parallel to the calcaneocuboid joint. When the beak of the navicular is unduly prominent medially, or when, in a varus foot, one cannot obtain adequate exposure of the talonavicular joint without excessive retraction, a second dorsomedial incision may be used to expose the talonavicular joint.

Plate C. Triple Arthrodesis

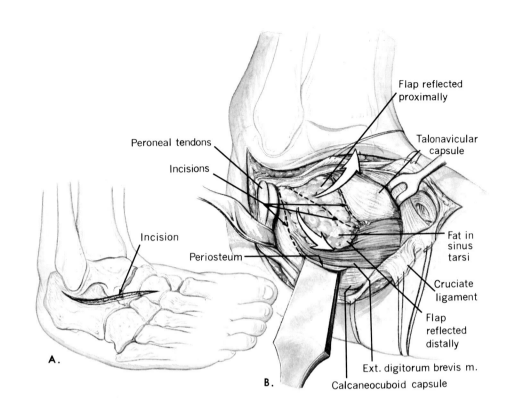

Flap reflected proximally

Talonavicular capsule

Peroneal tendons

Incisions

Incision

Periosteum

Fat in sinus tarsi

Cruciate ligament

Flap reflected distally

Ext. digitorum brevis m.

Calcaneocuboid capsule

A.

B.

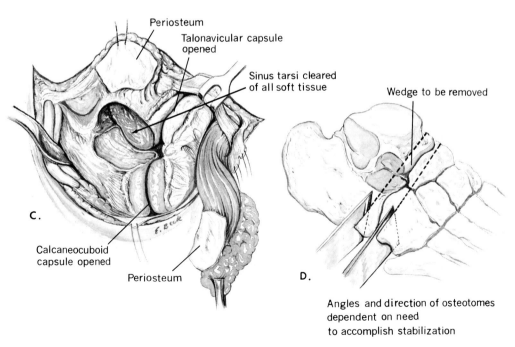

Periosteum

Talonavicular capsule opened

Sinus tarsi cleared of all soft tissue

Wedge to be removed

C.

Calcaneocuboid capsule opened

Periosteum

D.

Angles and direction of osteotomes dependent on need to accomplish stabilization

Triple Arthrodesis (Continued)

E to H. With a laminar spreader in the sinus tarsi, the subtalar joint is widely exposed and the cartilage of the anterior and posterior joints is excised. One should keep in mind the neurovascular structures behind the medial malleolus. The wedges of bone that must be removed to correct the deformity are excised in one mass with the articular cartilage. It is of great help to leave the osteotome used on the opposing articular surface in place and held steady by the assistant as a second osteotome or gouge is used to take contiguous cartilage and bone. The divided articular surfaces of the joints to be arthrodesed are "fish-scaled" for maximum raw cancellous bony contact.

The skin is closed with interrupted sutures. A well-molded long leg cast is applied, holding the foot in the desired position. The author has not found necessary and does not recommend fixation of the joints by staples. In foot stabilization in children with cerebral palsy, especially in the severely athetoid or spastic, secure criss-cross Kirschner wires are used to maintain position. These are removed in six to eight weeks.

Plate C. Triple Arthrodesis

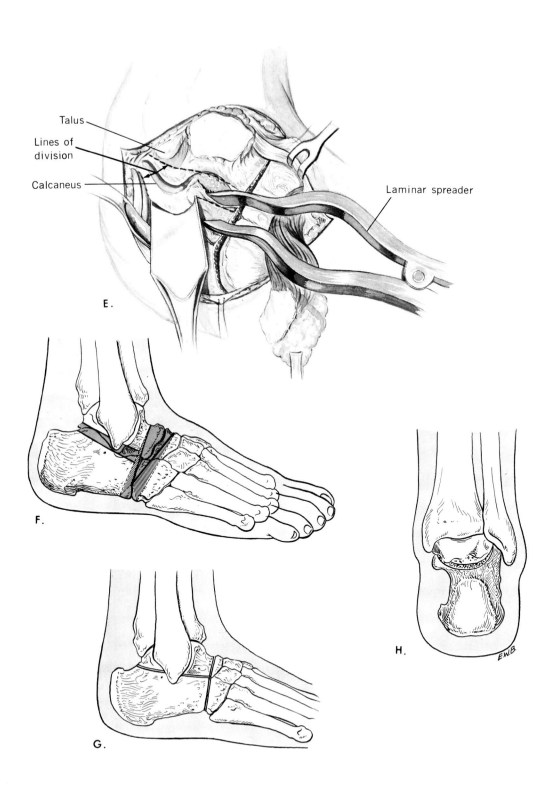

Talus

Lines of
division

Calcaneus

Laminar spreader

E.

F.

G.

H.

E.W.B.

Arthrodesis of Ankle Joint Through Anterior Approach Without Disturbing Distal Tibial Growth Plate

OPERATIVE TECHNIQUE

A and **B.** A longitudinal skin incision is made, beginning 7 cm. proximal to the ankle joint between the extensor digitorum longus and extensor hallucis longus tendons; it extends distally across the ankle joint in line with the third metatarsal and ends 4 cm. distal to the ankle joint.

The subcutaneous tissue is divided, and the skin flaps are mobilized and retracted to their respective sides. The veins crossing the field are clamped, divided, and coagulated. The intermediate and medial dorsal cutaneous branches of the superficial peroneal nerve are identified and protected by retraction to one side of the wound.

C. The deep fascia and transverse crural and cruciate crural ligaments are divided in line with the skin incision. The ligaments are marked with 00 silk suture for accurate closure later.

Plate D. Arthrodesis of Ankle Joint Through Anterior Approach Without Disturbing Distal Tibial Growth Plate

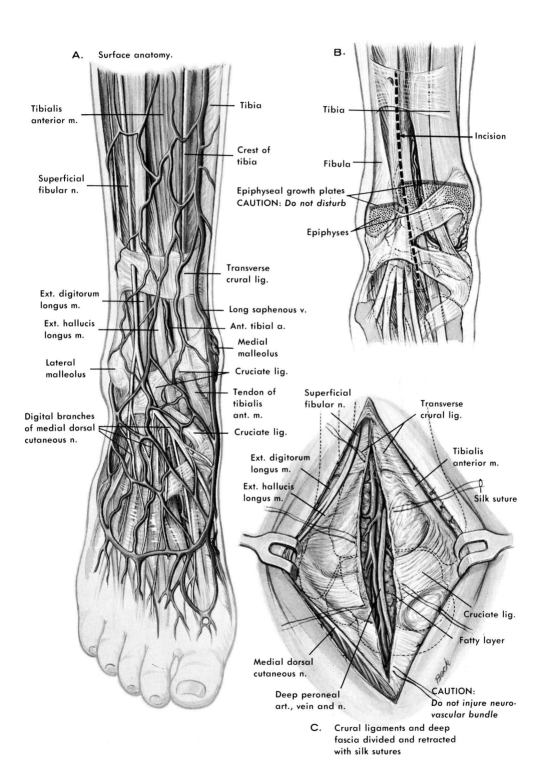

A. Surface anatomy.

Tibialis anterior m.

Tibia

Superficial fibular n.

Crest of tibia

Ext. digitorum longus m.

Transverse crural lig.

Ext. hallucis longus m.

Long saphenous v.

Ant. tibial a.

Lateral malleolus

Medial malleolus

Cruciate lig.

Digital branches of medial dorsal cutaneous n.

Tendon of tibialis ant. m.

Cruciate lig.

B.

Tibia

Incision

Fibula

Epiphyseal growth plates CAUTION: *Do not disturb*

Epiphyses

Superficial fibular n.

Transverse crural lig.

Ext. digitorum longus m.

Tibialis anterior m.

Ext. hallucis longus m.

Silk suture

Cruciate lig.

Fatty layer

Medial dorsal cutaneous n.

Deep peroneal art., vein and n.

CAUTION: *Do not injure neuro-vascular bundle*

C. Crural ligaments and deep fascia divided and retracted with silk sutures

2182O

Arthrodesis of Ankle Joint Through Anterior Approach
Without Disturbing Distal Tibial Growth Plate (Continued)

D. The neurovascular bundle (deep peroneal nerve, anterior tibial–dorsalis pedis vessels) is identified, isolated, and retracted laterally with the extensor hallucis longus, extensor digitorum longus, and peroneus tertius tendons. The anterolateral malleolar and lateral tarsal arteries are isolated, clamped, divided, and ligated. The distal tibia, ankle joint, and talus are identified. A transverse incision is made in the capsule of the talotibial joint from the posterior tip of the medial malleolus to the lateral malleolus. The edges of the capsule are marked with 00 silk suture for meticulous closure later.

E to G. The capsule is reflected and retracted distally on the talus and proximally on the tibia. The periosteum of the tibia should not be divided. The distal tibial and fibular epiphyseal plates should not be disturbed in growing children. With thin curved and straight osteotomes, the cartilage and subchondral bone are removed from the opposing articular surfaces of the distal tibia and proximal talus down to raw bleeding cancellous bone. Cartilage chips should not be left posteriorly.

H. Next, a large piece of bone for grafting is taken from the ilium and fashioned to fit snugly in the ankle joint. The graft should have both cortices intact and should be thicker at one end and wedge-shaped. The cortices of the graft are perforated with multiple tiny drill holes. The ankle joint is held in the desired position, and the bone graft is firmly fitted into the joint with an impacter. If any space is left on each side of the graft, it is packed with cancellous bone from the ilium. The graft in the ankle joint gives compressional force to the arthrodesis and adds to the height of the foot and ankle. The capsule of the ankle joint and the transverse crural and cruciate crural ligaments are closed carefully in layers. The deep fascia and the wound are closed in the usual manner. Radiograms are obtained in anteroposterior and lateral views to ensure that the ankle joint is in the desired position.

I. A long leg cast is applied with the ankle joint in the desired position of plantar flexion (boys, 10 degrees; girls, 15 to 20 degrees) and the knee in 45 degrees of flexion.

POSTOPERATIVE CARE

Periodic radiograms are obtained to determine the position of the graft and the extent of healing. Eight to ten weeks after surgery, the solid cast is removed and radiograms are obtained with the cast off. Ordinarily, by this time, the fusion is solid and the patient is gradually allowed to be ambulatory. Full weight-bearing is begun two to three weeks later.

Plate D. Arthrodesis of Ankle Joint Through Anterior Approach Without Disturbing Distal Tibial Growth Plate

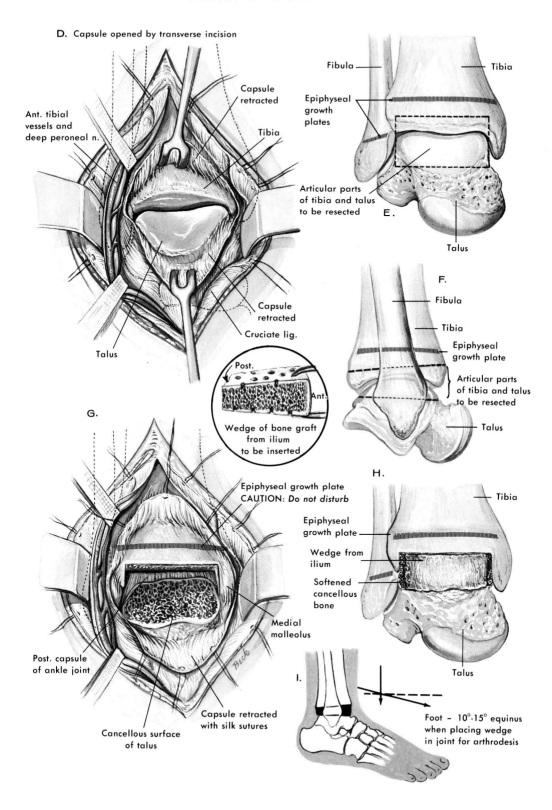

D. Capsule opened by transverse incision

Capsule retracted

Ant. tibial vessels and deep peroneal n.

Tibia

Capsule retracted

Cruciate lig.

Talus

Fibula

Tibia

Epiphyseal growth plates

Articular parts of tibia and talus to be resected

E.

Talus

F.

Fibula

Tibia

Epiphyseal growth plate

Articular parts of tibia and talus to be resected

Talus

Post.

Ant.

Wedge of bone graft from ilium to be inserted

G.

Epiphyseal growth plate CAUTION: *Do not disturb*

Epiphyseal growth plate

Wedge from ilium

Softened cancellous bone

H.

Tibia

Medial malleolus

Post. capsule of ankle joint

Cancellous surface of talus

Capsule retracted with silk sutures

Talus

I.

Foot – 10°-15° equinus when placing wedge in joint for arthrodesis

2182Q

Flexorplasty of the Elbow (Steindler)

OPERATIVE TECHNIQUE

A. With the elbow in extension, a curved longitudinal incision is made over the anteromedial side of the elbow, beginning approximately 3 inches above the flexion crease of the elbow joint over the medial intermuscular septum and extending distally to the anterior aspect of the medial epicondyle. At the joint level it turns anterolaterally on the volar surface of the forearm along the course of the pronator teres muscle for a distance of approximately 2½ inches.

B. The subcutaneous tissue and fascia are divided in line with the skin incision, and the skin flaps are widely mobilized and retracted. Next, the ulnar nerve is located posterior to the medial intermuscular septum and lying in a groove on the triceps muscle. It is isolated, and a moist hernia tape is passed around it for gentle handling. The ulnar nerve is traced distally to its groove between the posterior aspect of the medial epicondyle of the humerus and the olecranon process. The fascial roof over the ulnar nerve is carefully divided under direct vision over a grooved director.

C. The ulnar nerve is dissected free distally to the point where it passes between the two heads of the flexor carpi ulnaris muscle. Inadvertent damage to the branches of the ulnar nerve to the flexor carpi ulnaris muscle should be avoided. A second hernia tape is passed around the ulnar nerve in the distal part of the wound, and the nerve is retracted posteriorly.

Plate E. Flexorplasty of the Elbow (Steindler)

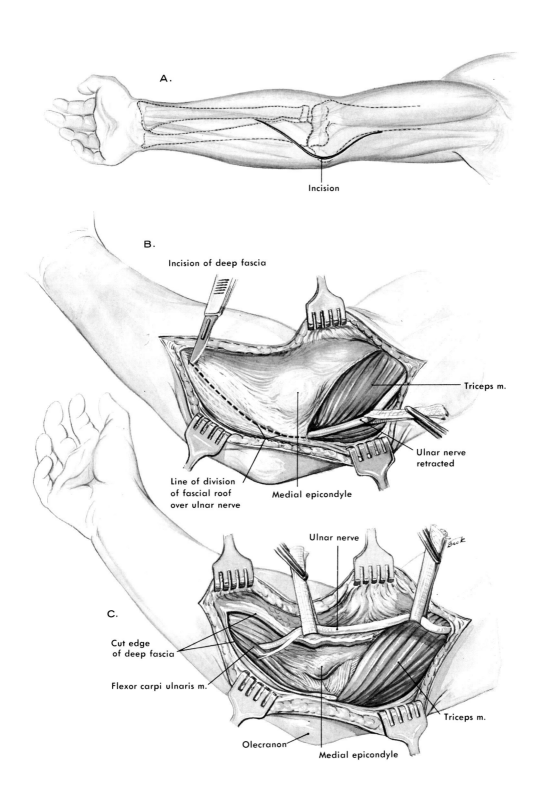

A.

Incision

B.

Incision of deep fascia

Triceps m.

Ulnar nerve retracted

Line of division of fascial roof over ulnar nerve

Medial epicondyle

C.

Ulnar nerve

Cut edge of deep fascia

Flexor carpi ulnaris m.

Triceps m.

Olecranon

Medial epicondyle

Flexorplasty of the Elbow (Steindler) (Continued)

D. Next, the biceps tendon is identified over the anterior aspect of the elbow joint. The deep fascia and the lacertus fibrosus are divided along the medial aspect of the biceps tendon.

E. By digital palpation, the interval between the biceps and pronator teres muscle is developed. The brachial artery with its accompanying veins runs along the medial side of the biceps tendon. The median nerve, lying medial to the brachial artery, is dissected free of the surrounding tissues and gently retracted anteriorly with a moist hernia tape. The branches of the median nerve to the pronator teres muscle must be identified and protected from injury.

F. Next, with an osteotome, the common flexor origin of the pronator teres, flexor carpi radialis, palmaris longus, flexor digitorum sublimis, and flexor carpi ulnaris is detached en bloc with a flake of bone from the medial epicondyle.

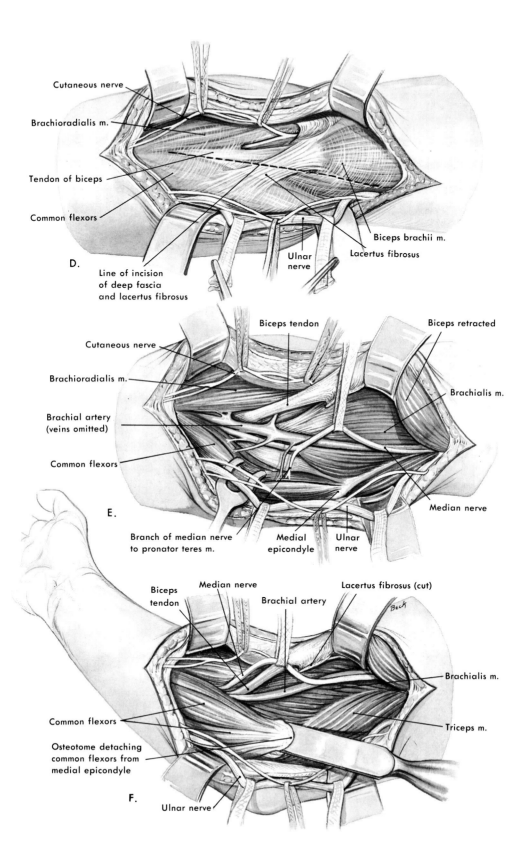

D.

Cutaneous nerve

Brachioradialis m.

Tendon of biceps

Common flexors

Line of incision
of deep fascia
and lacertus fibrosus

Ulnar nerve

Lacertus fibrosus

Biceps brachii m.

E.

Cutaneous nerve

Brachioradialis m.

Brachial artery
(veins omitted)

Common flexors

Biceps tendon

Biceps retracted

Brachialis m.

Median nerve

Branch of median nerve
to pronator teres m.

Medial epicondyle

Ulnar nerve

F.

Biceps tendon

Median nerve

Brachial artery

Lacertus fibrosus (cut)

Beck

Brachialis m.

Triceps m.

Common flexors

Osteotome detaching
common flexors from
medial epicondyle

Ulnar nerve

2182U

Flexorplasty of the Elbow (Steindler) (Continued)

G. By sharp and blunt dissection, the flexor muscle mass is freed and mobilized distally away from the joint capsule and the ulna as far as the motor branches of the median nerve and ulnar nerve will permit. A No. 1 silk whip suture is placed in the proximal end of the common flexors.

H. The biceps muscle, brachial vessels, and median nerve are retracted laterally, and the atrophied branchial muscle is split longitudinally. The periosteum is incised and stripped, exposing the anterior aspect of the distal humerus.

The elbow is then flexed to 120 degrees to determine the site of attachment of the transfer (usually 2 inches proximal to the elbow). With a drill, a hole is made on the anterior surface of the humerus. The opening is enlarged with progressively larger diamond-head hand drills to receive the transferred muscle. The action of the transfer as a pronator of the forearm is decreased by transferring it laterally on the humerus. With smaller size drill points, two tunnels are made from the lateral and medial cortices of the humerus and are connected to the larger hole for passing the suture.

I and **J.** Because the elbow will be immobilized in acute flexion, it is best to close the distal half of the wound before anchoring the transplant to the humerus. The ends of the whip suture are brought out through the tunnels, and the common flexors and the origin are firmly secured in the larger hole. The periosteum is closed with interrupted sutures over the transferred tendon, thus reinforcing its anchorage. The proximal half of the wound is closed, and a long arm cast is applied with the elbow in acute flexion and the forearm in full supination.

For postoperative care, see the guidelines outlined in the text on principles of tendon transfer.

Plate E. Flexorplasty of the Elbow (Steindler)

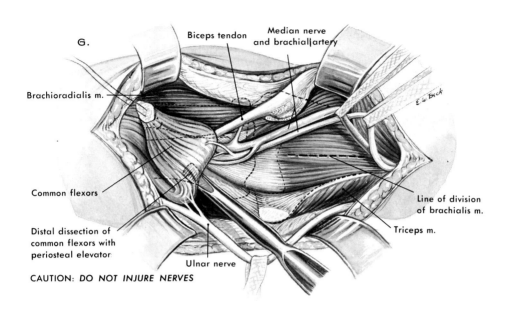

G.

Biceps tendon

Median nerve and brachial artery

Brachioradialis m.

Common flexors

Distal dissection of common flexors with periosteal elevator

Ulnar nerve

CAUTION: DO NOT INJURE NERVES

Line of division of brachialis m.

Triceps m.

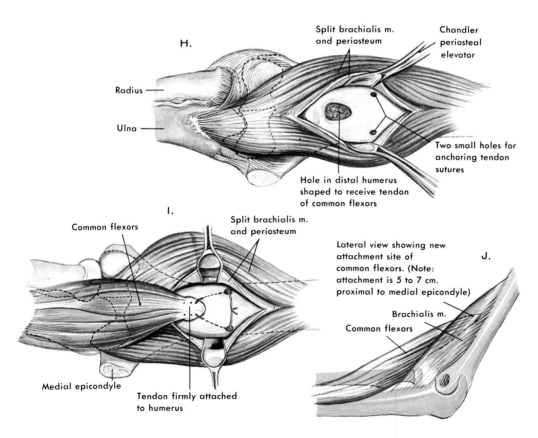

H.

Split brachialis m. and periosteum

Chandler periosteal elevator

Radius

Ulna

Two small holes for anchoring tendon sutures

Hole in distal humerus shaped to receive tendon of common flexors

I.

Common flexors

Split brachialis m. and periosteum

Lateral view showing new attachment site of common flexors. (Note: attachment is 5 to 7 cm. proximal to medial epicondyle)

J.

Brachialis m.

Common flexors

Medial epicondyle

Tendon firmly attached to humerus

6. The Spine

CLASSIFICATION OF SPINAL DEFORMITIES

Spinal deformity may be one or a combination of three basic types: scoliosis, kyphosis, and lordosis. The following classification of scoliosis by etiology, endorsed by the Scoliosis Research Society, is given to serve as a simple workable outline.

SCOLIOSIS
Structural scoliosis
  Idiopathic
    Infantile (0 to 2 years inclusive)
      Resolving
      Progressive
    Juvenile (3 to 10 years)
    Adolescent (10 years and older)
    Adult—after full skeletal maturity
  Neuromuscular
    Neuropathic
      Upper motor neuron lesion
        Cerebral palsy
        Spinocerebellar degeneration
          Friedreich's ataxia
          Charcot-Marie-Tooth disease
          Roussy-Lévy syndrome
        Syringomyelia
        Spinal cord tumor
        Spinal cord trauma
        Other
      Lower motor lesion
        Poliomyelitis
        Other viral myelitides
        Traumatic
        Spinal muscular atrophy
          Werdnig-Hoffmann disease
          Kugelberg-Welander disease
        Myelomeningocele (paralytic)
        Arthrogryposis (neuropathic)
        Dysautonomia (Riley-Day syndrome)
        Other
    Myopathic
      Arthrogryposis (myopathic)
      Muscular dystrophy
        Duchenne (pseudohypertrophic)
        Limb-girdle
        Fascioscapulohumeral
      Fiber type disproportion
      Congenital hypotonia
      Myotonia dystrophica
      Other
  Congenital
    Failure of formation
      Wedge vertebra
      Hemivertebra
    Failure of segmentation
      Unilateral bar (unsegmented)
      Bilateral (fusion)
      Mixed
    Associated with neural tissue defect
      Myelomeningocele
      Meningocele
      Spinal dysraphism
        Diastematomyelia
        Other
  Neurofibromatosis
  Mesenchymal disorders
    Marfan's syndrome
    Ehlers-Danlos syndrome
    Other

Traumatic
  Fracture or dislocation (nonparalytic)
  Postirradiation
  Surgical (postlaminectomy)
  Other
Extraspinal soft-tissue contracture
  Post empyema
  Post burn
  Other
Bone dysplasia
  Spondyloepiphyseal dysplasia
  Multiple epiphyseal dysplasia
  Mucopolysaccharidosis—such as Morquio's
  Diastrophic dwarfism
  Other
Metabolic related disorders
  Rickets
  Juvenile osteoporosis
  Osteogenesis imperfecta
  Homocystinuria
  Other
Related to spondylolysis or spondylolisthesis
Tumor
  Benign—such as osteoid osteoma, histiocytoma
  Malignant
Rheumatoid disease
Thoracogenic
  Post thoracoplasty
  Post thoracotomy
  Other
Nonstructural scoliosis
  Functional
  Postural
  Secondary to lower limb length inequality
  Due to pelvic obliquity (abduction or adduction contracture of the hips)
  Other
  Secondary to nerve root irritation
    Herniated nucleus pulposus
    Tumor
  Hysterical scoliosis
  (The so-called sciatic and hysterical scolioses are not true scolioses, as the deformity is in only one plane.)
  Inflammatory
KYPHOSIS
Kyphosis
  Postural
  Scheuermann's disease
  Congenital
    Defect of formation
    Defect of segmentation
    Mixed

Neuromuscular
Myelomeningocele
  Developmental (late paralytic)
  Congenital (present at birth)
Traumatic
  Due to bone or ligament damage or both without cord injury
  Due to bone or ligament damage or both with cord injury
Postsurgical
  Postlaminectomy
  Following excision of vertebral body
Postirradiation
Metabolic
  Osteoporosis
    Senile
    Juvenile
  Osteomalacia
  Osteogenesis imperfecta
  Other
Skeletal dysplasias
  Achondroplasia
  Mucopolysaccharidosis
  Neurofibromatosis
  Other
Collagen disease
  Marie-Strümpell disease
  Other
Tumor
  Benign
  Malignant
    Primary
    Metastatic
Inflammatory
Lordosis
  Postural
  Congenital
  Neuromuscular
  Postlaminectomy
  Secondary to hip flexion contracture
  Other

TERMINOLOGY

The Scoliosis Research Society has developed a glossary of terms to clarify the confusion that existed in the past in the description of curves and to make some sense in communication between surgeons.[1-3]

The term *idiopathic scoliosis* is used to denote scoliosis of unknown cause. This is further subdivided by the age of onset: *infantile*—developing during the first two years of life; *juvenile*—developing between three years of age and the onset of puberty; *adolescent*—developing after the onset of puberty and before skeletal maturity. *Adult* scoliosis is spinal curvature of any of the previous three types existing after closure of the physis. The curves are further described by the level of the apex of the curve; a spinal curve that has its apex between C-1 and C-6 is known as a *cervical curve*; one with the apex between C-7 and T-1, as a *cervicothoracic curve*; one with the apex between T-2 and T-11, as a *thoracic curve*; one with the apex at T-12 or L-1 or at the interspace between them, as a *thoracolumbar curve*; one with the apex between L-2 and L-4, as a *lumbar curve*; and one with the apex at L-5 or distal to it, as a *lumbosacral curve*. It should be noted that the term *dorsal* is not used for anatomic area; *thoracic* is substituted for it. *Dorsal* denotes the posterior aspect of the spine (i.e., spinous process, lamina); it is opposite to *ventral*, which means anterior. "Right" and "left" are used to indicate the direction of lateral angulation. The *apical vertebra* is the one most deviated from the vertical axis of the patient; it is also the most rotated vertebra. The *end vertebra* is the most *cephalad* vertebra of a curve whose upper surface tilts maximally toward the concavity of the curve or the most *caudal* vertebra whose inferior surface tilts maximally toward the concavity of the curve.

The term *structural curve* is used when the lateral curvature of the spinal segment is fixed, i.e., fails to be fully corrected on lateral side-bending supine radiograms—the normal flexibility of the spine is lost. A *nonstructural curve* does not have fixed rotation and lateral angulation; it can be fully corrected by traction or lateral bending. An *idiopathic* scoliosis that is minimal may be flexible and not fixed; when inspected from the dorsal view, it is characterized by rotation of the vertebrae to the convexity of the curve. A *postural* curve is always flexible, and when examined dorsally, the vertebrae are rotated to the concavity of the curve.

The term *congenital scoliosis* is used to describe curves caused by anomalous vertebral development. *Neuropathic* and *myopathic* scolioses are those due to neurologic or muscular disorders.

A *kyphos* is an abnormal posterior convexity (kyphosis) of a segment of the spine. *Lordosis* refers to anterior convexity (or posterior concavity) of a segment of the spine. The prefixes *hypo-* and *hyper-* are used to denote abnormalities of sagittal alignment. *Thoracic hypokyphosis* refers to abnormal diminution of the normal dorsal convexity of the thoracic spine; if

it is curved anteriorly the term *thoracic lordosis* is appropriate.

The terms *major* and *minor* applied to curves denote simply the larger and smaller degrees of angulation. Ordinarily the major curve is the more structural curve. The use of the terms *primary* (first to appear) and *secondary* when related to curves is discouraged, because it is difficult to identify when a curve actually first developed. *Double structural scoliosis* refers to two structural curves in the same spine; one curve balances the other. If both of these structural curves have their apex in the thoracic spine they are referred to as a *double thoracic curve*.

When the midline of the skull is aligned—centered—over the midline of the sacrum the curves are *compensated*; if it is not in the midline the scoliosis is *decompensated*. Clinically this is referred to as "balanced" or "out of balance" (or unbalanced) as the patient is inspected from the dorsal view in the erect position. A *compensatory* curve is one that tends to maintain normal body alignment. It is above or below a major curve and can be structural.

Lordoscoliosis is a lateral curvature of the spine associated with a decrease in the normal posterior convexity for that area; in the sagittal plane there may be hypokyphosis or true lordosis. *Kyphoscoliosis* is lateral curvature of the spine associated with increased posterior angulation in the affected segment of the spine; or there may be associated decrease in the anterior angulation in the sagittal plane normal for that area. A sharply angulated kyphos is referred to as a *gibbus*. Rotational prominence is determined in the forward bending position. Rotation of the thoracic vertebrae causes prominence of the ribs; in the lumbar region the rotation of vertebrae produces prominence of the paravertebral muscles. An *inclinometer* is an instrument used to measure the rib hump or the angle of thoracic rotation or inclination.

References

1. Goldstein, L. A., and Waugh, T. R.: Classification and terminology of scoliosis. Clin. Orthop., *93*:10, 1973.
2. McAlister, W. H., and Shackelford, G. D.: Classification of spinal curvatures. Radiol. Clin. North Am., *13*:93, 1975.
3. Terminology Committee, Scoliosis Research Society: A glossary of scoliosis terms. Spine, *1*:57, 1976.

Posture and Postural Defects[1-15]

Posture can be defined as the relationship of the parts of the body to the line of the center of gravity. The orthopedic surgeon is concerned with posture as a gauge of mechanical efficiency of the neuromusculoskeletal system in the erect position.

Development of Posture

In the uterus the fetus is almost invariably in a position of flexion, with the convex curve of the spine lying against the curve of the uterine wall. The head, arms, and legs of the fetus are flexed on the torso (Fig. 6–1). The entire fetus lies suspended in the amniotic fluid, which has a specific gravity similar to that of the fetus. Following birth the development of posture is affected by the constant forces exerted by gravity.

The newborn holds his shoulders, elbows, hips, and knees in flexion, with his limbs slightly bowed and rotated inward (Fig. 6–2 A). Fifteen to thirty degrees of flexion contracture of the knee is a normal physical finding. The infant lies in a nearly horizontal position, unable to support his head or trunk. In either the prone or the supine position, gravitational force is exerted on a horizontal plane and tends to unroll the "coiling" that was previously assumed within the uterus.

The rate of development of muscle strength varies in the different parts of the body. When the infant is in a horizontal position, the hip flexors, the anterior muscles of the neck, and the abdominal muscles are stretched and used minimally, whereas the extensors of the neck, back, and thigh are relaxed and are the first to increase their motor power. When the child is able to support his head and begins to sit up, the weight of the head, combined with the persistent flexion attitude of the hips and the associated flexion of the pelvis on the spine,

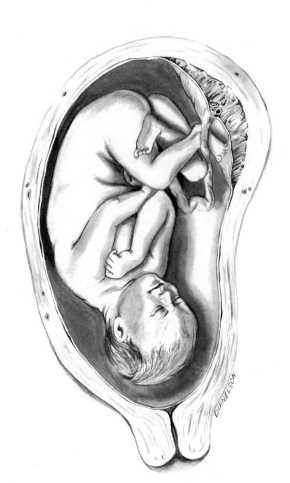

FIGURE 6–1. Posture of fetus in utero.

Note the position of flexion.

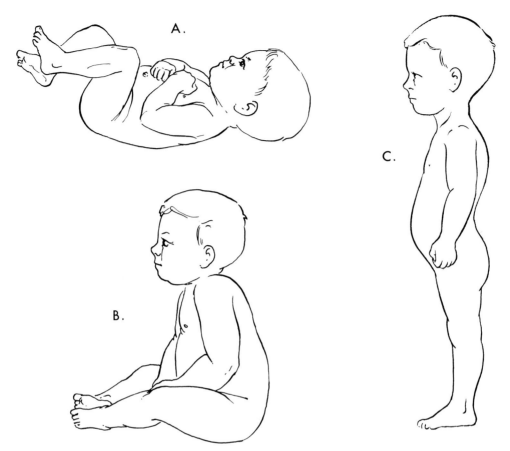

FIGURE 6–2. Development of posture.

A. In the newborn. Note the flexion attitude of the hips and knees. **B.** In the prestanding stage. Total convex curve of the spine is normal. **C.** In the 18-month-old child. A prominent abdomen and exaggerated lumbar lordosis are normal.

produces a long convex curve of the entire spine. In the prestanding stage, this total convex curve of the back is normal (Fig. 6–2 B).

When the child begins to stand and walk, the extensor muscles of the back, neck, and hips are well developed and the spine is usually straight. In the upright position, the force of gravity is exerted in a vertical direction, causing an exaggerated lumbar lordosis and a protuberant abdomen (Fig. 6–2 C). With further growth and development, the child improves his stance and becomes more agile in walking and running. In studying posture, one should bear in mind the interdependence of various parts of the body. For example, mild pronation of the feet is normal and common in a child of preschool age. The gastrocnemius-soleus muscles are long enough to allow dorsiflexion of the feet 20 to 30 degrees beyond neutral. In stance, mild genu valgum is common. These physical findings are normal and not pathologic.

Normal Posture

The posture of each person has characteristics that are uniquely his. Various factors affecting posture are:

Bony Contours. The shape of the vertebrae may be modified by diseases such as tuberculosis or Scheuermann's disease, which produce dorsal kyphosis.

Laxity of Ligamentous Structures. The degree of ligamentous laxity varies in different individuals, giving rise to looseness or tautness of the joints. The spine is composed of many joints, and is itself dependent upon the articulations inferior to it, such as those of the feet, knees, and hips.

Fascial and Musculotendinous Tautness. Tautness of soft-tissue structures, especially the fascia lata, hamstrings, anterior hip capsule, and pectorals, affect posture.

Muscle Strength. Particularly important is the

strength of the gluteus maximus, abdominal, erector spinae, and scapular adductor muscles.

Pelvic Inclination. The pelvis is the base upon which the vertebral column rests. Any change in its inclination will cause a corresponding change in the position of the fifth lumbar vertebra in relation to the sacrum, which in turn alters the posture of the entire spine. Inclination of the pelvis is ordinarily controlled by the muscles about the hip (Fig. 6–3). It is increased by contraction of the extensors of the hip, i.e., the glutei, hamstrings, and the posterior portion of the hip adductors, and it is decreased by contraction of the hip flexors, i.e., the iliopsoas, rectus femoris, pectineus, and the more anterior portion of the hip adductors. The spine is flexed by the iliopsoas and abdominal muscles, and is extended by the erector spinae. The abdominal muscles act synergetically with the glutei, the latter decreasing the pelvic inclination and the former reducing the lumbar lordosis. Motion of the vertebral column is greatest in the lumbar region; in the thoracic spine, however, rotation is of considerable magnitude, but flexion and extension are limited. The muscles of respiration (the diaphragm and intercos-

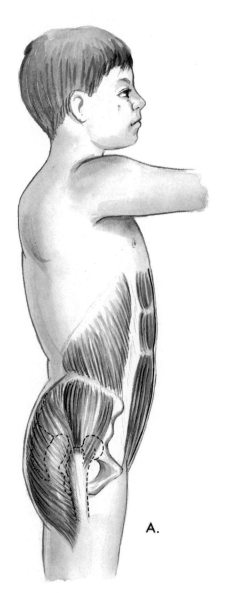 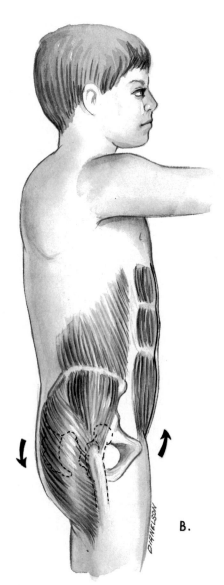

FIGURE 6–3. Pelvic tilt.

tals) produce a secondary effect on posture, as there is some extension of the dorsal spine with each inspiration.

In normal posture the body weight is carried forward on the balls of the feet, the lower limbs are straight with the hips and knees in neutral extension, the pelvic inclination is about 60 degrees to the vertical, the abdomen is retracted, the shoulders are level and flat, and the head is held erect. The line of the center of gravity of the body passes from the mastoid process to the cervicodorsal junction, crossing the bodies of the vertebrae at the dorsolumbar junction, and falling just anterior to the sacroiliac articulation and slightly posterior to the hip joint; it passes through the anterior knee joint and terminates at the front of the talus in the ankle.

Gradation of Posture

Posture can be classified into four grades (Fig. 6–4 A to D):

A—*excellent* or almost perfect posture
B—*good*, but not ideal posture
C—*poor*, but not the worst possible posture
D—*bad* and very possibly symptom-producing posture

In excellent *(A)* posture, the head and shoulders are balanced over the pelvis, hips, and ankles, with the head erect and the chin held in. The sternum is the part of the body farthest forward, the abdomen is drawn in and flat, and the spinal curves are within normal limits. In bad *(D)* posture, the head is held forward to a marked degree, the chest is depressed, the abdomen is completely relaxed and protuberant, the spinal curves are exaggerated, and the shoulders are held behind the pelvis.

Treatment of Postural Defects

Poor posture in children should be observed, and corrective measures taken to increase the strength of the back so that it will be less susceptible in adult life to fatigue, back strain, and injury. Children rarely complain of backache from poor posture. In adults, however, poor body mechanics and posture are frequent causes of low back strain.

Treatment consists of passive and active exercises (Figs. 6–5 and 6–6). First, if there are any contracted soft tissues—such as triceps surae, hamstrings, anterior hip structures, lumbosacral fascia, pectorals, and neck flexors—they should be passively stretched. The taut anterior neck and shoulder structures may be stretched by lying down with a small bolster between the two scapulae for 15 minutes twice a day. The child is also instructed to perform exercises to increase the motor strength of the key muscles affecting posture; namely, the ab-

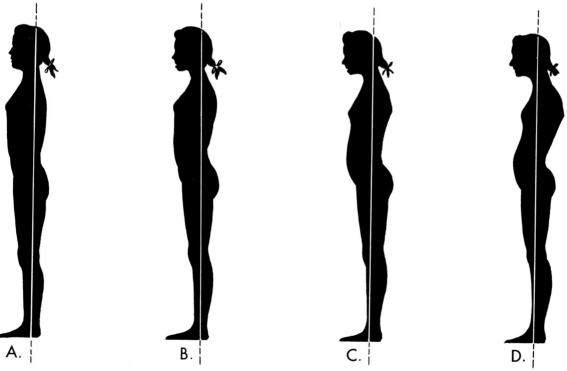

A.   B.   C.   D.

FIGURE 6–4. Gradation of posture (see text for explanation).

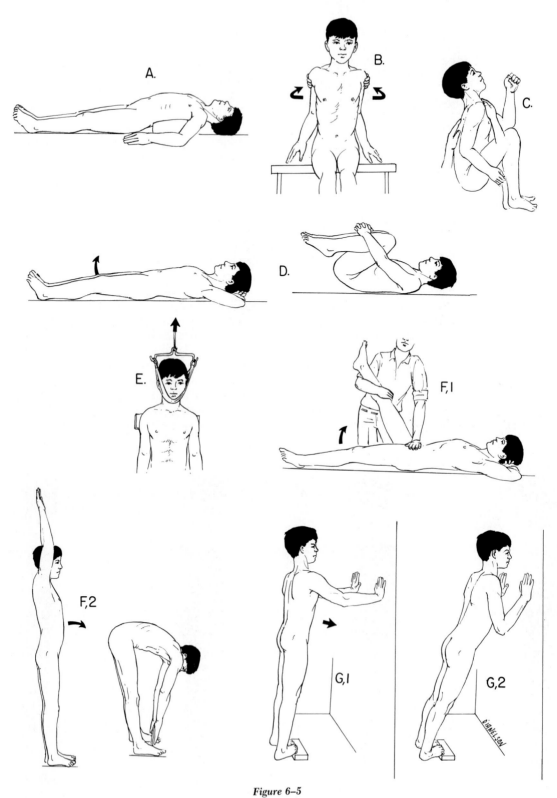

Figure 6–5

See legend on oppposite page

dominal muscles (sit-ups, flutter-kick, and bi-cycling), gluteus maximus (hip extension against gravity with knees in flexion), erector spinae (hyperextension of spine against gravity in prone position) and scapular adductors (bringing shoulder blades together in prone or sitting position).

The most important exercise is the pelvic tilt (Figs. 6–3 and 6–6 E). The patient is instructed to decrease the pelvic inclination by use of the abdominal and gluteus maximus muscles. Initially, he performs the pelvic tilt exercise in a supine position, then standing against the wall. By decreasing the pelvic tilt, all the exaggerated curves of the spine are decreased. The shoulders are brought over the pelvis with the head held erect and chin held in, thus correcting the poor posture. Postural exercises should be carried out until the individual is able to maintain the correct posture naturally. The patient should continue the exercises until they become part of his normal stance and gait.

NONSTRUCTURAL SCOLIOSIS

Postural Scoliosis

Poor posture may be associated with a mild scoliosis, which is a long thoracolumbar curve with no compensatory curves. There is no rotation of the vertebrae to the convexity of the curve revealed by clinical inspection of the patient bending forward and viewed from behind; there is neither rib hump nor unilateral prominence of paravertebral muscles on the convex side of the curve. The scoliosis is very flexible, disappearing on recumbency or when the patient is asked to stand straight and on

lateral trunk flexion to the convex side of the curve. Lumbar lordosis and dorsal roundback are usually exaggerated.

Postural scoliosis does not progress and does not become structural. It is of little clinical importance, and ordinarily no treatment is indicated. If it is marked, however, general postural exercises are in order.

Functional Scoliosis Due to Lower Limb Length Disparity

In this type of nonstructural scoliosis, the curve is a single long thoracolumbar curve, usually extending from the cervicodorsal junction to the sacrum. The convexity of the curve is toward the side of the depression of the pelvis, i.e., the side of the short lower limb (Fig. 6–7 A). Compensatory curves do not exist. It shows little rotation of the vertebrae, and as the spine is bent forward, the minimal rotation is toward the *concave* side of the curve, as opposed to structural scoliosis, in which rotation is to the convexity of the curve (Fig. 6–7 B). Curvature of the spine is present in the standing position; it disappears in recumbency and also on suspension. The spine bends equally well to both sides on lateral flexion of the trunk, with no fixed rotation or lateral angulation. The patient can voluntarily correct the lateral deviation of the spine and assume an erect posture. Correcting the lower limb length discrepancy with a lift under the foot levels the pelvis, and the scoliosis disappears (Fig. 6–7 C to E). In radiograms of the spine, there is no evidence of wedging or other structural changes in the vertebrae.

A short leg will not of itself cause a structural

Text continued on page 2196

FIGURE 6–5. *Passive exercises for poor posture.*

Stretching of contracted anterior neck and pectorals. **A.** The child lies supine with a bolster just distal to the apex of kyphosis for 15 minutes once or twice a day. **B.** With the child sitting on a chair, parent passively stretches the contracted pectorals by pushing the forward drooped shoulders posteriorly. **C.** The child lies on his side, knees flexed on the chest, while an assistant places one hand at the apex of the kyphosis with same forearm steadying the lower spine, and with the other hand, pushes the upper spine above the kyphosis into hyperextension.

Stretching of contracted lumbosacral fascia. **D.** Knee-chest exercises. Lying supine, bring knees on chest, flattening the lumbar spine and passively stretching the contracture of the lumbosacral fascia; count to 10 and lower legs to starting position.

Passive stretching of contracture of anterior soft tissues of the neck. **E.** Head-neck traction in a Sayre sling.

Hamstring stretching. **F-1.** The child lies supine; an assistant steadies the pelvis with one hand and, with the other hand, holds the leg in extension, raises the leg to a right angle, or as close to it as possible, then lowers it to starting position. The knee should always be in complete extension and the pelvis steadied flat on the floor. **F-2.** Toe-touching. Standing erect with the feet flat on the floor and 6 inches apart and the arms extended over the head; keeping the knees extended, bend forward to touch the floor between the feet, count to 5, and return to starting position.

Gastrocnemius-soleus stretching. **G-1.** Stand 2 to 3 feet away from the wall. Keep the feet, especially the heels, flat on the floor; curl the toes; the feet should be in slight inversion with the big toes pointing medially. Steady the trunk by placing hands against the wall. A wooden block may be used under the forefeet for more effective stretching. **G-2.** Keeping knees and hips in extension and the heels on the floor, carry the buttocks and trunk toward the wall. Count to 5 and return to starting position.

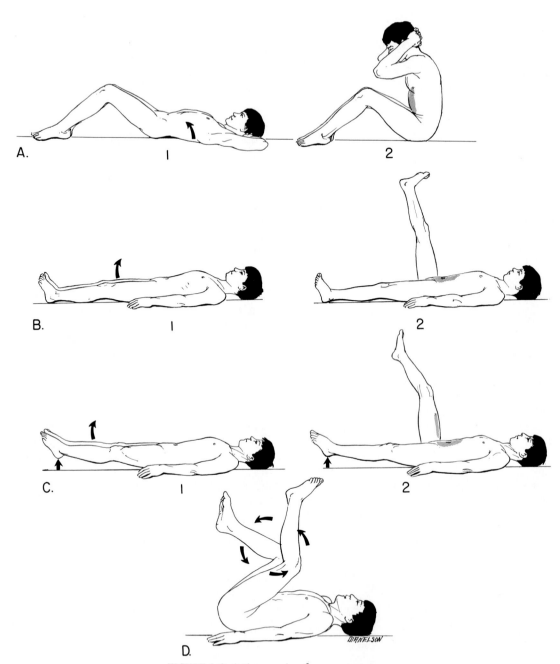

FIGURE 6–6. *Active exercises for poor posture.*

Abdominal exercises. **A.** Sit-ups. **1.** Lie supine, hips and knees flexed 30 degrees and in neutral rotation, hands clasped behind head, keeping the feet on the floor (support may be used if necessary) and the back straight. **2.** Move to sitting position to the count of 5, then lower body to starting position. **B.** Leg raising. **1.** Lie supine, legs together, knees and hips in extension, arms at the side and lumbar spine flat. **2.** Raise right leg until it is at a right angle to the trunk, or as close to this position as possible, then slowly lower it. Repeat the same with left leg. Continue the exercise by alternating legs. **C.** Flutter-kick. **1.** Same position as in **B,** but keep the feet off the floor to a height of 2 or 3 inches. **2.** Slowly raise the right leg until it is perpendicular to the trunk, or as close to this position as possible, then slowly lower the leg to the starting position. Repeat the same with left lower extremity. Always keep feet and legs off the floor. **D.** Bicycling.

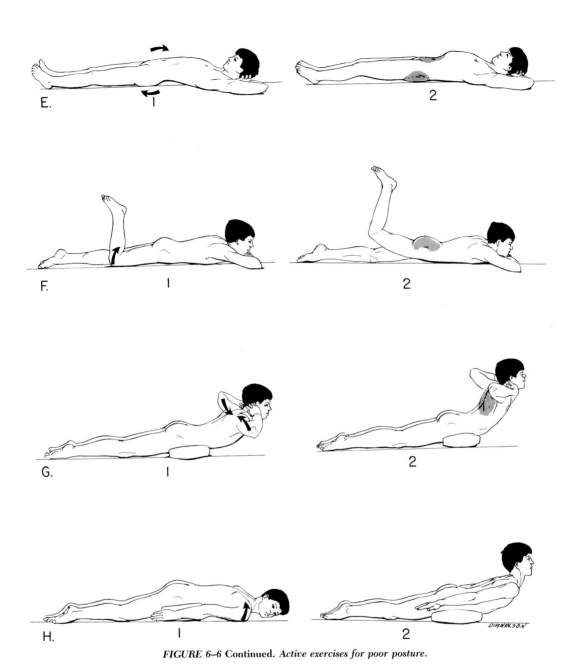

FIGURE 6–6 Continued. *Active exercises for poor posture.*

Pelvic tilt. **E-1.** Lying supine on the floor, pinch buttocks together and, without taking a deep breath, pull in abdominal muscles to flatten the lumbar spine. **E-2.** Graduate this exercise by performing the pelvic tilt exercise in stance while standing against the wall, and then in gait while walking away from the wall (Fig. 6–3).

Gluteus maximus exercises. **F-1.** Lie prone with knee flexed at right angle (to eliminate action of hamstrings) and arms under chin. **F-2.** Raise right thigh off floor as high as possible while keeping the knee flexed, count to 5, then lower it. Repeat the same with opposite side. Graduate this exercise to lifting both thighs off the floor at the same time.

Scapular adduction. **G-1.** Lying prone with one or two pillows under abdomen with shoulders abducted and hands clasped behind the neck, raise the head, neck, and upper trunk off the floor. **G-2.** Bring the shoulder blades together, count to 5, then return to starting position. The same exercise could be performed sitting on a chair with lower spine acutely flexed.

Thoracic hyperextension. **H-1.** Lie prone with the arms along the sides and the palms of the hands pressing against the thighs. **H-2.** Slowly raise the head, neck, and shoulders off the floor as high as possible, count to 5, then gradually return to starting position.

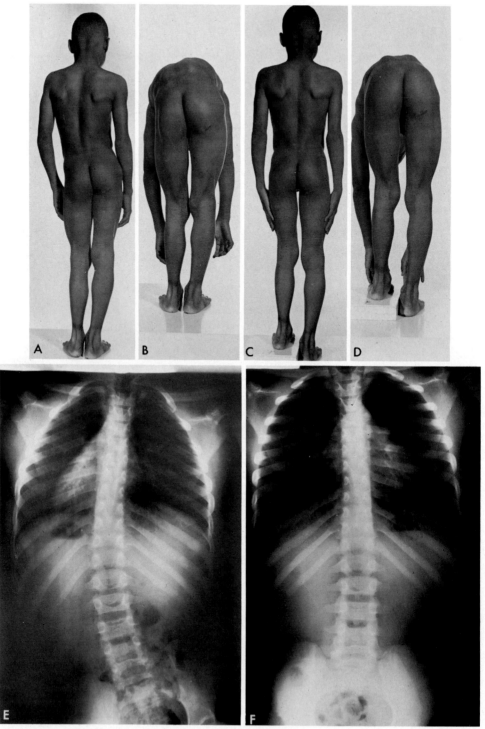

FIGURE 6–7. *The spine of a ten-year-old boy with functional scoliosis due to short left lower limb.*

A. Note the single long thoracolumbar scoliosis without compensatory curves. It is convex to the left. **B.** The rotation of the vertebrae is toward the concave side of the curve as the patient bends forward. **C.** Note the disappearance of the scoliosis when the pelvis is leveled by correction of the leg length shortening with a lift under the foot. **D.** With the pelvis level, note correction of rotation of vertebrae. **E.** Radiogram of the spine. The lateral curvature starts at the lumbosacral junction. There is no evidence of wedging or other structural changes in the vertebrae. **F.** Radiogram of the spine demonstrating the disappearance of scoliosis by correction of the leg length discrepancy with a lift under the left foot and leveling of the pelvis.

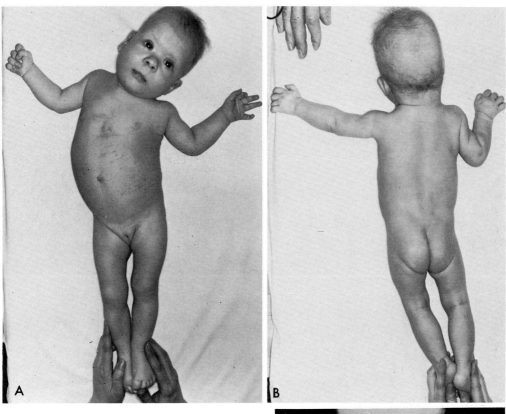

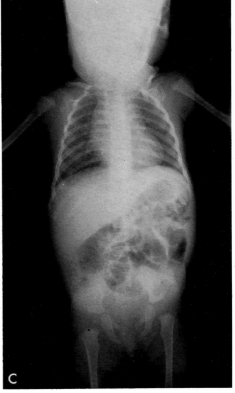

FIGURE 6–8. *Functional scoliosis due to congenital abduction contracture of the right hip.*

A and **B.** Clinical appearance of patient. **C.** Antero-posterior radiogram of the spine.

curve. Parents should be reassured of this to relieve them of many years of anxiety. Treatment consists of limb length equalization when the lower limb inequality, secondary scoliosis, and decompensation of the spine and trunk are significant.

Nonstructural Scoliosis due to Pelvic Obliquity

This nonstructural scoliosis is due to obliquity of the pelvis. It is commonly seen in infants due to either abduction or adduction contracture (or both) of the hips secondary to intrauterine malposture (Fig. 6–8). Treatment consists of passive stretching exercises to correct the contractural deformities of the hip. Occasionally surgical release of contracted soft tissues is indicated to correct pelvic obliquity.

Hysterical Scoliosis

The curvature is a long C-curve without rotation. This can occur in emotionally disturbed teenagers. The patient's trunk may twist into bizarre contortions. In the upright or sitting posture the scoliosis is present, but may or may not disappear in recumbency. There may be changing patterns or increase or decrease in the severity of the scoliosis from day to day. The scoliosis disappears during sleep or appropriate sedation.

Radiograms do not disclose any rigidity of the curve. One should be extremely cautious in diagnosing hysterical scoliosis. A thorough neurologic examination should be performed to rule out spinal cord tumor or other intraspinal pathologic conditions. Obtain a neurologic consultation! It is prudent to perform a bone scan with technetium-99m to rule out occult disease such as osteoid osteoma. Treatment of hysterical scoliosis is by psychotherapy; it is not orthopedic. Orthoses and exercises should not be prescribed, as they will aggravate the hysteric.

References

1. Adams, M. A., and Hutton, W. C.: The effect of posture on the lumbar spine. J. Bone Joint Surg., 67-B:625, 1985.
2. Browne, D.: Congenital postural scoliosis. Proc. R. Soc. Med., 49:395, 1956.
3. Dieck, G. S., Kelsey, J. L., and Goel, V. K.: An epidemiologic study of the relationship between postural asymmetry in the teen years and subsequent back and neck pain. Spine, 10:872, 1985.
4. Driscoll, D. M., Newton, R. A., and Lamb, R. L.: A study of postural equilibrium in idiopathic scoliosis. J. Pediatr. Orthop., 4:677, 1984.
5. During, J., Goudfrooij, H., and Keessen, W.: Toward standards for posture. Postural characteristics of the lower back system in normal and pathologic conditions. Spine, 10:83, 1985.
6. Hellebrandt, F. A., and Franseen, E. B.: Physiological study of the vertebral stance of man. Physiol. Rev., 23:220, 1943.
7. Howorth, B.: Dynamic posture. J.A.M.A., 131:1398, 1946.
8. Keith, A.: Man's posture: Its evolution and disorders. Br. Med. J., 1:451, 1923.
9. Klein, A.: Posture Clinics: Organization and Exercises. Washington, D.C., U.S. Department of Labor, Children's Bureau, 1931, Publication 164.
10. Liandres, Z. A., and Zaidel, O. P.: Posture defects and scoliosis in children, their prevention and functional treatment. Vopr. Kurortol. Fizioter. Lech. Fiz. Kult., 3:22, 1977.
11. Lowman, C. L., and Young, C. H.: Postural Fitness: Significance and Variances. Philadelphia, Lea & Febiger, 1960.
12. Phelps, W. M., Kiphuth, R. J. H., and Goff, C. W.: The Diagnosis and Treatment of Postural Defects. 2nd Ed. Springfield, Ill., Thomas, 1956.
13. Stotz, S.: Abnormal posture in children and adolescents. M.M.W., 121:165, 1979.
14. Williams, H. G., Fisher, J. M., and Tritschler, K. A.: Descriptive analysis of static postural control in 4, 6, and 8 year old normal and motorically awkward children. Am. J. Phys. Med., 62:12, 1983.
15. Wilner, S.: Spinal pantograph—a noninvasive anthropometric device for describing postures and asymmetries of the trunk. J. Pediatr. Orthop., 3:245, 1983.

Congenital Anomalies of the Spine

Congenital deformities of the spine are caused by anomalous vertebral development. They are relatively rare, being much less common than idiopathic scoliosis. A congenital anomaly of the spine may be *simple and benign*; it does not cause spinal deformity. Often such innocuous vertebral anomalies are discovered incidentally in a radiograph taken for some other reason. Conversely, a congenital spinal anomaly may be *complex and vicious* in its natural history, causing severe spinal deformity, even cor pulmonale or paraplegia. Some of these severe congenital spinal deformities are present at birth, whereas others develop during the juvenile or adolescent period, becoming progressively severe with abnormal growth of the spine. They may be associated with numerous other malformations.

A long C-curve in the newborn caused by pelvic obliquity and intrauterine malposture is not congenital scoliosis. Infantile idiopathic scoliosis may, however, develop during the first few months of life; it should not be mistaken for congenital scoliosis.

Classification

Congenital anomalies of the spine may be due to defects of segmentation or defects of formation. Frequently a congenitally deformed spine is the result of both pathogenic factors.

Defective segmentation produces an unsegmented bar. Two or more vertebrae may be affected, either the vertebral bodies, the posterior elements, or both being involved. Unsegmented unilateral bars have the worst prognosis for progression and deformity. When lateral, the resultant deformity is scoliosis (Fig 6–9 A). Anterior unsegmented bars cause kyphosis, whereas bilateral posterior unsegmented bars result in fixed lordosis, and unilateral posterior bar, lordoscoliosis (Fig 6–9 B and C). Circumferential symmetrical failure of segmentation results in the "bloc" vertebra, which does not cause angular or rotatory spinal deformity, but

vertical vertebral growth and segmental motion are lost (Fig. 6–9 D). Klippel-Feil syndrome is a severe form of failure of segmentation of the vertebrae.

Defects of formation may be partial or complete. Partial unilateral failure of formation of a vertebra produces a wedge and trapezoid shape of the vertebra. A small vestigial pedicle may be seen on the radiogram. Hemivertebrae, caused by failure of complete unilateral formation, can be nonsegmented, semisegmented, or segmented from the adjacent vertebrae. Hemivertebrae may be balanced or unbalanced.

A *segmented hemivertebra* is fully separated (with intact vertebral growth plate and disc) from the adjacent vertebra (Fig. 6–10 A). In such an anomaly scoliosis develops as a result of asymmetrical vertebral growth. If there are two or more hemivertebrae on one side of the spine the degree of asymmetry of vertebral

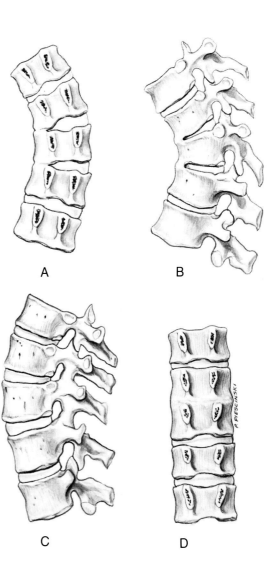

FIGURE 6–9. *Congenital deformities of the spine due to defective segmentation.*

A. Unilateral unsegmented bar. The defective segmentation is lateral and on only one side. The resultant deformity is severe progressive scoliosis. **B.** Anterior unsegmented bar. It leads to progressive kyphosis. **C.** Bilateral posterior failure of segmentation results in lordosis. **D.** "Bloc" vertebra due to bilateral and symmetrical failure of segmentation. Segmental motion is lost, and longitudinal vertebral growth does not take place. However, there is no angular or rotatory spinal deformity.

(Redrawn from Winter, R.B.: Congenital Deformities of the Spine. New York, Thieme-Verlag, 1983.)

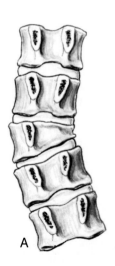
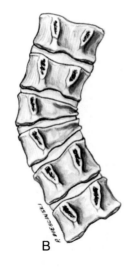

FIGURE 6–10. Segmental hemivertebra.

It is fully separated, with intact vertebral growth plate and disc. Asymmetrical vertebral growth causes progressive scoliosis. **A.** One hemivertebra. **B.** Two hemivertebrae on one side—the likelihood of severe scoliosis is greater. (Redrawn from Winter, R.B.: Congenital Deformities of the Spine. New York, Thieme-Verlag, 1983.)

growth is greater and the prognosis for severe spinal deformity is worse (Fig. 6–10 B). The scoliosis may be balanced if the two hemivertebrae are situated on opposite sides, but the degree of curvature may still be progressive.

A *semisegmented hemivertebra* is separated from one adjacent vertebra (superior or inferior) by a normal vertebral growth plate and disc, but fused to the other adjacent vertebra. Because of some asymmetry of growth there is likelihood of progressive spinal deformity (Fig. 6–11 A).

A *nonsegmented hemivertebra* is fused to both adjacent vertebrae (those above and below) with no discs or vertebral growth plates (Fig. 6–11 B). In absence of asymmetrical growth, a nonsegmented hemivertebra does not cause progressive spinal deformity.

Kyphosis will result when the anterior part of the vertebral body is aplastic or hypoplastic owing to failure of formation and the posterior elements are normally developed; one or more

vertebrae may be defective (Fig. 6–12). The resultant kyphosis is angular rather than rounded. Congenital absence of the sacrum and lumbar spine is an extreme form of failure of formation of the entire lower vertebral column.

Of the *mixed types* of congenital anomalies of the spine, the combination of segmented hemivertebra and unsegmented bar has the worst prognosis. The resultant scoliosis will be very severe.

There are some types of mixed segmentation and formation defects that result in a jumbled mass of abnormal bones and are not characterized by a single preponderant anomaly. They are unclassifiable. In such cases linear and computed tomography are indicated to delineate the pathologic anatomy.

Heredity

Hemivertebra occurs sporadically and there is no risk to subsequent siblings or offspring.

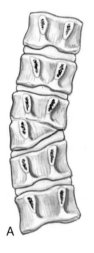
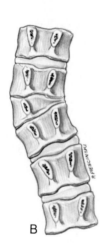

FIGURE 6–11. Semisegmental and nonsegmented hemivertebrae.

A. Semisegmented hemivertebra. It is fused to one adjacent vertebra (superior or inferior) but is separated from the other by normal vertebral growth plate and disc. Scoliosis develops, but it is less progressive than that of segmented hemivertebra. **B.** Nonsegmented hemivertebrae. It is fused to adjacent vertebra—the ones proximal and distal.

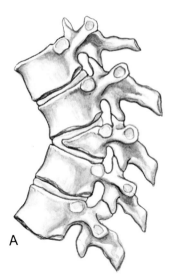
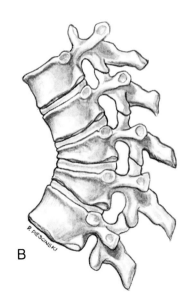

FIGURE 6–12. Failure of formation of the anterior part of the vertebral body with the posterior elements of the spine normally developed. The resultant deformity is kyphosis, which is angular.

A. Hypoplasia of anterior part of one vertebral body. **B.** Hypoplasia of anterior part of two adjacent vertebral bodies. (Redrawn after Winter, R.B.: Congenital Deformities of the Spine. New York, Thieme-Verlag, 1983.)

A   B

In *multiple congenital anomalies* of the vertebrae (excluding myelomeningocele) the risk to subsequent siblings is 5 to 10 per cent.[87] In Winter's extensive study the familial incidence of congenital anomalies of the spine was 1 per cent.[79] Reports of congenital malformation of the spine in identical twins vary—both twins may be involved, or one of the twins may have a congenital defect of the spine and the other may be normal.[2, 8, 36, 61]

The spondylothoracic dysplasia (Jarcho-Levin syndrome), consisting of multiple levels of nonsegmentation, multiple fused ribs, and frequently absence of segments, is hereditary with both autosomal dominant and recessive inheritance reported in the literature. Respiratory failure may cause premature death in some of these patients.[13, 41, 63]

Associated Anomalies

Congenital deformation of the spine may be associated with other congenital malformations.

Fusion of the Ribs. The ribs may be fused into a bony mass close to and continuous with the vertebrae (usually associated with an unsegmented bar). These curves do progress, and correction cannot be obtained unless rib resection and osteotomy of the bar are performed. The ribs may also be fused anteriorly at a distance from the vertebrae; this anomaly does not have a significant relationship to curvature of the spine.

Congenital Malformation of the Neural Axis (Spinal Dysraphism). In examination of the patient one should carefully examine the spine for external signs of spinal dysraphism—such as hair patches, lipomata, dimples, or nevi. Also, a thorough neurologic examination should always be performed to rule out neurologic deficit. Is there calf or thigh atrophy? Is one foot smaller than the other? Are the deep tendon reflexes normal? Is there any sensory disturbance? The presence of pes cavus requires a thorough diagnostic work-up to rule out neurologic impairment. Other possible neurogenic foot deformities are talipes equinovarus and congenital convex pes valgus.

Radiograms of the entire spine should be made, showing occiput to coccyx in both the anteroposterior and lateral projections. Oblique views are taken as indicated. Is there any spina bifida, midline bony defect, or widening of the intrapedicular distance in the anteroposterior projection or the spinal canal in the lateral view? When the routine radiographs suggest diastematomyelia or whenever there is evidence of neurologic deficit distal to an abnormal region of the spine, computed tomography and magnetic resonance imaging are performed to delineate the spinal cord and any pathology related to it. Myelography is an invasive procedure; it should be performed only when indicated. Diastematomyelia, when present, should be excised prior to spinal fusion or whenever it is associated with neurologic deficit.

Associated Congenital Anomalies Other than Those of the Vertebral Column or Ribs. These are not uncommon. Winter and associates found 115 associated anomalies in 73 of 234 patients having congenital scoliosis. In their series, some of the common ones were congenital heart disease (16 patients), Sprengel's deformity (14 patients), cleft palate (9 patients), hypoplasia of

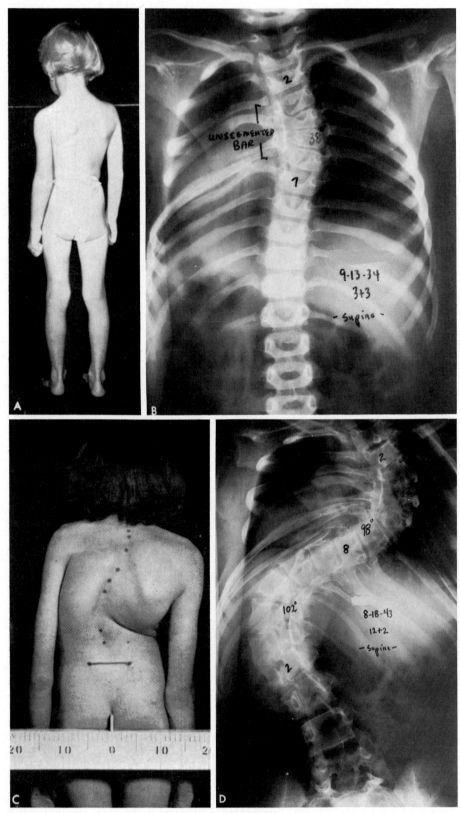

Figure 6–13

See legend on opposite page

one leg (9 patients), talipes equinovarus (6 patients), extra thumbs (4 patients), hypoplastic thumbs (4 patients), vertical talus (2 patients), pectus carinatum (2 patients), and cleft lip (2 patients).[82]

Other associated malformations are mandibular hypoplasia, ocular dermoids, preauricular skin tags, hypoplasia or aplasia of a kidney, horseshoe kidney, obstructive neuropathy, absence of uterus or atresia of the vagina. Genitourinary malformations are present in one fourth of the patients with congenital deformities of the spine; therefore it is vital that all patients with congenital spinal anomalies have thorough assessment of the genitourinary system by ultrasonography and intravenous pyelography.[51]

In general, the curves in the cervicothoracic area tend to be associated with cardiac anomalies, Sprengel's deformity, and congenital anomalies of the upper limb, such as partial amelia or congenital absence of the radius, whereas those in the lumbar area tend to be associated with anomalies of the genitourinary tract or the lower limbs. It should be noted, however, that urinary tract deformities are also frequent with malformations of the upper spine, particularly the Klippel-Feil syndrome.

CONGENITAL SCOLIOSIS
Natural History

In the past, it has been an unfortunate tendency of many physicians to assume that congenital scoliosis does not progress and therefore treatment is not indicated. Kuhns and Hormell, in a study of 165 patients with congenital scoliosis, were able to obtain data on 85 children followed to maturity without treatment. They found that 13 showed no progression, 40 showed moderate progression (5 to 30 degrees), and 32 showed progression of more than 30 degrees. Thoracic curves, particularly those with multiple unbalanced anomalies, had the worst prognosis.[43]

Unilateral unsegmented bars cause severe progression.[6] In the review of 88 patients with congenital scoliosis, the ten patients with unsegmented bar had average progression of 5 degrees per year; ordinarily the curves began at 30 degrees and progressed to about 100 degrees.[50] Shands and Bundens noted sudden progression during adolescence.[67]

In congenital scoliosis, when there is one hemivertebra, or two hemivertebrae are on the same side, the curve will be severe, whereas when double hemivertebrae are on opposite sides, they balance each other and result in a relatively mild deformity.

The natural history of congenital scoliosis was determined in 39 of 88 patients with congenital scoliosis by Rathke and Sun. They found one patient progressed more than 50 degrees, one up to 50 degrees, three up to 30 degrees, seven up to 20 degrees, eleven up to 10 degrees, and fourteen up to 5 degrees; only two patients showed no progression.[62]

The prognosis of congenital scoliosis has been reported by several investigators. Winter and associates, in a study of 234 patients, noted curve progression to 5 degrees or less in 18 per cent, 6 to 30 degrees in 37 per cent, and 37 or more degrees in 45 per cent. The curves with a poor prognosis were those due to a unilateral unsegmented bar and single or double unbalanced hemivertebrae. The thoracic curves resulted in severe deformity.[82] Again, these findings were noted by Tsou and associates, by Nasca and associates, by Touzet, and by McMaster and Ohtsuka.[54, 57, 71, 72]

In summary, the following factors affect the natural history of congenital scoliosis:

Specific Anomaly. Unilateral unsegmented bars, a common anomaly, are most often seen in the thoracic area and have the worst prognosis for progression and deformity (Fig. 6–13). The least progressive curves are those with bloc vertebrae.

A single hemivertebra or double unbalanced hemivertebrae progress slowly until the adoles-

---

FIGURE 6–13. *The natural history of an unsegmented unilateral bar in the thoracic area.*

A. Clinical appearance of a girl three years old. **B.** Radiogram of the spine of the same patient at three years of age. Note the unsegmented unilateral bar on the left side from the third through the six thoracic vertebrae. The right thoracic curve is 38 degrees. The beginning of a left thoracolumbar compensatory curve is apparent. This patient was treated ineffectively with a leather and steel underarm thoracolumbar orthosis (TLSO). **C.** Photograph of same patient at age of 12 years, showing the severe clinical deformity. **D.** Radiogram of same patient at the age of 12 years. Note the progression of the major curve from 38 to 98 degrees and the development of severe structural secondary curve from the eighth thoracic vertebra to the second lumbar curve. This child well demonstrates that unsegmented unilateral bars in the thoracic area have the worst prognosis for progression and deformity. (From Winter, R. B., Moe, J. H., and Eilers, V. E.: Congenital scoliosis. A study of 234 patients treated and untreated. J. Bone Joint Surg., 50-A:12, 1968. Reprinted by permission.)

cent growth spurt, and then they increase rapidly. Beware! They require close observation and follow-up.

Area of the Spine Involved. In general, cervicothoracic and lumbar curves are less progressive than are curves in the thoracic region. One should be cognizant of the fact that a mild cervicothoracic curve may produce an unsightly appearance because of head and neck tilt and asymmetry and depression of one shoulder. Lumbar curves do not tend to cause much cosmetic deformity unless decompensation or pelvic obliquity occurs. Thoracic curves are likely to be more progressive than those primarily in other areas. Congenital scoliosis in the thoracolumbar area is largely due to hemivertebrae, which may be located laterally, posterolaterally, or sometimes directly posteriorly. The more posterior the hemivertebrae, the worse the kyphosis and the more ominous the prognosis.

Balance and Pattern of the Curve. In general, multiple balanced anomalies throughout the spine do not progress, and there is a satisfactory cosmetic appearance (Fig. 6–14). The more unbalanced the anomalies, the more likely is progression of the scoliosis (Fig. 6–15).

Age of the Patient and Prognosis. Congenital scoliosis, like idiopathic scoliosis, tends to progress most rapidly during the preadolescent growth spurt. It is common, however, for most curves to progress slowly, even in infancy and throughout growth. Steady progression during the entire growth period is characteristic of curves due to unilateral unsegmented bars or to multiple unbalanced thoracic hemivertebrae. Once a curve begins to progress, it does so as long as there is growth.

Severity of the Curve. The severity of the curve and the rate of progression cannot be related, because some of the mild curves progress more rapidly than the severe ones.

Progression patterns in congenital scoliosis are shown in Figure 6–16.

Avoid the following pitfalls: (1) Accepting poor quality films. The radiographs should show detail and include the entire spine. In the uncooperative, wiggly child a supine film is made; this is preferrable to a poor standing film. (2) Failure to measure the curves accurately. (3) Failure to detect subtle but steady progression of the curvature. When one measures serial standing radiograms carefully and compares the most recent radiogram with the initial one, the slow and steady progression will become apparent. (4) Failure to assess secondary or compensatory curves. They may progress more and produce more deformity than the primary curve. (5) Failure to determine the growth pattern of one side versus the other. In congenital scoliosis curves progress because of asymmetrical growth.

Treatment

Nonoperative Treatment. Electrical stimulation, manipulation, and massage are ineffective; passive stretching exercises consisting primarily of lateral bending and head-neck traction are performed to keep the curve as flexible as possible. Exercises will improve poor posture but do not correct or prevent progression of congenital scoliosis. The only nonoperative method of treatment that has been shown to be of some value is spinal orthosis—specifically, the Milwaukee brace.[86] It may prevent progression of a long flexible curve. Short rigid curves do not respond to orthotic treatment. Flexibility of the curve is determined by bending and traction films. Orthotic treatment in congenital scoliosis is indicated in a child who has several more years of skeletal growth before the adolescent growth spurt; the one with a long (eight to ten vertebrae) curve, preferably with the apex at the thoracolumbar junction; and the one with a curve that is flexible and shows 50 per cent or more correction on bending or traction films. During orthotic treatment the curves (both primary and compensatory) should be carefully followed in order to detect progression. Often the objective of orthotic treatment is to buy time and delay spinal fusion until adequate vertebral growth has taken place. Progression of compensatory flexible curves may be checked by orthosis.

In high thoracic or cervicothoracic curves with head tilt, asymmetrical neckline, and elevation of one shoulder, some degree of balance and symmetry can be achieved by the addition of appropriate clavicular, shoulder, and head-neck pieces. Underarm thoracolumbar orthoses should not be used because they may cause constriction of the thoracic cage. The Milwaukee brace can be fitted to a young child, usually around two years of age.

Surgical Treatment. The modality of operative procedure employed depends on the type and severity of the spinal deformity, the natural history of the specific type of scoliosis, the anatomic area of the deformity, and the age of the patient.

In Situ Posterior Fusion. If the severity of the spinal deformity is minimal to moderate, cosmetically acceptable, and the natural history

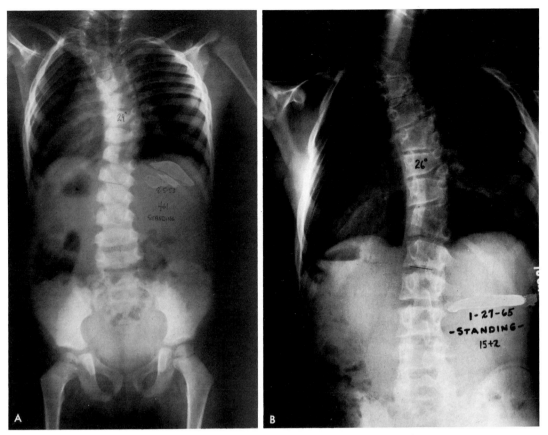

FIGURE 6–14. *The natural history of multiple balanced anomalies of the spine.*

A. Radiogram of the spine depicting multiple fairly well-balanced anomalies throughout the spine in a boy when he was four years old. Excellent clinical appearance. He received no treatment. **B.** Radiograms of the same boy at the age of 15 years. Note that the curve has not progressed. Cosmetic appearance and function of spine are excellent. (From Winter, R. B., Moe, J. H., and Eilers, V. E.: Congenital scoliosis. A study of 234 patients treated and untreated. J. Bone Joint Surg., 50-A:9, 1968. Reprinted by permission.)

of the deformity is relentless progression, stabilization of the spine by posterior fusion in situ is performed. Autogenous iliac bone is preferable to bone bank bone. The unilateral unsegmented bar is a typical example; in such a case the fused area should incorporate the entire bar and extend one mobile level above and one mobile segment distal to the bar.

Unilateral Epiphysiodesis—Anteriorly and Posteriorly—on Convex Side. When there is a possibility of vertebral growth on the concave side of a congenital curve and many years of vertebral growth are still to be expected, the convex side of the curve is fused both anteriorly and posteriorly. Unilateral epiphysiodesis (by anterior and posterior convex fusion) arrests the excessive growth on the convex side of the curve and allows vertebral growth to take place on the concave side.[5, 9, 56, 64, 65, 78] The presence of excessive kyphosis is a contraindication to such a procedure.[78, 79]

Correction of Curvature and Fusion. When a severe deformity is present it should be corrected prior to fusion. Modalities to obtain correction are cast, traction, and instrumentation. Instrumentation is the preferred method of correction; it may, however, be difficult or impossible if the bones are small and malformed. Correction by *instrumentation* always carries the risk of spinal cord damage and paraplegia. Correction by *cast* has little risk, and if the curve is flexible a great degree of correction can be achieved. Correction by *traction* is indicated when sudden elongation of the spine by stretching a curve by instrumentation is contraindicated.[15] When an unsegmented bar is osteotomized prior to fusion or when a tethering structure has been released prior to fusion, the curve should be corrected by traction. Gradual stretching of spinal cord and nerves prevents paraplegia. This is followed by fusion and internal fixation by instrumentation. The

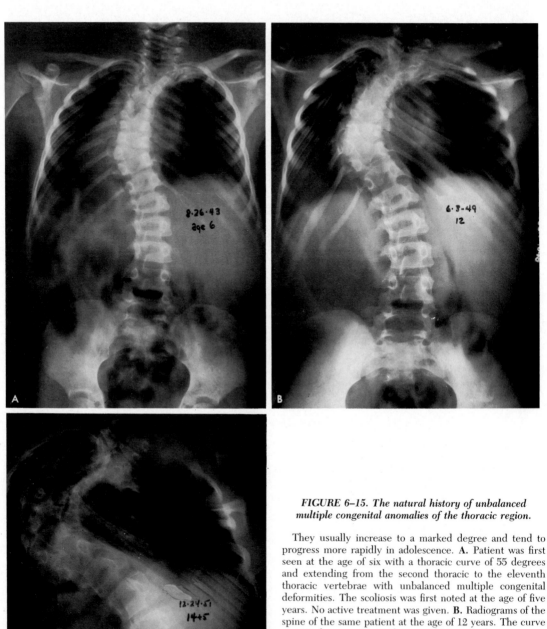

FIGURE 6–15. *The natural history of unbalanced multiple congenital anomalies of the thoracic region.*

They usually increase to a marked degree and tend to progress more rapidly in adolescence. **A.** Patient was first seen at the age of six with a thoracic curve of 55 degrees and extending from the second thoracic to the eleventh thoracic vertebrae with unbalanced multiple congenital deformities. The scoliosis was first noted at the age of five years. No active treatment was given. **B.** Radiograms of the spine of the same patient at the age of 12 years. The curve was 78 degrees. **C.** At the age of 14 years the curve was 120 degrees. Note the marked late progression. (From Winters, R. B., Moe, J. H., and Eilers, V. E.: Congenital scoliosis. A study of 234 patients treated and untreated. J. Bone Joint Surg., *50-A*:16–17, 1968. Reprinted by permission.)

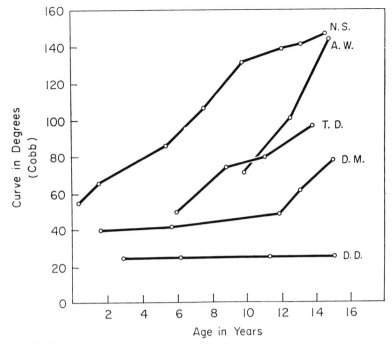

FIGURE 6–16. Progression pattern in congenital scoliosis in untreated patients.

N.S., a unilateral thoracic unsegmented bar; A.W., a single hemivertebra, third thoracic vertebra; T.D., multiple unbalanced thoracic anomalies; D.M., unbalanced anomalies, thoracolumbar junction; and D.D., multiple balanced anomalies in the entire space. (From Winters, R. B., Moe, J. H., and Eilers, V. E.: Congenital scoliosis. A study of 234 patients treated and untreated. J. Bone Joint Surg., 50-A:8, 1968. Reprinted with permission.)

type of instrumentation may be Harrington or Luque rods. Narrowness or absence of interlaminar spaces makes instrumentation with Luque rods difficult. Recently segmental instrumentation has been utilized for fixation.[70] When correcting congenital scoliosis by instrumentation, electronic cord monitoring and wake-up tests are mandatory.[11, 21, 28, 34, 58, 74]

Excision of Hemivertebrae. This is indicated when they are located at the lumbosacral junction, resulting in severe decompensation and tilting of the spine. It is best to perform this at a young age prior to development of structural changes in the secondary curves above. Following excision, correction is achieved and maintained by insertion of compression rods. When there is associated spina bifida or spinal dysraphism, a convex hemifusion between the fifth lumbar and first sacral vertebrae is performed first; this provides adequate bone stock for placing the hooks of spinal instrumentation.[14, 44, 66, 73, 75, 76]

Osteotomy of the Spine. This is ordinarily performed when there is a unilateral unsegmented bar in an older child or adolescent who has developed a rigid, severe, angular scoliosis and in whom other means to provide spinal

compensation are not available. Fused ribs on the concave side, if present, are resected at the same time. Anterior and posterior wedge resection osteotomy with correction and fusion is complex, difficult, and very risky; however, it is possible with the development of newer technology for anterior spinal surgery. It should be performed only by the very experienced spine surgeon. The high risk of neurologic complications should be fully understood by the patient and the parents.

References

1. Akbarnia, B. A., and Moe, J. H.: Familial congenital scoliosis with unilateral unsegmented bar. Case report of two siblings. J. Bone Joint Surg., 60-A:259, 1978.
2. Akbarnia, B. A., Heydarian, K., and Ganjavian, M. S.: Concordant congenital spine deformity in monozygotic twins. J. Pediatr. Orthop., 4:502, 1983.
3. Allen, B. L., Jr.: Segmental spinal instrumentation with L-rods. A.A.O.S. Instr. Course Lect., 32:202, 1983.
4. Anderson, P. R., Puno, M. R., Lovell, S. L., and Swayze, C. R.: Postoperative respiratory complications in non-idiopathic scoliosis. Acta Anaesthesiol. Scand., 29:186, 1985.
5. Andrew, T., and Piggott, H.: Growth arrest for progressive scoliosis: Combined anterior and posterior fusion of the convexity. J. Bone Joint Surg., 67-B:193, 1985.

6. Bairov, G. A., Ulrikh, E. V., and Krylova, L. P.: Therapeutic-preventive resection of lateral hemivertebrae in infants with congenital scoliosis. Vestn. Khir., *124*:91, 1980.

7. Blount, W. P.: Congenital scoliosis. *In* Huitieme Congres de la Societé International de Chirurgie Orthopédique et de Traumatologie, New York, 4–9 Septembre, 1960. Bruxelles, Imprimerie des Sciences, 1961, p. 748.

8. Bonicoli, F., and Delveccio, E.: Scoliosis in monochorionic twins. Chir. Organi Mov., *57*:178, 1968.

9. Bradford, D. S.: Partial epiphyseal arrest and supplemental fixation for progressive correction of congenital spinal deformity. J. Bone Joint Surg., *64-A*:610, 1982.

10. Browne, D.: Congenital postural scoliosis. Proc. R. Soc. Med., *49*:395, 1956.

11. Bunch, W. H., Scarff, T. B., and Trimble, J.: Current concepts review—spinal cord monitoring. J. Bone Joint Surg., *65-A*:707, 1983.

12. Carcassonne, M., Gregoire, A., and Hornung, H.: Excision of the "free" hemivertebra: Preventive treatment of congenital scoliosis. Chirurgie, *103*:110, 1977.

13. Castroviejo, I. P., Rodriquez-Costa, T., and Costillo, F.: Spondylothoracic dysplasia in three sisters. Dev. Med. Child Neurol., *15*:348, 1973.

14. Compere, E. L.: Excision of hemivertebrae for correction of congenital scoliosis. Report of two cases. J. Bone Joint Surg., *14*:555, 1932.

15. Dewald, R. L., and Ray, R. D.: Skeletal traction for the treatment of severe scoliosis. J. Bone Joint Surg., *52-A*:233, 1970.

16. Dubousset, J.: Congenital kyphosis. *In* Bradford, D. S., and Hensinger, R. M. (eds.): Pediatric Spine. New York, Thieme-Stratton, 1985, pp. 196–217.

17. Dubousset, J., and Gonon, E. P.: Cyphoses et cyphoscolioses angulaires. Rev. Chir. Orthop., Suppl. II:69, 1983.

18. Dwyer, A. F., and Shafer, M. F.: Anterior approach to scoliosis. J. Bone Joint Surg., *56-B*:218, 1974.

19. Eelen, H., and Fabry, G.: Congenital scoliosis. A follow-up study. Acta Orthop. Belg., *43*:585, 1977.

20. Eisenstein, S., and O'Brien, J. P.: Chylothorax—a complication of Dwyer anterior instrumentation. Br. J. Surg., *64*:339, 1977.

21. Engler, G. L., Spielholtz, N. I., Bernhard, W. N., et al.: Somatosensory evoked potentials during Harrington instrumentation for scoliosis. J. Bone Joint Surg., *60-A*:520, 1978.

22. Faust, D., and Happel, L. T.: Cortical evoked potentials in spinal surgery. Orthopedics, 7:44, 1984.

23. Fishchenko, V. I., Uleshchenko, V. A., and Sokoliuk, A. M.: Functional indices of external respiration in congenital scoliosis. Ortop. Travmatol. Protez., 5:45, 1982.

24. Friedman, R. J., and Micheli, L. J.: Acquired spondylolisthesis following scoliosis surgery. Clin. Orthop., *180*:132, 1984.

25. Garrett, A. L., Perry, J., and Nickel, V. L.: Stabilization of the collapsing spine. J. Bone Joint Surg., *43-A*:474, 1961.

26. Gaubert, J., Regnier, C., Rochiccioli, P., Gaillard, J., Rolland, M., Bardier, M., and Panques, L. P.: Major aplasia of the thoracic wall and congenital thoracic scoliosis (3 observations). Chir. Pediatr., *22*:389, 1981.

27. Gillespie, R., Faithfull, D. K., Roth, A., and Hall, J. E.: Intraspinal anomalies in congenital scoliosis. Clin. Orthop., *93*:103, 1973.

28. Ginsburg, H., Shetter, A., and Raudzens, P.: Postoperative paraplegia with preserved intraoperative somatosensory evoked potentials. Orthop. Trans., 8:161, 1984.

29. Gotze, H. G.: Prognosis and therapy of the congenital scoliosis. Z. Orthop., *116*:258, 1978.

30. Grimer, R. J., Milligan, P. J., and Thompson, A. G.:

31. Thoracic outlet syndrome following correction of scoliosis in a patient with cervical ribs. J. Bone Joint Surg., *65-A*:1172, 1983.

31. Grundy, B. L., Nash, C. L., and Brown, R. H.: Anterior pressure manipulation alters spinal cord function during correction of scoliosis. Anaesthesiology, *54*:249, 1981.

32. Hall, J. E.: Congenital scoliosis. *In* Bradford, D. S., and Hensinger, R. M. (eds.): Pediatric Spine. New York, Thieme-Stratton, 1985.

33. Hall, J. E., Herndon, W. A., and Levine, C. R.: Surgical treatment of congenital scoliosis with or without Harrington instrumentation. J. Bone Joint Surg., *63-A*:608, 1981.

34. Hall, J. E., Levine, C. R., and Sudhir, K. G.: Intraoperative awakening to monitor spinal cord function during Harrington instrumentation and spine fusion. J. Bone Joint Surg., *60-A*:533, 1978.

35. Harrington, P. R.: Treatment of scoliosis. Correction and internal fixation by spine instrumentation. J. Bone Joint Surg., *44-A*:591, 1962.

36. Hathaway, G. L.: Congenital scoliosis in one of monozygotic twins: A case report. J. Bone Joint Surg., *59-A*:837, 1977.

37. Hoffman, H. J., Hendrick, E. B., and Humphreys, R. P.: The tethered spinal cord: Its protean manifestations, diagnosis, and surgical correction. Childs Brain, 2:145, 1976.

38. Hood, R. W., Riseborough, E. J., Nehme, A. M., Micheli, L. J., Strand, R. D., and Neuhauser, E. B. D.: Diastematomyelia and structural spinal deformities. J. Bone Joint Surg., *62-A*:520, 1980.

39. James, C. C. M., and Lassman, L. P.: Diastematomyelia and the tight filum terminale. J. Neurol. Sci., *10*:193, 1970.

40. James, J. I. P.: Paraplegia in congenital kypho-scoliosis. J. Bone Joint Surg., *57-B*:261, 1975.

41. Jarcho, S., and Levin, P. M.: Hereditary malformations of the vertebral bodies. Bull. Johns Hopkins Hosp., *62*:215, 1938.

42. Kahanovitz, N., Brown, J. C., and Bonnett, C. A.: The operative treatment of congenital scoliosis. A report of 23 patients. Clin. Orthop., *143*:174, 1979.

43. Kuhns, J. G., and Hormell, R. S.: Management of congenital scoliosis. Review of one hundred and seventy cases. Arch. Surg., *65*:250, 1952.

44. Langenskiöld, A.: Correction of congenital scoliosis by excision of one-half of a cleft vertebra. Acta Orthop. Scand., *38*:291, 1967.

45. Leatherman, K. D.: Altering the forces of growth in the developing spine. *In* Zorab, P. A., and Siegler, D. (eds.): Scoliosis, 1979. London, Academic, 1980, pp. 97–101.

46. Leatherman, K. D., and Dickson, R. A.: Two-stage correction surgery for congenital deformities of the spine. J. Bone Joint Surg., *61-B*:324, 1979.

47. Letts, R. M., and Bobechko, W. P.: Fusion of the scoliotic spine in young children. Effect on prognosis and growth. J. Bone Joint Surg., *56-B*:589, 1974.

48. Lonstein, J. E., Winter, R., Moe, J., et al.: Neurologic deficits secondary to spinal deformity: A review of the literature and report of 43 cases. Spine, 5:331, 1980.

49. MacEwen, G. D.: Congenital scoliosis with a unilateral bar. Radiology, *90*:711, 1968.

50. MacEwen, G. D., Conway, J. J., and Miller, W. T.: Congenital scoliosis with a unilateral bar. Radiology, *40*:711, 1968.

51. MacEwen, G. D., Winter, R. B., and Hardy, J. H.: Evaluation of kidney anomalies in congenital scoliosis. J. Bone Joint Surg., *54-A*:1341, 1972.

52. McKinley, L. M., and Leatherman, K. D.: Idiopathic and congenital scoliosis in twins. Spine, 3:227, 1978.

53. McMaster, M. J.: Occult intraspinal anomalies and congenital scoliosis. J. Bone Joint Surg., *66-A*:588, 1984.

54. McMaster, M. J., and Ohtsuka, K.: The natural history of congenital scoliosis. A study of two hundred and fifty-one patients. J. Bone Joint Surg., 64-A:1128, 1982.

55. Mensink, J. H. A., and Rogge, C. W. L.: Congenital scoliosis. Arch. Chir. Neerl., 26:109, 1974.

56. Morscher, E.: Experiences with the transthoracic hemilateral epiphyseodesis in the treatment of scoliosis. In Operative Treatment of Scoliosis, 1971 Symposium, Nijmegan. Stuttgart, Thieme, 1975, pp. 135–137.

57. Nasca, R. J., Stelling, F. H., and Steel, H. H.: Progression of congenital scoliosis due to hemivertebrae and hemivertebrae with bars. J. Bone Joint Surg., 57-A:456, 1975.

58. Nash, C. L., Lorig, R. A., Schatzinger, L. A., and Brown, R. H.: Spinal cord monitoring during operative treatment of the spine. Clin. Orthop., 126:100, 1977.

59. Ominus, M., and Michel, C. R.: Problèmes posés par la resection des hemivertèbres lombosacrées. Chir. Pediatr., 19:119, 1978.

60. Owen, R.: The association of axial skeleton defects with gastro-intestinal and genito-urinary abnormalities. In Zorab, P. A. (ed.): Scoliosis. London, Academic, 1977.

61. Peterson, H. A., and Peterson, L. F. A.: Hemivertebra in identical twins with dissimilar spinal columns. J. Bone Joint Surg., 49-A:938, 1967.

62. Rathke, W. F., and Sun, H. Y.: Untersuchungen über Missbildungsskoliosen. Z. Orthop., 97:173, 1963.

63. Rimoin, D. L., Fletcher, B. D., and McKusick, V. A.: Spondylocostal dysplasia. A dominantly inherited form of short trunked dwarfism. Am. J. Med., 45:948, 1968.

64. Roaf, R.: The late results of unilateral growth arrest of the spine for scoliosis. Acta Orthop. Scand., 33:393, 1963.

65. Roaf, R.: The treatment of progressive scoliosis by unilateral growth arrest. J. Bone Joint Surg., 45-B:637, 1963.

66. Royle, N. D.: The operative removal of an accessory vertebra. Med. J. Aust., 1:467, 1928.

67. Shands, A. R., Jr., and Bundens, W. D.: Congenital deformities of the spine. An analysis of the roentgenograms of 700 children. Bull. Hosp. Joint Dis., 17:110, 1956.

68. Shapiro, F., and Eyre, D.: Congenital scoliosis. A histopathologic study. Spine, 6:107, 1981.

69. Sodha, U.: Congenital scoliosis. Nurs. Times, 76:1524, 1980.

70. Stoll, J., and Bunch, W. H.: Segmental spinal instrumentation for congenital scoliosis. A report of two cases. Spine, 8:43, 1983.

71. Touzet, P. C.: Les scolioses des hemivertèbres simples: Classification, histoire naturelle, et elements de pronostic. Doctoral Thesis, Hôpital de Enfants Malades, Prof. A. P. Rigaut, Paris, 1980.

72. Tsou, P., Yau, A., and Hodgson, A.: Congenital spinal deformities: Natural history, classification, and the role of anterior surgery. J. Bone Joint Surg., 56-A:1767, 1974.

73. Ulrikh, E. V., and Bairov, G. A.: Wedge resection method in treating congenital scoliosis in young infants. Klin. Khir., 6:24, 1982.

74. Vauzelle, C., Stagnara, P., and Jouvinroux, P.: Functional monitoring of spinal cord activity during spinal surgery. Clin. Orthop., 93:173, 1973.

75. Von Lackum, H. L., and Smith, A. DeF.: Removal of vertebral bodies in the treatment of scoliosis. Surg. Gynecol. Obstet., 57:250, 1933.

76. Wiles, P.: Resection of dorsal vertebrae in congenital scoliosis. J. Bone Joint Surg., 33-A:151, 1951.

77. Winter, R. B.: The effects of early fusion on spine growth. In Zorab, P. A. (ed.): Scoliosis and Growth. Edinburgh, Churchill-Livingstone, 1971.

78. Winter, R. B.: Convex anterior and posterior hemiarthrodesis and hemiepiphyseodesis in young children with progressive congenital scoliosis. J. Pediatr. Orthop., 1:361, 1981.

79. Winter, R. B.: Congenital Deformities of the Spine. New York, Thieme-Stratton, 1983.

80. Winter, R. B., Haven, J. J., Moe, J. H., and LaGaard, S. M.: Diastematomyelia and congenital spine deformities. J. Bone Joint Surg., 56-A:27, 1974.

81. Winter, R. B., and Moe, J. H.: The results of spinal arthrodesis for congenital spinal deformity in patients younger than five years old. J. Bone Joint Surg., 64-A:419, 1982.

82. Winter, R. B., Moe, J. H., and Eilers, V. E.: Congenital scoliosis. A study of 234 patients treated and untreated. J. Bone Joint Surg., 50-A:1, 1968.

83. Winter, R. B., Moe, J. H., and Lonstein, J. E.: The incidence of Klippel-Feil syndrome in patients with congenital scoliosis and kyphosis. Spine, 9:363, 1984.

84. Winter, R. B., Moe, J. H., and Lonstein, J. E.: Posterior spinal arthrodesis for congenital scoliosis. An analysis of the cases of two hundred and ninety patients five to nineteen years old. J. Bone Joint Surg., 66-A:1118, 1984.

85. Winter, R. B., Moe, J. H., and Wang, J. F.: Congenital kyphosis. J. Bone Joint Surg., 55-A:223, 1973.

86. Winter, R. B., Moe, J. H., MacEwen, G. D., and Peon-Vidales, H.: The Milwaukee brace in the nonoperative treatment of congenital scoliosis. Spine, 1:85, 1976.

87. Wynne-Davies, R.: Congenital vertebral anomalies. Etiology and relationship to spina bifida cystica. J. Med. Genet., 12:280, 1975.

CONGENITAL KYPHOSIS

Congenital kyphosis is acute posterior angulation of the spine due to localized congenital malformation of the vertebrae. It must be distinguished from the developmental kyphosis associated with bone dysplasias such as Morquio's disease and gargoylism. Only true congenital kyphosis is considered in this section.

Classification

Congenital kyphosis may be caused by either failure of formation or a failure of segmentation of the vertebral body. In *Type I* (failure of formation) there is hypoplasia or aplasia of a part or the entire vertebral body. One, two, or even three vertebral bodies may be affected. Kyphosis develops with preservation of the posterior elements of the vertebra and absence or hypoplasia of the vertebral body. The degree of kyphosis varies; the greater the failure of formation and the more vertebral bodies involved, the greater the severity of the deformity. Anatomically, failure of formation may result in one of the following types: absence of the body of the vertebra, absence of the body of the vertebra associated with microspondyly of a neighboring vertebra, microspondyly of one vertebra, or microspondyly of two neighboring vertebrae (Fig. 6–17 A to D). In the radiogram an anteriorly wedged vertebra gives a butterfly appearance in the anteroposterior projection

(Fig. 6–17 G and H). An anteriorly wedged vertebral body may have a deficient corner posteriorly in the lateral view (Fig. 6–17 F).

In *Type II*, there is failure of segmentation of the anterior part of two or more adjacent vertebral bodies resulting in an anterior unsegmented bar (Fig. 6–17 E). The kyphosis progressively increases as the vertebrae grow posteriorly but not anteriorly. In addition to asymmetry of growth of the vertebral bodies, pathomechanical forces of the kyphosis exert increased pressure, erode vertebrae, and cause progression of the deformity.

In order to classify congenital kyphosis accurately linear tomography and computed axial tomography are often performed to delineate in detail bone and joint pathologic anatomy.

Clinical Picture

The most common site of kyphosis is between the tenth thoracic and the second lumbar vertebrae; it has, however, been observed anywhere between the fourth thoracic and fourth lumbar segments.

The kyphotic deformity is usually noticed in

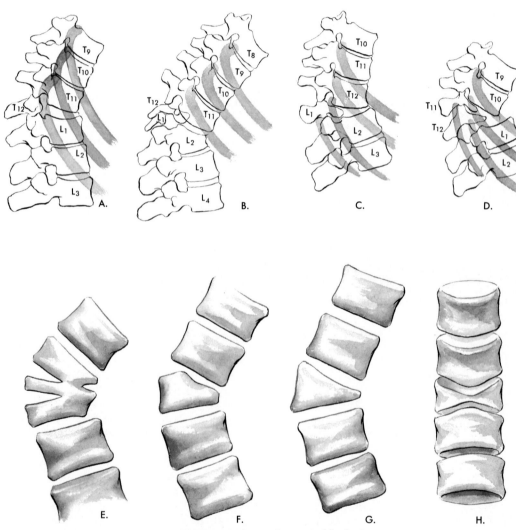

FIGURE 6–17. Types of congenital kyphosis.

A. Absence of the body of the vertebra (T12). **B.** Absence of the body of one vertebra (L1) and microspondyly of a neighboring vertebra (T12). Note that the pedicles are present. **C.** Microspondyly of one vertebra (L1). **D,** Microspondyly of two neighboring vertebrae (T11, T12). **E.** Type II congenital kyphosis due to failure of segmentation of the anterior part of three adjacent vertebrae. **F.** Absence of the superoposterior corner of a wedged vertebra. **G.** Wedged vertebra, lateral view. **H.** Wedged vertebra, anteroposterior view. Note its butterfly appearance. (Redrawn after Bingold, A.C.: Congenital kyphosis. J. Bone Joint Surg., 35-B:579, 1953.)

infancy and becomes more pronounced as the child starts to stand and walk (Fig. 6–18). With further growth of the spine the kyphosis usually increases. In children it is painless, and there is no local tenderness or muscle spasm; in the adult, however, pain may be a symptom when degenerative arthritic changes develop. Ordinarily, the total height of the patient is somewhat below normal.

Paraplegia due to compression of the spinal cord or cauda equina occurs frequently in congenital kyphosis. It is vital to perform sequential neurologic examinations. When neurologic deficit develops, magnetic resonance imaging of the entire spine is carried out. Myelography is performed as indicated. Paraplegia usually occurs during the adolescent growth spurt, but it may develop earlier. Paraplegia is common with anomalous vertebrae due to failure of formation (Type I) and very rare in deficits of segmentation (Type II).

Natural History

Congenital kyphosis tends to be relentlessly progressive when due to failure of formation (Type I), producing severe deformity and paraplegia, whereas kyphosis due to failure of segmentation is less progressive, produces mild or moderate deformity, and ordinarily does not cause paraplegia.

Clinically kyphosis due to anterior unsegmented bar when located in the thoracolumbar area (a common site) produces compensatory hyperlordosis below in the lumbar spine. Back pain develops because of the compensatory hyperlordosis and not because of the primary kyphosis.

Differential Diagnosis

When an infant or child presents with kyphosis, one should always rule out spinal cord tumor. Always perform a thorough neurologic evaluation! In the differential diagnosis one should consider tuberculous spondylitis and postirradiation or postlaminectomy kyphosis. Tuberculous spondylitis may be ruled out by a lack of systemic signs, a normal sedimentation rate, negative tuberculin skin tests, and the absence of bone or disc destruction, osteoporosis, and paravertebral abscess.

Treatment

The deformity cannot be corrected, and progression cannot be prevented by conservative measures. Nonoperative measures are ineffective. Treatment of congenital kyphosis is surgical; the timing and type of surgical procedure performed depend on the type of congenital kyphosis and its natural history, the severity of the deformity, and the age of the patient.

Anterior unsegmented bar is treated by simple local posterior spinal fusion if the degree of deformity is mild or moderate and of no clinical significance. The area of posterior fusion extends one vertebra proximal and one vertebra distal to the level of the unsegmented bar. Posterior spinal fusion will prevent further increase of the kyphosis; it will not, however, correct the degree of kyphosis. Ordinarily spinal instrumentation in the form of Harrington or Luque rods is not indicated when in-situ fusion is performed. The optimum age for a posterior fusion is between one and two years of age—definitely before three years of age.[38]

When the deformity is severe, *both anterior and posterior spinal fusions* are performed. Posterior fusion alone does not provide stability of the kyphotic spine where distraction forces are exerted on the posterior fusion mass. Pseudarthrosis develops, and the degree of kyphosis increases. As a rule, if the degree of kyphosis is over 50 to 60 degrees, the indication is for anterior fusion followed by posterior fusion that extends one level above and one level below the extent of the anterior fusion. With growth some degree of lordosis develops when the posterior fusion extent is greater than the anterior one.

Correction of severe kyphosis is indicated when it is severe and rigid. Before surgery a thorough neurologic examination should be performed, including computed axial tomography and magnetic resonance imaging. In the presence of paraparesis, spinal dysraphism should be ruled out. The site of cord compression should be determined. When there is no nerve tissue anomaly and no neurologic deficit, the first stage is osteotomy of the anterior unsegmented bar combined with disc excision and bone grafting. The second stage is posterior spinal fusion with Harrington compression rods, performed one to two weeks later. Between the two stages gentle skin traction may be applied for gradual correction of the kyphosis. Do not employ halo-femoral or halo-pelvic skeletal traction because of the high risk of paraplegia.

Treatment of Congenital Kyphosis Due to Defects of Formation. Early simple local posterior spinal fusion is paramount in this type of kyphosis because its natural history is one of steady progression into severe deformity and

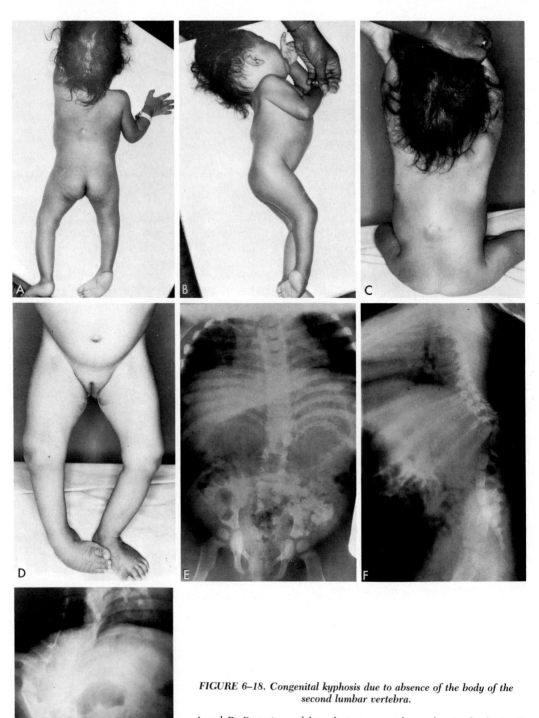

**FIGURE 6–18. Congenital kyphosis due to absence of the body of the
second lumbar vertebra.**

A and B. Posterior and lateral views, recumbent, showing kyphosis. C.
Sitting posterior view. D. Anterior view of lower limbs; note the talipes
equinovarus deformity of right foot. E and F. Anteroposterior and lateral
radiograms showing congenital absence of first lumbar vertebra. G. Oblique
lateral view one year postoperatively following local spinal fusion.

eventual paraplegia.[8] Perform posterior fusion between one and three years of age. Internal fixation by instrumentation is not necessary. Postoperatively the spine is supported in a hyperextension cast, a thoracolumbar underarm cast when the apex of the kyphosis is between T-10 and L-2, and a cervicothoracolumbar cast (full Risser including the neck) for thoracic kyphosis. The period of immobilization in the cast is six months. The cast is changed at intervals when soiled or when the child outgrows it. This is followed by support in a thoracolumbosacral orthosis (TLSO) for another six months. If pseudarthrosis develops it is repaired and reinforced with a bone graft. It is best not to perform anterior fusion in these young children because, with anterior vertebral growth and surgical cessation of posterior spinal growth, the angle of kyphosis gradually and steadily decreases.[38] Anterior spinal fusion will stop anterior vertebral growth and prevent this progressive correction of the kyphosis.

Anterior and posterior spinal fusions are indicated when the degree of kyphosis is greater than 55 degrees.[39] Both anterior and posterior fusions are indicated in the adult who requires surgical treatment regardless of the degree of kyphosis. The first step is the anterior procedure, releasing all anterior tethering structures, i.e., the thick contracted anterior longitudinal ligament, the annulus fibrosus, and vestigial cartilaginous tissues. These structures are thoroughly excised across right to left and all the way to the posterior annulus. The kyphosis is corrected with an anterior distractor if indicated and safe; next, autogenous bone grafts consisting of fibula and rib are utilized to maintain the correction. The second step is posterior spinal fusion with autogenous iliac bone grafting and fixation with internal instrumentation, consisting of Harrington compression or Luque rods.

When there is paraplegia, in addition to computed axial tomography and magnetic resonance studies, a myelogram should be performed to delineate the exact site of cord compression. In some cases, correction of the kyphosis removes the pressure from the cord, thus eliminating the necessity for exposure of the dura.[20] In severe cases a thorough anterior cord decompression is performed, followed by anterior and posterior spinal fusions.

The importance of early surgery by local posterior spinal fusion to prevent severe kyphosis and paraplegia cannot be overemphasized.

References

1. Adams, J. C.: Techniques, dangers and safeguards in osteotomy of the spine. J. Bone Joint Surg., *34-B*:226, 1952.
2. Adelstein, L. J.: Spinal extradural cyst associated with kyphosis dorsalis juvenilis. J. Bone Joint Surg., *23-A*:93, 1941.
3. Bingold, A. C.: Congenital kyphosis. J. Bone Joint Surg., *35-B*:579, 1953.
4. Bjerkreim, I., Magnaes, B., and Semb, G.: Surgical treatment of severe angular kyphosis. Acta Orthop. Scand., *53*:913, 1982.
5. Bradford, D. S., Ganjavian, S., Antonious, D., Winter, R. B., Lonstein, J. E., and Moe, J. H.: Anterior strut grafting for the treatment of kyphosis. J. Bone Joint Surg., *64-A*:680, 1982.
6. Chou, S. N.: The treatment of paralysis associated with kyphosis: Role of anterior decompression. Clin. Orthop., *128*:149, 1977.
7. Dubousset, J.: Congenital kyphosis. *In* Bradford, D. S., and Hensinger, R. M. (eds.): Pediatric Spine. New York, Thieme-Stratton, 1985.
8. Dubousset, J., and Gonon, E. P.: Cyphoses et cyphoscolioses angulaires. Rev. Cir. Orthop., Suppl. II:69, 1983.
9. Eisberg, C. A., Dike, C. G., and Brewer, E. D.: The symptoms and diagnosis of extradural cysts. Bull. Neurol. Inst., *3*:395, 1934.
10. Hallock, H., Francis, K. D., and Jones, J. B.: Spine fusion in young children. A long-term end-result study with particular reference to growth effects. J. Bone Joint Surg., *39-A*:481, 1957.
11. Herbert, J. J.: Ostéotomie pour cyphose congénitale. Rev. Chir. Orthop., *37*:506, 1951.
12. Hodgson, A. R., and Stock, F. E.: Anterior spine fusion. Br. J. Surg., *48*:172, 1960.
13. James, J. I. P.: Paraplegia in congenital kyphoscoliosis. J. Bone Joint Surg., *57-B*:261, 1975.
14. Kharrat, K., and Dubousset, J.: Bloc vertébral antérieur progressif chez l'enfant. Rev. Chir. Orthop., *66*:485, 1980.
15. Leatherman, K. D., and Dickson, R. A.: Congenital kyphosis in myelomeningocele. Vertebral body resection and posterior spine fusion. Spine, *3*:22, 1978.
16. Leatherman, K. D., and Dickson, R. A.: Two-stage corrective surgery for congenital deformities of the spine. J. Bone Joint Surg., *61-B*:324, 1979.
17. Lerner, D. J., and Riley, G.: Congenital kyphoscoliosis in a foal. J. Am. Vet. Med. Assoc., *172*:274, 1978.
18. Lindemann, K.: Zur Kasuistik der angeborenen Kyphosen. Arch. Orthop. Unfallchir., *30*:27, 1931.
19. Lombard, P., and Le Genissel: Cyphoses congénitales. Rev. Orthop., *25*:532, 1938.
20. Lonstein, J. E., Winter, R. B., Moe, J. H., Bradford, D. S., Chou, S. N., and Pinto, W.: Neurologic deficits secondary to spinal deformity, a review of the literature and report of 43 cases. Spine, *5*:331, 1980.
21. Lorenzo, R. L., Hungerford, G. D., Blumenthal, B. I., Bradford, B. F., Sanchez, F., and Haranath, B. S.: Congenital kyphosis and subluxation of the thoracolumbar spine due to vertebral aplasia. Skeletal Radiol., *10*:255, 1983.
22. Matthuas, H.: Treatment of congenital lumbar kyphosis. Z. Orthop., *112*:1312, 1974.
23. Mayfield, J. K., Winter, R. B., Bradford, D. S., and Moe, J. H.: Congenital kyphosis due to defects of anterior segmentation. J. Bone Joint Surg., *62-A*:129, 1980.
24. Montgomery, S. P., and Hall, J. E.: Congenital kyphosis. Spine, *7*:360, 1982.
25. Muller, W.: Die angeborene Gibbusbildung mit Wirbelkorrperspaltung an der unteren Brustwirbelsaule. Arch. Orthop. Unfallchir., *30*:319, 1931.
26. Nogami, H., Terashima, Y., Tamaki, K., and Oohira, A.: Congenital kyphoscoliosis and spinal cord lesion produced in the rat by beta-aminopropionitrile. Teratology, *16*:351, 1977.

27. Pinto, W. C., Avanzi, O., and Winter, R. B.: An anterior distractor for the intraoperative correction of angular kyphosis. Spine, 3:309, 1978.
28. Rivard, C. H., Nairbaitz, and Vithoff, H. K.: Congenital vertebral malformation. Orthop. Rev., 8:135, 1979.
29. Roaf, R.: Vertebral growth and its mechanical control. J. Bone Joint Surg., 42-B:40, 1960.
30. Schapira, C.: Su alcune forme rare di malformazioni congenite del rachide (sinostosi vertebrali-cifosi congenite). Chir. Organi Mov., 22:39, 1936.
31. Tsou, P. M.: Embryology of congenital kyphosis. Chir. Orthop., 128:18, 1977.
32. Tsou, P., Yau, A., and Hodgson, A.: Congenital spinal deformities: Natural history, classification, and the role of anterior surgery. J. Bone Joint Surg., 56-A:1767, 1974.
33. Van Assen, J.: Angeborene Kyphose. Acta Chir. Scand., 67:14, 1930.
34. White, A. A., Punjabi, M. M., and Thomas, C. L.: The clinical biomechanics of kyphotic deformities. Clin. Orthop., 128:8, 1977.
35. Winter, R. B.: Congenital kyphoscoliosis with paralysis following hemivertebra excision. Clin. Orthop., 119:116, 1976.
36. Winter, R. B.: Congenital kyphosis. Clin. Orthop., 128:26, 1977.
37. Winter, R. B.: Congenital deformities of the spine. New York, Thieme-Stratton, 1983.
38. Winter, R. B., and Moe, J. H.: The results of spinal arthrodesis for congenital spine deformity in patients younger than 5 years old. J. Bone Joint Surg., 64-A:419, 1982.
39. Winter, R. B., Moe, J. H., and Lonstein, J. E.: The incidence of Klippel-Feil syndrome in patients with congenital scoliosis and kyphosis. Spine, 9:363, 1984.
40. Winter, R. B., Moe, J. H., and Wang, J. F.: Congenital kyphosis. J. Bone Joint Surg., 55-A:223, 1973.

CONGENITAL ABSENCE OF THE SACRUM AND LUMBOSACRAL VERTEBRAE (LUMBOSACRAL AGENESIS)

Lumbosacral agenesis is a severe axial skeletal and neural deficiency characterized by absence of variable amounts of the sacrum and lumbar spine and associated neural elements. There are concomitant anomalies of the viscera, particularly of the genitourinary and lower gastrointestinal systems, with resultant impairment of bladder and bowel function.

The failure of development ranges from mere absence of the lower coccygeal segment to complete aplasia of vertebrae below the twelfth thoracic segment. The lesser degrees of involvement, such as absence of the lower coccygeal segments, often go unnoticed and are usually recognized fortuitously during unrelated radiographic studies, whereas the more extreme degrees of involvement may be incompatible with life and have been described in reports on stillbirths.

The first known case was described by Hohl in 1852, and since then a number of review articles and case reports have appeared in the literature.[1-74] Because of the wide range of possible vertebral anomalies, the recorded case presentations do not precisely depict the true incidence of the condition.

Etiology

In the human embryo, differentiation of the lumbar spine, sacrum, and coccyx occurs between the fourth and seventh postovulatory weeks. Duraiswami, in his study of insulin-induced skeletal abnormalities in developing chickens, found that vertebral changes often resulted from insulin injections made in the first two days of incubation, whereas other skeletal aberrations resulted from later injections, indicating that the part most affected was that which was in the most active stage of development or differentiation.[16] The noxious agent must exert its influence early in embryonic development if it is to cause congenital absence of the lumbosacral spine.

A higher than normal incidence of diabetes mellitus and spontaneous abortions among women having offspring with congenital absence of the sacrum is reported by Blumel and associates.[10]

Freedman suggested the theory of failure of provocative mechanisms during early embryonic differentiation.[25] Detwiler and Holtzer presented evidence of inductive and formative influence of the spinal cord upon the vertebral column.[13] Animal experiments have shown that many defects of the nervous system can result from a failure of inductive interaction between the presumptive notochord and neural ectoderm during very early embryonic stages.[28] One may attribute this failure to a genetically determined exaggeration of the pattern of ontogenic cellular death in mesodermal and neural elements of the posterior body regions.[59]

As to the importance of inheritable genetic factors, a single instance of congenital absence of the sacrum occurring in father and son was reported by Pouzet in 1938.[53] Absence of the rump in fowl, closely resembling similar human disorders, has been known for centuries. In fowls, the anomaly occurs as a hereditary anomaly as well as spontaneously as a mutation.[14, 15]

Pathologic Findings

The gross and histologic findings depend on the level of the lesion. In total absence of the lumbosacral spine, normal muscle tissue is replaced by large globules of soft, deep, yellow fat. Tendons are found as thin filaments, but have normal configuration. There is an abnormal nerve root pattern at the end of the spinal cord. Femoral vessels are very small. Femoral nerves are represented as gross fatty tissue adjacent to the small vessels. Afferent tracts are usually fairly well preserved, whereas efferent motor neuron pathways are impaired or missing.[62] The spinal cord does not disclose any lumbar enlargement or lumbosacral plexus, and terminates at a higher level than usual, for example, at the seventh thoracic vertebra when the vertebral column ends at the second lumbar segment; otherwise the anatomy of the spinal cord is normal above the lesion.

Classification

Lumbosacral agenesis, according to Renshaw, can be classified into four types.

Type I is either total or partial unilateral sacral agenesis (Fig. 6–19). *Type II* is partial sacral agenesis with a partial but bilaterally symmetrical defect and a stable articulation between the ilia and a normal or hypoplastic first sacral vertebra (Fig. 6–20). This is the most common type. *Type III* is variable lumbar and total sacral agenesis, with the ilia articulating with the sides of the lowest vertebra present (Fig. 6–21). *Type IV* is variable lumbar and total sacral agenesis, the caudal end-plate of the lowest vertebra resting above either fused ilia or an iliac amphiarthrosis (Fig. 6–22).

Clinical Picture

The appearance of the patient depends on the extent of spinal involvement and on the degree of concomitant neurologic deficit.

Type I. In total or partial unilateral sacral agenesis the pelvic ring and lumbosacral junction are intact; therefore, the vertebropelvic articulation is usually, but not always, stable. The unilateral absence of the sacrum results in an oblique lumbosacral joint and lumbar scoliosis. The scoliosis ordinarily is not progressive and does not require orthotic or surgical treatment. Hips and knees are usually normal; there may, however, be a calcaneovarus deformity of the foot. There is sensory loss corresponding to the distribution of the involved sacral roots.

Type II. The vertebropelvic junction is stable unless there is associated myelomeningocele. Some of the cases with associated myelomeningocele develop progressive kyphosis and paralytic scoliosis requiring surgical stabilization to facilitate sitting. There may be associated congenital anomalies of the spine (such as hemi-

vertebrae), which may cause progressive congenital scoliosis and require treatment by spinal fusion. There may be associated rib anomalies in the form of fusion of adjacent ribs or absence of ribs.

Motor paralysis is present; it corresponds within one level with the vertebral defect. *Sensation* is usually intact. There may be anesthesia at S-4 and distally. In those patients with associated myelomeningocele the level of paralysis may be higher than the level of vertebral deficit, and the sensory loss more extreme. *Hip dislocation* occurs in Type II and may be unilateral or bilateral. The pathogenesis of dislocation appears to be dynamic imbalance of muscles controlling the hip—absence or weakness of hip abductors-extensors versus normal motor strength of hip adductors-flexors. Foot deformities and flexion deformity of the knee are usually not marked. Most patients with Type II lumbosacral agenesis are ambulatory.

Type III. The lumbopelvic junction is relatively stable in this third type with entire absence of the sacrum and, in some, absence of the fifth lumbar vertebra. Progressive kyphosis and scoliosis may develop in these patients, particularly when there is associated myelomeningocele. The level of motor paralysis parallels the level of vertebral deficit within one segment. Sensation is intact at least down to the fourth sacral nerve root level. In total absence of the sacrum, the buttocks are flattened, the intergluteal cleft is shortened, and there is dimpling of each buttock lateral to the cleft. The normal posterior convexity of the sacrococcygeal region is lost; on rectal examination the concavity of the sacrum and coccyx is absent. Hip dislocation, knee contracture, and foot deformity are common in Type III and require treatment. Type III patients are unable to stand and walk without appropriate orthotic support or crutches (Fig. 6–23).

Type IV. In complete absence of the lumbar spine and sacrum, the patients are of short stature, having a characteristic cross-legged Buddha-like attitude (Fig. 6–24). The twelfth thoracic vertebra is dorsally prominent. There is marked disproportion between the thorax and the pelvis. The narrow, flat buttocks manifest a depressed dimpling 2 or 3 inches lateral to the gluteal cleft. The normal convexity of the sacrococcygeal region is lost, and the anus is horizontal. The pelvis is very unstable under the spine—it tends to roll up under the thorax and drops forward, seeming to rest anterior to the thoracic spine, where the patient tries to sit unsupported and is forced to support himself

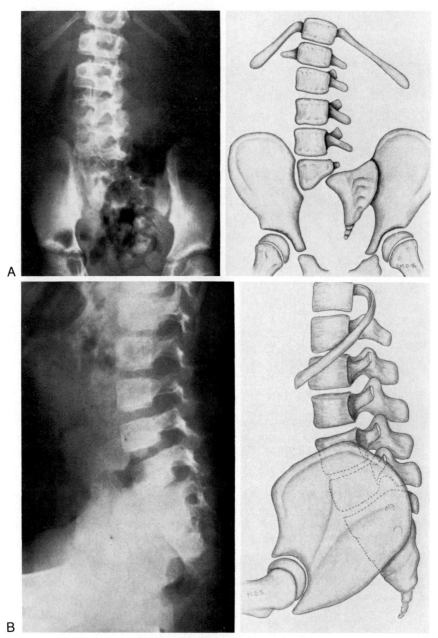

FIGURE 6–19. *Type I lumbosacral agenesis.*

Note the absence of the right hemisacrum. **A.** Anterior posterior radiogram and corresponding line drawing. **B.** Lateral radiogram of lumbosacral spine and corresponding line drawing. (From Renshaw, T.S.: Sacral agenesis. J. Bone Joint Surg., *60-A*:373, 1978. Reprinted by permission.)

on his hands. In the occasional case in which there is also absence of the twelfth thoracic vertebra, the opposing ribs articulate in the midline posteriorly. Almost all patients with Type IV lumbosacral agenesis develop progressive spinopelvic kyphosis and scoliosis; they do require stabilization of the spine by spinal fusion.

The hips have severe flexion (80 to 110 de-

grees) and abduction contracture. They may be dislocated but in most cases are not. The knees show 60 to 90 degrees of flexion contracture with large popliteal webs and heavily callused knee pads. Fixed calcaneus deformities of the feet are present.

There is muscle paralysis and atrophy of the lower limbs that is complete at and below the knees, with no voluntary or involuntary motor

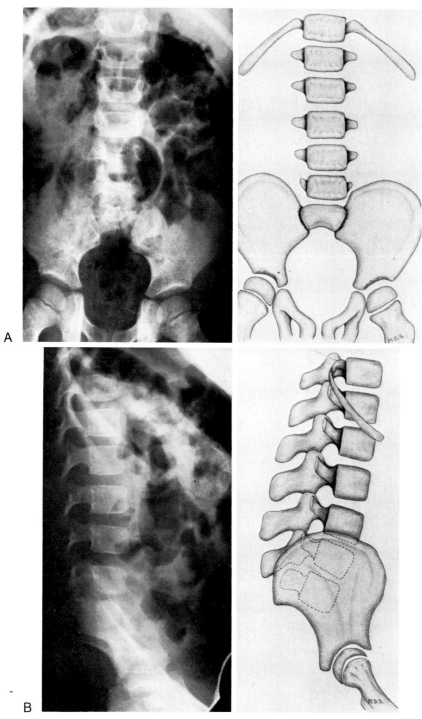

FIGURE 6–20. *Type II lumbosacral agenesis.*

Note the absence of the sacrum, with a hypoplastic first sacral vertebra providing a stable lumbopelvic articulation. **A.** Anterior posterior radiogram with corresponding line drawing. **B.** Lateral radiogram with corresponding line drawing. (From Renshaw, T.S.: Sacral agenesis. J. Bone Joint Surg., *60-A*:373, 1978. Reprinted by permission.)

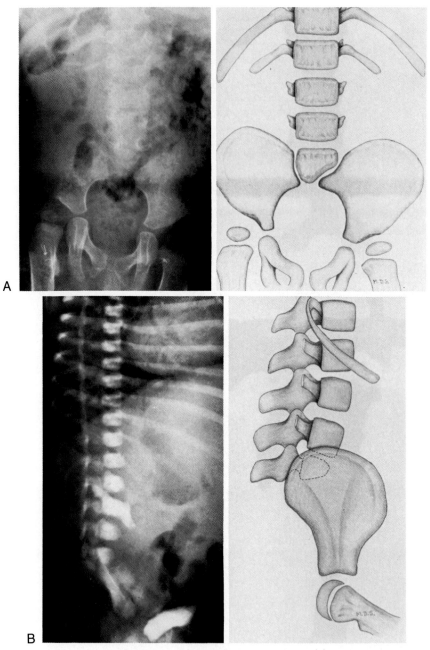

FIGURE 6–21. Type III lumbosacral agenesis.

Note the absence of the fifth and fourth lumbar vertebrae and the sacrum and coccyx. The sides of the third lumbar vertebrae are articulating in the ilia. **A.** Anterior posterior radiogram with corresponding line drawing. **B.** Lateral radiogram with corresponding line drawing. (From Renshaw, T.S.: Sacral agenesis. J. Bone Joint Surg., *60-A*:373, 1978. Reprinted by permission.)

or reflex movement. Because of marked muscle atrophy, the lower half of the body develops a cone-shaped appearance. In the very extreme case, a "mermaid" configuration develops that has merited the designation of "siren."

Sensation is usually normal down to the knees. Distally, there may be spotty areas of hypesthesia or anesthesia. Trophic changes are absent. The patients have no bladder or bowel control.

The severe pelvic outlet deformity may obstruct the lower intestinal tract, requiring co-

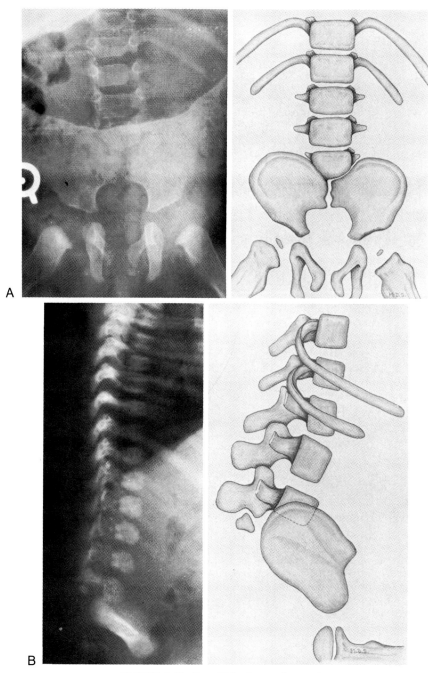

FIGURE 6–22. *Type IV lumbosacral agenesis.*

A. Anterior posterior radiogram with corresponding line drawing. **B.** Lateral radiogram with corresponding line drawing. (From Renshaw, T.S.: Sacral agenesis. J. Bone Joint Surg., 6-A:373, 1978. Reprinted with permission.)

lostomy (Fig. 6–25). In order to ambulate, Type IV patients require spinopelvic stabilization or extensive orthotic support.

Radiographic Findings

The rib cage is normal except for the absence of ribs or the fusion of adjacent ribs. In the thoracic and upper lumbar spine there may be hemivertebrae or segmental defects that may cause scoliosis or kyphosis or both. In total absence of the lumbosacral spine the twelfth thoracic vertebra is the most distal segment. The sacrum and coccyx are absent (see Fig. 6–24 I to K). The pelvis is narrow, with the ilia

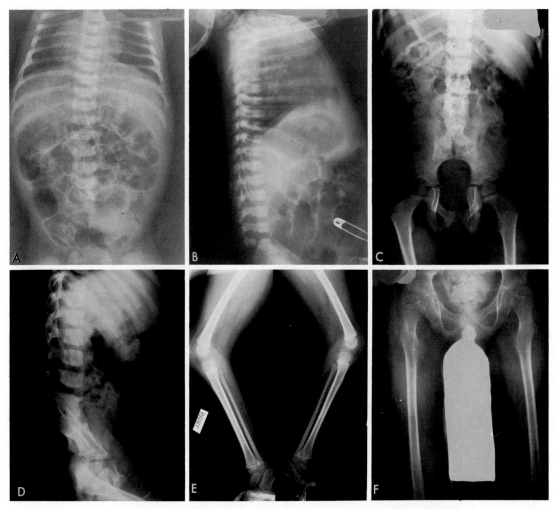

FIGURE 6–23. Congenital absence of sacrum and coccyx—Type III lumbosacral agensis.

A and **B.** Anteroposterior and lateral radiograms of the spine at birth. Note the absence of the sacrum and coccyx. **C** and **D.** Anteroposterior and lateral radiograms of the spine at three years of age. **E.** Lateral radiograms of the lower limbs, showing normally developed bones. There is 35 degrees of flexion deformity of the knees. **F.** Anteroposterior radiogram of the hips and femora at seven years of age. Note the severe coxa valga and subluxation of the hips. At this time bilateral varization osteotomy of the proximal femora was performed to correct the coxa valga deformity.

articulating amphiarthrodially. The femora and tibiae are atrophic but normally formed. The femoral heads may be well seated in normal acetabuli, or the hip joints may be dislocated. The knee joints are well defined, but are held in 45 to 90 degrees of flexion (Fig. 6–24 L and M). The feet and ankles exhibit calcaneus deformity. All patients with lumbosacral agenesis should have an intravenous pyelogram and other appropriate diagnostic tests to rule out associated anomalies of the genitourinary tract.

Treatment

Reconstruction of the lower limbs in total absence of the lumbosacral spine (Type IV) has

not been successful because of the absence of muscle fibers and major motor nerves.[62]

Russell and Aitken and Frantz and Aitken have reported the results of treatment by bilateral subtrochanteric amputation and fitting with a pelvic-thoracic bucket and Canadian hip disarticulation prosthesis. These patients were able to be partially self-sufficient and to walk with the swing-to or swing-through gait, as performed by paraplegics.[24, 62]

The one major problem that has not been dealt with in this procedure is that of spinopelvic instability. As long as this defect remains uncorrected, the patient is neither able to sit unsupported nor to ambulate without the aid of a cumbersome pelvic-thoracic bucket.

With increasing age and body mass Type IV

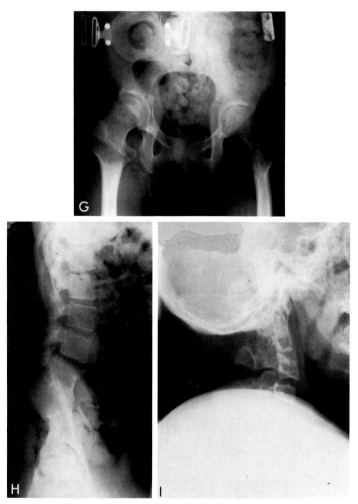

FIGURE 6-23 Continued. *Congenital absence of sacrum and coccyx.*

G. Postoperative radiograms of the hips. The femoral heads are well seated in the acetabula, and the coxa valga deformity is corrected. **H.** Lateral radiogram of the lumbosacral spine at age 17 years. Note the spur at the superior-anterior margin of the fifth lumbar vertebra. **I.** Lateral radiogram of cervical spine, showing congenital fusion of upper five cervical vertebrae (Klippel-Feil).

Illustration continued on following page

and some Type III patients develop severe spinopelvic kyphosis and require stabilization of the spine. Furthermore, orthotic devices extending proximally to the thoracic spine cause ureteral compression and severe hydrone-phrosis. Pelvicospinal stabilization by spinal fusion enables these patients to sit up unsupported and ambulate with knee-ankle-foot orthoses or prosthetic devices. The decision to be made is whether knee disarticulation should be performed and autogenous tibiae used for spinal fusion or allografts be used and the limbs

salvaged. Factors to be considered are the severity of the knee flexion and foot deformity and the desire and motivation of the patient. Knee disarticulation is a simple solution to the problem—such an illustrative case with the operative findings and preoperative and post-operative photographs is shown in Figure 6–24.

Often the knee flexion and foot deformities are corrected by surgical releases at an early age. A plantigrade foot can be provided for weight-bearing with orthotic support. The prob-

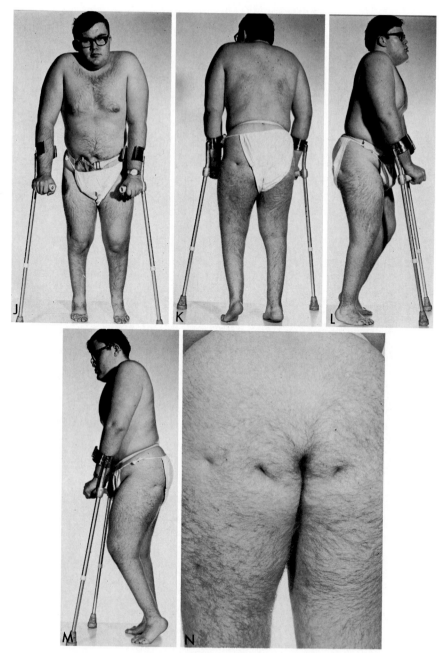

FIGURE 6–23 Continued. *Congenital absence of sacrum and coccyx.*

J to M. Clinical appearance of patient. He is able to walk with crutches. N. Close view of buttocks showing the gluteal dimples.

lem is recurrence of knee flexion deformity. These joints have been immobile in fetal life because of motor paralysis; the intra-articular and periarticular fibrosis is similar to that of arthrogryposis. The only difference is that in congenital absence of the lumbosacral spine the muscles are not as fibrotic as in arthrogryposis. This author recommends the intermittent part-

time use of continuous passive motion of the knees during the day and night-splinting to prevent recurrence of knee flexion deformity and to maintain functional range of knee flexion for sitting and other activities of daily living. Hip flexion deformity is treated by extension osteotomy of the proximal femur (Fig. 6–26).

With the motor paralysis the lower limbs will

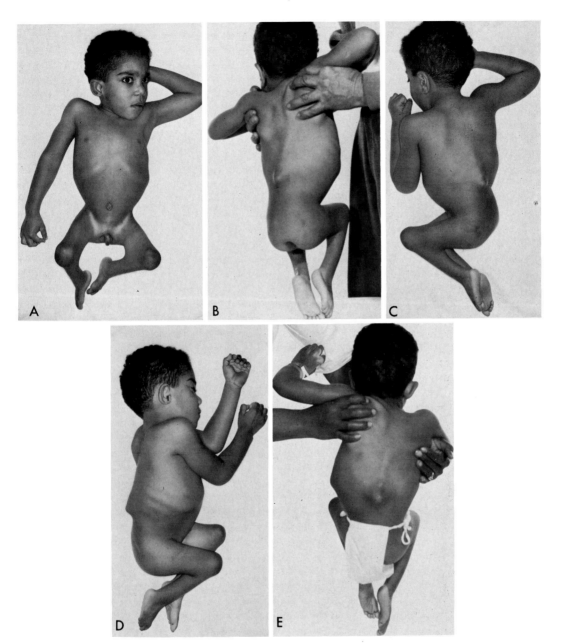

FIGURE 6–24. Congenital absence of the lumbosacral spine in a six-year-old child.

A to **E.** Clinical appearance of patient in the front, right and left oblique, lateral, and back views.

Illustration continued on following page

be short—the parents should understand that the end result at skeletal maturity will be disproportionate stature with short lower limbs.

Enlargement of the pelvic outlet may be necessary when the lower intestinal tract is obstructed; this is performed in collaboration with a pediatric surgeon.

The neuromuscular deficit is less in congenital absence of the sacrum and coccyx—Types I and II. These patients have spinopelvic stability; they can sit and walk. The foot and knee deformities should be corrected. Ankle-foot or-

thoses are provided as necessary. Crutches may be necessary for ambulation in Type II defects.

References

1. Abraham, E.: Lumbosacral coccygeal agenesis. Autopsy case report. J. Bone Joint Surg., 58-A:1169, 1976.
2. Abraham, E.: Sacral agenesis with associated anomalies (caudal regression syndrome): Autopsy case report. Clin. Orthop., 145:168, 1979.
3. Aitken, G. T., and Frantz, C. H.: Management of the child amputee. A.A.O.S. Instr. Course Lect., 17:246, 1960.

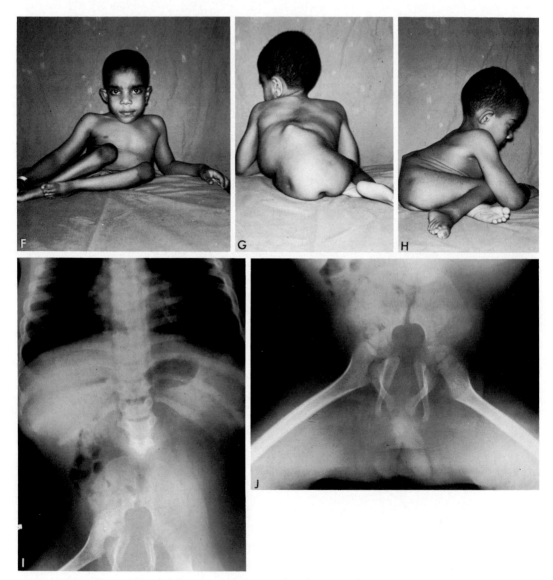

***FIGURE 6–24* Continued.** *Congenital absence of the lumbosacral spine in a six-year-old child.*

F to **H.** Note the sitting posture. He has to support himself on his hands. The pelvis seems to roll up under the thorax. **I** and **J.** Anteroposterior radiogram of the spine (**I**) and pelvis (**J**). Note the absence of sacrum, coccyx, and distal three lumbar vertebrae. The second lumbar vertebra is the most distal segment present. The pelvis is narrow, with the ilia articulating amphiarthrodially. The hips are dislocated.

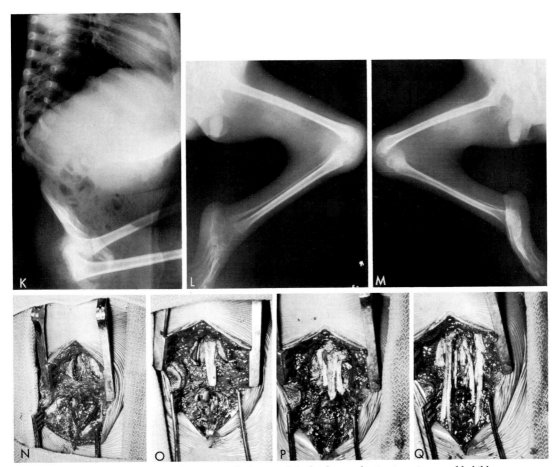

FIGURE 6–24 Continued. *Congenital absence of the lumbosacral spine in a six-year-old child.*

K. Lateral radiogram of the spine. **L** and **M.** Lateral radiograms of the lower extremities. Note the atrophy of the femora and tibiae. The knee joints are well formed but held in 120 degrees of flexion. **N.** Pathologic findings at operation. Note the absence of the spinal cord. There is no evidence of the lumbosacral plexus. **O.** The tibia of the patient's own amputated leg is used to stabilize the spine by grafting from the second lumbar vertebra to the pelvis. **P** and **Q.** Reinforcement of fusion by addition of large matchsticks of autogenous tibial graft.

Illustration continued on following page

4. Anderton, J. M., and Owens, R.: Absence of the pituitary gland in a case of congenital sacral agenesis. J. Bone Joint Surg., 65-B:182, 1983.
5. Andrish, J., Kalamchi, A., and MacEwen, G. D.: Sacral agenesis: A clinical evaluation of its management, heredity, and associated anomalies. Clin. Orthop., 139:52, 1979.
6. Araujo, A.: Distrofia cruro-vesico-glutea por agenesia total do sacro-coccyx. Arq. Bras. Cir. Ortop., 4:43, 1936.
7. Balinsky, B. I.: An Introduction to Embryology. 3rd Ed. Philadelphia, Saunders, 1970, p. 427.
8. Banta, J. V., and Nichols, O.: Sacral agenesis. J. Bone Joint Surg., 51-A:693, 1969.
9. Blumel, J., Butler, M. C., Evans, E. B., and Eggers, G. W. N.: Congenital anomaly of the saccrococcygeal spine. Report of eight cases of absence or malformation. Arch. Surg., 85:982, 1962.
10. Blumel, J., Evans, E. B., and Eggers, G. W. N.: Partial and complete agenesis or malformation of the sacrum with associated anomalies. J. Bone Joint Surg., 41-A:497, 1959.
11. Cohn, J., and Bay-Nielsen, E.: Hereditary defect of

the sacrum and coccyx with anterior sacral meningocele. Acta Paediatr. Scand., 58:268, 1969.
12. Cotel, Y., and Banai, M.: Congenital absence of the lumbar articular facets. Apropos of 2 cases. Rev. Chir. Orthop., 62:731, 1976.
13. Detwiler, S. R., and Holtzer, H.: The inductive and formative influence of the spinal cord upon the vertebral column. Bull. Hosp. Joint Dis., 15:114, 1954.
14. Dunn, L. C.: The inheritance of rumplessness in domestic fowl. J. Hered., 16:127, 1925.
15. Dunn, L. C., and Landauer, W.: The genetics of the rumpless fowl with evidence of a case of changing dominance. J. Genet., 29:217, 1934.
16. Duraiswami, P. K.: Insulin-induced skeletal abnormalities in developing chickens. Br. Med. J., 2:384, 1950.
17. Duraiswami, P. K.: Experimental causation of congenital skeletal defects and its significance in orthopaedic surgery. J. Bone Joint Surg., 34-B:646, 1952.
18. Elting, J. J., and Allen, J. C.: Management of the young child with bilateral anomalous and functionless lower extremities. J. Bone Joint Surg., 54-A:1523, 1972.
19. Feller, A., and Sternberg, H.: Zur Kenntnis der Fehlbildungen der Wirbesaule. III Mitteilung. Über den vollständigen Mangel der unteren Wirbelsaulenabschn-

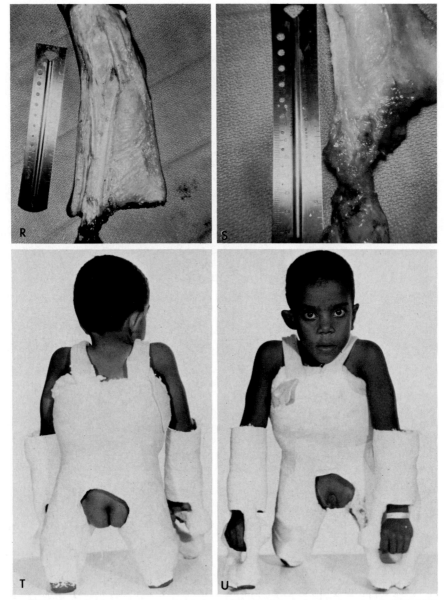

FIGURE 6–24 *Continued. Congenital absence of the lumbosacral spine in a six-year-old child.*

R and **S.** Gross appearance of the amputated legs. Normal muscle tissue is replaced by large globules of soft deep yellow fat. Tendons are thin filaments, and the vessels very small. **T** and **U.** Hip-body spica cast with especially made short cast crutches for ambulation in the immediate postoperative period.

itte und seine Bedeutung fur die formale Genese der Defektbildungen des hinteren Korperendes. Virchow. Arch. Pathol. Anat., *280*:649, 1931.

20. Fields, G. A., Schwarz, R. H., Dickens, H. O., and Tunnessen, W.: Sacral agenesis in the infant of a gestational diabetic. Surg. Gynecol. Obstet., *32*:778, 1968.

21. Fitch, R. R.: Congenital absence of vertebrae below the first sacral and malformation of the lower cervical and upper dorsal vertebrae. Am. Orthop. Surg., *7*:540, 1910.

22. Foix, C., and Hillemand, P.: Dystrophie cruro-vesico-fessière par agenesie sacro-coccygienne. Rev. Neurol., *40*:450, 1924.

23. Frantz, C. H.: Complete absence of the lumbar spine and sacrum. *In* Selected Lower Limb Anomalies: A

Symposium. Washington, D.C., National Academy of Sciences, 1971, pp. 29–48.

24. Frantz, C. H., and Aitken, G. T.: Complete absence of the lumbar spine and sacrum. J. Bone Joint Surg., *49-A*:1531, 1967.

25. Freedman, B.: Congenital absence of the sacrum and coccyx. Report of a case and review of the literature. Br. J. Surg., *37*:299, 1950.

26. Friedel, G.: Defekt der Wirbelsaule vom 10. Brustwirbel an abwärts bei einem Neugeborenen. Arch. Klin. Chir., *93*:944, 1910.

27. Fucera, J.: Exposure to fat solvents: A possible cause of sacral agenesis in man. J. Pediatr., *72*:857, 1968.

28. Gruneberg, H.: The Pathology of Development. Oxford, Blackwell, 1963.

29. Handelsman, J. E.: Lumbosacral Agenesis. Proc. 12th

Text continued on page 2229

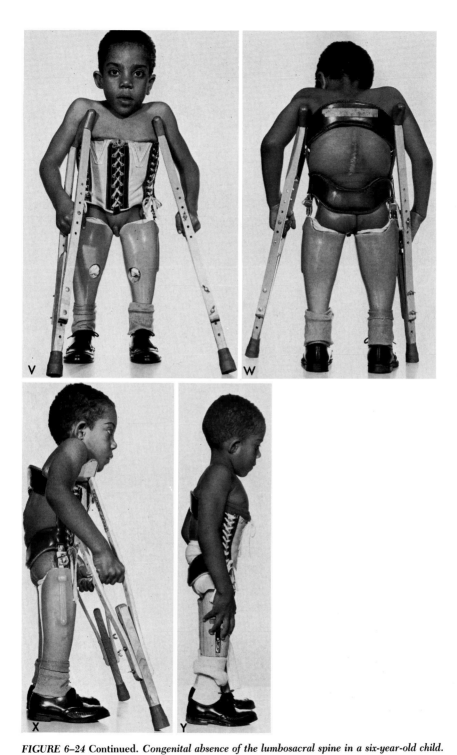

FIGURE 6–24 Continued. *Congenital absence of the lumbosacral spine in a six-year-old child.*

V to Y. Patient is able to walk with his prosthetic limbs and spinal brace. He even can stand without support.

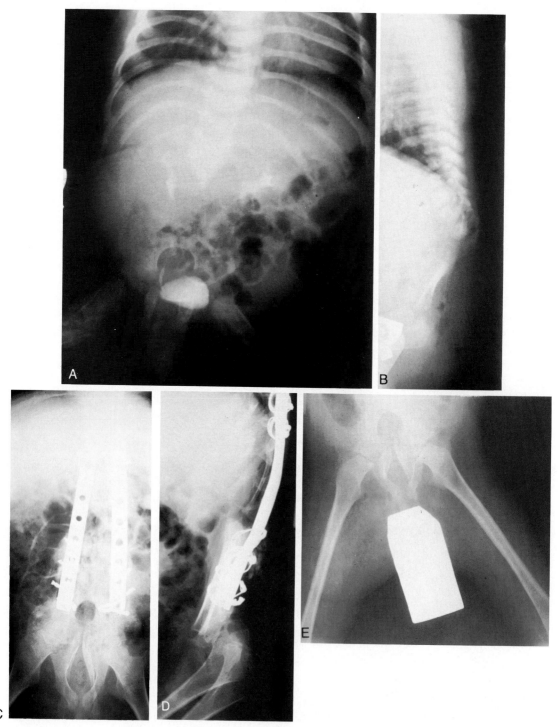

FIGURE 6–25. *Type IV lumbosacral agenesis in a six-year-old girl.*

   A and **B.** Initial AP and lateral radiograms of the spine at one month of age. When the patient was three years of age, her spine was stabilized with fusion and internal fixation. **C** and **D.** Postoperative radiograms at age five years. **E.** AP radiogram of the pelvis showing dislocation of both hips and marked constriction of the pelvic outlet. The latter was treated by osteotomy of the pelvic bones.

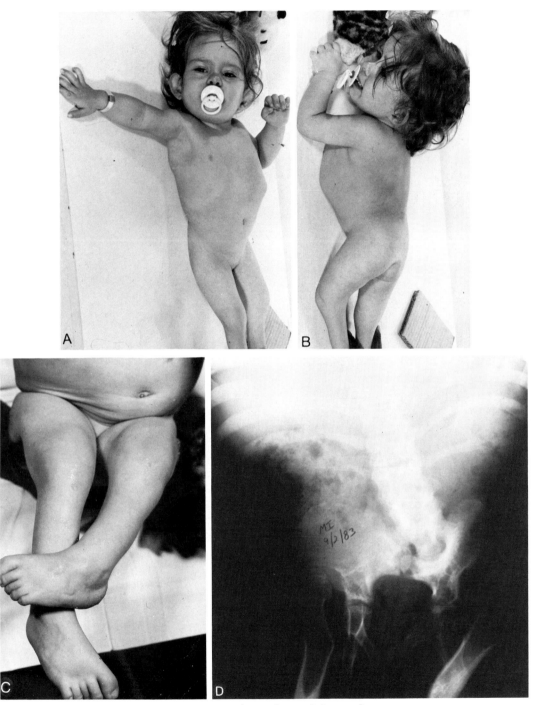

FIGURE 6–26. Lumbosacral agenesis in a newborn.

A to **C.** Initial photographs of the patient. **D.** Anteroposterior radiogram of the patient at age ten years. The lower spine was stabilized by fusion, and both hips are dislocated.

Illustration continued on following page

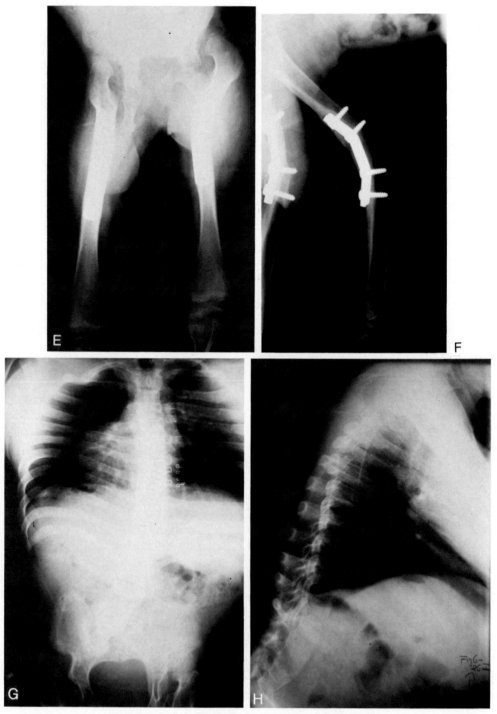

FIGURE 6–26 Continued. *Lumbosacral agenesis in a newborn.*

E and F. She had extension abduction osteotomy of both proximal femora performed to correct severe flexion and adduction deformity of both hips. G and H. AP and lateral films of lumbosacral spine showing the end result of spine stabilization by fusion at age 18 years. The patient is ambulatory and attending normal school.

Cong. Int. Soc. of Ortho. Surg., and Traumatology. Amsterdam, Excerpta Medica, 1972, p. 421.

30. Hilgenreiner, H.: Ein Fall von Anchypodie. Beitrag zum vollständigen Kreuzbein Defekt. Z. Orthop., 66:224, 1937.

31. Hohl, A. F.: Zur Pathologie des Beckens. I. Das schagovale Becken. Leipzig, Englemann, 1852, p. 61.

32. Ignelzi, R. J., and Lehman, R. A. W.: Lumbosacral agenesis: Management and embryological implications. J. Neurol. Neurosurg. Psychiatry, 37:1273, 1974.

33. Israel, J., Day, D. W., Hirschman, A., and Smith, G. F.: Sacral agenesis and associated anomalies. Birth Defects 12:45, 1976.

34. Kalitzki, M.: Congenital malformations and diabetes. Lancet, 2:641, 1965.

35. Katz, J. F.: Congenital absence of the sacrum and coccyx. J. Bone Joint Surg., 35-A:398, 1953.

36. Kenefick, J. S.: Hereditary sacral agenesis associated with pre-sacral tumours. Br. J. Surg., 60:271, 1973.

37. Klinghoffer, L., Murdock, M. G., and Hermel, M. B.: Congenital absence of lumbar articular facets. Report of two cases. Clin. Orthop., 106:151, 1975.

38. Kucera, J.: Exposure to fat solvents: A possible cause of sacral agenesis in man. J. Pediatr., 72:857, 1968.

39. Lichtor, A.: Sacral agenesis. Report of a case. Arch. Surg., 54:430, 1947.

40. Louri, H.: Sacral agenesis. Case report. J. Neurosurg., 38:92, 1973.

41. Macleod, S., and Hendry, G. M.: Congenital absence of a lumbar pedicle. A case report and a review of the literature. Pediatr. Radiol., 12:207, 1982.

42. Marsh, H. O., and Tejano, N. A.: Four cases of lumbosacral and sacral agenesis. Clin. Orthop., 92:214, 1973.

43. Mayfield, J. K.: Severe spine deformity in myelodysplasia and sacral agenesis: An aggressive surgical approach. Spine, 6:498, 1981.

44. Millar, E. A., and Lindquist, T. C.: Agenesis of the lumbo-sacral spine. Read at the Annual Meeting of The American Orthopaedic Association. San Francisco, California, June 13, 1974.

45. Mongeau, M., and LeClaire, R.: Complete agenesis of the lumbosacral spine. A case report. J. Bone Joint Surg., 54-A:161, 1972.

46. Moretti, M., Rigillo, N., and DeBlasio, A: Agenesia sacro coccigea nell infanzia. Pediatria, 69:1058, 1961.

47. Nicol, W. J.: Lumbosacral agenesis in a 60 year old man. Br. J. Surg., 59:577, 1972.

48. Nogami, H., and Ingalls, T. H.: Pathogenesis of spinal malformation induced in the embryos of mice. J. Bone Joint Surg., 49-A:1551, 1967.

49. Passarge, E., and Lenz, W.: Syndrome of caudal regression in infants of diabetic mothers: Observations of further cases. Pediatrics, 36:672, 1965.

50. Pearlman, C. K., and Bors, E.: Congenital absence of the lumbosacral spine. J. Urol., 101:374, 1969.

51. Perry, J., Bonnett, C. A., and Hoffer, M. M.: Vertebral pelvic fusions in the rehabilitation of patients with sacral agenesis. J. Bone Joint Surg., 52:288, 1970.

52. Phillips, W. A., Cooperman, D. R., Lindquist, T. C., Sullivan, R. C., and Millar, E. A.: Orthopedic management of lumbosacral agenesis. Long-term follow-up. J. Bone Joint Surg., 64-A:1282, 1982.

53. Pouzet, F.: Les anomalies du developpement du sacrum. Lyon Chir., 35:371, 1938.

54. Price, D. L., Dooling, E. C., and Richardson, E. P., Jr.: Caudal dysplasia (caudal regression syndrome). Arch. Neurol., 23:212, 1970.

55. Redhead, R. G., Vitali, M., and Trapnell, D. H.: Congenital absence of the lumbar spine. Br. Med. J., 3:595, 1968.

56. Redman, J. F.: Congenital absence of the lumbosacral spine. South. Med. J., 66:770, 1973.

57. Renshaw, T. S.: Sacral agenesis. A classification and review of twenty-three cases. J. Bone Joint Surg., 60-A:373, 1978.

58. Rochet, E., Gacon, G., Robert, J. M., and Grunthaler, C.: Dystocie osseuse par agénésie sacro-coccygienne. Observation familiale avec polyethalite d'origine malformative associée. Gynecol. Obstet., 65:115, 1966.

59. Rosenthal, R. K.: Congenital absence of the coccyx, sacrum, lumbar vertebrae and the lower thoracic vertebrae. Report of a case. Bull. Hosp. Joint Dis., 29:287, 1968.

60. Ruderman, R. J., Keats, P., and Goldner, J. L.: Congenital absence of the lumbo-sacral spine. A report of an unusual case. Clin. Orthop., 124:177, 1977.

61. Rusnak, S. L., and Driscoll, S. G.: Congenital spinal anomalies in infants of diabetic mothers. Pediatrics, 35:989, 1965.

62. Russell, H. E., and Aitken, G. T.: Congenital absence of the sacrum and lumbar vertebrae with prosthetic management. J. Bone Joint Surg., 45-A:501, 1963.

63. Saunders, J. W., Jr.: Death in embryonic systems. Science, 154:604, 1966.

64. Say, B., and Coldwell, J. G.: Hereditary defect of the sacrum. Humangenetik, 27:231, 1975.

65. Sinclair, J. G., Duren, N., and Rude, J. C.: Congenital lumbosacral defect. Arch. Surg., 43:474, 1941.

66. Smith, E. D.: Congenital sacral anomalies in children. Aust. N.Z. J. Surg., 29:165, 1959.

67. Stelling, C. B.: Anomalous attachment of the transverse process to the vertebral body: An accessory finding in congenital absence of a lumbar pedicle. Skeletal Radiol., 6:47, 1981.

68. Stern, L., Ramos, A., and Light, I.: Congenital malformations and diabetes. Lancet, 1:1393, 1965.

69. Tanaka, T., and Uhthoff, H. K.: The pathogenesis of congenital vertebral malformations. A study based on observations made in 11 human embryos and fetuses. Acta Orthop. Scand., 52:413, 1981.

70. Van, H., and Fourie, I. J.: Sacral agenesis and neurogenic bladder dysfunction. A case report and review of the literature. S. Afr. Med. J., 65:55, 1984.

71. White, R. I., and Klauber, G. T.: Sacral agenesis. Analysis of 22 cases. Urology, 8:521, 1976.

72. Williams, D. I., and Nixon, H. H.: Agenesis of the sacrum. Surg., Gynecol. Obstet., 105:84, 1957.

73. Yousfzadeh, D. K., El-Khoury, G. Y., and Lupetin, A. R.: Congenital aplastic-hypoplastic lumbar pedicle in infants and young children. Skeletal Radiol., 7:259, 1982.

74. Zeligs, I. M.: Congenital absence of the sacrum. Arch. Surg., 41:1220, 1940.

CONGENITAL LUMBAR PEDICLE APLASIA

Congenital absence of a lumbar vertebral pedicle is extremely rare. Survey of the English literature reveals isolated case reports.[1-16] It commonly occurs at the fourth lumbar (L-4) level. Only a few reports of cases occurring in the thoracic spine have been published.[7, 12] In a few cases the lumbar pedicle is hypoplastic rather than totally absent; this anomaly is slightly more prepoderant in the male. Age at its diagnosis ranges from 9 to 66 years.[1, 8]

The condition may be asymptomatic and incidentally discovered in radiographs made for other reasons, such as an intravenous pyelogram. About half the patients complain of backache, especially during exertion. The pain may radiate to the gluteal region on the affected side. On physical examination paravertebral muscle spasm may be evident. Radiograms will show absence of the pedicles of the involved vertebra. Misdiagnosis of this congenital anomaly for a neoplastic or inflammatory lesion is a problem. Computed tomography is of great value in delineation of the nature of the lesion.[2] A bone scan with technetium-99m may be performed if an inflammatory lesion is suspected; in congenital absence of the vertebral pedicles it will be normal. Associated radiographic findings that have been described are contralateral arch hypertrophy (sclerosis of the contralateral pedicle, isthmus, or lamina); deformity, obliquity, hypoplasia, or fusion of the ipsilateral superior articular facet; a corresponding abnormality of the inferior articular facet of the immediate cephalad vertebra; spinous process tilt of the immediately cephalad vertebra toward the deficient side; and anomalous attachment of the ipsilateral transverse process.* The lumbar transverse processes normally arise from the lateral aspect of the pedicle and are pointed laterally and slightly dorsally. In congenital absence of the lumbar vertebral pedicle the ipsilateral transverse process will be small and located in an anterior position at the posterior edge of the vertebral body. This is best visualized in the lateral and ipsilateral oblique projection.

Treatment

If absence of the pedicle is asymptomatic, no treatment is necessary. If symptomatic, the spine is supported in an orthosis, and physical exertion is curtailed. If conservative measures do not relieve symptoms, local spinal fusion is indicated.

---

*See references: contralateral arch hypertrophy, 1, 7, 9, 15; deformity . . . of ipsilateral superior articular facet, 7, 9, 14; abnormality of inferior articular facet of immediate cephalad vertebra, 9, 14; spinous process tilt of cephalad vertebra, 7.

References

1. Bardsley, J. L., and Hamelin, L. G.: The unilateral lumbar pedicle. Radiology, *101*:315, 1971.
2. DeBoeck, M., DeSmedt, E., and Potvliege, R.: Computed tomography in the evaluation of a congenital absent lumbar pedicle. Skeletal Radiol., 8:197, 1982.
3. Demos, T.: Radiologic case study: Congenital absence of lumbar vertebral pedicle. Orthopedics, 2:168, 1979.
4. Douillet, P., Lascaux, J. P., and Faure, C.: Absence congénitale d'un pédicule vertébral. J. Radiol., 58:459, 1977.
5. Klein, A.: Congenital absence of a lumbar vertebral pedicle: A report of three cases. S. Afr. Med. J., 50:1795, 1976.
6. Klinghoffer, L., Murdock, M. G., and Hermel, M. B.: Congenital absence of lumbar articular facets. Clin. Orthop., 106:151, 1975.
7. Maldague, B., and Malghem, J. J.: Unilateral arch hypertrophy with spinous process tilt: A sign of arch deficiency. Radiology, *121*:567, 1976.
8. Morin, M. E., and Palacios, E.: The aplastic hypoplastic lumbar pedicle. A.J.R., *122*:639, 1974.
9. Norman, W. J., and Johnson, C.: Case report: Congenital absence of a pedicle of a lumbar vertebrae. Br. J. Radiol., *46*:631, 1973.
10. Roche, M. B., and Rowe, G. G.: The incidence of separate neural arch and coincident bone variations. J. Bone Joint Surg., *34*:491, 1952.
11. Stelling, C. B.: Anomalous attachment of the transverse process to the vertebral body: An accessory finding in congenital absence of a lumbar pedicle. Skeletal Radiol., 6:47, 1981.
12. Tomsick, T. A., Lebowitz, M. E., and Campbell, C.: The congenital absence of pedicles in the thoracic spine: Report of two cases. Radiology, *111*:587, 1974.
13. Trotter, M., and Peterson, R. R.: Osteology. *In* Anson, B. J. (ed.): Morris' Human Anatomy. 18th Ed. New York, McGraw-Hill, 1966, p. 150.
14. Verhaak, R.: Congenital defect of a lumbar vertebral pedicle with dysplasia of the intervertebral joint. Radiol. Clin. (Basel), *43*:127, 1974.
15. Wilkinson, R. H., and Hall, J. E.: The sclerotic pedicle: Tumor or pseudotumor? Radiology, *111*:683, 1974.
16. Wilson, C., and Norell, H. A.: Congenital absence of pedicle in the cervical spine. A.J.R., 97:639, 1966.

Congenital Anomalies of the Occiput and Cervical Spine

Congenital anomalies of the occiput and cervical spine are formed during any of the four stages of development of this portion of the axial skeleton. Some remain asymptomatic and undetected, while others predispose the patient to mechanical or neurologic disorders or both. Many anomalies become apparent on radiograms taken for some other reason. Some of these anomalies are potentially serious to the patient; it is important that they be differentiated from those that are not.

Aberrations of the occiput and cervical spine are caused by failure of completion of one of the four stages of formation of the axial skeleton. These stages include formation of the notochord at about the fifteenth to sixteenth day of fetal life, progressive mesenchymal segmentation, chondrification and ossification of these mesenchymal segments, and fusion and union of the ossified mesenchymal segments into complete osseous structures.

In Stage I, the notochord develops as a flexible unsegmented rod, extending from the sphenoid base through the occipital region of the skull anterior to the future spinal cord, then caudally to the coccyx. It persists in the mature fetus as the nucleus pulposus of the intervertebral discs and as the apical and alar ligaments of the axis.

In Stage II, the paraxial mesoderm begins segmentation in the future occipital region at about the twenty-first day of fetal life. This segmentation proceeds caudally to completion in about ten days. There are 4 occipital somites and 8 cervical somites, the total number of human somites varying from 42 to 44 segments. Each somite differentiates into a dermatome, a myotome, and a sclerotome. The first occipital somite regresses and disappears by the time 20 somites have formed. Later, portions of the second and third occipital somites also regress and disappear, leaving only the fourth occipital somite to contribute to the formation of the axial skeleton. Each somite differentiates into a cranial and a caudal portion. The cranial half is composed of loosely packed, somewhat acellular tissue. The very densely cellular caudal half develops processes that eventually grow dorsally around the spinal tube, and also lateral processes that become the intersegmental septa. The caudal half of each somite shifts to unite with the cranial half of the adjacent somite, forming each provertebra. Symmetrical and asymmetrical disorders of segmentation occur during this second stage, since no further change in position of the anlage takes place after segmentation. Other anomalies occur during subsequent stages of chondrification, ossification, and fusion in each segment.

In Stage III, chondrification takes place in both halves of the provertebral body and the neural arch at the fifth or sixth week of fetal life. The centers of chondrification in the body fuse, and each half of the neural arch subsequently fuses with the body. That portion of the provertebral body that represents the centrum of the vertebra may have one or more centers of chondrification. Each half of the arch develops a transverse process directed toward the midline. These two processes finally fuse in the midline posteriorly at approximately the fourth month of fetal life.

In Stage IV, ossification begins with the invasion of the cartilaginous elements by blood vessels. The number and site of the ossification of each segment is, as yet, undefined. Certain congenital anomalies suggest that there are two centers in each vertebral body. It is generally accepted, however, that there is one center in each half of the neural arch from the third cervical vertebra caudally, and in some instances, there are costal processes that ossify separately and eventually fuse with the major portion of the vertebra. Ossification of the posterior arch and incorporation of the ringed epiphyses of the vertebral body are completed some time between the eighteenth and twenty-fifth years of life.

Only the common anomalies of the occiput and upper cervical spine are presented here.

OSSICULUM TERMINALE AND OCCIPITAL VERTEBRA

These two types of accessory ossicles are produced by an abnormality of segmentation around the fourth week of fetal life. They lie anterior to the spinal cord between the atlas and occiput, possibly representing an incompletely developed hypochordal bow of the fourth occipital somite. This segment may be represented by a third occipital condyle, an accentuation of the edges of the foramen magnum, a paramastoid process, or a separate small anterior ossicle. They are usually found incidentally on the radiograms and present no clinical disorder. Lanier, in a study of the size, shape, and anomalies of the presacral vertebrae, reported evidence of an occipital vertebra in only 13 of 1,246 skulls.[37] The existence of these ossicles is mentioned so that they may be distinguished from the other anomalies listed here.

BASILAR INVAGINATION, BASILAR IMPRESSION, AND PLATYBASIA

The term *platybasia* is used when the angle formed by the intersection of the plane of the anterior fossa with the plane of the clivus is flattened. The normal range of the basal angle (created by the intersection of the planes of the sphenoid bone and the clivus) is 115 to 145 degrees.[58] Platybasia is diagnosed if the basal angle is greater than 145 degrees. The existence of platybasia alone is of no clinical significance if it is not associated with symptoms of spinal cord or hindbrain compression. In nearly all cases of platybasia, atlanto-occipital motion can be demonstrated.

Basilar impression or invagination is not synonymous with, and should be distinguished from, platybasia. In the presence of basilar impression, the basal angle may remain normal or be increased, indicating that basilar impression may be present without platybasia, and vice versa. Basilar impression (invagination) may be congenital or acquired. The *congenital type*, or primary basilar impression, occurs in association with other vertebral defects, such as Klippel-Feil syndrome, abnormalities of the odontoid process, hypoplasia of the atlas, bifid posterior arch of the atlas, or atlanto-occipital synostosis. The *acquired type* is found in association with various types of rickets, osteomalacia, and the adult Paget's disease. The deformity is caused by softening of the cranial bones so they are no longer able to support the weight of the skull. The base of the skull is forced upward into the cranial vault. This upward displacement causes the odontoid peg, the rim of the invaginated foramen magnum, and the upper cervical vertebra to encroach on the brain stem and spinal cord. Frequently associated with this abnormality is a heavy posterior band of dura at the cranial vertebral junction, which may also produce signs and symptoms of spinal cord compression. Radiographically the diagnosis of basilar impression is made by determination of the position of the tip of the odontoid process in relation to the McGregor's line, which is drawn from the upper surface of the posterior edge of the hard palate to the most caudal point of the occipital curve of the skull. When the tip of the odontoid process is over 4.5 mm. above McGregor's line the diagnosis of basilar impression is made. Treatment and prognosis depend on the underlying disease. Any pressure from impinging structures should be relieved surgically.

CONGENITAL FUSION OF FIRST CERVICAL VERTEBRA AND OCCIPUT

In this malformation there is partial or complete synostosis between the atlas and the base of the occiput. It is also known as occipitalization of the atlas and assimilation of the atlas into the occipital bone. Only a few isolated reports of cranial cervical anomalies are to be found in the literature before the presentation of 25 cases of congenital fusion of the first cervical vertebra and the occiput by McRay and Barnum.[43] This report defines the anatomic variation and the clinical disorders with which it is associated.

Embryologic Data

During the stage of segmentation, the fourth occipital somite develops a dense posterior portion and a less dense anterior portion. Normally, the posterior portion does not unite with the anterior portion of the subjacent vertebra, as does happen in the spinal column below the cranial cervical junction. Rather, it remains in place and is assimilated into the occipital bone. When fusion of the occiput and atlas does occur, the posterior dense portion of the occipital fourth somite apparently joins with the anterior portion of the first cervical somite, and fusion is produced. Since the centrum and the hypochordal bow of the first cervical somite are formed separately (the anterior part included), the dense posterior portion is not incorporated in the occiput to first cervical fusions, but becomes a normal odontoid process.

Clinical Picture

Symptoms and signs may begin in early childhood and are usually of short duration before medical aid is sought. The age range of patients presenting with this anomaly is reported as being from 8 to 52 years. Some patients develop symptoms following mild trauma, while others remain entirely asymptomatic throughout life, the presence of the anomaly being discovered only incidentally on radiographs. It is important to note that one third of these cases are misdiagnosed as a neurologic disorder, usually multiple sclerosis. This anomaly should, therefore, be included in the differential diagnosis of spinal cord degenerative diseases.

Weakness and ataxia in the lower limbs, and occasionally in the upper limbs, are usually the primary complaints. In about half the cases, there is also numbness and pain. Headache and neck pain are occasionally present. Blurring of vision or diplopia may be caused by papilledema due to cerebrospinal fluid block at the foramen magnum. Dizziness, difficulty in swallowing, distorted phonation, and evidence of sympathetic pathway disturbance may also be present. Neurologic signs are those of long tract compression. Posterior column compression signs are less frequent, but may be seen when an associated dural band is present. The similarity between this clinical picture and that of several degenerative neurologic disorders should be evident. On inspection the patient has a short, broad neck and low hairline. Motions of the neck are restricted. There may be associated torticollis, high scapula, and other anomalies.

Radiographic Findings

Diagnosis is established in the radiographs with the demonstration of bony union between the occiput and the atlas. Absence of motion between the atlas and the skull on cervical flexion-extension films is not sufficient evidence. In most cases, bony union between the anterior edge of the foramen magnum and the anterior arch of the first cervical vertebra can be seen in overexposed lateral films of the cervical spine. If superimposed structures obstruct clear visualization of this area, linear and computed axial tomography may be necessary. Fusion of the posterior halves of the arches of the first cervical vertebra may be partial or complete. Anomalies of the transverse processes may also be present. Bony anomalies that may be visible include a backward tilt of the odontoid process, an articular facet between the anterior rim of the occiput and the odontoid process, asymmetrical atlantoaxial joints as seen on the anteroposterior view, and fusion of the body and lamina of the second to the third cervical vertebrae. Usually, the basal angle is normal or basilar impression is slight, although asymmetry of the foramen magnum may be noted. Intercranial anomalies associated with this fusion include the Arnold-Chiari malformation and posterior dural bands. Because of the associated anomalies, air myelography or magnetic resonance imaging may be of assistance in defining the entire picture.

The most frequent cause of symptoms is the malformed odontoid process, which is tilted and enlarged. Posterior displacement and posterior angulation are most frequently implicated when neurologic signs are present.

Treatment

Initially nonsurgical measures in the form of traction and support of the neck by an orthosis are carried out. If symptoms and neurologic deficit persist and increase, surgery is indicated.

Combined posterior laminectomy and C-1–C-2 spinal fusion are performed. Resection of dural bands and posterior fossa decompression for the Arnold-Chiari malformation are carried out when indicated. The risk of morbidity and death is high.

CONGENITAL ANOMALIES OF THE ODONTOID PROCESS

Anomalies of the odontoid process (dens axis) may range from complete absence (aplasia) to partial absence (hypoplasia) to separate odontoid process, or os odontoideum. These anomalies may lead to atlantoaxial instability and cause neurologic deficit and even death.

The Separate Odontoid Process

The separate odontoid process may be of either congenital or post-traumatic origin. Congenitally separate os odontoideum was first described by Giacomini, in 1886.[64] Both types may be associated with severe neurologic disturbances, but they must be treated differently.

The odontoid process is a separate ossicle in some lower vertebrate forms (reptiles) because of differences in the processes of segmentation and chondrification between reptilian and human embryos. In the human, after segmentation is complete, the body of the proatlas is joined to that of the proaxis by loose, mesenchymal tissue. Chondrification of this tissue normally joins the two segments; if chondrification fails to take place, however, the odontoid process remains a separate ossicle. A real joint is formed by traction and compression in the unchondrified mesenchymal tissue. The joint surfaces are covered by articular cartilage. The tip of the odontoid process is formed from a separate ossification center, which probably represents a portion of the fourth occipital somite; it chondrifies separately and ossifies separately. Ossification of the odontoid process begins in the second year of life, and bony union with the axis is complete by the twelfth year; that of the tip of the odontoid process appears between the second and fifth years, and union is complete by the twelfth year. The junction between the odontoid process ossification center and the axis ossification center lies above the plane between the superior articular processes of the axis. This point is useful in distinguishing a fracture of the odontoid process from a separate os odontoideum. The tip of the odontoid process may exist as a separate ossicle, usually sitting in the cup-shaped end of the odontoid process when this is present.

Clinical studies in the recent literature indicate that at least half the patients with this deformity have neurologic signs and symptoms.[30, 42, 64] A history of mild trauma with complaints and findings out of proportion to the degree of trauma is common. The severity of possible presenting complaints may range from pain and limitation of range of motion of the neck through transient signs of spinal cord compression to complete quadriplegia. The same clinical picture may be present following fracture of the odontoid process, in which the pathomechanics of signs and symptoms are the same. In the absence of stability between the axis and atlas, even slight flexion forces allow the atlas to ride forward on the axis, causing the anterior body of the axis and the base of the odontoid process to impinge on the spinal cord.

DIFFERENTIAL DIAGNOSIS

The diagnosis of congenitally separate os odontoideum is suggested by three findings on the anteroposterior view of the cranial cervical junction and on the lateral view of the cervical spine, as suggested by Wollin (Fig. 6–27). First, a space of varying height is seen between the base of the odontoid process and the separate os odontoideum. Second, the plane of this space lies above the plane of the superior articular processes of the axis, with the base of the odontoid process projecting above this line. Third, there are other associated bony abnormalities present.

The characteristic plane of a fracture of the odontoid process appears jagged and irregular and lies below the plane of the superior articular processes of the axis. A fracture may also be suggested if the inferior cortex of the separate ossicle cannot be demonstrated.

Linear and computed axial tomography may be useful for clarification. Instability may be demonstrated on upright flexion-extension views of the cervical spine, but this technique should be used with caution in cases presenting with a history of recent trauma.

The ossification center at the tip of the odontoid process has been mentioned to avoid confusion when this anomaly is present. It is possible for the odontoid process to be absent and this tip to be present. There is no report of this anomaly producing clinical signs or symptoms.

TREATMENT

If the presence of a fracture is established, immobilization in an extension Minerva jacket for three to four months should provide sufficient time for healing. If instability or neurologic signs or symptoms persist when the plaster is removed, as in the case of a symptomatic separate os odontoideum, a posterior cervical spinal fusion should be performed. If the congenitally separate os odontoideum remains asymptomatic, a posterior cervical spinal fusion should be completed if any physical or sports activity is anticipated that might predispose the patient to cervical trauma.

If the separate os odontoideum or the un-united fracture is allowed to remain untreated, it is mandatory that any activity that might place strain on the craniocervical junction be avoided. Even minor trauma might produce permanent quadriplegia.

Absence of the Odontoid Process

Partial or complete absence of the dens may also be either congenital or acquired.[22, 24] Congenital absence of the odontoid process appears to be compatible with normal life. Mild trauma may, however, precipitate instability, and severe neurologic deficit may result from subluxation and dislocation.[24] In the presence of instability, symptoms of cord compression may be found as early as two years of age or as late as the fifth or sixth decade of life. Dislocation may be anterior, posterior, or lateral, because ligamentous structures provide the only stability for the atlantoaxial joint. The odontoid process is not seen radiographically. The base of the odontoid process may be present, projecting above the plane of the superior articular processes of the axis. The remainder of the bony anatomy is usually normal.

Familial hypoplasia of the odontoid process has been reported by Shepard. Five subjects in three generations of the same family were studied. One sustained a fatal dislocation of the upper cervical spine, two had severe neurologic deficits resulting from spinal cord compression, and two remained asymptomatic.[55] When congenital absence or hypoplasia is discovered, investigation of other family members is advocated.

Acquired absence is also associated with instability of the atlantoaxial joint. This may be related to postfracture resorption, or may occur after osteomyelitis or in relation to inflammatory processes in the neck.[13, 24, 44, 60] Again, radiologically, the dens is absent. The ossification center at the tip of the odontoid process (contributed by the fourth occipital somite) may be present in either congenital or acquired absence of the body of the odontoid process. Differential diagnosis depends on evidence that the dens was present previously, on findings of associated infection or retropharyngeal abscess, and on the general radiologic appearance.

It is suggested that the risk of neurologic catastrophe stemming from the absence of the odontoid process warrants atlantoaxial fusion even in those patients who are asymptomatic.

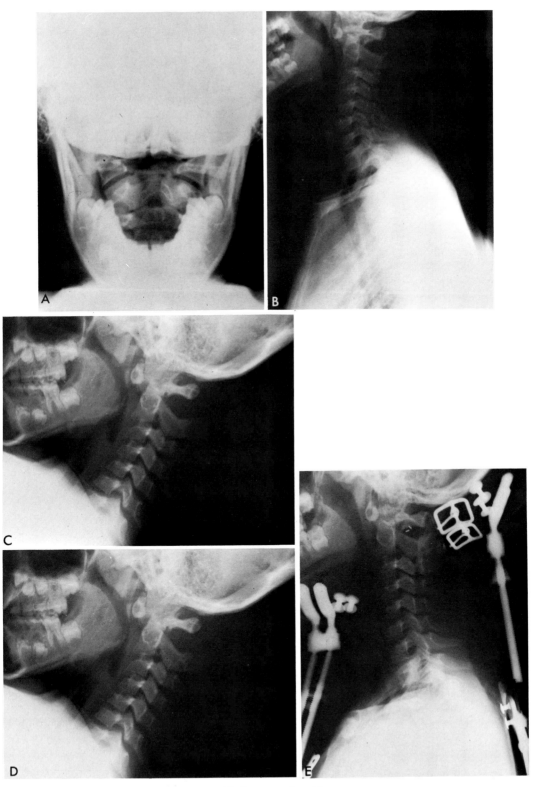

FIGURE 6–27. *Separate odontoid process.*

A to **D.** Open-mouth and lateral views of cervical spine in neutral, flexion, and extension positions, showing separate odontoid process. Note the instability. **E.** Postoperative lateral view in brace, showing fusion from the atlas to C3.

CONGENITAL ABSENCE OF PEDICLES AND FACETS IN THE CERVICAL SPINE

Congenital absence of these two components is discussed at the same time because if one is absent, the other is usually absent also. This abnormality probably originates in the chondrification stage, since the defect represents incomplete formation of the neural arch, caused by absence of the lateral chondrification center. Most of the patients are young adults with a history of mild trauma, neck stiffness, and neck pain. Radicular pain may be present with signs and symptoms of nerve root compression. One patient had reported intermittent numbness in her hand since childhood. The condition is not necessarily painful, and the physical examination is usually not remarkable unless there is associated trauma.

Radiologic Examination

For a definite diagnosis of this anomaly, stereoscopic 45-degree oblique views of the cervical spine are recommended. This view demonstrates the characteristic elongated intervertebral foramen extending the length of the involved segment. The transverse process is also deficient posteriorly. When associated with absence of the posterior facets on the same side, compensatory overgrowth of the inferior facet from the vertebra above and the superior facet from the vertebra below provides a bony bridge and some degree of stability for this segment of the cervical spine. The posterior neural arch may be present with both superior and inferior facets; in this case, the arch is sclerotic and enlarged. Because the defect is usually unilateral, there may be associated lateral angulation of the cervical spine at the level of the lesion.

Computed axial tomography and magnetic resonance imaging will depict the pathologic anatomy in detail.

Differential Diagnosis

The differential diagnosis is primarily concerned with erosive lesions (i.e., malignant tumors, neurofibromas) that may involve the pedicles and neural foramen of the cervical spine. Knowledge of this deformity may also prevent confusion concerning certain types of cervical spinal trauma. The radiographic appearance is most important, and comparative oblique views may be helpful. The presence of compensatory abnormalities of the neural arch and structural changes in the facets is of assistance in the differential diagnosis. These compensatory changes, which attempt to provide stability, would not be present if a neoplastic process had destroyed the pedicle. Additional information may be gathered by myelography, vertebral artery angiography, computed axial tomography, and magnetic resonance imaging.

Prognosis and Treatment

Since most of these patients are without symptoms throughout a significant portion of their life span, conservative management with external support is suggested. When present, symptoms are usually related to hypertrophic arthritis or the trauma that brought attention to the cervical spinal anomaly. None of the reported cases required fusion, though this may be necessary if symptoms persist or become severe. Appropriate diagnosis may prevent unwarranted surgical exploration.

SPONDYLOLISTHESIS OF THE CERVICAL SPINE

In this rare anomaly the presenting complaints are neck stiffness, aching in the back of the neck, minimally limited range of motion, and pain at the extremes of cervical motion. Often there is no previous history of trauma. Radicular pain and signs of spinal cord compression are absent. No muscle spasm in the cervical spine has been reported. A palpable step-off in the cervical spine at the level of the defect was present in one patient.

Radiographic Findings

Forward displacement of the affected vertebra is demonstrated on the lateral radiograph, and a bilateral defect in the lamina is shown on oblique projection of the cervical spine.

Treatment

Treatment depends on the persistence of symptoms and the demonstration of instability. If either is present, cervical spinal fusion may be carried out.

References

1. Ahlback, I., and Collert, S.: Destruction of the odontoid process due to axial pyogenic spondylitis. Acta Radiol. (Diagn.) (Stockh.), *10*:394, 1970.

2. Bailey, D. K.: The normal cervical spine in infants and children. Radiology, *59*:712, 1952.
3. Bassett, F. H., and Goldner, J. L.: Aplasia of the odontoid process. J. Bone Joint Surg., *50-A*:833, 1968.
4. Bharucha, E. P., and Dastur, H. M.: Craniovertebral anomalies (a report on 40 cases). Brain, *87*:469, 1964.
5. Caffey, J.: Paediatric X-ray Diagnosis. Chicago, Year Book, 1967.
6. Chamberlain, W. E.: Basilar impression (platybasia). Yale J. Biol. Med., *11*:487, 1939.
7. Corner, E. S.: Rotary dislocations of the atlas. Ann. Surg., *45*:9, 1907.
8. DeBarros, M. C., Farias, W., Ataide, L., and Lins, S.: Basilar impression and Arnold-Chiari malformation: A study of 66 cases. J. Neurol. Neurosurg. Psychiatry, *31*:596, 1968.
9. Durbin, F. C.: Spondylolisthesis of the cervical spine. J. Bone Joint Surg., *38-B*:734, 1956.
10. Epstein, B. S., and Epstein, J. A.: The association of cerebellar tonsillar herniation with basilar impression incident to Paget's disease. A.J.R., *107*:535, 1969.
11. Evarts, C. M., and Lonsdale, D.: Ossiculum terminale—an anomaly of the odontoid process: Report of a case of atlantoaxial dislocation with cord compression. Cleveland Clin. Q., *37*:73, 1970.
12. Fielding, J. W.: Normal and selected abnormal motion of the cervical spine from the second cervical vertebra based on coneroentgenography. J. Bone Joint Surg., *46-A*:1779, 1964.
13. Fielding, J. W.: Disappearance of the central portion of the odontoid process. J. Bone Joint Surg., *47-A*:1228, 1965.
14. Fielding, J. W.: The cervical spine in the child. Curr. Pract. Orthop. Surg., *5*:31, 1973.
15. Fielding, J. W., and Griffin, P. P.: Os odontoideum: An acquired lesion. J. Bone Joint Surg., *56-A*:187, 1974.
16. Fielding, J. W., Hawkins, R. J., and Ratzan, S. A.: Spine fusion for atlanto-axial instability. J. Bone Joint Surg., *58-A*:400, 1976.
17. Fielding, J. W., Hensinger, R. N., and Hawkins, R. J.: Os odontoideum. J. Bone Joint Surg., *62-A*:376, 1980.
18. Fiorani-Gallotta, G., and Luzzatti, G.: Sublussazione laterale e sublussazione rotatoria dell-atlanta. Arch. Ortop., *70*:467, 1957.
19. Fischgold, H., and Metzger, J.: Etude radiotomographique de l'impression basilaire. Rev. Rhum. Mal. Osteoartic., *19*:261, 1952.
20. Ford, F. K.: Syncope, vertigo, and disturbances of vision resulting from intermittent obstruction of the vertebral arteries due to a defect in the odontoid process and excessive mobility of the axis. Bull. Johns Hopkins Hosp., *91*:168, 1952.
21. Frank, T. J. F.: Osteomyelitis of the odontoid process of the axis. Med. J. Aust., *1*:198, 1944.
22. Freiberger, R. H., Wilson, P. D., Jr., and Nicholas, J. A.: Acquired absence of the odontoid. J. Bone Joint Surg., *47-A*:1231, 1965.
23. Fromm, G. H., and Pitner, S. E.: Late progressive quadriparesis due to odontoid agenesis. Arch. Neurol., *9*:291, 1963.
24. Garber, J. N.: Abnormalities of the atlas and axis vertebrae—congenital and traumatic. J. Bone Joint Surg., *46-A*:1782, 1964.
25. Giannestras, N. J., Mayfield, F. H., Provencio, F. P., and Maurer, J.: Congenital absence of the odontoid process. J. Bone Joint Surg., *46-A*:839, 1964.
26. Gillman, C. L.: Congenital absence of the odontoid

process of the axis: Report of a case. J. Bone Joint Surg., *41-A*:340, 1959.
27. Greeley, P. W.: Bilateral (90 degrees) rotatory dislocation of the atlas upon the axis. J. Bone Joint Surg., *12*:958, 1930.
28. Greenberg, A. D.: Atlantoaxial dislocations. Brain, *91*:655, 1968.
29. Greenberg, A. D., Scovillo, W. P., and Davey, L. M.: Transoral decompression of atlantoaxial dislocation due to odontoid hypoplasia: Report of two cases. J. Neurosurg., *28*:266, 1968.
30. Greenfield, J. G.: Malformations et dégénérescence des disques intervertébraux de la région cervicale. Rev. Med. Suisse Rom., *73*:229, 1953.
31. Gwinn, J. L., and Smith, J. L.: Acquired and congenital absence of the odontoid process. A.J.R., *88*:424, 1962.
32. Hadley, L. A.: Congenital absence of pedicle from the cervical vertebrae. A.J.R., *55*:193, 1946.
33. Hawkins, R. J., Fielding, J. W., and Thompson, W. J.: Os odontoideum: Congenital or acquired. A case report. J. Bone Joint Surg., *58-A*:413, 1976.
34. Hinck, V. C., Hopkins, C. E., and Savara, B. S.: Diagnostic criteria of basilar impression. Radiology, *76*:572, 1961.
35. Hohl, M., and Baker, H. R.: The atlantoaxial joint. Roentgenographic and anatomical study of the normal and abnormal motion. J. Bone Joint Surg., *46-A*:1739, 1964.
36. Jackson, H.: Diagnosis of minimal atlanto-axial subluxation. Br. J. Radiol., *23*:672, 1950.
37. Lanier, R. R., Jr.: Presacral vertebrae of white and Negro males. Am. J. Phys. Anthropol., *25*:341, 1966.
38. Locke, G. R., Gardner, J. I., and van Epyrs, E. F.: Atlas-dens interval (ADI) in children: A survey based on 200 normal cervical spines. A.J.R., *97*:135, 1966.
39. MacAlister, A.: Notes on the development and variations of the atlas. J. Anat. Physiol., *27*:519, 1892.
40. McGregor, M.: The significance of certain measurements of the skull in the diagnosis of basilar impression. Br. J. Radiol., *21*:171, 1948.
41. McRae, D. L.: Bony abnormalities in the region of the foramen magnum: Correlation of the anatomic and neurologic finds. Acta Radiol., *40*:335, 1953.
42. McRae, D. L.: The significance of abnormalities of the cervical spine. A.J.R., *84*:3, 1960.
43. McRae, D. L., and Barnum, A. S.: Occipitalization of the atlas. A.J.R., *70*:23, 1953.
44. Makins, G. H., and Abbott, F. C.: An acute primary osteomyelitis of the vertebrae. Ann. Surg., *23*:510, 1926.
45. Marar, B. C., and Balachandran, N.: Non-traumatic atlanto-axial dislocation in children. Clin. Orthop., *92*:220, 1973.
46. Michaels, L., Prevost, M. J., and Crong, D. F.: Pathological changes in a case of os odontoideum (separate odontoid process). J. Bone Joint Surg., *51-A*:965, 1969.
47. Michie, I., and Clark, M.: Neurological syndromes associated with cervical and craniocervical anomalies. Arch. Neurol., *18*:241, 1968.
48. Minderhoud, J. M., Braakman, R., and Penning, L.: Os odontoideum: Clinical, radiological, and therapeutic aspects. J. Neurol. Sci., *8*:521, 1969.
49. Nicholson, J. S., and Sherk, H. H.: Anomalies of the occipitocervical articulation. J. Bone Joint Surg., *50-A*:295, 1968.
50. Overton, L. M., and Grossman, J. W.: Anatomical variations in articulation between second and third cervical vertebrae. J. Bone Joint Surg., *34-A*:155, 1952.

51. Perlman, R., and Hawes, L. E.: Cervical spondylolisthesis. J. Bone Joint Surg., *38-B*:734, 1956.
52. Roach, J. W., Duncan, D., Wenger, D. R., Maravilla,
A., and Maravilla, K.: Atlanto-axial instability and
spinal cord compression in children—Diagnosis by
computerized tomography. J. Bone Joint Surg., *66-
A*:708, 1984.
53. Rowland, L. P., Shapiro, J. H., and Jacobsen, H. G.:
Neurological syndromes associated with congenital absence of the odontoid process. Arch. Neurol. Psychiatry, *80*:286, 1958.
54. Schiller, F., and Nieda, I.: Malformations of the odontoid process. Report of a case and clinical survey. Calif.
Med., *86*:394, 1957.
55. Shepard, C. N.: Familial hypoplasia of the odontoid
process. J. Bone Joint Surg., *48-A*:1224, 1965.
56. Sherk, H. H., and Nicholson, J. L.: Ossiculum terminale and mongolism. J. Bone Joint Surg., *51-A*:957,
1969.
57. Spierings, E. L. H., and Braakman, R.: The management of os odontoideum. Analysis of 37 cases. J. Bone
Joint Surg., *64-B*:422, 1982.
58. Spillane, J. D., Pallis, C., and Jones, A. M.: Developmental anomalies in the region of the foramen magnum. Brain, *80*:11, 1956.
59. Steinback, H. L., Boldrey, E. B., and Sooy, F. A.:
Congenital absence of the pedicle and superior facet
from a cervical vertebra. Radiology, *59*:838, 1952.
60. Sullivan, A. W.: Subluxation of the atlanto-axial joint:
Sequel to inflammatory process of the neck. J. Pediatr.,
35:451, 1949.
61. Sullivan, C. R., Brewer, A. J., and Harris, L. E.:
Hypermobility of the cervical spine in children: Pitfall
in the diagnosis of cervical dislocation. Am. J. Surg.,
95:636, 1958.
62. von Torklus, D., and Gehle, W.: The Upper Cervical
Spine. New York, Grune & Stratton, 1972.
63. Watson-Jones, R.: Spontaneous hyperaemic dislocation
of the atlas. Proc. R. Soc. Med., *25*:586, 1932.
64. Wollin, D. G.: The os odontoideum. J. Bone Joint
Surg., *45-A*:1459, 1963.

Spondylolisthesis

History and Terminology

The term *spondylolisthesis* is derived from the Greek word *spondylos*, meaning "spine," and *olisthanein*, meaning "to slip." The condition originally attracted the attention of obstetricians as a cause of obstruction in labor, although in 1741 André had already described the cause of a "hollow back" as inward warping of the spine.[8, 114] During the early part of the nineteenth century, it was described as a luxation of the lumbosacral joint. The term *spondylolisthesis* was coined in 1854 by Kilian, who pointed out that it represented a slow displacement of the last lumbar vertebra due to superimposed body weight.[138] Robert, in 1855, was the first to focus attention on a lesion of the neural arch. By careful dissection and freeing of the fifth lumbar vertebra of all soft tissues, he demonstrated that it was impossible for the vertebra with an intact neural arch to slip. If the neural arch was cut, however, the vertebra was free to slip.[234] The discontinuity in the pars interarticularis was demonstrated by Lambl in 1858.[148] Neugebauer studied anatomic specimens of vertebral columns and discovered in some a lesion of continuity in the pars interarticularis, with or without forward displacement of the vertebral body.[200]

When there is a defect in the pars interarticularis with no forward slipping, the term *spondylolysis* is applied (formed by combining *spondylo* with *lysis*, "to disintegrate"). *Spondyloschisis*, schisis meaning "cleavage, crack, or fissure," is another term that has been used.

Junghanns used the term *pseudospondylolisthesis* to describe spondylolisthesis between the fourth and fifth lumbar vertebrae with an intact neural arch. He preferred to reserve the term *spondylolisthesis* for slipping caused by any lesion of the pars interarticularis.[133] The term *spondylolisthesis*, however, originally introduced by Kilian in 1854, referred to slipping of a vertebra, not to a lesion of continuity in the neural arch. This is significant when considering the true nature of spondylolisthesis and the different types that occur.

Spondylolisthesis was considered comparatively rare until the discovery of roentgen rays in 1895 made it a common diagnostic entity.

The term *neural arch defect* is a general one that can refer to several defects. "Pars defect," "interarticular defect," or "isthmal defect" all refer to a defect in that portion of the lamina located between the superior and inferior articular processes called the pars interarticularis. "Pedicle defect" refers to a bony discontinuity in that portion of the arch extending from the body of the vertebra to the lamina. Defects of the lamina may occur near the midline, thus involving the spinous process as well.

Types of Spondylolisthesis

Newman described five different types of spondylolisthesis encountered in a study of 319 patients. In classifying these various groups, he considered the three main possible causes of spondylolisthesis; namely, a defect of the facets, which may be congenital or acquired; a defect of the neural arch or pedicle, congenital or acquired; and structural inadequacy of bone.[202] Wiltse, Newman, and MacNab classified five types of spondylolysis and spondylolisthesis as (1) dysplastic; (2) isthmic (including pars defect, due to lytic [stress] factor, pars elongation [but intact pars interarticularlis], and acute pars fracture); (3) degenerative; (4) traumatic; and (5) pathologic.[319] The salient features of the five types are shown in Figure 6–28.

Type I. Dysplastic Spondylolisthesis. In this type, slipping at the lumbosacral junction is due to a congenital dysplasia of the upper sacrum and fifth lumbar vertebra. The pars interarticularis may remain intact; often, however, it is attenuated and elongated and undergoes a secondary break in continuity. The degree of slip is usually severe, and neurologic deficit is not uncommon because the lamina of L-5 is pulled against the dural sac. The dysplastic type of spondylolisthesis is twice as frequent in girls as in boys.

Type II. Isthmic Spondylolisthesis. In this type slipping of the vertebra is due to elongation or, more commonly, a break of the *pars interarticularis*, or a combination of both with the facets remaining intact. The basic pathologic event is a stress or fatigue fracture of the pars interarticularis. Elongation of the pars is secondary to repeated stress fractures that heal with the pars in attenuated-elongated position. An acute pars fracture may cause isthmic spondylolisthesis.

Type III. Traumatic Spondylolisthesis. Slipping in this type is due to instability caused by an acute fracture of the pedicle, lamina, or facet; the pars interarticularis is intact.

Type IV. Degenerative Spondylolisthesis. This type is also known as pseudospondylolisthesis, so called by Junghanns in 1931, and spondylolisthesis with intact neural arch, the term used by MacNab in 1950.[133, 166] Slipping is due to facet deficiency caused by degenerative joint changes. It almost always occurs at the fourth lumbar level. It is three times as common in women as in men, and has not been encountered in patients under 40 years of age. In this type there is high incidence of involvement of nerve tissue, such as the fifth lumbar root or the cauda equina.

Type V. Pathologic Spondylolisthesis. This is rare and is characterized by forward slipping of one or more vertebrae due to insufficiency of the bone structure. Bone weakness may stem from a developmental defect such as osteogenesis imperfecta or Albers-Schönberg disease, or

from a local disease such as neurofibromatosis or a neoplastic lesion.

Because degenerative spondylolisthesis is not seen in children, and because of the rarity of the traumatic and pathologic forms, they are not discussed in this book. The natural history of spondylolisthesis in children is different from that of the adult.[62, 104, 113, 153]

DYSPLASTIC (CONGENITAL) SPONDYLOLISTHESIS

This type of spondylolisthesis was recognized and carefully described at postmortem examination by investigators prior to the discovery of roentgen rays.

It is more common in the female with 2 : 1 female to male ratio.[317] The degree of slip is likely to be severe, and occasionally it is likely to cause obstruction during labor and delivery.

A sacral spina bifida is present, especially in the first sacral vertebra, and development of the superior sacral facets is deficient. Because of the constant downward and forward thrust of the trunk toward the lower lumbar vertebrae in erect posture, the lumbosacral facets give way, and the last lumbar vertebra gradually slips forward and downward over the top of the sacrum. The inferior facets of the last lumbar vertebra wear away the remnants of the superior sacral facets. The spinous process of the last lumbar vertebra is displaced forward and rests on the fibrous defect of the first sacral neural arch (Fig. 6–29). The pars interarticularis is attenuated and bent downward, but generally remains intact. Occasionally it may break under stress. The degree of slip is usually marked, and in very severe cases, the body of the last vertebra may come to lie anterior to the sacrum.

In severe spondylolisthesis, the cauda equina and the first sacral nerve root in particular are likely to be stretched in an elongated S-bend between the neural arches of the last two lumbar vertebrae anteriorly and the protuberance of the back of the first sacral body posteriorly. Ground between the vertebrae, the lumbosacral disc degenerates and is destroyed. The cartilage of the apophyseal joints wears down. Occasionally, spontaneous bony fusion takes place during this period of instability—an attempt of nature to stabilize the process and prevent further slipping. A similar reaction is the formation of a buttress of bone from the anterior aspect of the first sacral vertebra (Fig. 6–30).

When there has been a sudden increase in

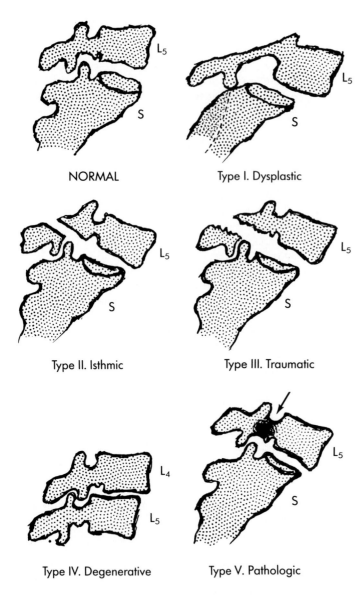

NORMAL

Type I. Dysplastic

Type II. Isthmic

Type III. Traumatic

Type IV. Degenerative

Type V. Pathologic

FIGURE 6–28. *Types of spondylolisthesis.*

Normal. Type I, dysplastic spondylolisthesis. Note the deficient development of the sacral neural arches with deficiency of the superior sacral facets. The pars interarticularis is attenuated and bent downward, but usually remains intact. Type II, isthmic spondylolisthesis (true spondylolisthesis). Note the break in the pars interarticularis. Type III, traumatic spondylolisthesis. Note the fracture of the neural arch. Type IV, degenerative spondylolisthesis. The slipping is due to degenerative joint changes causing facet deficiency. It is not seen in patients under 40 years. There is a high incidence of nerve root involvement, almost always at the fourth lumbar level. Type V, pathologic spondylolisthesis. Forward slipping is caused by insufficiency of bone structure from neoplasm or developmental defects such as osteogenesis imperfecta. (Redrawn from Newman, P. H.: The etiology of spondylolisthesis. J. Bone Joint Surg., *45-B*:41, 1963.)

FIGURE 6–29. *Findings at operation in a case of congenital spondylolisthesis.*

Note the fibrous defect in the uppermost neural arches of the sacrum. The spinous process of the last lumbar vertebra lies on the fibrous defect. The lumbosacral apophyseal joints have given way. (From Newman, P. H., and Stone, K. H.: The etiology of spondylolisthesis. J. Bone Joint Surg., *45-B*:47, 1963. Reprinted by permission.)

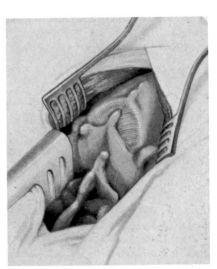

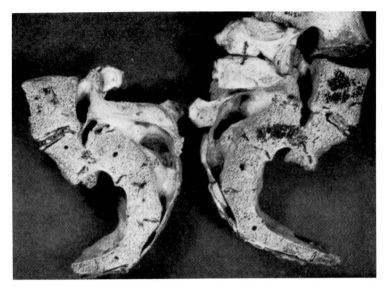

FIGURE 6–30. *Stabilization in spondylolisthesis by the formation of the buttress of bone from the anterior aspect of the first sacral vertebra.*

(From Newman, P. H., and Stone, K. H.: The etiology of spondylolisthesis. J. Bone Joint Surg., 45-B:45, 1963. Reprinted with permission.)

the degree of slip, owing to trauma or a rapid spurt of growth, the presenting complaint may be acute low back pain. On examination, one will find a rigid lumbar spine, spastic hamstrings, and often, scoliosis (Fig. 6–31). This has been described as the "clinical crisis" and "spondylolisthesis with tight hamstrings." It is due to stretching of nerve tissues.[207, 218]

ISTHMIC SPONDYLOLISTHESIS

This is the most common type of the disorder and is sometimes referred to as true spondylolisthesis. It apparently occurs only in man, who has a true upright stance, lumbar lordosis, and a bipedal gait.

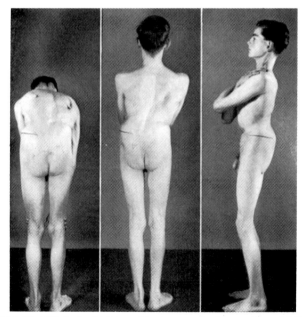

FIGURE 6–31. *"Clinical crisis" in sudden increase in degree of spondylolisthesis.*

Note the tightness of the hamstrings, the rigid lumbar spine, and the scoliosis. (From Newman, P. H., and Stone, K. H.: The etiology of spondylolisthesis. J. Bone Joint Surg., 45-B:46, 1963. Reprinted by permission.)

The total incidence of isthmic spondylolisthesis varies in different races. Absolutely accurate studies are unavailable. The overall incidence in white Americans and Europeans is approximately 4 to 5 per cent. Roche and Rowe, in a study of 4,200 skeletons, found a total incidence of 4.2 per cent. On the basis of sex and ethnic groups, however, the incidence was found to be 6.4 per cent in the white male, and 2.3 per cent in the white female; in the Negro male it was 2.8 per cent, and in the Negro female 1.1 per cent.[240] Willis, in 1923, in 1,520 unselected skeletons, found an incidence of 5.2 per cent.[309] Bailey, in 1947, reported the results of 2,080 radiographic examinations of army draftees in which he found neural arch defects in 4.4 per cent.[12] Runge, in 1954, noted an incidence of 3.09 per cent in 4,654 radiograms made in unselected pre-employment examinations, with an occurrence of actual spondylolisthesis of 2.08 per cent.[248]

In the Japanese, the incidence was reported to be 5.5 per cent in 125 skeletons studied by Hasebe in 1912.[109] Stewart, in 1953, described the Eskimos as having by far the highest incidence (24 per cent). Even more striking were the differences recorded among three groups of Eskimos according to geographic location, indicating more penetrance of hereditary factors by inbreeding. South of the Yukon River, 18.8 per cent of the individuals examined had arch defects; 31.6 per cent of the Kodiak and Aleutian Islanders were affected; and north of the Yukon River, the incidence increased to 52.6 per cent.[284]

Age Incidence

Isthmic spondylolisthesis is not present at birth and seldom before the age of four years.[13] The youngest patient reported in the literature is that of a 3½-month-old infant with spondylolisthesis between L-4 and L-5 with no history of birth trauma.[28] There are several other case reports of spondylolisthesis in young children—in a ten-month-old infant, a 17-month-old, two two-year-olds, and two three-year-olds.*

The acquired nature of isthmic spondylolisthesis is supported by the report of Wertzberger and Peterson. They reported a normal radiogram of the spine in a 7½-month-old infant who had developed spondylolisthesis at 18 months of age when re-examined.[308] Also, there

are case reports of intact but elongated neural arches in children who later exhibited spondylolisthesis with a defect in the pars interarticularis.[28, 40, 83, 142, 234, 252, 303]

Defects in the pars interarticularis appear most frequently between the ages of seven and ten years. The incidence increases with age until adulthood, but not thereafter. In 1953, Stewart reported the age incidence of neural arch defects in Alaskan natives as 5 per cent at the age of 6 years; 17 per cent at the age of 30 years; 34 per cent between 30 and 40 years of age; and no increase after the age of 40, a striking example of the increase in incidence with age.[284]

Slipping occurs before the age of 20 years. The period of most rapid olisthy is between 10 and 15 years. Unless there has been surgical intervention, slipping rarely, if ever, increases after the age of 20.

Etiology

The true etiology of isthmic spondylolysis has given rise to much controversy. Its pathogenesis is not yet established. Wiltse and Newman, in reviews of the etiology of spondylolisthesis, refuted several of the theories that had been advanced over the years.[202, 311, 313]

Abnormal Ossification. This theory was one of the first to be presented. It proposed that, in patients with spondylolisthesis, each lateral mass, which normally ossifies from one center, instead ossified from two centers. The origin of the defect was thought to be a lack of fusion between two separate centers of ossification. Anatomic sections of over 700 fetuses have shown neither separate ossification centers nor any defect in the pars interarticularis.[17, 20, 50, 51, 83, 171, 208, 238, 261] Radiograms of newborns have not shown any evidence of spondylolisthesis nor any defect in the pars interarticularis.[13, 116]

Acute Trauma. This has been eliminated as a causative factor, at birth or during postnatal life, by the failure of Rowe and Roche to produce a fracture of the pars interarticularis in experiments on stillborn infants.[247] Unquestionable fractures of the pars interarticularis, as reported in the literature, have healed.[239, 311] Studies by Stewart did not show the evidence of repair that one normally observes in fractures.[282, 284] In histologic sections of the defect there was neither evidence of callus formation nor anything that would seem to suggest an acute fracture.[238, 310]

Pinching-off of Pars Interarticularis by Impingement of Articular Process. In 1885, Lane

---

*See references: ten-month-old, 84; 17-month-old, 143; two-year-olds, 253; three-year-olds, 40, 304.

suggested that the defect in the pars interarticularis of the fifth lumbar vertebra is produced by downward pressure of the inferior articular process of the fourth lumbar vertebra and upward pressure of the superior articular process of the sacrum eroding through the pars interarticularis (Fig. 6–32).[151] This theory has been supported by Capener in 1931 and 1960, by Meyer-Burgdorff in 1931, and by Nathan in 1959.[47, 48, 176, 195] The pinching-off process, however, is not seen in radiograms of children and adolescents.

Following an extensive study of the etiology of spondylolisthesis, Wiltse formulated the theory that the defect is caused by two factors: an inherited dysplasia or defect present in the cartilage model of the arch of the affected vertebra, and a strain on tne weakened pars interarticularis from physical forces resulting from man's characteristic upright stance and lumbar lordosis. He believes that stress and strain on the pars interarticularis will not in itself produce the defect unless the dysplasia or hereditary weakness is already present. Dysplasia is characterized by lack of normal ability of the bone to repair itself. The result is bone resorption rather than new bone formation, and the production of the characteristic defect.[313]

Instability in the lumbosacral region due to weakness of the supporting structures and a deficiency of the lumbosacral fascia, the posterior spinal ligaments, and the intervertebral disc were suggested by Newman as being contributory factors. He believed that the defect in the pars interarticularis is not the cause of spondylolisthesis, but rather, is a result of the instability, which produces so much stress on the once normal pars that it undergoes a stress fracture.[202] Roberts advanced the idea that the defect is a stress fracture.[235]

Repetitive stress and microtrauma are major factors in the pathogenesis of the pars interarticularis elongation and defect. This is suggested by the high incidence of spondylolysis and spondylolisthesis in adolescents who take part in certain sports such as weight-lifting, wrestling, gymnastics, high-jumping, diving, rowing, and American football.[119, 126, 184, 245, 290, 320]

In the literature there are several reports of spondylolisthesis occurring immediately above the level of fusion in the lumbosacral area secondary to stress fracture due to the deranged biomechanics of the spine.[7, 59, 65, 107, 287, 300] Spondylolisthesis has also been observed in association with a congenitally fused segment of the spine and as a sequel to a disc space infection.[59, 256]

In species other than *Homo sapiens* spondylolisthesis is not recorded. Man's upright posture is a requisite for the causation of the pars interarticularis defect. In a study of 143 non-ambulatory cerebral palsy patients with an average age of 27 years, Rosenberg and associates did not find a single case of spondylolysis or spondylolisthesis.[243]

When upright the pars interarticularis is the anatomic site of greatest stress. Lumbar lordosis aggravates the stress forces across it, and the incidence of spondylolysis becomes greater with increase in the lordotic angle. The forces that cause lysis of the pars interarticularis and spondylolisthesis are flexion overload, unbalanced stress force, and forced rotation.[75] The extended posture of the spine increases the strain from the forces that cause fatigue fracture.

Genetic Factors

There is definite evidence that defects in the pars interarticularis have a familial incidence.[13, 14, 83, 152, 281, 282, 313] The incidence, as reported in the literature, varies from 28 to 69 per cent.*

Baker and McHollick studied the radiograms of 400 unselected six- to seven-year-old children (225 boys and 175 girls) and found defects in the pars interarticularis in 18 of them (12 males and 6 females). Radiograms of these children's parents revealed defects in 28 per cent of them.[13] Wiltse studied 36 families in which one member had spondylolisthesis. He found a parental incidence of 26 per cent (26 of 101 individuals).[313]

Familial incidence is higher in dysplastic than in isthmic spondylolisthesis. In a radiographic survey of families of patients with spondylolisthesis, Wynne-Davies and Scott reported 33 per cent of relatives of patients with dysplastic spondylolisthesis were affected, whereas the familial incidence in isthmic spondylolisthesis was 15 per cent.[325] Associated with the dysplastic form there is also a higher incidence of sacral spina bifida and deficient development of the superior facets of the upper sacrum. Spondylolisthesis has been described in identical twins.[293, 306]

The mode of inheritance that is consistent with the data and that explains most of the pedigrees is that there is a single recessive gene with incomplete penetrance. There is a suggestion, however, that the involved gene sometimes shows incomplete dominance when nei-

---

*See references 13, 83, 137, 213, 265, 282, 290, 297, 311, 312, 325.

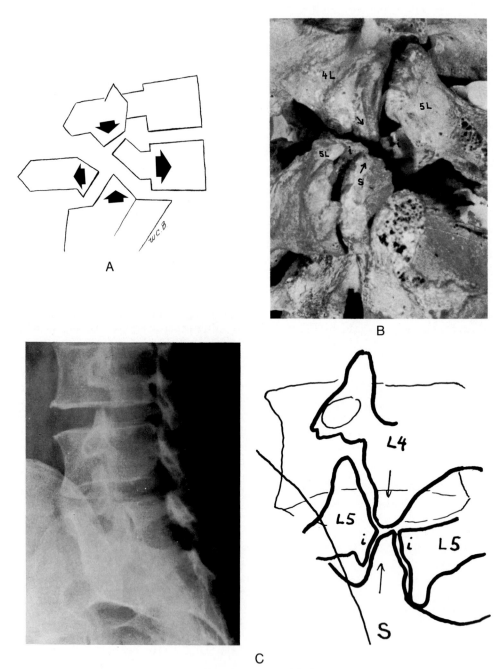

FIGURE 6–32. *Spondylolisthesis.*

A. Diagrammatic lateral view of the lower lumbosacral spine showing the wedgelike eroding forces on the defective pars interarticularis produced by downward pressure of the superior articular process of the first sacral vertebra. (Redrawn from Capener, N.: Spondylolisthesis. Brit. J. Surg., *19*:374, 1931.)

B. Gross specimen of typical spondylolisthesis of the fifth lumbar vertebra. Right lateral view of the articulated fourth lumbar vertebra, fifth lumbar vertebra, and sacrum. Note the cleft between the articular process of the fourth lumbar vertebra (*4L arrow*) and the articular process of the sacrum (*S arrow*). The cleft isthmus (*i., i.*) is thinner than normal. **C.** Left oblique radiogram and diagrammatic tracing of the radiogram of the lower spine with bilateral spondylolysis of the fifth lumbar vertebra. Note the articular process of the sacrum (*S arrow*) projects upward and penetrates deeply into the cleft, meeting the downward-projecting inferior articular process of the fourth lumbar vertebra (*L4 arrow*). (From Nathan H: Spondylolysis: Its anatomy and mechanisms of development. J. Bone Joint Surg., *41-A*:305, 310, 1959. Reprinted by permission.)

ther parent is affected but four of five siblings of the propositus are affected.

Pathology

The pathologic anatomy of the defect has been described by a number of observers.[30, 90, 227, 238, 310, 313] No evidence of callus formation was revealed by any of the studies, nor were there histologic findings to suggest fracture healing. The pathologic picture is not identical in every case, however. The tissue in the defect is more fibrous in nature when there is a wide gap. In some cases there may be a mass of fibrocartilage that appears to press on the nerve roots. When the gap is narrow, the bone ends tend to be smooth, blunt, and eburnated, or even to have some hyaline cartilage on each side of the defect. There is no periosteum over them; the transition from fibrous tissue to bone is usually abrupt. In some specimens they taper out at the defect.

The body of the fifth lumbar vertebra in the adult afflicted with spondylolisthesis is slightly trapezoid, its anterior border being longer than the posterior one (Fig. 6–33). It tends to become more trapezoid in shape as slipping takes place. To delineate this anatomic peculiarity, Vallois and Lozarthes described a lumbar index.

Lumbar index =

$$\frac{\text{Height of posterior border of body in millimeters} \times 100}{\text{Height of anterior border of body in millimeters}}$$

An index of less than 100 means that the height of the posterior border of the vertebral body is less than the anterior. They found the average lumbar index to be 89 in 500 normal spines, 83 in 41 spines with spondylolysis, and 76 in 65 spines with spondylolisthesis.[301]

In spines with severe slipping of the fifth lumbar vertebra, the top of the sacrum is dome-shaped.[189] The dome-shaped sacrum and severely trapezoid shape of the body of the vertebra represent secondary changes that are not present in the very young child following the first appearance of the defect.

The 1962 study of Wiltse showed spina bifida to be 13 times as frequent in persons with a defect in the pars interarticularis as in those with normal spines. A severe degree of idiopathic structural scoliosis was noted to be four times more common in spondylolysis than in normal spines.[313]

Level of Involvement

The fifth lumbar vertebra is most commonly involved (103 of 115 defects in the series of Bosworth and associates), and the next in frequency is the fourth (10 out of 115 defects).[30] The third may be involved. Several vertebrae may be affected, usually two, including the fourth and fifth lumbar segments.[225] Spondylolisthesis may also occur in the cervical vertebrae.[73, 93, 100, 136, 210] The defect in the cervical spine is in the pedicle, however, and not in the pars interarticularis.

Forward Slipping

The degree of severity of anterior displacement of spondylolisthesis is classified by Meyerding, according to the percentage of slippage, into Grade I, Grade II, Grade III, and Grade IV (Fig. 6–34).[177, 178] The superior border of the anteroposterior diameter of the subjacent vertebra is divided into four equal parts; in Grade I, the displacement is 25 per cent or less, i.e., the posteroinferior angle of the anteriorly displaced vertebra lies within the first segment; in Grade II, between 25 and 50 per cent; in Grade III, between 50 and 75 per cent; and in Grade IV, more than 75 per cent.

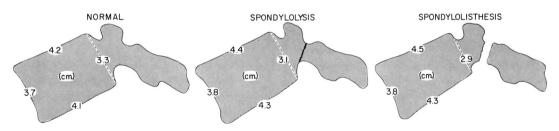

FIGURE 6–33. *Average dimensions of the adult fifth lumbar vertebra.*

Shown with no defects in the pars interarticularis, with spondylolysis, and with spondylolisthesis. Note the trapezoid shape of the fifth lumbar vertebra with spondylolisthesis. (Redrawn after Wiltse, L. L.: The etiology of spondylolisthesis. J. Bone Joint Surg., *44-A*:548, 1962.)

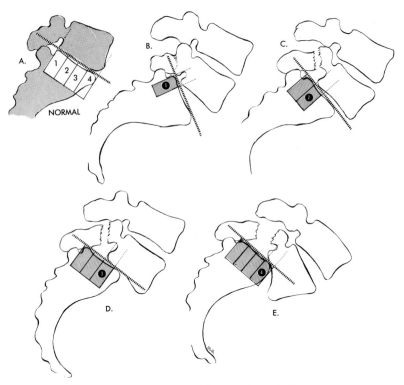

FIGURE 6–34. Gradation of degrees of spondylolisthesis.

A. Normal. The superior border of the anteroposterior diameter of the subjacent vertebra is divided into four equal parts. **B.** Grade I: The anterior displacement is 25 per cent or less, i.e., the posteroinferior angle of the displaced vertebra lies within the first segment. **C.** Grade II: The displacement is between 25 and 50 per cent. **D.** Grade III: The displacement is between 50 and 75 per cent. **E.** Grade IV: The displacement is greater than 75 per cent. (Redrawn from Meyerding, H. W.: Spondylolisthesis. Surg. Gynecol. Obstet., 54:371, 1932.)

In the Meschan method of measuring the degree of spondylolisthesis on the lateral radiogram, shown in Figure 6–35, the first line extends between the posterior lip of the vertebral body below (points A and B), and the second line is drawn between the posterior upper and lower lips of the slipped vertebral body (points C and D). The lines are extended; if not parallel, they will meet and form an angle, which is measured with a protractor. If the lines are parallel (very occasionally this may occur in spondylolisthesis), the linear distance between the lines is measured. When the angle is as much as 10 degrees, the spondylolisthesis can be called slight; 11 to 20 degrees, moderate; and greater than 20 degrees, severe. When the two lines are parallel, a distance of more than 3 mm. is abnormal. The degree of displacement should be reported accurately by stating, ". . . spondylolisthesis with a displacement through an angle of x degrees"; or, if the lines are parallel, ". . . a distance of x mm."[175]

The degree of spondylolisthesis may also be measured by comparing the anteroposterior diameter of the slipped vertebra with the one above it (Fig. 6–36).[47] Ullman's sign is demonstrated by drawing a line at a right angle to the upper border of the sacrum at its anterior edge; in the normal spine, the fifth lumbar vertebra lies entirely behind this line, whereas in spondylolisthesis the perpendicular line is intersected by the slipped vertebral body.

In the method of Marique and Taillard the displacement is measured as a percentage of the anteroposterior diameter of the subjacent vertebral body (Fig. 6–37).[280] A similar but slightly modified technique is utilized by Bradford (Fig. 6–38).[38, 39] First, a line is drawn along the posterior aspect of the body of the first sacral vertebra—this serves as a consistent reference point for future measurements. Second, a perpendicular line is drawn from the posteroinferior cortex of the fifth lumbar vertebra, and the amount of anterior displacement is measured in millimeters (A). Third, the greatest dimension of the width of the sacrum is measured—this serves as the denominator (B). The percentage of slippage is:

$$\frac{\text{A (The amount of anterior displacement in millimeters)}}{\text{B (The dimension of the greatest width of the body of the sacrum)}}$$

This author recommends use of the *percentage of slip* as the method for quantitating the severity of the slip.

The *slip angle* is the angular relationship between the fifth lumbar and first sacral vertebrae.[318] In the literature it is also referred to as the angle of lumbosacral kyphosis.[278] The term *slip angle* is preferred by most authors.[31, 38, 39, 62] The slip angle is the angle formed between lines drawn on the superior surface of the endplate of the fifth lumbar vertebral body and the inferior surface of the end-plate of the first sacral vertebra (Fig. 6–39). This author prefers these two surfaces because frequently the endplates of the L-5–S-1 disc are distorted. Bradford favors measuring the slip angle by first drawing a line perpendicular to a line drawn along the posterior aspect of the first sacral vertebral body and, second, drawing a line parallel to the inferior end-plate of the fifth lumbar vertebral body. The angle formed between these two lines is the slip angle, and this method reflects its true magnitude.[39]

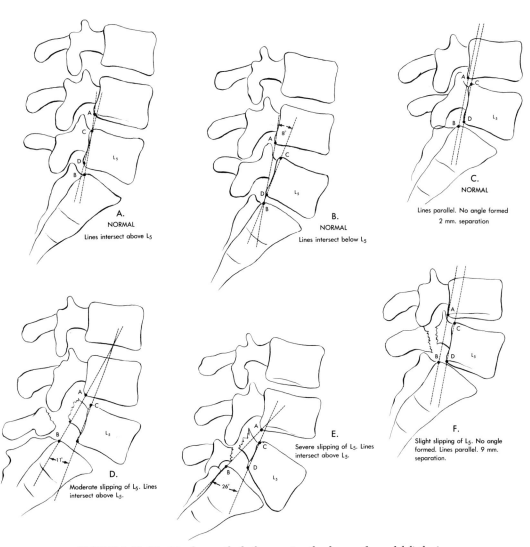

FIGURE 6–35. *The Meschan method of measuring the degree of spondylolisthesis.*

A to **C.** The three general types of normal lumbosacral spine. Note the position of the apex of the angles made by intersecting lines are at L5 in Figure 6–19 A or below L5 in Figure 6–19 B. **D** to **F.** Note the arrangement of the lines in cases of spondylolisthesis. See text for explanation. (Redrawn after Meschan, I.: Spondylolisthesis. A.J.R., 53:230–243, 1945.)

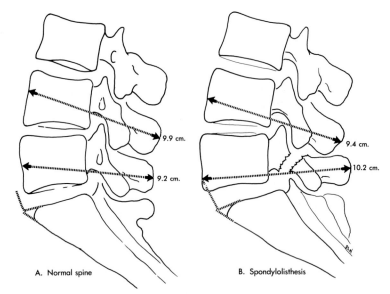

9.9 cm.

9.2 cm.

9.4 cm.

10.2 cm.

A. Normal spine

B. Spondylolisthesis

FIGURE 6–36. *Capener's method of determining the degree of spondylolisthesis.*

Displacement is measured by comparison of anteroposterior diameters of the spondylolytic vertebra and the normal vertebra above it. Ullman's sign is demonstrated by drawing a line at right angles to the upper border of the sacrum at its anterior edge. Note in the normal spine (**A**) the fifth lumbar vertebra lies entirely behind this line, whereas in spondylolisthesis, the perpendicular line is intersected by the slipped vertebral body. (Redrawn after Capener, N.: Spondylolisthesis. Brit. J. Surg., *19*:374, 1931.)

Clinical Features

In spondylolisthesis the defects are often discovered incidentally on radiograms taken for some other reason. Usually the condition is asymptomatic.[80] In Lafond's series of 415 patients with spondylolisthesis, only 9 per cent had enough pain to seek medical attention during childhood or adolescence.[147]

The clinical picture depends on the age of the patient and the severity of the slipping. In children under ten years of age, it does not usually cause symptoms; poor posture and increasing lumbar lordosis may be the only presenting complaint.

Symptoms usually begin insidiously in the second decade of life, at the adolescent growth spurt. Initially the pain is a dull low backache during standing or walking and is usually relieved by rest. Later, pain may develop in the buttocks and posterior parts of the thighs. Pain of this pattern results from instability of the fifth lumbar segment. The second pattern of pain is radicular pain radiating distally to one or both lower limbs along the course of the sciatic nerve, especially into the distribution of the fifth lumbar or first sacral dermatomes. Sciatica may be accompanied by sensory or motor disturbances and is caused by irritation of the nerve roots caused by the fibrocartilaginous mass at the defects in the pars interartic-

ularis (Figs. 6–40 and 6–41). In the adult, very occasionally, the sciatica may be caused by protrusion of an intervertebral disc (usually the one at the L-4–L-5 level). Complaints of weakness and stiffness of the lower back are common. Trauma, as from a fall or a twisting strain, may aggravate the symptoms of spondylolisthesis.

Physical findings depend on the extent of slipping and the presence or absence of nerve root irritation. In asymptomatic Grade I and II slips the only positive physical finding will be exaggeration of lumbar lordosis. In prone position on hyperextension of the lumbosacral spine and deep palpation, there may be local tenderness at the L-5–S-1 level. There may be mild scoliosis, which may be structural or due to reflex spasm.

In most symptomatic and some asymptomatic slips there is hamstring tautness or spasm, as shown by a decrease in range of straight leg raising and limitation of forward flexion of the trunk. Hamstring tautness is often a compensatory mechanism to provide some degree of stability to an unstable L-5–S-1 articulation; the center of gravity is readjusted by the increase in the degree of lumbar lordosis and hip and knee flexion. In severe spondylolisthesis, traction on the cauda equina may cause hamstring spasm.

In cases of severe spondylolisthesis, the torso is shortened, and transverse skin creases are

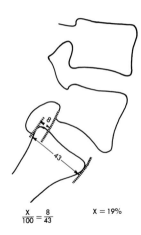

FIGURE 6–37. *The method of Marique and Taillard for measuring the degree of slipping.*

The olisthy is measured as a percentage of the subjacent vertebral body. (Redrawn after Taillard, W.: Le spondylolisthesis chez l'enfant et l'adolescent: Étude de 50 cas. Acta Orthop. Scand., *24*:115, 1954.)

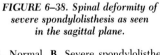

$$\frac{X}{100} = \frac{8}{43} \qquad X = 19\%$$

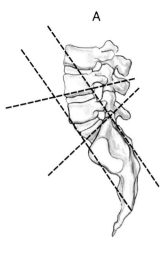

A

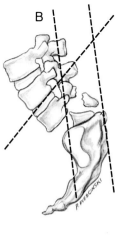

B

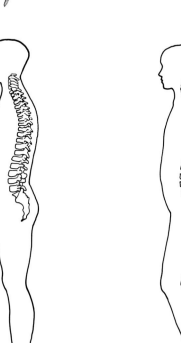

FIGURE 6–38. *Spinal deformity of severe spondylolisthesis as seen in the sagittal plane.*

A. Normal. **B.** Severe spondylolisthesis. Note the vertical sacrum, the severe lumbosacral kyphosis, the forward displacement of the lumbar spine, and the compensatory lordosis. (Redrawn from Bradford, D. S.: Spondylolysis and spondylolisthesis. *In* Moe, J. H.: Textbook of Scoliosis and Other Spinal Deformities. 2nd Ed. Philadelphia, W.B. Saunders, 1987, p. 418.)

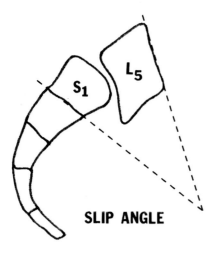

SLIP ANGLE

FIGURE 6–39.

The slip angle is the angle between lines drawn on the superior surface of L5 and inferior surface of S1 vertebral bodies. This determination should be made on true spot lateral radiograms of L5–S1 spine taken with the patient standing. (From Amundson, G. M., and Wenger, D. R.: Spondylolisthesis—natural history and treatment. Spine: State of the Art Reviews. Vol. 1, No. 2, January 1987, Reprinted by permission.)

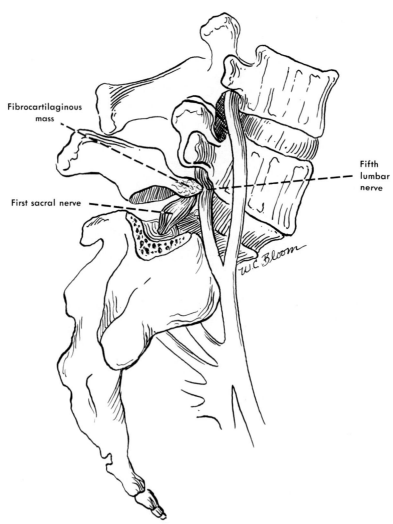

FIGURE 6–40. Pathologic anatomy of spondylolisthesis at L5–S1 level.

Note the impingement upon the first sacral and fifth lumbar nerve roots by the fibrocartilaginous mass at the defect and the freely moveable fifth lumbar lamina. (Redrawn after Woolsey, R. D.: Mechanism of neurological symptoms and signs in spondylolisthesis at the fifth lumbar, first sacral level. J. Neurosurg., *11*:67, 1954.)

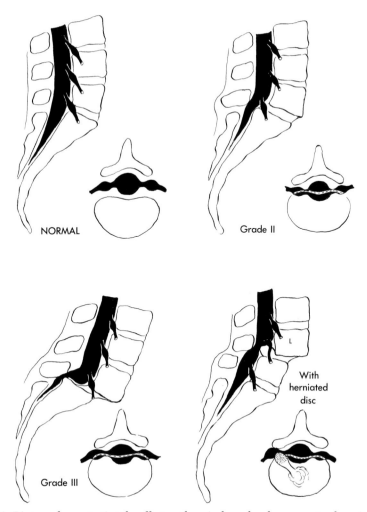

NORMAL

Grade II

Grade III

With herniated disc

L

FIGURE 6–41. *Diagram demonstrating the effect on the spinal canal and nerve roots of varying degrees of spondylolisthesis and herniated disc.*

seen between the rib cage and the iliac crests. The distances between the xiphoid cartilage and the pubis and between the ribs and the iliac crests are diminished. The spine gives the appearance of having been telescoped into the pelvis. The sacrum is prominent and more vertical than normal. On palpation and inspection, the spinous process of the detached neural arch is prominent, and there is a depression just above it. The bi-iliac diameter, which is normally less than the bitrochanteric diameter, becomes greater in severe spondylolisthesis. The pelvic inclination is increased, and there is exaggeration of the normal lumbar lordosis. There may be spasm of the erector spinae and marked tautness of the hamstring muscles. The spine of the involved vertebra will be tender on deep palpation.

The body of the slipped lumbar vertebra may be palpable on abdominal or pelvic examination

or both. The gait will be awkward, with a waddle characterized by shortened stride length, wide base of support, and limited hip flexion. Neurologic findings depend on the level and the degree of nerve root irritation or compression.

Radiographic Findings

When spondylolysis or spondylolisthesis is suspected clinically, anteroposterior, lateral, and right and left oblique (45-degree) views of the lumbosacral spine and a spot lateral view of the fifth lumbar and first sacral vertebrae are made. The lateral radiographs should be made standing because in an upright posture the percentage and angle of slip increase.[31]

Spondylolysis is best shown by a 25- to 45-degree oblique view of the lumbosacral joint. In this view the lamina will flatten out, and an outline resembling a Scottish terrier can easily be seen, the dog's "neck" being formed by the pars interarticularis in which the defect is shown as a break or a separation (Fig. 6–42). In one fifth of cases of spondylolysis the defect is unilateral; therefore, it is important to take both right and left oblique projections of the lumbosacral spine.

In unilateral spondylolysis there may be reactive sclerosis of the opposite pars interarticularis.[269] Asymmetry of the neural arch and unilateral wedging of the vertebral body are other radiographic findings sometimes associated with spondylolysis.

In spondylolisthesis and sometimes in spondylolysis the defect in the pars interarticularis may be seen in the lateral projection. In clinically suspected cases of spondylolysis in which routine radiographs appear to be normal, oblique linear tomography and computed axial tomography (CT scan) will clearly depict the defect.

In spondylolisthesis, forward displacement of the vertebra is seen in the lateral radiograph. In the normal spine a straight line placed along the shadow of the anterior border of the body of the first sacral vertebra will project upward and forward well to the front of the shadow of the fifth lumbar body, whereas in spondylolisthesis the straight edge will transect the body of the fifth lumbar vertebra (Ullman's sign).

In the anteroposterior view a "bowline" appearance of the slipped fifth lumbar vertebra has been described by Brailsford; it represents convergence of the vertebra's inferior and lateral aspects with the inferior and lateral aspects of its transverse processes (Fig. 6–43).[40] It is seen clearly in advanced cases, and it is of value in diagnosis.

In severe spondylolisthesis, in the anteroposterior radiograph, the slipped fifth lumbar vertebra is visualized "end-on," overlapping the first sacral vertebra—this is referred to as the "reverse Napoleon hat sign"—the hat is upside down.

In symptomatic spondylolisthesis, mobility at the defect between L-5 and S-1 is determined by supine hyperextension and hyperflexion true lateral spot radiographs of the lumbosacral spine. Traction in hyperextension will further increase the percentage of a hypermobile slip.

Bone Imaging With Technetium-99m. The affected pars interarticularis will show increased uptake of the radionuclide. This is particularly true in "acute" cases when there is reparative response to the stress fracture.[86] In the early acute stages the bone scan with SPECT pinhole

imaging is much more sensitive than the plain oblique radiographs in the detection of spondylolysis. It will assist in distinguishing the acute from the chronic lesions; thereby, it is of value in determining when to treat spondylolysis with support in a lumbosacral orthosis. With early adequate treatment, healing of the defect in the pars interarticularis may occur.[80]

Myelography is ordinarily not performed in symptomatic spondylolisthesis with radicular pain. Associated disc herniation is extremely rare in children and adolescents.[1, 30, 180] When sciatic pain is out of proportion and persists despite bed rest, and neurologic findings suggest the possibility of a coexisting lesion such as a spinal cord tumor or other intraspinal disease, metrizamide myelography is indicated with computed axial tomography scanning. Recently magnetic resonance imaging is being performed first because it is not an invasive procedure.

Treatment

The modality of treatment depends on the absence or presence of the following clinical and radiographic *risk factors* for progressive slippage and disability (Table 6–1).

Age of the Patient. Except in rare cases, spondylolisthesis does not usually appear until the age of four or five years. Progressive displacement of the vertebrae may occur during periods of rapid growth spurts in childhood and adolescence, but once the age of 20 years is reached, further slipping usually does not take place unless there has been surgical intervention in the form of extensive laminectomy. As a rule adolescents during their growth spurt are at risk for increase in slip.

Symptoms. Asymptomatic spondylolysis has a better prognosis than the symptomatic one. Adolescents with back pain tend to have recurring episodes of symptoms.

Sex. Girls are at greater risk for progressive slip than boys; this is particularly true in the dysplastic type of spondylolisthesis.

Marked Ligamentous Hyperlaxity. Such laxity, as seen in children with Marfan's or Down's syndrome, is a poor prognostic sign. The probabilities are great for further slip.

Type of Spondylolisthesis. Dysplastic lesions have a greater tendency for progressive olisthy than the isthmic type.

Degree of the Slip. Simple spondylolysis or minimal spondylolithesis in an adolescent is very unlikely to show further displacement,

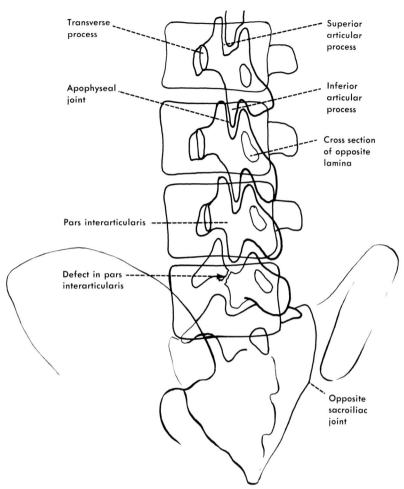

Transverse process

Superior articular process

Apophyseal joint

Inferior articular process

Cross section of opposite lamina

Pars interarticularis

Defect in pars interarticularis

Opposite sacroiliac joint

FIGURE 6–42. *Spondylolisthesis.*

Diagram of oblique view in radiogram shows the defect in the pars interarticularis.

FIGURE 6–43.

The anteroposterior radiographic appearance of the spondylolisthetic vertebra.

The outline of the vertebra is that of a bow—the anterior convex outline of the body merges imperceptibly on each side by a gradual concavity into the outline of the lumbar transverse process. This outline is projected into the shadows of the first and second sacral vertebral bodies. (Redrawn after Brailsford, J.: Spondylolisthesis. Brit. J. Radiol., 6:666, 1933.)

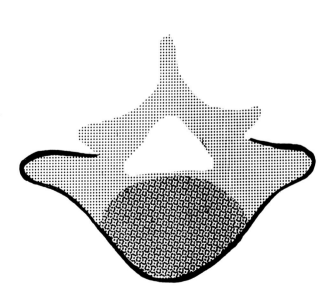

Table 6–1. *Risk Factors for Progression of Spondylolisthesis*

Clinical

Age—young child, under ten years
Sex—females at greater risk
Symptomatology—children with backache have greater likelihood.
Excessive ligamentous hyperlaxity

Radiologic

Type of spondylolisthesis—dysplastic lesions have greater tendency than isthmic defects.
Degree of slip. Simple spondylolysis, minimal chances; 50 per cent and over, olisthesis is greater probability.
High slip angle—40–50 and over
Mobility at L5–S1 indicates instability and greater possibility for progression.
Anatomic stability—a trapezoid or wedge-shaped body of the fifth lumbar vertebra and a dome-shaped top of the first sacral vertebra means instability and greater likelihood of progression. An anterior lip of the sacrum and narrowed L5–S1 disc interspace indicates stability and minimal chance of further slip.

whereas a child with 50 per cent slippage is at great risk for progression.

Slip Angle. When a child presents with a high slip angle (over 40 to 50 degrees) there is greater probability of progression of the anterior displacement.

Mobility of the Defect. Revealed by dynamic radiographs, such mobility indicates instability and the possibility of increase in the degree of spondylolisthesis.

Anatomic Stability at L-5 and S-1. The chances of progressive slippage are great when the superior surface of the sacrum is perpendicular and dome-shaped and the fifth lumbar vertebra is trapezoid. Conversely, a buttress of the anterior lip of the sacrum and narrowed disc interspace between L-5 and S-1 indicates stability.

SPONDYLOLYSIS

Most children with spondylolysis do not develop backache; these asymptomatic cases do not require treatment. The patients are allowed to take part in normal activities with no restriction. Both the parents and patient are informed of the defect and the risk factors as to progression.

If the child remains asymptomatic he is reexamined in 3 to 6 months, but repeat radiographs are unnecessary unless symptoms such as increasing hamstring tautness and gait disturbance develop.

If the patient has exaggerated lumbar lordosis and an increase in pelvic tilt, postural exercises are in order. They consist of gluteus maximus, abdominal, and pelvic tilt exercises. Acute flex-

ion of the trunk in abdominal exercises should be avoided. Pelvic tilt exercises are first done supine and then standing against the wall, rolling the buttocks under.

Symptomatic spondylolysis is treated conservatively. When the child or adolescent presents with acute pain and a positive bone scan indicates stress fracture, the lumbosacral spine is supported in a brace in the form of reverse (anterior closure) Boston thoracolumbosacral (TLSO) orthosis. In a noncompliant adolescent a plaster of Paris body cast may be employed. In the initial very acute phase, bed rest and traction with the hips and knees in a comfortable degree of flexion may be appropriate. With such rest and support, the symptoms ordinarily will subside, the hamstring tautness will improve, and gradually the patient will become asymptomatic. With early diagnosis and effective treatment some of these stress fractures (spondylolysis) of the pars interarticularis do heal in six months as shown by negative follow-up bone scans and normal radiographs.

For patients with symptomatic spondylolysis, physical activities such as contact sports or those in which there is risk of trauma to the spine should be curtailed. The patients should be advised against participation in weight-lifting and cautioned against becoming overweight.

Symptomatic spondylolysis that does not respond to conservative orthotic treatment for a period of 12 months and is disabling, interfering with activities of daily living, should be treated by spinal fusion. If the spondylolysis is between L-5 and S-1 the posterolateral fusion extends between the fifth lumbar vertebra and the mid-sacrum. The transverse process of L-5 is often small; it is important not to mistake the transverse process of L-4 for it and not to include L-4 in the fusion area.

If the pars defect is between L-4 and L-5, direct repair of the defect is performed. By not extending the fusion across normal joints, normal motion of the lumbar spine is preserved. The Scott technique of internal fixation with wire from the transverse process to the spinous process and autogenous iliac bone grafting of the pars defect is recommended by Bradford.[37] Internal fixation by a screw across the defect is technically demanding and has the potential of causing neurologic deficit.[44]

SPONDYLOLISTHESIS

When the disorder is *asymptomatic* and the percentage of slip is less than 50 per cent, treatment is conservative. Patients with asymptomatic spondylolisthesis are checked clinically and radiographically every six months during childhood and adolescence. When the percentage of slip is less than 25 per cent, normal physical activity is allowed; if the percentage of slip is greater than 25 per cent, however, the patient should be restricted from strenuous physical activity such as weight-lifting and contact sports and should be advised to refrain from heavy labor.

Patients with *symptomatic spondylolisthesis* of less than 25 per cent usually respond to conservative management in the form of orthotic support to the lumbosacral spine. They ordinarily do not require stabilization by fusion. If symptoms recur after resumption of strenuous activity, the brace is reapplied. *Symptomatic spondylolisthesis* greater than 25 per cent and less than 50 per cent is initially treated conservatively; however, these patients, during the growing years of childhood and adolescence, require close observation and reassessment. If symptoms keep recurring and disability is great, it is best to perform simple posterolateral transverse alar fusion.

OPERATIVE TREATMENT

Indications. Operative intervention is indicated (1) when there is persistent back pain and marked disability interfering with activities of daily living despite conservative management, i.e., temporary support to the spine, activity restriction, and physical therapy for a period of six months to a year; (2) in severe slip—greater than 50 per cent—with severe tautness of the hamstrings, postural deformity, and abnormal gait unresponsive to aggressive physical therapy; (3) when there is progression of the slip beyond 25 to 50 per cent owing to marked instability at the defect; (4) in the presence of neurologic deficit that does not improve with conservative management and may or may not progress; and (5) when persistent sciatic scoliosis is unresponsive to rest, physical therapy, and support of the spine.

When the spondylolisthesis is 50 per cent or more and the slip angle is over 50 degrees in a growing child or adolescent, the period of conservative management should not be prolonged if the symptoms and disability persist. Results of surgical stabilization are excellent; the parents and patient should be informed of the psychosocial importance of normal physical activity for an adolescent.

Objectives. The goals of surgery are (1) to stabilize the unstable spondylolytic segment; (2) to prevent further slip; (3) to relieve any nerve root irritation and prevent further neurologic deficit; and (4) to correct hamstring tautness, poor posture, and abnormality of gait.

In Situ Fusion. The most effective method is posterolateral alar transverse process fusion, extending from the fourth or fifth lumbar vertebra to the midsacrum. The fusion extends to the tips of the transverse processes. Because of the high angle L-4–L-5 disc space and the small size of the transverse processes of the fifth lumbar vertebra, often the arthrodesis is extended to the fourth lumbar vertebra in order to prevent pseudarthrosis. Facet joint fusion is performed. The bone graft is autogenous, obtained from the ilium. Postoperative immobilization in a brace is adequate. When there is *neurologic deficit* (motor and sensory) due to nerve root involvement, thorough neurologic assessment and magnetic resonance imaging or CT scanning with metrazimide myelography are performed to delineate the pathologic anatomy. The fifth lumbar nerve root is the one most often involved because of compression by the upper segment of the pars interarticularis of L-5 as it is tilted anteriorly by the displaced body of the vertebra. The loose lamina of L-5 is not the cause of nerve root compression. Occasionally sacral nerve roots are involved, as shown by bladder sphincter tone weakness. Hamstring spasm is not ordinarily a sign of nerve root compression. In severe spondylolisthesis, Boxall and associates could not demonstrate any correlation between hamstring tautness and objective signs of neurologic deficit.[31] Clinical experience has shown that in cases with hamstring spasm that have been treated by in situ fusion without decompression the hamstring tautness resolves spontaneously six to eight months postoperatively, corresponding to the period of consolidation of the fused area.[317]

Decompression is indicated when there is unquestionable motor deficit or bladder or bowel dysfunction, and when computed tomography scanning with myelography or magnetic resonance imaging clearly demonstrates the cause of nerve involvement. As stated, the loose unstable lamina is not the cause of nerve irritation. The offending structures are the proximal part of the pars interarticularis or the hypertrophied fibrocartilaginous mass at the site of the deficit when the fifth lumbar nerve root is involved and the prominent portion of the body of the first sacral vertebra when sacral nerve roots are affected.

In the literature several reports of treatment of spondylolisthesis with decompression alone by removal of the loose lamina and the fibrocartilaginous mass have appeared.[89, 128, 140, 324]

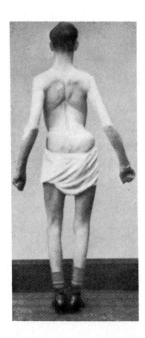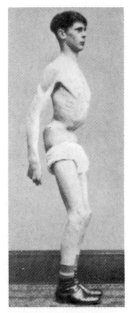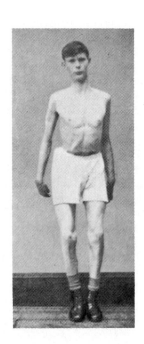

A

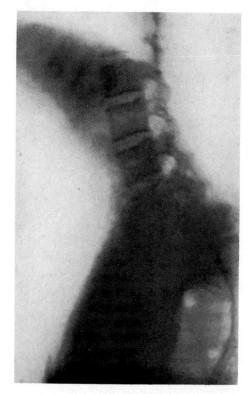

B

FIGURE 6–44. Severe spondylolisthesis with complete displacement of the fifth lumbar vertebra over the sacrum.

A. Clinical appearance of patient. Note severe compensatory lordosis. The posterior projection of the pelvis makes walking difficult. **B.** X-ray appearance. (From Jenkins, J. A.: Spondylolisthesis. Brit. J. Surg., *24*:80–85, 1936.)

C

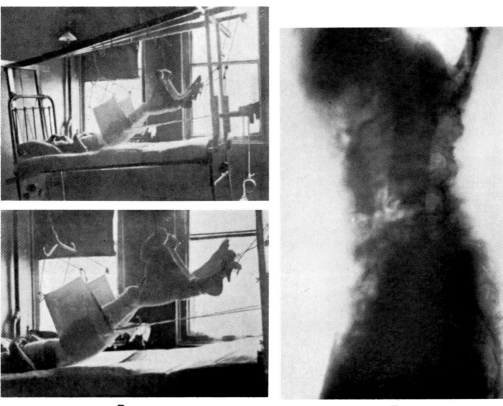

D   E

FIGURE 6–44 Continued. *Severe spondylolisthesis with complete displacement of the fifth lumbar vertebra over the sacrum.*

C and **D.** Method of reduction. (The author recommends direct skeletal traction with Steinmann pins through the distal femur and wires through both iliac wings.) **E.** Radiogram showing reduction. (From Jenkins, J. A.: Spondylolisthesis. Brit. J. Surg., *24*:80–85, 1936.)

Illustration continued on following page

Decompression alone, without fusion, has no place in the treatment of spondylolisthesis in children or adolescents, as it leads to increased instability, progression of forward slip, and greater lumbar kyphosis and deformity. Even a defective neural arch provides some support to the slipped vertebrae. Further olisthy can and does occur after removal of the arch. In Bosworth's series of 64 patients who had the arch removed and subsequent fusion, 19 (30 per cent) had measurable progression of the olisthy. Pseudarthrosis was present in only 5 of these patients, while the remaining 14 suffered slipping during the four to five months required for solidification of the fusion.[30]

Anterior Fusion. Anterior fusion or interbody arthrodesis was first performed by Burns in 1933.[46] Since then it has been advocated by several authors. Freebody and associates reported the results of 252 anterior fusions through the transperitoneal approach. Clinically, 92 per cent were rated as excellent or good, and radiologically, 84 per cent had

solid fusion.[82] Excellent results were also reported by Van Rens and Van Horn, and by Verbeist.[302, 304]

Posterior fusion is preferred because it is less hazardous. An anterior approach to the lumbosacral joint can injure the sympathetic nerve plexus and result in sterility secondary to retrograde ejaculation.[132] In the hands of an experienced spine surgeon the possibility of such a complication is extremely slight, but it can occur. The patient and parents should be forewarned preoperatively of such a possible complication. The posterior approach allows exploration of nerve roots and decompression if indicated, whereas anterior fusion will not relieve nerve entrapment. Bohlman and Cook have described a one-stage decompression and interbody fusion for lumbosacral spondyloptosis through the posterior approach.[27] Previously Cloward had described treatment of spondylolisthesis by laminectomy and posterior interbody fusion.[53]

Reduction of the Spondylolisthesis. Reduc-

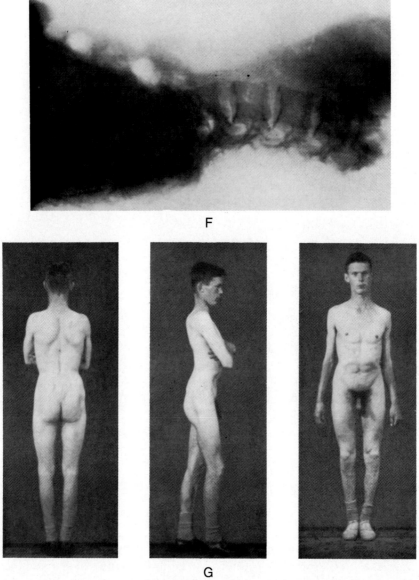

FIGURE 6–44 Continued. *Severe spondylolisthesis with complete displacement of the fifth lumbar vertebra over the sacrum.*

F. Postoperative radiogram. **G.** Photographs a year after operation showing clinical improvement. (From Jenkins, J. A.: Spondylolisthesis. Brit. J. Surg., *24*:80–85, 1936. Reprinted by permission.)

tion of the slipping was first described by Scherb in 1921.[250] Since then it has been reported by numerous authors using posterior, anterior, or combined surgical approaches.*

Reduction of spondylolisthesis is indicated in cases with almost complete olisthy. The sacrum is in vertical position; the resultant severe lumbosacral kyphosis "displaces" the lumbar spine forward, leading to marked lumbar compensatory lordosis (Fig. 6–44).

References

1. Adkins, E. W. O.: Spondylolisthesis. J. Bone Joint Surg., *37-B*:48, 1955.
2. Albanese, M., and Pizzutillo, P. D.: Family study of spondylolysis and spondylolisthesis. J. Pediatr. Orthop., *2*:496, 1982.
3. Allen, M. L., and Lindem, M. C.: Significant roentgen findings in routine pre-employment examination of the lumbosacral spine: A preliminary report. Am. J. Surg., *80*:762, 1950.

*See references 33, 66, 68, 103, 104, 105, 130, 149, 160, 188, 189, 204, 209, 249, 273, 274, 275.

4. Amundson, G. M., and Wenger, D. R.: Spondylolisthesis: Natural history and treatment. Spine, *1*:323, 1987.

5. Amuso, S., and Mankin, H.: Hereditary spondylolisthesis in spina bifida. J. Bone Joint Surg., *49-A*:507, 1967.

6. Amuso, S. J., Neff, R. S., Coulson, D. B., and Laing, P. G.: The surgical treatment of spondylolisthesis by posterior element resection. J. Bone Joint Surg., *52-A*:529, 1970.

7. Anderson, C. E.: Spondylolisthesis following spine fusion. J. Bone Joint Surg., *38-A*:1142, 1956.

8. André, N.: L'Orthopédie. Paris, La Veuve Gilx, 1741; English edition, London, Millar, 1743.

9. Arden, G. P.: Spondylolisthesis with bilateral drop foot. Proc. R. Soc. Med., *42*:601, 1949.

10. Azouz, E. M., Chan, J. D., and Wee, R.: Spondylolysis of the cervical vertebrae. Report of three cases, with review of the English and French literature. Radiology, *111*:315, 1974.

11. Bailey, W.: Persistent vertebral process epiphysis. A.J.R., *42*:85, 1939.

12. Bailey, W.: Observations on the etiology and frequency of spondylolisthesis and its precursors. Radiology, *48*:107, 1947.

13. Baker, D. R., and McHollick, W.: Spondyloschisis and spondylolisthesis in children. J. Bone Joint Surg., *38-A*:933, 1956.

14. Bakke, S. N.: Roentgenologische Beobachtungen über die Bewegungen der Wirbelsaule. Acta Radiol., *13*:Suppl., 1931.

15. Balderston, R., and Bradford, D.: Technique for achievement and maintenance of reduction for severe spondylolisthesis using spinous process traction wiring and external fixation of the pelvis. Spine, *10*:377, 1985.

16. Barash, H. L., Galante, J. O., Lambert, C. N., and Ray, R. D.: Spondylolisthesis and tight hamstrings. J. Bone Joint Surg., *53-A*:1319, 1970.

17. Bardine, C. R.: Numerical vertebral variations in the human adult and embryo. Anat. Anz., *25*:497, 1904.

18. Barnes, D. A., Borns, P., and Pizzutillo, P. D.: Cervical spondylolisthesis associated with the multiple nevoid basal cell carcinoma syndrome. Clin. Orthop., *162*:26, 1982.

19. Barr, J. S.: Spondylolisthesis. J. Bone Joint Surg., *37-A*:878, 1955.

20. Batts, M., Jr.: The etiology of spondylolisthesis. J. Bone Joint Surg., *21*:879, 1939.

21. Beeler, J. W.: Further evidence on the acquired nature of spondylolysis and spondylolisthesis. A.J.R., *108*:796, 1970.

22. Bellamy, R., Leiber, A., and Smith, S. D.: Congenital spondylolisthesis of the sixth cervical vertebra. Case report and description of operative findings. J. Bone Joint Surg., *56-A*:405, 1974.

23. Birch, J. G., Herring, J. A., and Maravilla, K. R.: Splitting of the intervertebral disc in spondylolisthesis: A magnetic resonance imaging finding in two cases. J. Pediatr. Orthop., *6*:609, 1986.

24. Bjerkreim, I.: Spondylolisthesis in children and adolescents. Tidsskr. Nor. Laegeforen., *101*:1653, 1981.

25. Blackburne, J. S., and Velikas, E. P.: Spondylolisthesis in children and adolescents. J. Bone Joint Surg., *59-B*:490, 1977.

26. Bleck, E. E.: Spondylolisthesis: Acquired, congenital or developmental. Dev. Med. Child Neurol., *16*:680, 1974.

27. Bohlman, H. H., and Cook, S. S.: One-stage decompression and posterolateral and interbody fusion for lumbosacral spondyloptosis through a posterior approach. J. Bone Joint Surg., *64-A*:415, 1982.

28. Borkow, S., and Kleiger, B.: Spondylolisthesis in the newborn. Clin. Orthop., *81*:73, 1971.

29. Bosworth, D. M.: Technique of spinal fusion in the lumbosacral region by the double clothespin graft (distraction graft, "H" graft) and results. A.A.O.S. Instr. Course Lect., *9*:44, 1952.

30. Bosworth, D. M., Fielding, J. W., Demarest, L., and Bonaquist, M.: Spondylolisthesis: A critical review of a consecutive series of cases treated by arthrodesis. J. Bone Joint Surg., *37-A*:767, 1955.

31. Boxall, D., Bradford, D. S., Winter, R. B., and Moe, J. H.: Management of severe spondylolisthesis in children and adolescents. J. Bone Joint Surg., *61-A*:479, 1979.

32. Bradford, D. S.: Spondylolysis and spondylolisthesis. *In* Chou, I. S. N., and Seljeskog, E. I. (eds.): Spinal Deformity and Neurologic Dysfunction. New York, Raven, 1978.

33. Bradford, D. S.: Treatment of severe spondylolisthesis: Combined approach for reduction and stabilization. Spine, *4*:423, 1979.

34. Bradford, D. S.: Spondylolysis and spondylolisthesis. Curr. Pract. Orthop. Surg., *8*:12, 1979.

35. Bradford, D. S.: Treatment of severe spondylolisthesis, a combined approach for reduction and stabilization. Orthop. Trans., *5*:3, 1981.

36. Bradford, D. S.: Management of spondylolysis and spondylolisthesis. A.A.O.S. Instr. Course Lect., *32*:151, 1983.

37. Bradford, D. S.: Repair of spondylolysis or minimal degrees of spondylolisthesis by segmental wire fixation and bone grafting. Spine, *10*:673, 1985.

38. Bradford, D. S.: Spondylolysis and spondylolisthesis in children and adolescents: Current concepts in management. *In* The Pediatric Spine. New York, Thieme, 1985, p. 403.

39. Bradford, D. S.: Spondylolysis and spondylolisthesis. *In* Moe, J. H.: Textbook of Scoliosis and Other Deformities. 2nd Ed. Philadelphia, Saunders, 1987, p. 403.

40. Brailsford, J.: Spondylolisthesis. Br. J. Radiol., *6*:666, 1933.

41. Briggs, D., and Evans, A.: Nursing care study: An 11-year-old girl with spondylolisthesis. Nurs. Times, *78*:483, 1982.

42. Briggs, H., and Keats, S.: Laminectomy and foraminotomy with chip fusion; operative treatment for relief of low-back pain and sciatic pain associated with spondylolisthesis. J. Bone Joint Surg., *29*:328, 1947.

43. Brocher, J. E. W.: L'etiologie du spondylolisthesis. Schweiz. Med. Wechenschr., *83*:788, 1953.

44. Buck, J. E.: Direct repair of the defect in spondylolisthesis. J. Bone Joint Surg., *61-A*:479, 1979.

45. Burns, B. H.: Two cases of spondylolisthesis. Proc. R. Soc. Med., *25*:571, 1932.

46. Burns, B. H.: An operation for spondylolisthesis. Lancet, *1*:1233, 1933.

47. Capener, N.: Spondylolisthesis. Br. J. Surg., *19*:374, 1931.

48. Capener, N.: The origins of spondylolisthesis. Bull. Hosp. Joint Dis., *21*:111, 1960.

49. Cedell, C., and Wiberg, G.: Longterm results of laminectomy in spondylolisthesis. Acta Orthop. Scand., *40*:773, 1970.

50. Chandler, F. A.: Lesions of the "isthmus" (pars interarticularis) of the laminae of the lower lumbar vertebrae and their relation to spondylolisthesis. Surg. Gynecol. Obstet., *53*:273, 1931.

51. Ciccone, R., and Richman, R. M.: Mechanism of injury and distribution of 3,000 fractures and dislocations caused by parachute jumping. J. Bone Joint Surg., *30-A*:77, 1948.

52. Cleveland, M., Bosworth, D. M., and Thompson, F. R.: Pseudarthrosis in the lumbosacral spine. J. Bone Joint Surg., *20-A*:302, 1948.

53. Cloward, R. B.: Spondylolisthesis: Treatment by lam-

inectomy and posterior interbody fusion. Clin. Orthop., *154*:74, 1981.

54. Colcher, A. E., and Hursh, A. M. W.: Pre-employment low-back x-ray survey; review of 1500 cases. Industr. Med. Surg., *21*:319, 1952.

55. Collingnon, J. C., and Flandroy, P.: Cervical spondylolisthesis. J. Belg. Radiol., *64*:495, 1981.

56. Colonna, P. C.: Spondylolisthesis; analysis of 201 cases. J.A.M.A., *154*:398, 1954.

57. Congdon, R. T.: Spondylolisthesis and vertebral anomalies in skeletons of American aborigines. With clinical notes on spondylolisthesis. J. Bone Joint Surg., *14*:511, 1932.

58. Cornish, B. L.: Traumatic spondylolisthesis of the axis. J. Bone Joint Surg., *50*:31, 1968.

59. Cozen, L.: The development of the origins of spondylolisthesis. J. Bone Joint Surg., *43-A*:180, 1961.

60. Crock, H. V.: Normal and pathological anatomy of the lumbar spinal nerve root canals. J. Bone Joint Surg., *63-B*:487, 1981.

61. Cyron, V. M., Hutton, W. C., and Stott, J. R. R.: Spondylolysis: The shearing stiffness of the lumbar intervertebral joint. Acta Orthop. Belg., *45*:459, 1979.

62. Dandy, D. J., and Shannon, M. J.: Lumbosacral subluxation (group I spondylolisthesis). J. Bone Joint Surg., *53-B*:578, 1971.

63. Davis, I. S., and Bailey, R. W.: Spondylolisthesis: Indications for lumbar nerve root decompression and operative technique. Clin. Orthop., *117*:129, 1976.

64. Dawley, J. A.: Spondylolisthesis of the cervical spine. J. Neurosurg., *34*:99, 1971.

65. DePalma, A. F., and Marone, P. J.: Spondylolysis following spinal fusion. Clin. Orthop., *15*:208, 1959.

66. DelTorto, U.: Surgical reduction and stabilization of spondylolisthesis. Clin. Orthop., *75*:281, 1971.

67. Devas, M. B.: Stress fracture in children. J. Bone Joint Surg., *45-B*:528, 1963.

68. DeWald, R. L., Faut, M., Taddonio, R. F., and Neuwirth, M. G.: Severe lumbosacral spondylolisthesis in adolescents and children: Reduction and stage circumferential fusion. J. Bone Joint Surg., *63-A*:619, 1981.

69. Deyerle, W. M.: Lumbar nerve root irritation in children. Clin. Orthop., *21*:125, 1970.

70. Dietrich, M., and Kurowski, P.: The importance of mechanical factors in the etiology of spondylolysis: A model analysis of loads and stresses in human lumbar spine. Spine, *10*:532, 1985.

71. Duncan, D.: Alterations in the structure of the nerves caused by restricting their growth with ligature. J. Neuropathol. Exp. Neurol., *7*:261, 1948.

72. Duncan, H. M., and Jonch, L. M.: The presacral plexus in anterior fusion of the lumbar spine. Suid-Afrikaanse Tydsk Chir., *3*:93, 1965.

73. Durbin, F. C.: Spondylolisthesis of the cervical spine. J. Bone Joint Surg., *38-B*:734, 1956.

74. Eisenstein, S.: Spondylolysis—a skeletal investigation of two population groups. J. Bone Joint Surg., *60-B*:488, 1978.

75. Farfan, H. F., Osteria, V., and Lamy, C.: The mechanical etiology of spondylolysis and spondylolisthesis. Clin. Orthop., *117*:40, 1976.

76. Faugeron, P.: Spondyloptosis lombo-sacré. Rev. Chir. Orthop., *37*:504, 1951.

77. Ferguson, R. J.: Low-back pain in college football linemen. J. Bone Joint Surg., *56-A*:1300, 1974.

78. Fisk, J., Moe, J., and Winter, R.: Scoliosis, spondylolysis, and spondylolisthesis. Spine, *3*:234, 1978.

79. Fredricksen, A., and Mangschau, A.: Neurogenic intermittent claudication in association with spondylolisthesis. Acta Neurol. Scand., *60*:385, 1979.

80. Fredrickson, B. E., Baker, D., McHollick, W. J., Yuan, H., and Lubicky, J.: The natural history of spondylolysis and spondylolisthesis. J. Bone Joint Surg., *66-A*:699, 1984.

81. Freebody, D.: Lumbosacral fusion by the transperitoneal approach. J. Bone Joint Surg., *44-B*:217, 1962.

82. Freebody, D., Bendall, R., and Taylor, R. D.: Anterior transperitoneal lumbar fusion. J. Bone Joint Surg., *53-B*:617, 1971.

83. Friberg, S.: Studies on spondylolisthesis. Acta Chir. Scand., *82*:Suppl. 56:1, 1939.

84. Gaines, R., and Nichols, W.: Treatment of spondyloptosis by two-stage L5 vertebrectomy and reduction of L4 onto L1. Spine, *10*:680, 1985.

85. Galluccio, A. C.: Spondylolisthesis: General considerations with emphasis on radiologic aspects. Radiology, *42*:143, 1944.

86. Gelfand, M. J.: Radionuclide bone imaging in spondylolysis of the lumbar spine in children. Radiology, *140*:191, 1981.

87. George, E. M.: Spondylolisthesis. Surg. Gynecol. Obstet., *68*:774, 1939.

88. Gill, G. G., and Binder, W. F.: Autoamputation of the first sacral nerve roots in spondyloptosis. Spine, *5*:3, 295, 1980.

89. Gill, G. G., Manning, J. G., and White, H. L.: Surgical treatment of spondylolisthesis without spine fusion. J. Bone Joint Surg., *37-A*:493, 1955.

90. Gill, G. G., Manning, J. G., and White, H. L.: Surgical treatment of spondylolisthesis treated by arthrodesis. J.A.M.A., *163*:175, 1957.

91. Glorieux, P., and Roederer, C.: La Spondylolyse et ses Consequences: Spondylolisthesis—Scoliose Listhesique. Etude Radiologique-Clinique-Medicolégale. Paris, Masson, 1937.

92. Goldberg, M. J.: Gymnastic injuries. Orthop. Clin. North Am., *11*:717, 1980.

93. Hadley, L. A.: Congenital absence of pedicle from the cervical vertebra; report of three cases. A.J.R., *55*:193, 1946.

94. Hadley, L. A.: Bony masses projecting into the spinal canal opposite a break in the neural arch of the fifth lumbar vertebra. J. Bone Joint Surg., *37-A*:787, 1955.

95. Hadley, L. A.: The Spine. Anatomico-Radiographic Studies. Development and the Cervical Region. Springfield, Ill., Thomas, 1956.

96. Hadley, L. A.: Secondary ossification centers and the intraarticular ossicle. A.J.R., *76*:1095, 1956.

97. Hallgrimsson, S.: Case of pseudospondylolisthesis with affection of spinal roots. Acta Orthop. Scand., *12*:309, 1941.

98. Halperin, N., Copeliovitch, L., and Schachner, E.: Radiating leg pain and positive straight leg raising in spondylolysis in children. J. Pediatr. Orthop., *3*:486, 1983.

99. Hammond, G., Wise, R. E., and Haggart, G. E.: Review of seventy-three cases of spondylolisthesis treated by arthrodesis. J.A.M.A., *163*:175, 1957.

100. Hanai, K., Miyashita, T., and Saburi, H.: Cervical spondylolisthesis. Acta Orthop. Scand., *47*:63, 1976.

101. Haraldsson, S., and Willner, S.: A comparative study of spondylolisthesis in operations on adolescents and adults. Arch. Orthop. Trauma. Surg., *101*:101, 1983.

102. Harnach, Z. G., Gotfryd, O., and Baudysova, J.: Spondylolisthesis with hamstring spasticity. A case report. J. Bone Joint Surg., *48-A*:878, 1966.

103. Harrington, P. R., and Dickson, J. H.: Spinal instrumentation in the treatment of severe progressive spondylolisthesis. Clin. Orthop., *117*:157, 1976.

104. Harrington, P. R., and Tullos, H. S.: Spondylolisthesis in children. Observation and surgical treatment. Clin. Orthop., *79*:75, 1971.

105. Harris, R. I.: Spondylolisthesis. Ann. R. Coll. Surg., *8*:259, 1951.

106. Harris, R. I., and Weinstein, S. L.: Longterm followup of spondylolisthesis 50% or greater treated with or without posterior fusion. Orthop. Trans., *8*:155, 1984.

107. Harris, R. I., and Wiley, J. J.: Acquired spondylolysis

as a sequel to spine fusion. J. Bone Joint Surg., 45-A:1159, 1963.

108. Hartmann, G.: Neuer Fall von Spondylolisthesis. Monatsschr. Gebuntsk., 25:465, 1865.

109. Hasebe, K.: Die Wirbelsaule der Japaner. Z. Morph. Anthrop., 15:259, 1912.

110. Haukipuro, K., Keranen, N., Koivisto, E., Lindholm, R., Norio, R., and Punto, L.: Familial occurrence of lumbar spondylolysis and spondylolisthesis. Clin. Genet., 13:471, 1978.

111. Henderson, E. D.: Results of the surgical treatment of spondylolisthesis. J. Bone Joint Surg., 48-A:619, 1966.

112. Hensinger, R. N.: Spondylolysis and spondylolisthesis in children. A.A.O.S. Instr. Course Lect., 52:132, 1983.

113. Hensinger, R. N., Lang, J. R., and MacEwen, G. D.: Surgical management of the spondylolisthesis in children and adolescents. Spine, 1:207, 1976.

114. Herbiniaux, G.: Traité sur Divers Accouchements Laborieux, et sur les Polypes de la Matrice. Bruxelles, DeBoubers, 1782.

115. Hirsch, C.: Anterior grafting in extensive spondylolisthesis. Arch. Orthop. Unfallchir., 60:46, 1966.

116. Hitchcock, H. H.: Spondylolisthesis: Observations on its development, progression and genesis. J. Bone Joint Surg., 22:1, 1940.

117. Hodgson, A. R., and Wong, S. K.: A description of a technique and evaluation of results in anterior spinal fusion for deranged intervertebral disc and spondylolisthesis. Clin. Orthop., 56:133, 1968.

118. Hoshina, H.: Spondylolysis in athletes. Physician Sports Med., 8:75, 1980.

119. Howorth, B.: Low backache and sciatica: Results of the surgical treatment. Part 3. Surgical treatment of spondylolisthesis. J. Bone Joint Surg., 46-A:1515, 1964.

120. Huizenga, B. A.: Reduction of spondyloptosis with two-stage vertebrectomy. Orthop. Trans., 7:21, 1983.

121. Hulbert, N. G.: Spondylolisthesis with cauda equina lesion. Proc. R. Soc. Med., 41:97, 1948.

122. Hutton, W. C., and Cyron, V. M.: Spondylolysis. Acta Orthop. Scand., 49:604, 1978.

123. Hutton, W. C., Stott, J. R. R., and Cyron, V. M.: Is spondylolysis a fatigue fracture? Spine, 2:202, 1977.

124. Inoue, S., Minami, S., Sho, E., and Ohki, I.: The results of anterior surgery in the treatment of spondylolisthesis. Presented at the 19th Annual Meeting of the Scoliosis Research Society, Orlando, Florida, Sept. 19–22, 1984.

125. Jacchia, G. E., Bartolozzi, P., and Petrucci, P.: Surgical stabilization of severe spondylolisthesis in adolescence (preliminary report). Arch. Putti Chir. Organi Mov., 30:33, 1980.

126. Jackson, D. W., Wiltse, L. L., and Cirincione, R. J.: Spondylolysis in the female gymnast. Clin. Orthop., 117:68, 1976.

127. Jaffer, Z., and Beighton, P.: Syndrome identification case report 98: Arachnodactyly, joint laxity, and spondylolisthesis. J. Clin. Dysmorphol., 1:14, 1983.

128. James, A., and Nisbet, N. W.: Posterior intervertebral fusion of lumbar spine: Preliminary report of new operation. J. Bone Joint Surg., 35-B:181, 1953.

129. Janos, K., Otto, B., and Arpad, B.: Simultaneous occurrence of Perthes' disease, spondylolysis—spondylolisthesis and other forms of aseptic necrosis. Magy. Traumatol. Orthop., 19:250, 1976.

130. Jenkins, J. A.: Spondylolisthesis. Br. J. Surg., 24:80, 1936.

131. Johnson, J. R., and Kirwan, E. O.: The long-term results of fusion in situ for severe spondylolisthesis. J. Bone Joint Surg., 65-B:43, 1983.

132. Johnson, R. M., and McQuire, E. J.: Urogenital complications of anterior approaches to the lumbar spine. Clin. Orthop., 154:114, 1981.

133. Junghanns, H.: Spondylolisthesen ohne Spalt im Zwischengelenkstuck. ("Pseudospondylolisthesen".) Arch. Orthop., 29:118, 1931.

134. Kahnovitz, N., Bullough, P., and Jacobs, R.: The effect of internal fixation without arthrodesis on human facet joint cartilage. Orthop. Trans., 7:14, 1983.

135. Kaneda, K., Satoh, S., Nohara, Y., and Oguma, T.: Distraction rod instrumentation with posterolateral fusion in isthmic spondylolisthesis: 53 cases followed for 18–89 months. Spine, 10:383, 1985.

136. Karasick, S., Karasick, D., and Wechsler, R. J.: Unilateral spondylolysis of the cervical spine. Skeletal Radiol., 9:259, 1983.

137. Kettelkamp, D. B., and Wright, D. G.: Spondylolysis in the Alaskan Eskimo. J. Bone Joint Surg., 53-A:563, 1971.

138. Kilian, H. F.: De Spondylolisthesis gravissmae Pelvangustiae caussa Nuper Detecta. Commentatio anatomico-obstetrica. Bonn, Georgii, 1854.

139. Kilian, H. F.: Schilderungen neuer Beckenformen und ihres Verhaltens in Leben. Mannheim, Bassermann & Mathey, 1854.

140. King, A., Baker, D. R., and McHollick, W. J.: Another approach to the treatment of spondylolisthesis and spondyloschisis. Clin. Orthop., 10:257, 1957.

141. Kirkaldy-Willis, W. H., Wedge, J. H., Yong-Hing, K., and Reilly, J.: Pathology and pathogenesis of lumbar spondylosis and stenosis. Spine, 3:319, 1978.

142. Kleinberg, S.: Spondylosthesis in an infant. J. Bone Joint Surg., 16:441, 1934.

143. Klenerman, L.: Posterior spinal fusion in spondylisthesis. J. Bone Joint Surg., 44-B:637, 1962.

144. Klinghoffer, L., and Murdock, M. G.: Spondylolysis following trauma: A case report and review of the literature. Clin. Orthop., 166:72, 1982.

145. Krenz, J., and Troup, J. D. G.: The structure of the pars interarticularis of the lower lumbar vertebrae and its relation to the etiology of spondylolysis. J. Bone Joint Surg., 55-B:735, 1973.

146. Labbe, A., Campagne, D., and Merle, P.: Congenital spondylolisthesis of the 6th cervical vertebra. Apropos of a pediatric case with a review of the literature. Ann. Radiol. (Paris), 26:691, 1983.

147. Lafond, G.: Surgical treatment of spondylolisthesis. Clin. Orthop., 22:175, 1962.

148. Lambl, W.: Beitrage Geburtsk Gynaekol von FWV Scanzoni, 1858.

149. Lance, E. M.: Treatment of severe spondylolisthesis with neural involvement: A report of two cases. J. Bone Joint Surg., 48-A:883, 1966.

150. Lane, W. A.: Case of spondylolisthesis associated with progressive paraplegia; laminectomy. Lancet, 1:991, 1893.

151. Lane, W. A.: Some of the changes which are produced by pressure in the lower part of the spinal column, spondylolisthesis, displacement backwards of the fifth lumbar vertebra, torticollis, etc. Trans. Pathol. Soc., 36:364, 1885.

152. Laurent, L. E.: Spondylolisthesis. Acta Orthop. Scand. (Suppl.), 35:7, 1958.

153. Laurent, L. E., and Einola, S.: Spondylolisthesis in children and adolescents. Acta Orthop. Scand., 31:45, 1961.

154. Laurent, L. E., and Osterman, K.: Spondylolisthesis in children and adolescents: A study of 173 cases. Acta Orthop. Belg., 35:717, 1969.

155. Laurent, L. E., and Osterman, K.: Operative treatment of spondylolisthesis in young patients. Clin. Orthop., 117:85, 1976.

156. Leger, J. L., Bouchard, R., and Maltais, R.: Etude radiologique de 305 cas de spondylolyse avec ou sans spondylolisthesis. J. Can. Assoc. Radiol., 46:573, 1946.

157. Lerner, H. H., and Gazin, A. L.: Interarticular isthmus hiatus (spondylolysis). Radiology, 46:573, 1946.

158. Lin, H. S., Liu, Y. K., and Adams, K. H.: Mechanical response of the lumbar intervertebral joint under physiologic (complex) loading. J. Bone Joint Surg., 60-A:41, 1978.

159. Lorenz, R.: Lumbar spondylolisthesis. Clinical syndrome and operative experience with Cloward's technique. Acta Neurochir. (Wien), 60:223, 1982.

160. Louis, R., and Maresca, C.: Stabilisation chirurgicale avec reduction des spondylolysis et des spondylolisthesis. Int. Orthop., 1:215, 1977.

161. Lowe, J., Schachner, E., Hirschberg, E., Shapiro, Y., and Libson, E.: Significance of bone scintigraphy in symptomatic spondylolysis. Spine, 9:653, 1984.

162. Lowe, R. W., Hayes, D. T., Kaye, J., Bagg, R. J., and Leukens, C. A., Jr.: Standing roentgenograms in spondylolisthesis. Clin. Orthop., 117:80, 1976.

163. Lusskin, R.: Pain patterns in spondylolisthesis. Clin. Orthop., 40:123, 1965.

164. McAfee, P. C., and Yuan, H. A.: Computed tomography in spondylolisthesis. Clin. Orthop., 166:62, 1982.

165. McKee, B. W., Alexander, W. J., and Dunbar, J. S.: Spondylolysis and spondylolisthesis in children: A review. J. Can. Assoc. Radiol., 22:100, 1971.

166. MacNab, I.: Spondylolisthesis with an intact neural arch—the so-called pseudo-spondylolisthesis. J. Bone Joint Surg., 32-B:325, 1950.

167. McPhee, I. B., and O'Brien, J. P.: Reduction of severe spondylolisthesis. A preliminary report. Spine, 4:430, 1979.

168. McPhee, I. B., and O'Brien, J. P.: Scoliosis in symptomatic spondylolisthesis. J. Bone Joint Surg., 62-B:155, 1980.

169. McQueen, M. M., Court-Brown, C., and Scott, J. H. S.: Stabilisation of spondylolisthesis using Dwyer instrumentation. J. Bone Joint Surg., 68-B:185, 1986.

170. Maldague, B., and Malghem, J.: Aspects radiologiques dynamiques de la spondylolyse lombaire. Acta Orthop. Belg., 47:441, 1981.

171. Mall, F. P.: On ossification centers in the human embryos less than one hundred days old. Am. J. Anat., 5:433, 1906.

172. Matsukura, M.: A mechanical investigation of the developing factors in spondylolysis. J. Physical Fitness Jpn., 31:112, 1982.

173. Mau, H.: Scoliosis and spondylosis—spondylolisthesis. Arch. Orthop. Trauma. Surg., 99:23, 1981.

174. Mercer, W.: Orthopaedic Surgery. Baltimore, Wood, 1936.

175. Meschan, I.: Spondylolisthesis; commentary on etiology and improved method of roentgenographic mensuration and detection of instability. A.J.R., 53:230, 1945.

176. Meyer-Burgdorff, H.: Untersuchungen über das Wirbelgleiten. Leipzig, Thieme, 1931.

177. Meyerding, H. W.: Spondylolisthesis. J. Bone Joint Surg., 13:39, 1931.

178. Meyerding, H. W.: Spondylolisthesis. Surg. Gynecol. Obstet., 54:371, 1932.

179. Meyerding, H. W.: Spondylolisthesis as an etiologic factor in backache. J.A.M.A., 111:1971, 1938.

180. Meyerding, H. W.: Low backache and sciatic pain associated with spondylolisthesis and protruded intervertebral disc: Incidence, significance and treatment. J. Bone Joint Surg., 23:461, 1941.

181. Meyerding, H. W.: Spondylolisthesis: Surgical treatment and results. J. Bone Joint Surg., 25:65, 1943.

182. Michel, C. R., and Caton, J.: Reduction of severe L-5 spondylolisthesis in children using the Harrington method. Acta Orthop. Belg., 47:479, 1981.

183. Micheli, L. J.: Low back pain in the adolescent: Differential diagnosis. Am. J. Sports Med., 7:362, 1979.

184. Monticelli, G., and Ascani, E.: Spondylolysis and spondylolisthesis. Acta Orthop. Scand., 46:498, 1975.

185. Moreton, R. D.: Spondylolisthesis. J.A.M.A., 195:671, 1966.

186. Moreton, R. D.: So-called normal backs. Indust. Med. Surg., 38:216, 1969.

187. Moseley, I.: Neural arch dysplasia of the sixth cervical vertebra. Congenital cervical spondylolisthesis. Br. J. Radiol., 49:81, 1976.

188. Mosimann, P.: Die Histologie der Spondylolyse. Arch. Orthop. Unfallchir., 53:264, 1961.

189. Mouchet, A., and Roederer, C.: Le spondylolisthesis. Presse Med., 39:569, 1931.

190. Munster, J. K., and Troup, J. D. G.: The structure of the pars interarticularis of the lower lumbar vertebrae and its relation to the etiology of spondylolysis. J. Bone Joint Surg., 55-B:735, 1973.

191. Murray, R. O., and Colwill, M. R.: Stress fractures of the pars interarticularis. Proc. R. Soc. Med., 61:555, 1968.

192. Mutch, J., and Walmsley, R.: The aetiology of cleft vertebral arch in spondylolisthesis. Lancet, 270:74, 1956.

193. Nachemson, A.: Repair of the spondylolisthetic defect and intertransverse fusion for young patients. Clin. Orthop., 117:101, 1976.

194. Nachemson, A., and Wiltse, L. L.: Editorial comment: Spondylolisthesis. Clin. Orthop., 117:4, 1976.

195. Nathan, H.: Spondylolysis: Its anatomy and mechanism of development. J. Bone Joint Surg., 41-A:303, 1959.

196. Neithard, F. B.: Scheuermann's disease and spondylolysis. Orthop. Trans., 7:103, 1983.

197. Neugebauer, F. L.: Die Entstehung der Spondylolisthesis. Zentralbl. Gynäk., 5:260, 1881.

198. Neugebauer, F. L.: Zur Entwicklungsgeschichte des Spondylolisthetischen Beckens und seiner Diagnose (mit Berücksichtigung von Körperhaltung und Gangspur). Casuistisch-Kritische Monographie. Halle, Niemeyer, 1882.

199. Neugebauer, F. L.: A New Contribution to the History and Etiology of Spondylolisthesis. The New Syndenham Society. Selected Monographs. London, New Sydenham Society, 1888.

200. Neugebauer, F. L.: The Classic: A new contribution to the history and etiology of spondylolisthesis. Clin. Orthop., 117:4, 1976.

201. Neuwirth, M.: Dysplastic and isthmic spondylolisthesis. Bull. Hosp. Joint Dis., 41:94, 1981.

202. Newman, P. H.: Spondylolisthesis, its cause and effect. Ann. R. Coll. Surg. Eng., 16:305, 1954.

203. Newman, P. H.: The etiology of spondylolisthesis. J. Bone Joint Surg., 45-B:39, 1963.

204. Newman, P. H.: A clinical syndrome associated with severe lumbo-sacral subluxation. J. Bone Joint Surg., 47-B:472, 1965.

205. Newman, P. H.: Surgical treatment for derangement of the lumbar spine. J. Bone Joint Surg., 55-B:7, 1973.

206. Newman, P. H.: Stenosis of the lumbar spine in spondylolisthesis. Clin. Orthop., 115:121, 1976.

207. Newman, P. H., and Stone, K. H.: The etiology of spondylolisthesis. J. Bone Joint Surg., 45-B:39, 1963.

208. Noback, C. R.: The developmental anatomy of the human osseous skeleton during the embryonic, fetal, and cirumnatal periods. Anat. Rec., 88:91, 1944.

209. Ohki, I., Inoue, S., Murata, T., Mikanagi, K., and Shibuya, K.: Reduction and fusion of severe spondylolisthesis using halopelvic traction with wire reduction device. Int. Orthop., 4:107, 1980.

210. Op Den Roth, J. O., Penning, L., and Kluft, O.: Lateral spondylolysis of the sixth cervical vertebra. J. Bone Joint Surg., 51-A:1379, 1969.

211. Orth, J. O., Penning, A., and Kluft, O.: Lateral spondylolysis of the sixth cervical vertebra. J. Bone Joint Surg., 51-A:1379, 1969.

212. Osterman, K., Lindholm, T. S., and Laurent, L. E.:

Late results of removal of the loose posterior element (Gill's operation) in the treatment of lytic lumbar spondylolisthesis. Clin. Orthop., *117*:121, 1976.

213. Ota, H.: Spondylolysis: Familial occurrence and its genetic implications. J. Jpn. Orthop. Assoc., *41*:931, 1967.

214. Padovani, J. P., and Rigault, P.: A technique for reducing a severely displaced lumbosacral spondylolisthesis in children and adolescents. Chirurgie, *106*:751, 1980.

215. Pease, C. N., and Najat, H.: Spondylolisthesis in children. Special reference to the lumbosacral joint and treatment by fusion. Clin. Orthop., 52:187, 1967.

216. Perlman, R., and Hawes, L. E.: Cervical spondylolisthesis. J. Bone Joint Surg., 33-A:1012, 1951.

217. Pfeil, E.: Conservative treatment of spondylolysis and spondylolisthesis in childhood. Beitr. Orthop. Traumatol., 22:238, 1975.

218. Phalen, G. S., and Dickson, J. A.: Spondylolisthesis and tight hamstrings. J. Bone Joint Surg., 43-A:505, 1961.

219. Pizzutillo, P. D.: Spondylolisthesis: Etiology and natural history. *In* Bradford, D., and Hensinger, R. (eds.): The Pediatric Spine. New York, Thieme, 1985, p. 395.

220. Pizzutillo, P. D., Mirenda, W., and MacEwen, G. D.: Posterolateral fusion for spondylolisthesis in adolescence. J. Pediatr. Orthop., 6:311, 1986.

221. Porter, R. W., and Park, W.: Unilateral spondylolysis. J. Bone Joint Surg., 64-B:344, 1982.

222. Post, M. J. D.: Computed Tomography of the Spine. Baltimore, Williams & Wilkins, 1984.

223. Potter, R. M., and Norcross, J. R.: Spondylolisthesis without isthmus defect. Radiology, 63:678, 1954.

224. Pouliquen, J. C., and Pennecot, G. F.: Lumbosacral spondylolisthesis in children. Surgical treatment and therapeutic indications. Ann. Pediatr. (Paris), 27:203, 1980.

225. Privett, J. T. J., and Middlemiss, J. H.: Multiple lower lumbar spondylolysis. Br. J. Radiol., 48:866, 1975.

226. Rambaud, A., and Renault, C.: Origine et developpment des os. Paris, Chamerot, 1864.

227. Raney, R. B.: Isthmus defects of the fifth lumbar vertebra. South. Med. J., 38:166, 1945.

228. Reynolds, J. B., and Wiltse, L.: Surgical treatment of degenerative spondylolisthesis. Spine, 4:148, 1979.

229. Rhodes, M. P., and Colangelo, C.: Spondylolysis and its relation to spondylolisthesis. Am. J. Surg., 72:20, 1946.

230. Richardson, H. D., and Brown, C. W.: Surgical treatment of spondylolisthesis. J. Med. Assoc. Ga., 69:193, 1980.

231. Rigault, P., Pouliquen, J. C., Beneux, J., Padovani, J. P., Guyonvarch, G., and Durand, Y.: Reduction of lumbosacral spondylolisthesis with major displacement in children, using Harrington's instruments followed by intersomatic L-5–S-1 arthrodesis. Apropos of 6 cases. Chirurgie, 102:829, 1976.

232. Riley, P., and Gillespie, R.: Severe spondylolisthesis: Results of posterolateral fusion. Orthop. Trans., 9:119, 1985.

233. Risser, J. C., and Norquist, D. M.: Sciatic scoliosis in growing children. Clin. Orthop., 21:137, 1961.

234. Robert (zu Coblenz): Einbe eigenthümliche angeborene Lordose, wahrscheinlich bedingt durch eine Verschiebung des Korpers des letzten Lendenwirbels auf die vordere Fläche des ersten Kruezbeinwirbels (spondylolisthesis Kilian; bebst Bemerkungen über die Mechanik dieser Beckenformation). Geburtskunde Frauenk., 5:81, 1855.

235. Roberts, R. A.: Chronic Structural Low Back Ache due to Low Back Structural Derangements. London, Lewis, 1947.

236. Robson, M. J., Brown, L. M., and Sharrard, W. J.: Cervical spondylolisthesis and other skeletal abnormalities in Rubinstein-Taybi syndrome. J. Bone Joint Surg., 62-B:193, 1980.

237. Roche, M. B.: Bilateral fracture of the pars interarticularis of a lumbar neural arch. J. Bone Joint Surg., 30-A:1005, 1948.

238. Roche, M. B.: The pathology of the neural arch defects: A dissection study. J. Bone Joint Surg., 31-A:529, 1949.

239. Roche, M. B.: Healing of the bilateral fracture of the pars interarticularis of the lumbar neural arch. J. Bone Joint Surg., 32-A:428, 1950.

240. Roche, M. B., and Rowe, G. G.: The incidence of separate neural arch and coincident bone variations. J. Bone Joint Surg., 34-A:491, 1952.

241. Rombold, C.: Treatment of spondylolisthesis by postero-lateral fusion, resection of pars interarticularis and prompt mobilization of the patient. J. Bone Joint Surg., 48-A:1282, 1966.

242. Rosenberg, N. J.: Degenerative spondylolisthesis and surgical treatment. Clin. Orthop., *117*:112, 1976.

243. Rosenberg, N. J., Bargar, W. L., and Friedman, B.: The incidence of spondylolysis and spondylolisthesis in non-ambulatory patients. Spine, 6:35, 1981.

244. Rosomoff, H. L.: Lumbar spondylolisthesis: Etiology of radiculopathy and role of the neurosurgeon. Clin. Neurosurg., 27:577, 1980.

245. Rossi, F.: Spondylolysis, spondylolisthesis, and sports. J. Sports Med. Phys. Fitness, *18*:317, 1978.

246. Rothman, R. H., and Simeone, F. A.: The Spine. Philadelphia, Saunders, 1975.

247. Rowe, G. G., and Roche, M. B.: The etiology of separate neural arch. J. Bone Joint Surg., 35-A:102, 1963.

248. Runge, C. F.: Roentgenographic examination of the lumbosacral spine in routine pre-employment examinations. J. Bone Joint Surg., 36-A:75, 1954.

249. Scaglieti, O., Frontino, G., and Bartolozzi, P.: Technique of anatomical reduction of lumbar spondylolisthesis and its surgical stabilization. Clin. Orthop., *117*:164, 1976.

250. Scherb, R.: Zur Indikation und Technik der Albec de Quervain Operation. Schweiz. Med. Wochenschr., *20*:763, 1921.

251. Schluter, K.: Form und Struktur des normalen und des pathologisch veranderten Wirbels. Stuttgart, Hippokrates-Verlag, 1965.

252. Schmorl, G.: Beitrag zur Kenntnis der Spondylolisthese. Dtsch. Z. Chir., *237*:422, 1932.

253. Schmorl, G., and Junghanns, H.: Die gesunde und kranke Wirbelsäule. Leipzig, Thieme, 1932.

254. Schneck, C. D.: The anatomy of lumbar spondylolysis. Clin. Orthop., *193*:20, 1985.

255. Schneidau, A., and Kendall, B.: Neural arch dysplasia of the sixth cervical vertebra associated with spinal cord compression. Br. J. Radiol., 55:162, 1982.

256. Schneider, C. C., and Melamed, A.: Spondylolysis and spondylolisthesis: Case report clarifying the etiology of spondylolysis. Radiology, 69:863, 1957.

257. Schulitz, K., and Niethard, F. U.: Strain on the interarticular stress distribution. Arch. Orthop. Trauma. Surg., 96:197, 1980.

258. Schults, A.: Age changes and variability in gibbons. A morphological study on a population sample of a manlike ape. Am. J. Phys. Anthropol., 2:11, 1944.

259. Schwegel, A.: Über Knochenmarietaten. Z. Rat. Med., 5:283, 1859.

260. Semon, R. L., and Spengler, D.: Significance of lumbar spondylolysis in college football players. Spine, 6:172, 1981.

261. Sensing, E. G.: The Early Development of the Human Vertebral Column. Contrib. to Embryology, Vol. 33:21. Washington Carnegie Institute, 1949.

262. Serre, H.: Spondylolyse traumatique vraie: Fracture isolée des isthmus de L-5 anterieurement normaux. Rev. Rhum., 23:44, 1956.

263. Seuzawa, Y., Jacob, H. A. C., and Bernoski, F. P.: The mechanical response of the neural arch of the lumbosacral vertebra and its clinical significance. Int. Orthop., 4:205, 1980.

264. Sevastikoglou, J. A., Spangfort, E., and Aaro, S.: Operative treatment of spondylolisthesis in children and adolescents with tight hamstring syndrome. Clin. Orthop., 147:192, 1980.

265. Shahriaree, H., Shjadi, K., and Rooholamini, S. A.: A family with spondylolisthesis. J. Bone Joint Surg., 61-A:1256, 1979.

266. Shands, A. R., Jr., and Bundens, W. D.: Congenital deformities of the spine. An analysis of the roentgenograms of 700 children. Bull. Hosp. Joint Dis., 17:110, 1956.

267. Sherk, H. H., and Howard, T.: Clinical and pathological correlations in traumatic spondylolisthesis of the axis. Clin. Orthop., 174:122, 1983.

268. Sherman, F. C., Rosenthal, R. K., and Hall, J. E.: Spine fusion for spondylolysis and spondylolisthesis in children. Spine, 4:59, 1979.

269. Sherman, F. C., Wilkinson, R. H., and Hall, J. E.: Reactive sclerosis of a pedicle and spondylolysis in the lumbar spine. J. Bone Joint Surg., 59-A:49, 1977.

270. Shore, L. R.: A report of a specimen of spondylolisthesis found in a skeleton of a Bantu native of South Africa; with further specimens illustrating an anomalous mode of development of the lower lumbar vertebrae. Br. J. Surg., 16:431, 1929.

271. Sicard, A., and Leca, A.: Les spondylolisthesis traumatiques. Presse Med., 60:914, 1952.

272. Siehl, D.: Heredity in spondylolisthesis and spondylolysis. J. Am. Osteopath. Assoc., 53:154, 1953.

273. Sijbrandij, S.: A new technique for the reduction and stabilization of severe spondylolisthesis. A report of two cases. J. Bone Joint Surg., 63-B:266, 1981.

274. Sijbrandij, S.: Reduction and stabilization of severe spondylolisthesis: A report of three cases. J. Bone Joint Surg., 65-B:40, 1983.

275. Silvello, L., and Vercellesi, E.: A case of spontaneous cure of spondylolisthesis in adolescence. Ital. J. Orthop. Traumatol., 6:235, 1980.

276. Snijder, J. G. N., Seroo, J. M., Snijer, C. J., and Schijvens, A. W. M.: Therapy of spondylolisthesis by repositioning and fixation of the olisthetic vertebra. Clin. Orthop., 117:149, 1976.

277. Southworth, J. D., and Bersack, S. R.: Anomalies of the lumbosacral vertebrae in five hundred and fifty individuals without symptoms referrable to the low back. A.J.R., 64:624, 1950.

278. Speck, G. R., McCall, I. W., and O'Brien, J. P.: Spondylolisthesis: The angle of kyphosis. Spine, 9:659, 1984.

279. Speed, K.: Spondylolisthesis: Treatment of anterior bone graft. Arch. Surg., 37:175, 1938.

280. Stauffer, R. N., and Coventry, M. B.: Posterolateral lumbar spine fusion. J. Bone Joint Surg., 54-A:1195, 1955.

281. Steiner, G.: Isolated fractures of the vertebral arch. A.J.R., 39:43, 1938.

282. Stewart, T. D.: Incidence of separate neural arch in the lumbar vertebrae of Eskimos. Am. J. Phys. Anthropol., 16:51, 1931.

283. Stewart, T. D.: Spondylolisthesis without separate neural arch (pseudo-spondylolisthesis of Junghanns). J. Bone Joint Surg., 17:640, 1935.

284. Stewart, T. D.: The age incidence of neural-arch defects in Alaskan natives considered from the standpoint of etiology. J. Bone Joint Surg., 35-A:937, 1953.

285. Stewart, T. D.: Examination of the possibility that certain skeletal characters predispose to defects in the lumbar neural arches. Clin. Orthop., 8:44, 1956.

286. Sugiura, Y.: Tricho-rhino-phalangeal syndrome associated with Perthes-disease-like bone change and spondylolisthesis. Jinrui Idengaku Zasshi, 23:23, 1978.

287. Sullivan, C. R., and Bickel, W. H.: The problem of traumatic spondylolysis; a report of three cases. Am. J. Surg., 100:698, 1960.

288. Taillard, W.: Le spondylolisthesis chez l'enfant et l'adolescent. Acta Orthop. Scand., 24:115, 1954.

289. Taillard, W.: Les Spondylolisthesis. Paris, Masson, 1957.

290. Taillard, W.: Etiology of spondylolisthesis. Clin. Orthop., 117:30, 1976.

291. Thieme, F. P.: Lumbar breakdown caused by erect posture in man; with emphasis on spondylolisthesis and herniated intervertebral disc. Anthrop. Papers, Museum of Anthrop., University of Michigan, Paper No. 4, 1950.

292. Tojner, H.: Olisthetic scoliosis. Acta Orthop. Scand., 33:291, 1963.

293. Toland, J. J.: Spondylolisthesis in identical twins. Clin. Orthop., 5:184, 1955.

294. Troup, J. D. G.: Mechanical factors in spondylolisthesis and spondylolysis. Clin. Orthop., 117:59, 1976.

295. Turner, H., and Markeloff, N.: Die Röntgendiagnostik der Spondylolysis im Lichte Experimenteller Forschung am Kadaver. Acta Chir. Scand., 67:914, 1930.

296. Turner, H., and Tchirkin, N.: Spondylolisthesis. J. Bone Joint Surg., 7:763, 1925.

297. Turner, R. H., and Bianco, A. J., Jr.: Spondylolysis and spondylolisthesis in children and teenagers. J. Bone Joint Surg., 53-A:1298, 1971.

298. Turney, J. P.: Cauda equina lesion due to spondylolisthesis. Br. Med. J., 2:1028, 1952.

299. Ullman, H. J.: Diagnostic line for determining subluxation of fifth lumbar vertebra. Radiology, 2:305, 1924.

300. Unander-Scharin, L.: A case of spondylolisthesis lumbalis acquista. Acta Orthop. Scand., 19:536, 1950.

301. Vallois, H. V., and Lozarthes, G.: Indices lombaires et indice lombaire totale. Bull. Soc. Anthropol., 3:117, 1942.

302. Van Rens, J. G., and Van Horn, J. R.: Long-term results in lumbosacral interbody fusion for spondylolisthesis. Acta Orthop. Scand., 53:383, 1982.

303. Velikas, E. P., and Blackburne, J. S.: Surgical treatment of spondylolisthesis in children and adolescents. J. Bone Joint Surg., 63-B:67, 1981.

304. Verbiest, H.: The treatment of lumbar spondyloptosis or impending lumbar spondyloptosis accompanied by neurologic deficit and/or neurogenic intermittent claudication. Spine, 4:68, 1979.

305. Vidal, J., Fassio, B., Buscayret, C., and Allieu, Y.: Surgical reduction of spondylolisthesis using a posterior approach. Clin. Orthop., 154:156, 1981.

306. Villiaumey, J.: Spondylolisthesis lombaire chez des jumeaux. Rev. Rhum. Mal. Osteoartic., 35:130, 1968.

307. Weitzman, G.: Dilatation of the common iliac vein and the inferior vena cava in spondylolisthesis. Report of a case with reference to three other cases. Clin. Orthop., 42:157, 1965.

308. Wertzberger, K. L., and Peterson, H. A.: Acquired spondylolysis and spondylolisthesis in the young child. Spine, 5:437, 1980.

309. Willis, T. A.: The lumbo-sacral vertebral column in man: Its stability of form and function. Am. J. Anat., 32:95, 1923.

310. Willis, T. A.: The separate neural arch. J. Bone Joint Surg., 13:709, 1931.

311. Wiltse, L. L.: Etiology of spondylolisthesis. Clin. Orthop., 10:48, 1957.

312. Wiltse, L. L.: Spondylolisthesis in children. Clin. Orthop., 21:156, 1961.

313. Wiltse, L. L.: The etiology of spondylolisthesis. J. Bone Joint Surg., 44-A:539, 1962.

314. Wiltse, L. L.: Classification and etiology. Symposium on the Spine. A.A.O.S., St. Louis, Mosby, 1969, p. 143.

315. Wiltse, L. L.: Spondylolisthesis. West. J. Med., 122:152, 1975.

316. Wiltse, L. L., and Hutchinson, R. H.: Surgical treatment of spondylolisthesis. Clin. Orthop., 35:116, 1964.
317. Wiltse, L. L., and Jackson, D. W.: Treatment of spondylolisthesis and spondylolysis in children. Clin. Orthop., *117*:92, 1976.
318. Wiltse, L. L., and Winter, R. B.: Terminology and measurement of spondylolisthesis. J. Bone Joint Surg., 65-A:768, 1983.
319. Wiltse, L. L., Newman, P. H., and MacNab, I.: Classification of spondylolysis and spondylolisthesis. Clin. Orthop., *117*:23, 1976.
320. Wiltse, L. L., Widell, E. H., Jr., and Jackson, D. W.: Fatigue fracture: The basic lesion in isthmic spondylolisthesis. J. Bone Joint Surg., 57-A:17, 1975.
321. Winter, R. B.: Severe spondylolisthesis in Marfan's syndrome: Report of two cases. J. Pediatr. Orthop., 2:51, 1982.
322. Winter, R. B., and Edwards, W. C.: Case report. Neurofibromatosis with lumbosacral spondylolisthesis. J. Pediatr. Orthop., *1*:91, 1981.
323. Woolsey, R. D.: Mechanism of neurological symptoms and signs in spondylolisthesis at the fifth lumbar, first sacral level. J. Neurosurg., *11*:67, 1954.
324. Woolsey, R. D.: Simple laminectomy for spondylolisthesis without spinal fusion. J. Int. Coll. Surg., 29:101, 1958.
325. Wynne-Davies, R., and Scott, J. H. S.: Inheritance and spondylolisthesis. J. Bone Joint Surg., 61-B:301, 1979.
326. Yano, T., Miyagi, S., and Ikari, T.: Studies of familial incidence of spondylolysis. Singapore Med. J., 8:203, 1967.
327. Zippel, H.: Pathogenesis of spondylolisthesis with reference to expert evaluation. Beitr. Orthop. Traumatol., 22:158, 1975.
328. Zippel, H., and Runge, H.: Morbid anatomy and pathogenesis of spondylolysis and spondylolisthesis in childhood. Z. Orthop., *114*:189, 1976.

Scoliosis

The word *scoliosis* (first used by Galen—A.D. 131–201) is derived from the Greek word meaning "crooked."[276] One of the most common deformities of the spine, it has been recognized since ancient times. Normal and abnormal spinal curves are described in the *Corpus Hippocraticum*. André devised the crooked spine as his symbol for orthopedics.[24]

During the past fifty years great strides have been made in the treatment of scoliosis. The Scoliosis Research Society, founded in 1966, has standardized and elevated the care of spinal deformity by stimulation of basic and clinical research and formation of scoliosis treatment centers. Two recently published textbooks present thorough discussion of spinal deformity: the first, *Scoliosis and Other Spinal Deformities* by Moe, Winter, Bradford, and Lonstein (published by W. B. Saunders Co., 2nd edition, 1987), and the second, *The Pediatric Spine*, edited by Bradford and Hensinger and published by Thieme Inc., New York, and Georg Thieme Verlag, Stuttgart, New York.[93, 517] In this book this author endeavors to be concise, stressing principles.

Definitions

The human spine is held erect by active muscular support and by the sense of balance. There is a definite inherent tendency for the spine to grow straight. There are normally physiologic curves in the sagittal plane, but the spine is straight when viewed in the frontal plane, i.e., some degree of lumbar lordosis or dorsal roundback is normal, but there is no lateral curvature of the normal spine.

Scoliosis may be defined as lateral deviation and rotation of a series of vertebrae from the midline anatomic position of the normal spinal axis. The deformity occurs in three planes—frontal, sagittal, and transverse. When the deviation cannot be corrected or the correction cannot be maintained, the scoliosis is considered pathologic. With progression of the curve, structural changes in the vertebrae occur, and deformity of the rib cage results from the rotation of the thoracic vertebral bodies. Associated pelvic deformity may take place. Relationships of intrathoracic and abdominal organs are distorted.

Scoliosis is a deformity that may have its genesis in fetal life, infancy, childhood, or adolescence, although the residual deformity persists throughout adult life.

IDIOPATHIC SCOLIOSIS

The term *idiopathic scoliosis* refers to a structural scoliosis whose etiology is unknown. This occurs in 80 per cent of patients with structural scoliosis. One should remember, however, that scoliosis is a physical sign and *not* a diagnosis. Ordinarily when neurologic and paralytic causes have been ruled out by a thorough physical examination, and congenital anomalies by a negative radiogram, the diagnosis of idiopathic scoliosis is made. Idiopathic structural scoliosis may have its onset at any age during growth, but usually it has three fairly well-defined peak periods: in the first year of life, at five to six years of age, and from after the eleventh year to the end of growth. Therefore, it is subdivided into three chronological age groups: *infantile* (from birth to three years of age); *juvenile* (from four years of age until the onset of puberty); and *adolescent* (at or about the onset of puberty and before closure of the physes). Adult scoliosis is spinal curvature existing after skeletal maturity—it may have had its onset in any of the three growth periods.

Prevalence

Prevalence of a disorder is the proportion of the population afflicted at a particular time. It should be distinguished from *incidence*; the latter refers to the rate of occurrence of new cases of a condition. Prevalence is determined by mass screening of unselected large population groups. In the literature two types of prevalence studies have been performed: first, school screening, and second, chest radiograms made for tuberculosis. The problems with chest radiogram screening are failure to visualize the lumbar spine adequately, underpenetration, and small size of the film.

Scoliosis is usually recognizable before the age of 14 years. In a survey taken in 1955 of 50,000 chest radiograms in a population over 14 years of age in Delaware, Shands and Eisberg found scoliosis of 10 degrees or more in 1.9 per cent and of 20 degrees or more in 0.5 per cent. The female to male ratio was 3.5 to 1.0.[680]

School screening is supposed to provide more accurate data as suspected cases are referred to orthopedic surgeons and have spine films made after thorough assessment. Wynne-Davies surveyed 10,000 children in Edinburgh whose ages ranged from two weeks to 18 years. Scoliosis was noted in 1.3 per 1,000 under age eight years (early onset) and 1.8 per 1,000 over age eight years.[802]

In North America the prevalence of curves of 10 degrees or less varies between 2 and 3 per cent; the prevalence, however, decreases with increasing magnitude of the curve—that of curves of 20 degrees or more is 0.2 to 0.3 per cent.[39, 454, 458, 637]

Sex Predilection

In the survey of Wynne-Davies, the female to male ratio was equal in children under eight years of age; in those over eight years the prevalence in females was 4.6 per 1,000 and in males 0.2 per 1,000.[802] Rogale and associates reported the sex prevalence of different curve magnitudes: the ratio of females to males was 1:1 for curves of 6 to 10 degrees, 1.4:1 for curves of 11 to 20 degrees, 5.4:1 for curves over 21 degrees, and 7.2:1 for curves under treatment.[637] This gender prevalence for idiopathic scoliosis—i.e., equal female to male prevalence

for small curves (less than 10 degrees) and increasing female prevalence for the larger and progressive curves—has also been reported by Asher and associates, by Drummond and associates, and by Lonstein and associates.[39, 206, 454, 458] The clinical significance of these observations is that curve progression is more common in girls.

School Screening

The value of massive school screening, first carried out in the state of Delaware in 1965, is well established and attested in the literature.[349] The objective of screening is early detection of spinal deformity in order to prevent its progression by effective treatment. Methods used for scoliosis detection are the Adams forward bend test, Bunnell's scoliometer for measurement of trunk rotation, various methods of rib hump measurement, and Moire topography.[10, 106, 107, 384] At present, low-dosage radiographic imaging is no longer performed. This author recommends the forward bending test and the use of the scoliometer (see the section on physical examination).

The first problem of school screening is overreferral, which takes place more commonly than missing a significant scoliosis. The use of Bunnell's scoliometer reduced over-referral by 50 per cent. The second problem is the risk and danger of diagnostic radiation. It is vital that a child suspected of having scoliosis be carefully examined by a competent orthopedic surgeon prior to making radiographs; the risks of diagnostic radiation are minimized by not making unnecessary ones. Initially, a single standing anteroposterior radiograph of the spine is made with the iliac crests as high as possible. Lateral, supine, and lateral bending anteroposterior views should not be made routinely. Radiation exposure can also be lowered by gonadal shielding, the use of high-speed rare earth intensifying screens, fast film, collimation, and beam filtration.[178, 542] The follow-up visits are timed according to the risk for progression (see Natural History and Risk Factors Related to Curve Progression). Small curves in boys are not likely to progress, whereas 15- to 20-degree curves in girls have a moderate risk for progression. The high-risk group is females with curves over 20 degrees. Routine follow-up radiographs should not be made; examine the child clinically before making x-rays. The third problem is lack of compliance by the parents. It is essential to educate students, parents, and primary care physicians. The fourth problem is cost effectiveness. School screening does diagnose scoliosis early. The number of children requiring surgery after screening programs have been established has diminished.[738] The question is whether conservative treatment with orthosis or lateral electrical surface stimulation can prevent curve progression. In the literature a 15 to 40 per cent failure rate has been reported.[203, 418, 500] Another fact to consider is that not all curves between 20 and 30 degrees do progress; therefore some of the good results of orthotic management can be accounted for by the favorable natural history of idiopathic scoliosis. Double-blind studies are needed to determine the effectiveness of nonsurgical treatment of scoliosis to prevent serious deformity. Despite all these problems this author concurs with Drummond that screening of children for scoliosis in the 10- to 12-year age group is justified and should be carried out.[203] Over-referral can be diminished by the combination of the Adams bending test with the use of Bunnell's scoliometer (or a similar device for measuring trunk rotation) and proper education of nurses, primary care physicians, and parents. Radiation hazard can be curtailed by making radiographs of the spine only after thorough examination by an orthopedic surgeon and by the use of appropriate radiographic techniques. All large curves were small initially. Early diagnosis of small curves will prevent much future embarrassment to the family physician and pediatrician if the curves are progressive. Also, it is appropriate to state that an orthopedic surgeon should always examine the spine of a child who presents with musculoskeletal deformity. Not infrequently this author sees a child referred for a foot or lower limb problem and finds that the referring physician has failed to examine the spine and missed spinal deformity. It is good medical practice to examine the entire child.

Genetic Aspects

Idiopathic structural scoliosis is a familial condition. There is, however, no single genetic basis for idiopathic scoliosis; this is shown in DeGeorge and Fisher's study of monozygotic and dizygotic twin pairs.[172] In the survey of Wynne-Davies it was found that the number of patients in whom onset of scoliosis was in adolescence who were the offspring of older mothers was significantly greater than the expected figure for the normal population.[802] Fisher and DeGeorge found a similar rise in the offspring of older mothers.[260] Therefore, daughters of mothers aged 30 to 39 years who have scoliosis

are at great risk for developing scoliosis, especially between the ages of 9 and 12 years.

The exact mode of inheritance is not known. The family studies of Wynne-Davies and of Riseborough and Wynne-Davies support a multifactorial mode; whereas that of Cowell and associates suggests a dominant mode.[160, 616, 802] In 1968, Wynne-Davies studied the family incidence of scoliosis in 114 patients by visiting and examining all their available relatives (well over 2,000 individuals), and compared these observations with the incidence of scoliosis in the general population (by examining a total of more than 10,000 children). For convenience in her genetic survey, Wynne-Davies divided scoliosis into two main groups: early-onset (under eight years of age) and late-onset (eight years of age and over). In the infants the great majority of curves were on the left side and thoracic (90 per cent). Late-onset scoliosis was more frequent in girls (seven girls to one boy). The early-onset type was slightly more common in boys (five boys to four girls), and the curve was either "resolving" or "progressive." In the late-onset type, structural scoliosis did not disappear spontaneously.[802] This survey indicates that, despite certain clinical differences, the infantile and adolescent types of scoliosis probably share the same basic etiology, as the families studied contain instances of each. The finding of plagiocephaly in all infants with scoliosis under one year of age suggests the action of an environmental factor in the infantile group (Fig. 6–45). Infants with resolving-type scoliosis had affected relatives in the same proportion as children with infantile progressive scoliosis, suggesting that this may be a mild form of the same disorder.

Comparison of the incidence of scoliosis in the general population and among the relatives of scoliotic patients is shown in Figure 6–46. There is undoubtedly a greater incidence of scoliosis among the families of patients when compared with the general population. There is a marked rise in incidence (scoliosis 20 times more common than in the general population) in the families of those girls with late-onset scoliosis. This strong evidence for a genetic factor suggests either a dominant or multiple gene inheritance.

In 1973 Riseborough and Wynne-Davies studied the families of 207 index patients in Boston and compared the results with those of the 1968 Edinburgh study. The Boston study revealed a marked drop in proportions of affected first-, second-, and third-degree relatives (11.1 per cent, 2.4 per cent, and 1.4 per cent

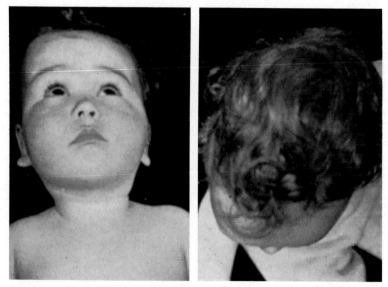

FIGURE 6–45. *Left-sided plagiocephaly associated with left thoracic scoliosis in infants.*

(From Wynne-Davies, R.: Familial (idiopathic) scoliosis. A family survey. J. Bone Joint Surg., *50-B*:24–30, 1968. Reprinted by permission.)

respectively) compared with the Edinburgh survey (7.0 per cent, 3.7 per cent, and 1.6 per cent respectively).[616] The findings of the comparison supported a multifactorial mode of inheritance.

In the study of Cowell and associates of 590 parents and siblings of an unselected group of 110 scoliosis patients, a dominant mode of in-

heritance was suggested; in 20 per cent of the cases the incidence was sporadic.[160]

Etiology

The exact cause of idiopathic scoliosis is unknown. A normal spine tends to grow straight. Irrespective of its pathogenesis, idiopathic sco-

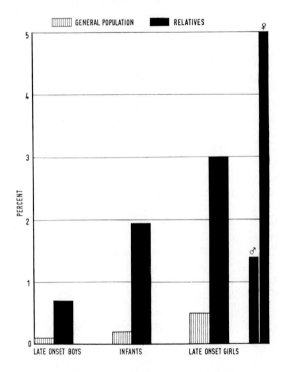

FIGURE 6–46. *Comparison of incidence of scoliosis in the general population and among the relatives of scoliotic patients.*

(From Wynne-Davies, R.: Familial (idiopathic) scoliosis. A family survey. J. Bone Joint Surg., *50-B*:24–30, 1968. Reprinted by permission.)

liosis represents a progressive structural deformity that is a product of abnormal and asymmetrical growth of the vertebral column.

A number of theories have been advanced to explain the mechanics of vertebral column failure and decompensation of the spine. Insufficiency of the costovertebral ligaments, asymmetrical weakness and muscle imbalance of the paraspinal musculature, unequal distribution of Type I and Type II muscle fibers, collagen abnormalities, and malfunction of the vestibular balancing system have been implicated as underlying factors in the pathogenesis of scoliosis.[255, 420, 611, 644, 647, 799]

The mechanics of scoliosis are still not entirely understood, but the following are important considerations.

The Law of Balance. Normally there is no lateral curvature of the human spine. Because of a natural sense of balance and equilibrium, the muscles controlling the vertebral column tend to hold the spine straight with the head erect over the mid-pelvis and the body in balance. When a curvature is initiated, compensatory curves promptly develop in an instinctive effort to maintain erect posture with the center of body mass located over the body midline.

Structure of the Spine. The human spine is not a straight rod, but consists of a series of jointed segments that are arranged in an anteroposterior curve in the sagittal plane. It is a physical necessity that, if a lateral curve (frontal plane) is imposed upon a rod already bent in an anteroposterior direction (sagittal plane), a rotation in the third direction (transverse plane) must take place. Thus, any lateral motion in the spine is accompanied by rotation of the vertebrae and their attached appendages, the ribs. Conversely, rotary displacement of the vertebrae is accompanied by lateral inclination. Loss of normal thoracic kyphosis is common in thoracic scoliosis. The resistance of the vertebrae to deforming rotational forces is decreased by the thoracic lordosis.[189]

Intrinsic Equilibrium. In the normal spinal column there is an intrinsic equilibrium produced by the elasticity of the longitudinal ligaments on one side, which presses the vertebrae together, and the expansile force of the discs on the other, which tends to separate the vertebrae. These elastic forces acting on the vertebral segments provide such a degree of stability that only a minimal amount of muscular force is necessary to maintain the spine in the erect position.

Inclinatory and Translatory Factors. The forces that produce scoliosis operate both in the inclinatory and translatory sense. It is important to make a distinction between the two, as they vary in importance and sequence in different types of scoliosis. The inclinatory factor is resisted normally by the muscle equilibrium; it is *intersegmental*, producing a contractural deformity between sections of the spine; it is characterized by a long-arc curve. The inclinatory factor is in the foreground and is the only one present in the earliest stages of paralytic scoliosis. The translatory factor is resisted normally by the intrinsic equilibrium of the spine; it is *intrasegmental*, producing a collapse between vertebrae; it is characterized by a short-arc curve. In idiopathic structural scoliosis the translatory factor is effective earlier than the inclinatory factor.[705, 706]

Experimental Scoliosis. As studies of scoliosis in man have not elucidated the pathogenesis of scoliosis, many authors have investigated the problem by animal experiments in an attempt to understand the normal processes of vertebral growth and the factors that may interfere with them. Scoliosis has been produced in animals by several means: excision or denervation of muscles, resection of ribs, division of posterior costotransverse ligaments, fixation of vertebrae or ribs to each other, operations on growth zones of vertebrae, radiation, and feeding of *Lathyrus odoratus* seeds to produce lathyrism.*

The experimental work of Ponseti and his co-workers is important, as it is the first example of scoliosis induced by metabolic changes.[589, 590, 593] The basic substance in sweet pea seeds is an amino nitrite, glutamyl-amino propionitrite, a metabolic poison interfering with chondroitin sulfate. Feeding the rat *Lathyrus odoratus* causes slipping of epiphyses, ligamentous detachment, scoliosis, and aneurysm of the aorta. A biochemical cause of scoliosis may be conjectured, as metabolic abnormalities are commonly inherited and idiopathic scoliosis is familial.

The results of Langenskiöld and Michelsson correspond well with the general anatomic findings in human scoliosis. They found that excision of the posterior costotransverse ligaments produced a scoliosis with the convexity toward the side of the operation. They proposed that the costotransverse ligament transfers the forces of the spinal muscles from the ribs to the

---

*See references: excision or denervation of muscles, 668; resection of ribs, 71; division of costotransverse ligaments, 428, 429; fixation of vertebrae or ribs, 502; operations on growth zones, 72, 317, 534, 535; radiation, 33, 235; lathyrism, 589, 590, 593.

vertebrae, and functional insufficiency of this ligament allows the spinal muscles on the opposite side to be overactive, producing rotation and lateral flexion deformity.[428, 429] Michelsson induced scoliosis in pigs by resection of the ribs and found that the neurocentral junction on the concave side remains open and grows, this being contrary to expectation based on human scoliosis.[502]

Pathology

The extent of structural changes varies with the degree of scoliosis.[237, 391, 424, 633] They are greatest at the apex of the curve, diminishing toward either end. In structural scoliosis, rotation of the vertebrae is to the convex side of the lateral curvature so that the spinous processes of the vertebrae are rotated toward the concavity of the curve.

Compressional and distractional forces act on the growing spine and produce changes in the vertebrae, which become wedge-shaped, higher on the convex side and lower on the concave side (Fig. 6–47). The vertebral body becomes condensed on the concave side as a result of the greater pressure, and is expanded and thinned on the convex side. The vertebrae always rotate toward the convexity of the curve in structural scoliosis.

There are associated changes in the neural canal and posterior arch. The laminae on the convex side are broad and widely separated, and those on the concave side are narrow and close together (Fig. 6–48). The pedicles are shorter and stubbier on the concave side. The transverse processes more closely approach the sagittal plane on the convex side and are more in the frontal plane on the concave side. The intraspinal canal becomes distorted because of the misshapen pedicles and articular processes (Fig. 6–49).

The intervertebral discs on the concave side, as a result of pressure, are compressed and show degenerative changes. The adjoining portion of the vertebra reacts with sclerosis and marginal lipping. Later in life degenerative arthritic changes take place. The muscles and ligaments are thickened and contracted on the concave side, consituting a primary obstacle to correction, and they become thin and atrophied on the convex side. Later, in severe curves, calcification of the ligamentous tissues and synostosis between the arches and intervertebral articulations may take place.

The thoracic cage is also affected by deformity. Because of rotation and translatory shift

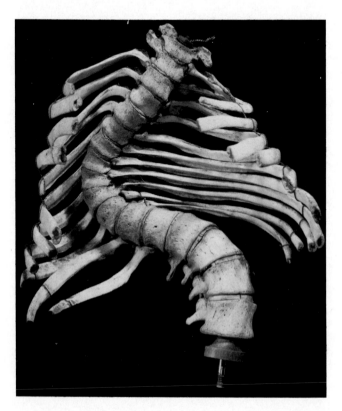

FIGURE 6–47. Gross anatomic specimen of the spine demonstrating structural changes of right thoracic scoliosis.

Note the wedging of the vertebrae on the concave side and rotation of the vertebral bodies to the convexity of the curve. The ribs on the concave side are rotated forward and on the convex side are thrust backward. (From James, J. I. P.: Scoliosis. Baltimore, Williams & Wilkins Co., 1967, p. 13. Reprinted by permission.)

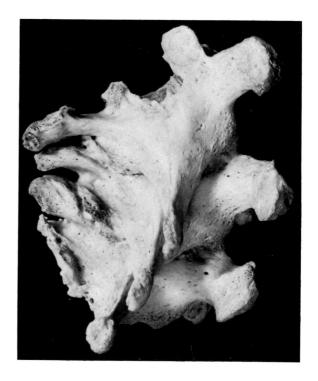

FIGURE 6–48. *Posterior view of the neural arch, showing the narrow laminae close together on the concave side.*

(From James, J. I. P.: Scoliosis. Baltimore, Williams & Wilkins Co., 1967, p. 15. Reprinted by permission.)

of the dorsal vertebrae, the ribs on the convex side are thrust backward, producing a posterior rib hump that is aptly described as a "razor back" in severe cases. On the concave side, the ribs are rotated forward, producing prominence of the anterior chest wall and the breast. The sternum rotates on a vertical axis in response to the change of position of the ribs; thus, in a right thoracic curve, the left border is in front of the right border. Also, the sternum may be laterally displaced from the median line.

With the translatory shift of the spine side-ward, the thorax is divided into two asymmetrical halves. Its capacity is diminished on the convex side and increased on the concave side. In severe cases, with marked angulation of the ribs posteriorly, the aeration of lung tissue is reduced on the convex side. The abnormal pressure and stresses exerted on the heart may disturb cardiac function.[355]

In severe scoliosis with distortion of the shape of the intraspinal canal the spinal cord will be angulated and stretched, but any interference with its function is very rare. Cord compression

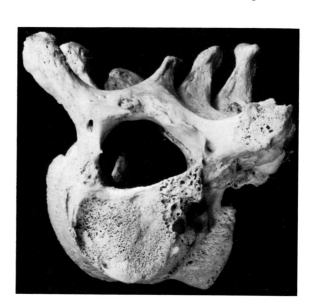

FIGURE 6–49. *Superior view of the vertebra with structural scoliosis.*

Note that on the concave side the pedicle is short and stubby and the intraspinal canal is narrowed. (From James, J. I. P.: Scoliosis. Baltimore, Williams & Wilkins Co., 1967, p. 15. Reprinted by permission.)

Table 6–2. *Curves at Risk for Progression in the Skeletally Immature Patient*

Age—in the young, particularly during periods of rapid growth

Risser sign—low grade, zero to two

Menarche—curves detected prior to menarche

Curve magnitude—the large curves

Curve pattern—double curves, particularly double thoracic. Lumbar curves have the least risk.

Rotation—Mehta's RVAD of greater than 20 degrees and transition from Phase I to Phase II in infantile and juvenile scoliosis. In adolescent, thoracic curves when rotation is 33 per cent or more.

Sex—girls ten times more at risk than boys

Positive family history—probably at greater risk

is due to an unusually tight dura mater and occurs only in severe deformities, especially in cases associated with marked dorsal kyphosis.

Natural History and Risk Factors Related to Curve Progression

It is important to know the natural history of scoliosis as it is a guide to prognosis and selection of patients for treatment.

Curve progression is defined as a sustained increase of 5 or more degrees (as measured by the Cobb method) on two or more consecutive examinations. Some curves wax and wane in magnitude from one examination to the next; it is important that in curve progression the increase in the degree of curvature be permanent.[203]

A *progressive curve* is one that if untreated increases in adult life; in general these are curves that are greater than 30 degrees.[766]

The following factors are related to curve progression (Table 6–2).

Age of Onset and Maturity: Growth Potential. Scoliosis is likely to be progressive as long as there is potential for growth. Historically, in 1824, Bampfield observed that increasing scoliosis appeared only during growth of the body, and he thought it was due to increased growth on one side of the vertebral bodies with progressive absorption from pressure on the other side.[49] Bradford, in 1890, described scoliosis as having three stages: initial, developmental, and stage of arrest. He stated that the stage of arrest occurred when all possible alteration in the shape of the bone had taken place with completion of ossification and when the vertebrae were sufficiently strong to sustain permanent weight without yielding laterally in the direction of torsion.[95]

Curve progression varies directly with growth potential. This direct relationship between vertebral growth and increasing scoliotic deformity is well documented by the study of Risser and Ferguson. The spine grows slowly in children from about seven to ten years of age, as indicated by comparison of vertical standing and sitting heights of the patients. In this age period the increase in scoliosis ranged from 3 to 5 degrees a year. In the preadolescent age of from 10 to 13 years, there was rapid growth of the spine and the scoliosis increased about 1 degree a month. It became essentially static after completion of vertebral growth, as shown by cessation of increase in sitting height. The spine stopped growing at an average age of 14½ years in girls and 16½ years in boys, the extremes being 13 and 16 years and 14½ and 17 years respectively.[623]

Curve progression takes place most during periods of rapid skeletal growth, especially during the adolescent growth spurt. It ordinarily coincides with the appearance of secondary sex characteristics with a Tanner grading of pubertal stage two. (In *girls* the breast begins to bud with enlargement of the areolar diameter and elevation of the breast and papilla as a small mound; girls in the second pubertal stage also grow long, slightly pigmented, downy pubic hair, appearing primarily around the labia. In *boys*, Tanner's second pubertal stage is characterized by enlargement of the testes and scrotum with change in the texture of the scrotal skin, and pigmented downy hair begins to grow at the base of the penis).[721] In girls a curve detected prior to menarche is at greater risk for progression (65 per cent) than one detected postmenarche (33 per cent). Scoliosis is more likely to progress in young children than in older children. With increasing age the incidence of progression decreases. In the study of Lonstein and Carlson the incidence of curve progression was 67 per cent in children under nine years of age and 11 per cent in adolescents over 15 years of age.[456] At present no studies are available that correlate curve progression with skeletal age.

Data are available, however, pertaining to curve progression in relation to skeletal maturity of the spine as determined by the Risser sign. In Lonstein's study, when the Risser sign was between 0 and 1 in children with curves of less than 20 degrees, curve progression occurred in 22 per cent with an average progression of 1 degree per month during an average year of observation, whereas when the Risser sign was between 2 and 4 it occurred in only 1.6 per cent.[455] In the study of Rogala and associates, the Risser sign was 3 or less in 40 per cent of the 41 patients with progressive curve when they were first examined.[637] Therefore, the lower the Risser grade at curve detection, the greater the chance of progression.

The Magnitude of the Curve. The larger the curve at initial detection, the greater the risk for progression.[190, 455, 637]

Curve Pattern. Double curve patterns, particularly double thoracic curves, have greater risk for progression than single curve patterns. Lumbar curves are least likely to progress.[455]

Sex. With comparable curves, progression is about ten times more likely in girls than in boys.

Infantile and juvenile scoliosis curves are at risk for progression when Mehta's rib-vertebral angle difference (RVAD) is greater than 20 degrees and when there is transition from Phase I to Phase II.

Rotation. In adolescent scoliosis, rotation is of no prognostic value in small curves. In thoracic curves, however, when rotation is 33 per cent or more the risk for progression is great.[766] The relation of body habitus and positive family history to curve progression is not clear. Drummond and Rogala noted a higher incidence of positive family history in progressive curves.[204]

Clinical Features

Patients with scoliosis usually seek medical attention with presenting complaints of a high shoulder, prominent shoulder blade or breast, high or prominent hip, asymmetry of flank creases and trunk, poor posture, and curvature. The deformity of scoliosis is the symptom in children. A chest radiogram or intravenous pyelogram may reveal previously undetected scoliosis.

It is very seldom that a child with scoliosis will complain of backache and fatigue. When pain is present as a clinical feature it is due to some other cause such as spondylolisthesis, Scheuermann's disease, bone lesions (such as osteoid osteoma or osteoblastoma), or spinal cord tumors. A painful spinal deformity in a child or adolescent should be thoroughly evaluated clinically. Is the pain in the curve area or in the lumbosacral region? Does it radiate to the gluteal region, thighs, or legs? Is the pain intermittent or constant? Is it increasing? What is its effect on activities of daily living? Has the patient taken any analgesics. It is important to know the type of analgesic, the dosage, and the frequency. Do salicylates relieve the pain? Has the patient taken any anti-inflammatory non-steroid drugs such as Naprosyn or Tolectin? Is the pain associated with sensory disturbance such as numbness of the toes? *A child with backache and spinal deformity* should have meticulous *clinical and neurologic examination, radiographs of the spine,* and *bone scan.* If indicated, computed tomography, magnetic resonance imaging, or both are performed.

In adults, particularly with lumbar scoliosis, backache is not uncommon and is due to degenerative arthritis in the posterior articulations; root pain may complicate local back pain. In very severe scoliosis, pressure of the ribs against the iliac crests may cause pain. Cardiorespiratory symptoms such as shortness of breath may occur in the severely scoliotic. Spinal cord compression is rarely encountered; it does occur during rapid growth periods of adolescence and is due to inability of the spinal cord to accommodate itself to structural changes in the intraspinal canal.

The examination of the child with scoliosis should follow a definite order. First, the patient is observed standing while clothed, and next, without clothing and properly draped. It is customary to use an examination gown open at the back; the underpants should be small, exposing the iliac crests and posterior superior iliac spines. First the standing (without shoes) and sitting heights are measured (Fig. 6–50). The general body habitus is noted. Next the posture and alignment of the spine are inspected from the front, side, and back (Fig. 6–51). Is there kyphosis or lordosis associated with the scoliosis? The deformity of lateral angulation is best seen from directly behind with the child standing. The level of the shoulders, position of the scapulae, and symmetry or asymmetry of the waistline are noted. Are the head, neck, and shoulders balanced over the pelvis? When a plumb line (string with a plumb bob or tape measure) is held over the spinous process of the seventh cervical vertebra, it should normally pass through the intergluteal cleft. When the spine is decompensated in scoliosis the plumb line will fall to the right or left of the intergluteal cleft. The amount of list of the trunk (the distance from the vertical plumb line to the intergluteal cleft) is measured and recorded in centimeters (Fig. 6–52). When the trapezius neckline is asymmetrical (indicating cervical or cervicothoracic scoliosis) the plumb line is projected from the occipital protuberance. Deviation of any number of spinous processes from this median line indicates a lateral curvature. The level and extent of lateral deviation should be recorded.

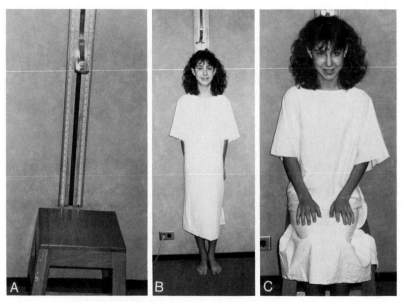

FIGURE 6–50. *Measurement of standing and sitting height.*

A. Measuring apparatus with a stool. **B.** Standing height. **C.** Sitting height.

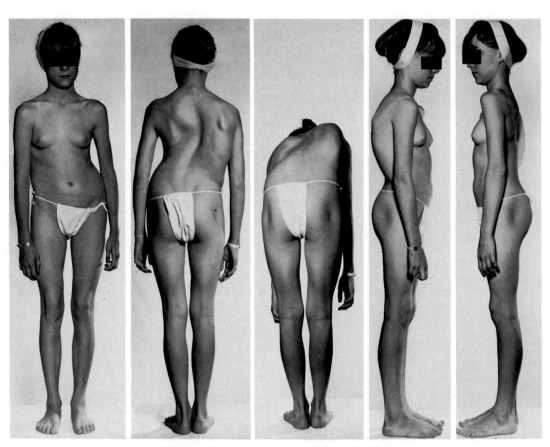

FIGURE 6–51. *Idiopathic structural thoracic scoliosis.*

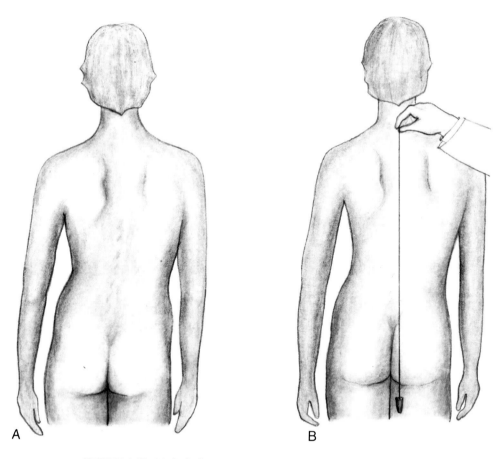

FIGURE 6–52. Method of measuring decompensation of the spine in scoliosis.

Normally, when a plumb line is dropped from the spinous process of the seventh cervical vertebra, it should fall in the intergluteal cleft. When the alignment of the spine is decompensated in scoliosis, the plumb line will fall to the right or left of the intergluteal cleft. Record the amount of list of the trunk by measuring the distance from the vertebral plumb line to the intergluteal cleft in centimeters. When there is cervicothoracic scoliosis (as shown by asymmetry of the trapezius neck line), drop the plumb line from the occipital protuberance.

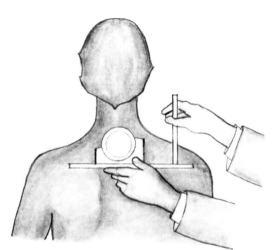

FIGURE 6–53. Method of measuring the level of the shoulders by the use of a level.

The level of the shoulders is inspected from the posterior view and measured with a level (Fig. 6–53). Place the horizontal level at the acromioclavicular joint of the lower shoulder and measure the vertical distance from the horizontal level to the top of the high shoulder in centimeters.

The degree and direction of associated rotation of the vertebrae are best seen by observing the child from the back as he bends forward at his waist (Adams' forward bending test).[10] The patient's knees should be straight, feet together, arms dependent, and palms in opposition. Inspect the patient head on (for cervical and thoracic rotation) and from the rear (for thoracolumbar and lumbar scoliosis). The right and left sides of the thoracic cage and paravertebral muscles in the lumbar area are compared for

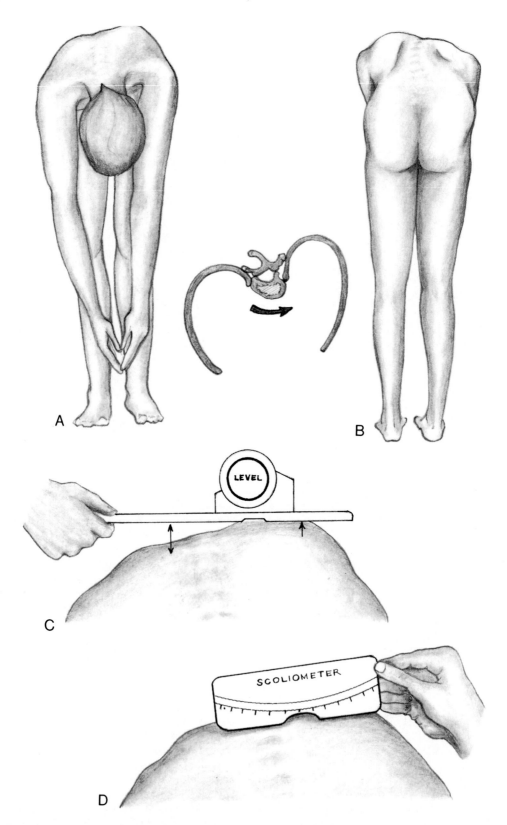

FIGURE 6–54. Adam's forward bending test.

A. Inspection of the patient cephalad (for cervical and thoracic rotation). **B.** Inspection of the patient from the posterior view for thoracolumbar and lumbar scoliosis. **C** and **D.** Clinical method of measuring vertebral rotation.

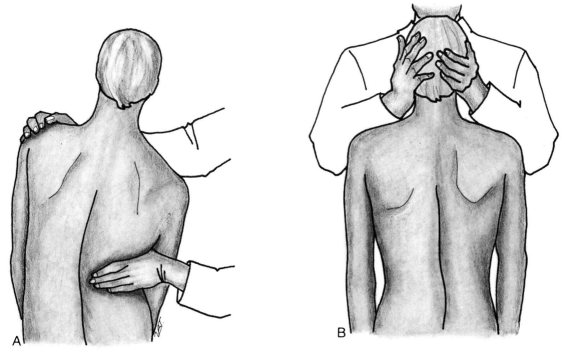

FIGURE 6–55. *Method of determining flexibility of the spine in scoliosis.*

A. Side bending. B. Head-neck traction.

symmetry. When the vertebrae are rotated one side will be higher than the other (Fig. 6–54).

In structural scoliosis, the rotation is to the convex side, whereas in postural scoliosis it is to the concave side of the curve. The degree of rotation can be measured by a scoliometer. An alternate way is to measure the height of the thoracic or paravertebral lumbar prominence in centimeters by use of a level.

At this point the patient is undraped and inspected from the anterior view for asymmetry of the pectoral regions, breasts, and rib cage.

Next, flexibility of each curve is studied. First, have the patient stand upright and perform right and left lateral bends. Next, apply longitudinal traction on the head (grasp the head at the mastoid area and lift the patient vertically upward) (Fig. 6–55).

The extent, degree, and rigidity of each curve are again evaluated with the patient in the prone position. Is there any paravertebral muscle spasm? Gently palpate the spine, and if any local tenderness is present, determine its exact site.

Next inspect the patient from the side and observe the general posture and sagittal contours of the spine. Is there excessive lordosis (hyperlordosis), or is the lumbar spine flat (hypolordosis)? Is the sagittal contour of the thoracic spine normal or is there hyperkyphosis or hypokyphosis? The flexibility of the sagittal curves is determined by prone hyperextension of the spine and the side view of forward bending test (Fig. 6–56). the normal dorsal roundback has a gentle contour. Structural fixed kyphosis (such as in Scheuermann's disease) has a sharp angulation. What are the degree of chest expansion and the anteroposterior diameter of the thoracic cage? Is there any pelvic obliquity? If present, is it flexible or fixed? Are there any contractures about the hips on the Thomas and Ober tests? How tight are the hamstrings? Actual and apparent leg lengths are recorded. Any discrepancy of foot lengths and thigh or calf circumferences are measured.

Ligamentous hyperflexibility is determined by thumb protrusion beyond the ulnar border of the palm (the Steinberg sign), the thumb to

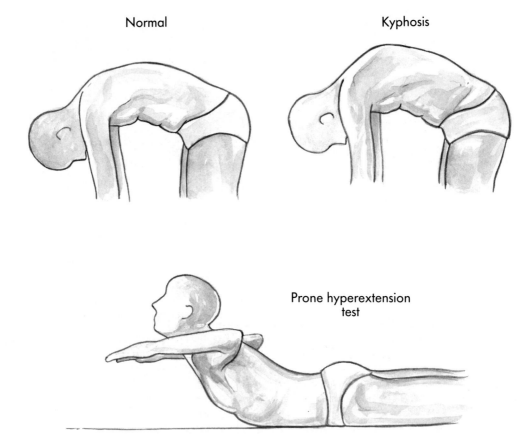

Normal   Kyphosis

Prone hyperextension
test

FIGURE 6–56. Method of determining mobility of sagittal curves of the spine.

A. Prone hyperextension test for thoracic hyperkyphosis. **B.** Side view of forward bending test.

Table 6–3. *Pubertal Stages in Girls and Boys**

Pubertal Stages in Girls	Pubertal Stages in Boys
Breast Staging	*Genitalia Ratings*
Stage 1. Pre-adolescent; elevation of papilla only.	Stage 1. Pre-adolescent; testes, scrotum and penis are of about the same size and proportion as in early childhood.
Stage 2. Breast bud stage; elevation of breast and papilla as a small mound, enlargement of areola diameter.	Stage 2. Scrotum and testes are enlarged with change in texture of the scrotal skin with slight reddening of the skin.
Stage 3. Further enlargement of breast and areola, with no separation of their contours.	Stage 3. Increase in size of the penis, in length mainly, but also in breadth, with continued growth of the testes and scrotum.
Stage 4. Projection of areola and papilla to form a secondary mound above the level of the breast.	Stage 4. Further enlargement of the testes, scrotum, and penis with development of the glans and darkening of the scrotal skin.
Stage 5. Mature stage; projection of papilla only, due to recession of the areola to the general contour of the breast.	Stage 5. Genitalia adult in size and shape.
Pubic Hair Stages	*Pubic Hair Stages*
Stage 1. Pre-adolescent; no pubic hair.	Stage 1. Pre-adolescent; no pubic hair.
Stage 2. Slight growth of long, slightly pigmented, downy hair, appearing chiefly along the labia.	Stage 2. Slight growth of long, slightly pigmented, downy hair, appearing chiefly at the base of the penis.
Stage 3. Darker, coarser hair that is more curled and spread sparsely over the junction of the pubes.	Stage 3. Darker, coarser hair that is more curled and spread sparsely over the junction of the pubes.
Stage 4. Hair is adult in type with no spread to medial surface of the thigh.	Stage 4. Hair is adult in type with no spread to medial surface of the thigh.
Stage 5. Adult in quantity and quality with no inverse triangle distribution and spread to the medial thighs.	Stage 5. Adult in quantity and quality with no inverse triangle distribution and spread to the medial thighs.

*Reprinted by permission from Tanner, J. M.: Growth and endocrinology of the adolescent. *In* Gardner, L. (ed.): Endocrine and Genetic Diseases of Childhood. Philadelphia, W. B. Saunders Co., p. 14, 1975.

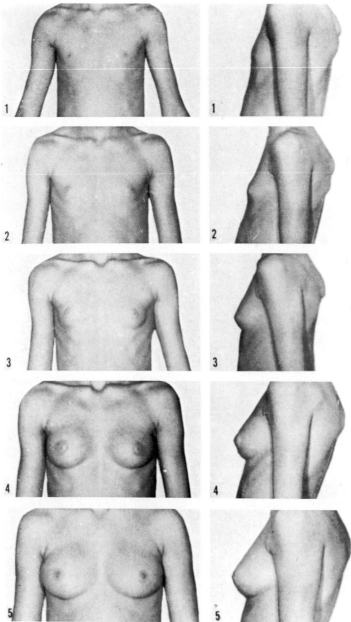

FIGURE 6–57. *Determination of sexual maturation according to Tanner system.*

A. Breast development in girls.

forearm test, and the degree of hyperextension of the elbows and knees.

Muscle power should be examined, especially of the anterior and lateral abdominal, erector spinae, quadratus lumborum, and thoracic groups. Is there any other muscle weakness? Are there any café-au-lait spots or subcutaneous or pedunculated tumors to suggest neurofibromatosis? The presence or absence of various skin lesions associated with congenital anomalies of the spine is significant—e.g., a hairy patch, a skin dimple, a hemangioma, a lipoma, or a myelomeningocele. Are there any deform-

ities of the foot? A pes cavus might suggest Friedreich's ataxia.

A thorough neurologic evaluation must always be part of the examination for scoliosis. Occasionally an intraspinal tumor or other neurologic disease may be the cause of the scoliosis. Also, all patients should have a complete physical examination, particular attention being paid to the cardiovascular and pulmonary systems. Any abnormalities of the mandible and teeth should be recorded.

Sexual maturity is determined according to the Tanner system by assessing breast and pubic

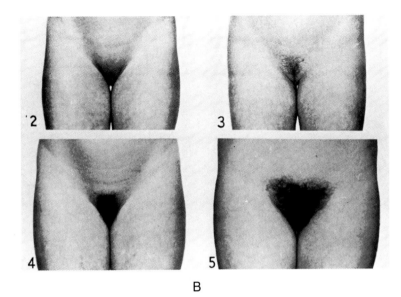

B

FIGURE 6–57 Continued.

B. Pubic hair development in girls. **C.** Genitalia development in boys. (*From* Moe, J. H.: Textbook of Scoliosis and Other Spinal Deformities. 2nd Ed. Philadelphia, W. B. Saunders, 1987. Reprinted by permission.)

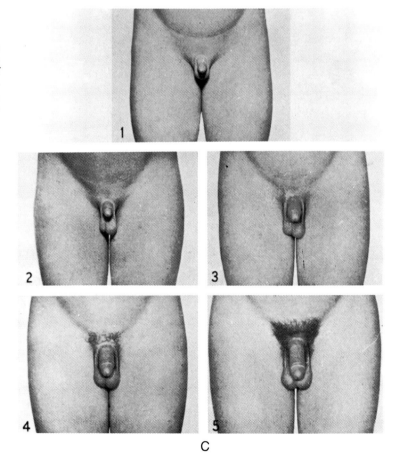

C

hair development in girls and genitalia and pubic hair development in boys (Table 6–3 and Fig. 6–57).

In management of spinal deformity in the adolescent girl it is also vital to assess her psychologic status and intellectual development. Is she mature enough to tolerate an orthotic device?

Routine photographs are made to provide an objective record of the deformity and body

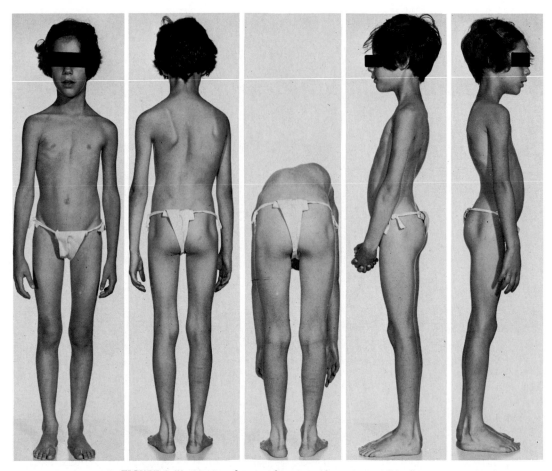

FIGURE 6–58. Routine photographic views of a patient with scoliosis.

posture, and to note any cosmetic improvement afforded by treatment. Photographic views should include front, back, right and left standing views, and a back view with the patient bending forward (Fig. 6–58).

Radiographic Assessment

At the initial examination of a patient with scoliosis radiographs of the entire spine are made to determine the type of scoliosis (such as congenital or idiopathic); the severity of the curvature; the curve pattern; the presence or absence of associated kyphosis or hypokyphosis of the thoracic spine, lordosis or hypolordosis, and spondylolisthesis (as observed in the lateral projection); and skeletal maturity. Evaluation of these radiograms will assist in decision making as to plan of treatment.

Radiation exposure of the patient should be minimized. The most important factor is the number of radiographs taken. *Routine views should not be made.* Order the radiograph after

examination of the patient at each visit! Ask the question, how will this radiographic examination assist you in decision-making! The gonads and the organs (thyroid, breast, and bone marrow) are at risk. Always shield the gonads with a lead screen covering the lower abdomen; the upper border of the gonad shield should extend to the anterior superior iliac spine. It is important not to obscure the iliac apophysis when making the upright films. Securing the gonad shield to an intravenous stand will allow it to be raised or lowered to the appropriate level as necessary. When making radiographs of the spine or pelvis of an adolescent girl, always inquire as to when the last menstrual period took place. When pregnancy is suspected do not make radiographs. In order to reduce radiation the techniques that should be used are collimation of the x-ray beam, use of antiscatter grids, beam filtration, use of intensifying screens (e.g., Quantum screens), and use of fast radiographic film. Radiation exposure of the breast can be minimized by using breast shields

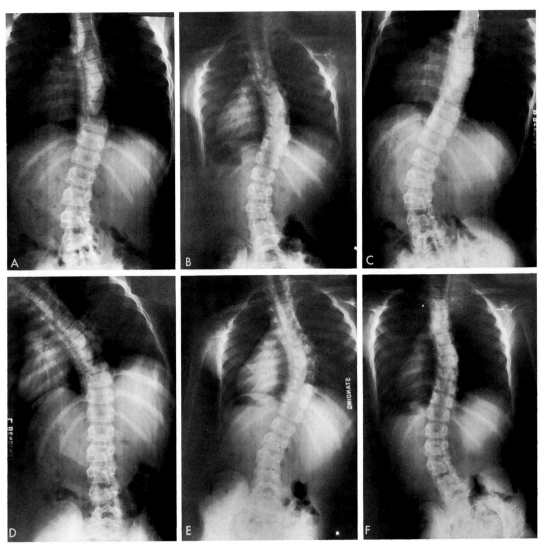

FIGURE 6–59. Radiographic views for structural scoliosis.

These are radiograms of patient shown in Figure 6–41. **A.** Recumbent. **B.** Standing. **C.** Right bend. **D.** Left bend. **E.** Left pelvic tilt. **F.** Right pelvic tilt.

and by making the radiographs in the antero-posterior instead of the posteroanterior position.

The entire spine should be radiographed on a single 14 × 36 inch (36 × 91 cm.) film. This enables one to assess the alignment of the entire spine and determine the relationship of the head, thorax, and pelvis. In children the use of a smaller film (14 × 17 inch or 36 × 43 cm.) is appropriate. Aluminum filters will give a uniform radiographic density of the vertebral column.

Spinal deformity in scoliosis is three dimensional. At the initial examination, upright posteroanterior and lateral projections of the entire spine are made. The patient stands as erect as possible with the knees straight and the feet together. It is best that the patient be barefoot; in case of lower limb length inequality the appropriate lift is worn under the short limb. Unsupported sitting views are made in patients who are unable to stand. Proper posturing is important. There should be no list or twisting of the trunk. The upper limit of the casette should extend to the external auditory meatus. In this upright lateral projection the shoulders are flexed forward 90 degrees with the arms supported on an intravenous stand.

Supine views of the spine are made in infants and patients who are unable to sit. In some

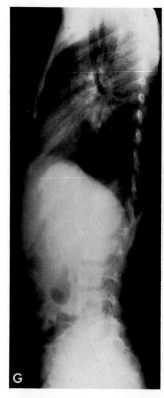
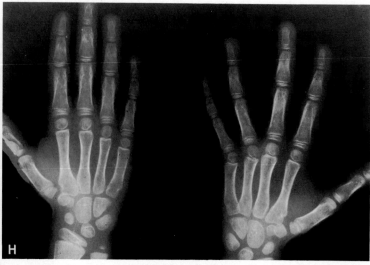

FIGURE 6–59. Continued. Radiographic views for structural scoliosis.

G. Lateral view of dorsolumbar spine. **H.** Anteroposterior view of hands and wrist for skeletal age.

cases of congenital scoliosis, recumbent views provide better visualization of bone detail. Side bending and traction views are ordinarily not indicated except in preoperative assessment when deciding on the level and extent of fusion.

Skeletal age determination by anteroposterior views of the left hand and wrist are made in some cases in order to determine bone maturity. The various radiographic views are illustrated in Figure 6–59.

In following the scoliotic child it is best to evaluate the patient clinically before taking radiographs. Unless the scoliosis is increasing or there is a change in the treatment, one upright radiogram of the spine made every three to six months is adequate.

Measurement of the Degree of the Curve. The angle of the curve is usually measured by the *Cobb method.* The first step is to determine the *end vertebrae*—in a curve these are the ones at each end of the curve nearest to the center and least rotated. The *top vertebra* of the curve is the highest one whose superior surface tilts to the side of the concavity of the curve to be measured. The superior surface of the vertebra above it usually tilts in the opposite direction to the side of the convexity, but it may be horizontal. The intervertebral space on the concave side is usually wider above the top

vertebra and narrower below it, but if there is vertebral wedging, the width of this intervertebral space may vary. The same applies to the inferior surface of the bottom vertebra. Cobb draws intersecting perpendicular lines from the superior surface of the top and the inferior surface of the bottom vertebrae of the curve. The angle formed by these perpendicular lines is the "angle of the curve" (Fig. 6–60).[138] In large curves it is possible to measure the angle formed by the end vertebral lines directly.

The *Ferguson method* of curve measurement is employed when the end-plates of the vertebral bodies are difficult to determine, as in congenital scoliosis with multiple anomalies. Mark a dot in the center of the shadow of the body in each of the three vertebrae—the two end and the apical ones. (The apical vertebra is the one that is most rotated at the crest of the curve.) Lines are drawn from the apex to each end. The angle of the curve is the divergence of these two lines from 180 degrees (Fig. 6–61).[249–251]

Recently the Oxford Cobb meter has simplified curve measurement (Fig. 6–62). The Cobb technique of curve measurement is accurate with an error of 3 degrees or less.

Vertical Wedging and Rotation. Wedging of vertebral bodies, according to Cobb, may be

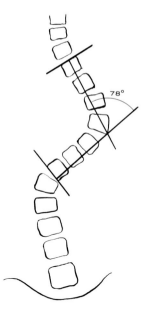

FIGURE 6–60. *Cobb's method of measuring of the angle of the curve in scoliosis (see text for explanation).*

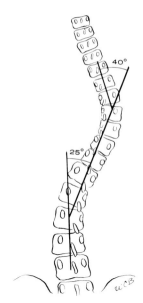

FIGURE 6–61. *Ferguson's method of measuring the angle of the scoliotic curve (see text for explanation).*

graded as follows: one plus (+), up to one sixth decrease in height of vertebral body; two plus (++), one sixth to one third; three plus (+++), one third to one half; and four plus (++++), more than one half (Fig. 6–63 A).[138]

Vertebral rotation can be measured either according to the Cobb or Nash and Moe methods. In the Cobb method the relationship of the spinous process to the center of the vertebral body is noted in the anteroposterior radiograph (Fig. 6–63 B).[138] In the Nash and Moe method the relationship of the pedicle to the center of the vertebral body is observed in the anteroposterior radiograph, and rotation is divided into five grades: zero (0) when both pedicles are symmetrical; Grade I when the convex pedicle has moved away from the side of the vertebral body; Grade III when the convex pedicle is in the center of the vertebral body; Grade II when rotation is between Grades I and III; and Grade IV when the convex pedicle has moved past the midline (Fig. 6–64).[539] Other methods of measuring vertebral rotation, such as that of Pedriolle, have been described.[577] Its evaluation on the plain radiograph is not very accurate and not of great value in decision-making. Therefore it is not commonly done.

Mehta's Rib-Vertebral Angle (RVA). The rib-vertebral angle of Mehta is measured as follows: First, determine the vertebra at the apex of the curve and draw a line perpendicular to the end-plate of the apical vertebra; second, draw lines bisecting the head and neck of the ribs on each side of the apical vertebra (Fig. 6–65). The rib-vertebral angle (RVA) is the angle formed by the intersection between the perpendicular line and the angle bisecting the ribs. In scoliosis the measurement is more acute on the convex side than on the concave side of the curve. The rib-vertebral angle difference (RVAD) is the difference of the angles between the two sides of the apical vertebra.

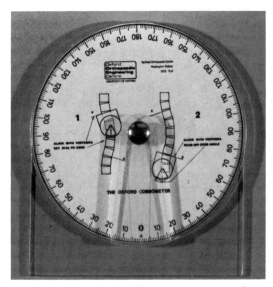

FIGURE 6–62. *Oxford Cobb meter to measure scoliosis.*

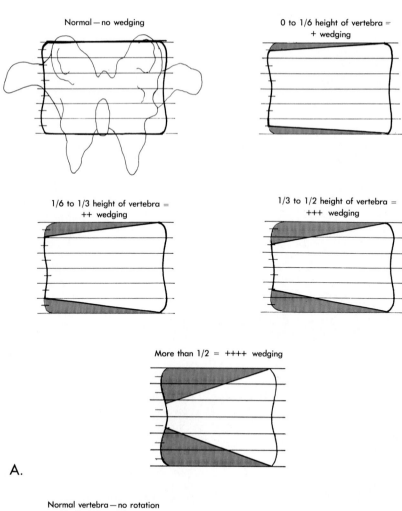

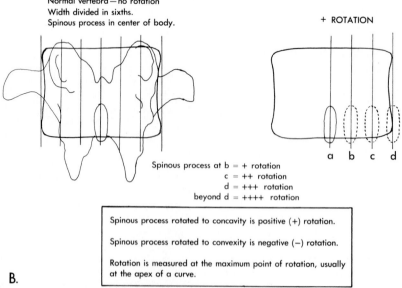

FIGURE 6–63. *Method of determination of degree of wedging* (A) *and rotation* (B) *of vertebrae in scoliosis.*

(Redrawn from Cobb, J. R.: A. A. O. S. Instructional Course Lectures, 5:261, 1948.)

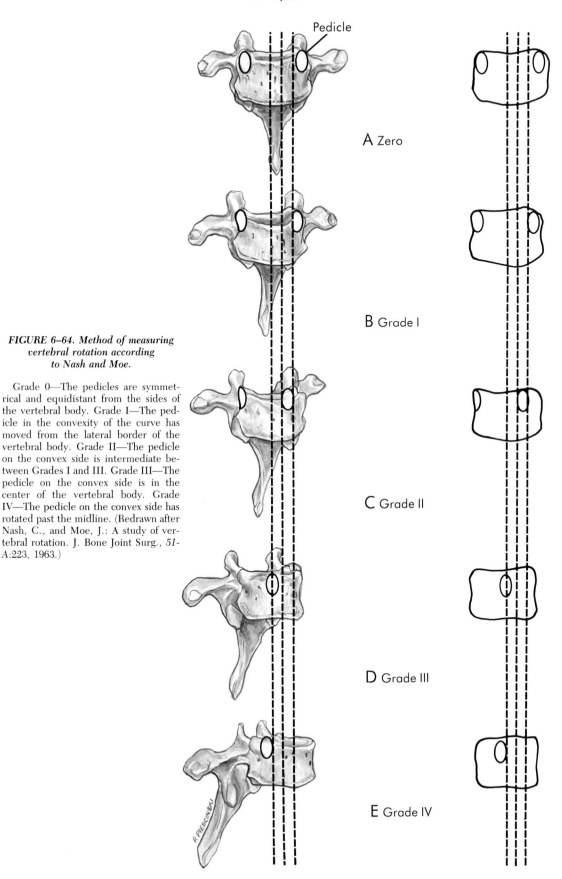

FIGURE 6–64. Method of measuring vertebral rotation according to Nash and Moe.

Grade 0—The pedicles are symmetrical and equidistant from the sides of the vertebral body. Grade I—The pedicle in the convexity of the curve has moved from the lateral border of the vertebral body. Grade II—The pedicle on the convex side is intermediate between Grades I and III. Grade III—The pedicle on the convex side is in the center of the vertebral body. Grade IV—The pedicle on the convex side has rotated past the midline. (Redrawn after Nash, C., and Moe, J.: A study of vertebral rotation. J. Bone Joint Surg., *51-A*:223, 1963.)

A Zero

B Grade I

C Grade II

D Grade III

E Grade IV

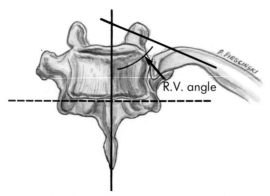

R.V. angle

FIGURE 6–65. Method of measurement of Mehta's rib vertebral angle (RVA).

First, draw a perpendicular line to the end-plate of the apical vertebra. Second, draw lines bisecting the head and neck of the ribs on each side of the apical vertebra. The angle formed by the intersection of these two lines is the RVA.

The value of Mehta's rib-vertebral angle difference is in prediction of whether infantile scoliosis is the resolving or progressive type. According to Mehta if the angle difference is greater than 20 degrees, there is an 80 per cent chance that the scoliosis is progressive.[497]

In addition Mehta describes two phases in the course of infantle scoliosis. In *Phase I* (noted in the early stage) the rib head on the convex side of the curve does not overlap (is separated from) the vertebral body in the posteroanterior radiograph. *In Phase II*, with progression of the curve, the rib head overlaps the vertebral body (Fig. 6–66). According to Mehta the transition from Phase I to Phase II indicates a progressive curve.[497] Further studies by Thompson and Bentley, and by Ceballos and associates have confirmed the prognostic value of Mehta's observations.[130, 732] Also, Tolo and Gillespie observed similar prognostic usefulness of Mehta's rib-vertebral angle difference in juvenile scoliosis.[736]

Measurement of Kyphosis and Lordosis in the Lateral Radiograph. The end vertebrae are the last vertebrae that are maximally tilted into the concavity of the curve. Perpendicular lines are drawn to the inferior and superior end-plates. The angle formed between the two perpendicular lines is the degree of kyphosis or lordosis; kyphotic curves are given a positive (+) value, whereas lordotic ones are given a negative (−) value (Fig. 6–67).

When hemivertebrae are present in congenital scoliosis all the vertebrae, including the hemivertebrae, are numbered from the first cervical vertebra to the sacrum. For example,

a hemivertebra at the thoracolumbar junction is described as a hemivertebra on the right at L-1 and not as a hemivertebra between T-12 and L-1. Associated anomalies of the ribs should also be noted. Soft-tissue shadows are observed.

Skeletal Maturity. Chronological age is not an accurate guideline for skeletal maturation. Risser utilized the ossification of the iliac apophysis as a criterion of maturation of vertebral growth. The ossification of the iliac apophysis begins near the anterior superior iliac spine and extends backward to the posterior iliac spine. The iliac apophysis is divided into four quarters. Risser one is 25 per cent excursion, Risser two is 50 per cent, Risser three is 75 per cent, and Risser four is complete excursion (Fig. 6–68). After complete excursion the ossified iliac apophysis fuses to the body of the ilium—this is graded as Risser five. Growth in height of the vertebral column ceases at Risser five. Risser observed that the completion of excursion of ossification of the iliac apophysis occurred simultaneously with completion of vertebral growth, and with it the scoliosis became static.[621]

The average ages at which the iliac apophyses completed their excursion of ossification across the iliac crests were 14 years in girls and 15½ years in boys. The average period of ossification excursion was one year from the first appearance of capping on the outer anterior border of the iliac crests to final completion, when the apophysis dipped down to come in contact with the ilium near the sacroiliac junction. The shortest period was seven months and the longest, more than two years. Occasionally, fragmentary development of the iliac apophysis occurs. Asymmetrical development of the two sides of the pelvis is seen in a number of cases.

Zaoussis and James, in a statistical study of patients with mature curves, confirmed that the cessation of spinal growth and curve progression coincides with the completion of growth in the iliac apophyses.[811] Their findings are shown in Figure 6–69.

Another parameter to determine skeletal maturity of the vertebral column and potential for further growth is ossification of the *vertebral ring* apophyses, which are situated at the superior and inferior margins of the vertebral body end-plates. They are least visible in the lateral projection, but can be seen in the posteroanterior view of the spine. Initially they appear as an irregular ossification center, then they become a complete ring that eventually fuses with the vertebral end-plate (Fig. 6–70). Like fusion of the iliac apophysis, fusion of the

Phase 1

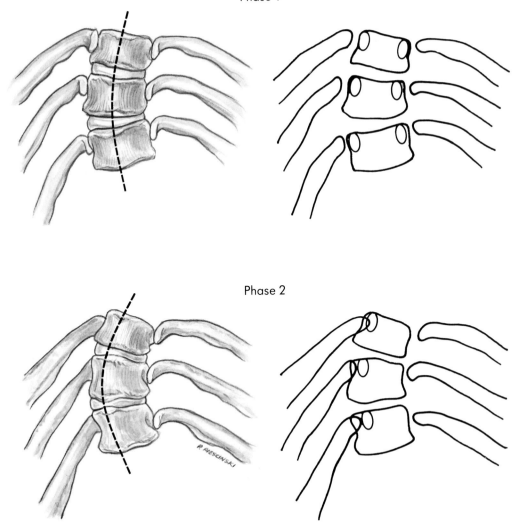

Phase 2

FIGURE 6–66. The two phases in progression of infantile scoliosis as seen in the posteroanterior radiogram.

Phase I—The rib head on the convex side does not overlap the vertebral body. Phase II—The rib head on the convex side overlaps the vertebral body.

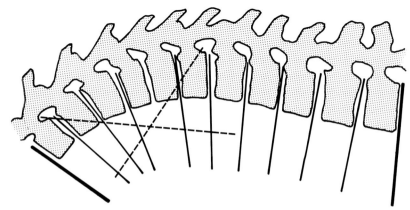

FIGURE 6–67. Measurement of the degree of kyphosis and lordosis.

First, determine the end vertebrae, which are the last ones tilted to the convexity of the curve. Second, draw perpendicular lines to the inferior and superior vertebral end-plates. The angle formed between these two lines is the degree of kyphosis (positive value) or lordosis (negative value).

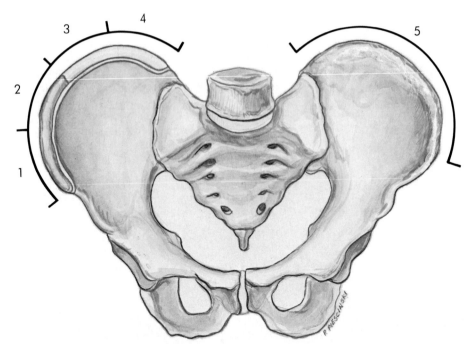

FIGURE 6–68. *Risser sign—ossification of the iliac apophysis as a method to assess maturation of the vertebral column.*

The ossification begins at the anterior superior iliac spine. After completion of its excursion, the ossified iliac apophysis fuses to the body of the ilium. **A.** Risser 1—25 per cent excursion. **B.** Risser 2—50 per cent excursion. **C.** Risser 3—75 per cent excursion. **D.** Risser 4—Complete excursion. **E.** Risser 5—Iliac crest fuses to the ilium.

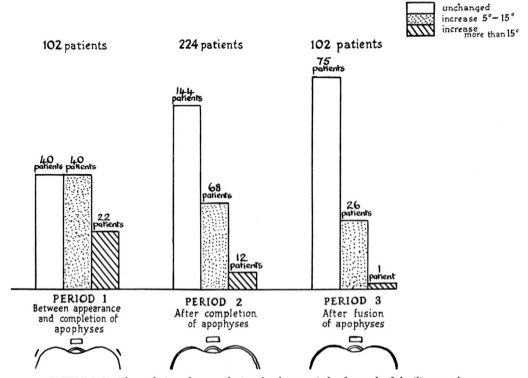

FIGURE 6–69. *The evolution of curves during the three periods of growth of the iliac apophyses.*

(From Zaoussis, A. L., and James, J. I. P.: The iliac apophysis and evolution of curves in scoliosis. J. Bone Joint Surg., 40-B:442, 1985. Reprinted by permission.)

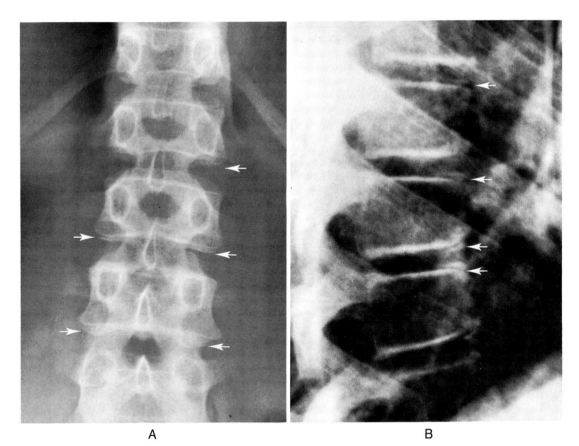

A   B

FIGURE 6–70. Ossification of the ring apophysis as depicted in the anteroposterior and lateral radiograms of the spine.

The arrows point to the ossified vertebral end-plates. Note that the ossification is more clearly visualized on the lateral projection. (From Bradford, D. S., Lonstein, J. E., Ogilvie, J. W., and Winter, R. B. (eds): Moe's Textbook of Scoliosis and Other Spinal Deformities, 2nd Ed. Philadelphia, W. B. Saunders, 1987. Reprinted by permission.)

vertebral ring apophysis indicates the end of growth of the vertebral column.

A third method utilized to determine skeletal age is to make an anteroposterior radiograph of the left hand and wrist and compare it with the standards in the Greulich and Pyle atlas. Ordinarily skeletal maturity is assessed by the ossification of the iliac apophysis and vertebral ring apophysis. Routine radiography of the hand and wrist is not recommended; it is done only in especially complex problems to aid in decision-making.

Special Studies. In complex cases, especially in congenital scoliosis or severe scoliosis with suggestion of spinal cord compression or spinal dysraphism, computed tomography and magnetic resonance imaging may be indicated. They will depict the spinal cord and nerves in detail and rule out spinal cord tumors, diastematomyelia, and osseous lesions. A plain laminagram may be performed when an ordinary radiograph does not show good bony detail. Occasionally, a myelogram is performed to delineate the

cause of neurologic deficit. Invasive procedures should be a last resort.

Curve Pattern

The location of the apical vertebra determines the site of the curve: *cervical*, when the apex is between C-1 and C-6; *cervicothoracic*, apex between C-7 and T-1; *thoracic*, apex between T-2 and T-11; *thoracolumbar*, apex at T-12 and L-1; *lumbar*, apex between L-2 and L-4; *lumbosacral*, apex between L-5 and S-1.

In idiopathic scoliosis, most of the characteristics of the curve or curves are present at the onset of the deformity and rarely change. The curvature may progress considerably, and during the later stages, one or two vertebrae may be added to the original extent of the curve; the apex, direction of rotation, and location of the curve do not change, however. Only in very exceptional cases does a change in pattern occur during the development of scoliosis.

Any angular deviation of the spine in one

direction causes an opposite angular deviation when the erect position is assumed, so that the head is balanced above the pelvis. This secondary deviation is compensatory. Structural changes, such as wedging and rotation, tend to develop in these secondary compensatory curves, which may make them difficult to distinguish from primary curves. In the past these curves were described by the terms *primary* and *secondary*. Such usage of terminology implies that the larger curve is a primary pathologic curve and the smaller secondary curve is compensatory. In order to avoid such inaccuracy of presumption the terms *major* and *minor* should be used as advocated by the Scoliosis Research Society.

The following criteria are helpful in identifying the major curve:

1. A major curve will deform and become fixed simultaneously, and will show no tendency to reverse itself or to retain any correction that has been mechanically obtained. Compensatory curves, on the other hand, only gradually become structural and tend to retain the power of spontaneous reversibility much longer. They are able to hold the reversed position after the primary correction. Therefore, the curve with the least flexibility and corrigibility is the major one; this is determined by the lateral bend and by the pelvic tilt test radiogram.

2. The greater curve, or that toward which the trunk is shifted, is the major curve.

3. In the case of three curves ("triple curve"), the middle one is always the major one; whereas in the case of four curves ("quadruple curve"), the two middle curves are usually major.

Thoracic curve convex to the right is the most common and clinically significant deformity (Fig. 6–71). Often the apex of the curve is at T-8 or T-9, with the upper end vertebra at T-5 or T-6 and the lower end vertebra at T-11 or T-12. *Double major right thoracic-left lumbar* is the second most common curve; in the thoracic component the apex is at T-7, the upper end vertebra is at T-5 or T-6, and the lower end vertebra is at T-10; in the lumbar component, the apex is at L-2 with the upper end vertebra at T-11 and the lower end vertebra at L-4. Next in order of decreasing frequency are single left lumbar, thoracolumbar, double thoracic, and right lumbar curves. Of the lumbar curves 70 per cent are convex to the left with the apex at L-1 or L-2, the upper end vertebra at T-11 or T-12, and the lumbar end vertebra at L-3 or L-4. Of the thoracolumbar curves 80 per cent are convex to the right with the apex at T-11 or T-12, the upper end vertebra at T-6 or T-7, and the lower end vertebra at L-1 or L-2. Left thoracic curves and cervical curves are extremely rare in idiopathic scoliosis—with these it is prudent to rule out congenital scoliosis, intraspinal or vertebral tumors, and other causes of scoliosis.

Moe and Kettleson studied 228 major idiopathic curves in 169 patients. They defined a *major curve* as one that produces a cosmetic deformity, includes major structural changes, and requires correction in order to regain com-

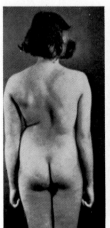 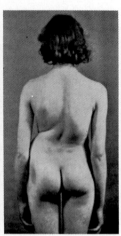 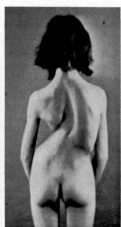 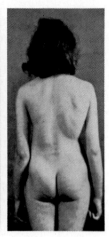

FIGURE 6–71. *Posterior view of four girls, each with 70 degrees of curvature.*

From left to right: lumbar, thoracolumbar, thoracic, and double major curves. It clearly shows that the thoracic curve is the most decompensated and deformed with the low shoulder, the severe razor-back deformity, and the asymmetrical flank creases. Thoracic scoliosis has the worst prognosis for the expected severity of the degree of curvature. Note that the girl with the double major curve is well balanced and least deformed. These photographs well illustrate that the deformity and prognosis in idiopathic scoliosis vary with the curve pattern. (From James, J. I. P.: Scoliosis. Baltimore, Williams & Wilkins Co., 1967, p. 53. Reprinted by permission.)

pensation and a satisfactory appearance. Thus, a patient may have a single major curve, or he may have double or even triple major curve patterns. The major curves were divided by Moe and Kettleson into three distinct groups: *high thoracic*, extending from the seventh cervical to the seventh thoracic vertebra; *thoracic*, extending from the third thoracic to the third lumbar vertebra; and *lumbar*, extending from the tenth thoracic to the fifth lumbar vertebra. Incidence of the major curves in the 169 patients was as follows: 17 per cent, high thoracic; 84 per cent, thoracic; and 33 per cent, lumbar. (The sum of these percentages is over 100 because of the occurrence of double and triple major curve patterns in a single spine.) A single major curve was found in 56.8 per cent of the patients; a double major curve pattern in 41.4 per cent; and a triple major curve pattern in 1.8 per cent. The right thoracic pattern was most common (43.2 per cent), followed in descending order of frequency by the double major right thoracic,–left lumbar curve (26 per cent); double major left high thoracic–right thoracic (14.2 per cent); and left lumbar, 7.1 per cent.[512]

Treatment

Uncertainty as to the future course of scoliosis necessitates its early and efficient treatment. Decisions about treatment must be individualized. It is vital to be cognizant of the natural history and possible course of the scoliosis.

In some cases, the curvature may arrest itself spontaneously and early; in others, the deformity may progress rapidly and become so extreme as to impair the cardiopulmonary function and health of the patient. The prime factors to consider in estimating the probability of curve progression are curve magnitude, curve pattern, skeletal maturity, and the age of the patient. With increased public awareness and screening, a greater number of patients with curves of small magnitude are referred to the orthopedic surgeon for treatment. Overdiagnosis and unnecessary treatment should be avoided. According to Weinstein and Ponseti, in the 10 to 16-year-old group of screened patients, only 0.6 per cent will require treatment, with a female to male ratio of 10:1. In screened children with curves greater than 10 degrees, active treatment is required in less than 10 per cent; and of these 85 to 90 per cent are effectively managed by nonoperative, i.e., orthotic, means.[766] The goals of scoliosis treatment are to correct the deformity and maintain the correction.

NONOPERATIVE TREATMENT

The realistic objectives of nonsurgical treatment of scoliosis are to arrest progression of scoliosis and in some cases to achieve minimal permanent correction. Nonoperative measures cannot provide normal alignment of the spine because of the inherent limitation of the corrective forces exerted by the nonsurgical methods. Nonoperative treatment can control curve progression in only 70 per cent of the cases with proved curve progression in growing (relatively immature) spines.

The nonsurgical modalities in the orthopedic armamentarium that are employed in treating scoliosis are: physical therapy, biofeedback, electrical stimulation, and orthosis—the last is the most effective and the most commonly used.

Physical Therapy. The purposes of exercises are to improve posture, to increase motor strength of the trunk and pelvifemoral muscles, and to maintain spinal flexibility.

Physical therapy per se is *ineffective* in the treatment of scoliosis; *it does not prevent progression* of the curvature. Derotation and lateral bending exercises do not improve rotatory and angular deformity. It is strongly recommended that children with scoliosis participate in normal physical activities. Swimming is the best exercise.

Commonly prescribed are: *general postural exercises* (abdominal, gluteus maximus, pelvic tilt, hyperextension, and bicycling); *asymmetrical exercises* (lateral bending toward the convexity of the greater curve, with derotation of the trunk if the patient has a list to one side); *trunk shift* to balance head and neck above the pelvis; *respiratory exercises* (such as blowing up balloons) to increase chest expansion and maximum breathing capacity in thoracic curves; and *stretching exercises* consisting of longitudinal head and neck traction applied by the parents in the infant and trapeze hanging in the older child.

Parents should be informed that a daily physical therapy regimen is not crucial; it does no harm but does not improve scoliosis deformity and does not prevent curve progression.

Physical therapy, however, is important as an adjunct to orthotic treatment. Exercises that should be performed several times a day in the brace are pelvic tilt, lateral shift, thoracic arching, and thoracic extension. If hamstrings are taut they should be stretched.

Biofeedback. Results of treatment by biofeedback, either by a trigger mechanism in the orthosis or in the form of an alarm mechanism in a harness when the trunk shortens, have been inconclusive.[524] At present, use of biofeed-back for the treatment of scoliosis is not recommended.

Electrical Stimulation. Experimental work in animals has shown that unilateral paraspinal muscle stimulation can cause scoliosis.[89, 569, 570] In computer-modeled human spines stimulation and contraction of muscles on the convex side of the scoliosis decreased the degree of scoliosis by compression. The biomechanical effectiveness of muscle contraction varied with the site of scoliosis—in thoracic curves the effective muscles were the intercostal, latissimus dorsi, and lateral erectors, whereas in lumbar curves the muscles exerting corrective forces were the lateral erectors and internal abdominal obliques. Electrical stimulation has no effect on vertebral rotation.[662]

At present in the United States, surface muscle stimulators are utilized in the treatment of scoliosis; implanted electrode muscle stimulation has been tried in Canada, but in the United States at this time it remains investigational. Surface muscle stimulators are marketed under the names of the EBI ScoliTron, Neuromuscular Stimulator and Medtronic Scoliosis System. The devices stimulate nerve fibers within the muscle and cause muscle contraction. The selection of stimulator parameters is such that they do not cause discomfort and muscle fatigue. Skin irritation is minimized by the use of an asymmetrical biphasic wave. In order to achieve adequate muscle contraction the intensity amplitude should be over 20 mA. and pulse width over 100 μsec.

The surface electrical stimulation is only used at night for a period of eight to ten hours. Appropriate instruction and supervision by a specially trained nurse clinician or physical therapist are crucial. Compliance by the patient appears to be 65 to 75 per cent, which is similar to that with orthoses. The use of minimally skin irritating coupling agents has relieved the problem of sleep disturbance.

Indications for electrical stimulation in treatment of idiopathic scoliosis are a progressive idiopathic curve of between 20 and 30 degrees, and initial presentation of a patient with scoliosis of 30 to 40 degrees. Contraindications are patients who are unable to operate the unit properly and those with mental illness, heart disease (especially arrythmias), curves greater than 40 degrees, and thoracic curves with hypokyphosis. The primary recommendation of the author in the nonoperative treatment of scoliosis is orthosis, not electrical stimulation, because reports of the latter's efficacy in control of progressive idiopathic scoliosis are conflicting. There is unanimity of opinion that electrical

stimulation should be tried only when curve correction during stimulation is demonstrated by supine anteroposterior radiographs of the spine with and without it. At best its results are similar to those of orthotic treatment, and several authors report that electrical stimulation has no or minimal effect on control of progressive scoliosis.[46, 99, 481] It appears that thoracolumbar and lumbar curves are better controlled than thoracic curves; orthoses utilized in treating these curves are, however, very well accepted by the adolescent patient. Psychologic studies by Kahanovitz and associates have shown that patients treated by electrical stimulation have higher self-esteem and are less hostile, less anxious and depressed, and more physically active than those treated by day-night orthosis.[403] It should be pointed out, however, that these observations may be inaccurate because in this study the patients did not undergo pre- and post-treatment psychologic testing, and criteria for patient evaluation and treatment of the two groups were not specified.[37] In this author's opinion, electrical stimulation for treatment of idiopathic scoliosis should be considered only for patients who do not emotionally accept and tolerate wearing an orthosis, and these adolescents should have psychologic assessment prior to beginning treatment.

ORTHOTIC TREATMENT

Historically Ambrose Paré is credited with being the first to use metal braces in the form of armor to treat scoliosis.[573, 574] Since then various types of braces and casts have been advocated, such as the suspensory plaster cast of Sayre and the hinge or turnbuckle cast of Hibbs and Risser.[359, 619, 654, 655] All these casts and the orthoses prior to the Milwaukee brace exerted passive corrective forces on the spine. In 1946 the Milwaukee brace was developed; in addition to passive forces it exerted dynamic active corrective forces.[83] In the 1960s thermoplastics were introduced in the manufacture of braces.

During the past three decades three types of orthosis that have proved effective in the treatment of scoliosis have evolved: (1) the cervicothoracolumbosacral orthosis (CTLSO), or the Milwaukee brace; (2) the thoracolumbosacral orthosis (TLSO), examples of which are the Boston brace, Wilmington brace (or DuPont jacket), Lyon brace, Miami brace, and Pasadena brace; and (3) various types of custom-fabricated braces and TLSOs. These braces have usually been named after the city of origin.

Biomechanics. The corrective forces exerted

by an orthosis that improve spinal deformity are longitudinal, transverse, and possibly active by muscle contraction (compression). It is questionable whether a spinal orthosis can relieve asymmetrical loading of the vertebral cartilaginous end-plates and decrease asymmetrical growth according to the Heuter-Volkmann law. It is a conjectural hope, but long-term results of orthotic treatment of scoliosis have shown that such biologic correction does not occur. Also, it is dubious whether any active correction of scoliotic deformity by muscle contraction takes place by orthotic treatment.

For orthotic treatment to be effective, the orthopedic surgeon must assess the anatomy and pathogenesis of spinal deformity; understand the geometry of the orthosis and the possible corrective forces that it can exert on the deformed spine, and the normal and abnormal growth mechanims of the vertebral column; and be knowledgeable as to the natural history of scoliosis. It is vital to select the patients carefully.

Indications. Orthotic treatment of scoliosis is primarily indicated when there is a *progressive* curve between 20 and 30 degrees in a *skeletally immature growing child.*[509] Progression should be documented. In the determination for necessity for bracing, the potential for future growth of the spine is the important consideration. It is important to assess skeletal age, Risser's sign, and status of appearance of ossification and fusion of the vertebral ring apophysis; other factors in potential of further growth are alteration in stature (increase in height), occurrence of menarche, breast development, and distribution of pubic hair. It is desirable that the Risser sign be two plus or less and the onset of menarche be no more than six months. In order to justify bracing there should be at least six to twelve months of skeletal growth remaining.[83]

The *magnitude of the curve* is the second consideration. Curves less than 15 degrees at presentation should be observed; they are braced when there is a documented progression of a minimum of 10 degrees. In curves between 25 and 40 degrees no documentation of progression is necessary—these curves are braced immediately. It is vital to individualize treatment of each patient.

Flexibility and compensation of the curves should be considered. This author recommends a more aggressive approach of orthotic treatment in the relatively inflexible and decompensated curves. Curves of less than 50 per cent flexibility are less likely to respond to orthotic treatment.

Another factor to assess is the *shape and size of the rib deformity*: the shape of the rib deformity should be round and not sharply angulated for orthotic treatment to be effective. Ribs that are angular and more vertical in position decrease the horizontal forces transmitted via the ribs to the spine, thereby lessening the potential of correction of scoliotic deformity. Computed tomography studies have shown that the forces exerted by the orthosis may increase the rib deformity in some severe cases. The height of the rib deformity should be less than 3 cm.; if the rib hump is greater than 3 cm., the brace is ineffective in correcting the large cosmetically unacceptable rib hump.

Should one brace a juvenile patient whose curve has shown rapid progression from 10 to 17 degrees? This decision as to treatment should be based on actual progression of the curve and not on risk factors based on natural history; the latter are only average estimates. Each child's natural history is unique. The actual course of an individual curve cannot be predicted accurately. It is important to have a frank discussion with the parents and explain the specificity of each curve in an individual patient; a 7-degree progressive curve in a nine-year-old girl may increase or stabilize. In such a case, this author will give the option to the parents for part-time orthotic treatment. *Progressive curves in the growing child* are the primary indication for orthotic treatment.

Contraindications. In idiopathic scoliosis orthotic treatment is contraindicated *first* when the curve is greater than 45 degrees. Flexible curves (i.e., greater than 50 per cent correction on lateral bending) of 40 to 45 degrees that are compensated in an adolescent can be treated by orthosis when only a year of future growth is remaining. Also, young children with a curve greater than 40 degrees can be treated in a brace in order to allow future vertebral growth before spinal fusion; however, in these children, the curve should be flexible and adequate initial correction should be obtained in the brace; the orthosis should control curve progression.

The *second* contraindication is patients who find the wearing of an orthosis emotionally intolerable. Appropriate psychologic counselling may be tried in these adolescents. It is surprising how often they change their negative attitude. The *third* contraindication is thoracic hypokyphosis. The *fourth* is the skeletally mature patient. The *fifth*, a relative contraindication, is the high thoracic and cervicodorsal curve because this ordinarily does not respond to orthotic treatment. When initial correction cannot be achieved, orthotic treatment should be abandoned.

The Milwaukee Brace

The Milwaukee brace was originated by Blount, Schmidt, and Bidwell, who presented a prototype of the orthosis in 1946 at the meeting of the American Academy of Orthopedic Surgeons in Chicago.[86] Since then, numerous changes have been made in the design of the brace.

The orthosis has three components (Fig. 6–72). (1) It has a *pelvic girdle* made of a thermoplastic material, which is waterproof and can be perforated for ventilation and remodeled to relieve areas of skin pressure. The plastic pelvic girdle provides total contact and is much better

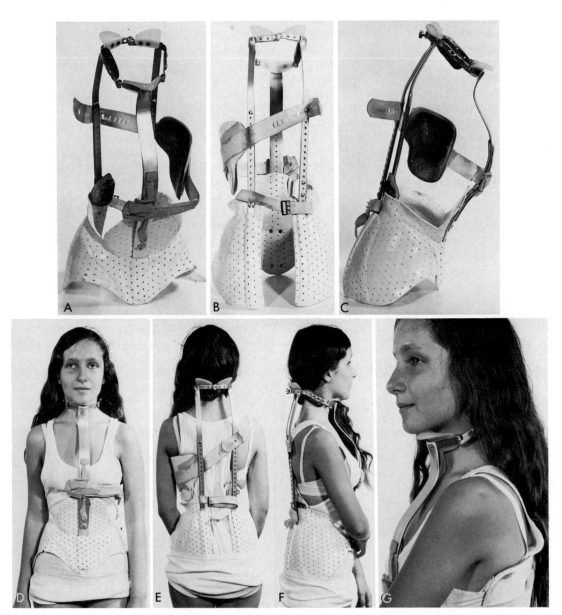

FIGURE 6–72. *The Milwaukee brace—the modern design.*

A to **C.** Anterior, posterior, and lateral views of the orthosis (see text for explanation). **D** to **G.** An adolescent girl wearing the Milwaukee brace. Note the following: (1) the *pelvic girdle* made of a thermoplastic material called Orthoplast. It is self-hinging, perforated for ventilation, light, and waterproof. It can be remolded by using a heat gun to relieve areas of skin pressure and accommodate the increasing size of the pelvis. Deterioration of the Orthoplast pelvic girdle is prevented by daily washing with soap and water. (2) The "throat mold" is snugly approximated and there is complete lack of pressure against the mandible. (3) The occipital pad fits the lower occiput accurately, following its contour. (4) The uprights fit closely to the torso, allowing room for deep breathing, lateral shift, pelvic tilt, and abdominal exercises.

tolerated than the older leather reinforced pelvic girdle. (2) It also has a *suprastructure* consisting of one anterior and two widely separated posterior uprights and a cervical ring with a throat mold and occipital piece, and (3) *lateral pads* that apply pressure on the apical vertebrae. Additional parts that are sometimes used include a chin stop to prevent turning of the head, an axillary sling to provide balancing forces against a double major thoracic curve pattern, and a padded plastic shoulder-clavicular mold, which exerts a comfortable downward and posterior pull against a high thoracic curve that deforms the neckline. It is recommended that the reader carefully study Blount and Moe's thorough monograph on the Milwaukee brace.[83]

The Milwaukee brace is designed to exert passive and active corrective forces on the spine in both longitudinal and tranverse planes. The orthosis was initially designed to apply passive longitudinal forces between the pelvic girdle and the mandibular-occipital pads; however, it soon became obvious that the exertion of passive longitudinal force on the mandible resulted in deformity of the mandible. The mandibular mold was therefore replaced by the throat mold and the occipital pads were lowered. This alteration of the design of the Milwaukee orthosis did not change the results of treatment because the transverse corrective forces are much more effective than the longitudinal forces in correcting scoliosis when the magnitude of the scoliosis is less than 50 degrees.[77] Also, in recumbency the cervical ring acts as a fulcrum for the head to distract the vertebral column; this mechanism is negated when the patient is upright and also by removal of the occipital piece.[26]

The pelvic girdle is designed to exert passive transverse corrective force by decreasing lumbar lordosis and by compressing the abdominal contents, which support the spine and diminish the load on the vertebral column. Gluteal extensions of the pelvic girdle tilt the pelvis and further reduce lumbar lordosis. Diminution of lumbar lordosis corrects lumbar scoliosis. Also, passive diminution of lumbar lordosis not only decreases lumbar scoliosis but also thoracic scoliosis.[743, 745, 771] The pads in the lumbar and thoracic areas at the apex of the curves also exert passive transverse corrective forces; however, three-point fixation is required for effective application of transverse forces: (1) the distal fixation is the pelvic girdle, (2) the proximal fixation is the cervical ring, and (3) the pads are at the center at the apex of the curve. The thoracic pad is placed over the ribs that articulate with the apex of the curve; it should

be remembered, however, that medially directed forces can deform the thoracic cage and the anteriorly directed forces can cause hypokyphosis. The use of the Milwaukee brace is therefore contraindicated when there is associated hypokyphosis or lordosis with the thoracic scoliosis and also in osteogenesis imperfecta—when the ribs are soft and malleable. Trunk decompensation can be corrected by greater trochanteric extension on the pelvic girdle. Active exercises in the brace in the form of pelvic tilt (which further decreases lumbar lordosis) and thoracic arching and lateral trunk shift (which push the deformed trunk further toward the pads) augment the passive transverse corrective forces. The patient is instructed to perform thoracic extension and elongation exercises within the confines of the brace's suprastructure.

Whether the Milwaukee brace exerts any active corrective force on the spine is conjectural; it has not been conclusively demonstrated. The righting reflex is the primary mechanism of application of active forces on the spine. In order to exert active muscle forces on the spine, the patient is instructed to perform pelvic tilt, lateral shift, thoracic arching, and thoracic extension in the Milwaukee brace. Normal neuromuscular function is a requisite for the use of the Milwaukee brace. In patients with neuromuscular disease and paralysis, the principle of active muscle contraction is not feasible; in these cases the orthotic devices therefore employ passive support but not corrective forces.

Orthopedic Evaluation of the Milwaukee Brace. This checklist, as outlined by Blount and Moe, is as follows:

Pelvic Girdle. This is the most important component in the successful fitting of the Milwaukee brace. It should be sufficiently long in the back, extending to about 1 inch above the seat of a hard chair when the patient is sitting; and in the front, the lower end of the pelvic girdle should extend to the pubis and should allow no lower abdominal protrusion. If the pelvic girdle is properly made, it is much lower posteriorly than anteriorly—the brace will not balance in an upright position on a flat surface. The pelvic girdle should be comfortably long in the groin and should be tight to a comfortable degree. The waistline should be at the proper level, not riding high on the ribs or low against the lateral margin of the iliac crests. The tightness of the pelvic girdle and the length of the uprights control the degree of constriction at the waist.

The tilt of the pelvic girdle and the posture of the lumbosacral spine are checked. A correctly fitted brace will hold the pelvis in a tilted position and flatten the lumbar spine. A common error is completion of the brace with a built-in lordosis. During preparation of the negative plaster model, the patient should tilt his pelvis and improve his posture. The lumbosacral lordosis can also be reduced by skiving the plaster mold in the abdominal and gluteal regions and extending the pelvic girdle posteriorly by gluteal extensions. During fitting of the brace, one can increase the tilt of the pelvic girdle and reduce the swayback by bending the vertical bars and adjusting their length.

Cervical Ring, Occipital Rest, and Throat Mold. In the past, the occipital pads were fitted snugly against the base of the occiput; at present, however, the occipital pads are lowered so that they are 2 cm. inferior to the base of the occiput, following the contour of the skull when the head is held in normal erect position. As stated before, this lowering of the occipital pads and reduction of the longitudinal force have not adversely affected the results of treatment. The occipital pad should not ride high on the back of the skull, as it will push the head forward, distraction force on the occiput will be lost, and excessive pressure will be exerted on the throat. The "throat mold" should be at a lower level than the occipital rest, the average angle being 30 degrees. In a properly fitted brace, the chin can be easily raised 3 cm. from the throat mold. When this is being checked, the pelvic girdle should be tight and accurately placed. One pitfall is to lengthen the anterior vertical bar without simultaneously lengthening the posterior bars. The head should be held in neutral comfortable position. The length of the cervical ring should be correct; if it is too short, it will choke, and if too long, pressure will be exerted on the mandible. Having the neck ring hinged anteriorly facilitates easy removal and reapplication of the brace. In infants, the neck ring is circularly padded and a throat mold is not used.

Placement of Lateral Pads. Thoracic and lumbar lateral pads help to stretch the spine and also press on the rotated areas, playing an important role in the effective use of the brace. The lateral pads are placed at sites where they will exert maximal corrective force on the apex of the deformity.[83] This is checked on the radiograms made with the brace on. Pads are selected according to curve pattern. With longitudinal growth and correction of the curve, it is necessary to change the sites of the pads. For a detailed discussion of this the reader is advised to consult the monograph by Blount and Moe.[83]

The Fit of the Uprights. The vertical uprights should fit the torso closely, leaving adequate room for deep breathing, lateral shift, pelvic tilt, and abdominal exercises. There should be no restriction of deep inspiration and no pressure by the upright against the chest wall. The exact position of the bars depends on the contours of the body. Leg length inequality, if present, should be corrected by appropriate lifts to correct listing of the upright.

In the Milwaukee brace, the patient should be comfortable and able to sit, stand, and walk with ease. There should be no problems with hygiene.

Orthopedic Follow-up of the Milwaukee Brace Patient. After checking the fit of the brace, a standing anteroposterior radiogram of the entire spine with the brace on is made. This permits visualization of the accurate placement of the pads and the degree of correction of the scoliosis obtained by the brace.

The long-term results of treatment of scoliosis by the Milwaukee CTLSO are directly proportional to the initial correction of the curve by the orthosis. If the Milwaukee brace does not improve the degree of curvature initially the result of orthotic treatment will be poor. Lack of correction may be due to inadequate fit of the orthosis; if this is the case, it should be fitted properly. Another cause of failure of correction is that the curve is so rigid that it does not respond to the forces applied by the orthosis. If the Milwaukee brace is properly fitted and does not correct greater than 35 per cent for a thoracic curve and 45 per cent for a lumbar curve, its use should be discontinued or the brace should be worn only eight hours a day, because a satisfactory long-term result cannot be obtained.

It should be emphasized that a tight pelvic girdle is more comfortable than a loose one, as the former presses into the soft tissues at the waist and causes fewer skin pressure problems than the latter, which rests on the sharp bony edges of the pelvis. The pelvic girdle is tightened as much as is comfortable for the patient and the strap is marked. Initially, the pelvic girdle may be loosened for short periods, but it should be retightened to maximal tolerance.

The patient is instructed gradually to increase periods of wearing the brace. Initially, it is worn for two to three hours and then is removed and the skin checked for pressure areas. Red pressure areas of the skin are treated by application of wet tea bags or alcohol sponges to toughen the skin. It is important that pressure sores do not develop. Contour fitting of the patient for the brace has been simplified by the use of thermoplastics. Brace adjustments are made as necessary. Gradually the period of brace wear is increased to four, then six, and then eight hours. The period of the day the brace is worn is individualized depending on the magnitude of the curve and the skeletal immaturity of the patient. In general the prepubescent patient with a progressive curve wears the brace 20 to 22 hours a day, whereas an older patient who is still skeletally immature wears the brace 10 to 12 hours a day. Adolescents are disturbed emotionally when they have to wear the brace to school. Green has shown that part-time bracing is effective in control of curve progression.[302] Kahanovitz and associates have also had success with part-time orthotic treatment provided the curves are less than 35 degrees and the rib-vertebral angle difference is less than 20 degrees.[402] This author recommends that adolescents, particularly the girls and boys with self-image consciousness, not wear the brace to school if the degree of curvature is less than 30 degrees; however, when a 25-degree curve progresses rapidly with part-time wearing of the brace, the brace should be worn for 20 to 22 hours a day. Another alternative is to use a removable suprastructure. Adolescents often object to wearing the uprights with the throat mold–cervical ring and occipital pads because it is cumbersome and esthetically unattractive. This author recommends that the removable suprastructure be worn during the evening and night, but not during school or social activities. This has diminished the emotional stress of wearing the Milwaukee orthosis. The use of polypropylene and other thermoplastics for the pelvic girdle has made the brace more form fitting, less cumbersome and visible, and easier to wear.

Exercises. Physical activities of the patient should remain as near normal as possible. The only games that are forbidden are body contact sports because of the danger to other players. There is no need for the patient to be excused from physical education classes at school. Participation in sports such as tennis, volleyball, or bicycling should be allowed. Swimming is an excellent sport for the scoliotic patient and should be encouraged, the patient being permitted to remove the brace and swim for an hour each day. When not in the water, the child must be recumbent and must not sit around the pool without wearing the brace.

The child should be taught general good posture by a physical therapist during the first week and at regular intervals of two to three months thereafter. Exercises are necessary to maintain muscle tone and proper body mechanics. Out of the brace the patient performs abdominal, dorsal hyperextension, gluteus maximus, lateral bend, and pelvic tilt exercises, the last-named exercise being the most important. The pelvic tilt exercises are done first with knees bent, later with knees straight and standing with the back against the wall, and last in stance and in gait. Contractural deformities such as taut hamstrings and hip flexion, if present, should be stretched by passive exercises.

Active corrective exercises for the scoliotic deformities are performed in the brace and consist of the following: *active distraction*—the patient pushes down on the anterior bar and then stretches up out of the brace as far as possible; *deep breathing*—the child inhales deeply and then exhales and arches the back like a cat against the major pad; *pelvic tilt and thoracic retraction*—while holding the position of pelvic tilt, the patient pulls away from the lateral pads and corrects the thoracic curve.

Recently the role of prescribed physical therapy in the Milwaukee brace treatment of scoliosis has been questioned.[127] Unless exercise is contraindicated by negative emotional response and triggering of parent and patient hostility because of demanding, strict parents, this author recommends a physical therapy program. Most adolescents cope with such a therapy regimen. It is important that the patient have supportive and understanding parents, a positive self-image, and a healthy outlook.

On subsequent office visits the standing and sitting heights are measured out of the brace. Has there been an increase in stature? Maturation of the patient should be determined—has the menarche commenced? The spine should be carefully examined. Is the scoliosis compensating? Where does the plumb line fall when dropped from the vertebra prominens or the midocciput? Is there any overcorrection? Are the shoulders level? Is the scapula prominent? Is there paravertebral muscle spasm? Are there any complications due to brace wear such as reddened pressure areas or pressure sores?

The brace is checked in an orderly fashion as to tautness of the pelvic girdle, throat mold–occiput fit, length of the brace, and location and proper fit of the pads.

As correction of scoliosis occurs, the child grows and the vertebral column lengthens, making the brace relatively shorter. The patient should be able to lift the chin at least one, but not more than three, fingerbreadths without pulling down on the ring. The orthosis is elongated both anteriorly and posteriorly and only one hole at a time. The neck ring may have to be adjusted. Review the prescribed exercises in and out of the brace! Are they being performed correctly? It is best for the patient to have an appointment with the physical therapist.

Progress in straightening of the scoliotic curve is checked by a standing radiograph of the spine out of the brace; the x-ray projection should include the iliac crests and extend as high as possible. Always examine the patient before ordering x-ray studies. Superfluous radiographs should be avoided. Frequency of radiographic examination varies depending on the magnitude of the curve and skeletal growth of the patient; ordinarily they are made at intervals of three months. It is vital to individualize each patient's care and to be constantly conscious of the hazards of radiation.

Weaning. In nonoperative treatment of scoliosis, the Milwaukee brace is worn until maximal correction is obtained. After the corrected spine is stable, gradual weaning from the brace may be started. Prior to weaning the following criteria of skeletal maturity should be met: (1) a Risser sign of at least four and beginning of fusion of the vertebral ring apophysis with the vertebral end-plates; and (2) no increase in stature of the trunk for at least four months. In other words, there should be no potential for further significant vertebral body growth. In the past, Blount recommended the Milwaukee brace to be worn until age 18 to 21 years, with the hope of achieving maintenance of correction.[76-78] At present, such a prolonged period of brace wear is not recommended because of the emotional scars and psychosocial disturbances provided by such long-term wear. As a rule the brace is worn for at least one year on a "maximum-time" basis prior to weaning. Too sudden weaning can cause substantial loss of correction.

The periods that the patient is permitted out of the brace depend on the patient's ability to maintain correction, as demonstrated by radiograms made after the patient has been out of the brace for a specific period. First, a standing radiogram of the spine is made after the patient has been out of the brace for four hours. If there is no loss of correction the patient is allowed gradually to remove the brace for four hours daily. These periods out of the brace are increased gradually to six, then eight hours daily. When the child is able to be out of the

brace for eight hours without loss of correction, or only 5 degrees as shown by standing radiographs of the spine, he is allowed to go to school without it. The brace is worn only during the night for the last three to six months.

Long-Term Results. Review of the literature discloses the following. (1) *Compliance rate* with the Milwaukee brace is only 75 per cent; (2) in the compliant skeletally immature patient the *control of curve progression* is only 80 per cent; (3) *permanent correction* five years after brace wear is discontinued is only 8 per cent in the coronal plane. In order to prevent disappointment to the patient and parents it is best to forewarn them of the fact that permanent correction of scoliosis by Milwaukee brace treatment is none or at best minimal. The primary goal of Milwaukee brace treatment is to prevent curve progression.

Thoracolumbosacral Orthoses (TLSO)

The Boston Brace. This is the most commonly used TLSO (Fig. 6–73). These prefabricated shells are vacuum-formed on a positive mold of a normal torso. The sites of corrective forces are prebuilt. A "blueprint" is made from the standing anteroposterior radiograph of the spine from which pad placement is determined. The Boston brace provides very effective derotation forces. Aaro and associates reported an average correction of vertebral rotation of 38 per cent with the Boston brace as compared with 28 per cent with the Milwaukee brace. The effectiveness of the derotation forces of the Boston brace has also been shown by computed tomography.[5]

Two types of Boston brace are used with or without Milwaukee suprastructure. For lumbar and thoracolumbar curves and thoracic curves with an *apex at T-8 or even T-7*, this author recommends *Boston brace without suprastructure*; in some of the thoracic curves an axillary support may have to be added. When the apex of a thoracic curve is *above T-7*, the use of *Boston brace with Milwaukee suprastructure* is recommended. A comparison of in-brace correction of thoracic curves (apex below T-7) with the Boston brace and with the Milwaukee brace is similar.[743]

The study of Uden and associates showed the Boston TLSO to be more effective than the Milwaukee CTLSO in holding thoracic curves with the apex below T-7. One third to one half of the correction achieved by the Boston TLSO appears to be due to the lumbar flexion that it produces.[743] Passive correction of lumbar lordosis decreases scoliosis both in the lumbar and thoracic spine. Other studies in the literature report the results of use of the Boston TLSO

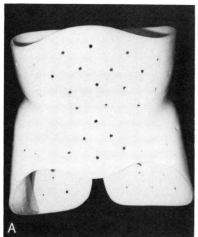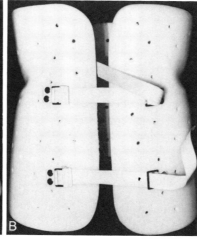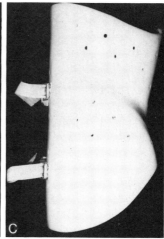

FIGURE 6–73. The Boston TLSO.

A. Anteroposterior view. **B.** Posteroanterior view. **C.** Lateral view.

for curves with an apex as high as T-7 to be similar to those of the Milwaukee CTLSO.[68, 324, 745] A double major thoracic-lumbar curve with the apex of the thoracic curve at T-7 or above requires the Milwaukee suprastructure with the Boston brace. Double thoracic and cervicothoracic curves are treated with the Milwaukee CTLSO; however, it is dubious whether a CTLSO can be effective in controlling these high curves. The short curves and interference from the scapula make it difficult to apply corrective forces on the apical vertebrae.

A definite advantage of the Milwaukee CTLSO with the anterior and posterior uprights is that it does not restrict chest expansion and pulmonary function; it permits the patient to pull away from the pads and straps, elongating the vertebral column. In contrast, the form-fitting Boston brace and other TLSOs interfere with chest expansion and pulmonary function. Posterior thoracic pads of the Milwaukee CTLSO can cause flattening of the rib cage and hypokyphosis; it is therefore important to make lateral radiographs of the spine at intervals—if thoracic hypokyphosis of 10 degrees or less begins to develop, the use of the Milwaukee CTLSO should be discontinued or the thoracic pads removed. It is appropriate to recall that James did not use thoracic pads.[391]

The Wilmington TLSO (or DuPont Jacket). This orthosis is manufactured of the thermoplastic Orthoplast, which has a working temperature of 140° F. or 60° C., permitting direct molding on the patient. The jacket opens anteriorly (Fig. 6–74). The patient is placed on the scoliosis traction casting (Risser) table and

the curvature is straightened by application of longitudinal traction and lateral corrective forces. The orthosis is custom made; the elimination of the necessity of a positive mold makes its fabrication simple and rapid.

The drawbacks of the Wilmington TLSO are compression of the thoracic cage, restriction of chest expansion, and interference with pulmonary function. Also, Orthoplast is not as durable as polypropylene and other thermoplastics. Bunell and associates reported the results in 48 patients treated with the Wilmington TLSO to

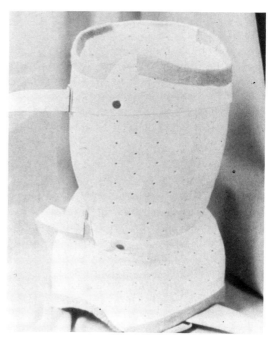

FIGURE 6–74. The Wilmington TLSO.

be similar to that of Milwaukee or Boston TLSO when the apex of the curve was below T-7.[109]

In the literature there are several reports of other TLSOs used for treatment of scoliosis, such as the Miami and Ponte.[482, 595]

Problems and Complications of Orthotic Treatment

Pressure sores. Skin irritation is a frequent problem; the undershirt should be wrinkle-free. Pressure sores should not occur under a properly made and fitted brace. If they are encountered, the brace is adjusted to relieve the pressure and daily skin care is given.

Orofacial deformities. Growing bone reacts to external pressure. The old Milwaukee brace with the chin piece exerted upward force on the mandible. It affected the dentition by extruding the incisors and depressing the molars. The effect was more pronounced in the lower molars. A shortening of the vertical dimension of the lower anterior face was found in all patients. Vertical growth seemed to be affected in the lower border of the body of the mandible.[16]

Since 1969, the chin piece has been eliminated and a throat mold has been substituted. This has eliminated the problem of dental and facial deformation by the Milwaukee brace. This author strongly recommends an examination of the teeth in order to rule out pre-existing malocclusion prior to initiation of treatment with the Milwaukee brace. If present, it should be recorded and an orthodontic consultation recommended. It is best to prevent future accusation by a dissatisfied patient and parents.

Nerve compression may cause neuralgia paresthetica. The brace is adjusted to relieve pressure on the nerve.

Fat thighs and stretch marks may develop. These resolve after discontinuing use of the brace.

Esophageal reflux may occur occasionally because of compression of the abdominal viscera and increased intragastric pressure. This may result in esophagitis. Occasionally the superior mesenteric artery may constrict the duodenum and cause acute gastric dilation.[310]

Sodium retention may occur because of decrease in glomerular filtration rate and effective renal blood flow following application of the TLSO.[1] This disturbance in renal function is reversible on removal of the brace; in some patients sodium retention has persisted for four to twelve months after brace removal.[59] However, this change in renal function is not permanent.

Thoracic cage compression, particularly by the form-fitting TLSO, restricts chest expansion and decreases vital capacity and pulmonary function. These changes in pulmonary function are not permanent. Long-term wear of form-fitting TLSOs can cause the thoracic cage to become tubular in shape. The pelvic girdle does not cause retardation of growth of the ilium and pelvic bones.

Compensatory curves may increase in magnitude. It is important to measure all of the curves and monitor changes in the compensatory curves.

Psychologic disturbances. Some patients react negatively to wearing the orthosis. (Emotional intolerance of these patients is a contraindication to orthotic treatment.) Some of these adolescents build a negative body image and even develop neuroses. Anorexia nervosa may develop in the emotionally disturbed patient after prolonged wear of the Milwaukee brace.[244, 299, 527, 657, 776]

Noncompliance. This obviously affects the final outcome of orthotic treatment. The percentage of spinal fusion in noncompliant patients is about five times higher than in compliant patients.[228, 229] The compliance rate is about 80 per cent. The patient acceptance of the Boston TLSO is better than the Milwaukee CTLSO; however, the compliance rate is the same for the two orthoses.

Curve progression. This problem occurs in about 20 per cent of the skeletally immature patients. Factors in failure of control of curve progression are inability of the orthosis to correct the curve initially, improper fit of the orthosis, noncompliance, curves greater than 40 degrees with severe structural changes, short rigid curves especially in the high thoracic and cervicodorsal region, and curves with thoracic hypokyphosis.

When scoliosis cannot be controlled by orthosis, orthotic treatment should be discontinued; the osteoporosis consequent to prolonged immobilization in a brace makes surgical fusion difficult to perform, less correction is achieved at surgery, and there is greater loss of correction postoperatively.

OPERATIVE TREATMENT

The indications for surgical management are (1) a cosmetically objectionable deformity with decompensation of the spine and asymmetry of the trunk in an adolescent or postadolescent patient, regardless of whether growth of the spine has ceased (Fig. 6–75); (2) a proved progressive curve in a young and growing child in whom conservative measures have failed; and

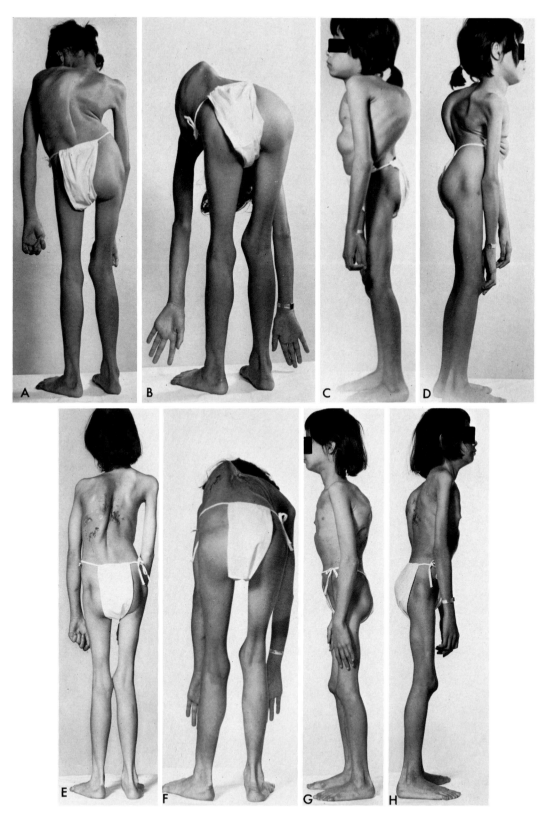

***FIGURE 6–75.** Severe structural scoliosis.*

A to **D.** Preoperative views. The spine is decompensated and the deformity is very severe. **E** to **H.** Postoperative views showing improvement of deformity.

(3) persistent backache that cannot be controlled by conservative means (seen especially in the adult patient with lumbar scoliosis or thoraco-lumbar scoliosis).

The primary purpose of operative treatment is to correct the scoliosis as much as possible and restore compensation of the spine with a symmetrical trunk and with head, neck, and shoulders centered over the pelvis; and to sta-bilize the spine and prevent curve progression.

Factors in decision-making in selection of a patient for surgical intervention are risk for progression, the degree of decompensation of the spine and trunk asymmetry, and whether the appearance is cosmetically objectionable or acceptable.

Surgery is ordinarily not indicated in curves less than 40 degrees, whereas curves greater than 50 degrees require operative treatment because they most likely will progress in adult life. Treatment of curves between 40 and 50 degrees should be individualized. In the skel-etally mature adolescent a 40-degree right tho-racic and 40-degree left thoracolumbar curve may be observed if the spine is compensated, the trunk is symmetrical, and the appearance of the patient is cosmetically acceptable; surgery is indicated in a 40-degree curve in a skeletally immature 11-year-old girl in whom the curve has not responded to orthotic treatment and has progressed from 30 to 40 degrees. Do not decide to operate based solely on the degree of the curvature! Consider the anteroposterior di-ameter of the chest and whether there is tho-racic lordosis. What are the risks for future cardiorespiratory compromise? A 35-degree thoracic curve with progressive thoracic lordosis should be corrected and stabilized by spinal fusion.

Preoperative Forcible Correction of Curves

In the past scoliotic curves were forcibly corrected prior to fusion by casts such as the turnbuckle cast, the Risser localizer cast, and the transection shift jacket of Von Lackum, or by distraction such as Cotrel traction.[155, 619, 757]

At present preoperative correction by casting and traction is not utilized because intraopera-tive correction of the curves by internal instru-mentation achieves equally good if not better correction and obviates complications of pres-sure sores and the inconvenience of wearing a cast. It also is evident that preoperative traction does not provide better correction than intra-operative internal instrumentation such as Har-rington instrumentation alone.[532]

In severe scoliosis preoperative distraction in the form of halo-gravity traction is occasionally employed in order to improve pulmonary func-tion.

Spinal Fusion

Stability to the curved spine and maintenance of correction can only be achieved by spinal fusion. Instrumentation without arthrodesis is not adequate to provide stability.

Hibbs, in 1911, reported the first spinal fu-sion procedure, which consisted of partially shearing off the base of the spinous processes, then breaking them down to bridge the inter-laminar spaces.[357] The spinal fusion was per-formed on three patients with Pott's disease. In this paper, Hibbs suggested that the procedure might well be used in scoliosis, which was first done in 1914. In 1924 Hibbs reported a series of 59 patients with scoliosis, in some of whom there was correction and in some, not.[358] Ho-worth has reviewed the history of the evolution of spinal fusion.[375]

The exact techniques of fusion vary with different surgeons. Any method in which frag-ments or leaves of bone are elevated from the laminae and spinous processes and are turned up and down so that they overlap is a modifi-cation of the Hibbs technique. Because it is used by every surgeon, a review of the Hibbs method of fusion, as described by him in 1924, is appropriate.

An incision is made through the skin and subcu-taneous tissue, from above downward, exposing the tips of the spinous processes of the vertebrae to be fused. The periosteum over the tips of these proc-esses is split longitudinally, and, with a periosteal elevator, pushed to either side, leaving them bare. The periosteum and interspinous ligaments in turn are still farther split and pushed forward a short distance from each spinous process as two lateral halves, gauze packs being inserted to prevent oozing. The dissection is carried farther and farther forward upon each vertebra in turn, until the spinous proc-esses, the posterior surfaces of the laminae, and the base of the transverse processes are bared, thereby exposing the ligamentum subflavum attached to the margins of the laminae and the articulations of the lateral processes.

The ligament is removed from the laminae with a curette, and the articulation of the lateral processes is destroyed in order to establish bone contact at this point. With a bone gouge, a substantial piece of bone is elevated from the adjacent edges of each lamina, of half its thickness and of half its width. The free end of the piece from above is turned down to make contact with the lamina below, and the free end of the piece from the lamina below is turned up to make contact with the lamina above. In transposing these pieces of bone from the laminae, it is better to avoid severing their continuity.

Each spinous process is then partially divided with

bone forceps and broken down, forcing the tip to come into contact with the bare bone of the vertebra below. The spinous process of the last vertebra below should be turned up to bring about contact with the next above. As the spinous processes of the lumbar region are wide, it is sometimes practicable to split them, turning one half up and the other half down. Thus is established contact of abundant cancellous bone at the articulations of the lateral processes, laminae, and spinous processes. The periosteum and ligament, which together have been pushed to either side and lie practically as an unbroken sheet, are brought together in the middle with interrupted sutures of ten-day chromic catgut.[358]

Details of the technique of spinal fusion as recommended by this author are described and illustrated in Plate 92.

Selection of Fusion Area. In order to provide a stable and balanced correction of scoliosis the fusion area should extend between stable vertebrae above and below the apex of the major curve or curves. Therefore, the *first step* in the determination of fusion level is to *identify the major curve*, which is the most deforming and obviously the part of the spine to be fused. This is determined in the anteroposterior radiographs of the standing patient, which is the position in which the deformity is most severe, and by determination of curve flexibility in supine side-bending anteroposterior radiographs of each curve. The percentage of correction of each curve is calculated next. The major curve is the least flexible as it is rigid because of greater structural changes. In double major curves both curves have the same degree of flexibility and structural deformation. As a rule the thoracic curve is more rigid, as wedging of the vertebral bodies occurs earlier in the thoracic than in the lumbar curves. Also, the thoracic curve, because of the associated rib rotation and "razor back," causes the greatest deformity. With double curves the thoracic curve is usually fused, as it is most deforming. Severe deformity and rigidity in both lumbar and thoracic curves is a difficult problem—it is best to refrain from extending the fusion to L-4 or L-5 as such a low lumbar fusion places high stresses on the remaining mobile lumbar discs. The *second step* is to *determine the end vertebrae*, which are neutrally rotated. As a general rule, the minimum fusion area should extend from end vertebra to end vertebra of the major curve. The end vertebrae are determined in the original standing films by the maximal vertebral tilting and paralleling or reversal of the intervertebral space wedging. On glancing at the radiographs one can easily locate the maximally tilted end vertebrae; the inexperienced may need to draw lines along the vertebral body margins in order to determine when these lines converge into the concavity of a curve and when they begin to diverge on the convex side of the adjacent curve. The intervertebral spaces within a curve will be wedge-shaped, with the lesser thickness of the wedge pointing into the concavity of a curve; the wedge will point in the opposite direction in the opposing curve.

An important factor in determining the fusion area is the extent of *rotation of the vertebral bodies* toward the convexity of the curve. The maximally tilted vertebra is still rotated to the convexity of the major curve, and such rotation may continue one or two vertebrae beyond the maximally tilted vertebra. In this event, it is essential to extend the fusion area beyond the major curve and to fuse all the vertebrae that are rotated toward the convexity of the major curve, including the neutrally rotated vertebrae above and below. Rotation is determined in the standing posteroanterior radiographs by the position of the spinous and pedicle shadows in relation to the vertebral body margins. In the neutrally rotated vertebra the spinous process is in the midline and the pedicle shadows are equidistant from the vertebral margins. In scoliosis with maximally tilted vertebra in the upper lumbar area and a short compensatory curve below, rotation may continue one or several vertebrae below so that the neutrally rotated vertebra is situated in the convexity of the lower curve. In such an instance one should disregard rotation persisting below the maximally tilted vertebra.

The *third step* is assessment of the relationship of a vertically drawn midsacral line to the major curve. Draw a line across the top of the iliac crests and then construct a perpendicular line from the midpart of the sacrum. The vertebra that lies closest to the end vertebra of the curve and is most closely bisected by the perpendicular midsacral line is the lower stable vertebra.[422] When the fusion area extends between the stable end vertebra there will be no additional vertebrae added to the curve beyond the fusion.

The age of the patient should be considered when determining the extent of the fusion. Errors in the young have arisen through failure to fuse a long enough portion of the spine. With growth of the spine, the original curve lengthens and the correction may be lost. Addition of one or two vertebrae will provide security of correction in the young.

Text continued on page 2316

Posterior Spinal Fusion for Scoliosis

OPERATIVE TECHNIQUE

Surgery is performed under general endotracheal anesthesia. The availability of blood should be double-checked before starting the operation. In order to replace blood adequately throughout the procedure the use of two large-gauge intravenous needles is mandatory.

A and **B**. Positioning of the patient. The operating surgeon himself should supervise the proper position of the patient. This is very important in order to minimize blood loss and to adequately expose the surgical field. The patient is turned in the prone position and placed on a four-poster or Relton-Hall frame. The abdomen should remain completely free—minimizing abdominal pressure decreases venous bleeding. There should be no pressure on the axillae. The upper pads should rest on the upper chest—manubrium, clavicles, and acromion. Shoulder abduction should be less than 90 degrees; elbows are flexed and placed over soft pads. Proper position of the upper limbs is vital; there should not be any stretch on the brachial plexus or pressure on the ulnar nerves.

The whole back is prepared and draped. The spinous process of the seventh cervical vertebra and the ilium on both sides should be in the sterile field. The use of a large self-adhering Betadine drape is of great value in ensuring asepsis.

The incision is made from above downward, initially through the dermis only from a level one vertebra superior to the proposed fusion area to a level one vertebra inferior to it. Next, in order to minimize bleeding the intradermal and subcutaneous tissues are infiltrated with an epinephrine solution (1:500,000). The direction of the skin incision is planned so that when the curve is maximally corrected by spinal instrumentation, the operative scar will be straight. This improves the appearance of the back and draws less attention to any residual curve.

C. The superficial and deep fasciae are divided in a straight line over the spinous processes to be fused. Three or four Wheatlander retractors are placed to spread the wound under tension.

Plate 92. Posterior Spinal Fusion for Scoliosis

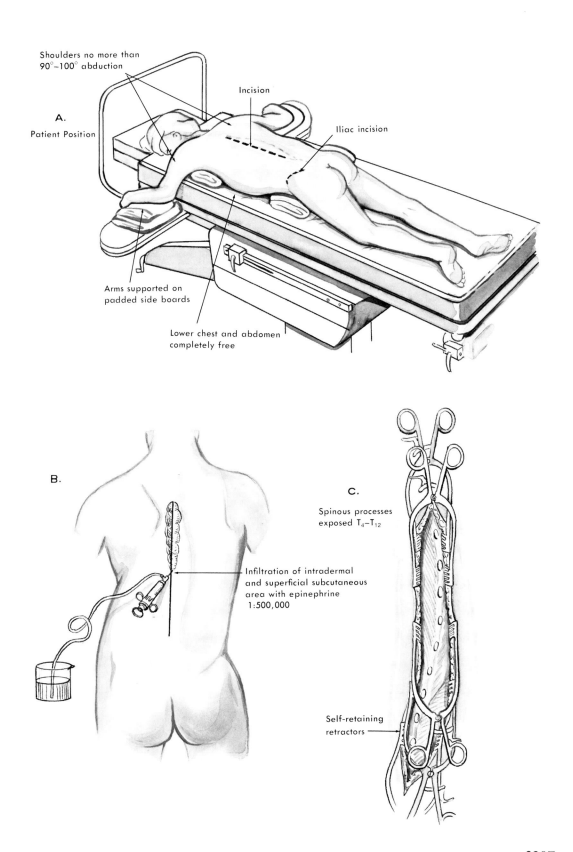

Shoulders no more than
90°–100° abduction

Incision

Iliac incision

A.

Patient Position

Arms supported on
padded side boards

Lower chest and abdomen
completely free

B.

Infiltration of intradermal
and superficial subcutaneous
area with epinephrine
1:500,000

C.

Spinous processes
exposed T₄–T₁₂

Self-retaining
retractors

Posterior Spinal Fusion for Scoliosis (Continued)

D. The median raphe is incised, exposing the tips of the spinous processes. Starting at the proximal end, the assistant presses down over the spinous process with a Kelly clamp, and the surgeon, with a scalpel or a Bovie's knife, splits the cartilaginous tip of the spinous process longitudinally in the midline down to bone. Dissection in this avascular plane minimizes blood loss.

E. Next, with Cobb periosteal elevators the spine is subperiosteally exposed as far laterally as the transverse process in the thoracic area and beyond the articular facets in the lumbar area. In the thoracic area begin dissection distally and proceed proximally—the inferosuperior dissection facilitates the subperiosteal elevation of the oblique attachments of short rotator muscles and ligaments from the lamina. Subperiosteal stripping of muscle and soft tissues from the spinous process, lamina, and transverse process should be meticulous. Avoid excessive force and muscle tearing. Use sharp dissection with a scalpel to detach tendons and ligaments, particularly the superior margin of the lamina.

F. As the subperiosteal dissection is carried out, each level is packed firmly with gauze to minimize bleeding. Dissect laterally with caution! A branch of segmented vessel lies immediately lateral to the facet joint—do not injure it! Be gentle—do not tear muscles laterally!

G. When this is completed, the packing is removed and Wheatlander retractors or laminectomy spreader retractors, or both, are placed deeply to spread the soft tissues out of the field. Next, with the scalpel, rongeurs, and curets the interspinous ligaments and all remaining soft tissue tags are removed from the spinous processes, laminae, facet joints, and transverse processes. The soft-tissue clean-up should be very thorough. Any bleeding, which may be vigorous in the intertransverse process spaces, is controlled with electrocautery. At this stage, radiopaque markers are placed in the spinous processes of the superior and inferior vertebrae to double-check and confirm the correct level of fusion.

Plate 92. Posterior Spinal Fusion for Scoliosis

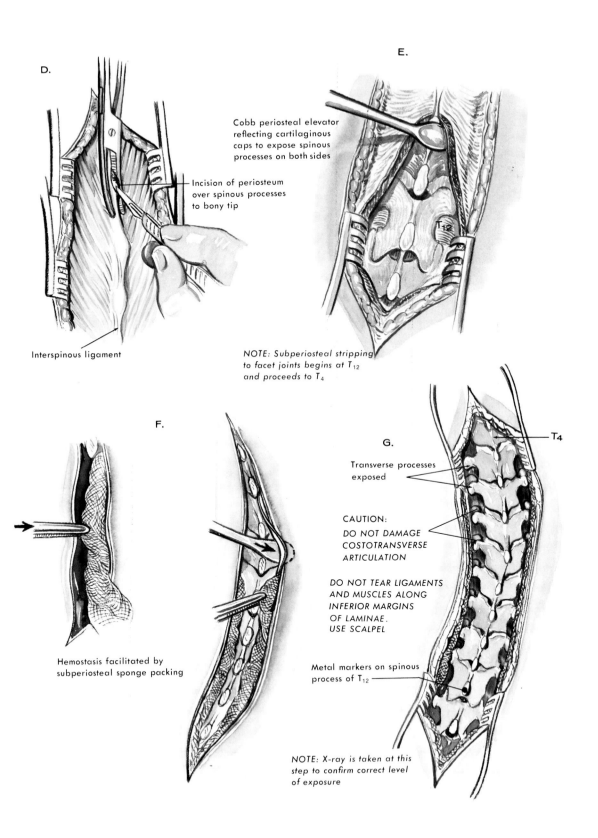

D.

Incision of periosteum over spinous processes to bony tip

Interspinous ligament

E.

Cobb periosteal elevator reflecting cartilaginous caps to expose spinous processes on both sides

T₁₂

NOTE: *Subperiosteal stripping to facet joints begins at* T₁₂ *and proceeds to* T₄

F.

Hemostasis facilitated by subperiosteal sponge packing

G.

T₄

Transverse processes exposed

CAUTION:

DO NOT DAMAGE COSTOTRANSVERSE ARTICULATION

DO NOT TEAR LIGAMENTS AND MUSCLES ALONG INFERIOR MARGINS OF LAMINAE. USE SCALPEL

Metal markers on spinous process of T₁₂

NOTE: X-ray is taken at this step to confirm correct level of exposure

Posterior Spinal Fusion for Scoliosis (Continued)

H to L. *Facet joint fusion* is performed by thorough excision of the cartilaginous material from the articular facet and firmly packing cancellous bone within the remaining space. Facet joint excision and grafting should be performed regardless of the type of spinal instrumentation. A variety of techniques of facet joint fusion have been described.

In the *Hibbs technique,*[357] in the thoracic area first, intra-articular fusion in the dorsal area is performed as follows: First, the posterior half of the facet joint is removed with a Hibbs or Cobb gouge. Then, with a curet, all of its articular cartilage is removed. Next, flaps of bone from the base of the transverse process are elevated and turned into the joint. The Hibbs technique is advocated by Risser and is simple and relatively quick.[618, 620, 622]

In the *Moe technique* of facet joint fusion, two hinged fragments of bone are elevated from adjacent transverse processes and tilted laterally to the intertransverse area. The facet joint is excised, removing all articular cartilage, and a block of cortical-cancellous bone is packed in the remaining defect. First, a cut is made at the base of the lamina of the superior articular process, carried along the transverse process to its tip, elevated leaving it attached to the tip of the transverse process, and then bent to lie between the transverse process. Second, the facet joint surface is resected with a separate cut and discarded; third, the articular cartilage is thoroughly curetted. Fourth, a hinged fragment of bone is elevated from the midportion of the inferior transverse process. Fifth, a cancellous-cortical bone graft is impacted in the defect of the previously resected facet joint. Moe's technique is time-consuming but achieves excellent facet joint fusion.[506, 517]

H. In the Hall technique the inferior facet joint is sharply cut with a semicircular gouge, removing the bone fragment with underlying articular cartilage in one piece.

I. This exposes the superior facet cartilage, which is removed with a sharp curet.

J to L. The outer cortex of the superior facet is resected, creating a trough into which cancellous bone from the outer wall of the ilium is layered and impacted.[91]

Plate 92. Posterior Spinal Fusion for Scoliosis

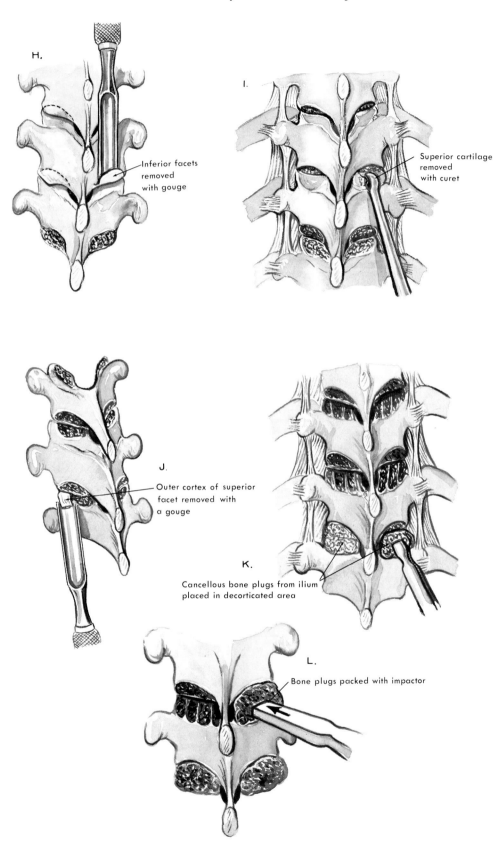

H.

Inferior facets removed with gouge

I.

Superior cartilage removed with curet

J.

Outer cortex of superior facet removed with a gouge

K.

Cancellous bone plugs from ilium placed in decorticated area

L.

Bone plugs packed with impactor

Posterior Spinal Fusion for Scoliosis (Continued)

M and **N.** In the lumbar area the articular facet joints are directed sagittally; they are best excised with small thin osteotomes. A spreader bar is applied between the spinous processes. The articular cartilage is curetted out, and into each joint a block of bone (obtained from the spinous processes or the ilium) is inserted and countersunk. The posterior elements of the spine should be thoroughly cleaned of all soft tissue.

O. Next, the spinous processes are resected with a bone cutter and saved for bone grafting. The spinous processes at the superior and inferior ends are left intact to facilitate secure internal fixation with either the Harrington rod or the L-rod.

P. Next, with sharp Hibbs or Cobb gouges, multiple flaps of bone, half of its thickness and half of its width, are elevated from the base of the spinous processes and laminae. The assistant, with a suction tip, keeps the edge of the bone gouge free of blood and clearly visible to the surgeon. It is easy to keep the flaps attached at their base by rotating the edge of the sharp gouge. The free end of the flap from the lamina below is turned up and locked under the laterally bent flap of the lamina above. The superior half of the spinous process of the most cephalic vertebra of the fusion area and the most inferior one are left intact. The facet joints at the extremes of the fusion area (i.e., between the superior vertebra and the one above, and the inferior vertebra and the one below) are not disturbed. Then the remaining portion of each spinous process is partially divided with a Hibbs bone cutter, broken down, and turned up to bring it in contact with the next above. Thus, when decortication is completed, there is contact of abundant cancellous bone at the laminae and spinous processes and at the facet joints.

The wound is copiously irrigated with antibiotic solution and is firmly packed with lap pads.

Plate 92. Posterior Spinal Fusion for Scoliosis

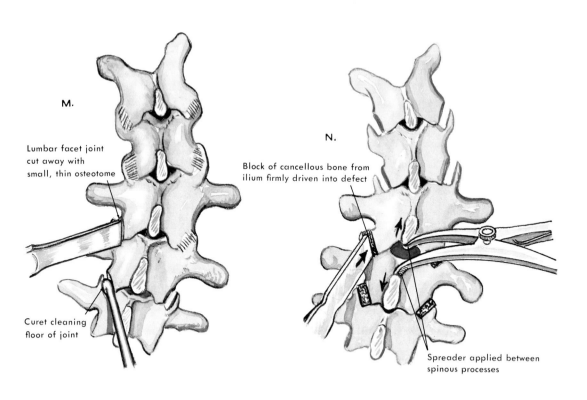

M.

Lumbar facet joint cut away with small, thin osteotome

Curet cleaning floor of joint

N.

Block of cancellous bone from ilium firmly driven into defect

Spreader applied between spinous processes

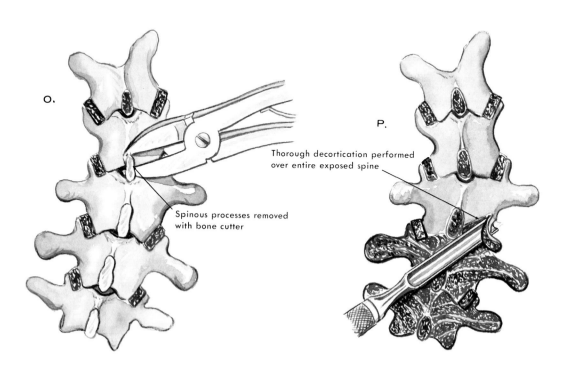

O.

Spinous processes removed with bone cutter

P.

Thorough decortication performed over entire exposed spine

Posterior Spinal Fusion for Scoliosis (Continued)

Q. *Bone grafting* is taken after decortication, to ensure surface cell biologic viability. The bone graft is usually autogenous and is taken from the outer table of the ilium. A separate vertical incision over the iliac crest is made; it is preferred over a curved incision made just distal to the posterior half of the iliac crest, because the operative scar is more pleasing. By sharp and dull dissection, over half of the posterolateral wall of the ilium is exposed. The most abundant and best quality of cancellous bone is adjacent to the upper part of the sciatic notch. By gentle dissection identify the sciatic notch; avoid injury to the superior gluteal vessels and nerve. With the help of gouges and osteotomes, cancellous cortical strips of bone graft are harvested in the usual fashion. Use bone wax for hemostasis. The cancellous and cortical bone grafts are placed over the facet joints and the laminae.

Occasionally bone graft is taken from the tibia. It is divided into two unequal pieces. The longer piece should reach the end vertebra of the fusion area. It is sutured to the base of the intact half of the spinous process of the inferior vertebra and placed snugly on the convex side of the curve. There should be adequate overlap of the two fragments. Fragments of autogenous bone from the tibia are laid down over the facet joint in the intertransverse process spaces and overlapping the laminae.

The retractors are removed, and the muscles are allowed to fall into place. The periosteum, with the deep layers of the muscle, is closed with interrupted sutures. The remaining wound is closed in layers in the usual manner. The skin is closed with subcutaneous 00 nylon suture.

Plate 92. Posterior Spinal Fusion for Scoliosis

Q.

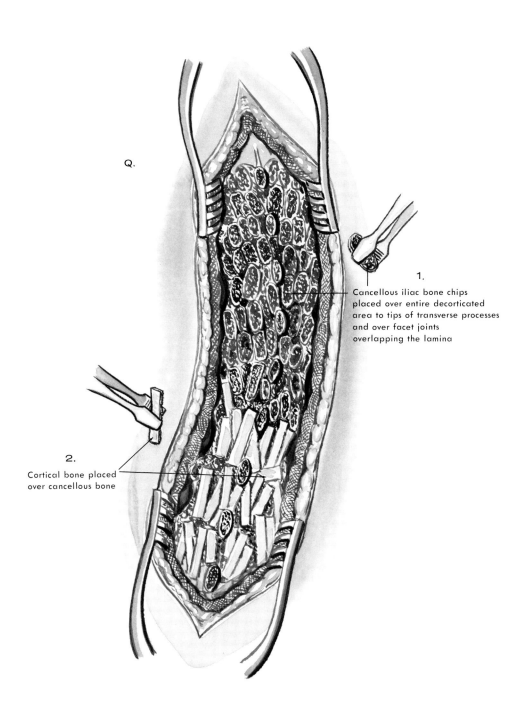

1.
Cancellous iliac bone chips placed over entire decorticated area to tips of transverse processes and over facet joints overlapping the lamina

2.
Cortical bone placed over cancellous bone

Fusion should not extend into compensatory curves if they are rigid and the vertebrae are structurally deformed. It is essential for the spine in the upright position to be symmetrical and in normal balance and equilibrium.

Selection of Spinal Instrumentation. The objectives of spinal instrumentation are, first, to correct the scoliotic deformity as much as possible and, second, to immobilize the spine internally until a solid fusion has taken place; the use of external immobilization such as body cast is thereby avoided.

During the past two decades several techniques of spinal instrumentation have been developed; each system has its advantages and disadvantages. When selecting the type of instrumentation, the following basic factors should be considered in the decision-making process: first, *stabilization of the spine by solid spinal fusion* is one of the major goals of surgical intervention; it is therefore important to perform a meticulous arthrodesis by thorough facetectomy, decortication, and autogenous iliac bone grafting. Initially, in the evolution of his instrumentation technique, Harrington did not perform a fusion, but he soon learned that a solid fusion was a requisite in order to maintain correction.[337, 343] Limited fusion technique with spinal instrumentation does not replace a solid spinal fusion. The problem is that some instrumentation systems occupy space where bone graft should be placed; thus, they prevent formation of massive fusion mass; conversely, decortication may weaken the stability of fixation by the instrument.

The second goal of surgery is to *correct the spinal curvature*. The scoliotic deformity is in three planes. Most thoracic curves are hypokyphotic or in lordosis at their apical segments. Any distraction instrumentation, particularly the Harrington rod, will produce a flat spine. The instrumentation system should restore the normal dorsal roundback and lumbar lordosis. The use of sublaminar wiring with a contoured rod will produce a thoracic kyphosis; therefore, it is used instead of distraction instrumentation when there is thoracic hypokyphosis or lordosis. In thoracolumbar and lumbar curves distraction instrumentation will decrease the normal lumbar lordosis and result in a flattened lumbar spine. Therefore, anterior instrumentation with Zielke or Dwyer instrumentation is utilized. Rotation is best corrected by the Cotrel-Dubousset system; it is used for instrumentation when the rotational prominence, especially in right thoracic curves, is disfiguring.

The third factor to consider is *mobility of the unfused segments of the spine*, which is particularly important in lumbar scoliosis. The level of spinal fusion should not extend distal to the fourth lumbar vertebra. When the fusion mass extends between L-4 and L-5 with added stress on the mobile L-5 to S-1 segments, degenerative arthritis will develop. When anterior instrumentation with the Zielke system is used, the extent of fusion is short, because the Zielke system achieves excellent correction and provides rigid stability; therefore, only the structural vertebrae in the curve, as determined by side-bending radiographs, are fused.

The fourth factor in decision-making in selection of instrumentation is the *potential of spinal cord injury*. This may be caused by direct cord trauma or by stretching when the vertebral column is distracted. Preoperatively it is crucial to rule out spinal cord pathology, particularly tethering. The newer instrumentation systems are powerful and obtain excellent correction. Rigid deformities should not be corrected excessively. Curve correction should be gently controlled with intraoperative assessment of spinal cord function. Sublaminar wires have a higher rate of neurologic complications. Do not sacrifice neurologic function for the sake of excellence of correction and stability of internal fixation.

The fifth factor to consider is the *strength of the bone*. The fixation device may come loose in atrophic vertebrae of paralytic scoliosis or osteogenesis imperfecta. Other causes of loss of fixation are improper placement of hooks, screws, or wires, and poor instrument design.

Segmental Spinal Instrumentation. In this technique of spinal instrumentation, vertebral components are interlocked and fixed at multiple levels. Historically the first segmental instrumentation was described in 1902 by Fritz Lange, who wired a rod to the spine.[92] Gruca, in 1958, developed a spring device to compress the ribs on the convex side of the curve, thereby attempting internal correction of scoliosis.[309] In 1962 Harrington reported a distraction-compression instrumentation system after correction and internal fixation of scoliosis; the Harrington instrumentation is segmental instrumentation.[337] Resina and Ferreira described a technique in which they fixed a rod to the spine with wires passed through the base of the spinous process at each vertebral level.[608] Luque first used sublaminar wires attached to Harrington rod and subsequently developed the more flexible L-rod.[468–470] Allen attached wires to Harrington rod and subsequently developed the more modified and standardized L-rod in strumentation technique.[18-20] During the past two decades several new techniques of segmental instrumentation have been developed. These procedures are technically difficult and demanding; they should be performed by surgeons who have had hands-on experience during a fellowship in spinal surgery centers.

Posterior Spinal Instrumentation

Harrington Instrumentation. Harrington developed his technique in the late 1950s and first reported it in 1962.[336, 337] In this system, bone-purchasing hooks are attached to posterior elements of the spine—facets, laminae, and transverse processes. Through these hooks *distraction forces* are applied to the *concave* side of the spinal curve by the *ratchet* principle, and *compression* forces are applied on the *convex* side of the thoracic curve at the base of the transverse processes and adjusted by the *threadnut* principle. As the distraction is the major corrective force, recently the tendency has been to use distraction instrumentation without the compression system.

Harrington instrumentation has stood up to the test of time over the past three decades and has become the standard by which other forms of spinal instrumentation are assessed. The met-als have excellent biocompatibility. In idiopathic scoliosis the correction rate is about 55 per cent in flexible curves and the fusion rate is 95 per cent. Metal failure is due to failure of fusion. It is vital to have solid fusion in order to maintain correction.

Harrington instrumentation has the following drawbacks. (1) Failure of derotation of the spine as the distraction force straightens the lateral curvature; as a result the rib hump is not corrected. (2) The distraction forces flatten the spine; as a result, lumbar lordosis is obliterated, producing a major deformity. (3) Instrumentation does not provide enough stability to the spine and therefore postoperative immobilization is required in the form of a cast or a spinal orthosis. The operative technique of Harrington instrumentation is described and illustrated in Plate 93 and an illustrative case is shown in Figure 6–76.

Harrington Rods With Sublaminar Wires. Sublaminar wire fixation augmenting Harrington distraction should not be used because of the high incidence of neurologic damage following the procedure. This is caused by overstretching the tenuous blood vessels of the spinal cord by the combination of distraction

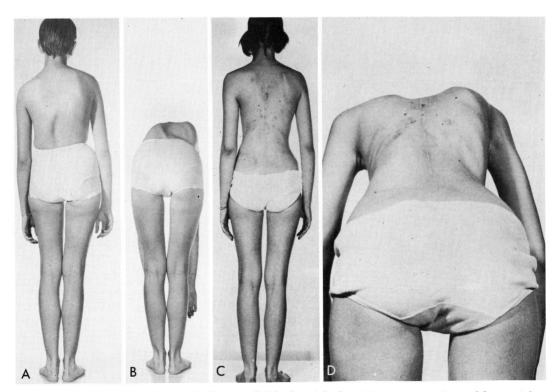

FIGURE 6–76. *Idiopathic scoliosis—double major (left lumbar right thoracic) curve pattern in an adolescent girl.*

A and **B.** Preoperative photographs. **C** and **D.** Following correction in the cast, spinal fusion, and Harrington instrumentation, showing improvement in deformity.

Illustration continued on following page

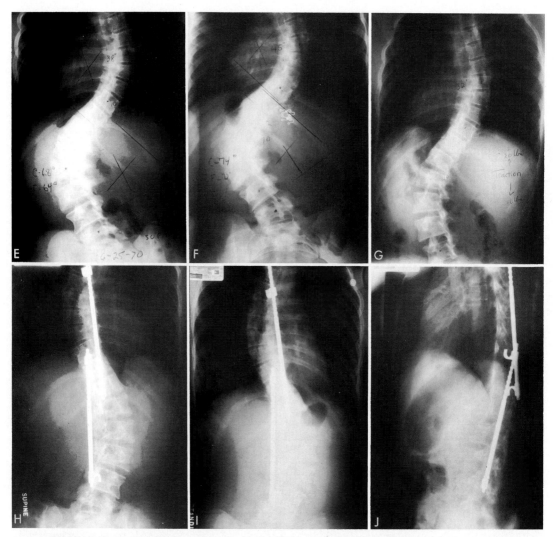

FIGURE 6–76 Continued. Idiopathic scoliosis—double major (left lumbar right thoracic) curve pattern in an adolescent girl.

E to G. Preoperative radiograms, supine, standing, and in traction. H to J. Postoperative radiograms showing degree of correction.

and transverse forces, by direct contusion of the spinal cord during insertion of the sublaminar wires, and by the anterior pulling of the hook into the spinal canal by the sublaminar wires. Broken wires in the epidural space present additional major problems. There are other less invasive systems that provide better fixation and correction without entering the neural canal.

Drummond System.[203] In this segmented spinal instrumentation technique the double wires are passed through a hole from one side to the other at the base of the spinous process, utilizing special awls. The wires are deep in the laminae but do not enter the neural canal. The wires are fixed to a Harrington distraction rod on the concavity and a Luque type rod on the convexity. The rods are contoured into the postural curves of dorsal roundback and lumbar lordosis, thereby avoiding flattening the spine. The distraction rod is fixed to a bifid Harrington hook superiorly and an André hook distally. The ³⁄₁₆-inch stainless steel Luque type rod is contoured to the shape of the desired final correction of the curvature and bent at both ends, lying across the interspace beyond the hooks. By tightening the convex and concave wires to the rods the scoliosis is corrected to the desired degree. Decortication and facet fusion are performed in the routine fashion.

Postoperative immobilization is not required as the segmented fixation is stable.

The Drummond system has the distinct advantage of not invading the neural canal and the double rod wire fixation provides adequate stability. Technically the procedure is relatively simple and not time consuming. Its disadvantage is that it does not derotate the spine.[203]

Cotrel-Dubousset (C-D) Instrumentation.[157] This segmented system, developed in 1981 by Cotrel and Dubousset in Paris, France, is very versatile and safe. It achieves correction of the scoliotic spine in three planes—anteroposterior, lateral, and axial. Its ability to derotate the spine produces normal thoracic roundback and lumbar lordosis; this is not possible with other posterior systems. In addition, the design of the system provides secure stability to the spine so that external fixation after surgery in the form of an orthosis or cast is not required. The patient is allowed to be up and around, resuming normal activities in the immediate postoperative period. The instrumentation system is versatile with powerful corrective forces, allowing its use in complex problems. So far the Cotrel-Dubousset system has an excellent safety record.

The disadvantages of the Cotrel-Dubousset system are that it is complex and cumbersome, with too many "moving parts." The system consists of two 7-mm. diamond-surfaced rods that are contoured to the spinal curve. The rods are connected to distraction and compression hooks that are designed either as laminar or pedicle. Seating collars firmly stabilize the hooks. The upper end of the pedicle hook is closed, and thereafter the hooks are open. The rods are passed through an opening in the hooks. The screw on the hook is tightened, thereby fixing the hook on the rod. The use of "C" clamps permits rotation of the hooks on the rod.

Illustrative cases of Cotrel-Dubousset instrumentation are shown in Figures 6–77 and 6–78. The operative technique is not described in detail here because of its complexity. It is vital to have hands-on experience and special spinal surgery training prior to using the Cotrel-Dubousset instrumentation system.

Luque Double L-Rod Segmented Instrumentation. In this system two contoured ³⁄₁₆- or ¼-inch stainless steel rods are wired to the spine at every vertebral level by sublaminar wires. The two rods are bent to a right angle at one end and wired transversely to one another. The rods are contoured to restore normal postural

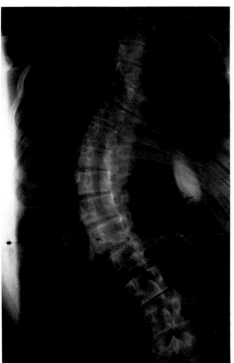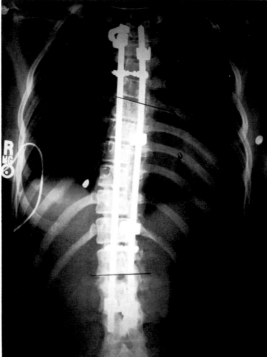

FIGURE 6–77. Cotrel-Dubousset instrumentation.

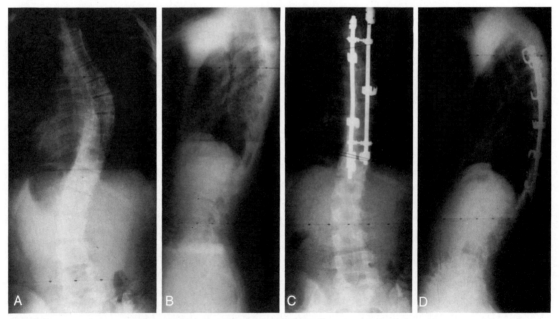

FIGURE 6–78. *Cotrel-Dubousset instrumentation.*

A and **B.** Preoperative radiograms. **C** and **D.** Postoperative anteroposterior and lateral radiograms of the spine. Note the excellent correction.

curves of dorsal roundback and lumbar lordosis. Prebending a single ¼-inch rod into a "U" shape superior prevents the problems of rod migration and rotation.

Determination of the extent and level of instrumentation is vital; it should extend end vertebra to end vertebra, determined by neutral rotation, and the end vertebra should be transected by the vertical seventh cervical midsacral line.[422]

In the Galveston modification, the rods are fixed to the pelvis by passing them through a hole made in the longitudinal axis of the ilium, immediately above the acetabulum. The rods are contoured to maintain normal lumbar lordosis. An example of double L-rod instrumentation in paralytic scoliosis is illustrated in Figure 6–79.

The advantage of double L-rod instrumentation is the provision of secure fixation, eliminating the need for postoperative cast or orthosis; this is a tremendous benefit to patients with paralytic deformity and insensitive skin. It also provides secure pelvic fixation, which is a definite advantage in the management of severe curves with pelvic obliquity, particularly in the osteopenic spine. Even in bones with poor stock the instrumentation provides adequate stability. The double L-rod can correct thoracic lordosis and restore normal postural curves.

The disadvantage of L-rod instrumentation is the risk of neurologic damage. Often this damage is relatively minor in the form of sensory

dysesthesias that resolve within two to three weeks. Major complications in the form of partial or total paralysis can occur.

Anterior Segmental Instrumentation. This was originally developed by Dwyer, and other techniques later followed with development of several compression implants.[222] The technique of Dwyer instrumentation is described and illustrated in Plate 94. However, with the advent of the Zielke instrumentation, the use of the Dwyer implant has been almost abandoned.

Disadvantages of the Dwyer system are inability to control the correction of each segmental level, difficulty in derotating the spine, and a high incidence of postinstrumentation kyphosis. The Zielke system blocks open the disc spaces anteriorly and maintains lordosis by the use of a flexible rod system, a derotating bar, and threaded nuts at each screw site. In both systems, major vessels should not lie on the implants in order to prevent erosion and rupture of vessels. The Zielke instrumentation system is illustrated in Figure 6–80.

Associated Procedures for Scoliosis. Rotational and angular deformities of the spine may be so fixed that it may be impossible to effect any correction. Under these circumstances, operations to improve external appearance may be indicated. The two available surgical procedures are resection of the prominent rib hump and subtotal scapulectomy. These two procedures may be combined.

Resection of Prominent Rib Hump. Preoper-
Text continued on page 2354

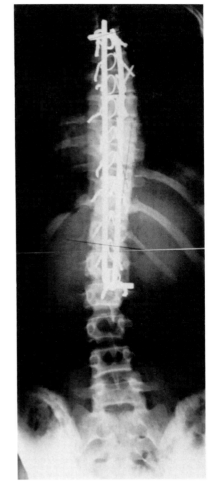

FIGURE 6–79. *Double Luque L-rod instrumentation for segmental instrumentation of the spine.*

Anteroposterior radiogram of the spine, showing the device.

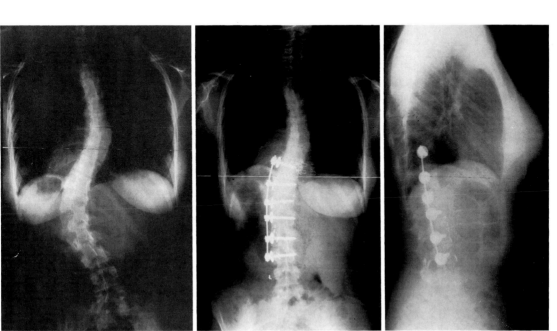

A

B

C

FIGURE 6–80. *Anterior instrumentation of the spine by the Zielke technique.*

A. Preoperative anteroposterior radiogram. **B** and **C.** Postoperative anteroposterior and lateral radiograms. Note the extent of correction and derotation.

Posterior Spinal Instrumentation by the Harrington System

OPERATIVE TECHNIQUE

The posterior spine is exposed as described in Plate 92 for spinal fusion. There should be meticulous subperiosteal exposure out to the tip of the transverse processes. The first stage of Harrington instrumentation is the *placement of the hooks*. In order to provide a normally aligned spine it is vital to select the correct level for the purchase site for the superior and inferior distraction hooks: The *superior distraction hook* should be anchored at or one vertebra above the superior end vertebra, whereas the inferior distraction hook should be at one or two vertebrae below the inferior end vertebra *within the stable zone*. The inferior distraction hook rarely, if ever, is placed distal to the fourth lumbar vertebra.

A and **B.** The superior distraction hook is seated in a facet joint. The purchase site is prepared as follows: First, all ligamentous and capsular tissue is removed from the lamina. The direction of the facet joint is determined by tapping a narrow periosteal elevator in the facet joint. Next, with a ¼-inch osteotome or a Capener gouge the inferior facet joint is squared off. The direction of the osteotomy is oblique, with the medial border directed more superiorly than the lateral margin.

C. Next, a No. 1251 sharp hook is inserted into the facet interspace with the hook tilted anteriorly at a driving angle of 45 degrees; this forward tilting of the hook is important in order to prevent fracturing of the lamina. Once the hook has engaged the pedicle, it is impacted with a mallet.

D. Then the No. 1251 sharp hook is removed and replaced with a dull No. 1262 flanged hook or a dull No. 1253 unflanged hook. This author prefers a flanged hook, as it will firmly grip the bone and will not fracture the lamina. It is best to place the medial one third of the hook medial to the facet joint in order to prevent lateral hook displacement or dislodgment. The hook should be firmly impacted into the pedicle.

Plate 93. Posterior Spinal Instrumentation by the Harrington System

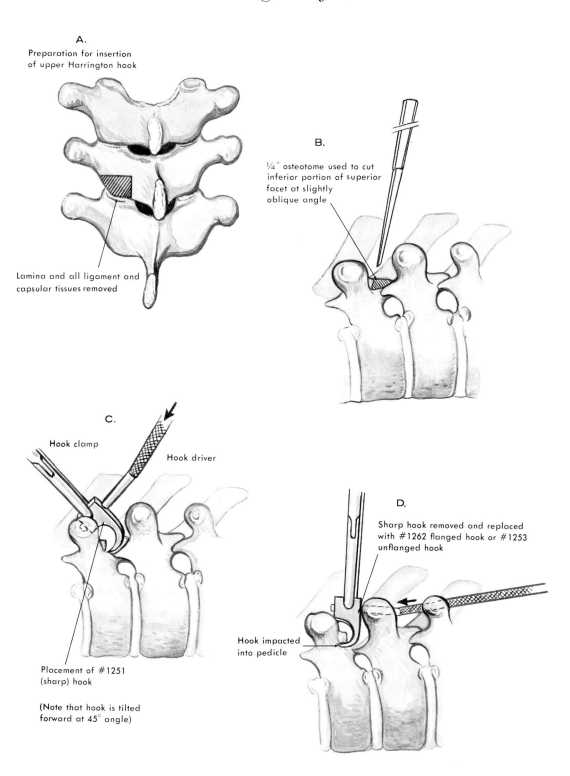

A.

Preparation for insertion of upper Harrington hook

Lamina and all ligament and capsular tissues removed

B.

¼″ osteotome used to cut inferior portion of superior facet at slightly oblique angle

C.

Hook clamp

Hook driver

Placement of #1251 (sharp) hook

(Note that hook is tilted forward at 45° angle)

D.

Sharp hook removed and replaced with #1262 flanged hook or #1253 unflanged hook

Hook impacted into pedicle

Posterior Spinal Instrumentation by the Harrington System (Continued)

E. The *inferior distraction hook* is seated underneath the superior border of the selected vertebra. First, remove a portion of the lamina and adjacent inferior facet with a Kerrison rongeur, producing a flat margin that extends to pars interarticularis. In order to facilitate hook insertion, distract the spinous processes of the adjacent vertebra with a Blount or laminar spreader.

F. Then insert a No. 1254 hook under the lamina. The shoe of the hook is in the epidural space.

G. Prior to placing the Harrington outrigger or rod, cancellous bone is packed at the lower hook site.

Plate 93. Posterior Spinal Instrumentation by the Harrington System

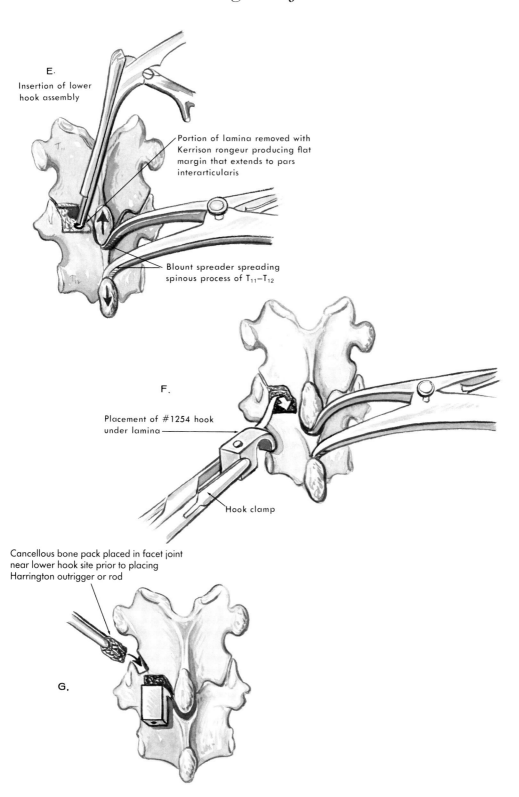

E.

Insertion of lower hook assembly

Portion of lamina removed with Kerrison rongeur producing flat margin that extends to pars interarticularis

Blount spreader spreading spinous process of T_{11}–T_{12}

F.

Placement of #1254 hook under lamina

Hook clamp

Cancellous bone pack placed in facet joint near lower hook site prior to placing Harrington outrigger or rod

G.

Posterior Spinal Instrumentation by the
Harrington System (Continued)

H and **I.** Next, the Harrington outrigger is inserted between the superior and inferior distraction hooks. Passive force is applied to the apex of the convexity of the curve, and the screw device on the outrigger is tightened, distracting and correcting the curve. The use of the Harrington outrigger is optional. It is recommended by this author because it facilitates exposure and correction; with the spine in the corrected position it is easier to perform decortication and spinal fusion; it also assists in choosing a rod of proper length.

J. Next, decortication of the posterior elements of the spine and facet fusion is carried out (see Plate 92). The posterior elements upon which the hooks are seated should be left intact.

K. The outrigger is removed, and the distraction rod is placed between the superior and inferior hooks. Then, using the Harrington spreader, gradual distraction is carried out, stopping short of rod bending or bone disruption. The degree of maximum distraction that can be performed safely depends upon the experience of the surgeon. It is best to perform a Stagnara wake-up test and determine neurologic status by asking the patient to actively move the foot, ankle, and knee.[751] If spinal cord and nerve function is intact, anesthesia is deepened and surgery continued. It is best to insert a C-ring or thread an 18-gauge wire around the superior ratchet of the rod immediately inferior to the hook in order to checkrein telescoping of the rod within the hook.

In the lumbar spine, contoured square-end rods should be used in order to preserve lumbar lordosis. In double major curves, a single distraction rod provides better balance to the spine than two overlapping distraction rods.

Application of the Harrington Compression Instrumentation on the Convex Side of the Curve. This is used when kyphosis is associated with scoliosis in the thoracic region. Some surgeons prefer to use compression in conjunction with distraction because it provides more stable fixation and increases the degree of correction (an average of 10 degrees).[342] The use of the compression assembly is contraindicated when the thoracic spine is hypokyphotic.

The compression assembly comes in two sizes: ⅛ inch and 5⁄11 inch. Ordinarily, the small size with the No. 1259 hook is used because it is flexible, contouring easily to the dorsal roundback. In the proposed fused area, the lamina and facet joint should be thoroughly cleared of all soft tissue.

Plate 93. Posterior Spinal Instrumentation by the Harrington System

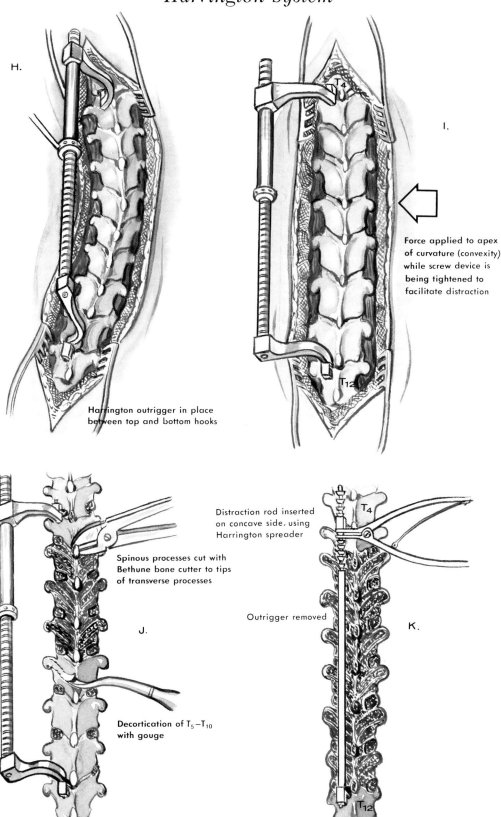

H.

Harrington outrigger in place between top and bottom hooks

I.

T₄

Force applied to apex of curvature (convexity) while screw device is being tightened to facilitate distraction

T₁₂

J.

Spinous processes cut with Bethune bone cutter to tips of transverse processes

Decortication of T₅–T₁₀ with gouge

K.

Distraction rod inserted on concave side, using Harrington spreader

T₄

Outrigger removed

T₁₂

Posterior Spinal Instrumentation by the Harrington System (Continued)

L. to N. The upper hooks (usually three in number) are inserted under the selected transverse processes at the junction of the transverse process and lamina. The shoe of the hook has a sharp edge that sections the costotransverse ligament. It is important that the edge of the hook not cut into the transverse process. Insert the hooks in a horizontal direction. Do not tilt the hook to slide under the transverse process. The upper three hooks are placed temporarily.

O to Q. The lower hooks (usually three in number) are inserted underneath the lamina as close to the facet joint as possible. This is because the transverse process of T11 and caudally are not suitable for hook purchase. The laminae of the selected distal vertebrae are prepared for hook placement. With an osteotome or Kerrison rongeur, an adequate amount of bone is resected from the laminae and inferior facet. Next, the two adjacent spinous processes are spread apart with a Blount or laminectomy spreader and the hook is inserted underneath the lamina in a horizontal fashion.

Plate 93. *Posterior Spinal Instrumentation by the Harrington System*

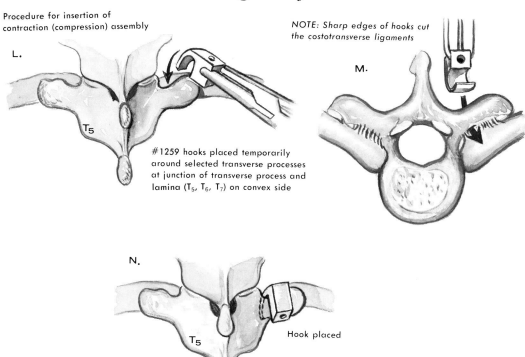

Procedure for insertion of
contraction (compression) assembly

L.

T₅

#1259 hooks placed temporarily
around selected transverse processes
at junction of transverse process and
lamina (T₅, T₆, T₇) on convex side

NOTE: *Sharp edges of hooks cut
the costotransverse ligaments*

M.

N.

T₅

Hook placed

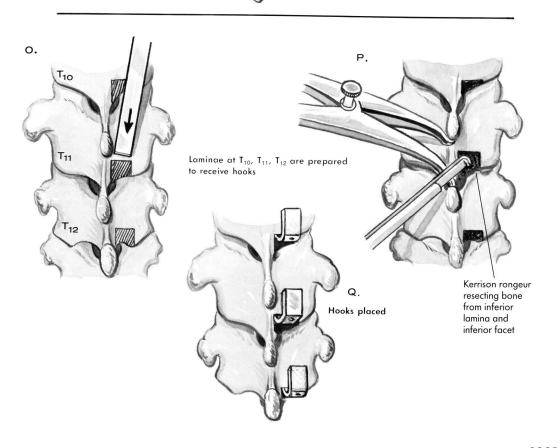

O.

T₁₀

T₁₁

T₁₂

Laminae at T₁₀, T₁₁, T₁₂ are prepared
to receive hooks

P.

Q.

Hooks placed

Kerrison rongeur
resecting bone
from inferior
lamina and
inferior facet

Posterior Spinal Instrumentation by the Harrington System (Continued)

R and **S.** Three hooks are placed under the transverse processes of the upper thoracic vertebrae and three hooks under the laminae of the lower thoracic and/or upper lumbar vertebrae. Next, a threaded rod with the hooks attached to it is inserted. Cranially directed hooks are inserted first, followed by the caudally directed hooks. Once the hooks are firmly secured in place, the compression assembly is tightened, using wire holders and Harrington spreader and spinning the nut around the hook using a Penfield. Finally, the nut is tightened with a wrench.

T. Next, the lower three hooks are tightened as in **R.** After maximal contraction is achieved, the central threads adjacent to the nuts are stripped (damaged) with a clamp as close to the nut as possible in order to prevent unwinding and loosening.

In kyphosis without scoliosis two compression rods are used, one on each side.

Plate 93. Posterior Spinal Instrumentation by the Harrington System

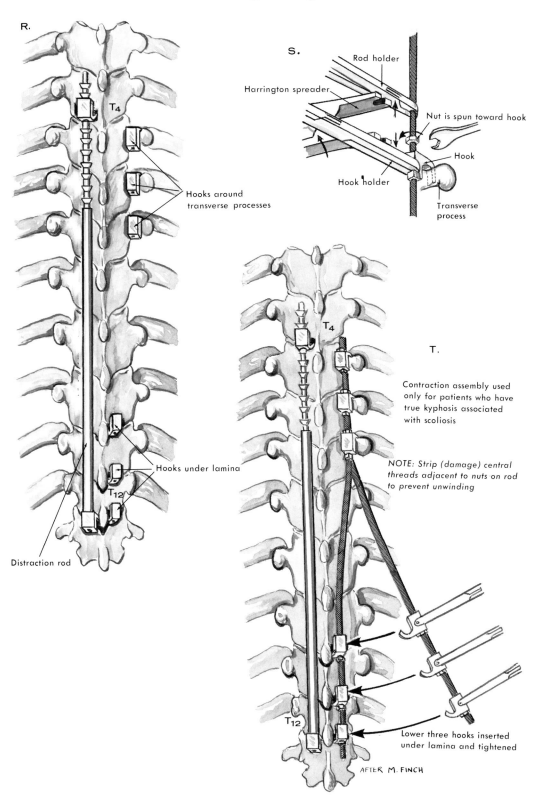

R.

T₄

Hooks around transverse processes

Hooks under lamina

T₁₂

Distraction rod

S.

Rod holder

Harrington spreader

Nut is spun toward hook

Hook

Hook holder

Transverse process

T.

T₄

Contraction assembly used only for patients who have true kyphosis associated with scoliosis

NOTE: Strip (damage) central threads adjacent to nuts on rod to prevent unwinding

Lower three hooks inserted under lamina and tightened

T₁₂

AFTER M. FINCH

2331

Anterior Instrumentation of the Spine (Thoracoabdominal Approach)

OPERATIVE TECHNIQUE

A and **B.** The patient is placed in the lateral decubitus position with the convex side of the curve upward. The upper arm is flexed forward and abducted to rotate the scapula away from the vertebral column. At the apex of the curve the table is elevated, in order to facilitate excision of the intervertebral discs.

It is necessary to remove a rib for exposure of the spine; the rib that is removed is the one immediately superior to the most cephalic vertebral body to be exposed; for example, for exposure from T5 or T6 to T11, the fifth rib is removed. Removal of the tenth rib allows exposure of the spine from T10 to the sacrum. The costal cartilage of the tenth rib is split longitudinally for exposure of the retroperitoneal plane and diaphragm. The attachments of the diaphragm to the rib cage are sectioned. In this plate, the thoracoabdominal approach for exposure of the lower thoracic and lumbar spine is described.

Skin Incision

A and **B.** It begins at the spinous process of T10 (or T9) and extends along the course of the tenth rib to the costocartilaginous junction, across the upper abdomen to the lateral edge of the rectus abdominus. At this point the incision is carried distally toward the symphysis pubis. This single incision allows exposure of the spine all the way to the sacrum.

Plate 94. Anterior Instrumentation of the Spine
(Thoracoabdominal Approach)

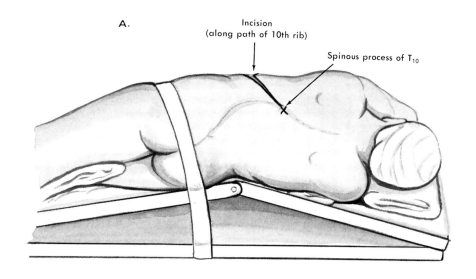

A.

Incision
(along path of 10th rib)

Spinous process of T_{10}

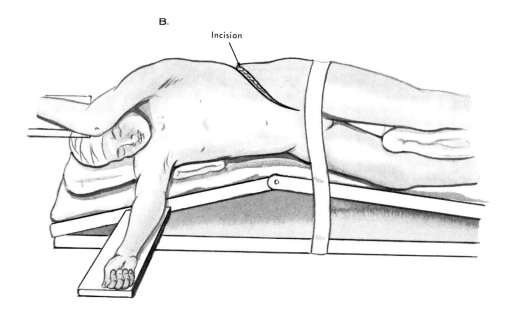

B.

Incision

Anterior Instrumentation of the Spine (Thoracoabdominal Approach) (Continued)

C. The tenth rib is freed by sharp and dull dissection, divided at its costocartilaginous junction, and excised. Removal of the rib permits a larger working aperture, and also the rib is used as autogenous bone graft.

D and **E.** The costal cartilage of the tenth rib is split longitudinally with a scalpel. It is best to place stay sutures on either side of the costal cartilage so that the tissue plane is easily identifiable for later closure.

Plate 94. Anterior Instrumentation of the Spine (Thoracoabdominal Approach)

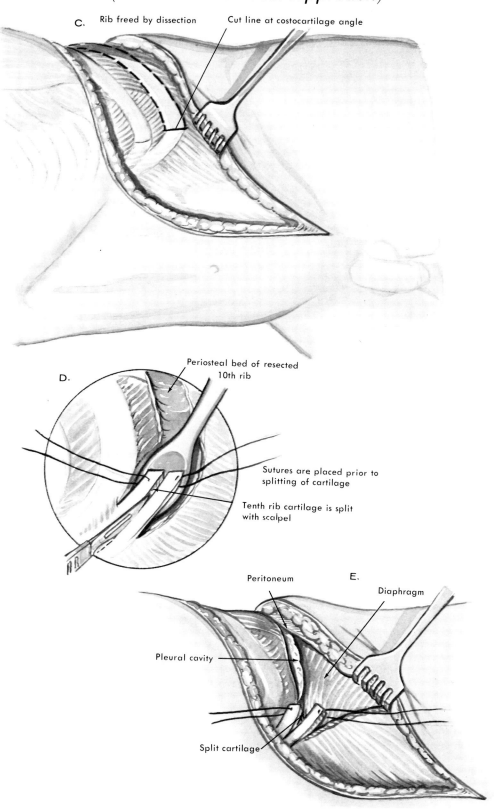

C. Rib freed by dissection   Cut line at costocartilage angle

D.

Periosteal bed of resected 10th rib

Sutures are placed prior to splitting of cartilage

Tenth rib cartilage is split with scalpel

Peritoneum   E.   Diaphragm

Pleural cavity

Split cartilage

Anterior Instrumentation of the Spine (Thoracoabdominal Approach) (Continued)

F. By blunt dissection the peritoneum is gently peeled off from the underside of the diaphragm. Upon freeing of the peritoneum, the viscera will fall anteriorly away from the vertebral bodies. Stay sutures are placed on either side of the intended line of division of the diaphragm, which is 1/2 to 3/4 inch from the site of attachment of the diaphragm. This will facilitate closure of the diaphragm later on.

G. The diaphragm is sectioned from its costal attachments. An alternative method of detachment of the diaphragm is to perform it from the thoracic side along its costal attachment using a Bovie knife (not illustrated). By this technique, bleeding is minimized and the problem of postoperative atelectasis is less common.

Plate 94. Anterior Instrumentation of the Spine (Thoracoabdominal Approach)

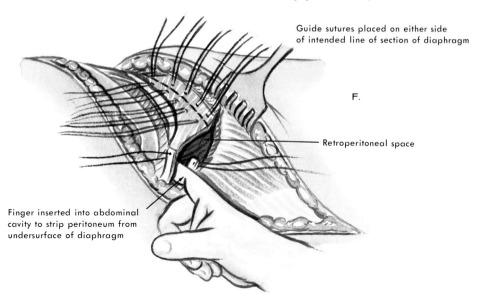

Guide sutures placed on either side of intended line of section of diaphragm

F.

Retroperitoneal space

Finger inserted into abdominal cavity to strip peritoneum from undersurface of diaphragm

Diaphragm (free from peritoneum on undersurface) is divided circumferentially 1.5 cm. from its costal attachment

G.

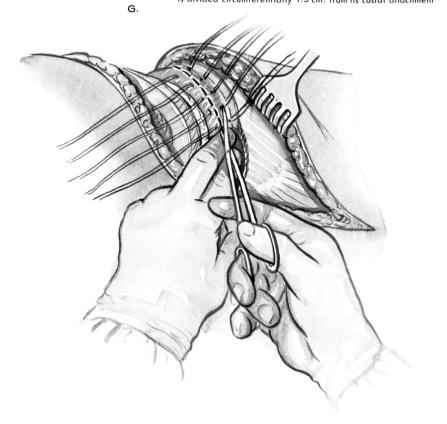

Anterior Instrumentation of the Spine (Thoracoabdominal Approach) (Continued)

H. Next, the parietal pleura is incised along the vertebral bodies throughout the extent of the vertebrae to be exposed.

I. In the lumbar region, the psoas muscle is gently elevated off the vertebral bodies and intervertebral discs. The segmented vessels are ligated either close to their origin from the aorta or in the middle of the vertebral body; thereby the vital vascular anastomosis near the intervertebral foramen is avoided and potential vascular infarct of the cord obviated.

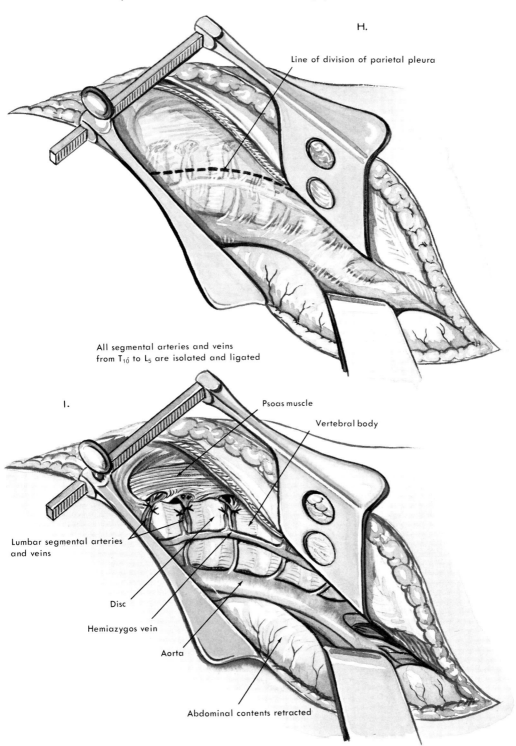

H.

Line of division of parietal pleura

All segmental arteries and veins
from T₁₀ to L₅ are isolated and ligated

I.

Psoas muscle

Vertebral body

Lumbar segmental arteries
and veins

Disc

Hemiazygos vein

Aorta

Abdominal contents retracted

Anterior Instrumentation of the Spine (Thoracoabdominal Approach) (Continued)

Interbody Fusion

J and **K.** The annulus is exposed anteriorly from the margin of one intervertebral foramen to the contralateral foramina. The aorta and vena cava are protected, and the anterior longitudinal ligament is incised with a sharp scalpel. Next, with a duck-billed rongeur, the discs are excised. Once the discs are excised, the posterior annulus and posterior longitudinal ligaments are visualized.

Plate 94. Anterior Instrumentation of the Spine (Thoracoabdominal Approach)

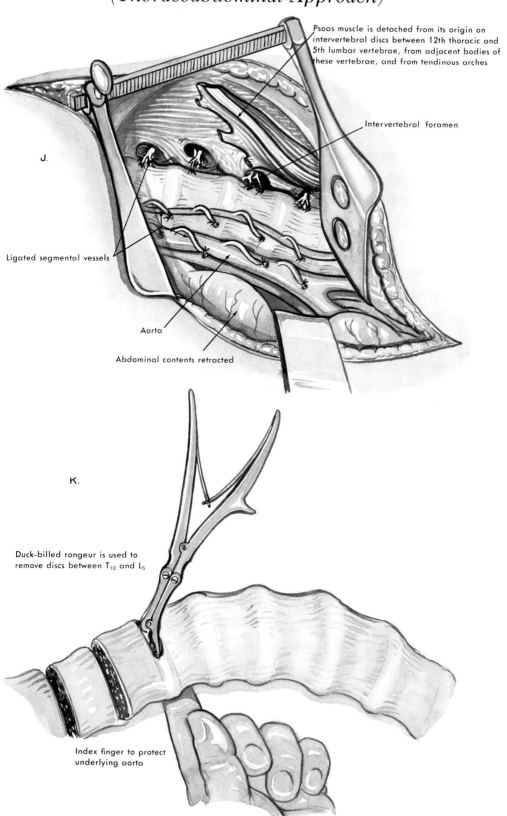

Psoas muscle is detached from its origin on intervertebral discs between 12th thoracic and 5th lumbar vertebrae, from adjacent bodies of these vertebrae, and from tendinous arches

Intervertebral foramen

J.

Ligated segmental vessels

Aorta

Abdominal contents retracted

K.

Duck-billed rongeur is used to remove discs between T_{10} and L_5

Index finger to protect underlying aorta

Anterior Instrumentation of the Spine (Thoracoabdominal Approach) (Continued)

L. The aorta and vena cava are protected with Chandler or other appropriate elevator-retractors. With a sharp osteotome and mallet, the vertebral end-plates are removed.

M. With a curet, any retained disc and vertebral end-plates are removed. In correction of kyphosis, all annular ligamentous tissue down to the posterior longitudinal ligament is removed; in scoliosis, however, the outer annular fibers on the concave side are preferably left intact. For hemostasis, the excised disc interspaces are packed with Gelfoam soaked in thrombin solution.

Plate 94. Anterior Instrumentation of the Spine (Thoracoabdominal Approach)

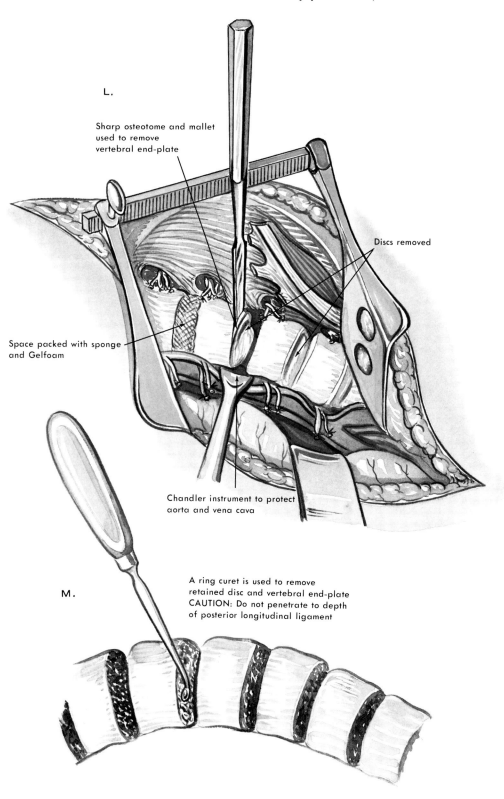

L.

Sharp osteotome and mallet used to remove vertebral end-plate

Discs removed

Space packed with sponge and Gelfoam

Chandler instrument to protect aorta and vena cava

M.

A ring curet is used to remove retained disc and vertebral end-plate
CAUTION: Do not penetrate to depth of posterior longitudinal ligament

Anterior Instrumentation of the Spine (Thoracoabdominal Approach) (Continued)

Dwyer Instrumentation for Anterior Vertebral Compression

In this textbook, Dwyer instrumentation is discussed and illustrated because it was the first compression spinal implant described. Zielke instrumentation has replaced the Dwyer technique, because the Dwyer instrumentation produces kyphosis, cannot modulate correction at each segmented level, and cannot derotate the spine effectively. These drawbacks of the Dwyer system are overcome by the Zielke instrumentation, as the latter utilizes a flexible rod system, a derotating bar, and threaded nuts at each screw site.

N to P. Select the appropriate-sized Dwyer staple; the calibrations in the staple starter determine the proper size. Secure the staple on a special staple introducer by tightening the handle.

Q. The staple is impacted in place with the flanges of the staple gripping immediately over the end-plates.

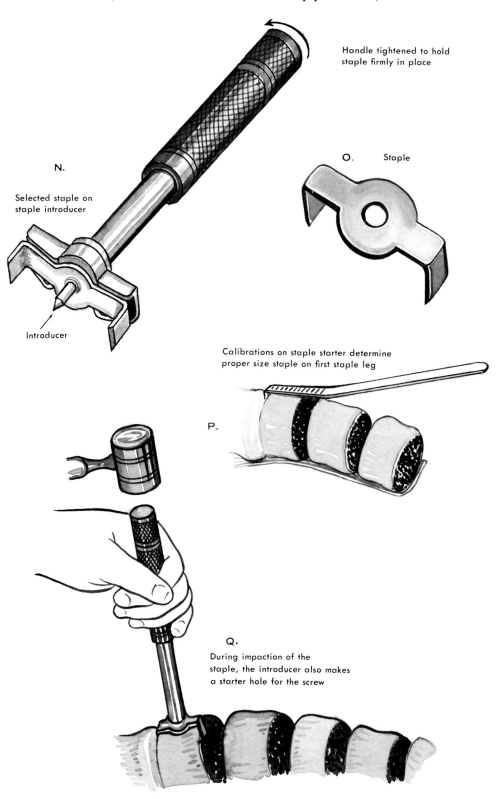

Handle tightened to hold staple firmly in place

O. Staple

N.

Selected staple on staple introducer

Introducer

Calibrations on staple starter determine proper size staple on first staple leg

P.

Q.

During impaction of the staple, the introducer also makes a starter hole for the screw

Anterior Instrumentation of the Spine (Thoracoabdominal Approach) (Continued)

R to **T**. An appropriate-sized cannulated cancellous screw is inserted into the vertebral body. The proper length of the screw is the one that engages the opposite cortex of the vertebra. The alignment of the screw is horizontal, parallel with the posterior longitudinal ligament and in front of the neural foramen; thereby the spinal canal is not entered and possible mechanical damage to the spinal cord is avoided.

U. Next, cable is passed through the cannulated screw heads. Instrumentation proceeds superoinferiorly on the convex side of the curve.

Plate 94. Anterior Instrumentation of the Spine (Thoracoabdominal Approach)

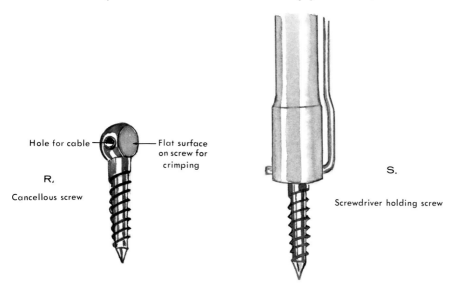

Hole for cable — Flat surface on screw for crimping

R.
Cancellous screw

S.
Screwdriver holding screw

Proper length screw must be used to engage opposite cortex of vertebra. Proper alignment is essential through center of vertebral body

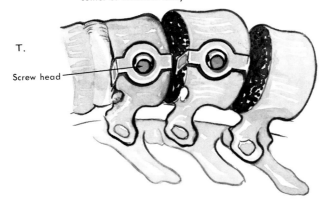

T.

Screw head

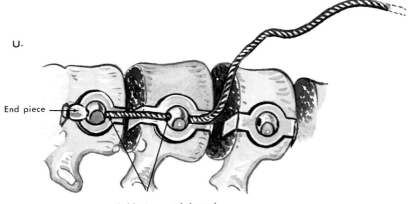

U.

End piece

Cable is passed through cannulated screw heads

Anterior Instrumentation of the Spine (Thoracoabdominal Approach) (Continued)

V. Bone chips (obtained from the resected rib and autogenous ilium) are placed between the vertebral bodies.

W. Tension is applied on the cable, shortening the distance between the screws. *Do not* apply tension on the cable until the operating table has been straightened.

Plate 94. Anterior Instrumentation of the Spine (Thoracoabdominal Approach)

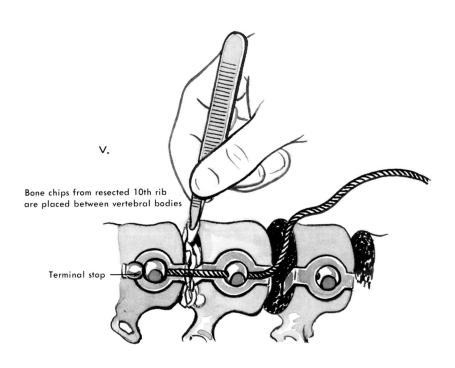

V.

Bone chips from resected 10th rib are placed between vertebral bodies

Terminal stop

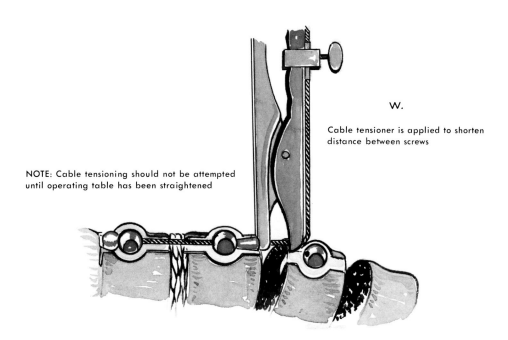

W.

Cable tensioner is applied to shorten distance between screws

NOTE: Cable tensioning should not be attempted until operating table has been straightened

Anterior Instrumentation of the Spine (Thoracoabdominal Approach) (Continued)

X and **Y**. When appropriate correction of scoliosis is achieved, the screw head is crimped onto the cable. Carry out same maneuvers for each succeeding vertebra and disc interspace.

Z. Below the final screw an extra collar is crimped on the cable. The cables are covered by suturing over the pleura and the psoas muscle. It is vital that vessels not lie on the implant; the vessels may rupture if meticulous attention is not paid to this important detail. The diaphragm is sutured, and the wound is closed in the usual fashion.

POSTOPERATIVE CARE

The spine is supported in a thoracolumbar body cast until fusion has taken place. Immobilization is ordinarily for six to nine months. Ambulation is allowed.

Plate 94. Anterior Instrumentation of the Spine (Thoracoabdominal Approach)

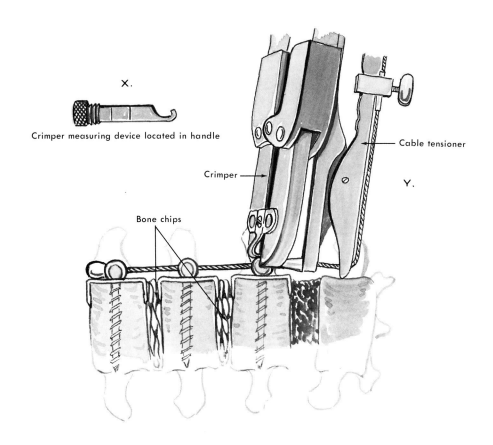

X.

Crimper measuring device located in handle

Cable tensioner

Crimper

Y.

Bone chips

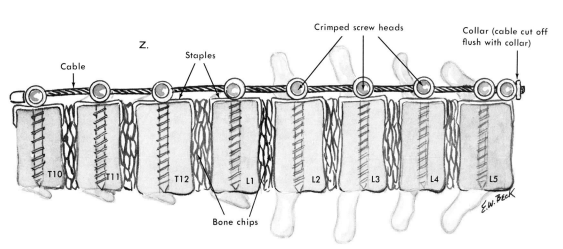

Crimped screw heads

Collar (cable cut off flush with collar)

Z.

Staples

Cable

T10   T11   T12   L1   L2   L3   L4   L5

Bone chips

E.W. BECK

Anterior Instrumentation of the Spine (Thoracoabdominal Approach) (Continued)

Zielke Instrumentation—Ventral Derotation Spondylodesis

AA. The anterior aspect of the vertebrae is exposed, and the discs are excised as described previously. The outer annular fibers on the concave side are left intact. Intraoperative radiograms of the spine are made with radiopaque markers to ensure that the exposed vertebrae correspond to the proposed level and extent of fusion. Begin instrumentation with the most cephalic vertebra.

First, with a caliper measure the diameter of the vertebral body. The length of the screw should be such that its tip perforates the opposite vertebral cortex. The thickness of the washers and angle plates should be taken into consideration; therefore, the selected screw will be 5 to 9 mm. longer than the diameter of the vertebral body as measured by caliper. It is vital to have bicortical fixation.

The threads of the Zielke screws are broad and self-cutting for firm anchoring in cancellous bone. The pressure force of the screws is distributed by angle plates and washers. Double-bladed angle plate (similar to Dwyer staples) is used for the end vertebrae, whereas washers are used for the intervening vertebrae. The screw heads have either lateral or upper slits, through which the compression rod is passed. The notches (slits) of the most cephalic and caudal screws are side-opening; whereas the intervening screws are top-opening.

Make a borehole for the screw with an awl; then insert the Zielke screw of appropriate length with an attached blade or washer across the center of the vertebral body. At the end vertebrae, the flanges of the staples should be in the vertebral body only; they should not penetrate the normal intervertebral disc. The screws should not penetrate the intraspinal canal. The screw in the apical vertebrae should now be posterolateral, with the most proximal and distal screws being 1 cm. anterior to the apical screws. From the lateral projection the line drawn between the screw heads should form a gentle C-curve. When the spine derotates and straightens, the rod will be straight.

BB. Next, insert a flexible stainless steel threaded rod of appropriate length into the notches of each screw head. The compression mechanism of ventral derotation spondylodesis (VDS) is similar to the Harrington compression rod; it is transmitted by similar hex nuts that have a central threaded hole fitting the threads of the compression rod. The cylindrical process of the nuts is received by bilateral cuttings of the screw heads. The nuts are advanced into screw heads manually. The terminal screws are fitted with two hex nuts, one facing the other, for locking. The intervening screws are fitted with only one locking nut, facing the apex of the scoliosis. With appropriate fitting of the hex nuts into the screw heads, the threaded compression rod is tautly anchored in the screw head, checkreining it from slipping out.

Next, the derotation bar is installed by fitting its shoes upon the ends of the compression rod. Using the handle bar, the convexity of the curve is gently pulled anteriorly. Simultaneously the force on the tension screw is adjusted. Avoid sudden maneuvers because they may rupture the vertebral body or fracture the pedicle. Normal lordosis is produced by derotating the spine.

CC and **DD.** After desired derotation is achieved, the intervertebral spaces are packed with autogenous bone obtained from the resected rib and ilium. Bone graft wedges of 1 to 2 cm. are placed anteriorly; small pieces of bone graft are placed posteriorly. It is vital to have complete bone-to-bone contact, in order to ensure solid fusion. Next, the hex nuts are tightened to achieve compression correction of the scoliotic deformity. After the desired degree of correction is achieved, the screws at the end of the system are firmly locked. The threads of the proximal and distal parts of the compression rod are destroyed by a mallet and impactor; this step will ensure that the lock nuts do not unwind. The wound is closed as described in Dwyer instrumentation of the spine.

POSTOPERATIVE CARE

After routine care in the intensive care unit, removal of the chest tube and the return of bowel and bladder function, a plaster-of-Paris body jacket is applied. Cast immobilization is usually for a period of four months; this is followed by support of the spine in a TLSO for an additional six months. Solid interbody fusion should be documented by tomography before orthotic support to the spine is discontinued.

Plate 94. Anterior Instrumentation of the Spine (Thoracoabdominal Approach)

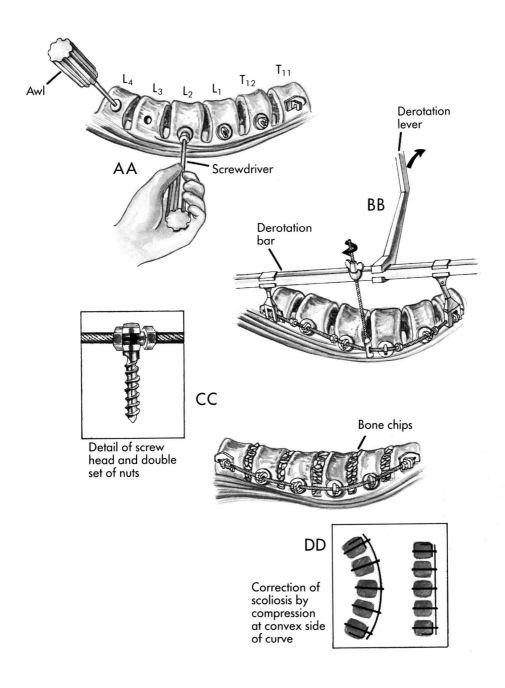

Awl

L4 L3 L2 L1 T12 T11

AA Screwdriver

Derotation lever

BB

Derotation bar

Detail of screw head and double set of nuts

CC

Bone chips

DD

Correction of scoliosis by compression at convex side of curve

ative studies should be undertaken to determine the cause of the razor-back deformity. Where is the site of angulation of the ribs? Careful clinical palpation and tangential radiographic views of the spine in the forward-bent position are of some help. If the prominence of the ribs is a few inches away from the transverse processes, a pleasing cosmetic improvement will be obtained by resection of the prominent posterior third and ends of the ribs (Fig. 6–81); however, if the main causes of razor-back deformity are rotated transverse processes and vertebral bodies with the rib angulation very close to the transverse process, improvement will be slight (Fig. 6–82). Pulmonary function

studies should be performed before advising such an operation.

The surgical approach is through the old midline spinal fusion incision with transverse lateral extensions for 3 to 4 inches along the lowest and highest rib to be resected. Resection of the supraspinous portion of the scapula is of great help in obtaining adequate access to the upper ribs. The skin, subcutaneous tissues, and deep fascia are divided in the line of incision. From the lateral border of the erector spinae muscles, parallel incisions are made along the center of each rib with a diathermy knife, the periosteum is stripped off the ribs, and the posterior inner 4 or 5 inches of each rib is

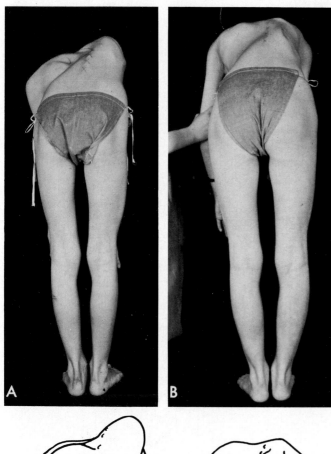

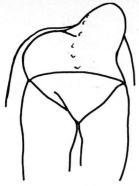
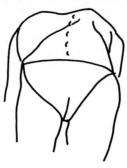

FIGURE 6–81. Forward bend photographs and sketches of patient before and after rib resection.

Note the marked improvement in razor-back deformity in severe structural scoliosis. (From Roaf, R.: Scoliosis. Baltimore, Williams & Wilkins Co., 1966. Reprinted by permission.)

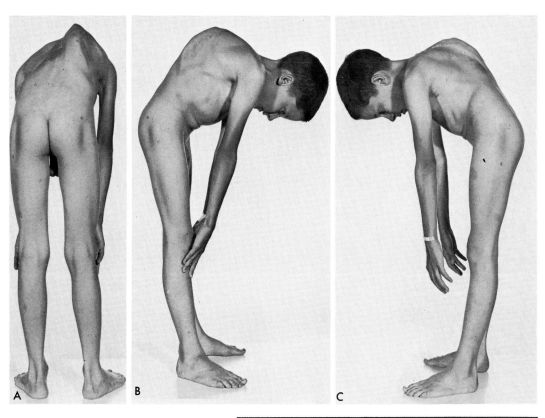

FIGURE 6–82. *Razor-back deformity in a ten-year-old boy with multiple neurofibromatosis and severe structural scoliosis.*

Note the café-au-lait spots. Spinal fusion was performed at four years of age. **A to C.** Forward bend and side views showing the severe razor-back deformity. **D.** Tangential radiogram of the spine in forward bend position. Note that the principal cause of razor-back deformity is the rotated transverse processes and the vertebral bodies with the rib angulation very close to the transverse processes. Improvement following rib and transverse process resection will be slight.

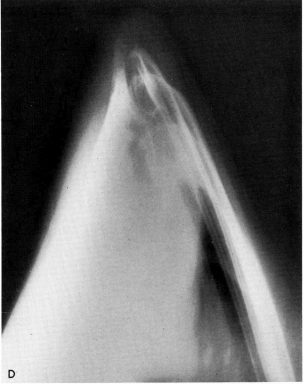

resected, including the transverse processes up to their base and the necks of the ribs up to the heads. The pleura should not be opened. Roaf recommends stabilization of the chest wall with No. 1 Mersilene sutures inserted through a hole (made with a rib punch) in each of the free ends of the resected ribs and secured to the corresponding interspinous ligaments.[633] It is desirable to drain the extrapleural space with closed-suction Hemovac drainage for a period of 24 to 48 hours. If the pleura is inadvertently opened, a separate intrapleural underwater drain is inserted, which is removed as soon as lung expansion is demonstrated in the postoperative radiograms.

Cosmetic improvement is usually satisfactory in the carefully chosen patient.

Subtotal Scapulectomy. This is indicated when there is marked protrusion of the vertebral border and prominence of the scapula. It is advisable to excise most of the blade of the scapula, because, with limited excisions, one often finds that part of the stump now appears to protrude and a further procedure is necessary.

Equalization of Apparent Lower Limb Length Inequality. If there is fixed lumbosacral scoliosis with marked tilting of the pelvis, the patient will have a noticeable list to one side. To compensate for the imbalance of the spine, the patient may stand with the knee flexed on the convex side and the ankle in equinus position on the concave side. The apparent leg length discrepancy may be corrected by a suitably built-up shoe, but many girls will not accept a raised shoe permanently. On such occasions, equalization of the apparent inequality in limb length can be achieved by epiphysiodesis at the appropriate age in a young child or by shortening of the femur over an intramedullary rod on the long side in the skeletally mature patient. The femur can also be shortened in the subtrochanteric region and internally fixed with a large blade plate. Lengthening of the tibia or the femur on the short side in a mature person is a complex procedure fraught with problems and complications. It should not be undertaken unless the patient fully understands the problem and the possible risks.

INFANTILE IDIOPATHIC SCOLIOSIS

This structural scoliosis develops in the first three years of life without evident cause. Clinically there is no neuromuscular disorder and radiologically the vertebrae are normal with no congenital or developmental abnormalities.[335]

Infantile idiopathic scoliosis is more common in boys and frequently the curve is left thoracic. The majority of the curves (about 85 per cent) are of the *resolving type*, disappearing spontaneously without treatment; 15 per cent are of the *progressive type*, increasing steadily into severe curves.[451]

Prevalence

Infantile idiopathic scoliosis is rare in North America, whereas in Europe it is relatively common. In a genetic survey of 208 patients in Boston, Massachusetts, Riseborough and Wynne-Davies found 89 per cent with adolescent curves, 10.5 per cent with juvenile curves, and 0.5 per cent with infantile curves.[616] The prevalence of infantile idiopathic scoliosis in Great Britain has markedly declined in recent years. In the four-year span from 1968 to 1971, the relative frequency, i.e., the percentage of the total number of patients with idiopathic scoliosis, was 41 per cent infantile versus 52 per cent adolescent and 7 per cent juvenile; whereas in a three-year span (1980 to 1982), the relative frequency of infantile scoliosis declined to 4 per cent versus 89 per cent adolescent and 7 per cent juvenile.[485] This change of relative frequency is most possibly the result of alteration of the position in which the infant is laid to sleep from supine to prone posture. In North America the newborn infant is commonly placed in prone position, which is an advantageous posture for the spine—as the infant cannot roll onto his side, preventing asymmetrical molding of the thorax; it also enhances early development of trunk extensor muscles. In the past, in Great Britain, the infants were placed supine and wrapped tightly in blankets. The natural tendency of the child is to roll to the right side when laid supine. This "side-lying" posture promotes plagiocephaly and plastic deformation of the skeletally immature thorax due to the influence of gravity and consequent scoliosis (Fig. 6–83). Plagiocephaly in infantile scoliosis is present in 86 per cent of the affected children and in 96 per cent of the cases under six months of age.

Axial rotation of the vertebrae can cause lateral curvature of the spine. Left thoracic scoliosis is produced by posterior vertebral rotation due to pressure from the mattress on the ribs (Fig. 6–84). The scoliosis resolves in most infants due to maturation of the central nervous system, increasing motor strength of the trunk

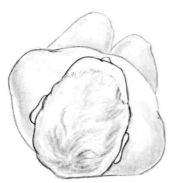

FIGURE 6–83. *Posturing molding of head and thorax in an infant who sleeps supine.*

musculature and mobility of the growing infant. If the spinal balance is irreversibly affected, the curve will progress instead of resolving.

Natural History—Prognosis

About 85 per cent of the cases of infantile scoliosis are of the resolving type and 15 per cent are of the progressive type; it is important to distinguish between the two types at an early age in order to initiate immediate treatment and prevent curve progression. Prognostic fac-

tors are rib-vertebral angle difference, age of onset, magnitude of the curve, and the presence or absence of secondary curves.

Rib-Vertebral Angle. Mehta studied the relationship between the rib and vertebral body in the thoracic region as depicted in the posteroanterior radiographs of patients with infantile structural scoliosis. On clinical and radiologic follow-up of 138 of these patients, he could distinguish the progressive from the resolving type by measuring the rib-vertebral angle difference (RVAD) of the apical vertebra of the

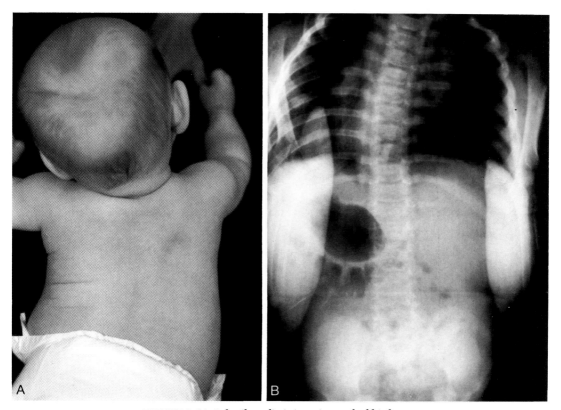

FIGURE 6–84. *Infantile scoliosis in a six-month-old infant.*

A. Photograph of the head showing plagiocephaly. **B.** Anteroposterior radiogram of spine showing scoliosis.

thoracic curve. In the normal spine, the RVAD is zero, whereas in scoliosis the ribs on the convex side of the spine are at a greater acute angle with the vertebrae than those on the concave side. In the course of progression of scoliosis, in the posteroanterior radiograph of the spine, initially the rib head does not overlap the vertebral body (Phase I); as the curve progresses the rib head overlaps the vertebral body (Phase II). In the progressive type of infantile scoliosis the rib-vertebral angle difference is greater than 20 degrees in 80 per cent of the patients; i.e., as a prognostic sign of curve progression rib-vertebral angle difference has 20 per cent inaccuracy.[497, 499] Overlap of the rib head on the vertebral body, which is caused by rotation of the curve (i.e., transition from Phase I to Phase II), is a sign of progressive type of infantile scoliosis.[497]

Age of Onset. In the study of Lloyd Roberts and Pilcher, when a curve develops during the first year of life, 92 per cent are of the resolving type.[451] In the experience of McMaster, 83 per cent of the curves that developed under one year of age resolved, whereas the curves that developed after one year of age have a poorer prognosis.[485]

Magnitude of the Curve. Curves greater than 35 degrees have a poor prognosis; they will usually progress. It should be noted, however, that a curve less than 20 degrees may also progress.

Presence of Secondary Curves. This signals a progressive type of infantile scoliosis.

Association With Developmental Anomalies. Connor has shown that the progressive type of infantile scoliosis has a higher incidence of associated developmental anomalies.[148]

Diagnosis

A meticulous neuromuscular examination is performed in order to rule out congenital hypotonia and other neurologic disorders. Radiographs are carefully scrutinized for the presence of congenital abnormalities such as unilateral unsegmented bars, which may not be visible in the plain radiographs because they are cartilaginous; it may take several years for these to ossify. Diagnosis of idiopathic infantile scoliosis is made by exclusion.

Treatment

Resolving infantile scoliosis is observed by clinical examination and radiographs of the spine performed every three to six months. No active treatment is indicated. It is strongly recommended that the infant be in prone posture when sleeping. Side-bending and head or arm suspension-distraction passive exercises are performed several times a day. Most of the resolving curves disappear by one or two years of age. Occasionally a resolving curve straightens slowly and does not fully correct until the child is eight years old. Lateral angulation straightens first; vertebral rotation resolves last. Once scoliosis has resolved, follow-up examinations are made at yearly intervals.

Occasionally a child with fully straightened resolving infantile scoliosis may develop scoliosis in adolescence.

Progressive infantile scoliosis requires immediate treatment as almost all of these curves will exceed 70 degrees and by the age of 10 years the majority will progress to more than 100 degrees.[393] The end result is a very deformed thoracic spine with an ugly unacceptable cosmetic appearance and cardiorespiratory embarrassment with cor pulmonale.

Nonoperative measures should be tried first; the objective is to control curve progression until sufficient skeletal growth is attained when spinal fusion is performed. It should be explained to the parents that spinal fusion will eventually be required. The reason for the delay in definitive treatment by spinal arthrodesis is to prevent a short vertebral column and trunk. Also, it should be clear to the parents that a short straight spine is better than a shorter curved one; i.e., when progression of scoliosis cannot be controlled nonoperatively, surgical measures should be employed.

It is difficult to fit a Milwaukee brace on an infant or a small chubby child; therefore, first a Risser scoliosis cast is applied using longitudinal traction and lateral pressure over the apex of the curve to correct the scoliosis. This is best done under general anesthesia. The cast is changed at two- to three-month intervals. With such serial plaster cast applications, moderate flexible curves can be fully corrected; however, correction of severe rigid curves is only partial—total correction is not possible.

Next the child is fitted with a Milwaukee CTLSO, which is worn full-time and then part-time until age 12 to 14 years as long as curve progression can be controlled. When a curve is fully corrected by the prepubertal growth spurt there is a good chance that it will not relapse during adolescence, whereas curves that cannot be fully corrected will relapse.[499]

Surgical treatment is indicated in curves that cannot be controlled by serial casts and orthotic treatment (Fig. 6–85). In children, flexible curves (as shown by traction and lateral bend-

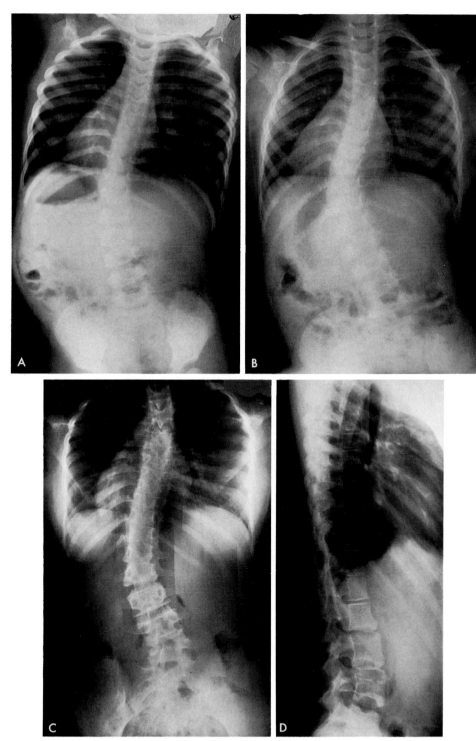

FIGURE 6–85. Infantile structural idiopathic left thoracolumbar scoliosis.

A. Anteroposterior standing radiogram of the spine at one and a half years. **B.** At three years of age. Note progression of the curve. Treatment consisted of intermittent use of a Risser localizer cast, which did not prevent progression of the scoliosis. Spinal fusion of the fifth dorsal to the second lumbar vertebrae, inclusive, was performed to stabilize the spine. **C** and **D.** Anteroposterior and lateral radiograms of the spine 11 years postoperatively at age 14 years. Stability and correction of the spine have been maintained, but note the retarded growth of the fused vertebrae.

ing) are treated by Harrington instrumentation without fusion. The distraction rod is placed within the paraspinal muscle or subcutaneously on the concave side. Subperiosteal exposure should not be performed because of the possibility of partial fusion on the concave side. Repeated distractions at intervals over a period of several years are carried out in an attempt to achieve maximal correction and to delay spinal fusion until a suitable skeletal age. Instrument failure, however, may necessitate earlier fusion.

Rigid curves are treated by posterior fusion. During the adolescent growth spurt a solidly fused spine can lose correction; therefore, be-

tween the ages of 10 to 14 years, it is good judgment to support these spines with a Milwaukee brace.

JUVENILE IDIOPATHIC SCOLIOSIS

One sixth to one eighth of idiopathic scoliosis cases develop between the ages of four and ten years. It is more common in girls than in boys. A scoliosis with its onset in infancy may be detected in a four- or five-year-old child, making it difficult to distinguish infantile from early juvenile scoliosis; also, many cases of adolescent

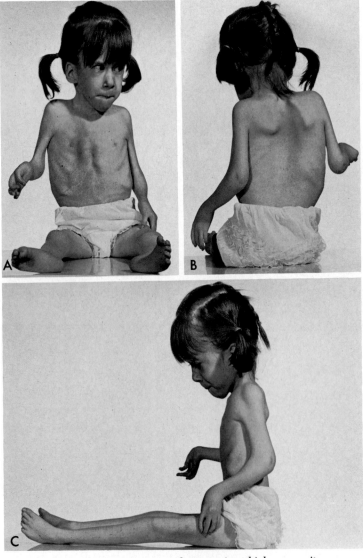

FIGURE 6–86. *Scoliosis in arthrogryposis multiplex congenita.*

A to C. Anterior, posterior, and lateral views of a three-year-old child with severe arthrogryposis multiplex congenita. Note the severe contractural deformities, hydrocephalus, and right thoracolumbar scoliosis. There is marked dorsal lordosis and decrease of anteroposterior diameter of the chest.

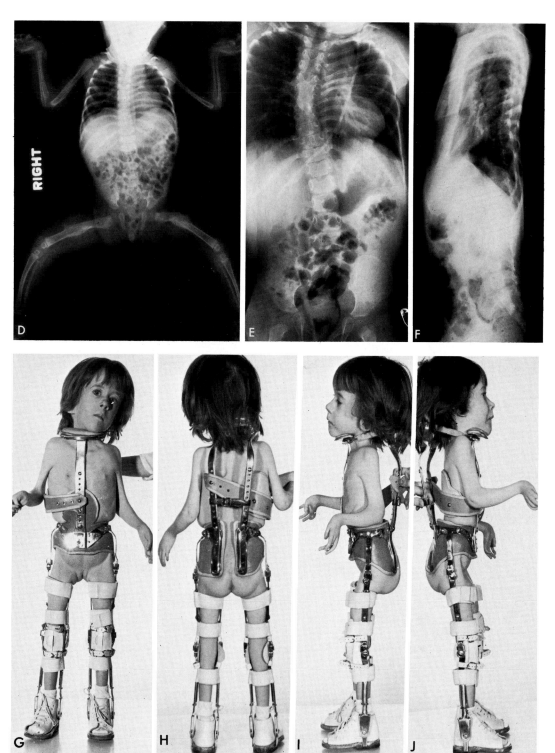

FIGURE 6–86 Continued. Scoliosis in arthrogyposis multiplex congenita.

D. Radiograms of spine, depicting the scoliosis at three months of age. **E** and **F.** Radiograms of spine, anteroposterior and lateral, at 18 months of age showing the increased scoliosis and the severe dorsal lordosis. **G** to **J.** Views of child in Milwaukee brace (old type). A chin guard was added to control rotation of neck. Long leg orthoses are used for ambulation.

scoliosis develop in children under ten years of age. A right thoracic curve is the more common curve pattern; next in frequency is a double curve pattern and then lumbar curves.

Treatment

It is vital to observe the patient closely for curve progression. Curves beyond 20 degrees require orthotic treatment. Approximately one half of the cases can be managed conservatively.

Surgical treatment is indicated when curve progression cannot be controlled by orthosis.[256, 736]

PARALYTIC SCOLIOSIS

This is encountered in cerebral palsy, spinal muscular atrophy, myelomeningocele, arthrogryposis multiplex congenita, and muscular dystrophy. The management of the spine in these various neuromuscular disorders is discussed in their appropriate sections. An illustrative case of scoliosis in arthrogryposis multiplex congenita is shown in Figure 6–86.

SCOLIOSIS IN NEUROFIBROMATOSIS

This is discussed in the section on neurofibromatosis. It is important to differentiate the dystrophic and nondystrophic curves. The former is treated like an idiopathic curve. The dystrophic scoliosis in neurofibromatosis progresses with nonoperative care and requires surgical management. Scoliotic curves with mild kyphosis are treated with posterior fusion, whereas those scoliotic curves with kyphosis greater than 50 degrees are stabilized by combined anterior and posterior fusion. Association with neurofibromas requires decompression and laminectomy followed by fusion. Failure to arthrodese the spine will result in severe kyphotic deformity and progressive neurologic deficit.

POSTIRRADIATION SCOLIOSIS

Radiation of the area of the spine for conditions such as Wilms' tumor or neuroblastoma may affect growth of the vertebral column asymmetrically, producing scoliosis.[33, 412, 774] In the young child, if the curve is flexible, the use of the Milwaukee brace is indicated; however, if progression cannot be controlled by conservative measures, early surgical fusion is required.

SCOLIOSIS IN THE MANAGEMENT OF BONE DYSPLASIAS

This is described in Chapter 3.

References

1. Aaro, S., and Berg, U.: The immediate effect of Boston brace on renal function in patients with idiopathic scoliosis. Clin. Orthop., *170*:243, 1982.
2. Aaro, S., and Dahlborn, M.: Vertebral rotation—estimation of vertebral rotation and spinal and rib cage deformity in scoliosis by computerized tomography. Spine, *6*:460, 1981.
3. Aaro, S., and Dahlborn, M.: The effect of Harrington instrumentation on the longitudinal axis rotation of the apical vertebra and on the spinal and rib-cage deformity in idiopathic scoliosis studied by computer tomography. Spine, *7*:456, 1982.
4. Aaro, S., and Ohlen, G.: The effect of Harrington instrumentation on the sagittal configuration and mobility of the spine in scoliosis. Spine, *8*:570, 1983.
5. Aaro, S., Burstrom, R., and Dahlborn, M.: The derotating effect of the Boston brace: A comparison between computer tomography and a conventional method. Spine, *6*:477, 1981.
6. Abbott, E. G.: Correction of lateral curvature of the spine. N.Y. Med. J., *95*:833, 1912.
7. Abbott, E. V.: Screening for scoliosis. A worthwhile preventive measure. Can. J. Pub. Health, *68*:22, 1977.
8. Abott, T. R., and Bentley, G.: Intra-operative awakening during scoliosis surgery. Anaesthesia, *35*:298, 1980.
9. Adair, I. V., Van Wijik, M. L., and Armstrong, G. W. D.: Moire topography in scoliosis screening. Clin. Orthop., *129*:165, 1978.
10. Adams, W.: Lectures on the Pathology and Treatment of Lateral and Other Forms of Curvature of the Spine. London, Churchill & Sons, 1865.
11. Agaiti, G., and Rastel Bogin, P.: Radiological aspects of scoliosis and kyphosis during growth stage. Minerva Pediatr., *32*:171, 1980.
12. Agostini, S., Taglialavoro, G., Fabris, D., Mammano, S., and Ferraro, C.: Relationship between rib hump deformity and vertebral rotation in idiopathic scoliosis. Ital. J. Orthop. Traumatol., *9*:387, 1983.
13. Akbarnia, B. A., and Rooholamini, S. A.: Scoliosis caused by benign osteoblastoma of the thoracic or lumbar spine. J. Bone Joint Surg., *63*-A:1146, 1981.
14. Akbarnia, B. A., Keppler, L., Price, E. A., and Gotz, T.: Lateral electrical surface stimulation (LESS) for the treatment of adolescent idiopathic scoliosis (AIS). An analysis based on progression risk. Orthop. Trans., *10*:3, 1986.
15. Alexander, M. A., and Season, E. H.: Idiopathic scoliosis: An electromyographic study. Arch. Phys. Med. Rehabil., *59*:314, 1978.
16. Alexander, R. G.: The effects of tooth position and maxillofacial vertical growth during treatment of scoliosis with the Milwaukee brace. Am. J. Orthod., *52*:161, 1966.
17. Allan, F. G.: Scoliosis operative correction of fixed curves. J. Bone Joint Surg., *37*-B:92, 1955.
18. Allen, B. L., Jr.: Segmental spinal instrumentation. A.A.O.S. Instr. Course Lect., *32*:202, 1983.
19. Allen, B. L., Jr.: Segmental instrumentation of the spine—indications, results and complications. *In* Dickson, R., and Bradford, D. (eds.): Management of Spinal Deformities. London, Butterworth, 1984. pp. 162–192.

20. Allen, B. L., Jr., and Ferguson, R. L.: The Galveston technique for L rod instrumentation of the scoliotic spine. Spine, 7:276, 1982.

21. American Orthopaedic Association Research Committee: End result study of the treatment of idiopathic scoliosis. J. Bone Joint Surg., 23:963, 1941.

22. Andersen, P. E., Jr., Andersen, P. E., and van der Kooy, P.: Dose reduction in radiography of the spine in scoliosis. Acta Radiol. (Diagn.), 23:251, 1982.

23. Anderson, M., Hwan, S., and Green, W. T.: Growth of the normal trunk in boys and girls during the second decade of life. J. Bone Joint Surg., 47-A:1554, 1965.

24. André, N.: L'Orthopaedia, ou l'Art de Prévenir et de Corriger dans les Enfants les Deformités du Corps. Paris, 1741.

25. Andrews, T., and Piggott, H.: Growth arrest for progressive scoliosis. Combined anterior and posterior fusion of the convexity. J. Bone Joint Surg., 67-B:193, 1985.

26. Andriacchi, T. P., Schultz, A. B., Belytschko, T. B., and DeWald, R. L.: Milwaukee brace correction of idiopathic scoliosis. J. Bone Joint Surg., 58-A:806, 1976.

27. Angevine, J. B.: Clinically relevant embryology of the vertebral column and spinal cord. Clin. Neurosurg., 20:95, 1973.

28. Apter, A., Morein, G., Munitz, H., Tyano, S., Maoz, B., and Wijsenbeck, H.: The psychosocial sequelae of the Milwaukee brace in adolescent girls. Clin. Orthop., 131:156, 1978.

29. Archer, I. A., and Dickson, R. A.: Stature and idiopathic scoliosis. A prospective study. J. Bone Joint Surg., 67-B:185, 1985.

30. Ardran, G. M., and Dickson, R. A.: Reduction of radiation exposure during radiography for scoliosis (letter). J. Bone Joint Surg., 65-A:1206, 1983.

31. Ardran, G. M., Coates, R., Dickson, R. A., Dixon-Brown, A., and Harding, F. M.: Assessment of scoliosis in children: Low dose radiographic technique. Br. J. Radiol., 53:146, 1980.

32. Arkin, A. M.: The mechanism of rotation in combination with lateral deviation in the normal spine. J. Bone Joint Surg., 32-A:180, 1950.

33. Arkin, A. M., and Simon, N.: Radiation scoliosis—an experimental study. J. Bone Joint Surg., 32-A:396, 1950.

34. Armstrong, G. W. D., and Connock, S. H. G.: A transverse loading system applied to a modified Harrington instrumentation. Clin. Orthop., 108:70, 1975.

35. Armstrong, G. W. D., Livermore, N. B., Suzuki, N., and Armstrong, J. G.: Nonstandard vertebral rotation in scoliosis screening patients: Its prevalence and relation to the clinical deformity. Spine, 7:50, 1982.

36. Ascani, E., Giglio, G. C., and Pagnotta, G.: Strumentazione precoce delle scoliosi infantili senza arthrodesi. Prog. Patol. Vertebrale, 3:247, 1980.

37. Asher, M. A.: Non-operative treatment of scoliosis. *In* Dickson, J. H. (ed.): Spinal Deformities, Vol. 1, No. 2. Philadelphia, Hanley & Belfus, 1987, p. 213.

38. Asher, M., and Whitney, W.: Orthotics for spinal deformity. *In* Redford, J. S. (ed.): Orthotics. 3rd Ed. Baltimore, Williams & Wilkins, 1986, pp. 153–197.

39. Asher, M., Greene, P., and Orrick, J.: A six year report. Spinal deformity screening in Kansas school children. J. Kans. Med. Soc., 81:568, 1980.

40. Ashworth, M. A., and Ersil, A. U.: The measurement of rib hump inclination—a potential aid in scoliosis screening. Orthop. Trans., 5:33, 1981.

41. Ashworth, M. A., Loewe, P. J., and Bryant, J. T.: A force-indicating spreader. Spine, 7:80, 1982.

42. Aulisa, L., Bartolini, F., Tamburrelli, F., and Valassina, A.: Early diagnosis of scoliosis: Methodologic problems. Arch. Putti Chir. Organi Mov., 32:129, 1982.

43. Avikainen, V. J., and Vaherto, H.: A high incidence of spinal curvature. A study of 100 female students. Acta Orthop. Scand., 54:267, 1983.

44. Axelgaard, J., and Brown, J. C.: Lateral electrical surface stimulation for the treatment of progressive idiopathic scoliosis. Spine, 8:242, 1983.

45. Axelgaard, J., Brown, J. C., and Swank, S.: Scoliosis treatment by lateral electrical surface stimulation. Orthop. Trans., 6:17, 1982.

46. Axelgaard, J., Nordwall, A., and Brown, J. C.: Correction of spinal curvatures by transcutaneous electrical muscle stimulation. Spine, 8:463, 1983.

47. Axelgaard, J., Brown, J. C., Hardya, Y., McNeal, D., and Nordwall, A.: Lateral stimulation for correction of scoliosis. Orthop. Trans., 2:267, 1978.

48. Bachmann, M.: Die Varanderungen des Innern Organe bei Hochgradiger Skoliosen und Kyphoskoliosen. Stuttgart, 1899.

49. Bampfield, R. W.: An Essay on Curvatures and Diseases of the Spine, Including All the Forms of Spinal Distortion. London, Longman, Hurst, Rees, Orme, Brown & Greene, 1824.

50. Bancet, P., Kallin, A., Hall, J., and Dubousset, J.: The Boston brace: Results of a clinical and radiologic study of 401 patients. Orthop. Trans., 8:33, 1984.

51. Barnes, J.: Rib resection in infantile idiopathic scoliosis. J. Bone Joint Surg., 61-B:31, 1979.

52. Barry, O. C., McManus, F., and Walshe, M.: Short term results of Cotrel traction in the treatment of idiopathic scoliosis. Ir. J. Med. Sci., 152:279, 1983.

53. Bartal, E., and Gage, J. R.: Idiopathic juvenile osteoporosis and scoliosis. J. Pediatr. Orthop., 2:295, 1982.

54. Bassett, G. S., and Bunnell, W. P.: Effect of a thoracolumbosacral orthosis in lateral trunk shift in idiopathic scoliosis. J. Pediatr. Orthop., 6:182, 1986.

55. Bassett, G. S., Bunnell, W. P., and MacEwen, G. D.: Treatment of idiopathic scoliosis with the Wilmington brace. Results in patients with a 20 to 39 degree curve. J. Bone Joint Surg., 68-A:602, 1986.

56. Bellyei, A., Czeizel, A., Barta, O., Nagda, T., and Molnar, L.: Prevalence of adolescent idiopathic scoliosis in Hungary. Acta Orthop. Scand., 48:177, 1977.

57. Belstead, J. S., and Edgar, M. A.: Early detection of scoliosis. Br. Med. J., 2:937, 1978.

58. Bengtsson, G., Fallstrom, K., Jansson, B., and Nachemson, A.: A psychological and psychiatric investigation of the adjustment of female scoliosis patients. Acta Psychiatr. Scand., 50:50, 1974.

59. Berg, U., and Aaro, S.: Long-term effect of Boston brace treatment on renal function in patients with idiopathic scoliosis. Clin. Orthop., 180:169, 1983.

60. Bergofsky, E. H., Turino, G. M., and Fishman, A. P.: Cardiorespiratory failure in kyphoscoliosis. Medicine, 38:263, 1959.

61. Bjerkreim, I., and Hassan, I.: Progression in untreated idiopathic scoliosis after the end of growth. Acta Orthop. Scand., 53:897, 1982.

62. Bernard, T. N., Jr., Johnston, C. E., II., Roberts, J. M., and Burke, S. W.: Late complications due to wire breakage in segmental spinal instrumentation. Report of two cases. J. Bone Joint Surg., 65-A:1339, 1983.

63. Bernstein, A., and Warner, G.: Onset of anorexia nervosa after prolonged use of the Milwaukee brace. Psychosomatics, 24:1033, 1983.

64. Bernstein, E.: Screening of school children for scoliosis (abstract). Acta Orthop. Scand., 53:312, 1982.

65. Bernstein, E., and Risgaard-Petersen, B.: Screening of school children for scoliosis. Examination of the back with Moire's topography and controlled forward bending test. Ugeskr. Laeger, 143:3373, 1981.

66. Bick, M., Copel, J. W., and Spector, S.: Longitudinal

growth of the human vertebra. J. Bone Joint Surg., 32-A:803, 1950.

67. Bigg, R. H.: Spinal Curvature. London, Churchill, 1882.
68. Bigos, S., Nachemson, A., Wortley, M. C., Anden, S., and Zeh, J.: Boston brace system for adolescent idiopathic scoliosis: A report of 111 cases followed for a minimum of 18 months. Orthop. Trans., 8:148, 1984.
69. Binstadt, D. H., Lonstein, J. E., and Winter, R. B.: Radiographic evaluation of the scoliotic patient. Minn. Med., 61:474, 1978.
70. Biscoping, J., and Weber, U.: Pulmonary complications following Harrington's operation. Z. Orthop., 121:741, 1983.
71. Bisgard, J. D.: Experimental thoracogenic scoliosis. J. Thorac. Surg., 4:435, 1935.
72. Bisgard, J. D., and Musselman, M. M.: Scoliosis. Its experimental production and growth; growth and fusion of vertebral bodies. Surg. Gynecol. Obstet., 70:1029, 1940.
73. Bjerkreim, I., and Hassan, I.: Progression in untreated idiopathic scoliosis after end of growth. Acta Orthop. Scand., 53:897, 1982.
74. Bjerkreim, I., Carlson, B., and Korsell, E.: Preoperative Cotrel traction in idiopathic scoliosis. Acta Orthop. Scand., 53:901, 1982.
75. Bjure, J., and Nachemson, A.: Non-treated scoliosis. Clin. Orthop., 93:44, 1973.
76. Blount, W. P.: Scoliosis and the Milwaukee brace. Bull. Hosp. Joint Dis., 19:152, 1958.
77. Blount, W. P.: Non-operative treatment of scoliosis. In A.A.O.S. Symposium on the Spine. St. Louis, Mosby, 1967, pp. 188–195.
78. Blount, W. P.: Use of the Milwaukee brace. Orthop. Clin. North Am., 3:3, 1972.
79. Blount, W. P.: The virtue of early treatment of idiopathic scoliosis (editorial). J. Bone Joint Surg., 63-A:335, 1981.
80. Blount, W. P., and Bidwell, T. R.: The Milwaukee brace principles and fabrication. In A.A.O.S. Atlas of Orthotics. St. Louis, Mosby, 1975.
81. Blount, W. P., and Bolinske, J.: Physical therapy in the non-operative treatment of scoliosis. Phys. Ther. Rev., 47:919, 1967.
82. Blount, W. P., and Mellencamp, D. D.: The effect of pregnancy on idiopathic scoliosis. J. Bone Joint Surg., 62-A:1083, 1980.
83. Blount, W. P., and Moe, J. H.: The Milwaukee Brace. 2nd. Ed. Baltimore, Williams & Wilkins, 1980.
84. Blount, W. P., and Schmidt, A. C.: The Milwaukee brace in the treatment of scoliosis. J. Bone Joint Surg., 39-A:693, 1957.
85. Blount, W. P., and Schmidt, A. C.: The Milwaukee brace in the treatment of scoliosis. J. Bone Joint Surg., 56-A:442, 1974.
86. Blount, W. P., Schmidt, A. C., and Bidwell, R. G.: Making the Milwaukee brace. J. Bone Joint Surg., 40-A:528, 1958.
87. Blount, W. P., Schmidt, A. C., Keever, E. D., and Leonard, E. T.: The Milwaukee brace in the operative treatment of scoliosis. J. Bone Joint Surg., 40-A:511, 1958.
88. Board, R.: Radiography of the scoliotic spine. Radiol. Technol., 38:219, 1967.
89. Bobechko, W. P., Herbert, M. A., and Friedman, H. G.: Electrospinal instrumentation for scoliosis: Current status. Orthop. Clin. North Am., 10:927, 1979.
90. Bonnett, C. A., and Tosoonian, R.: Results of Milwaukee brace treatment in seventy patients. Orthop. Rev., 7:79, 1978.
91. Bradford, D. S.: Anterior spinal surgery in the management of scoliosis—indications, techniques, results. Orthop. Clin. North Am., 10:801, 1979.

92. Bradford, D. S.: Techniques of surgery. In Bradford, D. S., Lonstein, J. E., Ogilvie, J. W., and Winter, R. B. (eds.): Moe's Textbook of Scoliosis and Other Spinal Deformities. Philadelphia, Saunders, 1987, p. 135.
93. Bradford, D. S., and Hensinger, R. W.: Pediatric Spine. New York and Stuttgart, Thieme, 1985.
94. Bradford, D. S., Tanguy, A., and Vanselow, J.: Surface electrical stimulation of idiopathic scoliosis: Preliminary results in 30 patients. Spine, 8:757, 1983.
95. Bradford, E. H.: Trans. Am. Orthop. Assoc., 3:125, 1890.
96. Bremberg, S., and Nilsson-Berggren, B.: School screening for adolescent idiopathic scoliosis. J. Pediatr. Orthop., 6:564, 1986.
97. Brinckman, P., Horst, M., and Polster, J.: Preoperative halo-gravity traction in scoliosis (author's transl.). Z. Orthop., 118:367, 1980.
98. Brown, C., Odom, J., Donaldson, D., and Tiefel, L.: Preliminary results of the treatment of scoliosis with an electrospinal orthosis. Orthop. Trans., 7:9, 1983.
99. Brown, J., Axelgaard, J., and Howson, D.: Multicenter trial of a noninvasive stimulation method for idiopathic scoliosis. Spine, 9:382, 1984.
100. Brown, M. P.: Segmental spinal instrumentation with the Harrington rod. Paper presented at the 17th Annual Meeting of Scoliosis Research Society, Denver, 1982.
101. Brown, R. A., and Nash, C. L.: Three-dimensional radiographic evaluation of spinal deformity. Paper presented at the 17th Annual Meeting of the Scoliosis Research Society, Denver, 1982.
102. Bunch, W. B.: Orthodontic positioner treatment during orthopedic treatment of scoliosis. Am. J. Orthod., 47:174, 1961.
103. Bunch, W. H., and Chapman, R. G.: Patient preference in surgery for scoliosis. J. Bone Joint Surg., 67-A:794, 1985.
104. Bunch, W. H., and Keagy, R. D.: Principles of Orthotic Treatment. St. Louis, Mosby, 1976.
105. Bunnell, W. P.: Treatment of idiopathic scoliosis. Orthop. Clin. North Am., 10:813, 1979.
106. Bunnell, W. P.: The angle of trunk rotation: An objective criterion for spinal screening. Paper presented at the 18th Annual Meeting of the Scoliosis Research Society, New Orleans, September, 1983.
107. Bunnell, W. P.: An objective criterion for scoliosis screening. J. Bone Joint Surg., 66-A:1381, 1984.
108. Bunnell, W. P.: Vertebral rotation—a simple method of measurement in routine radiographs. Orthop. Trans., 9:114, 1985.
109. Bunnell, W. P., MacEwen, G. D., and Jayakumar, S.: The use of plastic jackets in the non-operative treatment of idiopathic scoliosis. J. Bone Joint Surg., 62-A:31, 1980.
110. Buric, M., and Momcilovic, B.: Growth pattern and skeletal age in school girls with idiopathic scoliosis. Clin. Orthop., 170:238, 1982.
111. Burrington, J. D., Brown, C., Wayne, E. R., and Odom, J.: Anterior approach to the thoracolumbar spine: Technical considerations. Arch. Surg., 111:456, 1976.
112. Burwell, R. G., Dangerfield, P. H., and Vernon, C. L.: Anthropometry and scoliosis. In Zorab, P. A. (ed.): Scoliosis: Proceedings of the Fifth Symposium Held at the Cardiothoracic Institute, Brompton Hospital, London, September, 1976. London, Academic, 1977, pp. 123–164.
113. Burwell, R. G., Dangerfield, P. H., and Vernon, C. L.: Bone asymmetry and joint laxity in the upper limbs of children with adolescent idiopathic scoliosis. Ann. R. Coll. Surg., 63:209, 1981.
114. Burwell, R. G., Webb, J. K., and Moore, E. J.: School screening for scoliosis (letter). Lancet, 2:863, 1981.

115. Burwell, R. G., James, N. J., Johnson, F., and Webb, J. K.: The rib hump score: A guide to referral and prognosis? J. Bone Joint Surg., *64-B*:248, 1982.

116. Burwell, R. G., James, N. J., Johnson, F., Webb, J. K., and Wilson, Y. G.: Standardized trunk asymmetry scores. A study of back contour in healthy school children. J. Bone Joint Surg., *65-B*:452, 1983.

117. Burwell, R. G., Manning, C. W., Elves, M. W., Ali, S. Y., and Sayers, D. C. J.: A new method for studying the metabolic activity of the iliac crest growth-plate: Its relevance to scoliosis. J. Bone Joint Surg., *55-B*:428, 1973.

118. Burwell, R. G., Dangerfield, P. H., James, N. J., Johnson, F., Webb, J. K., and Wilson, Y. G.: Antropometric studies of normal and scoliotic children: Axial and appendicular skeletal asymmetry, sexual dimorphisms and age related changes. In Jacobs, R. R. (ed.): Pathogenesis of Idiopathic Scoliosis: Proceedings of an International Conference. Chicago, Scoliosis Research Society, 1984, pp. 27–44.

119. Burwell, W. P.: An objective criterion for scoliosis screening. J. Bone Joint Surg., *66-A*:1381, 1984.

120. Bushell, G. R., Ghosh, P., and Taylor, T. F.: Collagen defect in idiopathic scoliosis. Lancet, *2*:94, 1978.

121. Butterworth, T. R., Jr., and James, C.: Electromyographic studies in idiopathic scoliosis. South. Med. J., *62*:1008, 1969.

122. Calliet, R.: Scoliosis: Diagnosis and Management. Philadelphia, Davis, 1979.

123. Callis, D. K., and Ponseti, I. V.: Long-term follow-up of patients with idiopathic scoliosis not treated surgically. J. Bone Joint Surg., *51-A*:425, 1969.

124. Calot, F.: L'Orthopédie Indispensible aux Practiciens. Paris, Meloine, 1923.

125. Calvo, J. J.: Observations on the growth of the female adolescent spine and its relation to scoliosis. Clin. Orthop., *10*:40, 1957.

126. Cardoso, M. A., and Luque, E. R.: Instrumentacio segmentaria. Desarrollo de una tecnica. An. Ortop. Traumatol., *14*:2, 1978.

127. Carman, D., Roach, J. W., Speck, G., Wenger, D. R., and Herring, J. A.: Role of exercise in the Milwaukee brace treatment of scoliosis. J. Pediatr. Orthop., *5*:65, 1985.

128. Carr, W. A., Moe, J. H., Winter, R. B., and Lonstein, J. E.: Treatment of idiopathic scoliosis in the Milwaukee brace. J. Bone Joint Surg., *62-A*:599, 1980.

129. Cauchoix, J., and Binet, J. P.: Anterior approaches to the spine. Ann. R. Coll. Surg., *21*:237, 1956.

130. Ceballos, R., Ferrer-Torrelles, M., Castillo, F., and Fernandez-Paredes, E.: Prognosis in infantile idiopathic scoliosis. J. Bone Joint Surg., *62-A*:863, 1980.

131. Chan, F. L., and Chow, S. P.: Retroperitoneal fibrosis after anterior spinal fusion. Clin. Radiol., *34*:331, 1983.

132. Chmiel, J., Suszka, B., Pretczak, J., Ignatowicz, E., and Blazejewska, B.: Urinary glycosaminoglycans in children with idiopathic scoliosis. Chir. Narzadow Ruchu Ortop. Pol., *45*:37, 1980.

133. Chong, K. C., Letts, R. M., and Cumming, G. R.: Influence of spinal curvature on exercise capacity. J. Pediatr. Orthop., *1*:251, 1981.

134. Chopin, D., Briard, J. L., and Seringe, R.: Surgery for thoracic deformity in scoliosis. In Zorab, P. A., and Siegler, D. (eds.): Scoliosis, 1979. London, Academic, 1980, pp. 161–168.

135. Clarisse, P. H.: Prognostic evolutif des scolioses idiopathiques mineures de 10 degrees à 29 degrees, en periode de croissance. Thesis. Lyons, France, 1974.

136. Clark, S., Harrison, A., and Zorab, P. A.: One year's study of growth and total hydroxyproline excretion in scoliotic children. Arch. Dis. Child., *55*:467, 1980.

137. Cobb, J. R.: The treatment of scoliosis. Conn. Med. J., *7*:467, 1943.

138. Cobb, J. R.: Outline for the study of scoliosis. A.A.O.S. Instr. Course Lect., *5*:261, 1948.

139. Cobb, J. R.: Technique, after-treatment, and results of spine fusion for scoliosis. A.A.O.S. Instr. Course Lect., *9*:65, 1952.

140. Cobb, J. R.: Correction of scoliosis. In Poliomyelitis, Second International Poliomyelitis Congress. Philadelphia, Lippincott, 1953.

141. Cobb, J. R.: Spine arthrodesis in the treatment of scoliosis. Bull. Hosp. Joint Dis., *19*:187, 1958.

142. Cobb, J. R.: The problem of primary curve. J. Bone Joint Surg., *42-A*:1413, 1960.

143. Cochran, G. V. B., and Waugh, T. R.: The external forces in correction of idiopathic scoliosis. J. Bone Joint Surg., *51-A*:201, 1969.

144. Cochran, T., and Nachemson, A.: Long-term anatomic and functional changes in patients with adolescent idiopathic scoliosis treated with the Milwaukee brace. Spine, *10*:127, 1985.

145. Coetsier, M., Vercauteren, M., and Moerman, P.: A new radiographic method for measuring vertebral rotation in scoliosis. Acta Orthop. Belg., *43*:598, 1977.

146. Colletta, A. J., and Mayer, P. J.: Chylothorax: An unusual complication of anterior thoracic interbody spinal fusion. Spine, *7*:46, 1982.

147. Collis, D. K., and Ponseti, I. V.: Long-term follow-up of patients with idiopathic scoliosis not treated surgically. J. Bone Joint Surg., *51-A*:425, 1967.

148. Conner, A. N.: Developmental anomalies and prognosis in infantile idiopathic scoliosis. J. Bone Joint Surg., *51-B*:711, 1969.

149. Cooke, E. D., Carter, L. M., and Pilcher, M. F.: Identifying scoliosis in the adolescent with thermography: A preliminary study. Clin. Orthop., *148*:172, 1980.

150. Coonrad, R. W., and Feierstein, M. S.: Progression of scoliosis in the adult. J. Bone Joint Surg., *58-A*:156, 1976.

151. Cotrel, Y.: Correction-arthrodèse des scolioses graves par élongation pré-opératoire et greffon cortical encastré. Paper presented at the 40th Reunion Soc. Franc. Orthop., Paris, 1965.

152. Cotrel, Y.: Techniques nouvelles dans le traitement de la scoliose idiopathique. Int. Orthop., *1*:247, 1968.

153. Cotrel, Y.: Le corset de platre E.D.F. dans le traitement de la scoliose idiopathique. Med. Hyg., *28*:1032, 1970.

154. Cotrel, Y.: A new technique of correction and fusion. Isr. J. Med. Sci., *9*:759, 1973.

155. Cotrel, Y.: Traction in the treatment of vertebral deformity. J. Bone Joint Surg., *57-B*:260, 1975.

156. Cotrel, Y., and D'Amore, M.: Spinal traction in scoliosis. In Zorab, P. A. (ed.): Proceedings of a Second Symposium on Scoliosis. London, Livingstone, 1968, pp. 37–43.

157. Cotrel, Y., and Dubousset, J.: New segmental posterior instrumentation of the spine. Orthop. Trans., *9*:118, 1985.

158. Cotrel, Y., and Morel, G.: La technique de l'EDF dans la correction des scoliosis. Rev. Chir. Orthop., *50*:59, 1964.

159. Cotrel, Y., Seringe Plais, P. Y., and Palvzak, M.: Spinal traction in scoliosis. In Zorab, P. A., and Siegler, D. (eds.): Scoliosis 1979. New York, Academic, 1980.

160. Cowell, H. R., Hall, J. N., and MacEwen, G. D.: Genetic aspects of idiopathic scoliosis. Clin. Orthop., *86*:121, 1972.

161. Cronis, S., and Gleeson, A. W.: Orthopedic screening of school children in Delaware. Phys. Ther., *54*:1080, 1974.

162. Cronis, A., and Russell, A. Y.: Orthopaedic screening of children in Delaware public schools. Del. Med. J., *37*:89, 1965.

163. Cummine, J. L., Lonstein, J. E., Moe, J. H., Winter, R. B., and Bradford, D. S.: Reconstructive surgery in the adult for failed scoliosis fusion. J. Bone Joint Surg., 61-A:1151, 1979.

164. Curtis, R. C., Dickson, J. H., Harrington, P. R., and Wendell, D. E.: Results of Harrington instrumentation in the treatment of severe scoliosis. Clin. Orthop., 144:128, 1979.

165. Daruwalla, J. S., and Balasubramaniam, P.: Moire topography in scoliosis. Its accuracy in detecting the site and size of the curve. J. Bone Joint Surg., 67-B:211, 1985.

166. Daruwalla, J. S., Balasubramaniam, P., Chay, S. O., Rajan, U., and Lee, H. P.: Idiopathic scoliosis. Prevalence and ethnic distribution in Singapore school children. J. Bone Joint Surg., 67-B:182, 1985.

167. Daruwalla, J. S., Balasubramaniam, P., Tay, C. K., Chay, S. O., and Tow, S. H.: Moire contourgraphy in school screening for scoliosis: Preliminary report of first 327 cases. In Proceedings of the 9th Annual Meeting of the Japanese Society for Moire Contourgraphy, 1983, p. 42.

168. Dawson, E. G., Caron, A., and Moe, J. H.: Surgical management of scoliosis in the adult. J. Bone Joint Surg., 55-A:437, 1973.

169. Deacon, P., Berkin, C. R., and Dickson, R. A.: Combined idiopathic kyphosis and scoliosis. An analysis of the lateral spinal curvatures associated with Scheuermann's disease. J. Bone Joint Surg., 67-B:189, 1985.

170. Deacon, P., Flood, B. M., and Dickson, R. A.: Idiopathic scoliosis in three dimensions. J. Bone Joint Surg., 66-B:509, 1984.

171. Deane, G., and Duthie, R. B.: A new projectional look at articulated scoliotic spines. Acta Orthop. Scand., 44:351, 1973.

172. DeGeorge, F. V., and Fisher, R. L.: Idiopathic scoliosis: Genetic and environmental aspects. J. Med. Genet., 4:251, 1967.

173. Del Torto, U.: La correzione chirurgica delle deformita scoliotiche. Quad. Chir., 7:111, 1964.

174. Del Torto, U.: Rib resection with Marino-Zerco-Harrington instrumentation. Clin. Orthop., 65:191, 1969.

175. Del Torto, U.: Le Scoliosi. Rome, Verduci, 1975.

176. Dendy, J. M., Chase, S., and Determann, P.: School screening for scoliosis—organization of school and clinical procedure. Physiotherapy, 69:272, 1983.

177. DeSmet, A. A., and Ritter, E. M.: An improved film cassette for scoliosis radiography. Radiology, 141:249, 1981.

178. DeSmet, A. A., Fritz, S. I., and Asher, M. A.: A method for minimizing the radiation exposure from scoliosis radiographs. J. Bone Joint Surg., 63-A:156, 1981.

179. DeSmet, A. A., Tarlton, M. A., and Cook, L. T.: A radiographic method for three-dimensional analysis of spinal configuration. Radiography, 137:343, 1980.

180. DeSmet, A. A., Golin, J. E., Asher, M. A., and Scheuch, H. G.: A clinical study of the differences between the scoliotic angles measured on PA vs. AP radiographs. J. Bone Joint Surg., 64-A:489, 1982.

181. De Wald, R. L., and Ray, R. D.: Skeletal traction for the treatment of severe scoliosis. J. Bone Joint Surg., 52-A:233, 1970.

182. De Wald, R. L., Mulcahy, T. M., and Schultz, A. B.: Force measurement studies with the halo-hoop apparatus in scoliosis. Orthop. Rev., 2:17, 1973.

183. Dickson, J. H.: Twenty year follow-up on patients with idiopathic scoliosis having Harrington instrumentation and fusion. Paper presented at 19th Annual Meeting, Scoliosis Research Society, Orlando, Fla., 1984.

184. Dickson, J. H., and Harrington, P. R.: The evolution of the Harrington instrumentation technique in scoliosis. J. Bone Joint Surg., 55-A:993, 1973.

185. Dickson, R. A.: Screening for scoliosis. Br. Med. J., 289:269, 1984.

186. Dickson, R. A.: Conservative treatment for idiopathic scoliosis. J. Bone Joint Surg., 67-B:176, 1985.

187. Dickson, R. A., and Sevitt, E. A.: Growth and idiopathic scoliosis: A longitudinal cohort study. J. Bone Joint Surg., 64-B:385, 1982.

188. Dickson, R. A., Stamper, P., and Ardran, G. M.: A method for minimizing the radiation exposure from scoliosis radiographs (letter). J. Bone Joint Surg., 63-A:1499, 1981.

189. Dickson, R. A., Lawton, J. A., Archer, I. A., and Buxt, W. P.: The pathogenesis of idiopathic scoliosis. J. Bone Joint Surg., 66-B:8, 1984.

190. Dickson, R. A., Stamper, P., Sharp, A. M., and Harken, P.: School screening for scoliosis. Cohort study of clinical course. Br. Med. J., 73:265, 1980.

191. Dickson, R. A., Lawton, J. O., Archer, W. P., Butt, B., Jobbins, B., Berkin, C. R., Bliss, P., and Somerville, E. W.: Combined median and coronal plane asymmetry: The essential lesion of progressive idiopathic scoliosis. J. Bone Joint Surg., 65-B:368, 1983.

192. Doherty, J.: Complications of fusion in lumbar scoliosis. J. Bone Joint Surg., 55-A:438, 1973.

193. Dommisse, G. F.: The blood supply of the spinal cord. J. Bone Joint Surg., 56-B:225, 1974.

194. Dommisse, G. F.: The Arteries and Veins of the Human Spinal Cord from Birth. Edinburgh, Churchill-Livingstone, 1975.

195. Dommisse, G. F.: A survey of spinal deformity in the child. J. Bone Joint Surg., 61-B:259, 1979.

196. Donavan-Post, M. J.: Radiographic Evaluation of the Spine—Current Advances with Emphasis on Computer Tomography. New York, Masson, 1980.

197. Dorgan, J. C., Abbott, T. R., and Bentley, G.: Intraoperative awakening to monitor spinal cord function during scoliosis surgery. J. Bone Joint Surg., 66-B:716, 1984.

198. Dove, J., Hsu, L. C., and Yau, A. C.: The cervical spine following halo-pelvic traction. J. Bone Joint Surg., 62-B:158, 1980.

199. Dove, J., Hsu, L. C., and Yau, A. C.: Spontaneous cervical fusion. A complication of halo-pelvic traction. Spine, 6:45, 1981.

200. Dove, J., Lin, Y. T., Shen, Y. S., and Ditmanson, M. L.: Aortic aneurysm complicating spinal fixation with Dwyer's apparatus. Report of a case. Spine, 6:524, 1981.

201. Dove, J., Bottenburg, H. V., Arnold, P., Ali, M. S., and Elfakhri, T.: Biomechanical aspects of Luque segmental spinal instrumentation. Paper presented at the 18th Annual Meeting of the Scoliosis Research Society, New Orleans, 1983.

202. Driscoll, D. M., Newton, R. A., Lamb, R. L., and Nogi, J.: A study of postural equilibrium in idiopathic scoliosis. J. Pediatr. Orthop., 4:677, 1984.

203. Drummond, D. S.: The natural history of spine deformity. In Bradford, D., and Hensinger, R. (eds.): The Pediatric Spine. New York, Thieme, 1985, p. 167.

204. Drummond, D. S., and Rogala, E. J.: Growth and maturation of adolescents with idiopathic scoliosis. Spine, 5:507, 1980.

205. Drummond, D., Ranallo, F., and Lonstein, J. E.: Radiation hazards in scoliosis management. Spine, 8:741, 1983.

206. Drummond, D. S., Rogala, E., and Gurr, J.: Spinal deformity. Natural history and the role of school screening. Orthop. Clin. North Am., 10:751, 1979.

207. Drummond, D. S., Breed, A. L., Hoffman, J., and Engel, W. M.: The instaform mold: A rapid method of fabricating a scoliosis brace. Spine, 7:520, 1982.

208. Dubousset, A. M., Dubousset, J., and Loose, J. P.: Autotransfusion with acute hemodilution in the surgical treatment of scoliosis (author's transl.). Rev. Chir. Orthop., 67:609, 1981.

209. Duhaime, M., Poitras, B., and Archambault, J.: Depistage de la scoliose en millieu scolaire. Etude faite sur 14,886 radiographies. Union Med. Can., 105:886, 1976.

210. Duhaime, M., Lebel, M., Labelle, P., Simoneau, R., Poitras, B., Rivard, C. H., and Marton, D.: The evaluation of the Harrington technique in the treatment of double-curved scoliosis (author's transl.). Rev. Chir. Orthop., 67:99, 1981.

211. Dunn, B. H., Hakala, M. W., and McGee, M. E.: Scoliosis screening. Pediatrics, 61:794, 1978.

212. Dunn, H. K.: Spinal Instrumentation, Part I: Principles of posterior and anterior instrumentation. A.A.O.S. Instr. Course Lect., 32:192, 1983.

213. Dunn, H. K., and Bolstad, K. E.: Fixation of Dwyer screws for treatment of scoliosis. J. Bone Joint Surg., 59-A:54, 1977.

214. Dunoyer, J., de Leobardy, L., Valette, C., and Mechin, J. F.: Prognosis of infantile scoliosis (author's transl.). Rev. Chir. Orthop., 65:421, 1979.

215. Durand, Y., Rigault, P., Pooliquen, J. C., and Le-Hanaff, J. C.: Preoperative correction of severe scoliosis by halo and walking frame system. Chir. Pediatr., 21:215, 1980.

216. Durning, R. P., Scoles, P. V., and Fox, O. D.: Scoliosis after thoracotomy in tracheoesophageal fistula patients. A follow-up study. J. Bone Joint Surg., 62-A:1156, 1980.

217. Duval-Beaupere, G.: Les repères de maturation dans la surveillance des scoliosis. Rev. Chir. Orthop., 56:56, 1970.

218. Duval-Beaupré, G.: Pathogenic relationship between scoliosis and growth. In Zorab, P. A. (ed.): Scoliosis and Growth: Proceedings of the Third Symposium held at the Institute of Diseases of the Chest, Brompton Hospital, London. Edinburgh, Churchill-Livingstone, 1971.

219. Duval-Beaupere, G.: The growth of scoliosis patients. Hypothesis and preliminary study. Acta Orthop. Belg., 38:365, 1972.

220. Duval-Beaupere, G., Lespargot, A., and Grossiord, A.: Scoliosis and trunk muscles. J. Pediatr. Orthop., 4:195, 1984.

221. Dwyer, A. F.: Experience of anterior correction of scoliosis. Clin. Orthop., 93:191, 1973.

222. Dwyer, A. F., and Schafer, M. F.: Anterior approach to scoliosis: Results of treatment in fifty-one cases. J. Bone Joint Surg., 56-B:218, 1974.

223. Dwyer, A. F., Newton, N. C., and Sherwood, A. A.: An anterior approach to scoliosis. A preliminary report. Clin. Orthop., 62:192, 1969.

224. Dwyer, A. P.: A fatal complication of paravertebral infection and traumatic aneurysm following Dwyer instrumentation. J. Bone Joint Surg., 61-B:239, 1979.

225. Dwyer, A. P., O'Brien, J. P., Seal, P. P., Hsu, L., Yau, A. C. M. C., and Hodgson, A. R.: The late complications after the Dwyer anterior spinal instrumentation for scoliosis. J. Bone Joint Surg., 59-B:117, 1977.

226. Edgar, M. A.: To brace or not to brace? J. Bone Joint Surg., 67-B:173, 1985.

227. Edgar, M. A., Chapman, R. A., and Glasglow, M. M.: Preoperative correction in adolescent idiopathic scoliosis. J. Bone Joint Surg., 64-B:531, 1982.

228. Edmonsson, A. S., and Morris, J. T.: Follow-up study of Milwaukee brace treatment in patients with idiopathic scoliosis. Clin. Orthop., 126:58, 1977.

229. Edmonsson, A. S., and Smith, G. R.: Long-term follow-up study of Milwaukee brace treatment in patients with idiopathic scoliosis. Scoliosis Research Society Report, Denver, 1982.

230. Eisenstein, S., and O'Brien, J. P.: Chylothorax: A complication of Dwyer's anterior instrumentation. Br. J. Surg., 64:339, 1977.

231. Eismont, F. J., and Simeone, F. A.: Bone overgrowth (hypertrophy) as a cause of late paraparesis after scoliosis fusion. A case report. J. Bone Joint Surg., 63-A:1016, 1981.

232. Elfestrom, G., and Nachemson, A.: Telemetry recording of forces in the Harrington distraction rod: A method for increasing safety in the operative treatment of scoliosis patient. Clin. Orthop., 93:158, 1973.

233. Emans, J. B., Hall, J. E., and Koepfler, J. W.: Detection of progression in scoliosis by shadow Moire topography. Paper presented at the 18th Annual Meeting of the Scoliosis Research Society, New Orleans, September, 1983.

234. Emans, J. B., Kaelin, A., Bancel, P., and Hall, J. E.: Treatment of adolescent idiopathic scoliosis using the Boston brace system. Scoliosis Research Society Report, New Orleans, 1983.

235. Engel, D., and Richter, A.: Experiments on the production of spinal deformities by radium. A.J.R., 42:217, 1939.

236. Engler, G. L., Speilholz, N. I., Bernhard, W. N., Danziger, F., Merkin, H., and Wolff, E. E.: Somatosensory evoked potentials during Harrington instrumentation for scoliosis. J. Bone Joint Surg., 60-A:528, 1978.

237. Enneking, W. F., and Harrington, P.: Pathological changes in scoliosis. J. Bone Joint Surg., 51:165, 1969.

238. Erwin, W. D., and Dickson, J. H.: Utilization of Harrington Spinal Instrumentation and Fusion for Scoliosis. Zimmer Surgical Technique, 1984.

239. Erwin, W. D., Dickson, J. H., and Harrington, P. R.: The post-operative management of scoliosis patients treated with Harrington instrumentation and fusion. J. Bone Joint Surg., 58-A:479, 1976.

240. Erwin, W. D., Dickson, J. H., and Harrington, P. R.: Clinical review of patients with broken Harrington rods. J. Bone Joint Surg., 62-A:1302, 1980.

241. Eulert, J.: Scoliosis and kyphosis in dwarfing conditions. Arch. Orthop. Trauma, 102:45, 1983.

242. Evarts, C. M., Winter, R. B., and Hall, J. E.: Vascular compression of the duodenum associated with the treatment of scoliosis. J. Bone Joint Surg., 53-A:431, 1971.

243. Fabris, D., Trainiti, G., Di Comun, M., and Agostini, S.: Scoliosis due to rib osteoblastoma: Report of two cases. J. Pediatr. Orthop., 3:370, 1983.

244. Fallstrom, K., Nachemson, A. L., and Cochran, T. P.: Psychologic effects of treatment for adolescent idiopathic scoliosis. Orthop. Trans., 8:150, 1984.

245. Farady, J. A.: Current principles in the nonoperative management of structural adolescent idiopathic scoliosis. Phys. Ther. 63:512, 1983.

246. Farkas, A.: Basic factors in the development of scoliosis. Bull. Hosp. Joint Dis., 28:131, 1967.

247. Farren, J.: Routine radiographic assessment of the scoliotic spine. Radiography, 47:92, 1981.

248. Faut, M. M., and De Wald, R. L.: Restriction of cervical spine motion after Milwaukee brace treatment for idiopathic scoliosis. Orthop. Trans., 2:270, 1978.

249. Ferguson, A. B.: The study and treatment of scoliosis. South. Med. J., 23:116, 1930.

250. Ferguson, A. B.: Roentgen Diagnosis of the Extremities and Spine. New York, Hoeber, 1945.

251. Ferguson, A. B.: Roentgen interpretation and decisions in scoliosis. A.A.O.S., Instr. Course Lect., 7:160, 1950.

252. Ferguson, R. L., and Allen, B. L.: The technique of scoliosis revision surgery utilizing L rod instrumentation. J. Pediatr. Orthop., 3:563, 1983.

253. Fernand, R., Lombardi, S., and Avella, D.: Single distraction rod versus distraction, compression and transverse traction in the treatment of idiopathic sco-

liosis. Paper presented at the 17th Annual Meeting of the Scoliosis Research Society, Denver, 1982.

254. Ferreira, J. H., and James, J. I. P.: Progressive and resolving infantile idiopathic scoliosis. J. Bone Joint Surg., 54-B:648, 1972.

255. Fidler, M. W., and Jowett, R. L.: Muscle imbalance in the aetiology of scoliosis. J. Bone Joint Surg., 58-B:200, 1976.

256. Figueiredo, U. M., and James, J. I. P.: Juvenile idiopathic scoliosis. J. Bone Joint Surg., 63-B:61, 1981.

257. Fillio, N. A., and Thompson, M. W.: Genetic studies in scoliosis. J. Bone Joint Surg., 53-A:199, 1971.

258. Fishchenko, V. I.: Blood loss: Its prevention and correction in spinal operations for scoliosis. Ortop. Travmatol. Protez., 2:5, 1982.

259. Fishchenko, V. I.: Etiology and pathogenesis of scoliosis. Vestn. Khir., 129:111, 1982.

260. Fisher, R. L., and DeGeorge, F. V.: Idiopathic scoliosis: An investigation of genetic and enviromental factors. J. Bone Joint Surg., 49-A:1005, 1967.

261. Flatley, T. J.: Application of segmental spinal instrumentation. Orthopedics, 6:441, 1983.

262. Flinchum, D.: Rib resection in the treatment of scoliosis. South. Med. J., 56:1378, 1963.

263. Flynn, J. C., and Hoque, M. A.: Anterior fusion of the lumbar spine. J. Bone Joint Surg., 61-A:1143, 1979.

264. Flynn, J. C., and Price, C. T.: Sexual complications of anterior fusion of the lumbar spine. Spine, 9:489, 1984.

265. Flynn, J. C., Riddick, M. F., and Keller, T. L.: Screening for scoliosis in Florida schools. J. Fla. Med. Assoc., 64:159, 1977.

266. Fowles, J. V., Drummond, D. S., L'Ecuyer, S., Roy, L., and Kassab, M.: Untreated scoliosis in the adult. Clin. Orthop., 134:212, 1978.

267. Francis, M. J. D., Smith, R., and Sanderson, M. C.: Collagen abnormalities in idiopathic adolescent scoliosis. Calcif. Tissue Res., 22:381, 1977.

268. Freebody, D., Bendall, R., and Taylor, R. D.: Anterior transperitoneal lumbar fusion. J. Bone Joint Surg., 53-B:617, 1971.

269. Friedman, H. G., Herbert, M. A., and Bobechko, W. P.: Electrical stimulation for scoliosis. Am. Fam. Physician, 1982.

270. Frontino, G., and Lumini, A.: The surface electrical stimulation (L.E.S.S.) for the treatment of idiopathic progressive scoliosis. Orthop. Trans., 7:10, 1983.

271. Fustier, R.: Evolution radiologique spontanée des scolioses idiopathiques de moins de 45 degrées en periode de croissance. Etude graphique retrospective de cent dossiers du Centre de Readaptation Fonctionelle des Massues. Thesis. Université Claude-Bernard, Lyon, France, 1980.

272. Gaidukov, A. A.: Surgical treatment of progressive idiopathic scoliosis. Ortop. Travmatol. Protez., 2:17, 1981.

273. Gaidukov, A. A.: Surgical correction of curvatures of the lumbar spine in scoliosis. Ortop. Travmatol. Protez., 5:8, 1983.

274. Gaines, R. W., McKinley, L. M., and Leatherman, K. D.: Effect of the Harrington compression system on the correction of the rib hump in spinal instrumentation for idiopathic scoliosis. Spine, 6:489, 1981.

275. Galante, J., Schultz, A., DeWald, R. L., and Ray, R. D.: Forces acting in the Milwaukee brace on patients undergoing treatment for idiopathic scoliosis. J. Bone Joint Surg., 52-A:498, 1970.

276. Galen: De Moto Maerculorum (A.D. 131–201). Quoted by Moe, J. H.: Historical aspects of scoliosis. *In* Moe's Textbook of Scoliosis and Other Spinal Deformities. Philadelphia, Saunders, 1987, p. 1.

277. Garrett, A. L., Perry, J., and Nickel, V. L.: Stabili-

zation of the collapsing spine. J. Bone Joint Surg., 43-A:474, 1961.

278. Ghosh, P., Bushell, G. R., Taylor, T. K., Pearce, R. H., and Grimmer, B. J.: Distribution of glycosaminoglycans across the normal and the scoliotic disc. Spine, 5:310, 1980.

279. Gilsanz, V., Boechat, I. M., Birnberg, F. A., and King, J. D.: Scoliosis after thoracotomy for esophageal atresia. A.J.R., 141:457, 1983.

280. Ginsburg, H. H., Goldstein, L. A., Robinson, S., Haake, P. W., Devanny, J., Chan, D., and Suk, S.: Back pain in postoperative idiopathic scoliosis—long-term follow-up. Orthop. Trans., 3:50, 1979.

281. Gitelis, S., Whiffen, J., and DeWald, R. L.: The treatment of severe scoliosis in osteogenesis imperfecta. Case report. Clin. Orthop., 175:56, 1983.

282. Gittman, J. E., Buchanan, T. A., Fisher, B. J., Bergeson, P. S., and Palmar, P. E.: Fatal fat embolism after spinal fusion for scoliosis. J.A.M.A., 249:779, 1983.

283. Glasbey, J. A.: A study of vertebral body shape and skeletal shape in healthy and scoliotic children. Thesis, University of Nottingham, 1983.

284. Gold, L., Leach, D., and Kiefer, S. A.: Large volume myelography. Radiology, 97:531, 1970.

285. Goldberg, C., Dowling, F., Blake, N. S., and Regan, B. F.: A retrospective study of Cotrel dynamic spinal traction in the conservative management of scoliosis. Ir. Med. J., 74:363, 1981.

286. Goldberg, C., Thompson, F., Dowling, F., Regan, B. F., and Blake, N. S.: Pilot study for a scoliosis screening project in South Dublin. Ir. Med. J., 73:265, 1980.

287. Goldstein, L. A.: Results in the treatment of scoliosis with turnbuckle plaster cast correction and fusion. J. Bone Joint Surg., 41-A:321, 1959.

288. Goldstein, L. A.: Surgical management of scoliosis. J. Bone Joint Surg., 48-A:167, 1966.

289. Goldstein, L. A.: Treatment of idiopathic scoliosis by Harrington instrumentation and fusion with fresh autogenous iliac bone grafts. J. Bone Joint Surg., 51:209, 1969.

290. Goldstein, L. A.: The surgical treatment of idiopathic scoliosis. Clin. Orthop., 93:131, 1973.

291. Goldstein, L. A., and Waugh, T. R.: Classification and terminology of scoliosis. Clin. Orthop., 93:10, 1973.

292. Golomb, M., and Taylor, T. F. K.: Screening adolescent school children for scoliosis (letter). Med. J. Aust., 1:761, 1975.

293. Gonon, G. P., Perault, F., Michel, A., Butel, J., Stagnara, P., and De Mourgues, G.: Resultats de l'association Dwyer-Harrington dans le traitment de la scoliose. Rev. Chir. Orthop., 2:171, 1983.

294. Gonyea, W. J., Moore-Woodard, C., Moseley, B., Hollmann, M., and Wenger, D.: An evaluation of muscle pathology in idiopathic scoliosis. J. Pediatr. Orthop., 5:323, 1985.

295. Gore, D. R., Passehl, R., Sepic, S., and Dalton, A.: Scoliosis screening: Results of a community project. Pediatrics, 67:196, 1981.

296. Graf, H., Hecquet, J., and Dubousset, J.: 3-Dimensional approach to spinal deformities. Application to the study of the prognosis of pediatric scoliosis. Rev. Chir. Orthop., 69:407, 1983.

297. Granieri, U., Maiuri, F., Colantuono, C., and Maiuri, L.: Vertebral osteoid osteoma, rare causes of nerve root compression and scoliosis in childhood. Riv. Neurol., 50:278, 1980.

298. Gras, M., Bourbotte, G., Boluix, B., Castan, P., Pous, J. G., Dimeglio, A., and Frerebeau, P.: Scoliotic malformations with or without associated occult spinal dysraphia. A study in 82 children. Current radiological

techniques, indications and findings. J. Radiol., 63:383, 1982.

299. Gratz, R. R., and Papalia-Finlay, D.: Psychosocial adaptation to wearing the Milwaukee brace for scoliosis. J. Adolesc. Health Care, 5:237, 1984.

300. Gray, J., Hoffman, A. D., and Peterson, H. A.: Reduction of radiation exposure during radiography for scoliosis. J. Bone Joint Surg., 65-A:5, 1983.

301. Gray, S. W., Akin, J. T., Milsap, J. H., and SkanaLakis, J. E.: Vascular compromise of the duodenum. Contemp. Surg., 9:37, 1976.

302. Green, N. E.: Part-time bracing of adolescent idiopathic scoliosis. J. Bone Joint Surg., 68-A:738, 1986.

303. Greene, W. B., and McMillan, C. W.: Surgery for scoliosis in congenital factor VII deficiency. Am. J. Dis. Child., 136:411, 1982.

304. Gregg, E. C.: Radiation risks with diagnostic x-rays. Radiology, 123:447, 1977.

305. Gregoric, M., Pecak, F., Trontelj, J. V., and Dimitrijevic, M. R.: Postural control in scoliosis. A stato-kinesimetric study in patients with scoliosis due to neuromuscular disorders and in patients with idiopathic scoliosis. Acta Orthop. Scand., 52:59, 1981.

306. Grimer, R. J., Mulligan, P. J., and Thompson, A. G.: Thoracic outlet syndrome following correction of scoliosis in a patient with cervical ribs. A case report. J. Bone Joint Surg., 65-A:1172, 1983.

307. Gross, C., Gross, M., and Kuschner, S.: Error analysis of scoliosis curve measurement. Bull. Hosp. Joint Dis., 43:171, 1983.

308. Gruca, A.: L'alloplastie des muscles et myoplastie dans la scoliose idiopathique. Rev. Orthop., 42:916, 1956.

309. Gruca, A.: The pathogenesis and treatment of scoliosis. J. Bone Joint Surg., 40-A:570, 1958.

310. Gryboski, J. D., Kocoshis, S. A., Seashore, J. H., Gudjonsson, B., and Drennan, J. C.: "Body-brace" oesophagitis, a complication of kyphoscoliosis therapy. Lancet, 2:449, 1978.

311. Guadagni, J., Drummond, D., and Breed, A.: Improved postoperative course following modified segmental instrumentation and posterior spinal fusion for idiopathic scoliosis. J. Pediatr. Orthop., 4:405, 1984.

312. Gucker, T., III: Changes in vital capacity in scoliosis: Preliminary report on effects of treatment. J. Bone Joint Surg., 44-A:459, 1962.

313. Guerin, J.: Memoire sur les déviations simulées de l'épine et les moyens. Gaz. Med. Paris, 7:241, 1839.

314. Guerin, J.: Remarques préliminaires sur le traitement des déviations de l'épine par la section des muscles du dos. Gaz. Med. Paris, 10:1, 1842.

315. Gui, L., and Javani, R.: The surgical treatment of scoliosis in the adult. Ital. J. Orthop. Traumatol., 1:191, 1975.

316. Gui, L., and Savini, R.: Un tavolo di trazione per la chirurgia delle scoliosi. Chir. Organi Mov., 61:37, 1972.

317. Haas, S. L.: Experimental production of scoliosis. J. Bone Joint Surg., 21:963, 1939.

318. Haas, S. L.: Influence of fusion of the spine on growth of the vertebrae. Arch. Surg., 41:607, 1940.

319. Hall, J. E.: The anterior approach to spinal deformities. Orthop. Clin. North Am., 3:81, 1972.

320. Hall, J. E.: Combined anterior and posterior fusion in seventy-three spinally deformed patients: Indications, results and complications. Clin. Orthop., 164:110, 1982.

321. Hall, J. E., and Miller, W.: Prefabrication of Milwaukee braces. J. Bone Joint Surg., 56-A:1763, 1974.

322. Hall, J. E., Gray, J., and Allen, N.: Dwyer instrumentation and spinal fusion. A follow-up study. J. Bone Joint Surg., 59-A:117, 1977.

323. Hall, J. E., Levine, C. R., and Sudhir, K.: Intraoperative awakening to monitor spinal cord function during Harrington instrumentation and spine fusion. J. Bone Joint Surg., 60-A:533, 1978.

324. Hall, J. E., Emans, J. B., Kaelin, A., and Bancel, P.: Boston brace system treatment of idiopathic scoliosis. Follow-up in 400 patients finished treatment. Orthop. Trans., 8:148, 1984.

325. Hall, J. E., Miller, M. E., Shermann, W., and Stanish, W.: A refined conception in the orthotic management of scoliosis. Orthot. Prosthet., 29:7, 1975.

326. Hall, J. E., Mills, M. B., Lipton, H., and Gebhardt, M.: Treatment of hypokyphotic scoliosis: Nonoperative and operative. Orthop. Trans., 8:154, 1983.

327. Hamilton, F., Thomas, M. P., and Peralta, M. M., Jr.: Ventilation effects on the Harrington procedure for the treatment of scoliosis. Surg. Gynecol. Obstet., 130:1067, 1970.

328. Hancox, V.: Cotrel traction for patients with scoliosis. Physiotherapy, 67:71, 1981.

329. Hannon, K. M., and Wetta, W. J.: Failure of technetium bone scanning to detect pseudarthroses in spinal fusion for scoliosis. Clin. Orthop., 123:42, 1977.

330. Harada, Y., Takemitsu, Y., and Inai, M.: The role of contour line photography using the light cutting method and Moire topography in school screening for scoliosis. In Moreland, M. S., Pope, M. H., and Armstrong, G. W. (eds.): Moire Fringe Topography and Spinal Deformity. New York, Oxford, Toronto, Pergamon, 1983, pp. 113–121.

331. Hardy, J. H., and Dennis, M.: An evaluation of Milwaukee brace failures. J. Bone Joint Surg., 55-A:439, 1973.

332. Hardy, J. M., Cooke, R. W., and Einbund, M.: Hyperalimentation in the treatment of "cast syndrome." J. Bone Joint Surg., 54-A:200, 1972.

333. Hardy, R. W., Nash, C. L., and Brodkey, J. S.: Follow-up report: Experimental and clinical studies in spinal cord monitoring. The effect of pressure anoxia and ischaemia on spinal cord function. J. Bone Joint Surg., 55-A:435, 1973.

334. Hare, S.: Practical Observations on the Prevention, Causes and Treatment of Curvatures of the Spine. London, 1849.

335. Harrenstein, R. J.: Sur la scoliose des nourrissons et des jeunes enfants. Rev. Orthop., 23:289, 1936.

336. Harrington, P. R.: Surgical instrumentation for management of scoliosis. J. Bone Joint Surg., 42-A:1448, 1960.

337. Harrington, P. R.: Treatment of scoliosis. Correction and internal fixation by spine instrumentation. J. Bone Joint Surg., 44-A:591, 1962.

338. Harrington, P. R.: Scoliosis in the growing spine. Pediatr. Clin. North Am., 10:225, 1963.

339. Harrington, P. R.: The management of scoliosis by spine instrumentation. An evaluation of more than 200 cases. South. Med. J., 56:1367, 1963.

340. Harrington, P. R.: Nonoperative treatment of scoliosis. Tex. Med., 64:54, 1968.

341. Harrington, P. R.: Technical details in relation to the successful use of instrumentation in scoliosis. Orthop. Clin. North Am., 3:49, 1972.

342. Harrington, P. R., and Dickson, J. H.: An eleven year clinical investigation of Harrington instrumentation: A preliminary report on 578 cases. Clin. Orthop., 93:113, 1973.

343. Harrington, P. R., and Dickson, J. H.: The evolution of the Harrington instrumentation technique in scoliosis. J. Bone Joint Surg., 55-A:993, 1973.

344. Hassan, I., and Bjerkreim, I.: Progression in idiopathic scoliosis after conservative treatment. Acta Orthop. Scand., 54:88, 1983.

345. Hay, R. L.: Some clinical observations on the plasticity of the infant axial skeleton. In Zorab, P. A. (ed.):

Scoliosis and Growth. Edinburgh, Churchill-Livingstone, 1971, pp. 29–32.

346. Hefti, F. L., and McMaster, M. J.: The effect of the adolescent growth spurt on early posterior spinal fusion in infantile and juvenile idiopathic scoliosis. J. Bone Joint Surg., 65-B:247, 1983.

347. Heinig, C.: The egg shell procedure. In Luque, E. R. (ed.): Scoliosis Segmental Spine Instrumentation. Thorofare, N. J., Slack, 1984, pp. 221–230.

348. Hensinger, R. N., and MacEwen, G. D.: Evaluation of the Cotrel dynamic spine traction in the treatment of scoliosis: A preliminary report. Orthop. Rev., 3:27, 1974.

349. Hensinger, R. N., Cowell, H. R., MacEwen, G. D., Shands, A. R., Jr., and Cronis, S.: Orthopaedic screening of school age children. Review of a 10 year experience. Orthop. Rev., 4:23, 1978.

350. Herndon, W. A.: Scoliosis and maple syrup urine disease. J. Pediatr. Orthop., 4:126, 1984.

351. Herndon, W. A., Ellis, R. D., Hall, J. A., and Millis, M. G.: Correction with a transverse loading system in the operative management of scoliosis. Clin. Orthop., 165:168, 1982.

352. Herring, J. A., and Wenger, D. R.: Segmental spinal instrumentation: A preliminary report of 40 consecutive cases. Spine, 7:285, 1982.

353. Herring, J. A., Fitch, R., Wenger, D., Roach, J., Cook, J., and Frith, C.: Segmental spinal instrumentation—a review of early results and complications. Orthop. Trans., 8:172, 1984.

354. Herron, L. D., and Dawson, E. G.: Methylmethacrylate as an adjunct in spinal instrumentation. J. Bone Joint Surg., 59-A:866, 1977.

355. Heyman, C. H.: Spinal-cord compression associated with scoliosis. J. Bone Joint Surg., 19:1081, 1937.

356. Heyman, H. J., Ivankovich, A. D., Shulman, M., Millar, E., and Choudhry, Y. A.: Intraoperative monitoring and anesthetic management for spinal fusion in an amelic patient. J. Pediatr. Orthop., 2:299, 1982.

357. Hibbs, R. A.: An operation for progressive spinal deformities. A preliminary report of three cases from the service of the Orthopaedic Hospital. N.Y. State J. Med., 93:1013, 1911.

358. Hibbs, R. A.: A report of fifty-nine cases of scoliosis treated by the fusion operation. J. Bone Joint Surg., 6:3, 1924.

359. Hibbs, R. A., Risser, J. C., and Ferguson, A. B.: Scoliosis treated by the fusion operation. J. Bone Joint Surg., 13:91, 1931.

360. Hinck, V. C., Clark, W. M., and Hopkins, C. E.: Normal interpediculate distances (minimum and maximum) in children and adults. A.J.R., 97:141, 1966.

361. Hippocrates: On the Articulations. In Adams, F. (trans.): The Genuine Works of Hippocrates. Vol. 2. London, Sydenham Society, 1849.

362. Hirsch, C., and Waugh, T.: The introduction of force measurements guiding instrumental correction of scoliosis. Acta Orthop. Scand., 39:136, 1968.

363. Hodgett, S. G.: A radiological study of rotation, classification and height loss in idiopathic scoliosis. Thesis, University of Nottingham, 1985.

364. Hodgson, A. R., and Stock, F. E.: Anterior spinal fusion: A preliminary communication on the radical treatment of Pott's disease and Pott's paraplegia. Br. J. Surg., 44:266, 1956.

365. Hodgson, A. R., and Yau, A. C. M. C.: Anterior surgical approaches to the spinal column. In Apley, A. G. (ed.): Recent Advances in Orthopedics. London, Churchill, 1969.

366. Hoffa, A.: Operative Behandlung einer schweren Skoliose (Resection des Rippenbuckels). Z. Orthop. Chir., 4:402, 1896.

367. Hoffa, A.: Redression des Buckels nach der Methode von Calot. Dtsch. Med. Wochenschr., 1:3, 1898.

368. Hooper, G.: Congenital dislocation of the hip in infantile idiopathic scoliosis. J. Bone Joint Surg., 62-B:447, 1980.

369. Hopkins, R., Grundy, M., and Sherr-Mehl, M.: X-ray filters in scoliosis x-rays. Orthop. Trans., 8:148, 1984.

370. Hoppenfeld, S., Gross, A., and Andrews, C.: The ankle clonus test—an alternative to the Stagnara wake up test and somatosensory evoked potentials in the assessment of spinal cord damage in the treatment of scoliosis with Harrington rod instrumentation. Orthop. Trans., 9:118, 1985.

371. Houghton, G. R.: Cosmetic surgery for scoliosis. In Dickson, R., and Bradford, D. (eds.): Management of Spinal Deformities. London, Butterworth, 1984, pp. 237–251.

372. Houston, C. S.: Radiologists and thoughtful use of radiation. J. Can. Assoc. Radiol., 28:2, 1977.

373. Howard, C. C.: A preliminary report on infraocclusion of the molars and premolars produced by orthopedic treatment of scoliosis. Int. J. Orthodont., 12:434, 1926.

374. Howard, C. C.: A second report of infraocclusion of the molars and premolars produced by orthopedic treatment of scoliosis. Int. J. Orthodont., 15:329, 1929.

375. Howorth, M. B.: Evolution of spinal fusion. Ann. Surg., 117:278, 1943.

376. Hsu, L. C., Lee, P. C., and Leons, J. C.: Dystrophic spinal deformities in neurofibromatosis. Treatment by anterior and posterior fusion. J. Bone Joint Surg., 66-B:495, 1984.

377. Hsu, L. C., Zucherman, J., Tang, S. C., and Leons, J. C.: Dwyer instrumentation in the treatment of adolescent idiopathic scoliosis. J. Bone Joint Surg., 64-B:536, 1982.

378. Hughes, J. P., McEntire, J. D., and Setze, T. K.: Cast syndrome. Arch. Surg., 108:230, 1974.

379. Humbyrd, D. E., Latimer, R., Lonstein, J. E., and Samberg, L. C.: Brain abscess as a complication of halo traction. Spine, 6:365, 1981.

380. Hunter, R. E., Bradford, D. S., and Oegema, T. R.: Biochemistry of the intervertebral disc in scoliosis. Trans. Orthop. Res. Soc., 4:135, 1978.

381. Hyndman, O. R.: Transplantation of the spinal cord: The problem of kyphoscoliosis with cord signs. Surg. Gynecol. Obstet., 84:460, 1947.

382. Ibarra, G., Gaine, R. W., and Leatherman, K. D.: A new orthosis for immediate postoperative bracing in idiopathic scoliosis. Orthop. Trans., 3:56, 1979.

383. Inoue, S.: Screening of scoliosis among school children and the role of orthopedic surgeons. Nippon Seikeigeka Gakkai Zasshi, 54:701, 1980.

384. Inoue, S., Shinoto, A., and Ohki, I.: The Moire topography for early detection of scoliosis and evaluation after surgery. Orthop. Trans., 2:276, 1978.

385. Inoue, S., Utsuka, Y., and Shinoto, A.: Mass school screening for detection of scoliosis by use of Moire topography camera and low dose x-ray imaging. Fuginon Technical Information. Fuji Photo Optical Co., Japan, 1981.

386. Jackson, J. W.: Surgical approaches to the anterior aspects of the spinal column. Ann. R. Coll. Surg., 48:83, 1971.

387. Jackson, R. P., Simmons, E. H., and Stribnis, D.: Incidence and severity of back pain in adult idiopathic scoliosis. Spine, 8:749, 1983.

388. James, J. I. P.: Two curve patterns in idiopathic scoliosis. J. Bone Joint Surg., 33-B:399, 1951.

389. James, J. I. P.: Idiopathic scoliosis. The prognosis, diagnosis and operative indications related to curved patterns and the age at onset. J. Bone Joint Surg., 36-B:36, 1954.

390. James, J. I. P.: Infantile idiopathic scoliosis. Clin. Orthop., 21:106, 1961.

391. James, J. I. P.: Scoliosis. Baltimore, Williams & Wilkins, 1967.
392. James, J. I. P.: Scoliosis. 2nd Ed. New York, Churchill-Livingstone, 1976, pp. 203–205.
393. James, J. I. P., Lloyd Roberts, G. C., and Pilcher, M. F.: Infantile structural scoliosis. J. Bone Joint Surg., 41-B:719, 1959.
394. Jodoin, A., Hall, J. E., and Watts, H. G.: Treatment of idiopathic scoliosis by the Boston brace system. Early results. Orthop. Trans., 5:22, 1981.
395. Johnson, J. T. H., and Southwick, W. O.: Bone growth after spinal fusion. J. Bone Joint Surg., 42-A:1396, 1960.
396. Johnson, R. M., and McGuire, E. J.: Urogenital complications of anterior approaches to the lumbar spine. Clin. Orthop., 154:114, 1981.
397. Jonasson-Rajala, E., Josefsson, E., Lundberg, B., and Nilsson, H.: Boston thoracic brace in the treatment of idiopathic scoliosis. Initial correction. Clin. Orthop., 183:37, 1984.
398. Jones, E. T., Mathews, L. S., and Hensinger, R. N.: The wake-up technique as a dual protector of spinal cord function during spine fusion. Clin. Orthop., 168:113, 1982.
399. Jones, R. S., Kennedy, J. D., Hasham, F., Owen, R., and Taylor, J. F.: Mechanical inefficiency of the thoracic cage in scoliosis. Thorax, 36:456, 1981.
400. Kafer, E. R.: Respiratory and cardiovascular functions in scoliosis and the principles of anesthetic management. Anesthesiology, 52:339, 1980.
401. Kahanovitz, N., and Levine, D. B.: Iatrogenic complications of spinal surgery. Contemp. Orthop., 2:23, 1984.
402. Kahanovitz, N., Levine, D. B., and Lardone, J.: The part-time Milwaukee brace treatment of juvenile idiopathic scoliosis. Long-term follow-up. Clin. Orthop., 167:145, 1982.
403. Kahanovitz, N., Snow, B., and Pinter, I.: The comparative results of psychological testing in scoliosis patients treated with electrical stimulation or bracing. Spine, 9:442, 1984.
404. Kalamchi, A., Yau, A. C., O'Brien, J. P., and Hodgson, A.: Halo pelvic distraction apparatus. J. Bone Joint Surg., 58-A:1119, 1976.
405. Kane, W. J.: Scoliosis prevalence. A call for a statement of terms. Clin. Orthop., 126:43, 1977.
406. Kane, W. J.: A new challenge in scoliosis care (editorial). J. Bone Joint Surg., 64-A:479, 1982.
407. Kane, W. J., and Moe, J. H.: A scoliosis-prevalence study in Minnesota. Clin. Orthop., 69:216, 1970.
408. Kane, W. J., Moe, J. H., and Lai, C. C.: Halo-femoral pin distraction in the treatment of scoliosis. J. Bone Joint Surg., 49-A:1018, 1967.
409. Kane, W. J., Brown, J. C., Hensinger, R. N., and Keller, R. B.: Scoliosis and school screening for spinal deformity. Am. Fam. Physician, 17:123, 1978.
410. Karaharju, E. O.: Deformation of vertebrae in experimental scoliosis: The course of bone adaptation and modelling in scoliosis with reference to the normal growth of the vertebra. Acta Orthop. Scand., Suppl. 105, 1976.
411. Karroll, M., Hernandez, R. J., and Wessel, H. U.: Computed tomography diagnosis of bronchial compression by the spine after surgical correction of scoliosis. Pediatr. Radiol., 14:335, 1984.
412. Katzman, H., Waugh, T., and Berdon, W.: Skeletal changes following irradiation of childhood tumors. J. Bone Joint Surg., 51-B:825, 1969.
413. Kehl, D. K., Alsonso, J. E., and Lovell, W. W.: Scoliosis secondary to an osteoid osteoma of the rib. A case report. J. Bone Joint Surg., 65-A:701, 1983.
414. Keim, H. A., and Dwan, F. A.: Short term halo-femoral traction in the preoperative management of rigid and severe scoliosis. A review of 58 cases. Orthop. Rev., 10:57, 1981.
415. Keim, H. A., and Hilal, S. K.: Spinal angiography in scoliosis patients. J. Bone Joint Surg., 53-A:904, 1971.
416. Keim, H. A., and Reina, E. G.: Osteoid osteoma as a cause of scoliosis. J. Bone Joint Surg., 57-A:159, 1975.
417. Keim, H. A., and Weinstein, J. D.: Acute renal failure—a complication of spine fusion in the tuck position. J. Bone Joint Surg., 52-A:1248, 1970.
418. Keiser, R. P., and Shufflebarger, H. L.: The Milwaukee brace in idiopathic scoliosis: Evaluation of one hundred and twenty-three completed cases. Clin. Orthop., 118:19, 1976.
419. Keller, R. B., and Pappas, A. M.: Infection after spinal fusion using internal fixation instrumentation. Orthop. Clin. North Am., 3:99, 1972.
420. Khosla, S., Tredwell, S. J., Day, B., Shinn, S. L., and Ovalle, W. K., Jr.: An ultrastructural study of multifidus muscle in progressive idiopathic scoliosis. Changes resulting from a sarcolemmal defect at the myotendinous junction. J. Neurol. Sci., 46:13, 1980.
421. King, H. A., and Bradford, D. S.: Fracture-dislocation of the spine after spine fusion and Harrington instrumentation for idiopathic scoliosis. A case report. J. Bone Joint Surg., 62-A:1374, 1980.
422. King, H. A., Moe, J. H., Bradford, D. S., and Winter, R. B.: The selection of fusion levels on thoracic idiopathic scoliosis. J. Bone Joint Surg., 65-A:1302, 1983.
423. Kittleson, A. C., and Lim, L. W.: Measurement of scoliosis. A.J.R., 108:775, 1970.
424. Kleinberg, S.: Scoliosis: Pathology, Etiology and Treatment. Baltimore, Williams & Wilkins, 1951.
425. Kleinman, R. E., Csongradi, J. J., Rinsky, L. A., and Bleck, E. E.: A radiographic assessment of spinal flexibility in scoliosis. Clin. Orthop., 162:47, 1982.
426. Kling, T. F., Jr., Drennan, J. C., and Gryboski, J. D.: Esophagitis complicating scoliosis management with the Boston thoracolumbosacral orthosis. Clin. Orthop., 159:208, 1981.
427. Kristmundsdottir, F., Burwell, R. G., and James, J. I. P.: The rib-vertebra angles on the convexity and concavity of the spinal curve in infantile idiopathic scoliosis. Clin. Orthop., 201:205, 1985.
428. Langenskiöld, A., and Michelsson, J. E.: Experimental progressive scoliosis in the rabbit. J. Bone Joint Surg., 43-B:116, 1961.
429. Langenskiöld, A., and Michelsson, J. E.: The pathogenesis of experimental progressive scoliosis. Acta Orthop. Scand., 59:Suppl.:1, 1962.
430. Laulund, T., Sojbjerg, J. D., and Horlyck, E.: Moire topography in school screening for structural scoliosis. Acta Orthop. Scand., 53:765, 1982.
431. Laurnen, E. L., Tupper, J. W., and Mullen, M. P.: The Boston brace in thoracic scoliosis—a preliminary report. Spine, 8:388, 1983.
432. Lawton, L., and Moseley, C. F.: The use of the unit rod to control pelvic obliquity in segmental fixation of scoliosis. Paper presented at the 18th Annual Meeting of the Scoliosis Research Society, New Orleans, 1983.
433. Leatherman, K. D., Johnson, J. R., Holt, R. T., and Broadstone, P.: A clinical assessment of 357 cases of segmental spinal instrumentation. In Luque, E. R. (ed.): Segmental Spinal Instrumentation. Thorofare, N.J., Slack, 1984, pp. 165–184.
434. Leaver, J. M., Alvik, A., and Warren, M. D.: Prescriptive screening for adolescent scoliosis: A review of the evidence. Int. J. Epidemiol., 11:101, 1982.
435. Lehner, J., and Lorber, C.: A community experience with the Boston thoracolumbar spine orthosis: 130 consecutive cases. Orthop. Trans., 6:361, 1982.
436. Leider, L. L., Moe, J. H., and Winter, R. B.: Early ambulation after surgical treatment of idiopathic scoliosis. J. Bone Joint Surg., 55-A:1003, 1973.
437. Leong, J. C. Y., Low, W. D., Mok, C. K., Kung, L. S., and Yau, A. C. M. C.: Linear growth in southern

Chinese female patients with adolescent idiopathic scoliosis. Spine, 7:471, 1982.

438. Leslie, I. J., Dorgan, J. C., Bentley, G., and Galloway, R. W.: A prospective study of deep vein thrombosis of the leg in children with halo-femoral traction. J. Bone Joint Surg., 63-B:168, 1981.

439. Lespargot, A., and Grossiord, A.: Flexibility of scoliosis. What does it mean? Is this terminology appropriate? Spine, 10:428, 1985.

440. Lester, D. K., Painter, G. L., and Berman, A. T.: Idiopathic scoliosis associated with congenital upper limb deficiency. Clin. Orthop., 202:205, 1986.

441. Letts, M.: Scoliosis in children secondary to retroperitoneal fibrosis. Report of two cases. J. Bone Joint Surg., 64-A:1363, 1982.

442. Letts, R. M., and Bobechko, W. P.: Fusion of the scoliotic spine in young children. Clin. Orthop., 101:136, 1974.

443. Letts, R. M., and Hollenbert, C.: Delayed paresis following spine fusion with Harrington instrumentation. Clin. Orthop., 125:45, 1977.

444. Letts, R. M., Paiekar, G., and Bobechko, W. P.: Preoperative skeletal traction in scoliosis. J. Bone Joint Surg., 57-A:616, 1975.

445. Levacher, A. F. T.: Nouveau moyen de prévenir et de guérir la courbure de l'épine. Mem. Acad. R. Chir., 4:596, 1768.

446. Lezberg, S. F.: Screening for scoliosis. Preventive medicine in a public school. Phys. Ther., 54:371, 1974.

447. Lindahl, O., and Movin, A.: Measurement of the deformity in scoliosis. Acta Orthop. Scand., 39:291, 1968.

448. Lindh, M.: Energy expenditure during walking in patients with scoliosis. The effect of the Milwaukee brace. Spine, 3:313, 1978.

449. Lindh, M.: The effect of sagittal curve changes on brace correction of idiopathic scoliosis. Spine, 5:26, 1980.

450. Lindh, M., and Bjur, J.: Lung volumes in scoliosis before and after correction by Harrington instrumentation method. Acta Orthop. Scand., 46:934, 1975.

451. Lloyd Roberts, G. C., and Pilcher, M. F.: Structural idiopathic scoliosis in infancy. A study of the natural history of 100 patients. J. Bone Joint Surg., 47-B:520, 1965.

452. Lloyd Roberts, G. C., Pincott, J. R., McMeniman, P., Bayley, I. J., and Kendall, B.: Progression in idiopathic scoliosis: A preliminary report of a possible mechanism. J. Bone Joint Surg., 60-B:451, 1978.

453. Logan, W. R.: The effect of the Milwaukee brace on the developing dentition. Dent. Pract., 12:447, 1962.

454. Lonstein, J. E.: Screening for spinal deformities in Minnesota schools. Clin. Orthop., 126:33, 1977.

455. Lonstein, J. E.: Prognostication in idiopathic scoliosis. Orthop. Trans., 5:22, 1981.

456. Lonstein, J. E., and Carlson, J. M.: The prediction of curve progression in untreated idiopathic scoliosis during growth. J. Bone Joint Surg., 66-A:1061, 1984.

457. Lonstein, J. E., and Holter, A. R.: Complications of the anterior approach and the treatment of spinal deformities. In Proceedings of Scoliosis Research Society, 1985.

458. Lonstein, J. E., Bjorklund, S., Wanninger, M. H., and Nelson, R. P.: Voluntary school screening for scoliosis in Minnesota. J. Bone Joint Surg., 64-A:481, 1982.

459. Lonstein, J. E., Winter, R. B., Moe, J. H., and Gaines, D.: Wound infection with Harrington instrumentation and spine fusion for scoliosis. Clin. Orthop., 96:222, 1973.

460. Lonstein, J. E., Winter, R. B., Moe, J. H., Bianco, A. J., Campbell, R. G., and Norval, M. A.: School screening for the early detection of spine deformities. Progress and pitfalls. Minn. Med., 59:51, 1976.

461. Lovett, R. W.: The mechanism of the normal spine and its relation to scoliosis. Boston Med. Surg. J., 153:349, 1905.

462. Lovett, R. W., and Brewster, A. H.: Correction of the structural lateral curvature of spine. J.A.M.A., 82:1115, 1924.

463. Low, W. D., Chew, E. C., Kung, L. S., Hsu, L. C., and Leong, J. C.: Ultrastructures of nerve fibers and muscle spindles in adolescent idiopathic scoliosis. Clin. Orthop., 174:217, 1983.

464. Low, W. D., Mok, C. K., Leong, J. C. Y., Yau, A. C. M. C., and Lisowski, F. P.: The development of southern Chinese girls with adolescent idiopathic scoliosis. Spine, 3:152, 1978.

465. Lowe, R. W., and Jones, E. T.: Spinal screening in West Virginia. W. Va. Med. J., 78:243, 1982.

466. Luke, M. J., and McDonnell, E. J.: Congenital heart disease and scoliosis. J. Pediatr., 73:725, 1968.

467. Lukeschitsch, G., Meznik, F., and Feldner-Bustin, H.: Cerebral dysfunction in patients with idiopathic scoliosis. Z. Orthop., 118:372, 1980.

468. Luque, E. R.: Segmental spinal instrumentation: A method of rigid internal fixation of the spine to induce arthrodesis. Orthop. Trans., 4:391, 1980.

469. Luque, E. R.: Segmental spinal instrumentation for correction of scoliosis. Clin. Orthop., 163:192, 1982.

470. Luque, E. R.: The anatomic basis and development of segmental spinal instrumentation. Spine, 7:256, 1982.

471. Luque, E. R.: The correction of postural curves of the spine. Spine, 7:270, 1982.

472. Luque, E. R.: Vertebral column transposition. Orthop. Trans., 7:29, 1983.

473. Luque, E. R.: Anatomy of scoliosis and its correction. Clin. Orthop., 105:198, 1984.

474. Luque, E. R. (ed.): Segmental Spinal Instrumentation. Thorofare, N. J., Slack, 1984.

475. Luque, E. R., and Cardoso, A. M.: Treatment of scoliosis without arthrodesis or external support. Orthop. Trans., 1:37, 1977.

476. McAfee, P. C., Lubicky, J. P., and Weiner, F. W.: The use of segmental instrumentation to preserve longitudinal spinal growth. An experimental study. J. Bone Joint Surg., 65-A:935, 1983.

477. McAlister, W. H., and Shackelford, G. D.: Classification of spinal curvatures. Radiol. Clin. North Am., 13:93, 1975.

478. McAlister, W. H., and Shackelford, G. D.: Measurement of spinal curvatures. Radiol. Clin. North Am., 13:113, 1975.

479. McCall, I. W., Galvin, E., O'Brien, J. P., and Park, W. M.: Alteration in vertebral growth following prolonged plaster immobilization. Acta Orthop. Scand., 52:327, 1981.

480. McCarthy, R. E., Morrissy, R. T., and Dwyer, A. P.: Scoliosis school screening in Arkansas. J. Arkansas Med. Soc., 79:315, 1983.

481. McCollough, N., Friedman, H., and Bracale, R.: Surface electrical stimulation of the paraspinal muscles in the treatment of idiopathic scoliosis. Orthop. Trans., 4:29, 1980.

482. McCollough, N. C., III, Schultz, M., Javach, N., and Latta, L.: Miami TLSO in the management of scoliosis: Preliminary results in 100 cases. J. Pediatr. Orthop., 1:141, 1981.

483. MacEwen, G. D., and Cowell, H. R.: Familial incidence of idiopathic scoliosis and the implication in patient treatment. J. Bone Joint Surg., 52-A:405, 1970.

484. MacEwen, G. D., Bunnell, W. P., and Sriram, K.: Acute neurological complications in the treatment of scoliosis. J. Bone Joint Surg., 57-A:404, 1975.

485. McMaster, M. J.: Infantile idiopathic scoliosis: Can it be prevented? J. Bone Joint Surg., 65-B:612, 1983.

486. McMaster, M. J., and Macnicol, M. F.: The manage-

ment of progressive infantile idiopathic scoliosis. J. Bone Joint Surg., *61-B*:36, 1979.

487. McMaster, W. C., and Clayton, K.: Spinal bracing in the institutionalized person with scoliosis. Spine, 5:459, 1980.
488. Malcolm-Smith, N. A., and McMaster, M. J.: The use of induced hypotension in control of bleeding during posterior fusion for scoliosis. J. Bone Joint Surg., *65-B*:255, 1983.
489. Manning, C. W., Prime, F. J., and Zorab, P. A.: Partial costectomy as a cosmetic operation in scoliosis. J. Bone Joint Surg., *55-B*:521, 1973.
490. Manning, W. J., and Hardy, J. H.: Night bracing in idiopathic scoliosis. Orthop. Trans., 6:16, 1982.
491. Marchetti, P. G.: Le scoliosi. Bologna, Aulo Gaggi, 1968.
492. Marchetti, P. G.: Modificazioni ed usi speciali per lo strumentario di Harrington. Policlinico (Sez Chir.), 83:540, 1976.
493. Marshall, W. A., and Tanner, J. M.: Variation in patterns of pubertal changes in girls. Arch. Dis. Child., 44:291, 1969.
494. Mau, H.: Aetiology of idiopathic scoliosis. Reconstr. Surg. Traumatol., 13:184, 1972.
495. Mau, H.: The changing concept of infantile scoliosis. Int. Orthop., 5:131, 1981.
496. Mehta, M. H.: The natural history of infantile idiopathic scoliosis. *In* Zorab, P. A. (ed.): Scoliosis and Growth. London, Churchill-Livingstone, 1971, pp. 103–122.
497. Mehta, M. H.: The rib-vertebra angle in the early diagnosis between resolving and progressive infantile scoliosis. J. Bone Joint Surg., *54-B*:230, 1972.
498. Mehta, M. H.: Pain provoked scoliosis: Observations on the evolution of the deformity. Clin. Orthop., 135:58, 1978.
499. Mehta, M. H., and Morel, G.: The non-operative treatment of infantile idiopathic scoliosis. *In* Zorab, P. A., and Siezler, D. (eds.): Scoliosis. London, Academic, 1979, pp. 71–84.
500. Mellencamp, D. D., Blount, W. P., and Anderson, A. J.: Milwaukee brace treatment of idiopathic scoliosis. Late results. Clin. Orthop., 126:47, 1977.
501. Micheli, L. J., and Hood, R. W.: Anterior exposure of the cervicothoracic spine using a combined cervical and thoracic approach. J. Bone Joint Surg., *65-A*:992, 1983.
502. Michelsson, J. E.: The development of spinal deformity in experimental scoliosis. Acta Orthop. Scand., Suppl. 81, 1965.
503. Miles, M.: Vertebral changes following experimentally produced muscle imbalance. Arch. Phys. Med., 28:284, 1947.
504. Miller, D., and Lever, C. S.: Scoliosis screening: An approach used in the school. J. Sch. Health, 52:98, 1982.
505. Miller, J. A. A., Nachemson, A. L., and Schultz, A. B.: Effectiveness of braces in mild idiopathic scoliosis. Spine, 9:632, 1984.
506. Moe, J. H.: A critical analysis of methods of fusion for scoliosis: An evaluation of 276 patients. J. Bone Joint Surg., *40-A*:529, 1958.
507. Moe, J. H.: Complications of scoliosis treatment. Clin. Orthop., 53:21, 1967.
508. Moe, J. H.: The Milwaukee brace in the treatment of scoliosis. Clin. Orthop., 77:18, 1971.
509. Moe, J. H.: Indications for Milwaukee brace nonoperative treatment in idiopathic scoliosis. Clin. Orthop., 93:38, 1973.
510. Moe, J. H., and Denis, F.: The iatrogenic loss of lumbar lordosis. Orthop. Trans., 1:2, 1977.
511. Moe, J. H., and Gustilo, R. B.: Treatment of scoliosis: Results in 196 patients treated by cast correction and fusion. J. Bone Joint Surg., *46-A*:293, 1964.
512. Moe, J. H., and Kettleson, D. N.: Idiopathic scoliosis.

Analysis of curve patterns and the preliminary results of Milwaukee brace treatment in 169 patients. J. Bone Joint Surg., *52-A*:1509, 1970.
513. Moe, J. H., and Valuska, J.: Evaluation of treatment of scoliosis by Harrington instrumentation. J. Bone Joint Surg., *48-A*:1656, 1966.
514. Moe, J. H., Purcell, G. A., and Bradford, D. S.: Zielke instrumentation (VDS) for the correction of spinal curvature. Analysis of results in 66 patients. Clin. Orthop., *180*:133, 1983.
515. Moe, J. H., Sundberg, A. B., and Gustilo, R.: A clinical study of spine fusion in the growing child. J. Bone Joint Surg., *46-B*:784, 1964.
516. Moe, J. H., Kharrat, K., Winter, R. B., and Cummine, J. L.: Harrington instrumentation without fusion plus external orthotic support for the treatment of difficult curvature problems in young children. Clin. Orthop., *185*:35, 1984.
517. Moe, J. H., Winter, R. B., Bradford, D., and Lonstein, J.: Scoliosis and Other Spinal Deformities. 2nd Ed. Philadelphia, Saunders, 1987.
518. Monticelli, G., Ascain, E., Salsano, V., and Salsano, A.: Experimental scoliosis induced by prolonged minimal electrical stimulation of the paravertebral muscles. Ital. J. Orthop. Traumatol., *1*:39, 1975.
519. Moreland, M. S., Barce, C., and Pope, M. H.: Moire topography in scoliosis: Pattern recognition and analysis. *In* Moreland, M. S., Pope, M. H., and Armstrong, G. W. D. (eds.): Moire fringe topography and spinal deformity. New York, Oxford, Toronto, Pergamon, 1981, pp. 171–185.
520. Moreland, M. S., Cobb, L. C., Pope, M. H., and Stokes, A. F.: Pattern recognition in Moire topography. J. Pediatr. Orthop., 3:120, 1983.
521. Morgan, T. H., and Scott, J. C.: Treatment of infantile idiopathic scoliosis. J. Bone Joint Surg., *38-B*:450, 1956.
522. Mori, Y.: Evaluation of the rotational deformity in scoliosis. II. Application of laser torsography to the follow-up of the clinical course of rotation deformity during treatment. Nippon Seikeigeka Gakkai Zasshi, 57:703, 1983.
523. Morscher, E.: Experiences with the transthoracic hemilateral epiphyseodesis in the treatment of scoliosis. *In* Chapchal, G. (ed.): Operative Treatment of Scoliosis. Stuttgart, Thieme Stratton, 1973.
524. Mortensen, L.: Augmented feedback spinal orthosis. An introduction and preliminary report. Orthot. Prosthet., 36:56, 1982.
525. Moskowitz, A., Moe, J. H., Winter, R. B., and Binner, H.: Long-term follow-up of scoliosis fusion. J. Bone Joint Surg., *62-A*:364, 1980.
526. Mulcahy, T., Galante, J., DeWald, R., Schultz, A., and Hunter, J. C.: A follow-up study of forces acting on the Milwaukee brace on patients undergoing treatment for idiopathic scoliosis. Clin. Orthop., 93:53, 1973.
527. Myers, B. A., Friedman, S. B., and Weiner, I. B.: Coping with a chronic disability: Psychosocial observations of girl with scoliosis treated with a Milwaukee brace. Am. J. Dis. Child., *120*:175, 1970.
528. Nachemson, A.: A long-term follow-up study of nontreated scoliosis. Acta Orthop. Scand., *39*:466, 1968.
529. Nachemson, A., and Elfstrom, G.: A force-indicating distractor for Harrington-rod procedure. J. Bone Joint Surg., *51*:1660, 1969.
530. Nachemson, A., and Elfstrom, E.: Intravital wireless telemetry of axial forces in Harrington distraction rods in patients with idiopathic scoliosis. J. Bone Joint Surg., *53-A*:445, 1971.
531. Nachemson, A., and Nordwall, A.: The Cotrel dynamic spine traction—an ineffective method of preoperative correction of scoliosis. J. Bone Joint Surg., *58-A*:158, 1976.
532. Nachemson, A., and Nordwall, A.: Effectiveness of

preoperative Cotrel traction for correction of idiopathic scoliosis. J. Bone Joint Surg., 59-A:504, 1977.

533. Nachemson, A., Cochran, T. P., Fallstrom, K., and Irstam, L.: Somatic, social and psychologic effects of treatment for idiopathic scoliosis. Orthop. Trans., 7:508, 1983.

534. Nachlas, I. W., and Borden, J. N.: Experimental scoliosis—the role of the epiphysis. Surg. Gynecol. Obstet., 90:672, 1950.

535. Nachlas, I. W., and Borden, J. N.: The cure of experimental scoliosis by directed growth control. J. Bone Joint Surg., 33-A:24, 1951.

536. Naeye, R. L.: Kyphoscoliosis and cor pulmonale. Am. J. Pathol., 38:561, 1961.

537. Nakamura, T.: Histopathological study on the intervertebral discs of idiopathic scoliosis (author's transl). Nippon Seikeigeka Gakkai Zasshi, 54:523, 1980.

538. Nash, C. L., Jr.: Current concepts review: Scoliosis bracing. J. Bone Joint Surg., 62-A:848, 1980.

539. Nash, C. L., Jr., and Moe, J. H.: A study of vertebral rotation. J. Bone Joint Surg., 51-A:223, 1969.

540. Nash, C. L., Jr., Brodkey, J. S., and Croft, T. J.: A model for electrical monitoring of spinal cord function in scoliosis undergoing correction. J. Bone Joint Surg., 54-A:197, 1972.

541. Nash, C. L., Jr., Schatzinger, L., and Lorig, R.: Intraoperative monitoring of spinal cord function during scoliosis spine surgery. J. Bone Joint Surg., 56-A:1765, 1974.

542. Nash, C. L., Jr., Gregg, E. C., Brown, R. H., and Pillai, N. S.: Risk of exposure to x-rays in patients undergoing long-term treatment for scoliosis. J. Bone Joint Surg., 61-A:371, 1979.

543. Nash, C. L., Jr., Lorig, R. A., Schatzinger, L. A., and Brown, R. H.: Spinal cord monitoring during operative treatment of the spine. Clin. Orthop., 126:100, 1977.

544. Negri, V.: Incidence of scoliosis in adolescents of the schools of Parma. Acta Biomed. Ateneo Parmense, 53:41, 1982.

545. Neiman, I. Z.: Effectiveness of diskotomy in scoliosis in adolescents. Ortop. Travmatol. Protez., 5:22, 1980.

546. Nel, G., and Du Toit, G.: Congenital upper limb anomalies and scoliosis. S. Afr. Med. J., 63:893, 1983.

547. Neuhauser, E. B. D., Wittenborg, M. H., Berman, C. Z., and Cohen, J.: Irradiation effects of roentgen therapy on the growing spine. Radiology, 59:637, 1952.

548. Newman, D. C., and DeWald, R. L.: School screening for scoliosis. I.M.J., 151:31, 1977.

549. Nicastro, J. F., Traina, J., Lancaster, M., and Hartjen, C.: Sublaminar segmental wire fixation: Anatomic pathways during their removal. Orthop. Trans., 8:172, 1984.

550. Nickel, V. L., Perry, J., Garret, A., and Happenstall, M.: The halo: A spinal skeletal fixation device. J. Bone Joint Surg., 50-A:1400, 1968.

551. Nicolopoulos, K. S., Burwell, R. G., and Webb, J. K.: Stature of girls with adolescent idiopathic scoliosis: The importance of pelvic height and its sexual dimorphism in health. J. Bone Joint Surg., 66-B:289, 1984.

552. Nicolopoulos, K. S., Burwell, R. G., and Webb, J. K.: Stature and its components in adolescent idiopathic scoliosis. Cephalo-caudal disproportion in the trunk of girls. J. Bone Joint Surg., 67-B:594, 1985.

553. Nillius, A., Willner, S., Arborelius, M., and Nylander, G.: Combined radionucleotide phlebography and lung scanning in patients operated on for scoliosis with Harrington procedure. Clin. Orthop., 152:241, 1980.

554. Nilsonne, U.: Long-term prognosis in idiopathic scoliosis. Acta Orthop. Scand., 39:456, 1968.

555. Nilsonne, U., and Lundgren, K. D.: Long-term prog-

556. Nogami, H., Ogasawara, N., Kasai, T., Oki, T., and Murachi, S.: Lipid storage myopathy associated with scoliosis and multiple joint contracture. Acta Neuropathol. (Berl.), 61:305, 1983.

557. Nordwall, A.: Studies in idiopathic scoliosis relevant to etiology, conservative and operative treatment. Acta Orthop. Scand. (Suppl.), 150:1, 1973.

558. Nordwall, A.: Mechanical properties of tendinous structures in patients with idiopathic scoliosis. J. Bone Joint Surg., 56-A:443, 1974.

559. Nordwall, A., and Wilner, S.: A study of skeletal age and height in girls with idiopathic scoliosis. Clin. Orthop., 110:6, 1975.

560. Notage, W. M., Waugh, T. R., and McMaster, W. C.: Radiation exposure during scoliosis screening radiography. Spine, 6:456, 1981.

561. O'Brien, J. F.: The halo-pelvic apparatus: A clinical bioengineering and anatomical study. Acta Orthop. Scand. (Suppl.), 163:1, 1975.

562. O'Brien, J. F., Gillespie, R., McNeice, G. M., and Raso, J. V.: Instrumentation without fusion. A clinical experience of sixteen cases. Paper presented at the 14th Annual Meeting of the Scoliosis Research Society, Seattle, 1979.

563. O'Brien, J. P., and van Akkerveeken, P. F.: School screening for scoliosis. Results of a pilot study. Practitioner, 219:739, 1977.

564. O'Brien, J. P., Yau, A. C., Smith, T. K., and Hodgson, A. R.: Halo pelvic traction. J. Bone Joint Surg., 53-B:217, 1971.

565. Oda, M., Rauh, S., Gregory, P. B., Silverman, F. N., and Bleck, E. E.: The significance of roentgenographic measurement in scoliosis. J. Pediatr. Orthop., 2:378, 1982.

566. Ogden, J. A.: The development and growth of the musculoskeletal system. In Albright, J. A., and Brand, R. A. (eds.): The Scientific Basis of Orthopaedics. New York, Appleton-Century-Crofts, 1979, pp. 41–103.

567. Ogilvie, J. W., and Millar, E. A.: Comparison of segmental spinal instrumentation devices in the correction of scoliosis. Spine, 8:416, 1983.

568. Ollier, M.: Techniques des platres et corsets des scolioses. Paris, Masson, 1971.

569. Olsen, G., Rosen, H., Hohn, R., and Slocum, B.: Electrical muscle stimulation as a means of correcting induced canine scoliotic curves. Clin. Orthop., 125:227, 1977.

570. Olsen, G., Rosen, H., Stoll, S., and Brown, G.: The use of muscle stimulation for inducing scoliotic curves. A preliminary report. Clin. Orthop., 113:198, 1975.

571. Owen, R., Taylor, J. F., McKendrick, O., and Dangerfield, P.: Current incidence of scoliosis in school-children in the City of Liverpool. In Zorab, P. A., and Seigler, D. (eds.): Scoliosis 1979: Proceedings of the Sixth Symposium Held at the Cardiothoracic Institute, Brompton Hospital, London. London, Academic, 1980, pp. 31–34.

572. Paling, M. R., and Spasovsky-Chernick, M.: Scoliosis in cystic fibrosis—an appraisal. Skeletal Radiol., 8:63, 1982.

573. Paré, A.: Opera Ambrosil Parel. Paris, Apud Jacobum Du-Puys, 1582.

574. Paré, A.: Collected Works. Trans. Johnson, T. London, 1634.

575. Pasteyer, J., Jean, N., Merckx, J., et al.: Accidents de l'anesthésie au cours de la chirurgie des scolioses. Anaesth. Analg. Rev., 33:47, 1976.

576. Paul of Aegina: Collected Works. Adams, F. (trans.). London, Sydenham Society, 1834, et seq.

577. Pedriolle, R.: La Scoliose. Maloine S. A. (ed.). Paris, Masson et Cie, 1979.

578. Pedriolle, R., and Vidal, J.: Thoracic idiopathic curve evolution and prognosis. Spine, 10:785, 1985.

579. Pelker, R. P., and Gage, J. R.: The correlation of idiopathic lumbar scoliosis and lumbar lordosis. Clin. Orthop., 163:199, 1982.

580. Perricone, G., Luppis, F., and Parrilla Paricio, P.: Electromyographic research in idiopathic scoliosis. Chir. Organi Mov., 65:147, 1979.

581. Perry, J.: The halo in spinal abnormalities. Orthop. Clin. North Am., 3:69, 1972.

582. Perry, J., and Nickel, V. L.: Total cervical spine fusion for neck paralysis. J. Bone Joint Surg., 41-A:37, 1959.

583. Piggott, H.: Posterior rib resection in scoliosis: A preliminary report. J. Bone Joint Surg., 53-B:663, 1971.

584. Pin, L. H., Mo, L. Y., Lin, L., Hua, L. K., Hui, H. P., Hui, D. S., Chang, B. D., and Chang, Y. Y.: Early diagnosis of scoliosis based on school-screening. J. Bone Joint Surg., 67-A:1202, 1985.

585. Pincott, J. R., Davies, J. S., and Taffs, L. F.: Scoliosis caused by section of dorsal spinal nerve roots. J. Bone Joint Surg., 66-B:27, 1984.

586. Pink, P.: Harrington's surgical treatment of scoliosis. Wien. Med. Wochenschr., 132:515, 1982.

587. Pinto, W. C.: Complications of surgical treatment of scoliosis. Isr. J. Med. Sci., 9:837, 1973.

588. Ponder, R. C., Dickson, J. H., Harrington, P. R., and Erwin, W. D.: Results of Harrington instrumentation and fusion in the adult idiopathic scoliosis patient. J. Bone Joint Surg., 57-A:797, 1975.

589. Ponseti, I. V.: Experimental scoliosis. Bull. Hosp. Joint Dis., 19:216, 1958–1959.

590. Ponseti, I. V., and Baird, W. A.: Scoliosis and dissecting aneurysm of the aorta in rats fed with Lathyrus odoratus seeds. Am. J. Pathol., 28:1059, 1952.

591. Ponseti, I. V., and Friedman, B.: Prognosis in idiopathic scoliosis. J. Bone Joint Surg., 32-A:381, 1950.

592. Ponseti, I. V., and Friedman, B.: Changes in scoliotic spine after fusion. J. Bone Joint Surg., 32-A:751, 1950.

593. Ponseti, I. V., and Shepard, R. S.: Lesions of the skeleton and other mesodermal tissues in rats fed with sweet-pea (Lathyrus odoratus) seeds. J. Bone Joint Surg., 36-A:1031, 1954.

594. Ponte, A.: Postoperative paraplegia due to hypercorrection of scoliosis and drop in blood pressure. J. Bone Joint Surg., 56-A:444, 1974.

595. Ponte, A.: An orthopaedic brace for the non-operative treatment of lumbar and thoracolumbar scoliosis. J. Bone Joint Surg., 56-A:1764, 1974.

596. Ponte, A.: Prognostic evaluation of vertebral rotation in small idiopathic curves. Orthop. Trans., 6:6, 1982.

597. Portillo, D., Sinkora, G., McNeill, T., Spencer, D., and Schultz, A.: Trunk strengths in structurally normal girls and girls with idiopathic scoliosis. Spine, 7:551, 1982.

598. Powers, T. A., Haher, T. R., Devlin, V. J., Spencer, D., and Millar, E. A.: Abnormalities of the spine in relation to congenital upper limb deficiencies. J. Pediatr. Orthop., 3:471, 1983.

599. Pratt, W. B., Schader, J. B., and Phippen, W. G.: Elevation of hair copper in idiopathic scoliosis. Spine, 9:540, 1984.

600. Quick, M. M., and Highriter, M. E.: Is privacy important in scoliosis screening? J. Sch. Health, 51:458, 1981.

601. Raia, T. J., and Kilfoyle, R. M.: Minimizing radiation exposure in scoliosis screening. Appl. Radiol., 11:45, 1982.

602. Ransford, A. O., and Edgar, M. A.: A transverse bar system to supplement Harrington distraction instrumentation in scoliosis. A radiological study during operation. J. Bone Joint Surg., 64-B:226, 1982.

603. Ransford, A. O., and Manning, C. W. S. F.: Complications of halo-pelvic distraction for scoliosis. J. Bone Joint Surg., 57-B:131, 1975.

604. Ransford, A. O., Pozo, J. L., Hutton, P. A. N., and Kirwan, E. O. G.: The behaviour pattern of the scoliosis associated with osteoid osteoma or osteoblastoma of the spine. J. Bone Joint Surg., 66-B:16, 1984.

605. Raphael, B. G., Llackner, H., and Engler, G. L.: Disseminated intravascular coagulation during surgery for scoliosis. Clin. Orthop., 162:41, 1982.

606. Redford, J. B., Butterworth, T. R., and Clements, E. L., Jr.: Use of electromyography as a prognostic aid in the management of idiopathic scoliosis. Arch. Phys. Med., 50:433, 1969.

607. Relton, J. E., and Hall, J. E.: An operation frame for spinal fusion. A new apparatus designed to reduce haemorrhage during operation. J. Bone Joint Surg., 49-A:327, 1967.

608. Resina, J., and Ferreira, A.: A technique of correction and internal fixation for scoliosis. J. Bone Joint Surg., 59-B:159, 1977.

609. Reuben, J. D., Brown, R. H., Nash, C. L., Jr., and Brower, E. M.: In vivo effects of axial loading on double-curve scoliotic spines. Spine, 7:440, 1982.

610. Reuber, M., Schultz, A., McNeill, T., and Spencer, D.: Trunk muscle myoelectric activities in idiopathic scoliosis. Spine, 8:447, 1983.

611. Riddle, H. F. V., and Roaf, R.: Muscle imbalance in the causation of scoliosis. Lancet, 1:1245, 1955.

612. Rinsky, L., Kane, N., Bleck, E., Gamble, J., and Kalen, V.: Treatment of idiopathic scoliosis with SSI. Preliminary report. Paper presented at the 18th Annual Meeting of the Scoliosis Research Society, New Orleans, 1983.

613. Riseborough, E. J.: Treatment of scoliosis. N. Engl. J. Med., 276:1429, 1967.

614. Riseborough, E. J.: The anterior approach to the spine for the correction of deformities of the axial skeleton. Clin. Orthop., 93:207, 1973.

615. Riseborough, E. J., and Herndon, J. H.: Scoliosis and Other Deformities of the Axial Skeleton. Boston, Little, Brown, 1975.

616. Riseborough, E. J., and Wynne-Davies, R.: A genetic survey of idiopathic scoliosis in Boston, Massachusetts. J. Bone Joint Surg., 55-A:974, 1973.

617. Riska, E. B.: End results in the treatment of scoliosis. A survey of 57 cases. Acta Orthop. Scand. (Suppl.), 102:7, 1967.

618. Risser, J. C.: Important practical facts in the treatment of scoliosis. A.A.O.S. Instr. Course Lect., 5:248, 1948.

619. Risser, J. C.: The application of body casts for the correction of scoliosis. A.A.O.S. Instr. Course Lect., 12:255, 1955.

620. Risser, J. C.: Modern trends in scoliosis. Bull. Hosp. Joint Dis., 19:166, 1958.

621. Risser, J. C.: The iliac apophysis: An invaluable sign in the management of scoliosis. Clin. Orthop., 2:111, 1958.

622. Risser, J. C.: Scoliosis: Past and present. J. Bone Joint Surg., 46-A:167, 1964.

623. Risser, J. C., and Ferguson, A. B.: Scoliosis: Its prognosis. J. Bone Joint Surg., 18:667, 1936.

624. Risser, J. C., and Norquist, D. M.: A follow-up study of the treatment of scoliosis. J. Bone Joint Surg., 40-A:555, 1958.

625. Risser, J. C., Agostini, S., De Alvargenga Sampaio, J. R., and Garibald, C. A. H.: The sitting-standing height ratio as a method of evaluating early spine fusion in the growing child. Clin. Orthop., 24:7, 1973.

626. Risser, J. C., Iqbal, Q. M., Nagata, K., and Azevedo, G.: Early non-operative diagnosis of spinal pseudarthrosis. Int. Surg., 67:181, 1982.

627. Risser, J. C., Lauder, D. H., Norquist, D. M., and Craig, W. A.: Three types of body casts. A.A.O.S. Instr. Course Lect., 10:131, 1953.

628. Ritter, E. M., Wright, C. E., Fritz, S. L., Kirchmer,

N. A., and De Smet, A. A.: Use of a gradient intensifying screen for scoliosis radiography. Radiology, *135*:230, 1980.

629. Roaf, R.: Wedge resection for scoliosis. J. Bone Joint Surg., *37-B*:97, 1955.

630. Roaf, R.: Rotational movements of the spine with special reference to scoliosis. J. Bone Joint Surg., *40-B*:312, 1958.

631. Roaf, R.: Vertebral growth and its mechanical control. J. Bone Joint Surg., *42-B*:40, 1960.

632. Roaf, R.: The treatment of progressive scoliosis by unilateral growth arrest. J. Bone Joint Surg., *45-B*:637, 1963.

633. Roaf, R.: Scoliosis. Baltimore, Williams & Wilkins, 1966.

634. Roaf, R.: The basic anatomy of scoliosis. J. Bone Joint Surg., *48-A*:786, 1966.

635. Roaf, R.: Spinal Deformities. 2nd Ed. Turnbridge Wells, Pitman, 1980, p. 337.

636. Rogala, E., and Drummond, D. S.: The Shriner's flexicurve asssessment of scoliotic hump deformities. J. Bone Joint Surg., *61-B*:245, 1979.

637. Rogala, E. J., Drummond, D. S., and Gurr, J.: Scoliosis: Incidence and natural history. A prospective epidemiological study. J. Bone Joint Surg., *60-A*:173, 1978.

638. Rothman, R. H., and Simeone, F. A.: The Spine. 2nd Ed. Philadelphia, Saunders, 1982.

639. Rudicel, S., and Renshaw, T. S.: The effect of the Milwaukee brace on spinal decompensation in idiopathic scoliosis. Spine, *8*:385, 1983.

640. Saarrtok, T., Dahlberg, E., Bylund, P., Eriksson, E., and Gustafsson, J.: Steroid hormone receptors, protein and D.N.A. in erector spinae muscle from scoliotic patients. Clin. Orthop., *183*:197, 1984.

641. Sahgal, V., Shah, A., Flanagan, N., Schaffer, M., Kane, W., Subramani, V., and Singh, H.: Morphologic and morphometric studies of muscle in idiopathic scoliosis. Acta Orthop. Scand., *54*:242, 1983.

642. Sahlstrand, T.: An analysis of lateral predominance in adolescent idiopathic scoliosis with special reference to convexity of the curve. Spine, *5*:512, 1980.

643. Sahlstrand, T., and Lidstrom, J.: Equilibrium factors as predictors of the prognosis in adolescent idiopathic scoliosis. Clin. Orthop., *152*:232, 1980.

644. Sahlstrand, T., and Petruson, B.: A study of labyrinthine function in patients with adolescent idiopathic scoliosis. An electro-nystagmographic study. Acta Orthop. Scand., *50*:759, 1979.

645. Sahlstrand, T., and Sellden, U.: Nerve conduction velocity in patients with adolescent idiopathic scoliosis. Scand. J. Rehabil. Med., *12*:25, 1980.

646. Sahlstrand, T., Ortengren, R., and Nachemson, A.: Postural equilibrium in adolescent idiopathic scoliosis. Acta Orthop. Scand., *49*:354, 1978.

647. Sahlstrand, T., Petruson, B., and Ortengren, R.: Vestibulospinal reflex activity in patients with adolescent idiopathic scoliosis. Postural effects during caloric labyrinthine stimulation recorded by stabilometry. Acta Orthop. Scand., *50*:275, 1979.

648. Sahlstrand, T., Nachemson, A., Lidstrom, J., and Ortengren, R.: Postural control in scoliosis (letter). Acta Orthop. Scand., *54*:329, 1983.

649. Salanova, C.: Les resultats lointans du corset de Milwaukee: Les indications. Acta Orthop. Belg., *43*:606, 1977.

650. Savini, R., Cervellati, S., and Boroaldo, E.: Spinal deformities in Marfan's syndrome. Ital. J. Orthop. Traumatol., *6*:19, 1980.

651. Savini, R., Parisini, P., and Vincenzi, G.: Respiratory function in severe scoliosis before and after treatment. A review of 76 cases. Ital. J. Orthop. Traumatol., *2*:247, 1976.

652. Savini, R., Parisini, P., Cervellati, S., and Gualdrini,

G.: Surgical treatment of vertebral deformities in neurofibromatosis. Ital. J. Orthop., *9*:13, 1983.

653. Sayre, L. H.: Orthopedic Surgery and Disease of the Joints. New York, Appleton, 1876.

654. Sayre, L. H.: Spinal Disease and Spinal Curvature: Their Treatment by Suspension and the Use of Plaster of Paris Bandage. London, Smith, Elder, 1877.

655. Sayre, L. H.: History of treatment of spondylitis and scoliosis by partial suspension and retention by means of plaster of Paris bandages. N.Y. State Med. J., *11*:12, 1895.

656. Schafer, M. F.: Dwyer instrumentation of the spine. Orthop. Clin. North Am., *9*:115, 1978.

657. Shatzinger, L., Nash, C., Drotar, D., and Hall, T.: Emotional adjustment in scoliosis. Clin. Orthop., *125*:145, 1977.

658. Schmidt, A. C.: Fundamental principles and treatment of scoliosis. A.A.O.S. Instr. Course Lect., *16*:184, 1959.

659. Schmitt, E. W.: Post-instrumentation paraplegia and a negative Stagnara test—a case report. Presented at the Annual Meeting of the Scoliosis Research Society, Boston, Massachusetts, 1978.

660. Schmorl, G., and Junghans, H.: The Human Spine in Health and Disease. New York, Grune & Stratton, 1971.

661. Schultz, A. B.: A biomechanical view of scoliosis. Spine, *1*:162, 1976.

662. Schultz, A. B., and Andersson, G. B. J.: Analysis of loads on the lumbar spine. Spine, *6*:76, 1981.

663. Schultz, A. B., and Hursch, C.: Mechanical analysis of techniques for improved correction of scoliosis. Clin. Orthop., *100*:66, 1974.

664. Schultz, A. B., Haderspeck, K., and Takashima, S.: Correction of scoliosis by muscle stimulation. Biomechanical analysis. Spine, *6*:468, 1981.

665. Schultz, A. B., Sorenson, S., and Andersson, G. B. J.: Measurement of spine morphology in children ages 10–16. Spine, *9*:70, 1984.

666. Schultz, A. B., Ciszewski, D. J., DeWald, R. L., and Spencer, D. L.: Spine morphology as a determinant of progression tendency in idiopathic scoliosis. Orthop. Trans., *3*:52, 1979.

667. Schutt, R. C., Jr., Brown, C. W., Tiefel, L. C., Odom, J. A., and Donaldson, D. H.: Surface electrical stimulation for the treatment of scoliosis. Biomed. Sci. Instrum., *18*:83, 1982.

668. Schwartzmann, J. R., and Miles, M.: Experimental production of scoliosis in rats and mice. J. Bone Joint Surg., *27*:59, 1945.

669. Scoliosis Research Society: Spinal Screening Program Handbook. Chicago, Scoliosis Research Society, 1980.

670. Scott, J. C.: Scoliosis and neurofibromatosis. J. Bone Joint Surg., *47-B*:240, 1965.

671. Scott, M. M., and Piggott, H.: A short-term follow-up of patients with mild scoliosis. J. Bone Joint Surg., *63-B*:523, 1981.

672. Segil, C. M.: The incidence of idiopathic scoliosis in the Bantu and White population groups in Johannesburg. J. Bone Joint Surg., *56-B*:393, 1974.

673. Sensenig, E. C.: Early development of the human vertebral column. Contrib. Embryol., *33*:21, 1949.

674. Sevastikoglou, J. A., and Bergquist, E.: Evaluation of the reliability of radiological methods for registration of scoliosis. Acta Orthop. Scand., *40*:608, 1969.

675. Sevastikoglou, J. A., Aaro, S., and Normelli, H.: Scoliosis: Experimental and clinical studies. Clin. Orthop., *191*:27, 1984.

676. Sevastikoglou, J. A., Linderholm, H., and Lidgren, U.: Effect of the Milwaukee brace on vital and ventilatory capacity of scoliotic patients. Acta Orthop. Scand., *47*:540, 1976.

677. Sevastikoglou, J. A., Aaro, S., Elmstedt, E., Dahlborn, M., and Levander, R.: Bone scanning of the

spine and thorax in idiopathic thoracic scoliosis. Clin. Orthop., *149*:172, 1980.

678. Shaffer, J. W.: Rib transposition and vascularized bone grafts—hemodynamics assessment of donor rib graft and recipient vertebral body. Orthop. Trans., 8:153, 1984.

679. Shalding, B.: The so-called superior mesenteric artery syndrome. Am. J. Dis. Child., *130*:1371, 1976.

680. Shands, A. R., Jr., and Eisberg, H. B.: The incidence of scoliosis in the state of Delaware, a study of 50,000 minifilms of the chest made during a survey for tuberculosis. J. Bone Joint Surg., *37-A*:1243, 1955.

681. Shannon, D. C., Riseborough, E. J., and Valenca, L. M.: The distribution of abnormal lung function in kyphoscoliosis. J. Bone Joint Surg., *52-A*:131, 1970.

682. Shaw, B., and Read, J.: Hypoxia and thoracic scoliosis. Br. Med. J., 2:1486, 1960.

683. Shneerson, J. M.: Cardiac and respiratory responses to exercise in adolescent idiopathic scoliosis. Thorax, 35:347, 1980.

684. Shufflebarger, H. L., Price, C. T., and Riddick, M.: L rod instrumentation and spinal fusion: The Florida experience. Paper presented at the 18th Annual Meeting of the Scoliosis Research Society, New Orleans, 1983.

685. Silber, I., and McMaster, W.: Retroperitoneal fibrosis with hydronephrosis as a complication of the Dwyer procedure. J. Pediatr. Surg., *12*:255, 1977.

686. Simmons, E. H.: Observations on the technique and indications for wedge resection of the spine. J. Bone Joint Surg., *50-A*:847, 1968.

687. Simurda, M. A.: Arteriovenous fistula and neurological sequelae of spinal fusion. J. Bone Joint Surg., *51-B*:193, 1969.

688. Skandalakis, J. E., Akin, J. T., Milsap, J. H., and Gray, S. W.: Vascular compression of the duodenum. Contemp. Surg., *10*:33, 1977.

689. Skogland, L. B., and Miller, J. A. A.: Growth related hormones in idiopathic scoliosis: An endocrine basis for accelerated growth. Acta Orthop. Scand., *51*:779, 1980.

690. Skogland, L. B., and Miller, J. A.: The length and proportions of the thoracolumbar spine in children with idiopathic scoliosis. Acta Orthop. Scand., *52*:177, 1981.

691. Skogland, L. B., Miller, J. A., Skottner, A., and Fryklund, L.: Serum somatomedin A and non-dialyzable urinary hydroxyproline in girls with idiopathic scoliosis. Acta Orthop. Scand., *52*:307, 1981.

692. Smith, A. DeF., Butte, F. L., and Ferguson, A. B.: Treatment of scoliosis by the wedging jacket and spine fusion: A review of 265 cases. J. Bone Joint Surg., *20*:825, 1938.

693. Smyrnis, P. N., Valavanis, J., Alexopoulos, A., Siderakis, G., and Giannestras, N. J.: School screening for scoliosis in Athens. J. Bone Joint Surg., *61-B*:215, 1979.

694. Somerville, E. A.: Rotational lordosis: The development of the single curve. J. Bone Joint Surg., *34-B*:421, 1952.

695. Span, Y., Robin, G., and Makin, M.: Incidence of scoliosis in school children in Jerusalem. J. Bone Joint Surg., *58-B*:379, 1976.

696. Stafford, R. A.: William Adams Lectures on the Pathology and Treatment of Lateral and Other Forms of Curvature of the Spine. 2nd Ed. London, Churchill, 1882, pp. 240–241.

697. Stagnara, P.: Traction cranienne par le halo de Rancho Los Amigos. Rev. Chir. Orthop., *57*:287, 1971.

698. Stagnara, P.: Utilization of Harrington Device in the Treatment of Adult kyphoscoliosis Above 100 Degrees. Fourth International Symposium, 1971, Nijnegen. Stuttgart, Thieme, 1973.

699. Stagnara, P.: Les Deformations du Rachis: Scolioses, Cyphoses, Lordoses. Paris, Masson, 1985.

700. Stagnara, P., Biot, B., and Fauchet, R.: Critical evaluation of the surgical treatment of vertebral lesions due to neurofibromatosis: 31 cases. Rev. Chir. Orthop., *61*:17, 1975.

701. Stagnara, P., DeMauroy, J. C., and Dran, G.: Reciprocal angulation of vertebral bodies in a sagittal plane: Approach to references for the evaluation of kyphosis and lordosis. Spine, 7:335, 1982.

702. Stagnara, P., Fleury, D., Fauchet, R., Mazoyer, D., Bict, B., Van Zelle, C., and Jouvinroux, R.: Major scoliosis over 100 degrees in adults, 183 surgically treated cases. Rev. Chir. Orthop., *61*:101, 1975.

703. Steel, H. H.: Rib resection and spine fusion in correction of convex deformity in scoliosis. J. Bone Joint Surg., *65-A*:920, 1983.

704. Steinberg, I.: Cor pulmonale in kyphoscoliosis. Angiocardiographic feature of a case. A.J.R., *97*:658, 1966.

705. Steindler, A.: Nature and course of idiopathic scoliosis. A.A.O.S. Instr. Course Lect., 7:150, 1950.

706. Steindler, A.: Kinesiology of the Human Body. Springfield, Ill., Thomas, 1955.

707. Stephen, J. P., Wilding, K., and Cass, C. A.: The place of Dwyer anterior instrumentation in scoliosis. Med. J. Aust., *12*:206, 1977.

708. Stillwell, D. L.: Structural deformities of vertebrae bone. Adaptation and modeling in experimental scoliosis and kyphosis. J. Bone Joint Surg., *44-A*:611, 1962.

709. Stone, B., Beckman, C., and Hall, V.: The effect of an exercise program on change in curve in adolescents with minimal idiopathic scoliosis: A preliminary study. Phys. Ther., *59*:759, 1979.

710. Sudhir, K. G., Smith, R. M., Hall, J. E., and Hansen, D. D.: Intraoperative awakening for early recognition of possible neurologic sequelae during Harrington rod spinal fusion. Anesth. Analg. (Cleve.), 55:526, 1976.

711. Sullivan, J. A., and Conner, S. B.: Comparison of Harrington instrumentation and segmental spinal instrumentation in the management of neuromuscular spinal deformity. Spine, 7:299, 1982.

712. Sullivan, J. A., Davidson, R., and Renshaw, T.: Observations on the use of the scolitron in the management of scoliosis. Paper presented at the 18th Annual Meeting of the Scoliosis Research society, New Orleans, 1983.

713. Sundaresan, N., Shah, J., and Feshali, J. G.: A transsternal approach to the upper thoracic vertebrae. Am. J. Surg., *148*:473, 1984.

714. Sundaresan, N., Shah, J., Foley, K. M., and Rosen, G.: An anterior surgical approach to the upper thoracic vertebrae. J. Neurosurg., *61*:686, 1984.

715. Swank, S., Lonstein, J. E., Moe, J. H., Winter, R. B., and Bradford, D. S.: Surgical treatment of adult scoliosis. A review of two hundred and twenty-two cases. J. Bone Joint Surg., *63-A*:268, 1981.

716. Taddonio, R. H., Weller, K., and Appel, M.: A comparison of patients with idiopathic scoliosis managed with and without post-operative immobilization following segmental spinal instrumentation with Luque rods: A preliminary report. Paper presented at the 18th Annual Meeting of the Scoliosis Research Society, New Orleans, 1983.

717. Takemistu, Y., Harada, Y., Ando, M., and Sato, K.: Incidence of scoliosis in Japan by mass screening examination of school children. Read at the Annual Meeting of the Scoliosis Research Society, Chicago, September 1980.

718. Tamari, T., Kobayashi, H., and Inoue, S.: The clinical value of evoked spinal cord potentials as a monitoring of hazardous effects on the spinal cord. Paper presented at the 15th Annual Meeting of the Scoliosis Research Society, Chicago, 1980.

719. Tamborino, J. M., Armbrust, E. N., and Moe, J.: Harrington instrumentation in correction of scoliosis:

A comparison with cast correction. J. Bone Joint Surg., 46-A:313, 1964.

720. Tanner, J. M.: Growth at Adolescence. Oxford, Blackwell, 1962.

721. Tanner, J. M., and Whitehouse, R. H.: Clinical longitudinal standards for height, weight, height velocity, weight velocity and stages of puberty. Arch. Dis. Child., 51:170, 1976.

722. Tanner, J. M., Whitehouse, R. H., and Takaishi, M.: Standards from birth to maturity for height, weight, height velocity and weight velocity: British children. Arch. Dis. Child., 41:454, 1966.

723. Tavares, J., Puavilai, G., and MacEwen, G. D.: Early ambulation with localizer cast following posterior spinal fusion without internal fixation. J. Pediatr. Orthop., 2:492, 1982.

724. Taylor, J. R.: Growth of human intervertebral discs and vertebral bodies. J. Anat., 120:49, 1975.

725. Taylor, J. R.: Scoliosis and growth. Patterns of asymmetry in normal vertebral growth. Acta Orthop. Scand., 54:596, 1983.

726. Taylor, J. R., and Slinger, B. S.: Scoliosis screening and growth in Western Australian students. Med. J. Aust., 1:475, 1980.

727. Taylor, T. K., Ghosh, P., and Bushell, G. R.: The contribution of the intervertebral disk to the scoliotic deformity. Clin. Orthop., 156:79, 1981.

728. Telfer, R. B., Hoyt, W. F., and Schwartz, H. S.: Crossed eyes and halo pelvic traction (letter to editor). Lancet, 2:922, 1971.

729. Terminology Committee, Scoliosis Research Society: A glossary of scoliosis terms. Spine, 1:57, 1976.

730. Terver, S., Kleinman, R., and Bleck, E. E.: Growth landmarks and the evolution of scoliosis. Dev. Med. Child Neurol., 22:675, 1980.

731. Thompson, F., Walsh, M., Colville, J., and Willner, S.: An evaluation of Moire Topography as a method of screening for adolescent idiopathic scoliosis. J. Bone Joint Surg., 63-B:641, 1981.

732. Thompson, S. K., and Bentley, G.: Prognosis in infantile idiopathic scoliosis. J. Bone Joint Surg., 62-B:151, 1980.

733. Thulbourne, T., and Gillespie, R.: The rib hump in idiopathic scoliosis. Measurement, analysis and response to treatment. J. Bone Joint Surg., 58-B:64, 1976.

734. Tietjen, R., and Morgenstern, J. M.: Spondylolisthesis following surgical fusion for scoliosis. Clin. Orthop., 117:176, 1976.

735. Tolo, V. T.: Progression in scoliosis. A 360 degree change in 75 years. Spine, 8:373, 1983.

736. Tolo, V. T., and Gillespie, R.: The characteristics of juvenile idiopathic scoliosis and results of its treatment. J. Bone Joint Surg., 60-B:181, 1978.

737. Tolo, V., and Gillespie, R.: The use of shortened periods of rigid postoperative immobilization in the surgical treatment of idiopathic scoliosis. J. Bone Joint Surg., 63-A:1137, 1981.

738. Torelli, G., Nordwall, A., and Nachemson, A.: The changing pattern of scoliosis treatment due to effective screening. J. Bone Joint Surg., 63-A:337, 1981.

739. Tredwell, S. J., and O'Brien, J. P.: Apophyseal joint degeneration in the cervical spine following halo pelvic distraction. Paper presented at the Annual Meeting of the Scoliosis Research Society, Louisville, Kentucky, 1975.

740. Tredwell, S. J., and O'Brien, J. P.: Avascular necrosis of the proximal end of the dens: A complication of halo-pelvic distraction. J. Bone Joint Surg., 57-A:332, 1975.

741. Tronteji, J. V., Pecak, F., and Dimitrijevic, M. R.: Segmental neurophysiological mechanism in scoliosis. J. Bone Joint Surg., 61-B:310, 1979.

742. Uden, A.: Thromboembolic complications following scoliosis surgery in Scandinavia. Acta Orthop. Scand., 50:175, 1979.

743. Uden, A., and Willner, S.: The effect of lumbar flexion and Boston thoracic brace on the curves in idiopathic scoliosis. Spine, 8:846, 1983.

744. Uden, A., Nilsson, I. M., and Willner, S.: Bleeding time and scoliosis. Acta Orthop. Scand., 53:73, 1982.

745. Uden, A., Willner, S., and Peterson, H.: Initial correction with the Boston thoracic brace. Acta Orthop. Scand., 53:233, 1982.

746. Ulin, R. I., and McGinniss, G. H.: Segmental spinal instrumentation at the Mount Sinai Hospital. Mt. Sinai J. Med. (N.Y.), 50:348, 1983.

747. VanGrouw, A., Hadel, C. I., Weierman, R. J., and Lowell, H. A.: Long-term follow-up of patients with idiopathic scoliosis treated surgically: A preliminary subjective study. Clin. Orthop., 117:197, 1976.

748. VanLoon, L., and Hoogmartens, M.: Technique of combined anterior and posterior wedge resection for fixed lumbar scoliosis. Acta Orthop. Belg., 42:75, 1976.

749. Vanzelle, C., Stagnara, P., and Jouvinroix, P.: Functional monitoring of spinal cord during spinal surgery. Clin. Orthop., 93:173, 1973.

750. Veliskakis, K., and Levine, D.: Effects of posterior spine fusion on vertebral growth in dogs. J. Bone Joint Surg., 48-A:1367, 1967.

751. Vercauteren, M., and DeGroot, W. F.: A "mobile" halo. Spine, 5:297, 1980.

752. Vesely, D. G., and Blaylock, H. I.: Results of Milwaukee brace treatment in idiopathic scoliosis. J. Med. Assoc. State Ala., 50:18, 1980.

753. Victor, D. I., Bresman, M. J., and Keller, R. B.: Brain abscess complicating the use of halo traction. J. Bone Joint Surg., 55-A:635, 1973.

754. Vidal, J., Connes, H., Perdriolle, R., and Lamolinerie, G.: Treatment of scoliosis at the onset with braces. Acta Orthop. Belg., 48:529, 1982.

755. Vinke, T. H.: A skull traction apparatus. J. Bone Joint Surg., 30-A:522, 1948.

756. Volkman, R.: Resektion von Rippenstücker bei Skoliose. Berl. Klin. Wochenschr., 26:1097, 1889.

757. Von Lackum, W. H.: The surgical treatment of scoliosis. A.A.O.S. Instr. Course Lect., 5:236, 1948.

758. Von Lackum, W. H., and Miller, J. P.: Critical observations of the results of the operative treatment of scoliosis. J. Bone Joint Surg., 31-A:102, 1949.

759. Walker, A. P., and Dickson, R. A.: School screening and pelvic tilt scoliosis. Lancet, 2:152, 1984.

760. Warren, M., Leaver, J., and Alvik, A.: School screening for scoliosis (letter). Lancet, 2:522, 1981.

761. Watts, H. G.: Bracing spinal deformities. Orthop. Clin. North Am., 10:769, 1979.

762. Watts, H. G., Hall, J. E., and Stanish, W.: The Boston brace system for the treatment of low thoracic and lumbar scoliosis by the use of a girdle without superstructure. Clin. Orthop., 126:87, 1977.

763. Waugh, T. R.: Intravital measurements during instrumental correction of idiopathic scoliosis. Acta Orthop. Scand. (Suppl.), 93:1, 1966.

764. Waugh, T. R.: The biomechanical basis for the utilization of methylmethacrylate in the treatment of scoliosis. J. Bone Joint Surg., 53-A:194, 1971.

765. Waugh, T. R., Tamborino, J. M., Armbrost, E. N., and Moe, J. H.: Harrington instrumentation in correction of scoliosis. J. Bone Joint Surg., 46-A:313, 1964.

766. Weinstein, S. L., and Ponseti, I. V.: Curve progression in idiopathic scoliosis. J. Bone Joint Surg., 65-A:447, 1983.

767. Weinstein, S. L., Zavala, D. C., and Ponseti, I. V.: Idiopathic scoliosis. J. Bone Joint Surg., 63-A:702, 1981.

768. Weisl, H.: Unusual complications of skull caliper traction. J. Bone Joint Surg., *54-B*:143, 1972.

769. Wenger, D., and Carollo, J.: Biomechanics of segmental spinal instrumentation. *In* Luque, E. R. (ed.): Segmental Spinal Instrumentation. Thorofare, N.J., Slack, 1984, pp. 31–48.

770. Westgate, H. D., Fisch, R. O., and Langer, L. O., Jr.: Pulmonary function in kyphoscoliosis before and after correction by the Harrington instrumentation method. J. Bone Joint Surg., *51-A*:935, 1969.

771. White, A. A., III, and Panjabi, M. M.: The clinical biomechanics of scoliosis. Clin. Orthop., *118*:100, 1976.

772. White, A. A., and Panjabi, M. M.: Clinical Biomechanics of the Spine. Philadelphia, Lippincott, 1978.

773. White, A. A., and Panjabi, M. M.: The basic kinematics of the human spine: A review of past and current knowledge. Spine, *3*:12, 1978.

774. Whitehouse, W. M., and Lampe, I.: Osseous damage in irradiation of renal tumors in infancy and childhood. A.J.R., *70*:721, 1953.

775. Whittle, M. W., and Evans, M.: Instrument for measuring Cobb angle in scoliosis. Lancet, *1*:414, 1979.

776. Wickers, F. C., Bunch, W. H., and Barnett, P. M.: Psychological factors in failure to wear the Milwaukee brace for treatment of idiopathic scoliosis. Clin. Orthop., *126*:62, 1977.

777. Willner, S.: A growth study in girls with adolescent idiopathic structural scoliosis. Clin. Orthop., *101*:129, 1974.

778. Willner, S.: The proportion of legs to trunk in girls with idiopathic structural scoliosis. Acta Orthop. Scand., *46*:84, 1975.

779. Willner, S.: Moire topography—a method for school screening of scoliosis. Arch. Orthop. Trauma. Surg., *95*:181, 1979.

780. Willner, S.: A comparative study of the efficiency of different types of school screening for scoliosis. Acta Orthop. Scand., *53*:769, 1982.

781. Willner, S.: Moire topography—a non-invasive method for diagnosis and documentation of scoliosis in screening of children. Lakartidningen, *79*:2233, 1982.

782. Willner, S.: Spinal pantography—a noninvasive anthropometric device for describing postures and asymmetries of the trunk. J. Pediatr. Orthop., *3*:245, 1983.

783. Willner, S.: Development of trunk asymmetries and structural scoliosis in prepubertal scoliosis children in Malmo: Follow-up of children 10–14 years of age. J. Pediatr. Orthop., *4*:452, 1984.

784. Willner, S.: Effect of the Boston thoracic brace on the frontal and sagittal curves of the spine. Acta Orthop. Scand., *55*:457, 1984.

785. Willner, S., and Johnson, B.: Thoracic kyphosis and lumbar lordosis during the growth period in children. Acta Paediatr. Scand., *72*:873, 1983.

786. Willner, S., and Uden, A.: A prospective prevalence study of scoliosis in Southern Sweden. Acta Orthop. Scand., *53*:233, 1982.

787. Willner, S., and Willner, E.: The role of Moire photography in evaluating minor scoliotic curves. Int. Orthop., *6*:55, 1982.

788. Wilson, M. S., Stockwell, J., and Leedy, M. G.: Measurement of scoliosis by orthopaedic surgeons and radiologists. Aviat. Space Environ. Med., *54*:69, 1983.

789. Wilson, R. L., Levine, D. B., and Doherty, J. H.: Surgical treatment of idiopathic scoliosis. Clin. Orthop., *81*:34, 1971.

790. Winter, R. B.: The effects of early fusion on spine growth. *In* Zorab, P. A. (ed.): Scoliosis and Growth. London, Churchill-Livingstone, 1971, pp. 98–104.

791. Winter, R. B.: Scoliosis and spinal growth. Orthop. Rev., *6*:17, 1977.

792. Winter, R. B.: Posterior spinal fusion in scoliosis: Indications, techniques, and results. Orthop. Clin. North Am., *10*:787, 1979.

793. Winter, R. B.: Evolution in the treatment of idiopathic scoliosis in Minnesota. A family report. Minn. Med., *65*:627, 1982.

794. Winter, R. B., and Carlson, J. M.: Modern orthotics for spinal deformities. Clin. Orthop., *126*:74, 1977.

795. Winter, R. B., and Moe, J. H.: Orthotics for spinal deformity. Clin. Orthop., *102*:72, 1974.

796. Winter, R. B., and Moe, J. H.: A plea for the routine school examination of children for spinal deformity. Minn. Med., *57*:419, 1974.

797. Winter, R. B., Lovell, W. W., and Moe, J. H.: Excessive thoracic lordosis and loss of pulmonary function in patients with idiopathic scoliosis. J. Bone Joint Surg., *57-A*:972, 1975.

798. Wolf, A. W., Brown, J. C., Bonnett, C. A., Nordwall, A., and Sanderson, R.: Transverse traction in the treatment of scoliosis. A preliminary report. Spine, *6*:134, 1981.

799. Wolfe, E., Robin, G. C., Yarom, R., and Gonen, B.: Myopathy of deltoids in patients with idiopathic scoliosis. Electromyogr. Clin. Neurophysiol., *22*:357, 1982.

800. Wullstein, L., and Schulthess, W.: Die Skoliose in inner Behandlung und Entschung nach klinischen und experimentellen Studien. Z. Orthop. Klin., *10*:178, 1902.

801. Wyburn, G. M.: Observations on the development of the human vertebral column. J. Anat., *78*:94, 1944.

802. Wynne-Davies, R.: Familial (idiopathic) scoliosis. A family survey. J. Bone Joint Surg., *50-B*:24, 1968.

803. Wynne-Davies, R.: Genetic and other factors in aetiology of scoliosis. Ph.D. Thesis, University of Edinburgh, 1973.

804. Wynne-Davies, R.: The aetiology of infantile idiopathic scoliosis. J. Bone Joint Surg., *56-B*:565, 1974.

805. Wynne-Davies, R.: Infantile idiopathic scoliosis. Causative factors, particularly in the first six months of life. J. Bone Joint Surg., *57-B*:138, 1975.

806. Yamanoto, H., Tani, T., MacEwen, G. D., and Herman, R.: An evaluation of brainstem function as a prognostication of early idiopathic scoliosis. J. Pediatr. Orthop., *2*:521, 1982.

807. Yau, A. C. M. C., Hsu, L. C. S., O'Brien, J. P., and Hodgson, A. R.: Correction with spinal osteotomy, halo-pelvic distraction and anterior and posterior fusion. J. Bone Joint Surg., *56-A*:1419, 1974.

808. Yekutiel, M., Robin, G. C., and Yarom, R.: Proprioceptive function in children with adolescent idiopathic scoliosis. Spine, *6*:560, 1981.

809. Yong-Hing, K., and MacEwen, G. D.: Scoliosis associated with osteogenesis imperfecta. J. Bone Joint Surg., *64-B*:36, 1982.

810. Young, L. W., Oestreich, A. E., and Goldstein, L. A.: Roentgenology in scoliosis: Contribution to evaluation and management. A.J.R., *108*:778, 1970.

811. Zaoussis, A. L., and James, J. I. P.: The iliac apophysis and the evaluation of curves in scoliosis. J. Bone Joint Surg., *40-B*:442, 1958.

812. Zetterberg, C., Aniansson, A., and Grimby, G.: Morphology of the paravertebral muscles in adolescent idiopathic scoliosis. Spine, *8*:457, 1983.

813. Zielke, K., and Pellin, B.: Neue Instrumente und Implantate zur Erganzung des Harrington Systems. Z. Orthop. Chir., *114*:534, 1976.

814. Zorab, P.: The lungs in kyphoscoliosis. Dev. Med. Child Neurol., *4*:339, 1962.

815. Zorab, P. A.: The medical aspects of scoliosis. *In* James, J. I. P. (ed.): Scoliosis. Edinburgh, Churchill-Livingstone, 1976, pp. 334–343.

816. Zorab, P. A., Prime, F. J., and Harrison, A.: Lung function in young persons after fusion for scoliosis. Spine, *4*:22, 1978.

Scheuermann's Juvenile Kyphosis

Definition

Scheuermann's juvenile kyphosis is an arcuate and fixed kyphosis developing around the time of puberty. It is caused by a wedge-shaped deformity of one or more vertebrae that show certain radiographic changes. This characteristic wedging of the vertebral bodies with diminished anterior height was first described in 1920 by Scheuermann, who emphasized that a definite diagnosis is possible only by means of radiographic study.[100] In his original description, Scheuermann nearly always found three abnormal wedge-shaped vertebrae in each case, but he reported in 1936 that the number might vary from one to five.[101] The presence of wedge-shaped vertebrae is an important sign, and according to measurements of vertebral wedging, the limit between abnormal and normal appears to be in the vicinity of a wedging of 5 degrees.[33, 48] The radiographic definition of Scheuermann's juvenile kyphosis (according to Sørensen) is a kyphosis including at least three adjacent vertebrae with wedging of each vertebra of 5 degrees or more.[107]

Incidence

The exact prevalence of Scheuermann's disease in the general population is not known. According to Sørensen it varies from 4 to 8 per cent (6 per cent in soldiers and 8 per cent in men working in industry).[107] Ascani and associates screened about 20,000 subjects and found an incidence of about 1 per cent in the screened population.[4] Radiologic diagnosis of Scheuermann's disease is made after 11 to 12 years of age because its typical changes of vertebral wedging and kyphosis are not evident before 10 years of age. There is no sex predilection according to Sørensen; however, Bradford and associates reported a higher incidence in the female, with a female to male ratio of 2:1, and Ascani and co-workers reported a female to male ratio of 1.4:1.[3, 6, 23–26, 107]

Etiology and Pathogenesis

The cause of Scheuermann's disease is still unknown despite the many theories advanced in the literature. Initially, Scheuermann, in 1920, considered the changes to be caused by aseptic necrosis of bone of the same nature as that of Legg-Perthes disease.[100] The wedging of the vertebrae was explained as the result of aseptic necrosis of the cartilage of the ring apophysis, which disturbed the growth of the height of the vertebral body anteriorly, it being assumed that this growth took place from the limbus. In the beginning this theory was widely accepted, but later on it was refuted by the work of Bick and Copel and associates, who demonstrated that the limbus (or the ring apophysis) does not contribute to the longitudinal growth of the vertebral body.[14, 15] Later Scheuermann withdrew his theory of avascular necrosis and emphasized that the changes must be caused by an unknown basic factor.[101]

Pathologic studies on patients with Scheuermann's juvenile kyphosis disclosed limbi that were grossly as well as microscopically normal.[103] Wedging in patients as young as nine years, even before onset of ossification of the limbus, was found by Scheuermann in radiographic studies.[101] These findings tend to refute the theory of aseptic necrosis of the limbus.

Some authors proposed damage to the limbus primordium by inflammation or mild infection (epiphysitis). The theory that proposed epiphysitis to be the etiologic factor could not be accepted by others because inflammatory changes could not be demonstrated.[69, 70, 77]

Schmorl performed autopsies on six patients, aged 16 to 24 years, with Scheuermann's kyphosis. He advanced the theory that juvenile kyphosis was due to changes of the discs in the middle and lower thoracic spine. The bulged discs would rupture into the spongiosa through preformed or traumatic tears in the end-plates, with resultant diminution in mass and deformity of the discs. At the site of the perforation of the cartilage plates, enchondral skeletal growth was inhibited. Growth would also be delayed in the anterior part of the vertebral bodies, which were exposed to relatively great pressure because of the kyphosis. Schmorl claimed that these changes were not present in types of kyphosis other than the juvenile one.[103]

Schmorl's theory, however, was challenged by the finding of such changes in the vertebrae outside the area of kyphosis in patients with Scheuermann's kyphosis, and even in persons who did not have Scheuermann's disease.[101, 121]

Mechanical and static forces have been considered to be of etiologic importance. Taut hamstrings and contracture of the iliopsoas muscle have been proposed as causative factors. Ferguson implicated the anterior groove as a causative factor. He reviewed unselected normal lateral chest films in the age group from 6 to 11 years and observed the anterior vascular groove to close with anterior wedging and the development of a roundback in preadolescents.[44] On dissection, it was found that the indentation in the anterior border of the vertebra, as seen on the radiogram, was occupied by a large endothelium-lined vascular lake formed by the confluence of veins at this point. The stresses of upright posture and reduction of the spring action of the spine were implicated by Lambrinudi as a cause of wedging of the vertebrae.[70] This was supported by the reported high incidence of Scheuermann's disease in young agricultural workers who are involved in heavy labor; however, Scheuermann's disease occurs in normal healthy adolescents who are not involved in strenuous exercise or weightlifting.

Injuries prior to clinical onset of Scheuermann's kyphosis have been described in only 5 to 12 per cent of the cases.[70, 101]

The theory of mechanical factors as a cause of Scheuermann's kyphosis does not have an experimental basis. Investigators inserted steel wires subcutaneously into the tails of castrated and noncastrated male rats, fixing the steel wires to subcutaneous tissues and bending them to create a fixed kyphotic position that was maintained for a period of three to six months. Even at the end of six months histologic studies did not reveal any pressure necrosis or areas of degeneration in the cartilage or bone. Radiograms did not disclose wedging of the vertebral bodies in any case.[78]

The studies of Sørensen showed a very high familial occurrence of Scheuermann's kyphosis, but could not demonstrate any mode of inheritance.[107] Bradford and associates proposed osteoporosis as a primary cause of Scheuermann's disease. They based their theory on the common finding of dietary deficiency of calcium in these patients. In addition, they cited clinical and radiographic similarities between kyphosis of Scheuermann's disease and kyphosis in malabsorption syndromes such as cystic fibrosis.[27]

Pathology

The ultrastructural and histochemical studies of Ippolito and Ponseti have shown changes in the growth plate cartilage and matrix of the vertebral plate with an increase in the proteoglycans in the collagen-proteoglycan ratio. As a result enchondral ossification and longitudinal growth of vertebrae are disturbed. They could not show necrosis of the ring apophysis or abnormalities of the intervertebral discs.[58]

Accumulated data of pathologic findings in the early stages of the disease are very meager because of the rarity of the opportunity to perform postmortem studies. In the advanced case the anterior longitudinal ligament is contracted and thickened, acting as a bowstring across the kyphosis. The vertebral body is wedged anteriorly to a varying extent. The disc interspaces are of normal width initially. The vertebral end-plates are disrupted, with escape of disc material into the spongiosa of the vertebral bodies. Histologically there is no evidence of avascular necrosis or infection.

Clinical Features

The age of clinical manifestation is from 13 to 17 years, i.e., around puberty, occurring somewhat earlier in girls than in boys. In a few cases, it has been observed as early as nine years of age. As mentioned above, the radiographic findings typical of Scheuermann's disease are not apparent until age ten years. Therefore, in the juvenile period, cases of Scheuermann's disease may be misdiagnosed as postural roundback. The importance of following poor posture and "postural roundback" cannot be overemphasized. Some of these children may develop wedging of vertebrae and severe Scheuermann's disease. At present, solid data of the natural course of poor posture and progression into Scheuermann's disease are not available.

The patient is usually presented with the complaint of poor posture. He may complain of fatigue or pain in the region of the kyphosis. The aching sensation is aggravated after standing in the same position for a long time and is relieved by lying down.

The physical findings depend on the location of the apex of kyphosis. Its site is purely thoracic in about three fourths of the patients, thoracolumbar in nearly one fourth, and lumbar in only a few. If the summit is in the thoracic area, there is marked accentuation of the normal dorsal kyphosis, increased lumbar lordosis, and a protuberant abdomen (Fig. 6–87). The upper trunk and drooping shoulder are held backward, with the center of gravity falling behind the sacrum, and the normal pelvic tilt is exaggerated. As a rule, the cervical lordosis also becomes increased. The exaggerated cervical and lumbar lordosis is a compensatory phenomenon. The pectoralis major and minor muscles are shortened, with the shoulders protruding anteriorly.

If the apex is at the thoracolumbar level, the

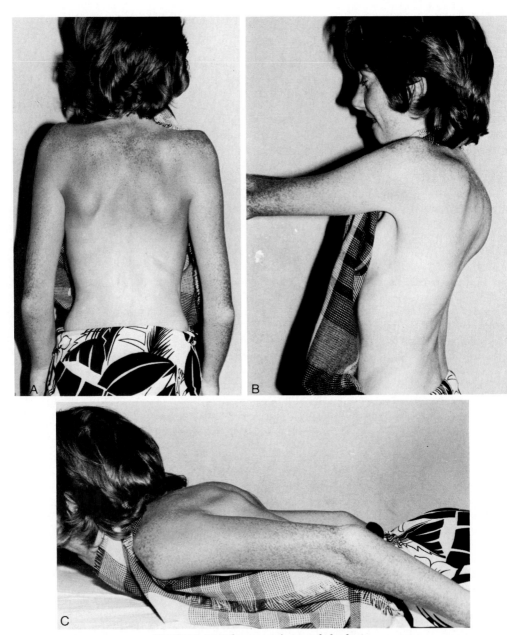

FIGURE 6–87. *Scheuermann's juvenile kyphosis.*

Photographs showing acute accentuation of dorsal kyphus. **A.** Posteroanterior view. **B.** Lateral view. **C.** Dorsal hyperextension.

result is a long kyphosis and a short, low lumbar lordosis. If the lesion is purely lumbar, the postural defect is that of a straight back with a flat thoracic spine and an angular transition between the kyphosis and the sacrum.

In the beginning stages, the postural defect may be corrected both actively and passively, but gradually, within a period of six to nine months, the kyphosis becomes fixed.

A minimal structural scoliosis in the area of kyphosis is present in about 30 to 40 per cent of patients.

Local tenderness on direct manual pressure or light percussion may be present. Muscle and neurologic examination is usually within normal limits. The hamstrings are commonly shortened, as shown by limitation of straight leg raising and in ability to touch the floor on forward flexion of the spine. In severe kyphosis, spinal cord compression may be present on very rare occasions; it manifests by spastic paraparesis and hyperreflexia.

Radiographic Findings

A positive diagnosis of Scheuermann's juvenile kyphosis is only possible by means of radiography. In the lateral view the constant finding is the wedge shape of the affected vertebrae (Fig. 6–88). The wedging is most marked in the central area of the kyphosis and diminished cephalad and caudad. Vertebral wedging is due to retardation of longitudinal growth of the anterior part of the vertebra; it is not due to stress fracture and collapse of the vertebra. Measurement of the vertebral wedging (vw) is carried out on the lateral radiogram by drawing lines through the levels of the two end-plates and determining the angle between the two lines with an ordinary goniometer (Fig. 6–89). The limit between abnormal and normal vertebral wedging appears to be 5 degrees. The kyphotic angle (kw) is the angle between the upper end-plate of the cranial vertebra in the kyphosis and the lower end-plate of the caudal vertebra in the kyphosis. Assessment of the degree of kyphosis should be made in a standing lateral 2-meter radiogram of the spine; the upper limbs are flexed forward 90 degrees so that they are parallel to the floor, with the hands supported on a stand, and the head of the patient held erect. The upper limit of normal dorsal roundback is 35 to 40 degrees.

Disc protrusions into the spongiosa of the vertebra described by Schmorl, and known as Schmorl's nodules, are frequently found on x-rays in the lateral views.[103] The Schmorl's nodules may be single or paired in the two vertebrae on either side of the disc and are delimited from the spongiosa by a narrow, more or less dense osseous zone.

Irregularity of the end-plates, which may be "moth-eaten," frayed, or indented, is often seen. These changes are frequently observed in the vertebrae that are deformed by Schmorl's nodules. These irregularities of vertebral end-plates are the result of growth disturbance and not caused by bone destruction. The *intervertebral discs* are normal in the early stage of the disease, maintaining their height between the wedged vertebrae; later they narrow, particularly in the central area of kyphosis. The anteroposterior diameter of wedged vertebrae may be increased.

The vascular groove from the anterior border into the body has been reported by Ferguson to be visibly longer than normal; however, this finding has not been confirmed by others.[44, 107]

It appears persistence of vascular grooves is a reflection of skeletal maturity of the spine. Scoliosis, if present, is depicted in a standing 2-meter anteroposterior radiogram. The curves, rarely exceeding 25 degrees, are short, with the apex usually at the apex of the kyphosis; rotation is minimal. The flexibility of the kyphosis should be assessed. It is measured on a supine lateral view of the maximally hyperextended spine with a polyurethane plastic wedge placed at the apex of the kyphosis.

Toward the end of the growth period the anterior corners of the kyphotic vertebrae may be sharpened. Later in adult life osteophytes may develop at the anterior border of the deformed vertebral bodies.

In summary the radiographic findings typical of Scheuermann's disease are anterior wedging of vertebrae 5 degrees or more; increase in thoracic kyphosis of more than 40 degrees; irregular vertebral end-plates; and apparent narrowing of disc interspace.

Differential Diagnosis

Postural roundback deformity should be distinguished from Scheuermann's disease. In postural roundback deformity the posterior convexity of the spine has a smooth symmetrical contour, whereas in Scheuermann's disease the kyphotic angulation is acute, usually at T-7 to T-8 level; this is easily detected from the side view with the patient bending forward. In *postural roundback deformity* the posterior convexity of the spine is mobile; it can be easily corrected on hyperextension of the spine; the hamstrings are usually not taut and there is no flexion deformity of the hips due to contracture of iliopsoas. In Scheuermann's disease, however, the kyphosis is fixed; it cannot be reduced on hyperextension of the spine, and straight leg raising is restricted due to tautness of the hamstrings and the iliopsoas is contracted. In the radiograms of the spine in postural roundback deformity there is no anterior wedging of the vertebral bodies (less than 5 degrees), no irregularity of vertebral end-plates, and no narrowing of intervertebral disc interspaces. These changes are characteristic of Scheuermann's disease. In borderline cases, lateral tomograms of the affected vertebrae should be performed to delineate changes in the vertebral end-plates. In postural roundback the degree of kyphosis is usually minimal to moderate—i.e., 40 to 60 degrees of the above criteria of differential. In Scheuermann's disease the kyphotic deformity is fixed.

Kyphosis may be present in other affections

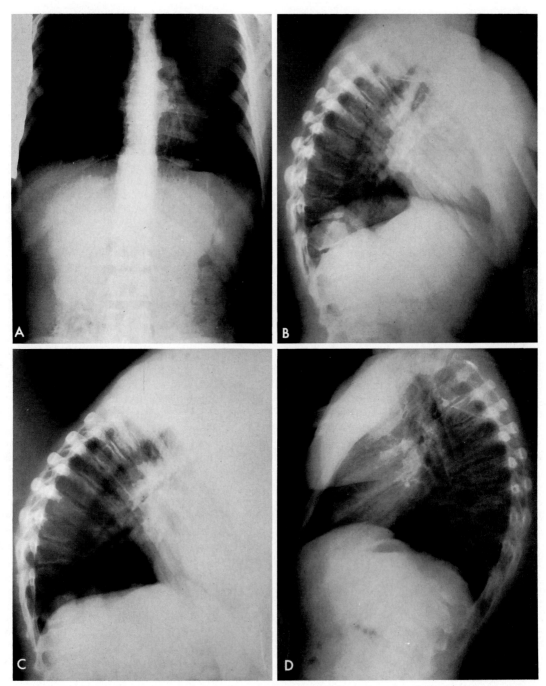

FIGURE 6–88. *Scheuermann's juvenile kyphosis involving the eighth, ninth, and tenth thoracic vertebrae.*

A and **B.** Anteroposterior and lateral views of dorsal spine. **C** and **D.** Flexion and extension views.

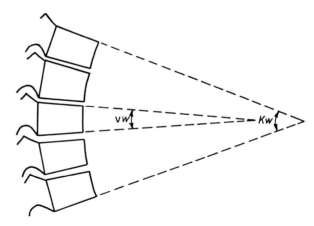

FIGURE 6–89. The method of measuring the degree of vertebral wedging (vw) and of kyphosis (kw). See text for explanation.

(From Sørensen, H. K.: Scheuermann's Juvenile Kyphosis. Copenhagen, Munksgaard, 1964. Reprinted by permission.)

of the spine. *Congenital kyphosis* (Type II) is distinguished from Scheuermann's disease by the spontaneous development of interbody fusion; in untreated Scheuermann's disease, osteophytes may arise anteriorly late in the course, but interbody vertebral fusion across the disc space does not occur. In *bone dysplasias* involving the spine, such as Hurler's syndrome or Morquio's disease, kyphosis may be a feature, but the other characteristic radiographic and clinical findings will establish the diagnosis. A thorough history, clinical examination, and radiographic assessment will rule out other conditions causing kyphosis—such as traumatic compression fractures of one or more vertebrae, infectious spondylitis, postlaminectomy kyphosis, ankylosing spondylitis, neoplasms, and postirradiation kyphosis.

Natural History, Course, and Prognosis

From the onset of the disease until the cessation of growth the radiographic changes have been divided into several stages. Mau, in 1925, grouped them as follows:

I. Stage of irritation (limbus changes)
II. Stage of deformation (development of wedging)
III. Stage of repair (epiphyseal synostosis at cessation of growth)
IV. Stage of proliferation (development of exostosis)[77]

Nathan and Kuhns classified the course into the early stage, the healing stage, and the healed stage, corresponding approximately to the classification of Mau. They noted that during the healing stage there was no progression of the wedge deformity and the structural changes present in the healed stage remained constant throughout life.[86]

A combined clinical-radiographic course of the disease was subdivided into the following stages by Brocher:

I. *Functional phase*, characterized clinically by poor posture from the age of nine or ten years. There may be some exaggeration of dorsal kyphosis, but there is not pain or other clinical symptom. It is rare, however, that one diagnoses Scheuermann's kyphosis in this stage. It is usually found accidentally while studying radiograms of the chest or spine that were taken for other reasons, or by examining the younger siblings of patients with known Scheuermann's kyphosis. In the radiogram, this phase is characterized by regular but abnormal wedging of several vertebrae.

II. *Florid stage*, which represents the typical clinical picture in the age range of 12 to 18 years. There is fixation of the kyphosis and possible minimal scoliosis in the area. Pain and fatigue in the back are usual complaints. Radiologically, this phase is characterized by abnormal wedging of the vertebrae with irregular end-plates, and not infrequently by Schmorl's nodules.

III. *Late stage*, seen in adult life. There is wedge deformity of the vertebrae with more regular end-plates, narrowing of the discs, and development of osteophytes. Local back pain is common. The muscles at the site of the kyphosis are poorly developed and may be the site of fibrositis.[30, 31]

Sørensen, in his long-term study, came to the following conclusions: (1) Back pain and fatigue are less common after the completion of growth than before its completion, having no effect on the working capacity of the patient. (2) One half of the patients develop low back pain later in life, and about one quarter of the patients develop low lumbar disc degeneration. In general, the extent and severity of kyphosis could not be correlated with low back pain, low lumbar disc degeneration, or strenuosity of the patient's work. (3) When the site of kyphosis was low or when it was long, involving the second lumbar vertebra caudally, the incidence of low lumbar disc degeneration causing pain was very high. (4) Radiologically, there will be a slow progression of the kyphosis due to very slight increase in vertebral wedging and to narrowing of the discs. (5) The prognosis appears to be most favorable in the classic type of Scheuermann's kyphosis confined to the thoracic spine.[107]

Treatment

The objectives of treatment are to relieve pain, correct the degree of kyphosis and thereby improve cosmetic appearance, and prevent increase of the degree of kyphosis. In decision-making as to method of treatment to be employed, the following factors are considered: (1) age of patient; (2) the stage in the course of the disease; (3) the degree and structural rigidity of the kyphosis; (4) the location of the posterior convexity; (5) the presence of symptoms such as pain; (6) whether there is associated scoliosis; and (7) psychosocial factors and compliance by the patient. Not all patients with Scheuermann's disease require treatment. A skeletally mature patient with an asymmetrically acceptable kyphosis and with no symptoms can be observed without treatment. General postural exercises are performed to improve posture; it should be clear to the patient that exercises alone have no effect on correction of vertebral wedging or on decreasing the degree of fixed kyphosis.

The effectiveness of surface electrical stimulation in treatment of kyphosis is dubious and not recommended by the author.

There are three modalities of treatment that are effective in treatment of Scheuermann's disease: (1) orthosis (Milwaukee brace), which was developed and is widely used in North America; (2) initial use of antigravity plaster of Paris cast to correct the kyphosis and later maintenance of correction by Plexidur spinal orthosis—the Lyon method developed by Stagnara and used extensively in France and other European countries;[109] and (3) surgery, which is very rarely indicated. The biomechanical principle of both orthotic and cast methods of treatment is the exertion of corrective forces: one posteriorly at the apex of the kyphosis and the other two to the end vertebrae at the extremities of the curve. In both methods, with dorsal kyphosis and exaggerated lumbar lordosis, the orthosis is manufactured (and the cast is applied) to decrease lumbar lordosis. The objective is to relieve compressive forces on the anterior part of the vertebrae and improve longitudinal vertebral growth anteriorly.

ORTHOTIC TREATMENT

The most effective method of treatment is the Milwaukee brace with two posterior kyphosis pads and a neck ring that is centered above the thorax (Fig. 6–90). It is important to correct the anterior jutting of the head and bring the head back centered over the sacrum (forward placement of the neck ring of the orthosis keeps the head forward; it does not improve the kyphosis). The abnormal pelvic tilt and exaggerated lumbar lordosis also should be corrected; pelvic tilt exercises are performed in and out of the brace. The brace is worn continuously (23 of 24 hours) for at least 12 and preferably 18 months. Within four to six weeks, significant correction can be achieved; with decrease of kyphosis, trunk height is increased, requiring adjustment of the orthosis. Usually within a few weeks the back pain is alleviated. Exercises to decrease lumbar lordosis and increase strength of thoracic extension are performed daily. Radiologic evidence of healing and correction of wedging usually takes place within one year; then the patient is gradually weaned from the brace during the ensuing 12 months, wearing the orthosis only at night for the last four to six months. Weaning from the brace in Scheuermann's disease can be commenced prior to completion of spinal growth. If there is any loss of correction during the weaning period, the orthosis is worn full-time and six months later the weaning is resumed, depending on the radiographic findings.

The results of treatment of Scheuermann's disease by the Milwaukee brace have been excellent. Bradford and associates, in a series of 75 patients, reported 40 per cent average correction of the kyphosis, 41 per cent average correction of vertebral wedging, and 36 per cent improvement of lumbar lordosis.[23, 24] Adequate duration of treatment is crucial. Short periods of orthotic wear will result in loss of initial correction. Montgomery and Erwin reported 15 degrees of loss of correction after 18 months of brace wear, whereas Bradford and associates reported only 6 degrees of loss of correction after 34 months of brace wear.[23, 24]

CAST TREATMENT—THE LYON METHOD

Several antigravity hyperextension casts are applied, usually during a total period of 4 to 12

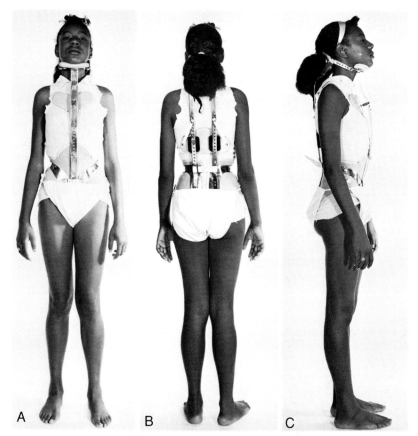

FIGURE 6–90. Milwaukee brace for Scheuermann's juvenile kyphosis.

A. Anteroposterior view. **B.** Posteroanterior view. **C.** Lateral view.

months, followed by full-time wear of a plastic spinal hyperextension orthosis until the wedging of the vertebrae is corrected; then the patient is weaned from the brace during the ensuing three months.[109]

Hyperextension cast may be applied in two stages. In the first stage the lordosis is corrected by positioning the patient bent forward when the lower part of the cast is applied; then, in the second stage, the patient stands erect, extending the cast to the upper part of the trunk, correcting the kyphosis. A simpler way is to apply the cast on a Risser scoliosis table with the patient supine; the lower part of the cast is applied first with the hips flexed to correct lumbar lordosis; then the upper part of the cast is applied with a vertical suspension strap at and below the kyphosis.

The use of the Milwaukee brace is recommended by this author and preferred to that of cast, because the orthosis is cosmetically more accepted by the adolescent and less objectionable socially; it can be removed for bathing and hygiene, and the patient can be gradually weaned from the orthosis.

The results of cast treatment are good; initially there is 30 to 40 per cent correction of the kyphotic curve and 40 to 50 per cent correction of vertebral wedging. However, similar to orthotic treatment, if the cast is discontinued too soon, there will be 50 to 60 per cent loss of the initially achieved correction. It is therefore important to follow the cast method with a period of brace treatment to minimize loss of correction.

SURGICAL CORRECTION

Operative correction of kyphotic deformity in Scheuermann's disease is rarely indicated. It is performed only in a skeletally mature patient with chronic local pain and kyphotic curves of 60 to 70 degrees or more and vertebral wedging of 10 degrees or more. Both anterior and posterior spinal fusion is necessary to achieve permanent correction. Posterior Harrington instrumentation with arthrodesis will achieve excellent correction, but the problem is maintenance of correction. Anterior approach (through a left thoracotomy incision) allows sectioning or excision of the thickened and hypertrophied anterior longitudinal ligament, which rigidly checkreins corrections of the kyphosis. The anterior anulus is released. The intervertebral discs at the apex of the convexity (four to six levels) are completely removed; it is important to leave the posterior anulus and posterior longitudinal ligament intact. Small autogenous corticocancellous grafts (obtained from the ilium and/or the excised rib) are packed into the disc interspaces. Occasionally an anterior strut graft is used. The wound is closed. Two weeks later posterior spinal fusion with internal fixation with Harrington instrumentation (two heavy compression rods) is carried out. When there is significant associated scoliosis, a distraction rod is used on the concave side and a compression rod on the convex side. Postoperatively the spine is supported in a hyperextension body cast or spinal orthosis for a period of nine to twelve months.

Some surgeons may prefer other methods of internal fixation such as Luque rods or segmental wiring with the Harrington rods.

Complications

Spinal cord compression is a rare complication of severe Scheuermann's disease. It may be due to traumatic disc herniation, direct mechanical compression of the cord at a narrow spinal canal at the apex of the kyphosis, or presence of associated intradural cysts. The pathology should be delineated by appropriate tomography, computed tomography, magnetic resonance imaging, and myelography studies. Anterior decompression is carried out, followed by anterior and posterior stabilization.

Atypical forms of Scheuermann's disease can occur; these usually manifest in two forms: *first*, vertebral body changes (irregularity of endplates, intervertebral disc space narrowing, Schmorl's nodules) without wedging or increased kyphosis; and *second*, increased kyphosis with anterior vertebral body wedging but no other vertebral body changes. These atypical forms most probably are variants of Scheuermann's disease, the growth disturbance exhibiting in less florid form.

References

1. Adelstein, L. J.: Spinal extradural cyst associated with kyphosis dorsalis juvenilis. J. Bone Joint Surg., 23:93, 1941.
2. Albanese, A.: Le cifosi dell'adolescenza. Arch. Orthop., 52:189, 1936.
3. Ascani, E., and Montanaro, A.: Scheuermann's disease. *In* Bradford, D., and Hensinger, R. (eds.): The Pediatric Spine. New York, Thieme, 1985, p. 307.
4. Ascani, E., Giglio, G., and Salsano, V.: Scoliosis screening in Rome. *In* Zorab, P. A., and Siegler, D. (eds.): Scoliosis 1979. New York, Academic, 1979, p. 39.
5. Ascani, E., Ippolito, E., and Montanaro, A.: Scheuermann's kyphosis: Histological, histochemical and ultrastructural studies. Paper presented at the 17th Meeting of Scoliosis Research Society, Denver, 1982.
6. Ascani, E., Salsano, V., and Giglio, G.: The incidence and early detection of spinal deformities. J. Ital. Ort., 3:111, 1977.
7. Ascani, E., Montanaro, A., La Rosa, G., and Crostelli, M: Malattia di Scheuermann II: Studio istologico, istochimico, e ultrastrutturale. Progressi in patologia vertebrale. Le cifosi. Vol. 5. Bologna, Gaggi, 1982, p. 105.
8. Ascani, E., Borelli, P., La Rosa, G., Montanaro, A., and Turturro, F.: Malattia di Scheuermann. I: Studio ormonale. Progressi in patologia vertebrale. Le cifosi. Vol. 5. Bologna, Gaggi, 1982, p. 97.
9. Aufdermaur, M.: Zur Pathogenese der Scheuermannschen Krankheit. Dtsch. Med. Wochenschr., 89:73, 1964.
10. Aufdermaur, M.: Juvenile kyphosis (Scheuermann's disease): Radiography, histology and pathogenesis. Clin. Orthop., 154:166, 1981.
11. Axhausen, G.: Über den Abgrenzungvorgang am epiphysaren Knochen (Osteochondritis dissecans König). Virchows. Arch., 252:458, 1924.
12. Becker, K. J.: Über die Behandlung jugendlicher Kyphosen mit einem aktiven bzw., einem kombinierten zweiteiligen akitv-passiven Reklinationskorsett. Z. Orthop., 89:464, 1958.
13. Beyeler, J., Reichmann, B., Schneider, W., and Schweizer, A.: 13. Scheuermann's disease. b). Thoracic Scheuermann's disease: 10- and more years' results of surgically and conservatively treated patients. Orthopaede, 8:180, 1979.
14. Bick, E. M., and Copel, J. W.: The ring apophysis of the human vertebra. Contribution to human osteogeny II. J. Bone Joint Surg., 33-A:783, 1951.
15. Bick, E. M., Copel, J. W., and Spector, S.: Longitudinal growth of the human vertebra. A contribution to human osteogeny. J. Bone Joint Surg., 32-A:803, 1950.
16. Bjersand, A. J.: Juvenile kyphosis in identical twins. A.J.R., 134:598, 1980.
17. Blount, W. P., Schmidt, A. C., Albert, C., and Bidwell, R. G.: Making the Milwaukee brace. J. Bone Joint Surg., 40-A:523, 1958.
18. Bradford, D. S.: Neurological complications in Scheuermann's disease. J. Bone Joint Surg., 51-A:657, 1969.
19. Bradford, D. S.: Vertebral osteochondrosis (Scheuermann's kyphosis). Clin. Orthop., 158:83, 1981.
20. Bradford, D. S., and Garcia, A.: Neurological complications in Scheuermann's disease. A case report and review of the literature. J. Bone Joint Surg., 51-A:567, 1969.
21. Bradford, D. S., and Moe, J. H.: Scheuermann's juvenile kyphosis: A histologic study. Clin. Orthop., 110:45, 1975.
22. Bradford, D. S., Moe, J. H., and Winter, R. B.: Kyphosis and postural roundback deformity in children and adolescents. Minn. Med., 56:114, 1973.
23. Bradford, D. S., Moe, J. H., Montalvo, F. J., and Winter, R. B.: Scheuermann's kyphosis and roundback deformity, results of Milwaukee brace treatment. J. Bone Joint Surg., 56-A:749, 1974.
24. Bradford, D. S., Moe, J. H., Montalvo, F. J., and Winter, R. B.: Scheuermann's kyphosis and roundback deformity, results of Milwaukee brace treatment in twenty-two patients. J. Bone Joint Surg., 56-A:749, 1975.
25. Bradford, D. S., Moe, J. H., Montalvo, F. J., and Winter, R. B.: Scheuermann's kyphosis. Results of

surgical treatment by posterior spinal arthrodesis in twenty-two patients. J. Bone Joint Surg., 57-A:439, 1975.

26. Bradford, D. S., Ahmed, K. B., Moe, J. H., Winter, R. B., and Lonstein, J. E.: The surgical management of patients with Scheuermann's disease. A review of twenty-four cases managed by combined anterior and posterior spinal fusion. J. Bone Joint Surg., 62-A:705, 1980.

27. Bradford, D. S., Brown, D. M., Moe, J. H., Winter, R. B., and Jowsey, J.: Scheuermann's kyphosis, a form of juvenile osteoporosis? Clin. Orthop., 118:10, 1976.

28. Bradford, D. S., Khalid, B. A., Moe, J. H., Winter, R. B., and Lonstein, J. E.: The surgical management of patients with Scheuermann's disease. A review of twenty-four cases managed by combined anterior and posterior spine fusion. J. Bone Joint Surg., 62-A:705, 1980.

29. Brocher, J. E. W.: Die Scheuermannsche Krankheit und ihre Differentialdiagnose. Basel, Schwade, 1946.

30. Brocher, J. E. W.: Die Wirbelsaulentuberkulose und ihre Differentialdiagnose. Stuttgart, Thieme, 1953.

31. Brocher, J. E. W.: Die Prognose der Wirbelsaulenleiden. Stuttgart, Thieme, 1957.

32. Buchman, J.: Vertebral epiphysitis: Cause of spinal deformity. J. Bone Joint Surg., 7:814, 1925.

33. Burdzik, G., and Wuensch, K.: Beitrag zum Röntgenbild der Brustkyphose und seiner Deutung. Z. Orthop., 84:591, 1954.

34. Burner, W. L., III, Badger, V. M., and Sherman, F. C.: Osteoporosis and acquired back deformities. J. Pediatr. Orthop., 2:383, 1982.

35. Cleveland, R. H., and Delong, G. R.: The relationship of juvenile lumbar disc disease and Scheuermann's disease. Pediatr. Radiol., 10:161, 1981.

36. Cloward, R. A., and Bucy, P. C.: Spinal extradural cyst and kyphosis dorsalis juvenilis. A.J.R., 38:681, 1937.

37. Dameron, T. B., and Gulledge, W. H.: Adolescent kyphosis. U.S. Armed Forces Med. J., 4:871, 1953.

38. Deacon, P., Berkin, C. R., and Dickson, R. A.: Combined idiopathic kyphosis and scoliosis. An analysis of the lateral spinal curvature associated with Scheuermann's disease. J. Bone Joint Surg., 67-B:189, 1985.

39. Denischi, A., Medrea, O., Antonescu, D., Roventa, N., and Gorun, N.: Orthopedic treatment of Scheuermann's juvenile kyphosis. Rev. Chir. (Chir.), 25:335, 1976.

40. De Smet, A., Fabry, G., and Mulier, J. C.: Milwaukee brace treatment of Scheuermann's kyphosis. Acta Orthop. Belg., 41:597, 1975.

41. Dittmar, O.: Die Rundrückenbildung der Jugendilcher (Kyphos juvenilis). Med. Klin., 35:1203, 1939.

42. Edgren, W.: Osteochondrosis juvenilis lumbalis. Acta Chir. Scand., (Suppl.), 227:1, 1957.

43. Elsberg, C. A., Dike, C. G., and Brewer, E. D.: The symptoms and diagnosis of extradural cysts. Bull. Neurol. Inst., 3:395, 1934.

44. Ferguson, A. B., Jr.: The etiology of pre-adolescent kyphosis. J. Bone Joint Surg., 38-A:149, 1956.

45. Ferguson, A. B., Jr.: Roundback in children. J. Med. Assoc. Ga., 45:458, 1956.

46. Fisk, J. W., Baigent, M. L., and Hill, P. D.: Incidence of Scheuermann's disease. Preliminary report. Am. J. Phys. Med., 61:32, 1982.

47. Fitzsimons, R. B.: Idiopathic scoliosis, Scheuermann's disease and myopathy: Two case reports. Clin. Exp. Neurol., 16:303, 1979.

48. Fletcher, G. H.: Anterior vertebral wedging—frequency and significance. A.J.R., 57:232, 1947.

49. Gardemin, H., and Herbst, W.: Wirbeldeformierung bie den Adoleszenten Kyphose und Osteoporose. Arch. Orthop. Unfallchir., 59:134, 1966.

50. Greene, T. L., Hensinger, R. H., and Hunter, L. Y.: Back pain and vertebral changes simulating Scheuermann's disease. J. Pediatr. Orthop., 5:1, 1985.

51. Guntz, E.: Kyphosis juvenilis sive Adolescentium. Z. Orthop., 65:53, 1937.

52. Hafner, R. H.: Localized osteochondritis. Scheuermann's disease. J. Bone Joint Surg., 34-B:38, 1952.

53. Halal, F., Gledhill, R. B., and Fraser, F. C.: Dominant inheritance of Scheuermann's juvenile kyphosis. Am. J. Dis. Child., 132:1105, 1978.

54. Hefti, F., and Jani, L.: The treatment of Scheuermann's kyphosis with the Milwaukee brace (author's transl.). Z. Orthop., 119:185, 1981.

55. Herndon, W. A., Emans, J. B., Micheli, L. J., and Hall, J. E.: Combined anterior and posterior fusion for Scheuermann's kyphosis. Spine, 6:125, 1981.

56. Heuck, F.: Letter: Roentgen diagnosis of Scheuermann's disease. Dtsch. Med. Wochenschr., 101:761, 1976.

57. Hodgen, J. T., and Frantz, C. H.: Juvenile kyphosis. Surg. Gynecol. Obstet., 72:798, 1941.

58. Ippolito, E., and Ponseti, I. V.: Juvenile kyphosis. Histological and histochemical studies. J. Bone Joint Surg., 63-A:175, 1981.

59. Ippolito, E., Bellocci, M., Montanaro, A., Ascnai, E., and Ponseti, I. V.: Juvenile kyphosis: An ultrastructural study. J. Pediatr. Orthop., 5:315, 1985.

60. Junghanns, H.: Fur Ätiologic, Prognose und Therapie des M. Scheuermann. Medizinische, 1:300, 1955.

61. Kemp, F. H., and Wilson, D. C.: Some factors in the aetiology of osteochondritis of the spine. Br. J. Radiol., 20:410, 1947.

62. Kemp, F. H., Wilson, D. C., and Emrys-Roberts, E.: Social and nutritional factors in adolescent osteochondritis of the spine. Br. J. Soc. Med., 2:66, 1948.

63. Kharrat, K., and Dubousset, J.: Bloc vertébral antérieur progressif chez l'enfant. Discussion des blocs vertébraux acquis au cours de la maladie de Scheuermann. Rev. Chir. Orthop., 66:485, 1980.

64. Kling, T. F., Jr., and Hensinger, R. N.: Scheuermann's disease: Natural history, current concepts and management. *In* Dickson, R. A., and Bradford, D. S. (eds.): Management of Spinal Deformities. (Butterworths International Medical Reviews: Orthopaedics 2.) London, Butterworths, 1984.

65. Knutson, F.: Observations on the growth of the vertebral body in Scheuermann's disease. Acta Radiol., 30:97, 1948.

66. Kosova, Z.: Observation of the activity of Scheuermann's disease (author's transl.). Acta Chir. Orthop. Traumatol. Cech., 42:154, 1975.

67. Kostuik, J., and Lorenz, M.: Longterm follow-up of surgical management in adult Scheuermann's kyphosis. Paper presented at the 17th Meeting of Scoliosis Research Society, Denver, 1982.

68. Kuhlenbaumer, C.: Sibling studies in Scheuermann's syndrome. Z. Orthop., 116:573, 1976.

69. Lachapele, A. P., and Lagarde, C.: De la maladie de Scheuermann (dite épiphysite vertébrale). J. Radiol. Electr., 28:10, 1947.

70. Lambrinudi, C.: Adolescent and senile kyphosis. Br. Med. J., 2:800, 1934.

71. Larsen, E. H., and Nordentaft, E. L.: Growth of the epiphyses and vertebrae. Acta Orthop. Scand., 32:210, 1962.

72. Leger, W.: X-ray diagnosis of Scheuermann's disease (author's transl.). Monatsschr. Kinderheilkd., 122: L784, 1974.

73. McCallum, M. J.: Scheuermann's disease the result of emotional stress? (letter). Med. J. Aust., 140:184, 1984.

74. Mallet, J., Rey, J. C., Raimbeau, G., and Senly, G.: Scheuermann's disease. Spinal growth dystrophy? Rev. Pract., 34:29, 1984.

75. Marciniak, R.: Scheuermann's disease. Pol. Tyg. Lek., 33:447, 1978.

76. Marciniak, R.: Characteristic radiological signs of Scheuermann's syndrome of the thoracic spine (author's transl.). Pol. Przegl. Radiol., 43:49, 1979.

77. Mau, C.: Die Kyphosis dorsalis adolescentium im Rahmen er Epiphysen und Epiphysentinienkrankungen des Wachstumsalters. Z. Orthop. Chir., 46:145, 1925.

78. Mau, C.: Tierexperimentelle Studien zur Frage der pathologischen Anatomie der Adoleszentenkyphose. Z. Orthop. Chir., 51:106, 1929.

79. Mau, H.: Differential diagnosis of early scoliosis in Scheuermann's disease and idiopathic scoliosis (author's transl.). Z. Orthop., 120:58, 1982.

80. Michelle, A. A.: Osteochondrosis deformans juvenilis dorsi. N.Y. State J. Med., 61:98, 1961.

81. Moe, J. H.: Treatment of adolescent kyphosis by nonoperative and operative methods. Manitoba Med. Rev., 45:481, 1965.

82. Muhlbach, R.: Evaluation and therapy of juvenile kyphoses (Scheuermann's disease). Beitr. Orthop. Traumatol., 21:89, 1972.

83. Muhlbach, R., and Rink, B.: Incidence of malocclusion in patients with adolescent scoliosis and Scheuermann's disease. Beitr. Orthop. Traumatol., 24:20, 1974.

84. Muhlbach, von R., Hahnel, H., and Cohn, H.: Zur Bedeutung biochemischer Parameter bei der Beurteilung der Scheuermannschen Krankheit. Medizin und Sport, 10:331, 1970.

85. Muller, G., and Gschwend, N.: Endokrine Storungen und Morbus Scheuermann. Arch. Orthop. Unfallchir., 65:357, 1969.

86. Nathan, L., and Kuhns, J. G.: Epiphysitis of spine. J. Bone Joint Surg., 22:55, 1940.

87. Nicod, L.: Traitment de la maladie de Scheuermann et des dystrophies rachidiennes de croissance. Praxis, 46:1619, 1968.

88. Nuschenpickel, H., and Ackermann, H. J.: Expert testimony on accidents in Scheuermann's disease. Beitr. Orthop. Traumatol., 22:161, 1975.

89. Ober, F. R.: The clinical diagnosis, treatment and prognosis of epiphyseal disturbances in childhood. J.A.M.A., 127:320, 1945.

90. Orosz, M., and Tomory, I.: Scheuermann's kyphosis and its conservative treatment. Orv. Hetil., 123:2843, 1982.

91. Outland, T., and Snedden, H. E.: Juvenile dorsal kyphosis. Clin. Orthop., 5:155, 1955.

92. Overgaard, K.: Prolapses of nucleus pulposus and Scheuermann's disease. Nord. Med., 5:593, 1940.

93. Podesta, A. M.: Osteochondrosis of growth: Scheuermann's disease. Minerva Med., 69:3133, 1978.

94. Rathke, F. W.: Pathogenese und Therapie der juvenilen Kyphose. Z. Orthop., 102:16, 1966.

95. Roaf, R.: Vertebral growth and its mechanical control. J. Bone Joint Surg., 42-B:40, 1960.

96. Rogge, C. W., and Nieman, A.: Isolated and atypical manifestations of Scheuermann's disease. Arch. Chir. Neerl., 28:149, 1976.

97. Roth, M.: Idiopathic scoliosis and Scheuermann's disease: Essentially identical manifestations of neurovertebral growth disproportion. Radiol. Diagn. (Berl.), 22:380, 1981.

98. Ruckstuhl, J., Scheier, H., and Gschwend, N.: 13. Scheuermann's disease. a). Active-passive straightening of the Scheuermann kyphosis. Long-term results (author's transl.). Orthopaede, 8:176, 1979.

99. Ryan, M. D., and Taylor, T. K.: Acute spinal cord compression in Scheuermann's disease. J. Bone Joint Surg., 64-B:409, 1982.

100. Scheuermann, H. W.: Deforming osteochondritis of spine. Ugeskr. Laeger., 82:385, 1920.

101. Scheuermann, H. W.: Kyphosis juvenilis (Scheuer-mann's Krankheit). Fortschr. Geb. Rongenstr., 53:1, 1936.

102. Schmitt, E.: Clinical aspects and prognosis of Scheuermann's scoliosis. Z. Orthop., 113:573, 1975.

103. Schmorl, G.: Beitrage zur pathologischen Anatomie der Wirbelhandscheiben und ihre Beziehungen zur den Wirbelkorpern. Arch. Orthop. Unfallchir., 29:389, 1931.

104. Schulze, K. J., and Maetzel, H.: Results of redression and corset treatment in Scheuermann's disease. Beitr. Orthop. Traumatol., 25:528, 1978.

105. Simon, R. S.: The diagnosis and treatment of kyphosis dorsalis juvenilis (Scheuermann's kyphosis) in the early stage. J. Bone Joint Surg., 24:681, 1942.

106. Smyslova, A. V.: Preoperative treatment and postoperative management of patients with lumbar osteochondrosis. Med. Sestra., 38:25, 1979.

107. Sørensen, H. K.: Scheuermann's Juvenile Kyphosis. Copenhagen, Munksgaard, 1964.

108. Speck, G. R., and Chopin, D. C.: The surgical treatment of Scheuermann's kyphosis. J. Bone Joint Surg., 68-B:189, 1986.

109. Stagnara, P., DuPelous, J., and Fauchet, R.: Traitment orthopédique ambulatoire de la maladie de Scheuermann en periode d'évolution. Rev. Chir. Orthop., 52:585, 1966.

110. Stagnara, P., De Mauroy, J. C., Dran, G., et al.: Reciprocal angulation of vertebral bodies in a saggital plane: Approach to references for the evaluation of kyphosis and lordosis. Spine, 7:335, 1982.

111. Stein, H., and Von Zahn, L.: Zur Pathogenese, Frühdiagnose und Prophylaxe des Morbus Scheuermann. Dtsch. Med. Wochenschr., 81:200, 1965.

112. Stoddard, A., and Osborn, J. F.: Scheuermann's disease or spinal osteochondrosis. Its frequency and relationship with spondylosis. J. Bone Joint Surg., 61-B:56, 1979.

113. Tabjan, W., and Suchocka, J.: Treatment of Scheuermann's disease by means of elongation-extension casts. Chir. Narzadow Ruchu Ortop. Pol., 41:705, 1976.

114. Tada, S.: Radiographic image of Scheuermann's disease. Rinsho Hoshasen, 26:1429, 1981.

115. Taylor, T. C., Wenger, D. R., Stephen, J., Gillespie, R., and Bobechko, W. P.: Surgical management of thoracic kyphosis in adolescents. J. Bone Joint Surg., 61-A:496, 1979.

116. Travaglini, F., and Conte, M.: Cifosi 25 anni dopo. Progressi in patologia vertebrale. Le cifosi. Vol. 5. Bologna, Gaggi, 1982, p. 163.

117. Wassman, K.: Kyphosis juvenilis Scheuermann. Acta Orthop. Scand., 21:65, 1951.

118. Wespi, K.: Contribution to the question of treatment of Scheuermann's disease (author's transl.). Praxis, 65:44, 1976.

119. Williams, E. R.: Observations on the differential diagnosis and sequelae of juvenile vertebral osteochondrosis. Acta Radiol. (Suppl.), 116:293, 1954.

120. Willner, S.: Spinal pantograph: A non-invasive technique for describing kyphosis and lordosis in the thoraco-lumbar spine. Acta Orthop. Scand., 52:525, 1981.

121. Winter, W. A., Veraart, B. E., and Verdegaal, W. P.: Bone scintigraphy in patients with juvenile kyphosis. (M. Scheuermann). Diagn. Imaging, 50:186, 1981.

122. Wissing, O.: Prolapse of nucleus pulposus. Nord. Med., 2:1384, 1939.

123. Yucel, M., Breitenfelder, J., and Gadiel, H. E.: Treatment of florid dorsal Scheuermann's disease with two new breathable plaster-of-paris casts and their biochemical principles of action (author's transl.). Z. Orthop., 119:292, 1981.

124. Yucel, M., Winhart, R., and Breitenfelder, J.: A new cast for treating florid dorsal Scheuermann's disease (author's transl.). Z. Orthop., 116:753, 1978.

Disorders of Intervertebral Discs in Children

INTERVERTEBRAL DISC CALCIFICATION

Calcification of intervertebral discs was first described by Calvé and Galland in 1922.[7] It is common after the fifth decade of life, when, in most cases, it is an accidental radiographic finding, usually occurring in the thoracic or thoracolumbar region. In adults, it is thought to be a degenerative process.

In children, intervertebral disc calcification is rare, but in recent years has been recognized more frequently. It is commonly located in the cervical spine, but does occur in the thoracic or lumbar disc spaces. The comprehensive papers of Eyring and associates, Newton, Silverman and Weens have reviewed most of the cases.[16, 35, 46, 55]

Etiology

Despite many theories, the cause of this disease is uncertain. It has been suggested that disc calcification is the result of a metastatic infective process.[26] The normal adult disc is avascular, but in children the intervertebral disc is supplied by a number of blood vessels that penetrate the cartilage plate, connecting it with the general circulation. These vascular channels in the discs undergo degeneration early in life, gradually disappearing by the age of 20 or 30 years. Thus, the discs in children may be exposed to infectious agents carried in the blood stream. However, strong evidence against infection is the fact that in the majority of cases there is no sign of pyogenic infection and the course of the disease is not the same as in infectious discitis. Calcification of discs in children may represent a nonspecific inflammatory reaction.

Trauma has often been implied as a predisposing factor, but in many children with disc calcification, a definite history of preceding injury cannot be obtained. In children, it seems unlikely that degenerative and vascular disease processes are etiologic agents. Generalized metabolic diseases such as alkaptonuric ochronosis have been ruled out by the negative urinary studies for ochronosis. The multiple disc calcifications in ochronosis do not develop until middle age.

Clinical Picture

Intervertebral disc calcification in childhood presents a distinct clinical syndrome. It is more frequent in the male, approximately in the ratio of two to one. The average age at the time of initial symptoms and diagnosis is seven years. When calcification occurs in the cervical spine, almost all patients have complaints and positive findings consisting of (1) neck pain, local or referred; (2) limitation of neck motion associated frequently with varying degrees of torticollis; (3) local tenderness; and (4) evidence of inflammation, as shown by elevation of temperature, or erythrocyte sedimentation rate, and of white blood count. Most patients are symptom-free within 14 days; however, a few will continue to have occasional neck pain for one or two years.

Calcified thoracic and lumbar discs, often an incidental radiographic finding, are generally multiple, asymptomatic, and persistent (Fig. 6–91). A definite association of this condition with congenital heart disease has been reported.

Radiographic Findings

In the cervical spine, the highest incidence of calcification is in the lower cervical region, but it does occur in all interspaces from the second to the seventh cervical vertebrae. More than one disc may be calcified. The site of calcification is usually central in the disc, presumably in the nucleus pulposus. Usually radiographic appearance of calcium is seen from several days to three weeks after the onset of symptoms. However, there are reported cases in which intervertebral disc calcification was noted long prior to the onset of symptoms, as if they were lying dormant. Usually there is subsequent regression and disappearance of calcification following the onset of neck symptoms. Resolution of these calcifications supports the presence of the previously described blood vessels supplying the discs.

In long-term follow-up of some patients there has been persistence of residual calcification of the disc interspace, flattening of the vertebral bodies, and osteophytes.[16]

Treatment

Simple conservative measures such as neck traction, cervical collar, and analgesics are effective in controlling symptoms. The prognosis is good. The use of radiotherapy, chelating agents, and antibiotics is not justifiable. Occasionally, the involved disc may prolapse posteriorly or laterally.[39, 53] In such cases, appropriate treatment such as decompression and disc ex-

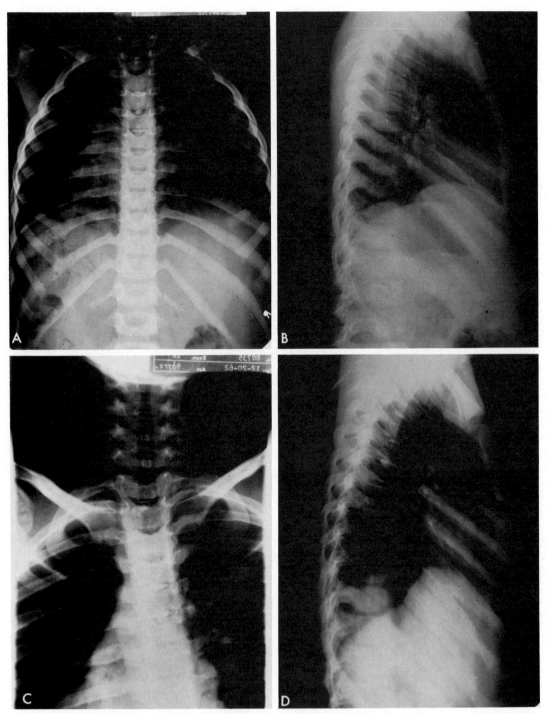

FIGURE 6–91. Intervertebral disc calcification in upper dorsal vertebrae.

A and B. Anteroposterior and lateral radiograms of dorsal spine. Note the calcified intervertebral discs between T3, T4, and T5 vertebrae. C and D. Anteroposterior and lateral radiograms of dorsal spine of same patient six years later. Note the persistence of calcification.

cision is carried out if persistence and severity of neurologic deficit and symptoms warrant it.

References

1. Asadi, A.: Calcification of intervertebral discs in children. Am. J. Dis. Child., *97*:282, 1959.
2. Barchman, L., Fossgreen, J., Matzen, P., and Moller, J. C.: Rheumatic torticollis in a child due to cervical intervertebral disc calcification. Ugeskr. Laeger., *137*:794, 1975.
3. Baron, A.: Über eine neue Erkrankung der Wirbelsaule. Z. Kinderheilk., *104*:357, 1924.
4. Bjelkhagen, I., and Gladnikoff, H.: Calcified disc protrusion in children. Acta Radiol., *48*:151, 1957.
5. Bohmig, R.: Die Blutgefassversorgung der Wirbelbandscheiben, das Verhalten des intervertebralen Chordasegments und die Bedeutung beider für die Bandscheibendegeneration; Zugleich ein Beitrag zur enchondralen Ossification der Wirbelkoerper. Arch. Klin. Chir., *158*:374, 1930.
6. Calandriello, B.: Sulla calcificazione del nucleo polposo intervertebrale nell'infanzia. Arch. Putti Chir. Organi Mov., *9*:277, 1957.
7. Calvé, J., and Galland, M.: Sur une affection particulière de la colonne vertébrale simulant le mal de Pott. J. Radiol. Electr., *6*:21, 1922.
8. Chou, C. W.: Pathological studies on calcification of the intervertebral discs. Nippon Seikeigeka Gakkai Zasshi, *56*:331, 1982.
9. Cohen, R., Burhip, R., and Wagner, E.: Calcification of the intervertebral disc in a child; report of a case. Ann. West. Med. Surg., *3*:202, 1949.
10. Connell, M. C.: Calcification of intervertebral discs in children. Clin. Radiol., *14*:87, 1963.
11. Coventry, M. B., Ghormley, R. K., and Kernohan, J. W.: The intervertebral disc: Its microscopic anatomy and pathology. Part I. Anatomy, development and physiology. J. Bone Joint Surg., *27*:105, 1945.
12. Coventry, M. B., Ghormley, R. K., and Kernohan, J. W.: The intervertebral disc: Its microscopic anatomy and pathology. Part II. Changes in intervertebral disc concomitant with age. J. Bone Joint Surg., *27*:233, 1945.
13. Coventry, M. B., Ghormley, R. K., and Kernohan, J. W.: The intervertebral disc: Its microscopic anatomy and pathology. Part III. Pathologic changes in intervertebral discs. J. Bone Joint Surg., *27*:460, 1945.
14. Crosett, A. D., Jr.: Calcification of the intervertebral discs in a child. Report of a case following poliomyelitis. J. Pediatr., *47*:481, 1955.
15. Eeg-Olofsson, O., Hager, A., Morales, O., and Resjo, M.: Herniated intervertebral disk with calcification, causing torticollis in a 10 year old boy. Lakartidningen, *80*:3320, 1983.
16. Eyring, E. J., Peterson, C. A., and Bjornson, D. R.: Intervertebral disc calcification in childhood. J. Bone Joint Surg., *46-A*:1432, 1964.
17. Francon, F., and Legrand, P.: Deux cas de calcification cervicale du "nucleus pulposus." Presse Med., *62*:1841, 1954.
18. Furukawa, K., Hoshino, R., Hasue, M., and Kuramochi, E.: Cervical intervertebral-disc calcification in a child. J. Bone Joint Surg., *59-A*:692, 1977.
19. Henry, M. J., Grimes, H. A., and Lane, J. W.: Intervertebral disk calcification in childhood. Radiology, *89*:81, 1967.
20. Jespersen, N. B., Lund, H. T., and Egeblad, M.: Intervertebral disc calcification in childhood. Acta Paediatr. Scand., *62*:437, 1973.
21. Keyzer, J. L.: Calcinosis intervertebral. Maandschr. Kindergeneesk., *8*:467, 1939.
22. Kohlmann, G.: Röntgendiagnostik der Wirbelsaule. Verh. Dtsch. Rontgenges., *23*:48, 1931.
23. Lasserre, C., and Phelippot, G.: Discite calcificante intervertébrale. Rev. Orthop., *33*:494, 1947.
24. Legre, J., Padovani, J., and Merjanian, R.: Calcification de disque intervertébral cervical chez le jeune enfant. J. Radiol. Electr., *41*:194, 1960.
25. Lindberg, T.: Intervertebral calcinosis in childhood. Ann. Paediatr., *201*:172, 1963.
26. Lyon, E.: Kalkablagerungen in der Zwischenwirbelscheibe im Kindesalter. Z. Kinderheilkd., *53*:570, 1932.
27. MacCartee, C. C., Griffin, P. P., and Byrd, E. B.: Ruptured calcified thoracic disc in a child. J. Bone Joint Surg., *54-A*:1272, 1972.
28. McGregor, J. C., and Butler, P.: Disc calcification in childhood: Computed tomographic and magnetic resonance imaging appearances. Br. J. Radiol., *59*:180, 1986.
29. Mainzer, F.: Herniation of the nucleus pulposus: A rare complication of intervertebral disk calcification in children. Paediatr. Radiol., *107*:167, 1977.
30. Mann, M. B.: Calcification of intervertebral discs in children. Report of a case. N.C. Med. J., *18*:195, 1957.
31. Melnick, J. C., and Silverman, F. N.: Intervertebral disc calcification in childhood. Radiology, *80*:399, 1963.
32. Mikity, V. G., and Esenbarger, J.: Intervertebral disk calcification in children. A.J.R., *95*:200, 1965.
33. Morris, J., and Niebauer, J.: Calcification of the cervical intervertebral disc. Am. J. Dis. Child., *106*:295, 1963.
34. Mougenot, J. F., Pernin, J., and Herve, J.: Calcification and hernia of an intervertebral disc in a child. Sem. Hop. Paris, *55*:1445, 1979.
35. Newton, T. H.: Cervical intervertebral-disc calcification in children. J. Bone Joint Surg., *40-A*:107, 1958.
36. Ongaro, M., and Ronconi, G. F.: Rilievi clinico-radiological sulla calcificazione dei dischi intervertebrale nell'infanzia. Minerva Pediatr., *14*:846, 1962.
37. Orth, J. O.: Calcification and ossification of the posterior and longitudinal ligament of the cervical spine. Fortschr. Geb. Röntgenstr., *122*:442, 1975.
38. Peacher, W. G., and Storrs, R. P.: Cervical disc calcification in childhood. Radiology, *67*:396, 1956.
39. Peck, F. C., Jr.: A calcified thoracic intervertebral disc with herniation and spinal cord compression in a child; case report. J. Neurosurg., *14*:105, 1957.
40. Pierce, F. T., Jr., and Hanafee, W.: Calcified cervical discs in a child. Calif. Med., *92*:282, 1960.
41. Rechtman, A. M., Hermel, M. B., Albert, S. M., and Boreadis, A. G.: Calcification of the intervertebral disc: Disappearing, dormant and silent. Clin. Orthop., *7*:218, 1956.
42. Schechter, L. S., Smith, A., and Pearl, M.: Intervertebral disk calcification in childhood. Am. J. Dis. Child., *123*:608, 1972.
43. Schorr, S., and Adler, E.: Calcified intervertebral disc in children and adults. Acta Radiol., *41*:498, 1954.
44. Sherman, W. D., Mulfinger, G. L., Garner, J. T., and Jacques, S.: Calcified cervical intervertebral discs in children. Spine, *1*:155, 1976.
45. Sigman, C. C., Jr., and Silepstein, C. M.: Calcification of intervertebral discs in children. The report of a case and review of the literature. J. Med. Assoc. Ga., *551*:214, 1962.
46. Silverman, F. N.: Calcification of the intervertebral discs in childhood. Radiology, *62*:801, 1954.
47. Smith, R. A., Vohman, M. D., Dimon, J. D., III, Averett, J. E., Jr., and Milsap, J. H., Jr.: Calcified cervical intervertebral discs in children. Report of three cases. J. Neurosurg., *46*:233, 1977.
48. Sonnabend, D. H., Taylor, T. K., and Chapman, G. K.: Intervertebral disc calcification syndromes in children. J. Bone Joint Surg., *64-B*:25, 1982.
49. Stewart, P. E., Silbiger, M. L., and Wolfson, S. L.:

Intervertebral disc calcification in childhood. Clin. Paediatr., *13*:363, 1974.

50. Sutton, T. J., and Turcotte, B.: Posterior herniation of calcified intervertebral discs in children. J. Can. Assoc. Radiol., *24*:131, 1973.

51. Swick, H. M.: Calcification of intervertebral discs in childhood. J. Paediatr., *86*:364, 1975.

52. Von Held, H. J.: Zur Frage der Zwischenwirbelscheibenverkalkung. Ein röntgenologisch-klinischer Beitrag. Dtsch. Z. Chir., *242*:676, 1934.

53. Walker, C. S.: Calcification of intervertebral discs in children. J. Bone Joint Surg., *36-B*:601, 1954.

54. Wallman, I. S.: Radiological calcification of intervertebral discs in children. Arch. Dis. Child., *32*:149, 1957.

55. Weens, H. S.: Calcification of the intervertebral discs in childhood. J. Pediatr., *26*:178, 1945.

DISCITIS

Discitis is a *nonspecific inflammatory* or infectious lesion of the intervertebral disc characterized by narrowing of disc space with minimal or no evidence of primary bone involvement. It occurs primarily in infants and young children under the age of five years; occasionally it is observed in older children and adolescents. There is no sex predilection.

The spectrum of discitis ranges from frank pyogenic disc space infection with extension to adjacent bone as osteomyelitis, to a benign, self-limiting inflammation of the intervertebral disc interspace. The two entities are distinct; they should be differentiated.

Narrowing of the intervertebral disc due to infection or inflammation has been described under various names in the literature.[1-65] A. DeF. Smith, in 1933, described it under the title "A Benign Form of Osteomyelitis of the Spine."[53] Harbin and Epton observed that, in some patients with osteomyelitis of the spine, the infection involved only the intervertebral disc, without osseous involvement.[26] Ghormley and associates, in 1940, described 20 adult patients with narrowing of an intervertebral disc in a "Study of Acute Infectious Lesions of Intervertebral Discs"; they proposed that, if osseous involvement of the vertebrae was extensive, a diagnosis of osteomyelitis should be made; if absent or minimal, it should be assumed that the lesion represents an infection of the disc and not osteomyelitis.[22] In describing the clinical entity, the term "acute osteitis of the spine" was used by Bremner and Neligan, and "spondylarthritis" by Saenger.[8, 50] Mathews and co-workers reported on nine children, calling the condition a "destructive lesion involving the intervertebral disc in children," and proposed that the disorder is a primary disease of the intervertebral disc that is self-limited and has a good prognosis.[41] Doyle reported 16 children with this condition under the title "Nar-

rowing of the Intervertebral Disc Space in Children. Presumably an Infectious Lesion of the Disc."[17] DuPont and Anderson and Jamison and associates called it nonspecific spondylitis.[18, 30] Menelaus reported on 35 children and gave credit to Price for coining the word *discitis* to describe the disorder as essentially an inflammation affecting a disc with little or no evidence of primary bone involvement.[43] In the series of 35 children reported on by Menelaus, the lumbar spine was involved in 74 per cent, the thoracic spine in 24 per cent, and in one child, the cervical spine was affected. More than one intervertebral disc may be involved.[43]

Pathogenesis

In the embryo and the young child the intervertebral discs receive their blood supply from the surfaces of the adjacent vertebral bodies.[14, 53] The blood supply to the intervertebral disc in childhood makes it possible for bacteria to gain entrance into the disc through the hematogenous route, which is not possible in the adult. The vascular supply to the intervertebral discs is greater in early life, and it gradually decreases with advancing age. Böhmig states that infectious blood diseases could affect the disc up to the twentieth year of age.[4] Another source of infection of the intervertebral disc is by direct inoculation of the bacteria, as in lumbar puncture or myelography.

It should be noted that discitis is rarely associated with pyogenic osteomyelitis or septic arthritis elsewhere in the body, and pathogenic organisms are cultured in less than 50 per cent of the cases of discitis in aspiration or open biopsy.[63] Viral infection has been conjectured, but laboratory investigations have not shown a particular virus as the etiologic factor. Trauma has been proposed as a cause; however, history of definite injury is given only in a few cases.[1, 43] At present the cause of nonspecific inflammation of the discs is unknown.

Clinical Findings

The typical patient is a young child between two and seven years of age who is brought to the physician with a complaint of pain in the back of one or two weeks' duration. The backache is localized around the involved vertebral area, although it may radiate as vague pains in the buttock, hip, thigh, knee, or abdomen. However, it lacks any true radicular nature. Parents usually state that the child has a limp or refuses to sit, stand, or walk. The symptoms are often nebulous. An upper respiratory infec-

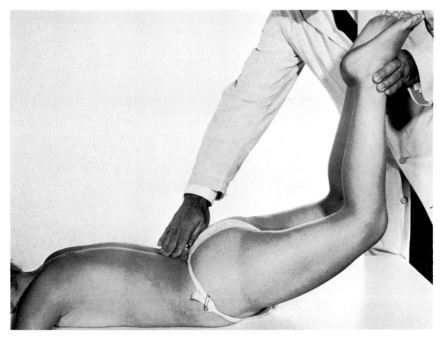

FIGURE 6–92. Method of demonstating paravertebral muscle spasm in the lumbar spine in a child.

tion or an episode of diarrhea may precede the onset of the illness.

On physical examination the child does not appear to be acutely ill, but is irritable and prefers the recumbent position. The temperature may be normal or slightly elevated, but generally not above 100° or 101° F. Paravertebral muscle spasm is the principal physical finding (Fig. 6–92). The normal lumbar lordosis may be lost. Hamstring muscle spasm, if present, will limit straight leg raising. In cervical or upper thoracic level lesions, Koenig's sign may be positive, with pain in the back on flexion of the neck. On careful examination, in a cooperative child, tenderness at the site of the lesion may be noted. There is no neurologic deficit; sensation, reflexes, and motor strength are normal.

Imaging Findings

Early in the course of the disease plain radiographs of the spine are normal. The first radiographic sign of the disease is intervertebral disc space narrowing (Fig. 6–93). This will develop two to three weeks after the onset of symptoms. Linear or computed tomography at this stage will show irregularity and erosion of the vertebral end-plates. Laminagrams will reveal more bone involvement than plain radiographs. Scintigraphy with technetium-99m will show increased uptake early in the course of the disease, prior to appearance of any radiographic

findings (Fig. 6–94). Bone imaging with technetium-99m is an invaluable tool for early diagnosis and localization of the lesion in discitis.[24, 65]

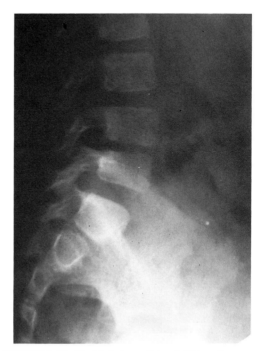

FIGURE 6–93. Discitis between L4 and L5 in a four-year-old child.

Note the narrowing of L4–L5 intervertebral disc interspace.

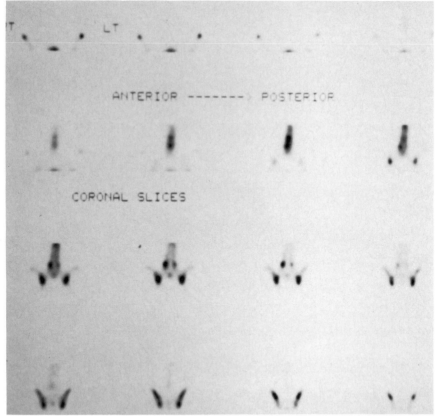

FIGURE 6–94. Bone imaging with technetium-99m in discitis.

Note the increased local uptake of the nucleotide.

Four to six weeks after onset of symptoms plain radiographs will show progressive narrowing of disc space and rarefaction and erosion of adjacent vertebral end-plates (Fig. 6–95). About eight weeks after onset of symptoms the plain radiographs will disclose paravertebral increased soft-tissue shadow due to abscess formation. Vertebral body "cavitation" may develop due to ballooning of disc material into it (Fig. 6–96) or due to bone destruction by the infectious process (Fig. 6–97).

Computed tomography will show erosion of vertebral end-plates, invagination of disc material into the body of the vertebra, and paravertebral abscess much earlier than the plain radiographs. When there is a question of pyogenic bacterial discitis, computed tomography scanning should be performed; however, if there are no systemic signs and laboratory studies do not suggest infection, one may withhold computed tomography study because of the considerable amount of radiation received by the patient during such scanning. Magnetic resonance imaging will depict the inflammatory swelling of the disc and associated pathology, and it does not involve radiation—with improved technology it is as effective a diagnostic tool as computed tomography. Its drawbacks are availability and cost.

Late in the course of discitis radiographic changes include (1) interbody fusion (partial or complete), (2) wedging of disc space (Fig. 6–98), (3) scoliosis and kyphosis, and (4) vertebral body enlargement (vertebra magna).

Laboratory Findings

At first, the erythrocyte sedimentation rate and white blood count are usually elevated, but they return to normal in four to six weeks. Initially, the possibility of tuberculosis should be considered, but the tuberculin skin test is negative in discitis. When radiologic features suggest the possibility of brucellosis or typhoid fever, routine febrile agglutination tests should be performed; they will be negative in discitis.

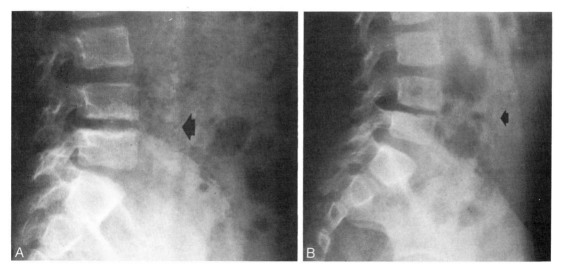

FIGURE 6–95. Progressive narrowing of disc interspace in discitis between L4 and L5.

A. Note the irregularity of the vertebral end-plates and narrowing of the disc interspace. **B.** Three months later. Note the progressive narrowing.

Diagnosis

In the differential diagnosis of discitis one should consider the following:

1. *Tuberculous spondylitis.* It is ruled out by negative skin test and normal chest radiographs. The level of the lesion in tuberculous spondylitis is more thoracic, whereas in discitis it is lumbar. In tuberculous spondylitis the course of the disease has a slower rate of progression with greater bone destruction and minimal reconstitution. Also, in tuberculous spondylitis there is a high incidence of paravertebral abscess formation, which is depicted early by computed tomography scan.

2. *Acute pyogenic vertebral oteomyelitis.* This is characterized by fulminating systemic signs, rapid progressive bone destruction (Fig. 6–99), and a very hot bone scan with technetium-99m, which on SPECT imaging will show bone involvement. Systemic signs in the form of high fever, elevated erythrocyte sedimentation rate, and leukocytosis are present. Computed tomography and magnetic resonance imaging are invaluable tools in delineation of pathology. Vertebral pyogenic osteomyelitis should be ruled out when the child is a severe diabetic!

3. In *salmonella and brucellar infectious spondylitis* blood, urine, or stool culture will be positive. The febrile agglutination tests will be positive. Salmonella osteomyelitis is more common in sickle cell disease and brucellar spondylitis in endemic areas.

4. *Other conditions to consider* in differential diagnosis are intervertebral disc calcification, localized form of Scheuermann's disease, traumatic spondylitis, spinal cord tumor, meningitis and other neurologic diseases, appendicitis, and pyelonephritis.

Attempts to obtain the bacterial organism and determine its sensitivity are made under the following circumstances: (1) presence of systemic signs, such as high fever, leukocytosis,

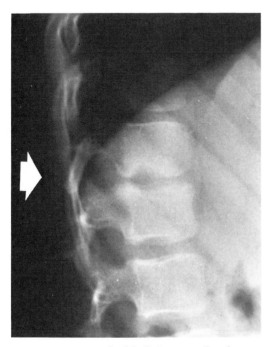

FIGURE 6–96. Vertebral body "cavitation" in discitis, most probably due to "ballooning" of the disc material into the vertebral body.

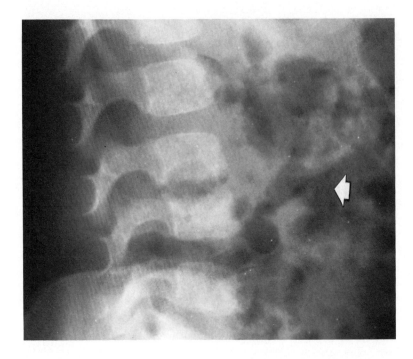

FIGURE 6–97. *Vertebral body cavitation in discitis due to bone destruction by infectious process.*

FIGURE 6–98. *Late residual changes in discitis showing wedging of vertebra, irregularity of ossification of anterior vertebral body, and kyphosis.*

A and **B.** Lateral radiograms of spine showing these changes.

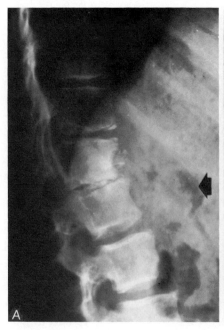
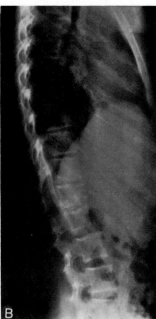

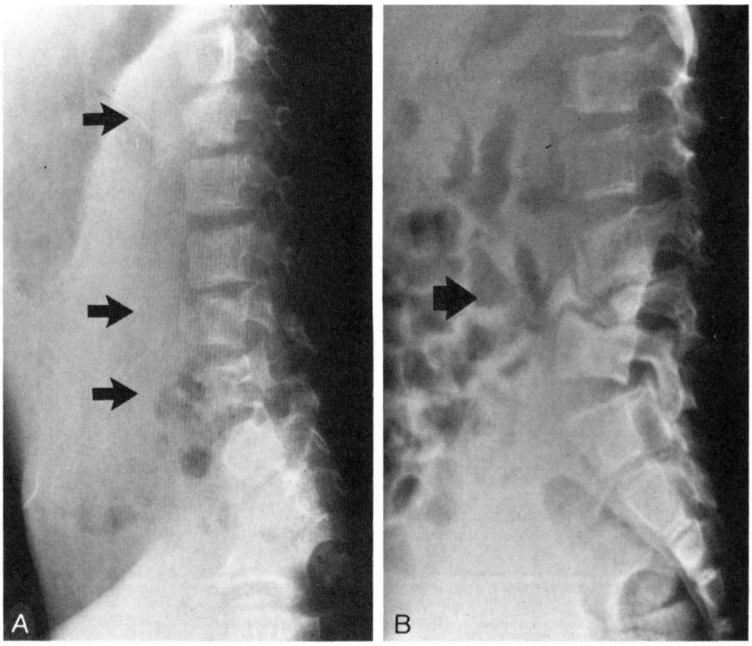

FIGURE 6–99. *Acute vertebral osteomyelitis in a child with diabetes mellitus with multiple-level involvement.*

A. Lateral radiogram of the spine five days after onset of infection. The arrows are pointing to the site of bone destruction. **B.** Three weeks later following antibiotic therapy. Note the fulminating course with the collapsed vertebra.

and elevated erythrocyte sedimentation rate—perform bone scan, computed tomography scan, or magnetic resonance imaging prior to needle aspiration; (2) presence of paravertebral abscess, particularly if it is enlarging; and (3) clinical and radiographic evidence of progression of the disease in spite of immobilization. Needle aspiration of the affected intervertebral space is performed under general anesthesia with the assistance of image intensifier x-ray control (Fig. 6–100). If no pus or sanguineous fluid is obtained, 1 ml. of normal saline solution is instilled and then reaspirated. Often these children have been given antibiotics for some reason before the diagnosis is made, and the condition is modified and organisms cannot be grown. In those with positive culture, *Staphylococcus aureus* is the most common pathogenic organism.

When computed tomography or magnetic resonance studies suggest a neoplastic or tumorous lesion because of marked bone destruction, biopsy should be performed to delineate the pathology. This author prefers open biopsy over closed Craig needle biopsy. The sequential steps of diagnostic assessment in discitis are summarized in Table 6–4.

Treatment

It is best to hospitalize a child who is suspected of having discitis for diagnostic work-up and initiation of treatment. The principle of

treatment is to rest the spine in recumbency in a plaster of Paris jacket, which includes the hips and thighs when the lumbar spine is affected, or the head and neck (Minerva jacket) when the thoracic or cervical spine is involved. An orthosis can be used instead of the plaster of Paris jacket in compliant patients with cooperative parents. Nonsteroid anti-inflammatory medication is given in appropriate dosage. A cooperative child with minimal signs and symptoms benefits from simple bed rest without external support. This treatment is continued until back pain, muscle spasm, or local tenderness has subsided, and until the blood sedimentation rate, temperature, and white blood count are normal and the radiograms indicate that bony erosion is not progressing. Healing is

Table 6–4. *Sequential Steps in Diagnostic Assessment of Discitis*

Plain radiograms
Laboratory studies—CBC with WBC differential, hemoglobin, ESR, and skin test for tuberculosis. Febrile agglutination when *Salmonella* or *Brucella* spondylitis suspected.
Bone scan with technetium-99m
Computed axial tomography and/or nuclear magnetic resonance imaging (NMR) to distinguish pyogenic spondylitis from nonspecific discitis.
Needle aspiration—when infection suspected with extensive destruction of vertebrae and paravertebral soft tissue mass
Biopsy—preferably open—if neoplasm or tumorous lesion suspected

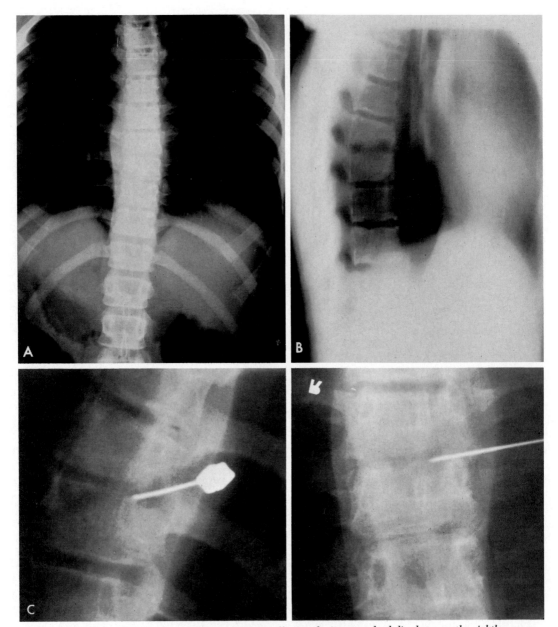

FIGURE 6-100. *Discitis—an infectious disease affecting the intervertebral disc between the eighth and ninth dorsal vertebrae.*

A and **B.** Anteroposterior and lateral (laminogram) radiograms of the dorsal spine. Note the erosion and partial wedging of the inferior surface of the eighth thoracic vertebra. **C.** Aspiration of the disc interspace between T8 and T9 under image intensifier radiographic control. The organism cultured was *Staphylococcus aureus.*

taking place as shown by the appearance of some sclerosis of the adjacent bony surfaces. This usually occurs in two months. These children are then gradually permitted to ambulate. A spinal hyperextension brace (TLSO) is used part-time for another one or two months if moderate narrowing of disc interspace is still present.

Antibiotics. When should they be given? Antibiotics are administered for a period of four to six weeks (1) when systemic signs (pyrexia, elevated erythrocyte sedimentation rate, and elevated white blood count) are present, (2) when there is positive blood or aspirate culture, and (3) when there is progression of the disease despite negative culture and adequate immobilization. Suppuration as a complication of discitis has been reported.[43] When a paravertebral abscess forms, it is surgically explored and drained by a closed suction-irrigation system.

References

1. Alexander, C. V.: The aetiology of juvenile spondiloarthritis (discitis). Clin. Radiol., *21*:178, 1970.
2. Ambrose, G. B., Alpert, M., and Neer, C. S.: Vertebral osteomyelitis—a diagnostic problem. J.A.M.A., *101*:1971, 1966.
3. Atkinson, R. N., Paterson, D. C., Morris, L. L., and Savage, J. P.: Bone scintigraphy in discitis and related disorders in children. Aust. N.Z. J. Surg., *48*:374, 1978.
4. Böhmig, R.: Die Blutgefässversorgung der Wirbelbandscheiben, das Verhalten des intervertebralen Chorda-segments und die Bedeutung beider für die Bandscheibendegeneration. Zugleich ein Beitrag zur enchondralen Ossification der Wirbelkorper. Arch. Klin. Chir., *158*:374, 1930.
5. Bolivar, R., Kohl, S., and Pickering, L. V.: Vertebral osteomyelitis in children: Report of four cases. Pediatrics, *62*:549, 1978.
6. Bonfiglio, M., Lange, T. A., and Kim, Y. M.: Pyogenic vertebral osteomyelitis. Disk space infections. Clin. Orthop., *96*:234, 1973.
7. Brass, A., and Bowdler, E. G.: Non-specific spondylitis of childhood. Ann. Radiol., *12*:343, 1969.
8. Bremner, A. E., and Neligan, G. A.: Benign form of acute osteitis of the spine in young children. Br. Med. J., *1*:856, 1953.
9. Butler, E. C. B., Blusger, I. N., and Perry, K. M. A.: Staphylococcal osteomyelitis of the spine. Lancet, *1*:480, 1941.
10. Bywaters, E. G.: Rheumatoid discitis in the thoracic region due to spread from costovertebral joints. Ann. Rheum. Dis., *33*:408, 1974.
11. Childe, A. E., and Tucker, F. R.: Spondylarthritis in infants and children. J. Can. Assoc. Radiol., *12*:47, 1961.
12. Compere, E. L., and Garrison, M.: Correlation of pathological and roentgenographic findings in tuberculosis and pyogenic infections of the vertebrae. Ann. Surg., *104*:1038, 1936.
13. Couture, A., Ferran, J. L., Blum, M., and Senac, J. P.: Discitis in small children. J. Radiol., *60*:743, 1979.
14. Coventry, M. B., Ghormley, R. K., and Kernahan, J. W.: Intervertebral disc: Its microscopic anatomy and pathology. J. Bone Joint Surg., *27*:105, 1945.
15. Craig, F. S.: Vertebral body biopsy. J. Bone Joint Surg., *38*-A:93, 1956.
16. Diament, M. J., Weller, M., and Bernstein, R.: Candida infection in a premature infant presenting as discitis. Pediatr. Radiol., *12*:96, 1982.
17. Doyle, J. R.: Narrowing of the intervertebral disc space in children. Presumably an infectious lesion of the disc. J. Bone Joint Surg., *42*-A:1191, 1960.
18. DuPont, A., and Anderson, H.: Non-specific spondylitis in children. Acta Pediatr., *45*:361, 1956.
19. Ferguson, W. R.: Some observations on circulation in foetal and infant spines. J. Bone Joint Surg., *32*-A:640, 1950.
20. Flemming, C.: Chronic staphylococcal osteomyelitis of the spine. Proc. R. Soc. Med., *28*:897, 1935.
21. Galil, A., Gorodischer, R., Bar-Ziv, J., Hallel, T., Malkin, C., and Garty, R.: Intervertebral disc infection (discitis) in childhood. Eur. J. Pediatr., *139*:66, 1982.
22. Ghormley, R. K., Bickel, W. H., and Dickson, D. D.: A study of acute infectious lesions of the intervertebral disks. South. Med. J., *33*:347, 1940.
23. Griffiths, H. E. D., and Jones, D. M.: Pyogenic infection of the spine. J. Bone Joint Surg., *53*-B:383, 1971.
24. Grunebaum, M., Horodniceanu, C., Mukamel, M., Varsano, I., and Lubin, E.: The imaging diagnosis of nonpyogenic discitis in children. Pediatr. Radiol., *12*:133, 1982.
25. Guri, J. P.: Pyogenic osteomyelitis of the spine. J. Bone Joint Surg., *28*:29, 1946.
26. Harbin, M., and Epton, J. W.: Osteomyelitis of the spine. Am. J. Surg., *22*:244, 1933.
27. Hensey, O. J., Coad, N., Carty, H. M., and Sills, J. M.: Juvenile discitis. Arch. Dis. Child., *58*:983, 1983.
28. Holliday, P. O., Davis, C. H., Jr., and Shaffner, L. S.: Intervertebral disc spine infection in a child presenting as a psoas abscess: Case report. Neurosurgery, *7*:395, 1980.
29. Horninge, H.: Discitis in children. Arch. Chir. Neerl., *24*:215, 1972.
30. Jamison, R. C., Heimlich, E. M., Miethke, J. C., and O'Loughlin, B. J.: Nonspecific spondylitis of infants and children. Radiology, *77*:355, 1961.
31. Kampmann, H.: Intervertebral discitis in a child. Ugeskr. Laeger, *137*:2282, 1975.
32. Keiser, R. P., and Grimes, H. A.: Intervertebral disk space infections in children. Clin. Orthop., *30*:163, 1963.
33. Keyes, D. C., and Compere, E. L.: The normal and pathological physiology of the nucleus pulposus of the intervertebral disc. J. Bone Joint Surg., *14*:879, 1932.
34. Knutsson, F.: Fusion of vertebrae following a noninfectious disturbance in the zone of growth. Acta Radiol., *32*:404, 1949.
35. Kulowski, J.: Pyogenic osteomyelitis of the spine. An analysis and discussion of 102 cases. J. Bone Joint Surg., *18*:343, 1936.
36. Lascari, A. D., Graham, M. H., and MacQueen, J. C.: Intervertebral disc infection in children. J. Pediatr., *70*:751, 1967.
37. Leigh, T. F., Kelley, R. P., and Weens, H. S.: Spinal osteomyelitis associated with urinary tract infections. Radiology, *65*:334, 1955.
38. Lopez Ros, S., and Navarro Gonzalez, J.: Intervertebral disk infection in children. An. Esp. Pediatr., *16*:176, 1982.
39. Martin, P.: Pyogenic osteomyelitis of the spine. Br. Med. J., *2*:688, 1946.
40. Marty, A. T., Kimura, R., and O'Reilly, R. R.: Idiopathic pyogenic osteomyelitis and discitis of the thoracic spine. Case report. Milit. Med., *143*:492, 1978.
41. Mathews, S. S., Wiltse, L. L., and Karbelnig, M. J.: A destructive lesion involving the intervertebral disc in children. Clin. Orthop., *9*:163, 1957.
42. Mau, G., Helbig, B., and Mann, M.: Discitis—a rare early symptom of ankylosing spondylitis. Eur. J. Pediatr., *137*:85, 1981.
43. Menelaus, M. B.: Discitis: An inflammation affecting the intervertebral discs in children. J. Bone Joint Surg., *46*-B:16, 1964.
44. Milone, F. P., Bianco, A. J., Jr., and Ivins, J. C.: Infections of the intervertebral disk in children. J.A.M.A., *181*:1029, 1962.
45. Moes, C. A. F.: Spondyloarthritis in childhood. A.J.R., *91*:578, 1964.
46. Petersen, V.: Diagnosis of discitis/spondylitis. Ugeskr. Laeger, *145*:3581, 1983.
47. Phemister, D. B.: Changes in articular surfaces in tuberculosis and in pyogenic infections of joints. A.J.R. *12*:1, 1924.
48. Pritchard, A. E., and Thompson, W. A. L.: Acute pyogenic infections of the spine in children. J. Bone Joint Surg., *42*-B:86, 1960.
49. Rocco, H. D., and Eyring, E. J.: Intervertebral disc

infections in children. Am. J. Dis. Child., *123*:448, 1972.

50. Saenger, E. L.: Spondylarthritis in children. A.J.R. *64*:20, 1950.
51. Scherbel, A. L., and Gardner, W. J.: Infections involving the intervertebral discs. Diagnosis and management. J.A.M.A., *174*:370, 1960.
52. Scoles, P. V., and Quinn, T. P.: Intervertebral discitis in children and adolescents. Clin. Orthop., *162*:31, 1982.
53. Smith, A. DeF.: A benign form of osteomyelitis of the spine. J.A.M.A., *101*:335, 1933.
54. Smith, N. R.: The intervertebral discs. Br. J. Surg., *18*:358, 1931.
55. Smith, R. F., and Taylor, T. K. F.: Inflammatory lesions of intervertebral discs in children. J. Bone Joint Surg., *49-A*:1508, 1967.
56. Spiegel, P. G., Kengla, K. W., Isaacson, A. S., and Wilson, J. C., Jr.: Intervertebral disc-space inflammation in children. J. Bone Joint Surg., *54-A*:284, 1972.
57. Stone, D. B., and Bonfiglio, M.: Pyogenic vertebral osteomyelitis. Arch. Intern. Med., *112*:491, 1963.
58. Sullivan, C. R.: Diagnosis and treatment of pyogenic infections of the intervertebral disc. Surg. Clin. North Am., *41*:1077, 1961.
59. Sullivan, C. R., and McCaslin, F. E., Jr.: Further studies on experimental spondylitis and intercorporeal fusion of the spine. J. Bone Joint Surg., *42-A*:1139, 1960.
60. Turner, P.: Acute infective osteomyelitis of the spine. Br. J. Surg., *26*:71, 1938.
61. Ubermuth, H.: Über die Altersveranderungen der menschlichen Zwischenwirbel-scheibe und ihre Beziehung zu den chronischen Gelenkleiden der Wirbelsaule. Ber. Verh. Sachs. Akad. Wissensch. Leipzig, Math.-phys. Klasse 81, 3, 1929.
62. Ubermuth, H.: Die Bedeutung der Altersveranderungen den menschlichen Bandscheiben für die Pathologie der Wirbelsaule. Arch. Klin. Chir., *156*:567, 1930.
63. Wenger, D. R., Bobechko, W. P., and Gilday, D. L.: The spectrum of intervertebral disc-space infection in children. J. Bone Joint Surg., *60-A*:100, 1978.
64. Wilensky, A. O.: Osteomyelitis of the vertebrae. Ann. Surg., *89*:561, 731, 1929.
65. Winter, W. A., Veraart, B. E., and Verdegaal, W. P.: Bone scintigraphy in patients with juvenile kyphosis (M. Scheuermann). Diagn. Imaging, *50*:186, 1981.

HERNIATED INTERVERTEBRAL DISC

Protruded intervertebral discs are rarely seen in children.[1-62] However, they should be considered in the differential diagnosis of low backache and sciatica in a child. They usually are encountered in the second decade of life and are equally common in boys and girls. The disorder seems to be more common in children with ligamentous hyperlaxity. The history and findings on neurologic examination do not differ from those in adults. Trauma such as heavy weight-lifting plays a definite role in the onset of complaints in the adolescent. The pain is increased with activity and relieved by rest in bed. Coughing and sneezing may aggravate the pain. Splinting and spasm of the paravertebral muscles may cause scoliosis. Neurologic deficit is ordinarily minimal, but abnormality of gait is not uncommon.

The plain radiographs usually are unremarkable—they do not show narrowing of intervertebral disc interspace. Diagnosis is readily made by magnetic resonance imaging (MRI). If the MRI is normal or inconclusive, first, bone scan with technetium-99m should be performed to rule out other causes of backache, such as discitis, tumors (such as osteoid osteoma, osteoblastoma, or eosinophilic granuloma), and trauma. Then a myelogram is performed for definitive diagnosis and localization of the lesion.

Treatment should be conservative with bed rest and traction, followed by orthotic support to the spine. If an adequate trial of conservative therapy fails to provide relief of symptoms, surgery is indicated. Chymopapain injection is carried out first; if it fails, excision of the disc is performed.

References

1. Barr, J. S., Kubik, C. S., Molloy, M. K., McNeill, J. M., Riseborough, E. J., and White, J. C.: Evaluation of end results in treatment of ruptured lumbar intervertebral disc with protrusion of nucleus pulposus. Surg. Gynecol. Obstet., *125*:250, 1967.
2. Beks, J. W., and terWeeme, C. A.: Herniated lumbar discs in teenagers. Acta Neurochir. (Wien), *31*:195, 1975.
3. Beks, J. W., and terWeeme, C. A.: Proceedings: Herniations of the lumbar intervertebral disc in children and adolescents. Acta Neurochir. (Wien), *31*:272, 1975.
4. Billot, C., Desgrippes, Y., and Bensahel, H.: Lumbar disc herniation in childhood. Rev. Chir. Orthop., *66*:43, 1980.
5. Borgesen, S. E., and Vang, P. S.: Herniation of the lumbar intervertebral disk in children and adolescents. Acta Orthop. Scand., *45*:540, 1974.
6. Boston, H. D., Jr., Bianco, A. J., Jr., and Rhodes, K. H.: Infections in children. Orthop. Clin. North Am., *6*:953, 1975.
7. Bradford, D. S., and Garcia, A.: Herniations of the lumbar intervertebral disc in children and adolescents. A review of thirty surgically treated cases. J.A.M.A., *210*:2045, 1969.
8. Bussiere, J. L., Leblanc, B., Lopitaux, R., Ristori, J. M., Chabannes, J., and Rampon, S.: Sciatica caused by disk herniation in children. Apropos of 4 cases. Rev. Rhum. Mal. Osteoartic., *48*:543, 1981.
9. Ciorba, E., Pezzella, F., Lancia, G., and Calzolari, P.: A case of herniated disk in childhood. Minerva Pediatr., *30*:567, 1978.
10. Cronqvist, S., and Mortensson, W.: Protrusion of calcified cervical discs into the spinal canal in children. A report of two cases. Neuroradiology, *9*:223, 1975.
11. Day, P. L.: The teenage disc syndrome. South. Med. J., *60*:247, 1967.
12. DeOrio, J. K., and Bianco, A. J., Jr.: Lumbar disc excision in children and adolescents. J. Bone Joint Surg., *64-A*:991, 1982.
13. Dilling-Ostrowska, E., and Wykrzykowska, L.: Clinicoetiological correlations in children with sciatica. Neurol. Neurochir. Pol., *17*:327, 1983.

14. Eeg-Olofsson, O., Hager, A., Morales, O., and Resjo, M.: Herniated intervertebral disk with calcification, causing torticollis in a 10 year old boy. Lakartidningen, *80*:3320, 1983.

15. Epstein, J. A., and Lavine, L. S.: Herniated lumbar intervertebral discs in teen-age children. J. Neurosurg., *21*:1070, 1964.

16. Epstein, J. A., Epstein, N. E., Marc, J., Rosenthal, A. D., and Lavine, L. S.: Lumbar intervertebral disk herniation in teen-age children: Recognition and management of associated anomalies. Spine, *9*:427, 1984.

17. Garrido, E., Humphreys, R. P., Hendrick, E. B., and Hoffman, H. J.: Lumbar disc disease in children. Neurosurgery, *2*:22, 1978.

18. Gurdjian, E. S., Webster, J. E., Ostrowski, A. Z., Hardy, W. G., Lindner, D. W., and Thomas, L. M.: Herniated lumbar intervertebral discs. An analysis of 1176 operated cases. J. Trauma, *1*:158, 1961.

19. Hall, B. B., and McCulloch, J. A.: Anaphylactic reactions following the intradiscal injection of Chymopapain under local anesthesia. J. Bone Joint Surg., *65*-A:1215, 1983.

20. Jaster, D.: Lumbar intervertebral disk prolapse in adolescents. Beitr. Orthop. Traumatol., *21*:389, 1974.

21. Kamel, M., and Rosman, M.: Disc protrusion in the growing child. Clin. Orthop., *185*:46, 1984.

22. Kelly, R. H.: Traumatic displacement of the cartilaginous vertebral rim: A sign of intervertebral disc prolapse. Radiology, *110*:21, 1974.

23. Key, J. A.: Intervertebral-disc lesions in children and adolescents. J. Bone Joint Surg., *32*-A:97, 1950.

24. Klug, N., and Smaii, M.: Herniation of an intervertebral disc with cauda compression syndrome in childhood. J. Neurol., *221*:209, 1979.

25. Koranda, I.: Herniated intervertebral disk in a child. Cesk. Pediatr., *38*:611, 1983.

26. Kozlowski, K.: Anterior intervertebral disc herniations in children. Report of four cases. Pediatr. Radiol., *6*:32, 1977.

27. Kozlowski, K.: Anterior intervertebral disc herniations (report of six cases). R.O.E.F.O., *129*:47, 1978.

28. Kurihara, A., and Kataoka, O.: Lumbar disc herniation in children and adolescents: A review of 70 operated cases and their minimum 5 year follow-up studies. Spine, *5*:443, 1980.

29. Lins, E., and Basedow, H.: Lumbar disc protrusion in childhood. Description of a case. Neuropaediatrie, *7*:122, 1976.

30. Lippitt, A. B.: Fracture of a vertebral body end plate and disk protrusion causing subarachnoid block in an adolescent. Clin. Orthop., *116*:112, 1976.

31. Lorenz, M., and McCulloch, J.: Chemonucleolysis for herniated nucleus pulposus. J. Bone Joint Surg., *67*-A:1402, 1985.

32. Lyons, H., Jones, E., and Quinn, F. E.: Changes in proteinpolysaccharide fractions of nucleus pulposus from human intervertebral disc with age and herniation. J. Lab. Clin. Med., *68*:930, 1966.

33. McCartee, C. C., Jr., Griffin, P. P., and Byrd, E. B.: Ruptured calcified thoracic disc in a child. J. Bone Joint Surg., *54*-A:1272, 1972.

34. MacNab, I.: Backache. Baltimore, Williams & Wilkins, 1977, p. 170.

35. Mixter, W. J., and Barr, J. S.: Rupture of the intervertebral disc with involvement of the spinal canal. N. Engl. J. Med., *211*:210, 1934.

36. Mougenot, J. F., Pernin, J., and Herve, J.: Calcification and hernia of an intervertebral disc in a child. Sem. Hop. Paris, *55*:1445, 1979.

37. Nashold, B. S., Jr., and Hrubec, Z.: Lumbar Disc Disease: A Twenty-year Clinical Follow-up Study. St. Louis, Mosby, 1971.

38. National Center for Health Statistics: NCHS Growth Charts, 1976. Monthly Vital Stat. Rep. Suppl., *25*:1, 1976.

39. O'Connell, J. E. A.: Intervertebral disk protrusions in childhood and adolescence. Br. J. Surg., *47*:611, 1960.

40. Otani, K., Nakai, S., Fujimura, Y., Manzoku, S., and Shibasaki, K.: Surgical treatment of thoracic disc herniation using anterior approach. J. Bone Joint Surg., *64*-B:340, 1982.

41. Paus, B., and Skalpe, I. O.: The recurrence of pain following operation for herniated lumbar disc: Fresh herniation or extradural scar tissue? Int. Orthop., *3*:133, 1979.

42. Peck, F. C.: A calcified thoracic intervertebral disk with herniation and spinal cord compression in a child. J. Neurosurg., *14*:105, 1957.

43. Plangger, C., Twerdy, K., Fischer, J., and Mohsenipour, I.: Four cases of intervertebral disc herniation in children. Neurochirurgia (Stuttg.), *25*:129, 1982.

44. Quattrini, M., and LaTerra, F.: Disk hernia in children: Observations of a case. Chir. Organi Mov., *66*:447, 1981.

45. Rand, R. W., and Rand, C. W.: Intraspinal Tumors of Childhood. Springfield, Ill., Thomas, 1960.

46. Resnick, D., and Niwayama, G.: Intravertebral disk herniations: Cartilaginous (Schmorl's) nodes. Radiology, *126*:57, 1978.

47. Rothman, R. H.: Indications for lumbar fusion. Clin. Neurosurg., *20*:215, 1973.

48. Rugtveit, A.: Juvenile lumbar disc herniations. Acta Orthop. Scand., *37*:348, 1966.

49. Russwurm, H., Bjerkreim, I., and Ronglan, E.: Lumbar intervertebral disc herniation in the young. Acta Orthop. Scand., *49*:158, 1978.

50. Schechter, L. S., Smith, A., and Pearl, M.: Intervertebral disk calcification in childhood. Am. J. Dis. Child., *123*:608, 1972.

51. Shannon, N., and Paul, E. A.: L4/5 and L5-S1 disc protrusions: Analysis of 323 cases operated on over 12 years. J. Neurol. Neurosurg. Psychiatry, *42*:804, 1979.

52. da Silva, V., Beyeler, F., Mumenthaler, M., Robert F., and Vassella, F.: Lumbar intervertebral disc herniation in children. A report of 16 cases. Ther. Umsch., *34*:405, 1977.

53. Smith, R. F., and Taylor, T. K. F.: Inflammatory lesions of intervertebral discs in children. J. Bone Joint Surg., *49*-A:1508, 1967.

54. Sonnabend, D. H., Taylor, T. K. F., and Chapman, G. K.: Intervertebral disc calcification syndromes in children. J. Bone Joint Surg., *64*-B:25, 1982.

55. Spiegel, P. G., Kengla, K. W., Isaacson, A. S., and Wilson, J. C., Jr.: Intervertebral disc-space inflammation in children. J. Bone Joint Surg., *54*-A:284, 1972.

56. Tadie, M., Helias, A., Thiebot, J., Rogler, P., Thorel, J. B., Creissard, P., Deshayes, P., and Benozio, M.: Lumbar phlebography without catheterization. Technic, indications and results in the diagnosis of intervertebral disk herniation. Rev. Rhum. Mal. Osteoartic., *46*:601, 1979.

57. Taylor, T. K. F.: Intervertebral disc prolapse in children and adolescents. J. Bone Joint Surg., *53*-B:357, 1971.

58. Techakapuch, S.: Rupture of the lumbar cartilage plate into the spinal canal in an adolescent. A case report. J. Bone Joint Surg., *63*-A:481, 1981.

59. Wahren, H.: Herniated nucleus pulposus in a child of twelve years. Acta Orthop. Scand., *16*:40, 1946.

60. Webb, J. H., Svien, H. J., and Kennedy, R. L. J.: Protruded lumbar intervertebral discs in children. J.A.M.A., *154*:1153, 1954.

61. Young, H. H., and Love, J. G.: End results of removal of protruded lumbar intervertebral discs with and without fusion. A.A.O.S. Instr. Course Lect. *16*:213, 1959.

62. Zamani, M. H., and MacEwen, G. D.: Herniation of the lumbar disc in children and adolescents. J. Pediatr. Orthop., *2*:582, 1982.

SLIPPED VERTEBRAL APOPHYSIS

This rare entity is a traumatic posterior displacement of the posteroinferior apophysis of a lower lumbar vertebra with its adjacent disc into the vertebral canal. The most common level of the lesion is the fourth lumbar vertebra, less commonly the fifth or third lumbar vertebra. Slipped vertebral apophysis is similar in its pathogenesis to that of slipped capital femoral epiphysis.

Slipped vertebral apophysis is uniquely encountered in adolescents, usually males, who complain of acute backache and sciatica immediately after heavy weight-lifting, shoveling snow, or gymnastics. Neurologic deficit in the form of muscle weakness or absent reflexes is common.

Radiographs and computed tomography studies will show the edge of the vertebral apophysis in the form of a small bony or osteocartilaginous fragment in the vertebral canal. Magnetic resonance imaging and contrast myelography will show the bony and cartilaginous mass producing an anterior extradural deficit or complete block.

It is vital to distinguish slipped vertebral apophysis from herniated disc. Chymopapain injection is contraindicated—it will not resolve the problem and will aggravate the symptoms. Treatment consists of surgical decompression in the form of laminectomy and excision of both the bony-cartilaginous mass and the extruded intervertebral disc. Results of surgery are excellent with complete relief of symptoms.

References

1. Handel, S. F., Twiford, T. W., Reigel, D. H., and Kaufman, H. H.: Posterior lumbar apophyseal fractures. Radiology, *130*:629, 1979.
2. Keller, R. H.: Traumatic displacement of the cartilaginous vertebral rim: A sign of intervertebral disc prolapse. Radiology, *110*:21, 1974.
3. Lippitt, A. B.: Fracture of a vertebral body end plate and disk protrusion causing subarachnoid block in an adolescent. Clin. Orthop., *116*:112, 1976.
4. Lowrey, J. J.: Dislocated lumbar vertebral epiphysis in adolescent children. Report of three cases. J. Neurosurg., *38*:232, 1973.
5. Techakapuch, S.: Rupture of the lumbar cartilage plate into the spinal canal in an adolescent. A case report. J. Bone Joint Surg., *63-A*:481, 1981.

Index

Index

Note: Page numbers in *italics* refer to illustrations; page numbers in boldface refer to surgical plates. Page numbers followed by the letter t refer to tables.

A

Abdominal circumference, in relation to age, in females, 78t
  in males, 77t
Abduction, definition of, 33
Abductor digiti quinti manus transfer of Littler, 2057, **2070–2071**
Abductor pollicis brevis, congenital absence of, *288–289*, 288–290
Abscess, in tuberculosis of spine, 1449, *1451*
Acetabular augmentation, Staheli's, in congenital dysplasia of hip in adolescent, 522–526, *524–525*
Acetabular index, in congenital dysplasia of hip, 322
  preoperative, in Salter's innominate osteotomy, 414–415
Acetabular torsion, computed tomography of, in congenital dysplasia of hip, 364, *366–367*
Acetabuloplasty, in congenital dysplasia of hip, 422–423
Acetabulum, in congenital dysplasia of hip in adolescent, 468, *469*
  labrum of, rose thorn in arthrography of, 351–352, *352*
    torn, in Legg-Calvé-Perthes disease, 988
  primary dysplasia of, in congenital dysplasia of hip, 302
  secondary dysplasia of, in congenital dysplasia of hip, 311–312
Achard's syndrome, Marfan's syndrome vs., 839
Achilles tendon, anterior advancement of, 1675, *1675*, **1678–1679**, 1680
  sliding lengthening of, 1666, *1667*, **1668–1669**, *1670*
  subcutaneous lengthening of, 1666, *1671*
  transfer of, in talipes equinovarus, 2512
  Z-lengthening of, 1666, *1671*
Achondrogenesis, 730
Achondroplasia, 720–727
  clinical picture in, 721, *722–725*, 726
  diagnosis in, 726–727
  etiology of, 721
  pathology in, 721
  prognosis and treatment in, 727

Achondroplasia *(Continued)*
  pseudoachondroplasia vs., 751t
  radiographic findings in, *722–727*, 726
Acidosis, in vitamin D refractory rickets, 908, 910
Acrocephalosyndactylism, 236–240, *237–239*
Acrocephalosyndactyly, 855–856
Acromioclavicular dislocation, 3041
Acromion process, fracture of, 3044
Actinomycosis, of bone, 1129
Adamantinoma, 1301–1304
  clinical features of, 1301
  differential diagnosis of, 1301
  pathologic findings in, 1301, 1303
  radiography in, 1301, *1302–1303*
  treatment of, 1303–1304
Adams' forward bending test, in scoliosis, 2275–2277, *2276*
Adduction, definition of, 33
Adductor longus, in gait, 14
Adductor magnus, in gait, 14
Adductor myotomy, and obturator neurectomy, of Banks and Green, **1638–1641**
Adductor pollicis, release of, **1726–1729**, 1730
Adiadochokinesia, in cerebral palsy, 1613
A-frame, in myelomeningocele, 1855, *1856*
Africoid talus, 2416, *2619*
Age, normal measurements in relation to, female, 78t
  male, 77t
Airway, in anesthesia, in juvenile rheumatoid arthritis, 69
Alpha-fetoprotein, in antenatal testing for myelomeningocele, 1776
Ambulation. See *Gait.*
Amikacin, in septic arthritis, 1424t
Aminoaciduria, in vitamin D refractory rickets, 908, 910
Amniocentesis, in myelomeningocele, 1776
Amphotericin B, in septic arthritis, 1424t
Ampicillin, in septic arthritis, 1424t
Amputation, below-knee, **1350–1353**
  elbow disarticulation, **1376–1379**
  forequarter (Littlewood), **1354–1367**
  hemipelvectomy (Banks and Coleman), **1318–1325**

Diastrophic dysplasia *(Continued)*
  radiography in, 756
  treatment in, 756
Digital gigantism, 277, *278*
Digitus minimus varus, congenital, 2653, 2655, *2658–2660*, 2661, **2662–2663**
Diplegia, 1606
  spastic, 1606, 1616–1617. See also *Cerebral palsy.*
Discitis, 2394–2401
  clinical findings in, 2394–2395, *2395*
  diagnosis of, 2397–2399, 2399t, *2400*
  imaging findings in, *2393–2398*, 2395–2396
  laboratory findings in, 2396
  pathogenesis of, 2394
  treatment of, 2399–2401
Discoid meniscus, 1539–1549. See also *Meniscus, discoid.*
Dislocation. See individual joint.
Down's syndrome, 890–895
  atlantoaxial instability in, 891–892
  dislocation of hip in, 892, *894*, 895
  maternal age and, 891t
  patellofemoral joint dislocation in, 895
  radiography in, 891, *891–893*
  treatment of, 891–895
Drooling, in cerebral palsy, 1756–1757
Drop-foot gait, 24
Drummond system, in scoliosis, 2318–2319
Duchenne muscular dystrophy. See *Muscular dystrophy, Duchenne.*
Dunn femoral head reduction by femoral neck shortening, in slipped femoral capital epiphysis, 1047, **1048–1055**, 1062
DuPont jacket, in scoliosis, *2301*, 2301–2302
Dwarfism, diastrophic, 752–756. See also *Diastrophic dysplasia.*
  dystrophic, talipes equinovarus in, 2452, *2454*, 2455
  pituitary, *926*, 926–927
  terminology in, 694
  thanatophoric, 730, *731*
Dwyer calcaneal lateral wedge resection, in pes cavus, 2700–2701, **2702–2703**
Dwyer calcaneal osteotomy, 1702–1703
  in talipes equinovarus, 2517, **2518–2519**, 2520–2521
Dwyer instrumentation, in scoliosis, 2320, **2332–2353**
Dyggve-Melchior-Clausen disease, 757–758
Dynamic stress method, in congenital dysplasia of hip, 324, *324*
Dysautonomia, familial, 1995, 1996t–1997t, 1998–1999
Dyschondroplasia, 1195, *1196–1198*
Dysdiadochokinesia, in cerebral palsy, 1613
Dysmetria, in cerebral palsy, 1613
Dysostosis multiplex, in mucopolysaccharidosis, 865–867, *866*
Dysplasia, congenital, of hip, 297–526. See also *Hip, congenital dysplasia of.*
  ectodermal, in Ellis–van Creveld syndrome, 736
  epiphyseal, multiple, 701–707. See also *Epiphyseal dysplasia, multiple.*
  fibrous, 1228–1239. See also *Fibrous dysplasia.*
  metaphyseal, 825–826, *826–828*
  osteopetrosis vs., 797
Dysplasia epiphysealis hemimelica, *712–714*, 716, *717–718*, 719
Dyssynergy, in cerebral palsy, 1613
Dystelephalangy, 287, *287*
Dystrophia myotonica, *2138–2140*, 2138–2141
Dystrophia ophthalmoplegia, progressive, 2138
Dystrophic gait, 26

E

Eccentric contraction, of muscle, 14
Ectodermal dysplasia, in Ellis–van Creveld syndrome, 736
Ectopia lentis, in Marfan's syndrome, 832
Ectromelia, 105
Egger's hamstring transfer, *1712*, 1712–1713
Ehlers-Danlos syndrome, 861–864, *862–863*
Elbow. See also individual disorders of.
  disarticulation of, in osteogenic sarcoma, **1376–1379**
  dislocation of, 3124–3134
    classification of, 3125t
    complications of, 3131–3134
      heterotopic bone formation and myositis ossificans as, 3133
      median nerve, *3132*, 3132–3133
      recurrence as, 3133–3134, *3134*
      ulnar nerve, 3131–3132
      vascular, 3131
    diagnosis of, 3125
    mechanism of injury and pathologic anatomy of, 3125, *3126–3130*
    treatment of, 3128–3131
  flexion deformity of, in cerebral palsy, 1746–1747
  in arthrogryposis multiplex congenita, 2101–2103, *2102*, **2104–2111**
  in hereditary onycho-osteodystrophy, 845, *846*
  in obstetrical brachial plexus palsy, 2022–2023, *2024–2025*
  in poliomyelitis, 1959, 1962–1971
  position of minimal intra-articular pressure for, 1410–1411
  pulled, 3148–3151
    diagnosis of, 3149–3150
    mechanism of injury and pathologic anatomy in, 3148–3149, *3149–3150*
    treatment of, 3150–3151
  range of motion of, 33, *34*
  Steindler flexorplasty of, 1959, *1962*, 1962–1963
  synostosis of, congenital, *177–179*, 179
Electrical current, faradic, 64
  galvanic, 64
Electrical stimulation, in congenital pseudarthrosis of tibia, 666–667, 678–681
Electrodiagnosis, 59, 64–65
Electromyography, 64–65
Elephantiasis, in neurofibromatosis, 1290, *1292*
Ellis test, 31
Ellis–van Creveld syndrome, 730, *731–753*, 736
Ely test, in spastic cerebral palsy, 1628, *1631*, 1714, *1715*
Enchondroma, solitary, 1191–1194
  clinical picture in, 1191, *1191*
  differential diagnosis of, 1193
  radiography in, *1192*, 1192–1193
  surgical pathology in, *1193*, 1193–1194
  treatment of, 1194
  unicameral bone cyst vs., 1264
Enchondromatosis, multiple, 1195, *1196–1198*
Endobone, in osteopetrosis, 796, *796*
Endocrinopathy, slipped femoral capital epiphysis due to, 1022
Engen's adjustable extension orthosis, in rheumatoid arthritis, 1482, *1483*
Englemann's disease, osteopetrosis vs., 797
Eosinophilic granuloma, of bone, 1278, 1281–1286
  age and sex in, 1278

Rheumatoid arthritis *(Continued)*
　　cervical fusion in, 1486
　　conservative, 1480–1482, *1481, 1483*
　　lower limb length disparity in, 1484–1485
　　soft-tissue release in, 1484
　　surgical, 1482–1486
　　synovectomy in, 1482–1484
　　total joint replacement in, 1485
　　total knee arthroplasty in, 1485–1486
　pathology in, 1467–1469, *1468–1469*
　pauciarticular, 1469–1470, *1471*
　polyarthritic, in minimal systemic manifestations, 1470–1472
　　in systemic manifestations, 1472–1473
　radiography in, *1472–1476,* 1473–1474
　rheumatoid nodule in, 1469, *1469*
　synovitis in, 1467, *1468*
　treatment of, 1477–1486
Rheumatoid arthritis cells, in joint fluid analysis, 1413
Rheumatoid nodule, 1469, *1469,* 1472
Ribs, fusion of, 2199
Rib-vertebral angle of Mehta, 2285, 2288, *2288–2289*
Rickets, 897–916
　genu varum vs., 2824, 2826
　pathogenesis of, 897–898
　vitamin D deficiency, 898–904
　　clinical findings in, 899, *900–902*
　　malabsorption syndrome and, 903–904
　　pathology of, 898–899, *899*
　　radiography in, 899, *901*
　　treatment of, 899, 903
　vitamin D refractory, 905–910
　　acidosis in, 908, 910
　　aminoaciduria in, 908, 910
　　biochemical findings in, 906
　　clinical features of, 905–906
　　cystine storage disease and, 910
　　heredity in, 905
　　hyperglycinuria and, 910
　　medical treatment of, 906–908
　　oculocerebral syndrome and, 910
　　orthopedic treatment of, 908
　　radiography in, 906, *907*
　　renal tubular acidosis and, 910
　　surgical treatment of, 908, *909*
Rifampin, in septic arthritis, 1424t
　in tuberculous arthritis, 1448
Righting reflex, 51–55
Riley-Day syndrome, 1995, 1996t-1997t, 1998–1999
Riordan thumb opposition restoration, 2057, **2062–2067**
Risser sign, 2288, *2290*
Roberts orthosis, in Legg-Calvé-Perthes disease, 973–974
Rocker-bottom foot, in talipes equinovarus, 2461–2462, *2464*
Rooting reflex, 55
Ropes test, 1413
Rose thorn, in arthrography of acetabular labrum, 351–352, *352*
Rubinstein-Taybi syndrome, 865
Russell skin traction, in femoral shaft fracture, 3264–3266, *3267*
Russell split traction, in congenital dysplasia of hip, 342–343, *343,* 345–346

S

Saber shin, in congenital syphilis, 1125, *1126*
Sacrum, congenital absence of, 2212–2228. See also *Lumbosacral agenesis.*

Saha trapezius transfer, in deltoid paralysis, 1958, *1958*
Salicylates, in rheumatoid arthritis, 1477–1479, 1478t
Salmonella osteomyelitis, 1120–1122, *1121–1122*
Salter's innominate osteotomy, in congenital hip dysplasia, 395–422
　advantages of, 404
　age limits in, 404–405
　complications of, 418–419
　drawbacks of, 405
　for acetabular antetorsion, 415, *415–417*
　in adolescent, 474
　increased intra-articular pressure in, 417
　increased pelvifemoral muscle tension in, 417
　indications for, 404
　ipsilateral limb elongation in, 417
　Kalamchi's modification of, 419–422, *421–423*
　limitations on degree of correction in, 405, 412–417, *412–417*
　objective of, 395, 404, *404*
　open reduction with, 405
　operative technique in, 404, **406–411**
　preoperative acetabular index in, 414–415
　preoperative radiographic assessment in, 412–414, *412–414*
　prerequisites for, 417–418
　Westin's modification of, 419, *419–420*
　in Legg-Calvé-Perthes disease, 979–981, *980–981*
Sanfilippo syndrome, 875
Sarcoma, Ewing's, 1387–1396. See also *Ewing's sarcoma.*
　osteogenic, 1305–1382. See also *Osteogenic sarcoma.*
　of fibula, 2780, *2788*
　synovial, 1598, *1599*
Sartorius, and tensor fasciae latae, posterior transfer of, 1650–1651, **1652–1657**
　in gait, 14
Scapula, aplasia of, 176
　congenital high, 136–168. See also *Sprengel's deformity.*
　embryologic development of, 137
　fracture of, 3042–3044
　　of acromion process, 3044
　　of body, 3043
　　of coracoid process, 3044
　　of glenoid cavity, 3044
　　of neck, 3043–3044
　nonunion of ossific centers of, 176, *177*
　ossification of, 3042–3043
　winging of, in Sprengel's deformity, 147
Scapulocostal stabilization, for scapular winging, **2146–2149**, 2151
Scapuloplasty, Green's, modified, in Sprengel's deformity, *147,* 148–160, **149–161**
Scheuermann's juvenile kyphosis, 2380–2388
　clinical features in, 2381–2383, *2382*
　definition of, 2380
　differential diagnosis of, 2383–2385
　etiology and pathogenesis of, 2380–2381
　incidence of, 2380
　natural history, course, prognosis of, 2385–2386
　pathology in, 2381
　radiography in, 2383, *2384–2385*
　treatment of, 2386–2388, *2387*
Sciatic nerve palsy, 2082–2084
　due to Chiari's innominate osteotomy, 506
　due to Salter's innominate osteotomy, 418
Sclera, in osteogenesis imperfecta, 763, 769
Sclerosis, multiple, differential diagnosis of, 1980t
Scoliosis, congenital, 2201–2205
　age of patient and prognosis in, 2202